THIRD EDITION

Biochemical Tests for Identification of Medical Bacteria

*Dedicated to my twin sister,
Joan M. Feustle*

Preface

Since the second edition of *Biochemical Tests for Identification of Medical Bacteria* was published (1980) the field of bacteriology has changed drastically in bacterial classification and nomenclature; however, biochemical methods for bacterial identification in the routine clinical laboratory have remained fairly constant throughout the years, with updating and introduction of new biochemical tests.

In the more than 19 years since the second edition, the most critical change is in nomenclature. DNA relatedness, rRNA sequence analysis, G + C ratios, and other sophisticated analytical methods have provided more in-depth information about many microorganisms. These advances resulted in reclassification and often transfer of species to different genera or renaming along with identification of new genera. A few years ago the genus *Micrococcus* had nine species, now there are only two; the other species were transferred to other genera. Also the number of species have multiplied enormously in some genera; e.g., *Staphylococcus* now has 44 species.

I have added nine new test chapters on widely used procedures: Bacitracin/Sulfamethoxazole-Trimethoprim (SXT) Tests; Indoxyl Substrate Hydrolysis Test; β-Lactamase Test; Lecithinase Test; Lipase Test; Lysostaphin Susceptibility Test; Porphyrin-δ-Aminolevulinic (ALA) Test; Pyrrolidonyl-β-Naphthylamide Hydrolysis (PYR) Test; and X and V Factors.

I have not changed the format but have updated previous test chapters where applicable, especially with current nomenclature. With the addition of new chapters I have retained old standard procedures that are in use in most working bacteriology laboratories and teaching facilities.

Identification tables have been divided into Gram-positive cocci/bacilli and Gram-negative cocci/bacilli, since many bacteria exhibit both coccal and bacillary forms. The *Enterobacteriaceae* are listed as a separate chapter. Many find flow charts for identification useful; therefore, I have retained the flow charts for those who may find them beneficial.

Genus and species classification (nomenclature) is listed according to the proposed 5 volumes of Bergey's *Manual*. I thank the Bergey's Trust for giving me the proposed outline to update all genera and species.

I especially want to thank Dr. David Power, BD Biosciences (formerly Becton Dickinson Microbiology Systems) for his invaluable help in references, test material, and photographs. Also, Scott Puyear, REMEL Laboratories, and Mike Cox, Anaerobe Systems, for providing me with photographs for the new test chapters.

Jean F. MacFaddin

THIRD EDITION

Biochemical Tests for Identification of Medical Bacteria

Jean F. MacFaddin
MS, MT(ASCP), SM(AAM)

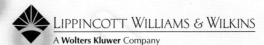

LIPPINCOTT WILLIAMS & WILKINS
A **Wolters Kluwer** Company
Philadelphia · Baltimore · New York · London
Buenos Aires · Hong Kong · Sydney · Tokyo

Editor: Lawrence McGrew
Managing Editor: Angela Heubeck
Marketing Manager: Debby Hartman
Project Editor: Karen Ruppert

Copyright © 2000 Lippincott Williams & Wilkins

227 East Washington Square
Philadelphia, PA 19106 USA

351 West Camden Street
Baltimore, Maryland 21201–2436 USA

All rights reserved. This book is protected by copyright. No part of this book may be reproduced in any form or by any means, including photocopying, or utilized by any information storage and retrieval system without written permission from the copyright owner.

The publisher is not responsible (as a matter of product liability, negligence or otherwise) for any injury resulting from any material contained herein. This publication contains information relating to general principles of medical care which should not be construed as specific instructions for individual patients. Manufacturers' product information and package inserts should be reviewed for current information, including contraindications, dosages and precautions.

Printed in the United States of America

Library of Congress Cataloging-in-Publication Data

MacFaddin, Jean F.
   Biochemical tests for identification of medical bacteria / Jean F. MacFaddin. — 3rd ed.
     p.   cm.
   Includes bibliographical references and index.
   ISBN (invalid) 0-683-05318-3
     1. Diagnostic bacteriology Laboratory manuals. 2. Pathogenic bacteria—
Identification Laboratory manuals. 3. Microbial metabolites—Analysis Laboratory
manuals. I. Title.
   [DNLM: 1. Bacteria—chemistry Laboratory Manuals.
   2. Bacteriological Techniques Laboratory Manuals. QW 25 M143b 1999]
   QR.2.M32   1999
   616.07′581—dc21
   DNLM/DLC
   for Library of Congress   99-30302
                                                                                                              CIP

The publishers have made every effort to trace the copyright holders for borrowed material. If they have inadvertently overlooked any, they will be pleased to make the necessary arrangements at the first opportunity.

To purchase additional copies of this book, call our customer service department at **(800) 638-3030** or fax orders to **(301) 824-7390**. For other book services, including chapter reprints and large quantity sales, ask for the Special Sales department.

Canadian customers should call **(800) 665-1148**, or fax **(800) 665-0103**. For all other calls originating outside of the United States, please call **(301) 714-2300** or fax us at **(301) 824-7390**.

Visit Lippincott Williams & Wilkins on the Internet: **http://www.lww.com** or contact our customer service department at **custserv@wwilkins.com**. Lippincott Williams & Wilkins customer service representatives are available from 8:30 am to 6:00 pm, EST, Monday through Friday, for telephone access.

                                                                                        99 00 01 02 03
                                                                   1 2 3 4 5 6 7 8 9 10

Contents

Preface vii
Color Figures 805

SECTION I. INDIVIDUAL BIOCHEMICAL TESTS

1. Bacitracin/Sulfamethoxazole-Trimethoprim (SXT) Tests 3
2. Bile Esculin (Aesculin) Hydrolysis Tests 8
3. Bile Solubility Test 27
4. CAMP/Reverse CAMP Tests (Reactions) and CAMP Inhibition (Phospholipase D Production) Test 35
5. Carbohydrate Fermentation Tests 57
6. Catalase-Peroxidase Tests 78
7. Citrate Test 98
8. Coagulase Test 105
9. Decarboxylase Tests (Lysine-Ornithine-Arginine) and Dihydrolase Test (Arginine) ... 120
10. Deoxyribonuclease (DNase) and Thermonuclease (TNase) Tests 136
11. β-Galactosidase (ONPG and PNPG) Tests 160
12. Gelatin Liquefaction Tests 170
13. Gluconate Oxidation Test 183
14. Hippurate Hydrolysis Test 188
15. Hydrogen Sulfide Test 205
16. Indole Test 221
17. Indoxyl Substrate Hydrolysis Tests 233
18. Kligler's Iron Agar/Triple Sugar Iron Agar Tests 239
19. β-Lactamase Test 254
20. Lecithinase Test 273
21. Leucine Aminopeptidase (Leucine Arylamidase) (LAP) Test 282
22. Lipase Test 286
23. Litmus Milk Test 294
24. Lysostaphin Susceptibility Test 303
25. Malonate Test 310
26. Methylene Blue Milk Reduction Test for Enterococci 316
27. Methyl Red Test 321
28. Motility Test 327
29. *Neisseria* Carbohydrate Utilization Tests 333
30. Nitrate/Nitrite Reduction Tests 348
31. Optochin Disk Test 363
32. Oxidase Test 368
33. Oxidation-Fermentation Test 379
34. Phenylalanine Deaminase Test 388
35. Phosphatase Test 394
36. Porphyrin-δ-Aminolevulinic (ALA) Test 403

37.	Pyrrolidonyl-β-Naphthylamide Hydrolysis (PYR) Test	407
38.	Starch Hydrolysis Test	412
39.	Urease Test	424
40.	Voges-Proskauer Test	439
41.	X and V Factors	451

SECTION II. MULTITEST SYSTEMS

| 42. | Multitest Systems | 457 |

SECTION III. IDENTIFICATION SCHEMAS

43.	Gram-Positive Bacteria	483
44.	Gram-Negative Bacteria	624
45.	Gram-Negative *Enterobacteriaceae* and Other Intestinal Bacteria	732

SECTION IV. APPENDICES

1.	Colored Photographic Results	805
2.	Metric System Units of Measure	818
3.	pH Indicators	819
4.	pH Adjustment	820
5.	McFarland's Nephelometer Standards	825
6.	Reagent Preparations	827
7.	Common Synonymous Terminology of Media	842
8.	Standard Test Tubes for Bacteria	843
9.	Temperature Conversions	844
10.	Culture Collections; Reference Cultures	845
11.	Addresses of Commercial Suppliers	851
12.	Glossary	861

SECTION V. INDICES

| 1. | General | 889 |
| 2. | Microorganisms | 901 |

SECTION I

Individual Biochemical Tests

1. Bacitracin/Sulfamethoxazole-Trimethoprim (SXT) Tests

I. PRINCIPLE

To determine an organism's susceptibility to bacitracin or bacitracin and sulfamethoxazole-trimethoprim (SXT)

II. PURPOSE

(Also see Chapter 43)
A. Presumptive differentiation of β-hemolytic group A streptococci from other β-hemolytic streptococci
B. Aid in screening out non-A, non-B streptococci that may be susceptible to bacitracin (5)

The accuracy of the bacitracin test is improved by using susceptibility to an SXT disk in combination with bacitracin. Adding SXT along with bacitracin increases the sensitivity and predictive value of the bacitracin test. Bacitracin/SXT susceptibilities are still in use where facilities for reliable serologic groups are not available. A more specific test to identify group A streptococci is the PYR test (pyrrolidonyl-β-napthylamide hydrolysis); it is best for production of the enzyme pyroglutamyl amidase (see Chapter 38).

III. BIOCHEMISTRY INVOLVED

Bacitracin

Bacitracin, an antibiotic originally isolated from *Bacillus licheniformis* (formerly *B. subtilis*), belongs to a class of antibiotics that inhibit bacterial cell wall synthesis. Bacitracin is a peptide antibiotic composed of peptide-linked amino acids.

Phe – phenylalanine
His – histidine
Asp – asparagine
Lys – lysine
Leu – leucine
Orn – ornathine

Bacitracin A
Isoleucine and cystein residue, condensed to form a thiazoline (A) ring rather than usual peptide linkage of a polypeptide

Bacitracin inhibits synthesis of the cell wall, a rigid structure that encloses the microbial cell. The fundamental structure consists of a complex three-dimensional structure containing peptidoglycan, a macromolecule (mucopeptide or glycopeptide or murien), and other polymers (e.g., polysaccharides, lipoproteins) that vary in different types of bacteria (7). Final cell wall rigidity is imparted by cross-linking of peptide chains, and the peptidoglycan layer is much thicker in the cell wall of Gram-positive bacteria. Bacitracin inhibits an early stage in the biosynthesis of peptidoglycan; inhibits dephosphorylation of a lipid pyrophosphate, a step essential for bacteria wall synthesis (10); and inhibits the recycling of certain metabolites required for maintaining peptidoglycan synthesis (7).

Peptidoglycans consist of long polysaccharide filaments interconnected by four amino peptides in which the third amino acid is variable. How peptide chains are interconnected differs among bacterial species.

There are two classes of inhibitors of cell wall synthesis: inhibitors of peptidoglycan synthesis (e.g., bacitracin) and inhibitors of synthesis or assembly of other components of the wall.

Bacitracin is (a) bactericidal, (b) **in**active against resting cells, and (c) inactive against bacteria that lack a cell wall. Bacitracin is bactericidal in that during growth, lytic enzymes active on the inner side of the cell wall break open the peptidoglycan chains to form "free ends." The cell wall then breaks, and cytoplasm flows out (7).

Bacitracin is inactive against resting cells. Lytic enzymes associated with cell wall synthesis are active **only** when cells are growing, **not** when they are resting (7); thus cell wall synthesis inhibitors are **inactive** against bacteria in the stationary phase (7).

Bacitracin A blocks phosphorylase that liberates one of the two terminal phosphates from the lipid carrier, which can then no longer function as an acceptor of muramylpentapeptide. Bacitracin is **not** specific, it can also inhibit other phosphorylase reactions (7).

Trimethoprim (TMP)

TMP (3,4,5-trimethoxybenzyl pyrimidine) inhibits dihydrofolic acid reductase. It is a pyrimidine structural analog of the pteridine portion of dihydrofolic acid that inhibits the enzyme reductase, thereby interfering with folic acid metabolism, subsequent pyrimidine synthesis, and one-carbon-fragment metabolism in the bacteria (10).

Trimethoprim

TMP inhibits the bacterial enzyme but **not** the mammalian enzyme.

Sulfonamides

Sulfonamides are derived from sulfanilamide.

Basic ring structure of sulfonamides

Sulfamethoxazole-Trimethoprim (SXT)

SXT competitively inhibits bacterial modification of *p*-aminobenzoic acid into dihydrofolate. Sequential inhibition of folate metabolism ultimately prevents synthesis of bacterial DNA (3).

Since sulfamethoxazole (SX) and TMP block the bacterial folic acid metabolic pathway at different sites, together they produce sequential blocking, resulting in a marked enhancement (**synergism**) of activity (3, 4).

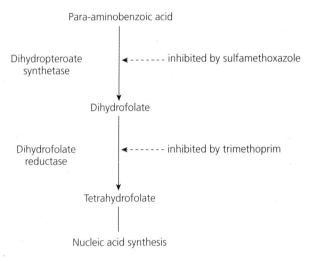

Mechanism of action of SMX-TMP (9). Bacterial folic acid pathway

When a homogeneous bacterial population is treated simultaneously with two antibiotics, three types of results can occur: (*a*) synergism, (*b*) additivity, and (*c*) antagonism. In synergism, the antibiotic effect of the combination is greater than the sum of the effects of each antibiotic alone. Synergism is due to so-called double metabolic block.

IV. REAGENTS EMPLOYED

A. **Bacitracin differential disks**
   1. Commercial Taxo A disks (BD Biosciences; see Appendix 12)
   2. 0.04 units; group A streptococci are susceptible to low concentration of bacitracin.
   3. Inhibit most oral bacteria
B. **SXT (cotrimoxazole) is a combination of two antibiotics**
   1. Commercial disks available
      a. SX: 23.75 µg
      b. TMP: 1.25 µg
   2. Suppresses most normal flora growth in throat cultures including viridans streptococci

V. PROCEDURES

A. **Procedure 1**
   1. Media: nonselective sheep blood agar (SBA) plates
   2. With an inoculating needle, pick 3–4 **pure** colonies of β-hemolytic streptococci.
   3. Streak inoculum down the center of one half of the Petri plate, and stab the medium deeply a few times for observation of subsurface hemolysis.
   4. With a **sterile** swab or bacteriological loop, spread inoculum over entire half of the plate.
   5. **Aseptically** place a bacitracin Taxo disk and an SXT disk on the inoculated area; place disks evenly.
   6. With **flamed** forceps, **gently** tap disks so they adhere to the agar.
   7. Incubate **inverted** (lids down), 18–24 h, 35°C, 5–10% CO_2; if results are negative, reincubate another 24 h.

B. **Procedure 2**
  1. Media: selective, Trypticase soy agar (TSA) (TSA-SXT) plates with sheep blood (SB)
  2. Formulation of Gunn, Ohashi, Gaydos, and Holt (2)
  3. Stock solutions
      a. Solution T: 0.125 g TMP in a few milliliters of 0.1 N HCl, brought to 50 mL with distilled water
      b. Solution SX: 2.375 g SX in a few milliliters 1.0 N NaOH, brought to 50 mL with distilled water
      c. Solution SXT: combine equal parts of solutions SX and T; final combined concentrations, 25 µg/mL. Store **un**sterilized in 6-mL aliquots; freeze at $-20°C$.
  4. Completed medium

      TSA   1000.0 mL
      SXT solution   1.0 mL
      after sterilization (121°C, 15 lb, 15 min) add
      Sheep blood, 7%, **sterile**, defibrinated, 70.0 mL

  5. Store in plastic bags in the refrigerator, 10–15°C for up to a week.

Kurzynski et al. (5, 6) state that TSA-SXT medium is superior to conventional nonselective medium for the recovery of group A streptococci within 18–24 h; it is acceptable for recovery of group A streptococci.

  6. Dispense Petri dishes; 15–20 mL/plate (15 × 100 mm)
  7. Pick 3–4 **pure** colonies of β-hemolytic streptococci.
      a. With **sterile** bacteriological loop or swab, streak for confluent growth; stab medium deeply several times for observation of subsurface hemolysis.
      b. **Aseptically** place a bacitracin Taxo A disk on the inoculated area.
      c. With **flamed** forceps, gently tap disk so it adheres to the agar.
  8. Incubate **inverted** (lids down), 35°C, 5–10% CO_2, 18–24 h; reincubate an additional 24 h if results are negative.

VI. QUALITY CONTROL MICROORGANISMS

A. Bacitracin susceptible (S): *Streptococcus pyogenes* ATCC 12344
B. Bacitracin resistant (R): *Streptococcus agalactiae* group B ATCC 13813

VII. RESULTS

> See Figures 1.1 and 1.2 (Appendix 1) for colored photographic results

VIII. INTERPRETATION—EITHER PROCEDURE

Bacitracin/SXT disks or bacitracin on TSA-SXT media
  1. **Sensitive** (S, Sen, susceptible)
      a. Any zone around disk; growth inhibited
      b. Report: β-hemolytic streptococci **presumptively** group A by bacitracin
  2. **Resistant** (R)
      a. No zone around disk; growth up to and around disk
      b. Report: β-hemolytic streptococci **presumptively** not group A by bacitracin

Table 1.1. Bacitracin/SXT Disk Interpretations

Bacitracin	SXT	Presumptive ID
S	R	Group A β-streptococci
R	R	Group B β-streptococci
R	S	**Not** group A or B β-streptococci
S	S	Rule out group A or B with serologic tests

(*Note:* Interpretation of SXT susceptibility may be difficult since the organism may grow **slightly** before total inhibition of growth occurs (4).) Anaerobic incubation increases the detection of group A streptococcal strains that only produce oxygen-labile streptolysin O and inhibits much of the normal flora (8). Zones of inhibition should **not** be measured. β-Hemolytic colonies on TSA/SXT medium and zones of hemolysis are smaller than when growth is on nonselective SBA.

IX. PRECAUTIONS

A. Some non–group A streptococci may also be inhibited by bacitracin; thus a test is frequently performed along with the SXT susceptibility test.
B. The bacitracin test is fairly accurate as a presumptive test but **not highly specific** (5). More than 10% of group C and G streptococci and 5% of group B strains are also susceptible to bacitracin (5).
C. Only β-hemolytic streptococci should be tested since many β-hemolytic streptococci (including *S. pneumoniae*) are susceptible to low concentrations of bacitracin (5). *Streptococcus cricetus, S. downei, S. ferus,* and *S. macacae* are also bacitracin sensitive but are seldom isolated from human infections.
D. Growth of the bacterial inoculum should be confluent; a too-light inoculum will cause non–group A streptococci to appear susceptible to bacitracin (1).
E. A throat culture is **not** recommended for inoculation since normal flora may partially inhibit growth of group A streptococci, especially in areas of more confluent growth (5).
F. Do not use positive (+) and negative (−) to indicate results; use S (sensitive, susceptible) and R (resistant). The terms *positive* and *negative* could denote grow/no growth on the plate but not necessarily around the disk.

REFERENCES

1. Facklam RR, Thacker LG, Fox B, Eriquez L. Presumptive identification of streptococci with a new test system. J Clin Microbiol 1982;15(6):987–990.
2. Gunn BA, Ohashi DK, Gaydos CA, Holt ES. Selective and enhanced recovery of group A and B streptococci from throat cultures with sheep blood agar containing sulfamethoxazole and trimethoprim. J Clin Microbiol 1977;5(6):650–655.
3. Hitchings GH. Mechanism of action of trimethoprim-sulfamethoxazole. Int J Infect Dis 1973;128(suppl):S433–S436.
4. Jawetz E, Melnick JL, Adelberg EA. Review of Medical Microbiology, ed 17. Los Altos, CA: Appleton & Lange, 1987.
5. Kurzynski TA, Meise CK. Evaluation of sulfamethoxazole-trimethoprim blood agar plates for recovery of group A streptococci from throat cultures. J Clin Microbiol 1979;9(2):189–193.
6. Kurzynski T, Meise C, Van Holten C. Evaluation of techniques for isolation of group A streptococci from throat cultures. J Clin Microbiol 1981;13(5):891–894.
7. Lancini G, Parenti F. Antibiotics An Integrated View. New York: Springer-Verlag, 1982:39, 46, 48.
8. Lauer BA, Reller LB, Mirrett S. Effect of atmosphere and duration of incubation on primary isolation of group A streptococci from throat cultures. J Clin Microbiol 1983;17(2):338–340.
9. Nagarajan R. Antibacterial activities and modes of action of vancomycin and related glycopeptides. Antimicrob Agents Chemother 1991;35:605–609.
10. Murray PR, Baron EJ, Pfaller MA, et al. Manual of Clinical Microbiology, ed 6. Washington, DC: American Society for Microbiology, 1995:1294, 1296.

Bile Esculin (Aesculin) Hydrolysis Tests

I. PRINCIPLE

To determine the ability of an organism to hydrolyze the glycoside esculin (aesculin) to esculetin (aesculetin) and glucose in the presence of bile; an aglycon test

II. PURPOSE

(See Chapters 43–45)
A. To aid in the identification and differentiation of group D *Enterococcus* spp. (+) (formerly *Streptococcus faecalis, S. faecium,* and *S. durans* plus new species) and group D nonenterococcal *Streptococcus* spp. (+) (e.g., *S. equinus, S. bovis,* and *S. bovis* variants) from other streptococci, not group D (−). It is a **presumptive** test (Table 2.1). The genus *Streptococcus* was split into three genera: *Enterococcus, Lactococcus,* and *Streptococcus* (68).

   It was previously accepted that growth in NaCl along with bile esculin would give a presumptive identification of *Enterococcus* spp. (29). However, now with isolation of *Pediococcus* and *Leuconostoc* spp. from human infections, such presumptive identification could be erroneous (29). Both *Pediococcus* and *Leuconostoc* spp. yield positive results with both NaCl and bile esculin (29).

B. To aid in the differentiation of the *Enterobacteriaceae,* primarily the *Klebsiella-Enterobacter-Serratia* (all V+) (K-E-S) division, *Kluyvera* (+), *Leclercia* (+), and *Cedecea* spp. (+) (21, 47) and serve as a taxonomic tool for classification of the family *Enterobacteriaceae* (22).
C. To aid in differentiation of *Listeria* species (+) from other Gram-positive facultatively anaerobic nonsporeforming bacilli (−) (71); e.g., morphologically similar *Erysipelothrix rhusiopathiae* and some diphtheroids (64).
D. Presumptive identification of *Bacteroides fragilis* group (see *Bacteroides* Bile Esculin (BBE) Agar (52) and Kanamycin-Bile-Esculin (KEB) Medium (11)).
E. Aid in identification of *Vibrio vulnificus* (81) (see Precautions).
F. Aid in identification of motile *Aeromonas eucrenophila* (+); differentiation of *Aeromonas* spp.: *A. caviae* (+), *A. veronii* (+), and *A. hydrophilia* (+) from *A. sobria* (−) (34). However, *Aeromonas* spp. **do not** grow at 10–45°C, a characteristic that may be used to differentiate them from enterococci.
G. Epidemiologic studies and presumptive identification of *Cryptococcus neoformans* from other *Cryptococcus* species by pigment production. This is not related to the brown-black color developed by the reaction of ferric ions with esculin (19). (See Esculin-Based Streptomycin-Chloramphenicol Agar Medium.)
H. Differentiation of *Fusobacterium* spp., primarily *F. mortiferum* (+) and *F. necrogenes* (+) from other *Fusobacterium* spp. (−) (2, 47).
I. Aid in differentiation of yellow-pigmented *Falvimonas oryzhabitans* (−) (formerly VE-2) from *Sphingomonas (Pseudomonas) paucimobilis* (+) and *Chryseomonas luteola* (+) (formerly VE-1) (47).

Table 2.1. *Enterococcus*[a] and *Streptococcus* Species Type Strain Classification

Group D *Enterococcus*:		
E. avium (13, 57)	ATCC 14025	
E. casseliflavus[b]	ATCC 25788	
E. columbae		
E. durans (13, 46)	ATCC 19432	
E. faecalis[c]	ATCC 19433	
E. faecium	ATCC 19434	
E. flavescens		
E. gallinarum (7, 13)	NCDO 2313	ATCC 49573
E. hirae (46)	NCDO 1258	ATCC 8043
E. malodoratus	NCDO 846	ATCC 43197
E. mundtii (12)	NCDO 2375	ATCC 43186
E. pseudoavium[d]	NCDO 2138	ATCC 49372
E. raffinose-variable[e]	CDC 1739-79	ATCC 49427
E. seriolicida	ATCC 49156	
E. solitarius[e]	CDC[f] 885-78	ATCC 49428
E. sulfureus		
Not Group D *Enterococcus*:		
E. cecorum	NCDO[g] 2674	ATCC 43198
E. dispar		
E. raffinose-variable		
E. saccharolyticus	NCDO 2594	ATCC 43076
Streptococcus:		
S. bovis	ATCC 33317	NCDO 597
S. equinus	ATCC 9812	

[a]Formerly in *Streptococcus* genus.
[b]Former *S. faecium* subsp. *casseliflavus* is now a separate species of *Enterococcus* (13, 83).
[c]Former subspecies: *Streptococcus faecalis* subsp. *liquefaciens*, *S. faecalis* subsp. *zymogens*, and *S. faecalis* subsp. *faecalis* are no longer recognized and are lumped into one species, *Enterococcus faecalis* (8, 44).
[d]Collins et al. submitted for publication (27).
[e]Collins MD, Facklam RR, Farrow JAE, Williams R submitted for publication (27).
[f]Centers for Disease Control.
[g]National Collection of Dairy Organisms.

III. BIOCHEMISTRY INVOLVED

Esculin is derived from the horse chestnut tree and has vitamin P activity (19). Esculin is a glucoside (glycoside general term), an acetal derivative of a simple monosaccharide (50). When a noncarbohydrate is linked to a sugar by an acetal linkage, the resulting acetal is called a *glycoside*, and the nonsugar moiety is called the *aglycon* (6) (or genin (33)); the steroid portion is linked to a carbon sugar residue. The aglycon is linked to the parent sugar through an oxygen atom (└O┘), a glycosidic link) (9). Two moieties of the molecule (glucose and 7-hydroxycoumarin) are linked together by an ester bond through oxygen (47).

The acetals are readily hydrolyzed by acids (9); the basis of the esculin test is hydrolysis at the β-linkage of esculin to esculetin by constitutive β-glucosidase (the enzyme esculinase), which frees the glucose molecule (33). Esculin, a coumarin derivative (6-β-glucoside-7-hydroxycoumarin) (47), is hydrolyzed to 6,7-dihydroxycoumarin and glucose.

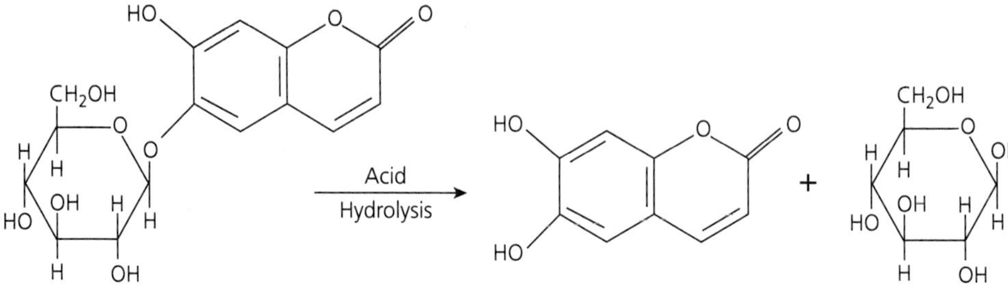

Esculin ($C_{15}H_{16}O_9$)
6, β-Glucoside-7-hydroxycoumarin

Esculetin (aglycone)
6, 7-Dihydroxycoumarin

β-D-Glucose

Esculin hydrolysis may be demonstrated by one of three means (14, 21–23, 55).

Routine

In the most commonly used method esculetin reacts with an iron (III) salt (ferric; Fe^{3+}) to form a dark brown or black phenolic complex. Ferric citrate ($FeC_6H_5O_7$) or ferric ammonium citrate (a 50/50 mixture of ferric citrate and ammonium citrate) is incorporated in bile esculin medium at a 0.05% concentration as an indicator of esculin hydrolysis and resultant esculetin formation. Routine esculin hydrolysis is a two-step procedure: the bacterial strain **must** (*a*) grow in the presence of a particular concentration of bile and (*b*) produce esculinase to hydrolyze esculin (22, 23).

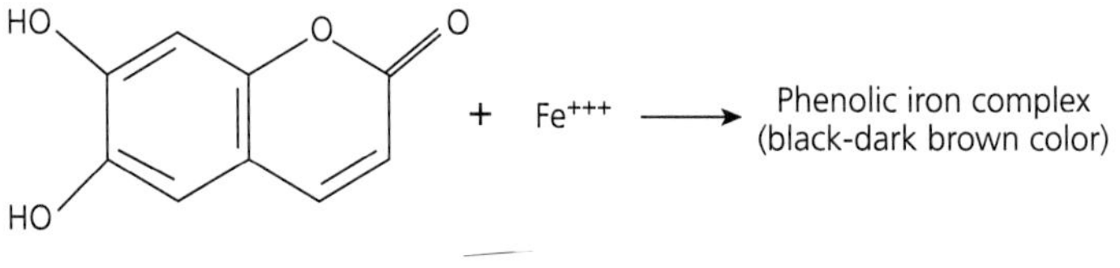

Esculin + Fe^{+++} → Phenolic iron complex (black-dark brown color)

Esculetin   Ferric ions

The exact mechanism is still not known, but it is hypothesized to be

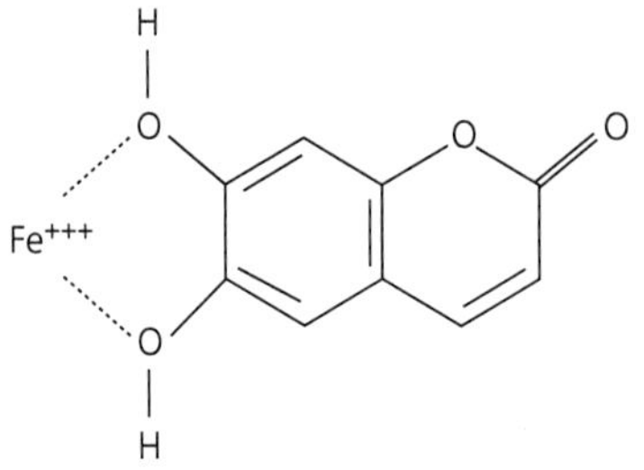

Alternatives

A. Measurement of acid production from the fermentation of the hydrolysis product, a glucose moiety, with or without gas formation (CO_2 and H_2S), with a resultant decrease in the

pH of the medium (14, 56). However, the relative insensitivity of secondary pH measurements with chemical indicators severely limits this glucose fermentation method (23).
B. Determination of a loss (decrease) of fluorescence (366 nm) as the intact esculin molecule is hydrolyzed; the β-D-glucosidic bond is broken (21, 23).

IV. MEDIA EMPLOYED

(*Notes:* Prolonged incubation is required because bacterial growth and multiplication must precede synthesis of the enzyme required for esculin hydrolysis (63).

Bile inhibits **non**–group D, esculin-hydrolyzing streptococci (22, 54); Oxgall 2%, a 10× concentration of bile, equals 20% bile salts, and 1–4% bile is equivalent to 10% and 40% bile. Bile inhibits Gram-positive bacteria other than enterococci.

Iron (III) is the new terminology for ferric (Fe^{3+}); iron (III) citrate is an indicator of esculin hydrolysis and resultant esculetin formation. Growth of enterococci can be optimized by the addition of horse serum.)

A. Formulations; growth-dependent media
   1. Bile esculin medium (BEM) agar (BEA); pH 7.1 ± 0.2

Casein peptone	5.0 g
Beef (meat) extract	3.0 g
Oxgall (bile)	40.0 g
Esculin powder, $C_{15}H_{16}O_9$,	1.0 g
Iron (III) citrate, $FeC_6H_5O_7$	0.5 g
or	
Iron (III) ammonium citrate, $(NH_4)_2HC_6H_5O_7$	
Agar **(solid medium only)**	15.0 g
Deionized water	1000.0 mL
After sterilization, add	
Horse serum, 5%, **sterile**	50.0 mL

   2. Modified bile esculin medium (MBEM): without horse serum
   3. Bile esculin azide agar/broth (Pfizer Selective Enterococcus Medium (PSE), selective enterococcus medium (SEM), Enterococcosel (BBL)
      a. Formulation of Isenberg, Goldberg, and Sampson (43); reduced concentration of bile and addition of sodium azide
      b. Ingredients; pH 7.1 ± 0.2

Casein peptone	17.0 g
Meat peptone	3.0 g
Yeast extract	5.0 g
Esculin	1.0 g
Oxgall (bile)	10.0 g
Sodium chloride, NaCl,	5.0 g
Sodium citrate, $C_3H_4OH(COO)_3Na_3$,	1.0 g
Iron (III) ammonium citrate (50/50)	0.5 g
Sodium azide, NaN_3,	0.25 g
Agar **(solid medium only)**	15.0 g
Deionized water	1000.0 mL

B. Inhibitors
   1. Bile inhibits growth of most Gram-positive cocci other than *Streptococcus* spp., and at a concentration of 20% it inhibits anaerobic bacteria other than the *B. fragilis* group as well as most facultative anaerobes.

2. Sodium azide (NaN$_3$) 0.25 g/L inhibits growth of Gram-negative bacteria, inhibits bacterial cytochromes (30), and reduces catalase activity. It permits growth of Gram-positive cocci (e.g., streptococci).
C. Method of preparation
 1. Weigh amount accurately as directed on the label; various company products may differ slightly.
 2. Rehydrate with distilled or deionized water; heat **gently** into solution.
D. Sterilization
 1. Media base: autoclave at 121°C, 15 lb, 15 min
 2. Horse serum: filtration (Millipore)
E. Dispense
 1. Petri dishes: 15–20 mL/plate (15 × 100 mm); dispense **after** sterilization
 2. Screw-cap tubes: 5.0 mL/tube (16 × 125 mm). Cool in a **slanted** position to yield **long slants.**
F. Finished/uninoculated medium appearance: cream colored (pale yellow), solid plate/tubed media
G. Storage
 1. Refrigerator, 2–8°C; plates inverted (**lids down**)
 2. Shelf life is approximately 3–4 weeks.
H. Method of inoculation
 1. Inocula
  a. Streptococci/enterococci testing
   (1) Growth from a 24-h pure culture in Todd-Hewitt broth (25)
   (2) Tubed medium: add 2 drops to the surface of the slant with either a Pasteur pipette or an inoculating loop; streak slant with an S-shaped motion (4).
   (3) Plate medium: add 2 **drops** to surface; use four-quadrant streaking for maximum isolation.
  b. *Enterobacteriaceae* testing
   (1) Growth from heart infusion agar (HIA), lysine iron agar (LIA), or Kligler iron agar/triple sugar iron agar (KIA/TSI); pure culture
   (2) Use a **heavy** inoculum (4-mm loopful) **except** when testing *Escherichia coli* (light inoculum) (20, 51, 85) (see Precautions).
I. Incubation: aerobically, 35°C
 1. Streptococci/enterococci: 48 h
  a. May check tubes periodically and if positive reaction, report result.
  b. Hold up to 72 h **before** reporting a negative result.
 2. *Enterobacteriaceae:* 18–24 h

An atmosphere with increased CO_2 increases the numbers of viridans streptococci that give a positive bile esculin reaction; group D streptococci and enterococci all grow well in an atmosphere **without** CO_2 (1).

V. RESULTS

See Figures 2.1–2.3 (Appendix 1) for colored photographic results

VI. INTERPRETATION

A. **Positive BE test result** (+) for esculin hydrolysis
 1. Slant (tubed medium)

a. A dark brown to black color diffuses onto the slant and onto translucent to white colonies.
   b. **Half or more** of the medium is blackened.
  2. Plate medium
   a. Any blackening is significant.
   b. Colonies are surrounded by black to dark brown halos.
  3. Plates or slants: blackening in any time interval (55).
 B. **Negative BE test result** (−): three possible readings
  1. **No** blackening of the medium.
  2. Blackening of **less than half** of tubed medium after a 72-h incubation (± reaction) (25).
  3. Growth may occur, but this **does not** indicate esculin splitting; it only indicates that the bile concentration did not inhibit the usual growth of organisms other than group D enterococci/streptococci.

VII. RAPID TESTS

(*Note:* Incubation for 4 h or less measures primarily **constitutive** esculinase (a β-glucosidase) (18). All rapid procedures use non-growth-supporting media.)

A. **Esculin spot test** (20, 21, 71)
  1. Hydrolysis is determined by loss of fluorescence measured with a 366-nm ultraviolet light generator. Loss of fluorescence indicates esculin hydrolysis. Esculin fluoresces, but neither glucose nor esculetin fluoresces at this wavelength.
  2. Esculin solution: pipette a 0.02% esculin solution onto filter paper on a microscope slide.
   a. Rub an isolated bacterial colony onto the test paper.
   b. Incubate at 35°C for 30 min.
  3. Interpretation
   a. Hydrolysis: darkening; loss of fluorescence
   b. No hydrolysis: no darkening; no loss of fluorescence
B. **Rapid buffered esculin solution (sodium chloride esculin hydrolysis test)**
  1. Procedure of Qadri, DeSilva, and Zubairi (61)
  2. Buffered esculin solution, adjust to pH 5.6 ± 0.2

Esculin powder, $C_{15}H_{16}O_9$	5.0 g
Iron (III) ammonium citrate (50/50)	0.5 g
Ferric citrate, $FeC_6H_5O_7$	
Ammonium citrate, $(NH_4)_3C_6H_5O_7$	
Monopotassium phosphate, KH_2PO_4	0.1 g
Dipotassium phosphate, K_2HPO_4	0.4 g
Sodium chloride, NaCl	50.0 g
Deionized water	1000.0 mL

  3. Dispensing/storage
   a. 0.5-mL/screw-cap tube (12 × 75 mm)
   b. Stable at least 8 weeks in refrigerator (4°C)
  4. Inoculum
   a. Density of McFarland standard #3 in 0.5 mL of buffered esculin solution (see Appendix 5).
   b. A **heavy** inoculum increases the rapidity of the test and makes it **un**necessary to use sterile materials, because the density of the organisms and the lack of appreciable carbon and nitrogen in the solution prevents overgrowth by contaminants within the time frame of the test.

5. Incubation: 35°C waterbath for up to 4 h
6. Interpretation
   a. Positive (+)
      (1) Color change of solution to dark brown to black
      (2) All enterococci show a 2+ to 4+ reaction within 2 h.
   b. Negative (−): no color change; solution remains colorless.

C. **Rapid bile esculin (RBE) reagent one-tube test**
   1. Procedure of Edberg, Trepeta, Kontnick, and Torres (23)
   2. Dual purpose
      a. To determine the production of esculinase in the presence of bile equivalent
      b. To determine the bile solubility of *Streptococcus pneumoniae*
   3. Principle: test is based on measurement of constitutive β-glucosidase (esculinase) with repression of enzyme by a bile equivalent (sodium desoxycholate).
   4. Reagent solution, pH 7.5
      a. Ingredients: to 0.05 M Sorensen phosphate buffer (pH 7.5) (see Appendix 6) add final concentrations (wt/vol) of
         (1) Sodium desoxycholate (deoxycholate), 2.5% (a substitute for bile salts)
         (2) *p*-Nitrophenyl-β-D-glucopyranoside, 0.5% (a hydrolyzable colorless esculinase substrate)
      b. Dissolve at 35°C
      c. Dispense 0.25 mL aliquots into screw-cap test tubes (12 × 75 mm)
      d. Storage: in the dark; stable at least 6 months
         (1) Liquid aliquots: refrigerate at 4–10°C.
         (2) Dehydrated aliquots: refrigerate at 4–10°C with desiccant.
   5. Inoculum: sufficient bacterial mass to produce a final turbidity of at least a 0.5 McFarland standard (see Appendix 5).
      a. **Liquid** reagent may gel on storage; bring to 35°C to reliquefy **before** use. Inoculate from bacterial **colonies.**
      b. **Dehydrated** reagent: inoculate with bacterial suspension in **distilled water.**
   6. Incubation: aerobically at 35°C; read at 5-min intervals for up to 30 min.
   7. Interpretation
      a. Yellow color (+)
         (1) Positive for esculin hydrolysis in presence of bile
         (2) Color equivalent to the dark brown to black color seen in the 40% bile esculin reaction
      b. **No** color change, **clearing** of turbidity
         (1) Bile solubility positive (sensitive, S)
            (a) Release of autolytic enzyme
            (b) *S. pneumoniae*
         (2) Esculin hydrolysis negative (−)
      c. **No** color change, no clearing of turbidity
         (1) Bile solubility negative (−)
         (2) Esculin hydrolysis negative (−)

Edberg and Bell (18) modified the procedure to differentiate *Bacteroides* (+) from *Fusobacterium* (−) on the basis of the presence of constitutive β-glucosidase. The **exceptions** to above procedure are

1. Dispense 0.30 mL aliquots.
2. Use a McFarland standard inoculum of 0.05 or **above** (see Appendix 5).
3. Incubate aerobically at room temperature (22–25°C).

VIII. ALTERNATIVE TESTS

A. **Anaerobic esculin broth**
   1. Heart infusion broth (HIB), 1 L, containing

Esculin	1.0 g
Agar	1.0 g
Hemin, 5 mg/mL (**optional**)	1.0 mL
Vitamin K_1 (**optional**)	1.0 mL

   2. Incubation: **anaerobically** at 35°C for 24–48 h or until good growth
   3. Add a few drops of 0.1% ferric ammonium citrate solution to each tube. Positive reaction: black color throughout medium.
   4. Alternatively, the tube may be observed under long-wave ultraviolet light (366 nm); loss of fluorescence indicates a positive result.

B. *Bacteroides* **bile esculin (BBE) agar (*B. fragilis* isolation agar, *B. fragilis* bile-esculin agar)**
   1. Medium of Livingston, Kominos, and Yee (52)
   2. Purpose: rapid selection and presumptive identification of *B. fragilis* group (76) (*B. fragilis, B. thetaiotaomicron, B. ovatus, B. distasonis, B. uniformis, B. caccae,* and *B. vulgatus* (60)) and selective medium for *Bilophila wadsworthia* (3)
   3. Selective and differential medium differentiates by the ability to hydrolyze esculin **and** produce catalase. A growth stimulator and hemin provide option of testing for catalase production (52). BBE may be used for the esculin reaction **if** the test organism is resistant to bile and gentamicin. Members of the *B. fragilis* group are almost always resistant to penicillin (36–38) and can protect penicillin-sensitive bacteria accompanying them in mixed infections (40).
   4. Ingredients
      a. Stock hemin solution: final concentration 5 g/mL. Hemin is required or markedly stimulates growth (72). To a 100-mL volumetric flask add

Hemin	0.5 g
Sodium hydroxide, NaOH, 1N	10.0 mL
Distilled water to 100.0 mL	

      b. Stock gentamicin solution
         (1) Gentamicin; Garamycine, 40 mg/mL solution, injectable. A broad-spectrum antibiotic that along with bile inhibits facultative anaerobes and **most** Gram-negative anaerobic bacteria, microorganisms other than esculin-positive *Bacteroides* that can tolerate bile (60).
         (2) Final concentration: 40 µg/mL
      c. Medium, pH 7.0 ± 0.2

Trypticase soy agar (TSA)	40.0 g
Bile, 20%	20.0 g
Esculin hydrate	1.0 g
Iron (III) ammonium citrate, (50/50)	0.5 g
Deionized water	1000.0 mL
No heating is required; swirl to dissolve and add	
Hemin, 5 µg/mL, **sterile** 2.5 mL	
Gentamicin solution, **sterile** 2.5 mL	

      d. Method of sterilization
         (1) Stock hemin and medium base: autoclave at 121°C, 121 lb, 15 min
         (2) Gentamicin: filtration (Millipore)

5. Dispense into Petri dish: 12–15 mL/plate (15 × 100 mm)
6. Uninoculated medium is a clear, slightly yellow, solid plate medium.
7. Storage
   a. Stock solutions and media: refrigerate at 2–8°C; plates inverted (**lids down**)
   b. Shelf life is approximately 3–6 weeks.
8. Method of inoculation
   a. Medium should be reduced immediately **before** inoculation by placing under anaerobic conditions for 18–24 h (16) or, e.g., GasPak anaerobic system (69). Regardless of which system is used, an indicator of anaerobiosis is needed.
   b. Direct specimen: use four-quadrant streaking for maximum isolation. Specimen should be streaked as soon as received in the laboratory.
9. Incubation: **anaerobically** at 35°C, plates inverted (**lids down**); read final results after 48 h.
10. Interpretation

(*Note:* Studies by Livingston et al. (52) showed three distinct types of colony morphology for the *B. fragilis* group. All were circular, raised, with entire margins and more than 1 mm in diameter, but specific differences cast them into three types.)

   a. Esculin hydrolysis
      (1) Positive (+)
         (a) Blackening of medium
            Type 1: 31% exhibited dull, opaque, brittle charcoal gray colonies surrounded by a dark zone with precipitated bile (52).
            Type 2: 68% exhibited glistening, butyrous, semitransparent, light to dark gray colonies surrounded by a gray zone with **no** precipitate (52).
         (b) **Presumptive** identification of *B. fragilis* group
      (2) Negative (−)
         (a) Growth but no change in color of medium
         (b) Esculin **not** hydrolyzed
         (c) *B. fragilis* group type 3; 1% exhibited glistening, butyrous, white colonies with no gray zone (52).
         (d) Rarely other microorganisms
   b. Catalase production
      (1) Expose growth on BBE plates to atmosphere for 30 min **before** addition of 3% hydrogen peroxide (H_2O_2).
      (2) Positive (+): evolution of bubbles
      (3) Negative (−): no bubbling
C. **Kanamycin-bile disk test**
   1. Procedure of Draper and Barry (17) modified by Vargo et al. (82)
   2. Screening test for *B. fragilis* group: bile stimulator test and kanamycin resistance test (82)
   3. Bile- and antibiotic-impregnated filter paper disk testing; *B. fragilis* group is the **only** species that can grow in the presence of bile and exhibit resistance to kanamycin (82).
      a. Bile 2% (Oxgall), 25 mg concentration
      b. Kanamycin, 1000 μg/mL
   4. Growth medium: thioglycollate broth (Thio); turbidity equal to McFarland 0.5 standard (see Appendix 5)
   5. Disk test medium: *Brucella* blood agar plates
   6. Incubation: **anaerobically** at 35°C for 24–48 h; all *B. fragilis* group organisms give positive result after 24 h.
   7. Interpretation
      a. Positive (+)

(1) Kanamycin resistant (R): zone of inhibition < 10 mm diameter
(2) Bile resistant (R): growth up to the edge of disk
b. Negative (−)
(1) Kanamycin sensitive (susceptible) (S): zone of inhibition > 12 mm diameter
(2) Bile sensitive (susceptible) (S): inhibition of growth, zones 17–30 mm in diameter

Bile disks are all surrounded by a large zone of hemolysis, and organisms that grow within this zone often produce a cloudy precipitate in agar; however, this phenomenon accentuates growth, making interpretation easier (17).

D. **Kanamycin-bile-esculin (KEB) medium**
   1. Medium of Chan and Porschen (11), based on medium of Swan (79)
   2. Screening to isolate and **presumptively** distinguish the *B. fragilis* group from other **anaerobic** Gram-negative bacilli (11, 17, 82) in specimens containing mixed flora.
   3. Test medium, Trypticase soy agar (TSA) containing

      Kanamycin, 1000 μg/mL, added **after** autoclaving
      Esculin, 5.0%
      Iron (III) ammonium citrate (50/50, ferric citrate and ammonium citrate)
      Bile, 20.0% (or Oxgall, 2%)

Kanamycin ensures selective isolation of members of the *B. fragilis* group and inhibits growth of Gram-negative facultative anaerobic and aerobic bacilli; 20% bile stimulates growth of the *B. fragilis* group but inhibits other anaerobic bacteria **except** *Fusobacterium mortiferum* (52).

   4. Incubation: **anaerobically** (e.g., GasPak, BBL) at 35°C for 24 h; an additional 24-h incubation is recommended when reactions are negative.
   5. Interpretation (60): examine colonies under a dissecting microscope with a long-wave UV lamp to detect fluorescence.
      a. Pigmented colonies of the *B. fragilis* group fluoresce orange to brick red. Fluorescence is visible **before** pigmentation.
      b. Bile esculin (+): growth with blackening in surrounding medium

Many investigators (5, 11, 17, 78, 82) have shown that the *B. fragilis* group is the **only** commonly encountered, anaerobic Gram-negative bacilli that are **not** inhibited by bile and are also resistant to high concentrations of kanamycin. On KEB medium, Chan and Porschen's studies (11) showed that 100% of *B. fragilis* organisms grew, with 97–100% hydrolyzing esculin, while selectively inhibiting growth of other Gram-negative anaerobes as well as most facultative anaerobes, thus no hydrolysis.

E. **Esculin-based streptomycin-chloramphenicol agar medium**
   1. Medium of Edberg, Chaskes, Alture-Werber, and Singer (19)
   2. Isolation and **presumptive** identification of *C. neoformans* (19) from other yeasts. Test is specific for *C. neoformans* (19).
   3. Principle: esculin or the esculetin component of esculin hydrolysis is converted to a melanin-like pigment.
      a. Developers (19) suspect that the reaction is similar to the conversion of diphenols, aminophenols, and diaminobenzenes to melanin.
      b. Pigment production is **not** related to the brown-black color produced by the reaction of ferric ions with esculin, although the colors produced by both mechanisms are similar. Studies do not determine whether the yeast can use the intact esculin molecule or hydrolysis is required. *C. neoformans* can produce melanin-like pigment from both esculin and esculetin. 6,7-Dihydroxycoumarin is structurally similar enough to diphenols to serve as an intermediate in the melanin biosynthetic pathway (19).

4. Medium, pH 7.1 ± 0.2
   a. Ingredients

Peptone	10.0 g
Yeast extract	1.0 g
Esculin powder	0.5 g
Glucose (dextrose)	5.0 g
Agar, purified	15.0 g
Deionized water	1000.0 mL
Autoclave at 121° C, 15 lb, for 15 min and add	
Gentamicin sulfate, filter sterilized (e.g., Millipore)	25.0 mg
Chloramphenicol, filter sterilized	10.0 mg

   b. Dispense/storage: 20-mL Petri dish (100 mm); refrigerate at 4–10°C; stable approximately 4–6 months
5. Interpretation
   a. Positive (+): brown-black pigmentation; *C. neoformans*
   b. Negative (−); two possible results
      (1) Pale yellow pigmentation
         (a) Designated "torpid"; weak pigmentation
         (b) *Cryptococcus* spp. other than *C. neoformans*
      (2) Colorless
         (a) No pigmentation
         (b) *Cryptococcus* spp. other than *C. neoformans* or *Candida* spp., *Torulopsis glabrata*, *Geotrichum* spp., or *Rhodotorula* spp.

IX. QUALITY CONTROL MICROORGANISMS

American Type Culture Collection (ATCC) strains; National Committee for Clinical Laboratory Standards (NCCLS) organisms

(*Note:* Always include an uninoculated plate/tube as a negative control.)

A. BE, BEM, MBEM
   1. Positive (+)
      Enterococcus faecalis ATCC 29212
   2. Negative (−)
      Streptococcus pyogenes ATCC 19615
      Streptococcus mutans ATCC 25175

B. BBE and KEB
   1. Positive (+)
      Bacteroides fragilis ATCC 25285
      Bacteroides thetaiotaomicron ATCC 29741
   2. Negative (−)
      Escherichia coli ATCC 25922
      Clostridium perfringens ATCC 13124
      Fusobacterium necrophorum ATCC 25286
      Proteus mirabilis ATCC 12453

C. Rapid bile esculin (RBE) reagent test
   1. Positive (+)
      a. Esculin hydrolysis: *Enterococcus faecalis* ATCC 29212
      b. Bile solubility: *Streptococcus pneumoniae* ATCC 49136
   2. Negative (−)
      Streptococcus pyogenes ATCC 12344

D. Esculin-based streptomycin-chloramphenicol *Cryptococcus* medium
   1. Positive (+)
      Cryptococcus neoformans ATCC 14116
   2. Negative (−)
      Cryptococcus albidus ATCC 10666
      Cryptococcus laurentii ATCC 18803
      Cryptococcus terreus ATCC 11799

X. PRECAUTIONS

A. **General**
   1. The bile esculin test was originally used to identify the enterococci (54); however, other group D streptococci and occasionally non–group D streptococci and other genera, *Aerococcus* (V, variable) (30, 34) and *Listeria* (71), can tolerate the bile concentration and split esculin. *Aerococcus* spp. do **not** grow at 10–45°C, a characteristic that may be used to differentiate them from the enterococci; they are α-hemolytic and are all variable with regard to bile esculin hydrolysis. Do a Gram stain to help; *Aerococcus* are usually Gram-positive cocci in tetrads. Confirm by serologically demonstrating the **lack** of group D antigen (42). Demonstration of group D antigen in extracts of culture is **not** specific for enterococci (27). **Some** strains of *Leuconostoc* and **most** strains of *Pediococcus* also have D antigen (29).

   The properties of growth on 1–4% bile media and acid from esculin (hydrolysis) are **not** unique to the group D streptococci; they are shared by most group D strains (24). Approximately 3% of viridans streptococci are bile esculin positive (47); e.g., *S. intermedius, S. mutans, S. uberis, S. sanguis,* and *S. constellatus* (2, 24, 26, 65). *S. intermedius* and *S. constellatus* are subjective synonyms of *Streptococcus anginosus*.

   The bile esculin test **alone** cannot be used to identify the enterococci, but a positive reaction can be used **in combination with other tests to presumptively** identify the *Enterococcus*. Facklam (24) and Facklam et al. (30) recommend a combination of bile esculin and salt tolerance (growth in 6.5% NaCl). It was previously accepted that growth in NaCl along with bile esculin gave a presumptive identification of *Enterococcus* spp. (29). However, with isolation of *Pediococcus* and *Leuconostoc* spp. from human infections, such presumptive identification could be erroneous (29). Both *Pediococcus* and *Leuconostoc* spp. yield positive results with both NaCl and bile esculin (29).

   Group D enterococci/streptococci differ in their susceptibility to antimicrobial agents (1), and for proper antimicrobic therapy to be administered, they **must** be differentiated. Enterococci are usually penicillin resistant, while nonenterococcal strains are usually penicillin susceptible (1). Serologic testing is the **only** way to **confirm** group D enterococci/streptococci identification (27).

   2. Differences in the formulation of bile esculin media account for the different reactions of microorganisms (25). Bile esculin medium (BEM) contains four times as much bile (40%) as does bile esculin azide (BEA) medium (10%).

   Nonenterococcal streptococci, such as some viridans streptococci, are capable of splitting esculin (e.g., *S. sanguis, S. mutans,* and *S. anginosus*), but these species **usually cannot** tolerate an increased concentration of 40% bile and hydrolyze esculin in combination. Studies by Sabbaj et al. (66) showed that all strains of *S. mutans* hydrolyze esculin; occasional strains could grow in 40% bile, but they could **not** grow in 6.5% salt. However, *S. mutans* colonies are easily distinguished as they are small and hard and tend to adhere to the agar surface. Another streptococcal species in the viridans group that could occasionally hydrolyze esculin and grow in an increased concentration of bile is *S. sanguis* (66).

   However, with the lower concentration of bile (10%) in BEA, some viridans streptococci may exhibit growth and hydrolysis (25); a lower concentration of bile is less inhibitory to non–group D enterococci/streptococci (24).

Therefore, azide-containing medium is a better selective primary medium, but one with an increased bile concentration (40%) and no azide is better for **differentiation.** Studies by Facklam (26) found SEM medium (Pfizer) unsatisfactory for accurate differentiation of group D from non–group D streptococci.

3. Wide discrepancies exist among studies of esculin hydrolysis in the family *Enterobacteriaceae*. Levine et al. (50) and Vaughn and Levine (84) rediscovered its value for differentiation among the *Enterobacteriaceae*. Wasilauskas (85) and Lindell and Quinn (51) showed that the *Enterobacteriaceae* will grow on bile-esculin growth medium (e.g., Vaughn-Levine (VL), BEM, MBEM) but that only certain members will hydrolyze esculin and produce the characteristic blackening upon reaction with iron. Edberg et al. (21) showed that the genera *Klebsiella* (V), *Enterobacter* (+), and *Serratia* (V+) and species *Proteus vulgaris* (V), *Proteus rettgeri* (V) (formerly *Providencia rettgeri*), and *Citrobacter koseri* (V) (formerly *C. diversus*) could hydrolyze esculin within 24 h. According to Edberg et al. (22), *Enterobacter cloacae* hydrolyzes esculin both variably and weakly; it either possesses small amounts of constitutive enzyme, produces it in inactive form, or contains it in a relatively inaccessible site, since it consistently produces a weaker positive reaction on both growth and nongrowth media, usually darkening only 2–5 mm below the slant into the butt.

Lindell and Quinn (51) found **100% positive** hydrolysis in 4 h with *Klebsiella pneumoniae* subsp. *pneumoniae, Enterobacter aerogenes,* and three species of *Serratia*; **100% negative** hydrolysis in 4 h with *Shigella sonnei, Salmonella* spp., *P. mirabilis, Morganella morganii,* and *Proteus inconstans* (formerly *Providencia alcalifaciens*), and *Providencia stuartii*; **70% negative** hydrolysis in **18 h** with *E. coli, Citrobacter freundii, C. koseri, Hafnia alvei,* and *P. vulgaris*; and obtained **equivocal** (±) results with *Pantoea agglomerans* (formerly *Enterobacter agglomerans*) and *P. rettgeri*. The glucosidase responsible for esculin hydrolysis in **all** *Enterobacteriaceae* **other than** *E. coli* is constitutive (55) and is readily detectable by rapid nongrowth esculin tests (21).

Edberg et al. (21) recommend BEM as the medium of choice for routine testing of *Enterobacteriaceae*. It is restricted in differentiation of the *Klebsiella-Enterobacter-Serratia* spp.

4. *E. coli* β-glucosidase is inducible, and the organism cannot produce constitutive enzyme (55). There is **no hydrolysis** in **nongrowth** tests (e.g., spot tests) (20, 21, 55); induction **does not** occur during such a short incubation period (20).

β-Glucosidase is not a normal component of *E. coli*; it is made as needed (e.g., when the bacterium must use lactose or another disaccharide or related compound as a source of carbon). Lactose acts as an inducer and allows production of the β-glucosidase encoded in the structural gene of *E. coli*. Therefore, one should use a **light inoculum** obtained by touching the top of a colony with a bacteriological **needle** (**not** a loop) when testing *E. coli* with a growth test medium (e.g., BEM, MBEM) and interpret the reaction within an 18-to 24-h incubation period (21, 55). Wasilauskas (85) suggests that the **time** required for an isolate to produce hydrolysis is **directly proportional** to the **size** of the inoculum. A heavy inoculum presents more cells for induction of β-glucosidase capable of hydrolyzing esculin and an incubation longer than 24 h results in more cells being induced with time; either or both (time/temperature) increase positivity (55). No other species in the family showed this marked increase in hydrolysis with time; however, after induction, the ability to hydrolyze is lost if organisms are subcultured on a non-glucoside-containing medium (55). Because *E. coli* β-glucosidase is induced, either use a light inoculum when using a growth medium with an incubation of 18–24 h or perform a rapid nongrowth strip or spot test (55).

5. Delayed pyocyanin production by *Pseudomonas aeruginosa* may darken BEA medium; this is **not** a "true" test reaction (58). Also, pyomelanine-producing strains may produce

intense blackening after a few days; this is **not** due to esculin hydrolysis since it **does not** fluoresce under ultraviolet light (58).
6. False-positive esculin hydrolysis may occur with H_2S-positive nonfermenting bacilli such as *Shewanella putrefaciens* (formerly *Pseudomonas putrefaciens*) (33).
7. Studies by Tison (81) showed that *V. vulnificus* hydrolyzes esculin in routine esculin-containing noninhibitory media (e.g., BEM, heart infusion esculin broth (HIE)) under standard incubation conditions. However, there are conflicting reports; *Bergey's Manual of Systematic Bacteriology,* vol. I (48), Baumann et al. (4), and Weaver et al. (86) report the species negative for esculin hydrolysis; other investigators (15, 53, 86) have reported varying positive results. Studies by Tison (81) also showed that some strains failed to hydrolyze esculin on media containing inhibitory compounds (e.g., BEA). According to Tison, failure of investigators to define conditions and variations in procedures may account for the conflicting reports in the literature of esculin hydrolysis by *V. vulnificus*.

B. **Bile esculin azide (BEA) agar medium**
1. Studies by Havelaar et al. (41) showed that BEA agar incubated at **44°C** for 48 h supports growth of group D enterococci/streptococci almost exclusively but is also the most inhibitory of all media tested (e.g., ethyl violet azide (EVA), azide dextrose broth, BEA, Kenner fecal (KF) broth) against group D streptococci. These authors recommend considering reactions on BEA positive **only** when dense growth **and** esculin hydrolysis are present (i.e., growth with brownish black halos around the colonies). Havelaar et al. (41) also found that strains other than group D streptococci could produce typical reactions on BEA when incubated at 37°C (the temperature recommended by Facklam (25)).
2. Some group B streptococci can grow on BEA agar, although they **do not** blacken the agar (59).
3. According to studies by Wasilauskas (85), esculin hydrolysis time and inoculum are related. The number of *E. coli* colonies able to hydrolyze esculin increases with time (55). Induction **does not** occur during a short incubation period (20). Wasilauskas (85) and Edberg et al. (20, 21) found that positivity increases with time.

C. **Anaerobes:** there are two main limitations to using bile-esculin media to identify Gram-negative anaerobic bacilli (52).
1. An anaerobic incubation period of 24–48 h is required.
2. One species, *Fusobacterium mortiferum,* is resistant to bile and can produce β-glucosidase (52) as **inducible** enzyme activity (18).

D. *Bacteroides* **bile esculin (BBE) agar**
1. Enterococci may grow weakly after prolonged incubation (2). They appear as small, transparent colonies and may stain Gram negative because of their damaged state (77).
2. Microorganisms in the *B. fragilis* group grow well; the **exception** is *B. vulgatus,* which usually does **not** hydrolyze esculin and thus exhibits **no** discoloration in the surrounding medium (60, 76). *Bacteroides splanchnicus* and *Bacteroides eggerthii,* which are not part of the *B. fragilis* group, are bile resistant and hydrolyze esculin (60); however, these species are rarely isolated and are part of the normal bowel flora (2).
3. Other anaerobes, *Enterobacteriaceae,* and enterococci that may grow on BBE fail to produce the characteristic morphology or blackening associated with the *B. fragilis* group.
4. Occasional *B. fragilis* strains fail to grow because of inhibition by 20% bile.
5. Occasionally *Fusobacterium* strains (e.g., *F. mortiferum* (2)) grow; however, this is predicted since fusobacteria are resistant to 20% bile (75). The colonies appear as "fried eggs" and are smaller than *Bacteroides* (<1 mm in diameter); their size is due to their relatively greater sensitivity to gentamicin (32). All are catalase negative (52).
6. Rare strains of *K. pneumoniae* subsp. *pneumoniae* can grow on BBE and blacken the medium (2); however, the colonies are easily distinguished by their pinpoint size and the less intense blackening that produces brownish black coloration rather than gray.
7. BBE medium fails to inhibit yeasts (52); however, no blackening occurs.

8. Medium will not permit detection of all penicillin-resistant *Bacteroides,* mainly those that are inhibited by bile (52). Examples: *B. melaninogenicus* and *Prevotella oralis* (formerly *Bacteroides oralis*) usually fail to grow on BBE (52).
9. Hemin has a dual function: growth stimulator and option for catalase testing. Many *Bacteroides* strains require hemin for growth (35, 87). The *B. fragilis* group **cannot** synthesize their own hemin and must transport preformed hemin to synthesize such heme proteins as cytochromes and catalase (73). A concentration of 1 μg/mL is required for optimal growth.
10. Studies by Wilkins et al. (88) showed that higher catalase activity was observed when hemin was added **after** autoclaving, indicating that hemin availability and not total hemin concentration determined catalase production. Catalase is **not** found consistently in all organisms of the *B. fragilis* group; however, *B. fragilis* specifically is the anaerobe organism most frequently isolated from clinical specimens, and it is usually catalase positive (88). The *B. fragilis* group and *B. putredinis* are the only Gram-negative anaerobic rods that are catalase positive (88).
11. Do not use a fermentable carbohydrate in base medium if you are determining catalase production. As little as a 0.5–1.0% concentration of glucose can cause immediate cessation of catalase production (39, 74). In a carbohydrate-containing medium little catalase is produced because cells continue to use glucose throughout growth cycle (88). Therefore, carbohydrate concentration and available hemin concentration can affect the catalase reaction (88).
12. Gentamicin prevents growth of most organisms other than esculin-positive *Bacteroides* that can tolerate bile. At a concentration of 10 μg/mL it suppresses facultative anaerobes while permitting growth of the *B. fragilis* group. *B. fragilis* group organisms have a minimal inhibitory concentration of 80 μg/mL or above (32). Gentamicin is heat stable and does not lose its activity with incubation; it may be added to the medium prior to sterilization (10).
13. Bile (Oxgall) inhibits almost all anaerobic, Gram-negative bacilli **except** those in the *B. fragilis* group (70).
14. Streak the specimen as soon as possible (ASAP) after it is received in the laboratory, as some strains of the *B. fragilis* group may not grow well because of the selective properties of the medium (60). It is advisable to also include a **non**selective blood agar medium such as CDC anaerobic blood agar (60).

E. *Bacteroides* **disk test**
1. The **reliability** of the disk test for *Bacteroides* screening depends on standardization of the inoculum density; if it is too dense, zones become much smaller and less distinct (17). Draper and Barry (17) standardized the procedure by adjusting the broth growth turbidity to match the McFarland 0.5 standard. Sutter et al. (75, 78) recommended that sensitive zones be >10 mm and resistant ones <10 mm; Vargo et al. (82), >12 mm and <12 mm; and Draper and Barry (17) standardized interpretations to sensitive, >12 mm, and resistant, <10 mm.
2. When testing for *B. fragilis* group organisms with a bile/antibiotic disk procedure (only a screening procedure), susceptibility to one or both disks indicates a need for further biochemical tests (17).

F. **Pigment production esculin-based medium for *C. neoformans***
1. Esculin hydrolysis by bacteria is a different reaction than pigment production directly from esculin **without** hydrolysis by *C. neoformans;* there is no iron (Fe^{3+}) in the medium, and the brown-black color produced is melanin, **not** the complex formed by esculin and ferric ions (19). Many *Cryptococcus* species hydrolyze esculin, and hydrolysis is variable among *Candida* spp. Esculin hydrolysis **cannot** be used to differentiate *Cryptococcus* species (19).

2. Pigment production by *C. neoformans* is **presumptive** evidence only, and further biochemical and serologic tests **must** be performed for confirmation (19).

G. **Rapid bile esculin (RBE) reagent test**
   1. At refrigerator temperature (4–10°C), the reagent may gel. It **must** be brought to 35°C to liquefy **before** use (23).
   2. A sodium deoxycholate concentration of 2.7% or above inhibits constitutive β-glucosidase of *Streptococcus bovis* (23). At a sodium deoxycholate concentration of 2.5% or less, the constitutive esculinase of *Streptococcus milleri* (current taxonomic status, *S. anginosus* (47)) and other members of the viridans group of streptococci begins to be detected (23).
   3. Most enterococci/streptococci **other than group D** are inhibited by sodium deoxycholate; however, bile-sensitive *S. pneumoniae* may also be identified within 30 min because of the autolytic induction by sodium deoxycholate (23).
   4. A pH of 7.5 is optimal for both color release and enzyme activity (23).
   5. The maximum incubation period is 30 min (23).

H. **Rapid esculin test of Qadri et al.** (57)
   1. A precipitate is formed in the solution during refrigeration; heat to 60–70°C to resuspend with **no** adverse effects (61).
   2. Studies by Qadri et al. (61) showed that among the Gram-negative bacilli, *Klebsiella* required up to 2–4 h for hydrolysis to occur; isolates of *Serratia marcescens* were slow to hydrolyze esculin, taking up to 4 h.
   3. One strain of *Streptococcus sanguis,* two strains of *S. salivaris,* and one strain each of *S. marcescens,* and *P. vulgaris* gave false-negative results compared with those in Vaughn-Levine broth medium (61).

I. **Sodium chloride esculin hydrolysis test**
   1. Terminating the test at 4 h will avoid any false-positive reactions by other streptococci (62).
   2. A pH below 5.4 will delay the reaction. Esculin hydrolysis is completely inhibited at a pH below 4.0, and a pH above 5.8 will cause a yellow discoloration of the medium that interferes with interpretation of results.

J. **Latex agglutination tests**
   1. There are many possible errors in the use of latex agglutination for group D streptococci identification. Facklam et al. (28) and Levchak and Ellner (49) recommend that **prior** to use of latex agglutination tests, microorganisms be biochemically separated into enterococcal and **non**enterococcal groups. Levchak and Ellner (49) recommend the following when using latex agglutination tests:
      a. Test only **pure** cultures because of occasional cross-reactions with Gram-negative bacilli.
      b. Trypsinize hemolytic colonies prior to testing.

REFERENCES

1. Balows A, Hausler WJ Jr, Herrmann KL, et al. Manual of Clinical Microbiology, ed 5. Washington, DC: American Society for Microbiology, 1991:246, 250.
2. Baron EJ, Finegold SM. Bailey & Scott's Diagnostic Microbiology, ed 8. Philadelphia: CV Mosby, 1990:90, 533, 538, 543.
3. Baron EJ, Summanen P, Downes J, et al. *Bilophila wadsworthia* gen. nov., sp. nov., a unique gram-negative anaerobic rod recovered from appendicitis specimens and human faeces. J Gen Microbiol 1989;135:3405–3411.
4. Baumann P, Furniss AL, Lee JV. Genus *Vibrio*. In: Holt JG, Krieg NR, eds. Bergey's Manual of Systematic Bacteriology, vol 1. Baltimore: Williams & Wilkins, 1984:518–538.
5. Bittner J. A simple method for rapid isolation and identification of *Bacteroides fragilis*. Arch Roum Pathol Exp Microbiol 1975;34:231.
6. Blazevic DJ, Schreckenberger PC, Matsen JM. Evaluation of the PathoTec "Rapid I-D System." Appl Microbiol 1973;26(6):886–889.
7. Bridge PD, Sneath PHA. *Streptococcus gallinarum* sp. nov. and *Streptococcus oralis* sp. nov. Int J Syst Bacteriol 1982;32:410–415.
8. Bridge PD, Sneath PHA. Numerical taxonomy of *Streptococcus*. J Gen Microbiol 1983;129:565–597.

9. Cantarow A, Schepartz B. Biochemistry, ed 3. Philadelphia: WB Saunders, 1962:10–11.
10. Casemore DP. Gentamicin as a bacterial agent in virology tissue culture. J Clin Pathol 1967;20(3):298–299.
11. Chan PCK, Porschen RK. Evaluation of Kanamycin-Esculin-Bile agar for isolation and presumptive identification of *Bacteroides fragilis* group. J Clin Microbiol 1977;6(5):528–529.
12. Collins MD, Farrow JAE, Jones D. *Enterococcus mundtii* sp. nov. Int J Syst Bacteriol 1986;36(1):8–12.
13. Collins MD, Jones D, Farrow JAE, et al. *Enterococcus avium* nom. rev., comb. nov.; *E. casseliflavus* nom. rev., comb. nov.; *E. durans* nom. rev., comb. nov., *E. gallinarum* comb. nov., and *E. malodoratus* sp. nov. Int J Syst Bacteriol 1984a; 43(2):220–223.
14. Cowan ST. Cowan & Steel's Manual for the Identification of Medical Bacteriology, ed 2. Cambridge: Cambridge University Press, 1974:29.
15. Desmond EP, Janda JM, Adams FI, Bottone EJ. Comparative studies and laboratory diagnosis of *Vibrio vulnifcus,* an invasive *Vibrio* sp. J Clin Microbiol 1984;19(2):122–125.
16. Dowell VR, Hawkins TM. Laboratory Methods in Anaerobic Bacteriology. CDC Laboratory Manual. Atlanta, GA: Centers for Disease Control, 1979.
17. Draper DL, Barry AL. Rapid identification of *Bacteroides fragilis* with bile and antibiotic disks. J Clin Microbiol 1977;5(4):439–443.
18. Edberg SC, Bell SR. Lack of constitutive β-glucosidase (esculinase) in the genus *Fusobacterium.* J Clin Microbiol 1985;22(3):435–437.
19. Edberg SC, Chaskes SJ, Alture-Werber E, Singer JM. Esculin-based medium for isolation and identification of *Cryptococcus neoformans.* J Clin Microbiol 1980;12(3):332–335.
20. Edberg SC, Gam K, Bottenbley CJ, Singer JM. Rapid spot test for the determination of esculin hydrolysis. J Clin Microbiol 1976;4(2):180–184.
21. Edberg SC, Pittman S, Singer JM. Esculin hydrolysis by *Enterobacteriaceae.* J Clin Microbiol 1977;6(2):111–116.
22. Edberg SC, Pittman S, Singer JM. The use of bile-esculin agar for the taxonomic classification of the family *Enterobacteriaceae.* Antonie van Leeuwenhoek 1977;43(1):31–35.
23. Edberg SC, Trepeta RW, Kontnick CM, Torres AR. Measurement of active constitutive β-D-glucosidase (esculinase) in the presence of sodium desoxycholate. J Clin Microbiol 1985;21(3):363–365.
24. Facklam RR. Recognition of group D streptococcal species of human origin by biochemical and physiological tests. Appl Microbiol 1972;23(6):1131–1139.
25. Facklam RR. Comparison of several laboratory media for presumptive identification of enterococci and group D streptococci. Appl Microbiol 1973;26(2):138–145.
26. Facklam RR. Physiological differentiation of viridans streptococci. J Clin Microbiol 1977;5(2):184–201.
27. Facklam RR, Collins MD. Identification of *Enterococcus* species isolated from human infections by a conventional test scheme. J Clin Microbiol 1989;27(4):731–734.
28. Facklam RR, Cooksey RC, Wortham EC. Evaluation of commercial latex agglutination reagents for grouping streptococci. J Clin Microbiol 1979;10(5):641–646.
29. Facklam R, Hollis D, Collins MD. Identification of gram-positive coccal and coccobacillary vancomycin-resistant bacteria. J Clin Microbiol 1989;27(4):724–730.
30. Facklam RR, Padula JF, Thacker LG, et al. Presumptive identification of group A, B, and D streptococci. Appl Microbiol 1974;27(1):107–113.
31. Farrow JAE, Collins MD. *Enterococcus hirae,* a new species that include amino assay strain NCDO 1258 and strains causing growth depression in young chickens. Int J Syst Bacteriol 1985;35(1):73–75.
32. Finegold SM, Sutter VL. Susceptibility of gram-negative anaerobic bacilli to gentamicin and other aminoglycosides. J Infect Dis 1971;124(suppl):S556–558.
33. Frank SK, von Riesen VL. Aglycon tests determine hydrolysis of arbutin, esculin, and salicin by nonfermentative gram-negative bacteria. Lab Med 1978;9(8):48–51.
34. George WL, Jones MJ, Nakata MM. Phenotypic characteristics of *Aeromonas* species isolated from adult humans. J Clin Microbiol 1986;23(6):1026–1029.
35. Gibbons RJ, MacDonald JB. Hemin and vitamin K compounds as required factors for the cultivation of certain strains of *Bacteroides melaninogenicus.* J Bacteriol 1960;80(2):164–170.
36. Gorbach SL, Bartlett JG. Medical progress. Anaerobic infections (part one). N Engl J Med 1974;290(21):1177–1184.
37. Gorbach SL, Bartlett JG. Medical progress. Anaerobic infections (part two). N Engl J Med 1974;290(21):1237–1245.
38. Gorbach SL, Bartlett JG. Medical progress: Anaerobic infections (part three). N Engl J Med 1974;290(21):1289–1294.
39. Gregory EM, Veltri BJ, Wagner DL, Wilkins TD. Carbohydrate repression of catalase synthesis in *Bacteroides fragilis.* J Bacteriol 1977;129(1):534–535.
40. Hackman AS, Wilkins TD. In vivo protection of *Fusobacterium necrophorum* from penicillin by *Bacteroides fragilis.* Antimicrob Agents Chemother 1975;7(5):698–703.
41. Havelaar AH, Tips PD, Engel HWB. Comparative study of confirmation media for detecting

group S streptococci. Water Res 1982;16(12): 1605–1609.
42. Howard BJ, Klaas J II, Rubin SJ, et al. Clinical and Pathogenic Microbiology. St. Louis: CV Mosby, 1987:251.
43. Isenberg HD, Goldberg D, Sampson J. Laboratory studies with a selective enterococcus medium. Appl Microbiol 1970;20(3):433–436.
44. Jones D, Sackin MJ, Sneath PHA. A numerical taxonomic study of streptococci of serological group D. J Gen Microbiol 1972;72:439–450.
45. Kalina AP. The taxonomy and nomenclature of enterococci. Int J Syst Bacteriol 1970;20(2): 185–189.
46. Knight RG, Shlaes DM. Deoxyribonucleic acid relatedness of Enterococcus hirae and Streptococcus durans homology group II. Int J Syst Bacteriol 1986;36(1):111–113.
47. Koneman EW, Allen SD, Janda WM, Schreckenberger PC, Winn WC Jr. Color Atlas and Textbook of Diagnostic Microbiology, ed 4. Philadelphia: JB Lippincott, 1992:155–156, 208–209, 271, 438, 459–460.
48. Krieg NR, Holt JG, eds. Bergey's Manual of Systemic Bacteriology, vol 1. Baltimore: Williams & Wilkins, 1984.
49. Levchak ME, Ellner PD. Identification of group D streptococci by SeroSTAT. J Clin Microbiol 1982;15(1):58–60.
50. Levine M, Vaughn R, Epstein SS, Anderson D. Some differential reactions in the Colon-Aerogenes group of bacteria. Proc Soc Exp Biol Med 1932;29(8):1022–1024.
51. Lindell SS, Quinn P. Use of Bile-Esculin agar for rapid differentiation of Enterobacteriaceae. J Clin Microbiol 1975;1(5):440–443.
52. Livingston SJ, Kominos SD, Yee RB. New medium for selection and presumptive identification of the Bacteroides fragilis group. J Clin Microbiol 1978;7(5):448–453.
53. Mertens A, Nagler J, Hansen W, Gepts-Friedenreich E. Halophilic, lactose-positive Vibrio in a case of fatal septicemia. J Clin Microbiol 1979; 9(2):233–235.
54. Meyer K, Schöenfeld H. Über die Unterscheidung des Enterococcus vom Streptococcus viridans und die Beziehunger beider zum Streptococcus lactis. Zentralbl Bakteriol Parasitenk d Infektionskr Hyg Abt I Orig 1926;99(6):402–419.
55. Miskin A, Edberg SC. Esculin hydrolysis reaction by Escherichia coli. J Clin Microbiol 1978; 7(3):251–254.
56. Norris JR, Ribbons DW. Methods in Microbiology, vol 6A. New York: Academic Press, 1971:11.
57. Nowlan SS, Deibel RH. Group Q streptococci. I. Ecology, serology, physiology, and relationship to established enterococci. J Bacteriol 1967;94: 291–296.
58. Oberhofer TR. Manual of Nonfermenting Gram-Negative Bacteria. New York: John Wiley & Sons, 1985:10.
59. Oberhofer TR. Manual of Practical Medical Microbiology and Parasitology. New York: John Wiley & Sons, 1985:128.
60. Power DA, McCuen PJ. Manual of BBL Products and Laboratory Procedures, ed 6. Cockeysville, MD: Becton Dickinson Microbiology Systems, 1988:108, 114.
61. Qadri SMH, DeSilva MI, Zubairi S. Rapid test for determination of esculin hydrolysis. J Clin Microbiol 1980;12(3):472–474.
62. Qadri SMH, Flournoy DJ, Qadri SGM. Sodium chloride-esculin hydrolysis test for rapid identification of enterococci. J Clin Microbiol 1987; 25(6):1107–1108.
63. Qadri SMH, Johnson S, Smith JC, Zubairi S, Gillum RL. Comparison of spot esculin hydrolysis with the PathoTec Strip Test for rapid differentiation of anaerobic bacteria. J Clin Microbiol 1981;13(3):459–462.
64. Qadri SMH, Smith JC, Zubairi S, DeSilva MI. Esculin hydrolysis by gram positive bacteria. A rapid test and its comparison with other methods. Med Microbiol Immunol 1981;169(2):67–74.
65. Rubin SJ. Species identification and clinical significance of viridans streptococci. Lab Med 1984;15(3):171–175.
66. Sabbaj J, Sutter VL, Finegold SM. Comparison of selective media for isolation of presumptive group D streptococci from human feces. Appl Microbiol 1971;22(6):1008–1011.
67. Schleifer KH, Kilpper-Bälz R. Transfer of Stretococcus faecalis and Stretococcus faecium to the genus Enterococcus nom. rev. as Enterococcus faecalis comb. nov. and Enterococcus faecium comb. nov. Int J Syst Bacteriol 1984;34(1):31–34.
68. Schleifer KH, Kilpper-Bälz R. Molecular and chemotaxonomic approaches to the classification of streptococci, enterococci, and lactococci. A review. Syst Appl Microbiol 1987;10:1–9.
69. Seip WF, Evans GL. Atmospheric analysis and redox potentials of culture media in the GasPak system. J Clin Microbiol 1980;11(3):226–233.
70. Shimada K, Sutter VL, Finegold SM. Effect of bile and desoxycholate on gram-negative anaerobic bacteria. Appl Microbiol 1970;20(5):737–741.
71. Smith PB, Rhoden DL, Tomfohrde KM. Evaluation of the Pathotec Rapid I-D System for identification of Enterobacteriaceae. J Clin Microbiol 1975;1(4):359–362.
72. Sneath PHA, Mair NS, Sharpe ME, Holt JG, eds. Bergey's Manual of Systemic Bacteriology, vol 2. Baltimore: Williams & Wilkins, 1986:611, 1085.
73. Sperry JF, Appleman MD, Wilkins TD. Requirement of heme for growth of Bacteroides fragilis. Appl Environ Microbiol 1977;34(4):386–390.
74. Stargel MD, Thompson FS, Phillips SE, et al. Modification of the Minitek miniaturized differential system for characterization of anaerobic bacteria. J Clin Microbiol 1976;3(3):291–301.
75. Sutter VL, Attebery HR, Rosenblatt JE, et al. Anaerobic Bacteriology Manual. Los Angeles:

Extension Division, University of California, 1972.
76. Sutter VL, Citron DM, Edelstein MAC, Finegold SM. Wadsworth Anaerobic Bacteriology Manual, ed 4. Belmont, CA: Star Publishing, 1985.
77. Sutter VL, Citron DM, Finegold SM. Wadsworth Anaerobic Bacteriology Manual, ed 3. St. Louis: CV Mosby, 1980:30.
78. Sutter VL, Finegold SM. Antibiotic disc susceptibility tests for rapid presumptive identification of gram-negative anaerobic bacilli. Appl Microbiol 1971;21(1):13–20.
79. Swan A. The use of a bile-aesculin medium and of Maxted's technique of Lancefield grouping in the identification of enterococci (group D streptococci). J Clin Pathol 1954;7(2):160–163.
80. Thiercelin E, Jouhaud L. Reproduction de l'enterocoque: Taches centrales; granulations peripheriques et microblastes. CR Seances Soc Biol Paris 1903;55:686–688.
81. Tison DL. Esculin hydrolysis by *Vibrio vulnificus*. Diagn Microbiol Infect Dis 1986;4(1):49–51.
82. Vargo V, Korzeniowski M, Spaulding EH. Tryptic soy bile-kanamycin test for the identification of *Bacteroides fragilis*. Appl Microbiol 1974;27(3):480–483.
83. Vaughan DH, Riggsby WS, Mundt JO. Deoxyribonucleic acid relatedness of strains of yellow-pigmented group D streptococci. Int J Syst Bacteriol 1979;29:204–212.
84. Vaughn RH, Levine M. Differentiation of the "intermediate" coli-like bacteria. J Bacteriol 1942;44(4):487–505.
85. Wasilauskas BL. Preliminary observations on the rapid differentiation of the *Klebsiella-Enterobacter-Serratia* group on Bile-Esculin agar. Appl Microbiol 1971;21(1):162–163.
86. Weaver RE, Hollis DG, Clark WA, Riley P. Revised tables from The Identification of Unusual Pathogenic Gram-Negative Bacteria by King EO. Atlanta, GA: Centers for Disease Control, US Dept Health and Human Services, 1983.
87. Wilkins TD, Chalgren SL, Jimenez-Ulate F, et al. Inhibition of *Bacteroides fragilis* on blood agar plates. J Clin Microbiol 1976;3(3):359–363.
88. Wilkins TD, Wagner DL, Veltri BJ Jr, Gregory EM. Factors affecting production of catalase by *Bacteroides*. J Clin Microbiol 1978;8(5):553–557.

Bile Solubility Test

I. PRINCIPLE

To test the ability of bacterial cells to lyse in the presence of bile salts within a specific time and temperature

II. PURPOSE

(Also see Chapter 43)
A. Used specifically to differentiate between bile-soluble *Streptococcus pneumoniae* and other bile-insoluble α-hemolytic *Streptococcus* spp.
B. May aid in species differentiation of bile-soluble *Haemophilus influenzae* and *Haemophilus aegyptius* from other bile-insoluble *Haemophilus* spp.

III. BIOCHEMISTRY INVOLVED

Bile Salts

Bile salts are sodium salts of bile acids that are all synthesized from a common compound, cholesterol (29). Downie et al. (11) separated bile acids into two categories: (*a*) uncombined acids, of which various types differ only in their chemical structure, and (*b*) choleic acids, which are addition compounds of deoxycholic that vary according to the type of additions.

Bile salts are bile acids conjugated with amino acids through amide linkages (C=O) between the carboxy group (COOH) of the acid and the amino group (NH_2) of either glycine (H_2NCH_2COOH) or taurine ($H_2NCH_2CH_2SO_3H$) (8, 26, 29).

The amino acid taurine is derived from another amino acid, cysteine (7), and its conjugated form with cholic acid is called taurocholic acid. Cholic acid conjugated with glycine is termed glycocholic acid.

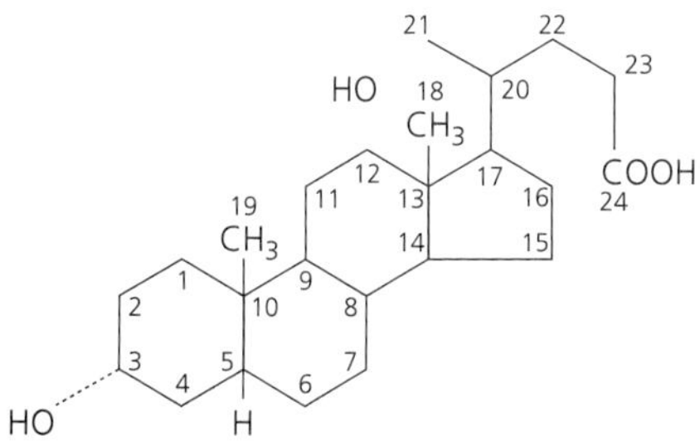

Deoxycholic acid

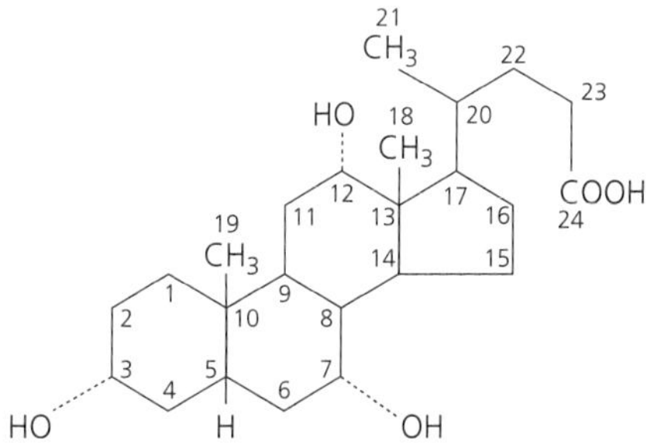

Cholic acid

[Structure: Taurocholic acid]

Taurocholic acid

Deoxycholic acid is a dihydroxy acid; cholic and taurocholic are trihydroxy acids. All bile acids have a common basic nucleus, the cyclopentanoperhydrophenanthrene ring (7).

[Structure: Cyclopentano-perhydrophenanthrene ring]

Cyclopentano-perhydrophenanthrene ring

Bile salts lacking hydroxyl groups (OH) are **inactive,** while salts of deoxycholic acid, a dihydroxy compound with hydroxyl groups at carbons 3 and 12, are more active than the trihydroxy acids, cholic or taurocholic, which possess hydroxyl groups at carbons 3, 7, and 12 in the basic nucleus (11). Downie et al. (11) state that rapid lysis of S. pneumoniae by bile acids is related to the number and position of the hydroxyl groups and their ability to form addition compounds with organic substances.

Bile salts used in bile solubility testing are usually either sodium deoxycholate (desoxycholate) or sodium taurocholate, since they are the most active lytic compounds among the various bile acids (11). These bile acids are present as anions at alkaline pH, thus the term *bile salts* (29). Deoxycholate, a monobasic acid, has a slight alkaline pH in an aqueous solution such as a sodium salt (20).

Sodium lauryl sulfate (2%), sodium dodecyl sulfate, saponins, white Dreft (1%), and other surface-lowering detergents may also be used to lyse *S. pneumoniae* (6, 16, 17, 31); however, sodium lauryl sulfate is less specific than sodium deoxycholate (16).

Cell Wall

Two major macromolecular components of the cell wall of *S. pneumoniae* constitute the species-specific substance (23): (*a*) **peptidoglycan** (murein), which is composed of amino acid sugars, glucosamine and muramic acid, lysine, alanine, glutamic, and muramic acid phosphate (23, 32), and (*b*) **teichoic acid,** which is rich in galactosamine, phosphate, and choline.

Peptidoglycan is a complex polymer consisting of three parts (18): (*a*) the backbone composed of alternating sequences of N-acetylglucosamine and N-acetylmuramic acid, (*b*) a set of identical tetrapeptide side chains attached to N-acetylmuramic acid, and (*c*) a set of identical peptide cross-bridges.

Cell wall **teichoic acid** is a water-soluble polymer of ribitol phosphate containing choline and galactosamine (23, 33). The choline component plays a key role in determining sensitivity to the autolytic enzyme (23). One function is to maintain a high concentration of divalent cations in the vicinity of the cell (15). Teichoic acid is covalently bound to the peptidoglycan layer by phosphodiester bridges (15).

Autolytic Enzyme

S. pneumoniae produces an autolytic intracellular enzyme, an amidase, (autolysin) that causes the organism to undergo rapid autolysis (lysis) when cultivated on artificial medium (8, 11, 12, 14).

Autolysis (Solubilization, Lysis)

The addition of bile salts (e.g., sodium deoxycholate) to a **neutralized** culture alters the surface of the pneumococci, which activates an autolytic amidase that cleaves the bond between muramic acid and alanine in the peptidoglycan portion of the cell wall (4, 9, 17, 23, 27). The autolytic enzyme acts on muramic acid of the cell wall only when normal choline-containing teichoic acid is present (23).

Bile salts lower surface tension at the medium-membrane interface (12, 28, 29) and also cause a cell membrane derangement (28). However, this lowering of surface tension is not the sole cause for lysis of *S. pneumoniae*; other, unexplained mechanisms are involved (11, 12, 28). Mair (22), Downie et al. (11), and Burrows et al. (6) state that the role of bile salts is to accelerate the natural autolytic process; the bile acids combine with the pneumococcal cells and activate the autolytic enzyme (8, 11, 12). Downie et al. (11) state that bile salts apparently do not lyse pneumococcal cells if the natural autolysin is absent; the two processes are similar (22). Goebel and Avery (14), however, state that the action of bile salts is independent of the autolytic enzyme. Burrows et al. (6), Cowan (8), and Dubos and Hirsch (12) state that if a culture of *S. pneumoniae* is heat killed (65°C, 30 min), which inactivates the autolytic enzyme, lysis does not occur either naturally or upon addition of bile salts. Goebel and Avery (14) also found that normal autolysis by *S. pneumoniae* may be inhibited if a high concentration of bile salts is used for testing bile solubility. Leifson (20) reported that some preliminary experiments indicated that other organisms besides *S. pneumoniae* subsp. *pneumoniae* are soluble in sodium deoxycholate.

IV. REAGENTS EMPLOYED

A. Sodium deoxycholate or sodium taurocholate (10%)
   1. Commercial products are available; commercial sodium taurocholate is a mixture of alcohol-soluble constituents of bile (35). Oxgall (BBL, Difco) (10, 30) is a dehydrated bile that may be substituted, but deoxycholate is preferred (5).
   2. Method of preparation
      a. Weigh amount of bile salt, 10 g/100 mL (10% concentration) and bring to 100 mL with distilled water. Both bile salts are readily soluble in distilled water (10).
         (1) Sodium deoxycholate: **colorless** solution (10)
         (2) Sodium taurocholate: clear **amber** solution (10)
      b. Commercial bile salts are neutral (pH 7.0) and require no pH adjustment (10). Commercial dehydrated bile salts are equivalent to fresh bile (8) and are preferred because they may be sterilized and the concentration can be controlled (6).
B. Phenol red pH indicator
   1. Alkaline: pinkish red color, pH 8.4
   2. Acid: yellow color, pH 6.8
C. Sodium hydroxide (NaOH), 10 N (40%).
   1. Ingredients

Sodium hydroxide, carbonate free, R. G. (reagent grade)	40.0 g
Distilled water	100.0 mL

   2. Method of preparation
      a. **Rapidly** weigh sodium hydroxide and dissolve in less than 100 mL of distilled water in a beaker. This reagent is highly hygroscopic.

b. Place beaker in a circulating water bath to control temperature.
c. Cool and transfer the sodium hydroxide solution to a 100-mL volumetric flask and bring to 100 mL with distilled water.
d. Store in a polyethylene- or paraffin-lined glass reagent bottle.
e. Label correctly.
   Sodium hydroxide is extremely caustic; avoid exposure to the skin because painful burns may occur.

D. Sodium hydroxide, 0.1 N
   1. Ingredients

Sodium hydroxide, 10 N	1.0 mL
Distilled water added to total	100.0 mL

   2. Method of preparation
      a. Using a pipette, transfer 1.0 mL of a 10 N NaOH solution to a 100-mL volumetric flask and bring to 100 mL with distilled water.
      b. Label correctly.

E. Sterile, physiologic saline (0.85% NaCl)

F. Storage: Store all reagents in a refrigerator (4°C) when not in use. Shelf life is approximately 6 months at room temperature (22–25°C) (3). Their stability varies; therefore, they should be checked periodically and discarded when they give a negative or weak reaction with a known positive organism.

V. QUALITY CONTROL MICROORGANISMS

(*Note:* All reagents must be tested with known positive and negative cultures before being put into general use.)

   Bile soluble: *Streptococcus pneumoniae* ATCC 12344, 49136
   Bile **in**soluble: other *Streptococcus* spp.; e.g., *Streptococcus mitis* ATCC 15909

VI. PROCEDURE

A. Bacterial inoculum-growth media: two selections
   1. Blood agar plate (BA) (5% sheep blood)
      a. Incubate at 35°C; 18–24 h
      b. Candle jar to increase CO_2 (2–3%)
   2. Todd-Hewitt broth (10, 23)
      a. Incubate at 35°C, 18–24 h
      b. Centrifuge, and discard the supernatant (8)

B. Method of utilization
   1. Prepare a **heavy** suspension of a **pure** culture in 1.0 mL of normal (physiologic) saline (NaCl, 0.85%).
   2. Add 1 drop of phenol red pH indicator and adjust to pH 7.0 (pink) by adding a few drops of 0.1 N NaOH, if required.
   3. Divide the neutral saline suspension of bacteria into two tubes (13 × 100 mm), 0.5 mL/tube. Label one **test**, the other **control**.
   4. Add 0.5 mL of 10% sodium deoxycholate (or sodium taurocholate) to tube marked "test."
   5. Add 0.5 mL of **sterile** normal saline to tube marked "control."
   6. Gently agitate **both** tubes to suspend bacteria.
   7. Incubation
      a. 37°C, incubator or water bath
      b. 3 h, checking hourly

8. Observe for clearing, which should occur within 3 h.

An actively growing culture of organisms to be tested may be used in place of a saline suspension; however, it **must** be buffered (3, 8). Todd-Hewitt broth contains glucose, and the acid produced by metabolizing organisms makes unbuffered medium too acidic to detect bile solubility. The pH of the medium must **not** be below 6.8 (8).

VII. RESULTS

> See Figure 3.1 (Appendix 1) for colored photographic results

VIII. INTERPRETATION

A. **Bile soluble:** solution clearing or clear (bile dissolved, solubilized) within 3 h; *S. pneumoniae*
B. **Bile insoluble:** solution remains turbid (cloudy); **same as** saline control; α-hemolytic *Streptococcus* spp. or other organism

IX. RAPID TESTS

A. **Plate technique**
   1. Screening method of Hawn and Beebe (16) who showed that the test can be accurately performed **directly** on isolated suspected colonies.
   2. Results within 30 min
   3. Procedure
      a. Inoculum: 18- to 24-h growth on 5% sheep blood agar (SBA) plate
         (1) Suspected *S. pneumoniae*
         (2) Well-isolated colonies

(*Note:* **Prior** to addition of the bile salt, circle the colony to be tested with a china marking pencil on the **bottom** of the Petri dish to help locate colony **after** testing.)

   b. Place a **loopful** (1 drop) of 2% deoxycholate (pH 7.0) **directly** on a **single** well-isolated colony.
   c. Incubation (3)
      (1) **Do not** invert plate; leave lid up.
      (2) 35°C, aerobically, 30 min
      (3) Bile soluble: colony disintegrates (disappears) under drop and leaves a partially hemolyzed area in medium where it had been located; area appears flat.
      (4) Bile insoluble: colony remains intact and visible.

B. **Rapid (modified) bile solubility–Gram stain procedure**
   1. Procedure of Murray (24), modified by Oberhofer (27)
   2. Purpose: rapid recovery and **presumptive** identification of *S. pneumoniae* from blood culture broths or on solid media; confirmed by conventional procedures
   3. Principle: combination of two procedures, bile solubility test and Gram stain, performed **directly** on isolated colonies
   4. Reagent: 2% sodium deoxycholate; pH 7.0
   5. Procedures
      a. Solid medium
         (1) Test 2–3 isolated colonies for catalase production
         (2) Catalase-negative isolates
            (a) Add loopful of reagent
            (b) Incubate 35°C, 30 min

(c) Results
1. Bile soluble: **presumptively** identified as *S. pneumoniae;* colony disappears, leaving partially hemolyzed medium
2. Bile insoluble: other streptococcal species; colony **un**affected
  b. Liquid (blood culture broth) medium
  (1) First do a Gram stain of **positive** blood cultures. Observe for Gram-positive cocci arranged in pairs or chains consistent with streptococci. **If found,** prepare a second slide.
  (2) Slide test
   (a) To one half of slide, mix 1 drop of broth with 1 drop of reagent. This is the **treated** portion of the slide.
   (b) To second half of slide mix 1 drop of broth with 1 drop of **water; control**
   (c) Air dry in ambient air; Gram stain slide and examine
  (3) Interpretation
   (a) **Presumptive** identification of *S. pneumoniae;* confirm by conventional test.
    1. Treated smear: **all cells** completely solubilized
    2. Control: **no** organisms on Gram stain
   (b) Suspicious
    1. If only partial reduction of cells on treated smear, **probably** *S. pneumoniae*
    2. If < 1–5 cocci per microscopic field are observed in control, repeat test with centrifuged (5 min at 2000 rpm) sediment of blood culture broth

X. PRECAUTIONS

A. **General**
1. The terms *soluble* or *insoluble* **must** be used for interpretations of the bile solubility test. Never use positive (+) or negative (−) to denote bile solubility results. The term *positive reaction* does not explain sufficiently; it could mean the organism is bile soluble or simply that the organism exhibits growth but no action with bile salts.
2. The bile solubility test is used only to differentiate between α-hemolyic *Streptococcus* spp. and *S. pneumoniae. S. pneumoniae* is the only streptococcus soluble in bile (25); other α-hemolytic streptococci **do not** possess active enzyme and will not dissolve in bile (3, 27). The effect of bile is to accelerate natural autolysis (22). If doubt exists about the hemolytic pattern exhibited by a possible *Streptococcus* spp., set up a bile solubility test. α-Hemolytic *Streptococcus* spp. and *S. pneumoniae* often are difficult to differentiate by Gram stain and colony morphology, and thus additional tests are needed (bile solubility and/or optochin tests). However, *S. pneumoniae* and all *Streptococcus* spp. are catalase negative, and this determination should be made prior to performing the bile solubility test.
3. Lysis by commercial sodium taurocholate is often variable; the most active lytic bile salt is sodium deoxycholate (17, 36).
4. A bile insoluble reaction can be confirmed by addition of a drop of dilute alkali (0.1 N NaOH) (36). Wilson and Miles (36) express doubt about whether solubility at alkaline pH depends completely on bile salts, since adding alkali alone to a suspension of *S. pneumoniae* causes lysis of most fresh isolates.
5. If a buffered broth culture is used for the bile solubility test procedure, avoid a dense culture; cell fragments may impart turbidity and mask a bile soluble reaction (3).
6. Downie et al. (11) report that variations in the bile solubility reaction of *S. pneumoniae* may at times indicate loss of the virulence factor, the capsule, which may alter the susceptibility of the organism to lysis by bile salts.
7. Downie et al. (11) state that temperature affects the natural autolytic property of *S. pneumoniae* and the lysis effected by bile salts. Goebel and Avery (14) report that lysis occurs

slowly at 0°C but increases at a higher temperature. The rate of lysis increases as the temperature reaches 37°C and then decreases as the temperature rises to 45°C (11).

8. Wilson and Miles (36) found that the salt concentration in bacterial suspensions affects the bile solubility of *S. pneumoniae*; addition of magnesium sulfate enhances lysis by bile salts. According to Falk and Yang (13), lysis is inhibited when monovalent chlorides are present in low concentration (0.004–1.0%) and is accelerated by a high concentration (2.0–4.0%). However, Anderson and Hart (1) found that there was a reciprocal relation between the concentration of bile salts required for lysis and the concentration of sodium chloride in the bacterial suspension. Sodium chloride showed no evidence of inhibiting lysis (1), and at the same time, in the absence of salt, lysis occurred. However, as the salt concentration increased (up to 5%), the concentration of bile salt required to produce lysis decreased (1). Salt content **must** be carefully controlled (36).
9. When performing the bile solubility test with either an actively metabolizing broth culture or a saline suspension, the pH **must** be adjusted to 7.0 before addition of the bile salts (8, 20, 27). In an acid suspension, sodium deoxycholate may form a precipitate or gel and give a false-negative result (3, 8, 20); an acid precipitate forms at about pH 6.4–6.5 (17, 20). Thus the pH **must** be carefully controlled (17, 36) and adjusted to pH 7.0 to prevent false-negative results (3). Test strains that are partially lysed are either mixed or the pH was not properly adjusted before addition of saline and bile salts (2). If organisms grown on agar are suspended in phosphate-buffered saline, pH 7.0, there is **no** need to adjust the pH (3).
10. If the solution has not cleared by the end of a 3-h incubation, the organism is bile insoluble.
11. α-Hemolytic *Haemophilus* spp. are also bile soluble. Branson (5) recommends that tubes be incubated at least 2 h if *Haemophilus* is present.
12. The test **must** be performed on young, viable cells. Older α-hemolytic streptococci cultures other than *S. pneumoniae* may give a false-positive result (complete solubilization (27)). Older cultures of *S. pneumoniae* may lose their active enzyme (3, 35); therefore, non–bile soluble streptococci that resemble pneumococci should be further identified by other methods (3).
13. An occasional rough *S. pneumoniae* isolate may fail to solubilize (27) or give equivocal results (21).
14. Pneumococci in which choline has been artificially replaced by ethanolamine in the teichoic acid are bile resistant and do not undergo autolysis (34).
15. Only 80% of *S. pneumoniae* will lyse completely, and additional tests (e.g., quellung reaction) may be required for the incompletely lysed strains (17).

B. **Spot bile solubility (plate) test**
   1. If blood agar is used for the test, a pronounced zone of hemolysis is produced around the drop of reagent. This reaction **must not** be confused with lysis of colonies (19), and the test is difficult to interpret (3).
   2. **Do not** move the plate around; some α-hemolytic colonies may be washed away (35). Keep the plate level to prevent reagent from running and washing away a nonpneumococcus colony, which produces a false-positive result (3). Ascertain that an α-hemolytic *Streptococcus* colony has **not** been washed to another portion of the plate by checking that blood under the drop becomes slightly hemolyzed (3).

C. **Rapid bile solubility–Gram stain procedure**
   1. For an isolate to be presumptively identified as *S. pneumoniae,* sodium deoxycholate treatment **must completely lyse all cocci,** and presumptive identification **must** be confirmed by conventional tests (24).
   2. The pH of the reagent **must** be neutral to prevent precipitation in an acid environment (27).

REFERENCES

1. Anderson AB, Hart PDA. The lysis of pneumococci by sodium deoxycholate. Lancet 1934; 2:359–360.
2. Balows A, Hausler WJ Jr, Herrmann KL, et al. Manual of Clinical Microbiology, ed 5. Washington, DC: American Society for Microbiology, 1991:249–250.
3. Baron EJ, Finegold SM. Bailey & Scott's Diagnostic Microbiology, ed 8. Philadelphia: CV Mosby, 1990:107–108.
4. Blazevic DJ, Ederer GM. Principles of Biochemical Tests in Diagnostic Microbiology. New York: John Wiley & Sons, 1975:7–11.
5. Branson D. Methods in Clinical Bacteriology. Springfield, IL: Charles C Thomas, 1972:9–10.
6. Burrows W, Lewert RM, Rippon JW. Textbook of Microbiology, vol II, ed 19. Philadelphia: WB Saunders, 1968:455.
7. Cantarow A, Schepartz B. Biochemistry, ed 3. Philadelphia, WB Saunders, 1962:40, 270–280.
8. Cowan ST. Cowan & Steel's Manual for the Identification of Medical Bacteria, ed 2. Cambridge: Cambridge University Press, 1974:11, 29, 169.
9. Davis BD, Dulbecco R, Eisen HN, Ginsberg HS. Microbiology, ed 3. Hagerstown, MD: Harper & Row, 1980:596.
10. Difco Manual, ed 10. Detroit: Difco Laboratories, 1984:872.
11. Downie AW, Stent L, White SM. The bile solubility of pneumococcus with special reference to the chemical structure of various bile-salts. Br J Exp Pathol 1931;12(1):1–9.
12. Dubos RJ, Hirsch JG, eds. Bacterial and Mycotic Infections of Man, ed 4. Philadelphia: JB Lippincott, 1965:392.
13. Falk IS, Yang SY. Studies on respiratory diseases. XXV. The influence of certain electrolytes and nonelectrolytes on the bile solubility of pneumococci. J Infect Dis 1926;38:1–7.
14. Goebel WF, Avery OT. A study of pneumococcus autolysis. J Exp Med 1929;49(2):267–286.
15. Gottschalk G. Bacterial Metabolism, ed 2. New York: Springer-Verlag, 1986:135.
16. Hawn CVZ, Beebe E. Rapid method for demonstrating bile solubility of *Diplococcus pneumoniae*. J Bacteriol 1965;90(2):549.
17. Howard BJ, Klaas J II, Weissfeld AS, Tilton RC. Clinical and Pathogenic Microbiology. St. Louis: CV Mosby, 1987:854.
18. Jawetz E, Melnick JL, Adelberg EA. Review of Medical Microbiology, ed 17. Los Altos, CA: Appleton & Lange, 1987:15.
19. Koneman EW, Allen SD, Dowell VR Jr, Janda WM, Sommers HM, Winn WC Jr. Color Atlas and Textbook of Diagnostic Microbiology, ed 3. Philadelphia: JB Lippincott, 1988:38–39, 450, 462.
20. Leifson E. New culture media based on sodium deoxycholate for the isolation of intestinal pathogens and for the enumeration of colon bacilli in milk and water. J Pathol Bacteriol 1935;40(3):581–599.
21. Lund E. Diagnosis of pneumococci by the optochin and bile tests. Acta Pathol Microbiol Scand 1959;47(3):308–315.
22. Mair W. System of bacteriology. Med Res Counc Spec Rep Ser (Lond) 1930;2:168.
23. Mosser JL, Tomasz A. Choline-containing teichoic acid as a structural component of pneumococcal cell wall and its role in sensitivity to lysis by an autolytic enzyme. J Biol Chem 1970; 245(2):287–298.
24. Murray PR. Modification of the bile solubility test for rapid identification of *Streptococcus pneumoniae*. J Clin Microbiol 1979;9(2):290–291.
25. Neufeld F. Über eine spezifische bakteriolytische Wirkung der Galle. Z Hyg Infektionskr 1900;34:454–464.
26. Noller CR. Chemistry of Organic Compounds, ed 3. Philadelphia: WB Saunders, 1965:973.
27. Oberhofer TR. Manual of Practical Medical Microbiology and Parasitology. New York: John Wiley & Sons, 1985:129–131.
28. Oginsky EL, Umbreit WW. An Introduction to Bacterial Physiology, ed 2. San Francisco: WH Freeman, 1959:104.
29. Oser BL, ed. Hawk's Physiological Chemistry, ed 14. New York: McGraw-Hill, 1965:28, 490–492.
30. Powers DA, McCuen PJ, eds. Manual of BBL Products and Laboratory Procedures, ed 6. Cockeysville, MD: Becton Dickinson Microbiology Systems, 1988:265.
31. Ragsdale AR, Sanford JP. Interfering effect of incubation in carbon dioxide on the identification of pneumococci by optochin discs. Appl Microbiol 1971;22(5):854–855.
32. Sneath PHA, Mair NS, Sharpe ME, Holt JG, eds. Bergey's Manual of Systemic Bacteriology, vol 2. Baltimore: Williams & Wilkins, 1986:1043.
33. Tomasz A. Choline in the cell wall of a bacterium: Novel type of polymer-linked choline in pneumococcus. Science 1967;157:694–697.
34. Tomasz A. Biological consequences of the replacement of choline by ethanolamine in the cell wall of pneumococcus: Chain formation, loss of transformability, and loss of autolysis. Proc Nat Acad Sci USA 1968;59(1):86–93.
35. Washington JA. Laboratory Procedures in Clinical Microbiology, ed 2. New York: Springer-Verlag, 1985:152–153.
36. Wilson G, Miles A, Parker MT, eds. Topley and Wilson's Principles of Bacteriology, Virology, and Immunology, vol 2, ed 7. Baltimore: Williams & Wilkins, 1983:196–197.

4 CAMP/Reverse CAMP Tests (Reactions) and CAMP Inhibition (Phospholipase D Production) Test

I. PRINCIPLE

A. To determine an organism's ability to produce and elaborate the CAMP factor, which acts synergistically with staphylococcal β-hemolysin (β-lysin) on ovine (sheep) or bovine (ox) erythrocytes to produce a lytic phenomenon (23) at the juncture of two organisms

B. Alternatives
  1. To determine the same phenomenon of synergistic hemolysis with CAMP factor and α-hemolysin (α-toxin) of *Clostridium perfringens* (41)
  2. To detect phospholipase D production, which inhibits the CAMP test reaction

The lytic phenomenon is called the CAMP test or reaction after the original authors: Christie, Atkins, and Munch-Petersen (18, 71). Later the term was given to other procedures. Murphy et al. (72) called lytic phenomenon the CAMP reaction and defined the CAMP test as a way to determine the ability of streptococci to produce a lytic agent (CAMP factor) that gives a hemolytic zone with staphylococcal β-lysin; hence, the acronym CAMP.

II. PURPOSE

(Also see Chapter 43)

A. **CAMP test**
  1. To differentiate and presumptively identify human or animal strains of group B *Streptococcus agalactiae* (+) from other *Streptococcus* spp. (−) when incubated aerobically or under reduced oxygen tension (candle extinction jar) (21, 23).
  2. To verify or identify hemolytic pathogenic species of *Listeria* along with acid production from D-xylose, L-rhamnoside, and α-methyl-D-mannoside (6, 57, 60, 83, 84, 91).
    a. **With *Staphylococcus aureus* subsp. *aureus***
      (1) To determine doubtful or weak ($+^w$) β-hemolytic reactions of *Listeria monocytogenes* (+) and *Listeria seeligeri* ($+^w$) (13, 40).
      (2) Aid in distinguishing *Propionibacterium acnes* (+) and *Propionibacterium granulosum* (variable) from other *Propionibacterium* spp. (−)
      (3) Aid in distinguishing *Actinomyces neuii* subsp. *anitratus* (+) and *A. neuii* subsp. *neuii* (+) from other *Actinomyces* spp. (−).
      (4) Aid in distinguishing *Corynebacterium auris* (+), *Corynebacterium bovis* (+), *Corynebacterium coylae* (strongly +), and *Corynebacterium glucuronolyticum* (+) from other *Corynebacterium* spp. (−). *Corynebacterium afermentans* subsp. *afermentans* and *Corynebacterium striatum* are variable for CAMP.
      (5) CAMP positivity is a key characteristic for *Turicella otitidis*.
      (6) *Micobacterium arborescens* is CAMP variable.
    b. **With *Rhodococcus equi*** (formerly *Corynebacterium equi*) to identify *Listeria ivanovii* (+) (52, 85).

B. **Reverse CAMP test**
  1. To presumptively distinguish *C. perfringens* (+) from other sulfite-reducing, nonspore-forming *Clostridium* spp. (−); it is highly specific for *C. perfringens* (42).

2. To help distinguish *Arcanobacterium haemolyticum* (+) from *Arcanobacterium pyogenes* (−) and *Arcanobacterium bernardiae* (−)
C. **Phospholipase D (PLD) production:** to distinguish *Corynebacterium pseudotuberculosis* (+) and *Corynebacterium ulcerans* (+) from other *Corynebacterium* spp. (−); a distinct marker within the genus (2)

III. BIOCHEMISTRY INVOLVED

The CAMP test (reaction) is based on the fact that group B streptococci produce a factor (CAMP factor) that acts synergistically with β-hemolysin of *S. aureus* subsp. *aureus* on either ovine or bovine blood agar medium (18, 23). *Synergism* is a coordinated or correlated action by two or more organisms; the synergist, CAMP factor, is an adjuvant that aids the action of another organism.

β-Lysin

Certain strains of *S. aureus* subsp. *aureus* produce a diffusible β-hemolysin (also called β-toxin, β-lysin, or β-staphylolysin) (37, 43, 44); it is produced primarily by staphylococci of animal origin and is uncommon in human strains (75). β-Lysin possesses phospholipase C (sphingomyelinase) activity (hemolysis, lysis) against ovine or bovine erythrocytes and hydrolyzes the sphingomyelin provided by the erythrocytes (67). The differences in susceptibility of erythrocytes from different species reflect substrate availability (29). Studies by Doery et al. (27) showed the existence of two phospholipases; one hydrolyzes phosphatidylinositol and lysophosphatidylinositol (which does not concern this case), the other sphingomyelin.

The existence of two components of phospholipase C (43, 44) was confirmed by Maheswaran et al. (68) and Chesbro et al. (17). The major one is a high concentration of cationic, hot-cold β-hemolysin, and the minor is a low concentration of anionic, hot-cold β-hemolysin. The anionic component is active only against sheep cells lysed in a "hot-cold" fashion (17, 68).

The major cationic component is a hot-cold lysin (15, 17, 29, 44, 68), a heat-labile (29, 96) macromolecule (44) produced aerobically and anaerobically (29, 96), with maximal activity at pH 7.0 (43) to 7.2 (27). Lysin acts on sheep but not rabbit erythrocytes (15, 70, 111) and exhibits only slight hemolytic activity against human cells (15, 70). Activity is slowest at 25°C and lost at 50°C (43); the optimal temperature is 37°C (43) to 40°C (27). Reaction activators magnesium (Mg^{2+}) or manganese (Mn^{3+}) ions are required for maximal activity (15, 29, 43, 67, 96, 113). These ions enhance release of organic phosphorus from sphingomyelin (43, 67). The requirement for Mg^{2+} ions led Wiseman (112) to state that β-lysin is definitely a phospholipase other than lecithinase, because Mg is a natural activator of most enzymes attacking phosphorylated substrates (e.g., sphingomyelin) and Turner (105) showed that sheep erythrocytes do not contain lecithins. The presence of 0.01 M Mg^{2+} or Mn^{3+} ions enhances the sensitivity of rabbit, human, and sheep erythrocytes to lysin; lysin preparations that lack these ions and give a negative reaction with rabbit and human cells can have their activity restored by addition of these ions (53, 113). Wiseman (112) found that cobalt (Co^{2+}) was equally effective; ferrous ions (Fe^{2+}) are less effective than Mg (43). Ethylenediaminetetraacetic acid (EDTA), citrate, or calcium ions (Ca^{2+}) inhibit hemolysis by preventing release of organic phosphorus from sphingomyelin (43, 53).

S. aureus subsp. *aureus* β-hemolysin is a hot-cold hemolysin for sheep cells; extensive lysis of erythrocytes does not occur during primary incubation at 37°C, but subsequent cooling to room temperature or 4°C reveals lysis by a clear zone of hemolysis central to the darkening area (15, 29, 43, 44, 68, 70, 111). The lysin-substrate reaction takes place at 37°C without lysis; cold shock at 25°C or below precipitates visible lysis (113). Hemolysis at 37°C is not characteristic of *S. aureus* subsp. *aureus* β-lysin, but it can be made to occur if the physical environment of β-lysin-sensitized red cells is altered (112). Wiseman (112) argues that this β-lysin is not a true hemolysin as are the staphylococcal α- and β-hemolysins, since the external environment of the erythrocyte must be altered before lysis occurs. β-Lysin reacts with substrate only indirectly implicated in preserving intact erythrocytes. The rate of reaction is directly proportional to the lysin concentration and temperature (112). In warm-phase incubation, β-lysin potentates lysis of sheep cells by certain other hemolysins (e.g., that of group B streptococci and β-staphylolysin (15).

Phospholipids

Phospholipids (phosphotides) are compound lipids containing various residues plus alcohols and fatty acids (75), a class of lipids concerned with structure and function of cell membranes by providing barriers to indiscriminate exchange of compounds with extracellular fluids (46). Phospholipids include sphingolipids (sphingomyelin) and phosphoglycerides (e.g., lecithin, cephalin). Sphingolipids are a heterogeneous collection of polar lipids that are partly soluble in water and nonpolar solvents (45), characterized by the presence of the long-chain amino alcohol sphingosine or a closely related substance (51, 69).

$$CH_3(CH_2)_{12}-CH=CH-\underset{OH}{\overset{H}{\underset{|}{C}}}-\underset{NH_2}{\overset{H}{\underset{|}{C}}}-\underset{OH}{CH_2}$$

Sphingosine (sphingol)
(*trans*-D-erythro-1,3-dihydroxy-2-amino-octadec-4-ene (66))
(dihydro sphinogosine)

In living materials, sphingosine does not exist in free form to any appreciable extent but occurs in one of three lipid subclasses: sphingomyelins, cerebrosides, and gangliosides (51, 69). Sphingosine is an unsaturated amino alcohol (51), a complex base (16).

$$CH_3(CH_2)_{12}-CH=CH-\underset{}{\overset{OH}{\underset{|}{CH}}}-\underset{CH_2}{\overset{H}{\underset{|}{CH}}}-\overset{H}{\underset{|}{N}}-\overset{O}{\underset{\|}{C}}-R$$

Sphingomyelin (43)

Ceramide residue = Sphingosine + Fatty acid (FA)
Phosphorylcholine residue (choline phosphate) = Phosphoric acid + Choline [$O=P(OH)-O-CH_2-CH_2-N^+(CH_3)_3$]

Phosphoglycerides (glycerophospholipids) include lecithin, cephalin, and phosphatidylserine, which differ only in the nitrogenous component attached to the phosphatidic acid component: choline in lecithin (phosphatidylcholine) is replaced by ethanolamine in cephalin (phosphatidylethanolamine) and the amino acid serine in phosphatidylserine (45).

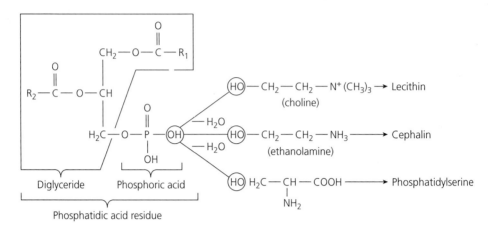

Phosphoglycerides are glyceryl esters of two fatty acid molecules attached to a phosphoric acid molecule and a nitrogenous base.

Erythrocytes

The erythrocyte membrane (stroma) is composed of lipid-protein molecules arranged in a bimolecular leaflet as originally proposed by Gorter and Grendel (39) and later emphasized by Danielli and Davson (22). The stromal network that holds hemoglobin and concentrates on the cell surface as a limiting membrane (cell wall) (16) is composed of approximately 50% proteins, 40% lipids, and 10% carbohydrates (11, 115). Phospholipids comprise approximately 50–70% of the total lipid content (74); the rest is glycolipids. The lipid bilayer (bileaflet) has asymmetric units composed of phospholipid and glycolipid layer components (11); this asymmetry means that the membrane always has a polarity, even in the absence of any associated proteins (11). The **outer** leaflet of lipid layer (external side) is composed of only choline-containing phospholipid sphingomyelin and choline-containing glycolipid lecithin (10, 11, 115), almost to the exclusion of other phospholipids (115). Sphingomyelin and lecithin can replace one another (11). Amino-containing phospholipids, phosphatidylethanolamine (cephalin), and phosphatidylserine mainly are present in the **inner** cytoplasmic half of the bileaflet (facing the cytoplasm), with possibly some choline-containing phospholipids, thus creating asymmetry (11, 115). There are more external than internal phospholipids (11). There is no lipid exchange ("flip-flop") across bilayers unless it is enzymatically catalyzed (11).

Phospholipids are important for permeability properties of the cell; plus they play a significant role in combination with proteins, in maintaining physical strength of cell membrane (20); they are involved with cell permeability (46) and control of the transfer of water and solutes (bicarbonate and chloride ions) between external and internal environment (45).

Lecithin and sphingomyelin do not bind Na^+ and K^+ ions (46). Observations by Nelson (74) suggest that the key to membrane function resides in protein-lipid interaction and that lipid-lipid or lipid-environment interactions have less physiologic significance (74).

Erythrocyte phospholipids common to all species are phosphatidic acid, phosphatidylethanolamine (cephalin), phosphatidylserine, sphingomyelin, and phosphatidylinositol (lipositol); however, the occurrence and quantities of these native phospholipids vary markedly among species (74). In general, lecithin and cephalin are most abundant (44). Cephalin or its vinyl or glycerol ether analogue is the major noncholine phospholipid in rat, rabbit, pig, dog, horse, sheep, cow, goat, cat, and guinea pig (74). The **inner** leaflet layers of sheep, guinea pig, and cow erythrocytes all consist mostly of cephalin and phosphatidylserine (11, 74, 115).

The ratio of lecithin to sphingomyelin in the outer leaflet varies considerably among ruminant species (115), as shown in Table 4.1. Sheep erythrocytes are composed almost entirely of sphingomyelin. The major lipid in human erythrocytes is lecithin, with a substantial amount of sphingomyelin. In guinea pig it is predominately lecithin, with a small amount of sphingomyelin (11, 74, 115). For all practical purposes, the most common CAMP substrates, sheep and bovine erythrocytes, do not contain any appreciable amount of lecithin (74).

CAMP Factor/Reaction

CAMP factor is a thermostable (heat-stable), extracellular (18), diffusible protein (molecular weight 23,500 (5)) product of group B streptococci (12), which lyses ruminant (cud chewers, e.g., sheep, cow) erythrocytes treated with staphylococcal β-hemolysin (54); it manifests specific synergism with sphingomyelinase C (41) on sheep and ox blood (18, 23). It is most effective when present before or nearly simultaneously with the enzymatic hydrolysis of sphingomyelin (41). Its action depends on a relatively high concentration of factor and the slower rate of degradation of substrate caused by dilution of sphingomyelinase (41). CAMP factor might interfere with precipitation of ceramide in situ (in position); removal of ceramide would leave wide spaces in the outer layer, rendering the inner layer in sheep cells susceptible to pressure from inside the cell and to possible enzymatic attack or enough open areas in the outer layer of human and guinea pig to expose the inner layer to action of a broader-spectrum phospholipase C (41).

Table 4.1. Lecithin: Sphingomyelin Ratios of Various Animals

Species	Lecithin:Sphingomyelin Ratio
Rats, dogs, guinea pig	4:1
Horse	3:1
Human, rabbit	3:2
Pig, cat	1:1
Bovine (cow, ox), sheep, goat	1:12

Enzymes act on the exterior membrane of intact erythrocytes, with three possible results from incubating cells with pure phospholipases (115): (*a*) no lipid hydrolysis—no hemolysis, (*b*) lipid hydrolysis—no hemolysis, or (*c*) lipid hydrolysis—hemolysis. Optimal activity of the sphingomyelin-cleaving enzyme occurs at pH 7.8–8.8 (77). The degradation of native sheep erythrocyte sphingomyelin is more rapid than that of purified sheep erythrocyte sphingomyelin (67). Dawson and Bangham (24) reported on the importance of the electrokinetic potential in some phospholipase-substrate interactions; native phospholipids possess favorable electrokinetic properties and are thus more susceptible to phospholipases than are purified phospholipids.

Sphingomyelinase C (sphingomyelin cholinephosphohydrolase (20)) from *S. aureus* subsp. *aureus* can attack the outer membrane of intact mammalian erythrocytes and produce water-insoluble ceramides and phosphorylcholine (20, 115). Studies by Colley et al. (20) showed that although sphingomyelinase produced no hemolysis, it causes 75–80% degradation of sphingomyelin, and prolonged incubation failed to break down sphingomyelin more extensively in intact cells. DeGier and van Deenen (25) suggested that sheep erythrocytes contain enough sphingomyelin to account for enough damage to cause hemolysis, and it may not be necessary to degrade all of the substrate to produce sufficient damage to allow eventual release of hemoglobin from erythrocytes. In the absence of hemolysis, enzymes can only act on the exterior of the cell membrane (115). The presence of sphingomyelinase in medium causes the reaction to occur.

Any observed changes in the molecular organization of the membrane should be considered in relation to the removal of the whole phospholipid molecule from the membrane structure, not just removal of the ionic end group (19). Ionic end groups that produce the main specificity of the substrate molecules are directed outward toward the membrane surface. Ceramides remain in position in the membrane, whereas enzymatically formed diglycerides migrate in discrete pools (20, 115). Removal of water-soluble phosphorylcholine (choline phosphate) on the exterior cell wall increases the susceptibility of sphingomyelinase-treated erythrocytes to osmotic shock after the action of β-hemolysin at 37°C, and ceramides thus produced retain a permeability barrier for hemoglobin even though the physical strength of membrane is definitely decreased (20, 115).

Sphingomyelin Degradation

After treatment with sphingomyelinase, lecithin molecules in the outer layer are readily attacked by phospholipase C, resulting in formation of diglycerides (115). The membrane structure must allow phospholipase C to interact specifically with the ionic end of phospholipid molecules (19). Sphingomyelin is more slowly hydrolyzed than lecithin (65).

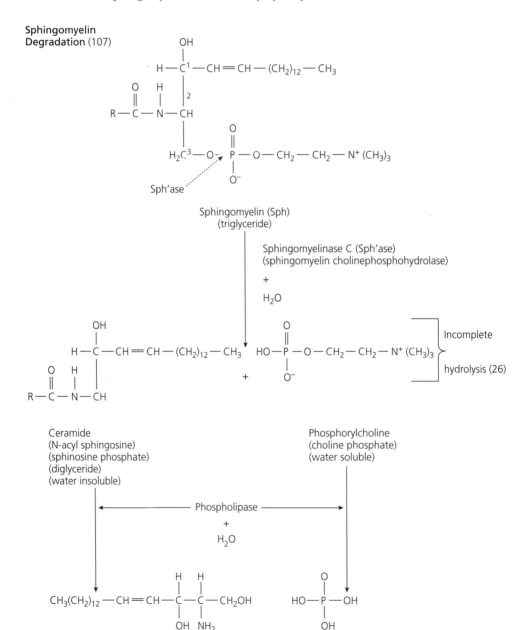

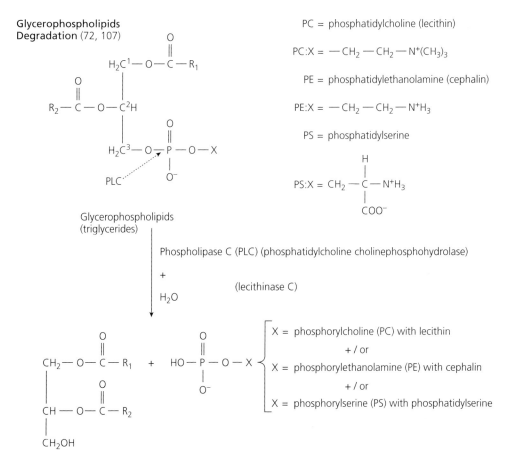

Phospholipase C (or lecithinase C (66); phosphatidylcholine cholinephosphohydrolase (69)) catalyzes the hydrolysis of phosphate bonds with liberation of phosphorylcholine from the phosphatides lecithin, cephalin, and sphingomyelin (66). The main products of hydrolysis are phosphorylcholine and phosphorylethanolamine and the neutral lipids, diglycerides, and ceramide (19). Phospholipase C does not hydrolyze glycerol phosphorylcholine (114). Phospholipases from different sources have different actions on the same membrane (e.g., phospholipases A_2 and D); lysis may be due to prior removal of choline phosphate from sphingomyelin (20).

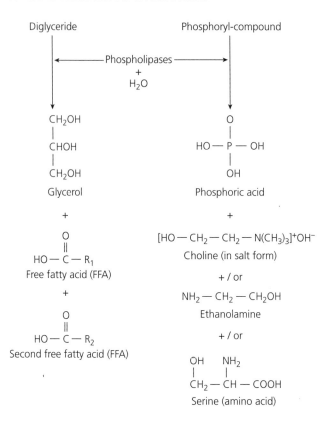

Glycerophospholipid Degradation

Ceramides and diglycerides may aggregate to form dense droplets (115). To compensate for the thermodynamically unfavorable interaction of water from the outside with the apolar part of inner lipid layers, phospholipid molecules of the inner layer (mainly choline and phosphatidylserine) may now "flip-flop" to the outer layer where they will be subsequently degraded by phosphorylase C, destroying membrane permeability with migration of diglycerides into pools and further weakening of the membrane structure (115). Sheep cells are resistant to phospholipase A_2 since they have little lecithin (11); lecithin is replaced by sphingomyelin (106). Erythrocytes from most other mammals are lysed by this enzyme (11). In sheep and bovine erythrocytes there is no breakdown of glycerophospholipids by the combined action of sphingomyelinase and phospholipase C and no hemolysis. Nonlytic degradation of phospholipids decreases the stability of the cell membrane (20, 115). Human and guinea pig erythrocytes incubated with a mixture of sphingomyelinase and phospholipase C produce complete hemolysis within 1 h, although neither of these enzymes produce lysis independently (20). When streptococci are grown near the edge of one of the uniform dark zones of staphylococcal β-lysin, the medium clears at the point nearest to the streptococcal colonies, suggesting that an invisible agent or products of such an agent have reached red cells already altered by staphylococcal β-lysin. Lysis is obtained with sheep or ox blood, not with horse, rabbit, human, or guinea pig (72). Phospholipase C from *Bacillus cereus* alone is not lytic; a combination of sphingomyelinase and phospholipase C produces hemolysis on human blood agar (HBA) and guinea pig blood agar (GPBA) (20). Hemolysis of erythrocytes is doubtless due to breakdown of lipoproteins, but other factors must also be involved because red cells of different species are not equally susceptible to hemolysis although phospholipids isolated from these cells are equally susceptible to hydrolysis (65).

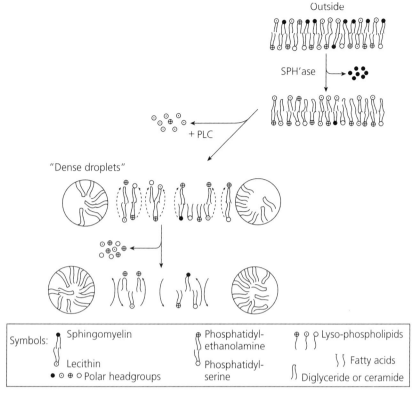

Highly schematized model of phospholipase attack on the outside of an asymmetric human red cell membrane. Abbreviations: PLC, phospholipase C; α SPH'ase, sphingomyelinase. (Redrawn in abbreviated form from Zwaal, R. F. A., Roelofsen, B., and Cooley, C. M. (1973). Localization of red cell membrane constituents. Biochim. Biophys. Acta, 300, 178, with permission of Elsevier/North Holland Biomedical Press, Amsterdam.)

IV. MEDIUM EMPLOYED: SHEEP BLOOD AGAR PLATES (SBA, SBAP)

Blood agar (BA) plate medium must be used to cultivate all *Streptococcus* spp. since they are fastidious and require additional enrichments for growth. Citrated or defibrinated sheep or ox blood **must** be used because **no** reaction occurs with horse, rabbit, guinea pig, or human blood (18). The presence of β-antitoxin in some batches of sheep blood will inhibit staphylococcal β-toxin production; to avoid this possibility use only cells (71).

V. QUALITY CONTROL MICROORGANISMS

(*Note:* Set up positive and negative controls simultaneously. Test both quality control strains (+ and −) each time the test is performed (4).)

A. **Standardized CAMP test**
   Streptococcus agalactiae (+) ATCC 27956
   Streptococcus pyogenes (−) ATCC 19615

B. ***Listeria* identification**
   1. With *S. aureus* subsp. *aureus*
      a. *Staphylococcus aureus* subsp. *aureus* ATCC 12600
      b. *Listeria monocytogenes* (+) ATCC 19112, NCTC 7973 (55). **Do not** use ATCC 15313; it does not produce β-hemolysin and **does not** produce hemolysis in the CAMP test (98).
      c. *Listeria seeligeri* (+) CIP 100100
      d. *Listeria welshimeri* (−) CIP 8149
   2. With *R. equi*

a. *Rhodococcus equi* NCTC 1621
b. *Listeria ivanovii* (+) ATCC 19119.
c. *Listeria monocytogenes* (−) NCTC 7973 (55)

VI. CAMP TESTS

A. **Standardized CAMP test**
  1. Original observations by Christie, Atkins, Munch-Petersen (18), and original test designed by Munch-Petersen, Christie, Simmons (71).
  2. Standardized procedure of Darling (23)
  3. β-Lysin substrate
     a. *S. aureus* subsp. *aureus* culture
     b. Any strain known to produce a high level of β-lysin (58) (exhibiting at least a 4-mm or larger band of β-lysin (darkening) activity and less than a 2-mm band of complete hemolysis on SBA (23))
  4. Test organism(s)
     a. Growth from an 18- to 24-h **pure** culture of **known** *Streptococcus* spp. (Todd-Hewitt, SBA)
     b. **Early stage of growth**
  5. **Before use**, plates and candle jar **must** be prewarmed to 37°C and be dry.
  6. Inoculations: **heavy inocula** (41, 110)
     a. With an inoculating needle or **edge** of loop, streak *Staphylococcus* **in a straight line across the center** of an SBA plate.
     b. Streak test organism(s) in a straight line 2–3 cm long and **perpendicular to** (i.e., at a right angle to) the staphylococcal inoculum **without touching the staphylococcal inoculum.**
     c. Four test organisms may be streaked per plate.
        (1) Label the test organisms (e.g., 1, 2, 3, 4) on the **bottom half** of the Petri dish **before** inoculation.
        (2) Streak two test organisms each side of the staphylococcal center inoculum.

(*Note:* This test is frequently used in conjunction with bacitracin and trimethoprim-sulfamethoxazole (TSM/SXT) tests on the same blood agar plate for presumptive identification of the streptococci (59) (Table 4.2.))

Table 4.2. *Listeria* **species Differentiation**

Species	β-Hemolysis	Pathogenic	CAMP with *S. aureus*	CAMP with *R. equi*	D-Xylose	L-Rhamnose	α-Methyl-D-Mannoside
L. monocytogenes[a]	+[a]	+	+[b]	−	−	A	A
L. seeligeri (104, 105)	+w	−	+	−	A	−	−
L. ivanovii[c]	+[d]	+	−	+[e]	A	−	−
L. innocua[f]	−	−	−	−	−	V	A
L. welshimeri (27, 86)	−	−	−	−	A	V	A

Data from refs 86 and 98; w, weakly positive.

[a]Not all strains of *L. monocytogenes* exhibit β-hemolysis; type strain ATCC 15313 is nonhemolytic (γ) on horse, sheep, and bovine blood (98); others produce a narrow zone, but this varies with blood species.
[b]ATCC 15313 negative reaction.
[c]*L. ivanovii* separated into *L. ivanovii* and *L. ivanovii* subsp. *londoniensis;* separated by two carbohydrates: *L. ivanovii* is ribose-positive (A) and mannosamine-negative (−); *L. ivanovii* subsp. *londoniensis* is ribose-negative (−) and mannosamine-positive (A).
[d]Wide zone or multiple zones usually exhibited (98).
[e]A positive CAMP result with *R. equi* is a specific marker to identify *L. ivanovii* (87).
[f]*L. innocua* may induce false-positive reactions when grown on blood agar with glucose (79, 93).

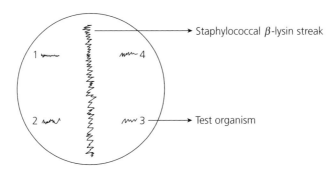

7. Incubation: plates **inverted** (lids down)
   a. **Recommended: no CO_2; 35°C**, 18–24 h. Air incubation (ambient air) increases the specificity of test because fewer **non–group B streptococci are positive in air** (4).
   b. **With a candle jar (reduced oxygen tension)**
      (1) **5–10% CO_2 or CO_2 incubator**
      (2) **35°C**; 5–6 h; if negative, continue incubating to 18 h. Some group A streptococci will be CAMP positive if incubated in a candle jar, in a CO_2 atmosphere, or under anaerobic conditions (59).
B. **CAMP test with *Listeria* species:** procedure the same as for *S. agalactiae* (group B streptococci)

L. monocytogenes sensu lato (broad sense) are now separated into five distinct species; differentiation is based on hemolysis in the CAMP test with either *S. aureus* subsp. *aureus* or *Rhodococcus equi* (formerly *Corynebacterium equi*) plus acid production from D-xylose, L-rhamnose, and α-methyl-D-mannoside (85). Based on observations by Fraser (33), the use of hemolytic synergism with *R. equi* proposed by other investigators (73, 90, 91) is explained by the presence of phospholipase C (91) (Table 4.2).

VII. RESULTS

> See Figures 4.1 and 4.2 (Appendix 1) for colored photographic results

VIII. INTERPRETATION

A. Positive CAMP reaction (+) (23)
   1. Production of a distinct **arrowhead** (⇑) zone (flare) of complete hemolysis (clear)
      a. Located at point of staphylococcal streak where diffusing products of the two organisms (CAMP factor and β-lysin) have converged and overlapped (12, 18, 23, 110), in the area between growth of the two strains (110).
      b. Synergistic hemolysis zone extends throughout the depth of the blood agar.
      c. Clear zone (synergistic hemolysis) is surrounded by a larger, darkened zone where staphylococcal β-lysin altered but not lysed by sheep erythrocytes (72).
   2. **Presumptive** group B *S. agalactiae* (Table 4.3)
B. Negative CAMP reaction (−) (23)
   1. **No** arrowhead phenomenon in candle jar or under aerobic conditions
   2. Possible increased hemolysis in zone of staphylococcal β-lysin activity
      a. Synergistic phenomenon; not CAMP reaction
      b. Bacteria **other than** group B *Streptococcus* spp. (e.g., group A streptococci)

In evaluating the CAMP test, Darling (23) incubated study organisms under all three types of atmospheric conditions and found that all known group B streptococci produced characteristic arrowhead positive reactions, usually within 5–6 h when incubated either anaerobically or in a candle extinction jar (reduced oxygen tension) and within 18 h aerobically. Group A streptococci produced an arrowhead positive reaction **only** anaerobically but exhibited increased hemolysis in the zone of staphylococcal β-lysin activity both in a candle extinction jar and aerobically. Under anaerobic conditions, arrowheads of group B were at least twice as large as those of group A. Groups C and G were negative under all three atmospheric conditions (Table 4.3).

Table 4.3. Atmospheric Conditions for CAMP Test

	Streptococci		
	Group B	Group A	Groups C + G
Anaerobic } 5–6 h	⇑	↑	—
Candle jar }	⇑	H	—
Aerobic 18 h	⇑	H	—

⇑, arrowhead positive CAMP reaction; ↑, smaller arrowhead positive CAMP reaction; H, increased hemolysis in zone β-lysin activity.

Darling (23) recommends that the acronym "CAMP test (reaction)" be reserved for the original observations of Christie et al. (18) and that the potentiation of hemolysis in a zone of staphylococcal β-lysin with other bacteria or their products be referred to **not** as "CAMP positive" but as "**synergistic hemolytic effect.**"

IX. REVERSE CAMP TEST (RCT)

A. This modification of the original CAMP test (18, 71) uses the α-toxin of *C. perfringens* (41).
   1. β-Lysin is replaced by α-toxin (α-lysin, α-hemolysin); alternate to Nagler test (α-lecithinase detection test)
   2. Use of human blood agar (HBA)
B. Purpose: **presumptive** discrimination of *C. perfringens* (+) from other sulfite-reducing, sporeforming *Clostridium* spp. (−); highly specific for *C. perfringens*
C. Biochemistry: phenomenon of synergistic hemolysis with the CAMP factor; α-toxin contains a sphingomyelinase C fraction similar to that of *S. aureus* subsp. *aureus* and a broader-spectrum phospholipase C (lecithinase) that hydrolyzes lecithin, sphingomyelin, and cephalin (19, 66).
D. Procedure of Hansen and Elliott (42)
   1. *Clostridium* spp. replace *S. aureus* subsp. *aureus* and a known group B streptococcus (*S. agalactiae*) is used.
   2. **Direct** inoculation of specimen
   3. Inoculate at right angles to within 1–2 mm of β-hemolytic group B streptococci on sheep blood agar (SBA).
      a. Four cultures may be tested per plate.
      b. Set up known positive and negative controls:

      | *Clostridium perfringens* (+) | ATCC 13124 |
      | *Clostridium bifermentans* (lecithinase-positive)(−) | ATCC 638 |
      | *Streptococcus agalactiae* NCTC | 8181 |

   4. Incubate **an**aerobically (GasPak), 35°C, 18–24 h; read under transmitted light (4).
E. Interpretation (42)
   1. RCT-positive: "bow-tie" or "reverse arrow" pattern of hemolysis at the juncture of the two cultures; the tip of the arrow points from *Streptococcus* sp. toward *C. perfringens* (59). A positive reaction indicates **only** *C. perfringens*.

2. RCT, ±: bullet-shaped zone of β-hemolysis
   a. May be due to less than optimal ratios of enzyme to CAMP factor or may be due to low levels of α-toxin (42)
   b. *C. perfringens,* other *Clostridium* spp. (42)

According to Buchanan (14) "free" hemolysin or lecithinase (or both) is required for a positive reverse CAMP reaction.

X. PHOSPHOLIPASE D (PLD) DETECTION BY CAMP TEST INHIBITION

A. Purpose: differentiation of *C. pseudotuberculosis* (*C. ovis*) (+) and *C. ulcerans* (+) from other *Corynebacterium* spp. (−) (4)
B. Principle: corynebacterial phospholipase D, "ovis toxin," is a sphingomyelinase (61, 62) that inhibits the enhanced hemolysis observed when the hemolysins of *S. aureus* subsp. *aureus* and *S. agalactiae* interact synergistically (positive CAMP) (4). PLD hydrolyzes sphingomyelins to N-acylsphingosyl phosphates (101, 102). The capacity of the products of these two species (*C. pseudotuberculosis* and *C. ulcerans*) to block the hemolytic activity of the β-lysin (phospholipase C of *S. aureus* subsp. *aureus* (18, 29, 34, 47) and that of the α-toxin of *C. perfringens* (99) and their PLD activity are all the same (38, 63, 100, 101).
C. Test microorganisms (4); fresh, 18- to 24-h cultures on sheep blood agar (SBA)
   1. *S. aureus* subsp. *aureus*: β-toxin-producing strain
   2. *S. agalactiae*: CAMP-positive strain
   3. Positive control: *C. ulcerans*; standard *C. ulcerans* has not yet been designated for this test (4).
   4. Unknown *Corynebacterium* strain
D. Procedure (4)
   1. Medium: 5% sheep blood agar (SBA) plate
   2. Inoculum: **Sterile,** cotton swabs of each microorganism
   3. Inoculation: (Fig. 4.8)
   4. Incubation: 35°C, 18–24 h
   5. Interpretation (4)
      a. PDL positive (+)
         (1) **Inhibition** of enhanced zone of hemolysis formed at the juncture of staphylococcal hemolysin and streptococcal hemolysis. **Constricted band** of enhanced hemolysis (Fig. 4.8)
         (2) *C. pseudotuberculosis* or *C. ulcerans*
      b. PDL negative (−): **no** constriction of band of enhanced hemolysis; other *Corynebacterium* spp.

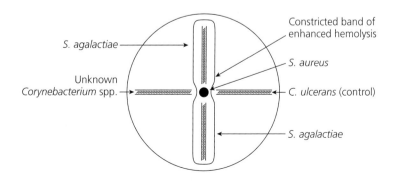

Barksdale et al. (2) found that all strains of *C. pseudotuberculosis* and *C. ulcerans* produce PLD **and urease** and that among the catalase-positive, pyrazinamidase-negative corynebacteria, they alone produce these two enzymes; the two can easily be distinguished on the basis of starch fermentation (*C. ulcerans* is positive; *C. pseudotuberculosis*, negative).

XI. ALTERNATIVE TESTS

A. **CAMP disk test**
   1. Procedure of Wilkinson (110), a modification of original CAMP test (18, 71), substitutes a staphylococcal culture with paper disks impregnated (i.e., saturated) with partially purified β-hemolysin of *S. aureus* subsp. *aureus*. It necessitates keeping a staphylococcal stock culture on hand.
   2. Commercial disks are available (REMEL)
   3. Storage: refrigerator or freezer, −20°C (31)
      a. Disks are **not** reliable if stored at 4–8°C, even for a short time
      b. Stable up to 1 month at −20°C
   4. Procedure
      a. Place the disk 1–2 mm from the end of a single *Streptococcus* streak.
      b. Incubate in a candle extinction jar, 35°C, 18–24 h.
   5. Interpretation
      a. Positive CAMP reaction: crescent-shaped area of increased lysis forms between the streptococcal streak and the β-lysin-containing disk
      b. Intermediate CAMP reaction: areas of increased lysis develop in shapes **other than** a crescent (or arrowhead); areas of lysis are usually smaller than those seen with the usual CAMP positive result and are quite distinctive (32)

B. **Spot CAMP test**
   1. Procedure of Ratner, Weeks, and Stratton (81); a rapid test that eliminates subculturing
   2. β-Lysin reagent
      a. Source: *S. aureus* subsp. *aureus* ATCC 12600 grown in Todd-Hewitt broth (THB); 35°C, 48 h
      b. Preparation: centrifuge and **aseptically** decant supernatant through a 0.45-μ bacteriological filter into a **sterile** container
      c. Storage: frozen, −70°C; thaw as needed
   3. Procedure
      a. Blood agar plates: trypticase soy agar (TSA) with 5% sheep blood
      b. With a Pasteur pipette, place a drop of β-lysin reagent next to the β-hemolytic colony(s)
      c. Hold at room temperature (22–25°C) (lid **up**), 20–30 min
   4. Positive CAMP reaction: arc or circle of enhanced hemolysis next to colony(s) where reagent dropped; group B streptococci

Ratner et al. (81) obtained spot test sensitivity of 99% and specificity of 100%. Similar results were obtained by other investigators (26, 31, 36, 54, 78).

XII. PRECAUTIONS

A. **General**
   1. The surface of agar plates **must** be absolutely dry; any condensation will facilitate spreading, running, and mixing of inocula (35).
   2. Citrated or defibrinated sheep or ox blood **must** be used; **no reaction** will occur with horse, human, rabbit, or guinea pig blood (18).
   3. Any size plate may be used; however, the depth of blood agar in **center must** be approximately **1.5 mm** (23). As the depth increases, arrowheads of hemolysis become less

distinct (23). The reaction is positive **only** if synergistic hemolysis in the β-lysin zone extends throughout the depth of blood agar.
4. The sheep blood plates **and** candle extinction jar **must** be prewarmed to 37°C **before use** (23) to avoid hot-cold lysis.
5. An accurate test is not ensured if the inocula intersect (23). Also, after inoculation, avoid tilting the plates until the inocula are absorbed into the agar; otherwise, inocula may run over plate (35) giving mixed and invalid results.
6. Avoid inoculating the test medium from the initial isolation medium; mixed cultures give invalid results.
7. Test plates should be read as soon as possible after the appropriate incubation period; if they are held at room temperature (25°C) for any period of time, interpretation is difficult because of hot-cold lysis of sheep erythrocytes (41).
8. The size of the zone depends on the amount of bacterial product and its diffusibility through the medium (41).
9. β-Lysin requires calcium (Ca) for its activity and is thus inactive in the presence of ions such as phosphate, citrate, or fluoride, which sequester this metal (66).

B. **Standard CAMP test with *S. aureus* subsp. *aureus***
1. Before being tested for CAMP reaction, a β-hemolytic organism(s) must be identified as a member of the genus *Streptococcus* by a catalase test and a Gram stain. All *Streptococcus* spp. are catalase-negative, Gram-positive cocci arranged in chains, pairs, or singly. Other Gram-positive cocci (e.g., some Gram-negative staphylococci) and some Gram-negative rods (48) can give a positive CAMP reaction.
2. This CAMP test is used to **aid** in identification of group B streptococci. No single test should be relied upon for **presumptive** identification of group B human or bovine organisms; a positive CAMP reaction must be used **in combination with other tests and criteria** (e.g., colony morphology, clinical source, bacitracin, PYR (L-pyrrolidonyl-β-naphthylamide)). However, there is **no** need to perform both hippurate hydrolysis and the CAMP test; use **only** one. A serologic test is the only means of confirming group B identification.

    Bacitracin or PYR, or trimethoprim-sulfamethoxazole (TSM or SXT) and the CAMP test, along with the hemolytic pattern should be used to identify the group B streptococci (Table 4.4).

    a. **Presumptive** group B by the CAMP test **if**

      Bacitracin resistant (R) (negative) or PYR negative, or TSM-SXT resistant (R)
      CAMP positive
      β-Hemolytic

    b. Group A or B streptococci separated by hemolytic pattern (group B hemolysis a smaller zone) **if**

      Bacitracin sensitive (S) (positive)
      CAMP positive
      β-Hemolytic

    c. **Presumptive** group A **if**

      Bacitracin sensitive (S) (positive) or PYR positive
      CAMP positive
      β-Hemolytic

    d. β-Hemolytic streptococci **not** group A or B **if**

      Bacitracin resistant (R) (negative) or PYR negative
      CAMP negative
      β-Hemolytic

Table 4.4. Identification of β-Hemolytic *Streptococcus* spp.

Microorganism	Bacitracin	TSM	CAMP	PYR
Presumptive Gp A	S	R	−	+
Presumptive Gp B	R	R	+	−
Non–gp A or B	R	S	−	−
Non–gp A or B	S	S	−	−

TSM, trimethoprim-sulfamethoxazole; PYR, pyrrolidonyl arylamidase hydrolysis; S, sensitive; R, resistant.
Data from reference 59.

3. Both human and bovine streptococci exhibit hemolysis (clear zone), but the human type shows larger hemolytic zones around colonies on blood agar plates after a 24-h incubation; group B zones are relatively narrow (small) and hazy (9).
4. This CAMP test is used primarily for identification within the genus *Streptococcus*; however, the synergistic hemolytic phenomenon is also found among **some species** of other genera and is used to differentiate species: *Pasteurella haemolytica* (+) from *P. multocida* (−) (8, 34) on sheep blood agar. Also some hemolytic strains of groups E, P, and U streptococci give a positive CAMP reaction (89) as do groups C, F, and G (98). Other organisms that are CAMP positive or said to produce a CAMP reaction with *S. aureus* subsp. *aureus* β-lysin include *L. monocytogenes* (34), *L. seeligeri* (83, 84), *Burkholderia pseudomallei* (34), *Corynebacterium renale* (34), *Mobiluncus mulieris*, and *Mobiluncus curtisii* (103), and *Propionibacterium* (56).

    Studies by Skalka et al. (94) showed that the purified β-lysin of *S. aureus* subsp. *aureus* and exotoxin of *C. pseudotuberculosis* gave synergistic lysis with the δ-hemolysin of *S. aureus* subsp. *aureus* and ε-hemolysin of coagulase-negative staphylococci.
5. A variation of the original CAMP reaction has led to confusion about how the test should be performed. Darling (23) has standardized the procedure and interpretation to avoid false positive results. Originally the CAMP test was considered 100% specific for group B streptococci, all strains, whether hemolytic or nonhemolytic on initial isolation (18, 71). Later studies, depending on cultural conditions and assessment of lytic zones, showed positive reactions for 20–100% of group A streptococci and a number of C and G stains, although many reactions were weaker than those of group B (41). At the same time, up to 5% of group B gave negative results (23, 30, 49, 54, 64, 95). Later studies by Barnum (3), Esseveld et al. (30), Biechteler (7), Pulverer (80), and Heeschen et al. (49) showed an average sensitivity of 98.4%. In 1976, studies by Jokipii and Jokipii (54) showed 95%.
6. A high concentration of β-antitoxin in some batches of sheep or ox blood and some other types will inhibit staphylococcal β-toxin (β-lysin) production and lead to false-negative results (23); this is avoided by using only erythrocytes (23, 71).
7. Darling (23) used *S. aureus* strain 681. Any viable strain that produces a 4-mm or **greater** band of β-lysin activity (darkening) and **less** than a 2-mm band of complete hemolysis on SBA is satisfactory for the CAMP test. However, an 18-h incubation may be required before a positive result is discernible (23). A narrow zone of complete hemolysis around the colony and a fairly broad outer zone of darkening (blackened) (partially hemolyzed erythrocytes) indicate good β-lysin production with minimal production of toxins (41).

    The type of medium used to maintain stock cultures affects β-lysin production. Nutrient broth is **not** suitable because hemolysin (lysin) is rapidly inactivated, but heart infusion (HI) and brain heart infusion (BHI) broths yield high titers (43). Haque and Baldwin (44) recommend maintaining *S. aureus* subsp. *aureus* on Trypticase soy agar (TSA) slants and **before** use, streaking it on SBA and picking a single isolated colony for the β-hemolysin streak on the CAMP plate. The staphylococcal strain **must** be free of spontaneous mutants capable of producing other hemolysins and interfering with the CAMP reaction (43). TSA slants suppress emergence of such mutants; agar protects the hemolysin molecule from denaturation; hence the stock culture β-hemolysin yield is high (43). However, continual propagation on TSA eventually reduces the yield of β-hemolysin, and Haque and Baldwin (43) recommend maintaining the culture by lyophilization.

8. Inocula should be sufficient to produce confluent growth (110); the extent and intensity of lysis depends on the size of the staphylococcal inoculum. If the inoculum is too light, so that growth is less than confluent, the reaction tends to be very weak, and test organisms should be retested with a heavier staphylococcal inoculum (41).
9. If the inocula are not perpendicular to each other, the production of arrowheads of hemolysis will **not** occur, and false-positive results will occur if the unknown is **not** a *Streptococcus* spp. (23) (e.g., δ-toxin producing *Staphylococcus epidermidis* produces synergistic hemolysis when inoculated perpendicular to a β-toxin-producing *Staphylococcus* (70)).
10. Prompt results are obtained when streptococcal and staphylococcal inocula are in an early stage of growth (23).
11. The reaction is positive only if synergistic hemolysis in the β-lysin zone **extends** throughout the depth of blood agar.
12. The agent produced by streptococcal cells (CAMP factor) **must** come in contact with sheep or ox red cells **before** staphylococcal β-hemolysin (21).
13. **Do not** incubate longer than 24 h; with longer incubation the reactive zones are so large that it is impossible to read neighboring reactions (35, 110).
14. Brown et al. (12) recommend substituting maltose for glucose in broth cultures of streptococci to enhance production of CAMP factor.
15. According to Oberhofer (76), β-hemolytic streptococci recovered from locations **other than** the throat **and all** nonhemolytic streptococci recovered from blood or spinal fluid (CSF) should be routinely tested for the CAMP reaction, since **not all** group B streptococci are hemolytic (31, 76, 110).
16. Synergistic hemolysis is seen with both hemolytic and nonhemolytic isolates of group B streptococci (59).
17. Other streptococci, mainly group A, may produce similar lysis of sheep erythrocytes (104), resulting in false-positive CAMP reactions (23, 30). The synergistic lytic factor of group A corresponds to streptolysin O (SO) of group A streptococci (104) produced during logarithmic growth phase, and Tapsall and Phillips (104) suggest that group A synergistic hemolysis is due to the action of small amounts of streptolysin that are unoxidized and thus can lyse fragile β-lysin-treated sheep erythrocytes.

Streptolysin O is a cytolysin capable of altering erythrocyte membranes and also affecting the permeability of membranes associated with subcellular organelles (97). The activity occurs in the reduced state, and SO is readily oxidized (50); thiol and other reducing agents are used to activate maximal activity. SO produced in broth cultures is not entirely oxidized, and some activity is present even in the absence of reducing agents (50). SO produced by group A streptococci in the CAMP test has enough activity to lyse fragile sheep blood cells (104).

The properties of SO are distinct from those of the CAMP protein of group B streptococci (104). CAMP factor leads to a nonenzymatic disruption of sphingomyelin-depleted bovine or sheep erythrocytes **only**, with **no** effect on erythrocytes of other species or on intact erythrocytes (6). Anaerobic conditions enhance SO activity (104).

The false-positive CAMP reaction due to group A streptococci can be eliminated by the use of SO inhibitors that **do not** simultaneously affect staphylococcal β-lysin or the CAMP factor of group B; this results in increased specificity without loss of sensitivity (104). To eliminate false-positive results, heat the culture supernatants; this inactivates the heat-labile SO of group A, with **no** inactivation of the heat-stable CAMP factor of group B streptococci (104).

C. *Listeria* **identification**
  1. The hemolytic pattern of *L. monocytogenes* varies (57, 91, 92); some strains produce weak hemolysis on blood agar plates that can easily be interpreted as a negative result (86). The hemolytic activity is a fundamental criterion for differentiation of *Listeria* species (86); nonhemolytic strains (apathogenic) are irrelevant (87). Not all strains of *L. monocytogenes* exhibit β-hemolysis; type strain ATCC 15313 is **non**hemolytic (γ) on horse, sheep, and bovine blood (98); others produce a narrow zone, but that varies with the source of the blood (species). Hemolysis of *L. monocytogenes* is enhanced when it is grown close to *S. aureus* subsp. *aureus* (13, 40); *L. monocytogenes* produces phospholipase C (57, 60).
  2. *Listeria* inocula may induce a false-positive CAMP result when they are grown on blood agar with glucose (79, 93).
  3. Rodríguez et al. (86) devised a microplate technique to determine the hemolytic activity of *Listeria* spp. for routine typing of *Listeria* strains in place of the CAMP test.
  4. A positive CAMP test result with *R. equi* is a specific marker to identify *L. invanovii* (87).
  5. In *Bergey's Manual* (88), CAMP-negative *L. monocytogenes* and CAMP-positive *L. ivanovii* have been adopted as the fundamental criteria for identification of hemolytic *Listeria* spp. (82). However, other investigators (1, 28, 33, 73, 82, 91, 107, 109) found *L. monocytogenes* strains that gave a CAMP-positive synergistic hemolysis reaction with *R. equi*. Vázquez-Boland et al. (107) showed that a circular or racket-shaped, well-defined zone of complete hemolysis develops from a streak of *L. monocytogenes* in the vicinity of *R. equi*, with differing intensity depending on the hemolytic activity of strain. The lytic phenomenon of *L. monocytogenes* could be distinguished from that of *L. ivanovii*, which was typically semicircular or shovel shaped (108). These studies also showed that in certain cases, especially when highly hemolytic *L. monocytogenes* strains are tested and when the test is performed on blood agar instead of washed erythrocytes, the *R. equi* CAMP reactions of both *Listeria* spp. are similar and often confused. Nakazawa and Nemoto (73) suggest that discordant results from various laboratories might be due to the fact that strains of *R. equi* may differ in their ability to interact with *L. monocytogenes*.

  Vázquez-Boland et al. (108) used the CIP (Collection de l'Institut Pasteur) 5869 strain of *R. equi*, which other investigators found to give negative results with *L. monocytogenes* (85). They also showed that both different strains and even subcultures of the same strain of *R. equi* differ in their CAMP property, which results in conflicting results. Thus it is recommended that the results of the CAMP test with *R. equi* as presently defined for *Listeria* identification (88) be interpreted with caution (108).

D. **Reverse CAMP test (RCT)**
  1. Group B streptococci exhibit some enhanced hemolysis with other clostridia; however, only *C. perfringens* produces the characteristic arrowhead form (4).
  2. Both false-positive and false-negative results may occur (59).

E. **Phospholipase D detection by CAMP test inhibition**
  Actinomyces pyogenes and *Aracnobacterium haemolyticum* are also PLD positive, pyrazinamidase negative, and catalase negative (4).

REFERENCES

1. Anonymous. Note de Service du 16/3/1987, DGAL/SVHA/N87/8041. Ministère de l'Agiculture, France.
2. Barksdale L, Linder R, Sulea IT, Pollice M. Phospholipase D activity of *Corynebacterium pseudotuberculosis* (*Corynebacterium ovis*) and *Corynebacterium ulcerans*, a distinctive marker within the genus *Corynebacterium*. J Clin Microbiol 1981;13(2):335–343.
3. Barnum DA. The use of the CAMP test for the rapid identification of *Streptococcus agalactiae*. Report of the Ontario Veterinary College. 1950: 120–125.
4. Baron EJ, Finegold SM. Bailey & Scott's Diagnostic Microbiology, ed 8. Philadelphia: CV Mosby, 1990:313, 343, 448, 466.
5. Bernheimer AW, Linder R, Avigad LS. Nature and mechanism of action of the CAMP protein of group B streptococci. Infect Immun 1979; 23(3):838–844.
6. Bernheimer AW, Linder R, Avigad LS. Stepwise degradation of membrane sphingomyelin by corynebacterial phospholipases. Infect Immun 1980;29(1):123–131.
7. Biechteler W. Beitrag zur Routine-Diagnostik hämolysierender Streptokokken (OBF-Test nach Guthoff, CAMP-test, Antibiogramm). Zentralbl Bakteriol 1964;193(1):48–56.
8. Bouley G. Épreuve de CAMP et distinction rapide entre *Pasteurella haemolytica*. Ann Inst Pasteur 1965;108(1):129–131.
9. Braunstein H, Tucker EB, Gibson BC. Identification and significance of *Streptococcus agalactiae* (Lancefield group B). Am J Clin Pathol 1969;51(2):207–213.
10. Bretscher MS. Phosphatidyl-ethanolamine: Differential labelling in intact cells and cell ghosts of human erythrocytes by a membrane-impermeable reagent. J Mol Biol 1972;71(3): 523–528.
11. Bretscher MS. Membrane structure: Some general principles. Science 1973;181:622–629.
12. Brown J, Farnsworth R, Wannamaker LW, Johnson DW. CAMP factor of group B streptococci: Production, assay, and neutralization by sera from immunized rabbits and experimentally infected cows. Infect Immun 1974;9(2): 377–383.
13. Brzin B, Seeliger HPR. A brief note on the CAMP phenomenon in *Listeria*. In: Woodbine W, ed. Problems of Listeriosis. Leicester, England: Leicester University Press, 1975:34–37.
14. Buchanan AG. Clinical laboratory evaluation of a reverse CAMP test for presumptive identification of *Clostridium perfringens*. J Clin Microbiol 1982;16(4):761–762.
15. Burrows W, Lewert RM, Rippon JW. Textbook of Microbiology. The Pathogenic Microorganisms, ed 19. Philadelphia: WB Saunders, 1968:418–419.
16. Cantarow A, Schepartz B. Biochemistry, ed 3. Philadelphia: WB Saunders, 1962:38, 802–803.
17. Chesbro WR, Heydrick FP, Martineau R, Perkins GN. Purification of staphylococcal β-hemolysin and its action on staphylococcal and streptococcal cell walls. J Bacteriol 1965; 89(2):378–389.
18. Christie R, Atkins NE, Munch-Petersen E. A note on lytic phenomenon shown by group B streptococci. Aust J Exp Biol Med Sci 1944; 22:197–200.
19. Coleman R, Finean JB, Knutton S, Limbrick AR. A structural study of the modification of erythrocyte ghosts by phospholipase c. Biochim Biophys Acta 1970;219:81–92.
20. Colley CM, Zwaal RFA, Roelofsen B, Van Deenen LLM. Lytic and non-lytic degradation of phospholipids in mammalian erythrocytes by pure phospholipases. Biochim Biophys Acta 1973;307:74–82.
21. Cowan ST. Cowan & Steel's Manual for the Identification of Medical Bacteria, ed 2. Cambridge, Cambridge University Press, 1974:30.
22. Danielli JF, Davson H. A contribution to the theory of permeability of thin films. J Cell Physiol 1935;5(4):495–508.
23. Darling CL. Standardization and evaluation of the CAMP reaction for the prompt, presumptive identification of *Streptococcus agalactiae* (Lancefield group B) in clinical material. J Clin Microbiol 1975;1(2):171–174.
24. Dawson RMC, Bangham AD. The importance of electrokinetic potentials in some phospholipase-substrate interactions. Biochem J 1961; 81:29P–30P.
25. DeGier J, van Deenen LLM. Some lipid characteristics of red cell membranes of various animal species. Biochim Biophys Acta 1961;49: 286–296.
26. DiPersio JR, Barrett JE, Kaplan RL. Evaluation of the Spot-CAMP test for the rapid presumptive identification of group B streptococci. Am J Clin Pathol 1985;84(2):216–219.
27. Doery HM, Magnusson BJ, Cheyne IM, Gulasekharam J. A phospholipase in staphylococcal toxin which hydrolyses sphingomyelin. Nature 1963;198:1091–1092.
28. Domínguez L, Rodríguez L, Vázquez Boland JA, et al. Microplate technique to determine hemolytic activity for routine typing of *Listeria* strains. J Clin Microbiol 1986;24(1):99–103.
29. Dubos RJ, Hirsch JG, eds. Bacterial and Mycotic Infections of Man, ed 4. Philadelphia: JB Lippincott, 1965:148, 418.
30. Esseveld HM, Daniëls-Basman SM, Leijnse B. Some observations about the CAMP reaction and its application to human β-haemolytic streptococci. J Microbiol Serol Leeuvenhock Med Tydschr 1958;24:145–156.
31. Facklam RR, Padula JF, Wortham EC, et al.

Presumptive identification of group A, B, and D streptococci on agar plate media. J Clin Microbiol 1979;9(6):665–672.
32. Facklam RR, Thacker LG, Fox B, Eriquez L. Presumptive identification of streptococci with a new test system. J Clin Microbiol 1982;15(6):987–990.
33. Fraser G. A plate method for the rapid identification of *Listeria* (*Erysipelothrix*) *monocytogenes*. Vet Rec 1962;74:50–51.
34. Fraser G. The effect on animal erythrocytes of combinations of diffusible substances produced by bacteria. J Pathol Bacteriol 1964;88(1):43–53.
35. Fuchs PC. The replicator method for identification and biotyping of common bacterial isolates. Lab Med 1975;6(5):6–11.
36. Fuchs PC, Christy C, Jones RN. Multiple-inocula (replicator) CAMP test for presumptive identification of group B streptococci. J Clin Microbiol 1978;7(2):232–233.
37. Glenny AT, Stevens MF. Staphylococcus toxins and antitoxins. J Pathol Bacteriol 1935;40(2):201–210.
38. Goel MC, Singh IP. Purification and characterization of *Corynebacterium ovis* exotoxin. J Comp Pathology 1972;82:345–353.
39. Gorter E, Grendel F. On bimolecular layers of lipoids on the chromocytes of the blood. J Exp Med 1925;41(4):439–443.
40. Groves RD, Welshimer HJ. Separation of pathogenic from apathogenic *Listeria monocytogenes* by three in vitro reactions. J Clin Microbiol 1977;5(6):559–563.
41. Gubash SM. Synergistic hemolysis phenomenon shown by an alpha-toxin-producing *Clostridium perfringens* and streptococcal CAMP factor in presumptive streptococcal grouping. J Clin Microbiol 1978;8(5):480–488.
42. Hansen MV, Elliott LP. New presumptive identification test for *Clostridium perfringens*: Reverse CAMP test. J Clin Microbiol 1980;12(4):617–619.
43. Haque R-U, Baldwin JN. Purification and properties of staphylococcal beta-hemolysin. I. Production of beta-hemolysin. J Bacteriol 1964;88(5):1304–1309.
44. Haque R-U, Baldwin JN. Purification and properties of staphylococcal beta hemolysin. J Bacteriol 1969;100(2):751–759.
45. Harper HA, Rodwell VW, Mayes PA. Review of Physiological Chemistry, ed 16. Los Altos, CA: Lange Medical Publications, 1977:111–112, 119.
46. Harrow B, Mazur A. Textbook of Biochemistry, ed 9. Philadelphia: WB Saunders, 1966:268, 315–316.
47. Hartwigk H. Antihämolysinbildung beim Tier vorkommender α-hämolytischer Corynebakterien. Hyg Abt I Orig 1963/1964;191:274–280.
48. Hébert GA, Hancock GA. Synergistic hemolysis exhibited by species of staphylococci. J Clin Microbiol 1985;22(3):409–415.
49. Heeschen W, Tolle A, Zeidler H. Zur Klassifizierung der Gattung Streptokokkus. Zentralbl Bakteriol I Abt Orig 1967;205(1–3):250–259.
50. Herbert D, Todd EW. Purification and properties of a haemolysin produced by group A haemolytic streptococci (streptolysin O). Biochem J 1941;35(10):1124–1139.
51. Holum JR. Elements of General and Biological Chemistry, ed 4. New York: John Wiley & Sons, 1975:340–341, 351.
52. Hunter R. Observations on *Listeria monocytogenes* type 5 (Iwanow) isolated in New Zealand. Med Lab Technol 1973;30(1):51–56.
53. Jackson AW, Little RM, Mayman D. Staphylococcal toxins. IV. Factors affecting hemolysis by β-lysin. Can J Microbiol 1958;4(5):477–486.
54. Jokipii AMM, Jokipii L. Presumptive identification and antibiotic susceptibility of group B streptococci. J Clin Pathol 1976;29(8):736–739.
55. Jones D, Seeliger HPR. Designation of a new type strain for *Listeria monocytogenes*. Int J Syst Bacteriol 1983;33(2):429.
56. Kar Choudhury TK. Synergistic lysis of erythrocytes by *Propionibacterium acnes*. J Clin Microbiol 1978;8(2):238–241.
57. Khan MA, Seaman A, Woodbine M. *Listeria monocytogenes* haemolysin: Lecithinase. Acta Microbiol Acad Sci Hung 1972;19:341–352.
58. Kleck JL, Donahue JA. Production of thermostable hemolysin by cultures of *Staphylococcus epidermidis*. J Infect Dis 1968;118(3):317–323.
59. Koneman EW, Allen SD, Janda WM, et al. Color Atlas and Textbook of Diagnostic Microbiology, ed 4. Philadelphia: JB Lippincott, 1992:447, 449, 459, 548.
60. Leighton I, Threlfall DR, Oakley CL. Phospholipase C activity in culture filtrates from *Listeria monocytogenes*. In: Woodbine M, ed. Problems of Listeriosis. Leicester, England, Leicester University Press, 1975:239–241.
61. Linder R, Bernheimer AW. Effect on sphingomyelin-containing liposomes of phospholipase D from *Corynebacterium ovis* and the cytolysin from *Stoichactis helianthus*. Biochim Biophys Acta 1978;530:236–246.
62. Linder RA, Bernheimer AW, Kim K-S. Interaction between sphingomyelin and a cytolysin from the sea anemone *Stoichactis helianthus*. Biochim Biophys Acta 1977;469:290–300.
63. Lovell R, Zaki MM. Studies on growth products of *Corynebacterium ovis*. II. Other activities and their relationship. Res Vet Sci 1966;7:307–311.
64. Lütticken R, Fritsche D. Identification of group B streptococci (*Streptococcus agalactiae*) by means of the "Triple-Test" Wallerström and

the CAMP-Test. Zentralbl Bakteriol I Abt Orig 1974;226(3):298–304.
65. MacFarlane MG. The biochemistry of bacterial toxins. 5. Variation in haemolytic activity of immunologically distinct lecithinases towards erythrocytes from different species. Biochem J 1950;47:270–279.
66. MacFarlane MG, Knight BCJG. The biochemistry of bacterial toxins. I. The lecithinase activity of Cl. welchii toxins. Biochem J 1941;35(8):884–902.
67. Maheswaran SK, Lindorfer RK. Staphylococcal α-hemolysin. II. Phospholipase C activity of purified α-hemolysin. J Bacteriol 1967;94(5): 1313–1319.
68. Maheswaran SK, Smith KL, Lindorfer RK. Staphylococcal α-hemolysin. I. Purification of α-hemolysin. J Bacteriol 1967;94(2):300–305.
69. Mahler HR, Cordes EH. Biological Chemistry. New York: Harper & Row, 1966:513, 638.
70. Marks J, Vaughan ACT. Staphylococcal δ-haemolysin. J Pathol Bacteriol 1950;62(4): 597–615.
71. Munch-Petersen E, Christie R, Simmons RT. Further notes on a lytic phenomenon shown by group B streptococci. Aust J Exp Biol Med Sci 1945;23:193–195.
72. Murphy JM, Stuart OM, Reed FI. An evaluation of the CAMP test for the identification of *Streptococcus agalactiae* in routine mastitis testing. Cornell Vet 1952;42:133–147.
73. Nakazawa M, Nemoto H. Synergistic hemolysis phenomenon of *Listeria monocytogenes* and *Corynebacterium equi*. Jpn J Vet Sci 1980;42: 603–607.
74. Nelson GJ. Lipid composition of erythrocytes in various mammalian species. Biochim Biophys Acta 1967;144:221–232.
75. Nussenbaum S. Organic Chemistry. Boston: Allyn & Bacon, 1963:418–419, 551.
76. Oberhofer TR. Manual of Practical Medical Microbiology and Parasitology. New York: John Wiley & Sons, 1985:133.
77. Pastan I, Macchia V, Katzen R. A phospholipase specific for sphingomyelin from *Clostridium perfringens*. J Biol Chem 1968;243 (13):3750–3755.
78. Phillips EA, Tapsall JW, Smith DD. Rapid tube CAMP test for identification of *Streptococcus agalactiae* (Lancefield group B). J Clin Microbiol 1980;12(2):135–137.
79. Pongratz G, Seeliger HPR. Hämolysewirkungen durch *Listeria* inocula auf Schaferythrozyten. Zentralbl Bakteriol Hyg I Abt Orig Reihe A 1984;257A(3):296–307.
80. Pulverer G. Gruppendifferenzierung beta-hämolysierender Streptokokken mit Hilfe des OBF-Testes nach Guthof und des CAMP-Tests. Zentralbl Bakteriol 1967;204(2):301–304.
81. Ratner HB, Weeks LS, Stratton CW. Evaluation of spot CAMP test for identification of group B streptococci. J Clin Microbiol 1986;24(2): 296–297.
82. Rocourt J. Identification of *Listeria* isolates. Vet Med Hefte 1987;5:134–145.
83. Rocourt J, Alonso JM, Seeliger HPR. Virulence compareé des cinq groupes génomiques de *Listeria monocytogenes* (*sensu lato*). Ann Microbiol Paris 1983;134A:3359–3364.
84. Rocourt J, Grimont PAD. *Listeria welshimeri* sp. nov. and *Listeria seeligeri* sp. nov. Int J Syst Bacteriol 1983;33(4):866–869.
85. Rocourt J, Schrettenbrunner A, Seeliger HPR. Différenciation biochimique des groupes génomiques de *Listeria monocytogenes* (*sensu lato*). Ann Microbiol Paris 1983;134A:65–71.
86. Rodriguez LD, Boland JAV, Garayzabal JFF, Tranchant PE, Gomez-Lucia E, Ferri EFR, Fernandez GS. Microplate technique to determine hemolytic activity for routine typing of *Listeria* strains. J Clin Microbiol 1986;24(1):99–103.
87. Seeliger HPR. Notion actuelle sur l'épidemiologie de la listériose. Med Mal Infect 1976;6:6–14.
88. Seeliger HPR, Jones D. Genus *Listeria* Pirie 1940 383[AL]. In: Sneath PAH, Mair NS, Sharpe ME, Holt JG, eds. Bergey's Manual of Systematic Bacteriology, vol 2. Baltimore: Williams & Wilkins, 1986:1235–1245.
89. Shuman RD, Nord N, Brown RW, Wessman GE. Biochemical and serological characteristics of Lancefield groups E, P, and U streptococci and *Streptococcus uberis*. Cornell Vet 1972;62:540–567.
90. Skalka B, Smola J. Selective diagnostic medium for pathogenic *Listeria* spp. J Clin Microbiol 1983;18(6):1432–1433.
91. Skalka B, Smola J, Elischerová K. Routine test for in vitro differentiation of pathogenic and apathogenic *Listeria monocytogenes* strains. J Clin Microbiol 1982;15(3):503–507.
92. Skalka B, Smola J, Elischerová K. Different haemolytic activities of *Listeria monocytogenes* strains determined on erythrocytes of various sources and exploiting the synergism of equifactor. Zentralbl Veterinaer Med Reihe B 1982;29:642–649.
93. Skalka B, Smola J, Elischerová K. Haemolytic phenomena under the cultivation of *Listeria inocula*. Zentralbl Bakteriol Mikrobiol Hyg Abt I Orig Reihe A 1983;253A:559–565.
94. Skalka B, Smola J, Pillich J. A simple method of detecting staphylococcal hemolysins. Zentralbl Bakteriol Hyg I Abt Orig A 1979;245A(3): 283–286.
95. Skorkovský B. KCNS (RK and RM)-Bacitracin and CAMP-tests for the identification of some groups of streptococci. Zentralbl Bakteriol Hyg I Abt Orig A 1974;226(3):305–313.
96. Smith DT, Conant NF, Willett HP. Zinsser's Microbiology, ed 14. New York: Appleton-Century-Crofts, 1968:459.

97. Smyth CJ, Duncan JL. Thiol-activated (oxygen-labile) cytolysins. In: Jeljaszewicz J, Wadstrom T, eds. Bacterial Toxins and Cell Membranes. New York: Academic Press, 1978:129–183.
98. Sneath PHA, Mair NS, Sharpe ME, Holt JG, eds. Bergey's Manual of Systemic Bacteriology, vol 2. Baltimore: Williams & Wilkins, 1986: 1241–1242.
99. Souček A, Součkov A, Patocka F. Inhibition of the activity of α-toxin of *Clostridium perfringens* by toxic filtrates of corynebacteria. J Hyg Epidemiol Microbiol Immunol 1967;11:123–124.
100. Souček A, Součkov A. Toxicity of bacteria sphingomyelinases D. J Hyg Epidemiol Microbiol Immunol 1974;18:327–335.
101. Součkov A, Souček A. Inhibition of the hemolytic action of α and β lysins of *Staphylococcus pyogenes* by *Corynebacterium haemolyticum*, *C. ovis*, *C. ulcerans*. Toxicon 1972;10:501–509.
102. Součkov A, Souček A. Two distinct toxic proteins in *Corynebacterium ulcerans*. J Hyg Epidemiol Microbiol Immunol 1974;18:336–341.
103. Spiegel CA, Roberts M. *Mobiluncus* gen. nov., *Mobiluncus curtisii* subsp. *curtisii* sp. nov., *Mobiluncus curtisii* subsp. *holmesii* supsp. nov., and *Mobiluncus mulieris* sp. nov., curved rods from human vagina. Int J Syst Bacteriol 1984; 34(2):177–184.
104. Tapsall JW, Phillips EA. *Streptococcus pyogenes* streptolysin O as a cause of false positive CAMP reactions. J Clin Microbiol 1984;19(4): 534–537.
105. Turner JC. Absence of lecithin from the stroma of the red cells of certain animals (ruminants), and its relation to venom hemolysis. J Exp Med 1957;105(3):189–193.
106. Turner JC, Anderson HM, Gandal CP. Species differences in red blood cells phosphatides separated by column and paper chromatography. Biochim Biophys Acta 1958;30:130–134.
107. Vázquez-Boland JA, Domínguez L, Fernández JF, et al. Revision of the validity of CAMP tests for *Listeria* identification. Proposal of an alternative method for the determination of hemolytic activity by *Listeria* strains. Acta Microbiol Hung 1990;37:201–206.
108. Vázquez-Boland JA, Domínguez L, Fernandez-Garayzábal JF, Suárez G. *Listeria monocytogenes* CAMP reaction [Letter]. Clin Microbiol Rev 1993;5(3):343.
109. Weaver RE. Morphological, physiological, and biochemical characterization. In: Jones GL, ed. Isolation and Identification of *Listeria monocytogenes*. Atlanta, Ga, Centers for Disease Control, 1989:39–43.
110. Wilkinson HW. CAMP-disk test for presumptive identification of group B streptococci. J Clin Microbiol 1977;6(1):42–45.
111. Williams REO, Harper GJ. Staphylococcal haemolysins on sheep-blood agar with evidence for a fourth haemolysin. J Pathol Bacteriol 1974;59(2):69–78.
112. Wiseman GM. Factors affecting the sensitization of sheep erythrocytes to staphylococcal beta lysin. Can J Microbiol 1965;11(3):463–471.
113. Wiseman GM. Some characteristics of the beta-haemolysin of *Staphylococcus aureus*. J Pathol Bacteriol 1965;89(1):187–207.
114. Zamecknik PC, Brewster LE, Lipmann F. A manometric method for measuring the activity of the *C. welchii* lecithinase and a description of certain properties of this enzyme. J Exp Med 1947;85(4):381–394.
115. Zwaal RFA, Roelofsen B, Colley CM. Localization of red cell membrane constituents. Biochim Biophys Acta 1973;300:159–182.

5 Carbohydrate Fermentation Tests

I. PRINCIPLE

To determine the ability of an organism to ferment (degrade) a specific carbohydrate incorporated in a basal medium and produce acid or acid with visible gas

II. PURPOSE

(See Chapters 43–45)

A. Fermentation patterns are generally characteristic for specific bacterial groups or species; all *Enterobacteriaceae* are glucose fermenters.
B. To aid in differentiation between genera: *Proteus penneri* (xylose A (acid)) from *Providencia* spp. (xylose −)
C. Carbohydrate utilization patterns may **aid** in species differentiation.
   1. **Gram-positive organisms**
      a. *Brochothrix campestris* (rhamnose A) from *Brochothrix thermosphacta* (rhamnose −)
      b. *Butyrivibrio fibrisolvens* (sucrose A) from *Butyrivibrio crossotus* (sucrose −)
      c. *Falcivibrio grandis* (glucose, galactose, fructose, maltose, ribose all A) from *Falcivibrio vaginalis* (all −)
      d. *Listeria grayi* (mannitol A) from other *Listeria* spp. (mannitol −)
      e. *Peptostreptococcus lactolyticus* (lactose A) from the *Peptostreptococcus* spp. *P. anaerobius, P. asaccharolyticus, P. hydrogenalis, P. indolicus, P. lacrimalis, P. magnus, P. micros, P. prevotii, P. tetradis,* and *P. vaginalis* (all lactose −)
      f. *Sarcina ventriculii* (melibiose A, xylose −) from *Sarcina maxima* (melibiose − and xylose A)
      g. *Staphylococcus aureus* subsp. *aureus* (xylose A), *S. arlettae* (xylose A), and *S. xylose* (xylose A) from other *Staphylococcus* spp. (xylose −)
   2. **Gram-negative organisms**
      a. *Alcaligenes xylosondans* (xylose A) from *A. faecalis, A. latus,* and *A. piechaudii* (all xylose −)
      b. *Comamonas acidovorans* (mannitol A) from *C. terrigena* and *C. testosteroni* (mannitol −)
      c. *Flavobacterium branchiophilum* (cellobiose A) from *F. aquatile* (cellobiose −)
      d. *Haemophilus ducreyi* (glucose −) from other *Haemophilus* spp. (glucose A)
      e. *Kingella kingae* (maltose A) from *K. denitrificans* (maltose −)
      f. *Neisseria lactamica* (lactose A) from other *Neisseria* spp. (lactose −)
   3. ***Enterobacteriaceae***
      a. *Escherichia fergusonii* (adonitol A, arabitol A) from other *Escherichia* spp. (adonitol −, arabitol −)
      b. *Morganella morganii* biogroup 2 (glycerol A) from *M. morganii* biogroup 1 (glycerol −)
      c. *Pantoea agglomerans* (salicin A) from *Pantoea dispersa* (salicin −)

d. *Proteus vulgaris* (maltose A) from *Proteus mirabilis* (maltose −) (21)
e. *Proteus penneri* (xylose A) from *P. inconstans, P. myxofaciens,* and *P. rettgeri* (all xylose −)

III. BIOCHEMISTRY INVOLVED

Carbohydrates are classified as (*a*) monosaccharides, polyhydroxylic aldehydes, or ketones; (*b*) polysaccharides or oligosaccharides, condensation products of two or more monosaccharides (polymers of monosaccharides); or (*c*) polyhydric alcohols and cyclitols, reduction products of monosaccharides (7). A monosaccharide or simple sugar usually contains 1–6 carbon atoms: erythrose is a 4-carbon sugar (tetrose, $C_4H_8O_4$); ribose, ribulose, xylose, and arabinose are 5-carbon sugars (pentoses, $C_5H_{10}O_5$); and glucose (dextrose), fructose (levulose), galactose, and mannose are 6-carbon sugars (hexoses, $C_6H_{12}O_6$) (9, 12). Among the pentoses, xylose, ribose, and arabinose are aldoses, while ribulose is a ketose (24). The hexose compounds glucose, galactose, and mannose are aldoses; fructose is a ketose compound (24).

Disaccharides ($C_6H_{22}O_{11}$) are polysaccharides (oligosaccharides) composed of two monosaccharide units, glucose plus another monosaccharide.

$$\text{Sucrose} \longrightarrow \text{Glucose + fructose}$$
$$\text{Maltose} \longrightarrow \text{2 Glucose units}$$
$$\text{Lactose} \longrightarrow \text{Glucose + galactose}$$

Glycoside is a general term that denotes a disaccharide regardless of the sugar present (13). The trisaccharide raffinose ($C_{18}H_{32}O_{16}$) contains three monosaccharides: glucose, fructose, and galactose.

An example of a polysaccharide is inulin, which is composed of many polymers of the monosaccharide fructose.

The alcohols that are collectively called "sugars" (9) are adonitol, dulcitol, mannitol, and sorbitol. All are polyhydric alcohols that are reduction products of a monosaccharide (7).

$$\text{Glucose} \xrightarrow{\text{reduction}} \text{Sorbitol (hexahydroxy alcohol)}$$

Inositol is a noncarbohydrate organic substrate (9).

Polysaccharides, trisaccharides, and disaccharides are too complex to enter a bacterial cell for degradation. If they can be metabolized by a particular bacterial species they are first catabolized to less complex monosaccharides by exocellular enzymes (permeases) so that they can be taken into the cell.

Fermentation is an **anaerobic** oxidation-reduction metabolic process in which an organic substrate serves as the final hydrogen acceptor (electron acceptor) instead of oxygen (31). Fermentation of organic substrates such as carbohydrates yields both reduced and oxidized end products (31). The end products produced by carbohydrate fermentations depend on several factors: (*a*) the organism conducting the fermentation process, (*b*) the substrate being fermented, and (*c*) at times, environmental factors such as temperature and acidity (31). Carbohydrates and alcohols, collectively termed "sugars" (9), have few fermentation end products: two gases, hydrogen and carbon dioxide; a few acids; a few alcohols; and one ketone (22).

Table 5.1. Classification of Most Frequently Used Carbohydrates (9)

Monosaccharides (simple sugars)
  Tetrose (4C), $C_4H_8O_4$
    Erythrose
  Pentoses (5C), $C_5H_{10}O_5$
    Arabinose
    Deoxyribose
    Ribose
    Ribulose
    Xylose
  Methylpentose
    Rhamnose (isodulcitol)
  Hexoses (6C), $C_6H_{12}O_6$
    Galactose
    Glucose (dextrose)
    Fructose (levulose)
    Mannose
    Sorbose
Disaccharides (glycosides), $C_{12}H_{22}O_{11}$
  Amygdalin
  Cellobiose
  Lactose (glucose + galactose)
  Maltose (glucose + glucose)
  Melibiose
  Salicin
  Sucrose (saccharose) (glucose + fructose)
  Threhalose
Trisaccharides, $C_{18}H_{32}O_{16}$
  Melezitose
  Raffinose (glucose + galactose + fructose)
Polysaccharides, $(C_6H_{10}O_5)_n$
  Cellulose
  Dextrins
  Glycogen
  Inulin
  Pectins
  Starch, soluble
Alcohols
  Adonitol
  Dulcitol
  Erythritol
  Glycerol
  Mannitol
  Sorbitol
Noncarbohydrate substrate
  Inositol

Data from reference 9.

Some bacteria can ferment glucose anaerobically; others oxidize glucose. Some can metabolize by both methods, while still others cannot use glucose by either method. Not all monosaccharides are degraded by all bacterial species; their fermentation patterns differ, aiding in group, genus, or species identification. Bacteria also differ in the pathways used to ferment the same substrate (25), resulting in different end products. The manner and extent to which a substrate is dissimulated depends upon the bacterial species and cultural conditions.

The most widespread fermentation process produces the end product lactic acid; however, other fermentation pathways occur, differing in respect to the substrate metabolized or the end product produced (31). One can use carbohydrate tests to reveal the fermentation patterns of a particular bacterial species by observing (*a*) the absence of glycosides and/or (*b*) the absence of monosaccharides in more complex disaccharides, trisaccharides, and polysaccharides (9), which show that glucose was metabolized.

Bacteria that ferment a carbohydrate are usually facultative anaerobes (16). In the fermentation process, a carbohydrate is degraded and split into two trioses (16) (carbon molecules) that are further degraded to a number of 1-, 2-, 3-, and 4-carbon compounds (6). The final end products vary with each bacterial species, depending upon the enzyme system present in the species and the environmental conditions. The important criterion is that before its breakdown glucose is phosphorylated to a glucose 6-phosphate compound (6). Fermentation requires an organic compound as the terminal electron acceptor.

The main fermentative pathway of glucose degradation is the Embden-Meyerhof-Parnas (EMP) pathway, although degradation may occur via or in combination with the pentose shunt (Warburg-Dickins pathway, hexose monophosphate (HMP) shunt) or the Entner-Doudoroff (ED) pathway (6). However, all three pathways require initial phosphorylation of glucose before degradation can occur.

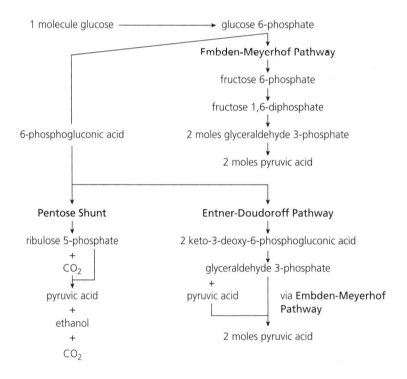

Three Phosphorylated Fermentation Pathways (5)

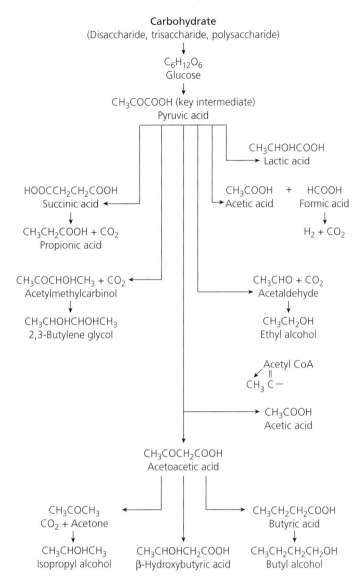

(Redrawn from Pelczar, M. J., and Reid, R. D. *Microbiology,* 2nd ed., 1965, p. 139, with permission of Mc-Graw-Hill Book Co., New York.)

Pyruvic acid ($CH_3COCOOH$) is the key intermediate in glucose degradation, and the dissimilation of pyruvic acid involves many different mechanisms that form a variety of end products characteristic of bacterial fermentations (6). Monosaccharides are catabolized as a result of oxidation to pyruvic acid through a sequence of stepwise processes mediated by specific enzymes. Bacteria may use different pathways to form pyruvic acid, and more than one pathway may occur simultaneously in the same organism (28).

The characteristic end products of bacterial fermentation are (*a*) lactic acid, (*b*) acetic and formic acids, (*c*) lactic acid and ethyl alcohol (ethanol), (*d*) ethanol, (*e*) acetylmethylcarbinol (acetoin) and CO_2, (*f*) succinic acid to propionic acid and CO_2, (*g*) CO_2 and acetone to isopropyl alcohol (isopropanol), and (*h*) butyric acid to butyl alcohol (butanol) (6, 25). Distinct classes of fermentation patterns are produced by bacteria, each dependent on characteristic end products formed. According to most authors, the most important groups of bacteria exhibit one of five main types of fermentation patterns.

Alcoholic Fermentation

$$\text{Glucose} \longrightarrow 2 \text{ ethanol} + CO_2$$

The alcoholic bacteria degrade glucose to pyruvic acid via the Embden-Meyerhof-Parnas pathway (6).

Lactic Acid Fermentation

The lactic acid bacteria may be further divided into two subgroups: homolactic and heterolactic fermenters. The homolactic acid, or simple lactic (22) acid, bacteria degrade glucose via the EMP pathway almost exclusively to lactic acid (6, 22, 25, 28), with only traces of other end products (28). The heterolactic acid fermenters are sometimes referred to as mixed lactic acid fermenters (7, 31). These organisms may catabolize glucose by one of three degradation pathways (EMP, pentose shunt, or the Entner-Doudoroff process (6)) to yield characteristic end products: lactic acid plus acetic acid and formic acids, ethanol, and CO_2 (6, 22, 25) and at times glycerol (22).

A single bacterial species may exhibit both homolactic and heterolactic acid fermentation. The controlling factors are the pH and the substrate present for bacterial activity (6).

Propionic Acid Fermentation

The chief end products from pyruvic acid are propionic acid (propionate) and CO_2 via succinic acid, although acetic acid may be produced (22, 25). Propionic fermentation is carried out by anaerobic organisms (31).

$$\text{Pyruvic acid} \begin{cases} \longrightarrow \text{acetaldehyde} \longrightarrow \text{acetic acid} \\ \longrightarrow \text{succinic acid} \longrightarrow \text{propionic acid} + CO_2 \end{cases}$$

Coliform Group Fermentations

The coliform group is often referred to as mixed-acid fermenters (28, 31), formic acid fermenters (28), or the colon-dysentery-typhoid bacteria (CDT group) (22, 25, 31). Mixed-acid fermentation is characteristic of the *Enterobacteriaceae,* and these organisms degrade glucose into a variety of end products.

The coliform group may be subdivided into two categories: (*a*) those that produce various mixed-acid products and (*b*) those that produce butylene glycol as the major end product. The type or combinations and amounts of end product produced depend on the genus or species being tested (25).

The mixed-acid organisms produce the following products: formic, acetic, lactic, and succinic acids; ethanol; and CO_2 and H_2; but **no** butylene glycol (butanediol) (6, 25, 28). Alcohol is formed by alcoholic fermentation; lactic acid, acetic acid, and CO_2 are formed by lactic fermentation through the dismutation of pyruvic acid (26). In the dismutation, one molecule of pyruvic acid is reduced to yield lactic acid, and the other molecule is oxidized, forming acetic acid and CO_2 (6). Among the *Enterobacteriaceae, Escherichia coli* exhibits this type of fermentation (6).

$$2 \text{ molecules pyruvic acid} \longrightarrow \text{acetic acid} + \text{lactic acid} + CO_2$$

The second group is composed of organisms whose major end product is butylene glycol (22, 28). Among the *Enterobacteriaceae,* the *Klebsiella-Enterobacter* groups exhibit this type of fermentation.

Butyl Alcohol (Butanol) Fermentation

Butanol fermentation is carried out by anaerobic bacteria such as *Clostridium* (6, 28). The various end products formed are acetic acid, formic acid, ethanol, butyric acid, butanol, acetone, isopropanol, and a large amount of CO_2 and H_2 (22, 25, 28, 31). The combination and amounts of end products formed depend upon the bacterial genus and species (25). Some organisms produce primarily butyric and acetic acid, CO_2 and H_2; others produce butylene glycol, acetone, butanol, and isopropanol (22). However, no lactic acid is formed.

IV. STANDARD BROTH BASE MEDIA

A. **Media**
1. With phenol red pH indicator (4, 11)
   a. **Broth**
      (1) Ingredients, pH 7.4± 0.2.

Peptone (proteose or pancreatic digest of casein)	10.0 g
Beef extract, **optional**	1.0 g
Sodium chloride, NaCl	5.0 g
Phenol red	0.018 g
Deionized water	1000.0 mL

      (2) pH indicator, phenol red
         (a) Acid: yellow color, pH 6.8
         (b) Alkaline: pinkish red color, pH 8.4
         (c) Uninoculated medium: reddish orange color; pH 7.4
      (3) Method of preparation
         (a) Weigh out amount accurately as directed on label. Various company products may differ slightly.
         (b) Rehydrate with distilled or deionized water.
         (c) Heat **gently** into solution.
   b. **With agar:** semisolid to solid phenol red broth base medium
      (1) Ingredients, pH 7.5 ± 0.2

Phenol red–carbohydrate broth medium	1000.0 mL
Agar, **semisolid only,** 4–6%	4.0–6.0 g
solid only, 15%	15.0 g

      (2) Method of preparation
         (a) Place flask containing the carbohydrate-base-agar mixture on a magnetic stirrer with a heat element.
         (b) Maintain a low temperature.
         (c) Add a magnet to the flask and keep medium in constant motion while dispensing into tubes (4.0–5.0 mL/tube).
      (3) A semisolid carbohydrate-base medium eliminates the use of Durham inserts for gas detection.
   c. **With serum**
      (1) Purpose: enrichment to promote growth of *Neisseria* spp. for fermentation studies
      (2) To 1 L of **sterile** base, **aseptically** add **sterile** 10% ascitic fluid, 10.0 g/L of base (18) (see Chapter 29, *Neisseria* Carbohydrate Utilization Tests).
2. With modified Andrade's pH indicator (1, 9).
   a. Alternate pH indicator replaces phenol red
   b. Recommended when carbohydrates are subjected to prolonged incubation; primarily used for aerobic, Gram-negative rods (e.g., the enterics).

c. Sodium hydroxide (NaOH) stock solutions.
   (1) NaOH (**10 N** or **40%**)
      (a) Ingredients

NaOH, carbonate-free, R. G. (reagent grade)	40.0 g
Distilled water	100.0 mL

      (b) Method of preparation
         1. **Rapidly** weigh out the NAOH and dissolve in less than 100 mL of distilled water in a beaker. *Caution:* this reagent is highly hygroscopic.
         2. Place beaker in a circulating cold water bath to control the temperature.
         3. Cool and transfer the NaOH solution to a 100-mL volumetric flask and bring to 100 mL with distilled water.
         4. Store in a polyethylene- or paraffin-lined glass reagent bottle and label correctly.
         5. *Caution:* sodium hydroxide is extremely caustic; avoid exposure to the skin as painful burns may occur.
   (2) NaOH (**1 N** or **4%**)
      (a) Ingredients

NaOH **10 N**	10.0 mL
Distilled water to bring to 100.0 mL	

      (b) Method of preparation: use a pipette (Pro or bulb type) to transfer 10 mL of 10 N NaOH to a 100-mL volumetric flask and bring to 100 mL with distilled water.

d. **Andrade's** indicator, 1.0% **working solution**
   (1) Ingredients, pH 7.1–7.2 ± 0.2

Acid fuchsin	0.5 g
Distilled water	100.0 mL
NaOH, 1 N	15.0–18.0 mL

   (2) Method of preparation (9)
      (a) Dissolve acid fuchsin in distilled water.
      (b) Add 15.0 mL of 1 N NaOH (4%).
      (c) Mix and let stand at room temperature (25°C) for 24 h (overnight) with frequent agitation. The red color **should** decolorize to brown. Decant supernatant to save and discard sediment (33).
         1. If decolorization is insufficient, add an additional 1.0 mL of NaOH (4%).
         2. Mix and let stand an additional 24 h.
         3. Addition of more alkali may be necessary to obtain the required **straw-yellow** color.
            a. Avoid adding excess NaOH.
            b. Add drop by drop until desired color is reached.

e. Completed medium

Broth base **without** phenol red, **sterile,** cooled (45–50°C)	1000.0 mL
Andrade's indicator solution, 1%	10.0 mL

   (1) Adjust to pH 7.1–7.2 with 1 N NaOH (9).
   (2) Add desired carbohydrate.

f. Andrade's color reactions: same as those for neutral red pH indicator (9)
   (1) Acid: pinkish-red color, pH 5.0
   (2) Alkaline: yellow to colorless, pH 12.0–14.0
   (3) Uninoculated: very slight pink color, pH 7.1–7.2

B. **Carbohydrates**
  1. Selection
     a. A variety of carbohydrates may be used depending on the difficulties encountered in identifying a particular microorganism.
     b. Generally use 8–10 sugars; those most commonly used are

adonitol	inositol	rhamnose
arabinose	inulin	sorbitol
cellobiose	lactose	sucrose
dulcitol	mannitol	trehalose
fructose (invert sugar)	melibiose	xylose
galactose	raffinose	
glucose	salicin	

     c. Add desired individual carbohydrates to aliquots of prepared broth base; final concentration
        (1) Salicin, 0.5%
        (2) All others, 1.0%
  2. Methods of addition of carbohydrates to broth base
     a. **Method 1**: add **directly** to base in desired concentration **before** sterilization
        (1) 0.5%: 5.0 g/L of base
        (2) 1.0%: 10.0 g/L of base
     b. **Method 2**: sugar solutions
        (1) Prepare a 5 or 10% concentration of desired sugar in distilled water.
        (2) Add **sterile** sugar solution to **sterile** base to give a final concentration of 0.5 or 1.0% (3); add 100 mL of a 0.5% solution or 1.0% solution to 1-L volumetric flask, bring to 1000 mL with phenol red broth base, and mix thoroughly.
     c. **Method 3**: carbohydrate differential disks are commercially available as stable, **sterile** paper disks impregnated with standardized concentrations of fermentable carbohydrates

Ad, adonitol	Mn, mannitol
Ar, arabinose	Ma, mannose
D, dextrose (glucose)	Me, melibiose
Du, dulcitol	Ra, raffinose
Ga, galactose	R(h), rhamnose
I, inositol	Sa, salicin
In, inulin	So, sorbitol
L, lactose	Su, sucrose
Le, levulose (fructose)	Tr, trehalose
M, maltose	X, xylose

        (3) Used in carbohydrate-free media: choices
           (a) Broth: phenol red broth
           (b) Semisolid: phenol red agar, tryptic agar base or cystine tryptic (Trypticase) agar (CTA)
        (4) Add disks **after** the medium has been autoclaved.
           (a) Disks are packaged in vials and are **sterile**.
           (b) Remove disks **aseptically** with **sterile** forceps (flamed in 95% ethanol); maintain sterility of vial cap and contents. A pH indicator and a specific carbohydrate may be used to determine whether a bacterium has degraded the carbohydrate to various end products by observation of a visible color change in the medium.

$$\text{pH indicator} + \text{CHO} \xrightarrow[\text{glycolysis, etc.}]{\text{bacterium}} CO_2, H_2, \text{aldehydes} + \text{color change}$$

Carbohydrate fermentation tests can be used to determine what end products have been formed but not the pathways used (22). Also, the medium contains other growth constituents that may be degraded to yield various end products similar to those produced by carbohydrate breakdown while the organism is using some of the carbon produced by carbohydrate degradation to produce new cells (22).

The pH indicator most commonly used to show carbohydrate fermentation is phenol red, since most of the end products of carbohydrate metabolism are organic acids. With phenol red the color change occurs near the original pH of the medium (pH 6.8 acid; medium pH 7.4).

The peptone in the medium is also degraded by the bacterial species and yields alkaline substances. The acid produced by the fermentation of a carbohydrate is observed by a pH change **only** when more acid is produced by carbohydrate degradation than alkaline substances by peptone degradation (9). Observation of a color change that denotes acidity is influenced by two factors: (*a*) the pH indicator used and (*b*) the buffering properties of the medium (9).

C. **Method of sterilization**
   1. Phenol red **broth** base **only**: autoclave 121°C, 15 lb, 15 min
   2. Phenol red broth base with carbohydrates added **directly**
      a. Autoclave **116–118°C, 10–12 lb,** 15 min
         (1) Certain carbohydrates can withstand autoclaving with little or no breakdown.
         (2) Autoclaving 15 min is not advisable for arabinose, lactose, maltose, salicin, sucrose, trehalose, and xylose.
      b. Autoclave 121°C, 15 lb, **3 min**
         (1) Used when time element is critical
         (2) Controls **must** be run **prior** to their use for diagnostic purposes to check for possible breakdown (see V. Quality Control Microorganisms).
   3. Broth base with Andrade's pH indicator
      a. Autoclave **115°C**, 15 lb, **20 min**
      b. Medium pink when hot; color disappears upon cooling (9)
   4. Carbohydrate solutions: membrane filtration (Millipore) with membranes 0.45-μ pore size. **Recommended method**

If **sterile** carbohydrate solutions or **sterile** disks are added to the sterilized base medium, cool sterilized broth in a 42–50°C water bath **before** adding carbohydrates.

D. **Dispense:** screw-cap tubes (13 × 100 mm)
   1. Agar (solid/semisolid): 8.0 mL/tube; cool in **upright** position
   2. Broth
      a. With carbohydrates added: 4–5 mL/tube
      b. With disks: 2.0 mL/tube
      c. To glucose tubes **only,** add inverted (bottom up, inverted position) Durham insert tubes **before** autoclaving.
      d. All media: cool before use and refrigerate for storage (4–10°C). Shelf life is approximately 6–8 weeks.
E. **Inoculation**
   1. Growth from an 18- to 24-h **pure** culture (Kligler's iron agar (KIA) or other suitable medium)
   2. **Heavy** inoculum
      a. A battery of carbohydrates may be inoculated with a single inoculum.
      b. Methods of inoculating carbohydrate broth/agar media

(1) Swab
  (a) Roll swab over the growth on KIA or other suitable culture. Swab may be first moistened with **sterile** saline or **sterile** broth if culture is grown on solid medium.
  (b) **Aseptically** roll swab against the side of each carbohydrate tube just above the liquid level.
  (c) Slant each carbohydrate tube to pick up inoculum.
  (d) Shake each tube **gently**. Do not slosh the liquid up into the cap (metal closure).
(2) Inoculating needle or loop
  (a) Roll needle or loop over the growth on a KIA or another suitable culture. Use an inoculating loop for a broth culture.
  (b) **Aseptically** dip needle or loop into each carbohydrate tube.
  (c) Shake each tube **gently**. Do not slosh the liquid up into the cap (metal closure).
(3) General, either inoculating method
  (a) A single inoculum **usually** suffices to inoculate 8–10 carbohydrate tubes.
  (b) When inoculating a battery there is no need to flame between inoculations. When using a needle or loop to inoculate a battery with a single inoculum, so little sugar is carried over from tube to tube that no tube contains a troublesome mixture of carbohydrates.
  (c) When inoculating a battery it is not necessary to actually observe an appreciable inoculum in each tube. A single heavy initial inoculum taken from a culture contains millions of bacteria, and each tube will receive enough bacteria to detect metabolism.
  (d) When testing a large battery of carbohydrates (e.g., 15–20 sugars), it may be necessary to use 2–3 separate culture inocula. In this case, always flame the needle or loop before reentering the growth culture. If using swabs, a new swab should be used for each reentry. These precautions avoid contaminating the growth culture, as it may be necessary to use it for further tests or for subculturing.
c. Carbohydrate semisolid/disk-containing media: Use a **heavy** inoculum. As the needle goes into the agar (stabbed), the disk is pushed aside and somewhat into the agar, but it stays fairly near the surface.

F. **Incubation:** aerobic or anaerobic depending on suspected microorganism(s), 35°C incubator
  1. Agar/broth with carbohydrates: 18–24 h. Incubation as long as 30 days may be needed to confirm a negative result.
  2. Semisolid agar with carbohydrate disks: read after 4–6 h and again after 18–24 h to detect any possible reversion of the initial reaction.

V. QUALITY CONTROL MICROORGANISMS

A. Glucose (dextrose)

  Positive controls (A/F):
  Escherichia coli (AG) ATCC 25922
  Klebsiella pneumoniae subsp. *pneumoniae* (AG) ATCC 13882
  Proteus vulgaris (AG) ATCC 6380
  Shigella flexneri (A) ATCC 12022
  Negative controls (−):
  Alcaligenes faecalis ATCC 8750
  Uninoculated

B. **Lactose**

Positive controls (A/F):
Escherichia coli ATCC 25922
Klebsiella pneumoniae subsp. *pneumoniae* ATCC 13883
Negative controls (−):
Proteus vulgaris ATCC 6380
Alcaligenes faecalis ATCC 8750
Uninoculated

VI. RESULTS

> See Figures 5.1 and 5.2 (Appendix 1) for colored photographic results

VII. INTERPRETATION

A. **Phenol red–carbohydrate broth medium**
  1. Positive (A/F)
     a. Acid: yellow color, pH 6.8
     b. Gas production variable
        (1) Positive for gas (G, Ⓐ)
            (a) Aerogenic: CO_2 + H_2 present
            (b) Gas bubbles present in Durham insert or medium is completely displaced by gas leaving a colorless portion in insert.
            (c) A **single** bubble in Durham insert is significant; record as gas production.
            (d) Record as acid and gas produced (AG, Ⓐ)
        (2) Negative for gas
            (a) **An**aerogenic
            (b) No gas bubbles present and medium in Durham insert remains yellow.
            (c) Record as only acid produced (A).
  2. Delayed: orange color. If unsure compare with an uninoculated tube and reincubate.
  3. Negative (−)
     a. Reddish pink color
     b. Peptones used with resultant alkalinity, pH 8.4
B. **Solid/semisolid phenol red–carbohydrate media**
  1. With carbohydrates added to medium
     a. **Positive (A/F)**
        (1) Acid: yellow color, pH 6.8
        (2) Gas production variable
            (a) Positive for gas (G, Ⓐ)
                1. Aerogenic: CO_2 + H_2 present
                2. Gas detection by a variety of means depending on the amount of gas produced.
                   a. Gas bubbles throughout medium
                   b. A slight indentation of medium away from side of the tube
                   c. Gas may lift medium from the bottom of tube, leaving a blank space. If a large amount of gas is produced, the medium may be pushed up into the tube closure or cap.
                   d. Splitting of medium
                   e. A **single** bubble in the medium is significant; record as gas production.
                   f. Record as acid and gas produced (AG, Ⓐ).

(b) Negative for gas: **an**aerogenic
  1. **No** gas bubbles and **no** splitting of medium
  2. Record as only acid produced (A).
 b. **Delayed:** orange color. If unsure compare with an uninoculated tube and reincubate.
 c. **Negative (−)**
  (1) Reddish pink color
  (2) Alkalinity, pH 8.4; use of peptones in the medium
 2. With carbohydrate disks
  a. **Bottom of the tube serves as a control.**
  b. Reactions begin near the disk, with formation of gas at surface, around disk, and/or along the line of inoculation.
  c. Motility (or its absence) may be determined simultaneously.
  d. Carbohydrate use with/without gas production: Same interpretation as semisolid medium with carbohydrates added (see above).
C. **Carbohydrate broth medium with Andrade's pH indicator** (9)
 1. **Positive (A/F)**
  a. Acid: pinkish red color, pH 5.0
  b. Gas production variable (see reactions for phenol red–carbohydrate broth medium.
 2. **Negative (−):** alkaline, yellow to colorless

VIII. ALTERNATIVE CARBOHYDRATE FERMENTATION MEDIA FOR SPECIFIC MICROORGANISMS

A. **Anaerobes; selections**
 1. **Peptone yeast (PY) broth with carbohydrates (peptone yeast fermentation media)**
  a. Medium ingredients
   (1) VPI salt solution (14); store in refrigerator (4–10°C).

Calcium chloride, anhydrous, $CaCl_2 \cdot 2H_2O$	0.2 g
Magnesium sulfate, anhydrous, $MgSO_4 \cdot 7H_2O$	0.2 g
Dipotassium phosphate, K_2HPO_4	1.0 g
Monopotassium phosphate, KH_2PO_4	1.0 g
Sodium chloride, NaCl	2.0 g
Sodium bicarbonate, $NaHCO_3$	10.0 g
Deionized water	1000.0 mL

   (2) Vitamin K–hemin solution; store in refrigerator (4–10°C) in a closed container protected from light.

Hemin, $C_{34}H_{32}O_4N_4FeCl$	0.5 g
Vitamin K_1 (phytomenadione)	0.05 g
Sodium hydroxide, NaOH	0.4 g
Ethanol, 95%	10.0 mL

   (3) Resazurin solution: 11 mg/44.0 mL deionized water (2) or one commercial resazurin tablet (Difco)/44.0 mL of water; E_h indicator (oxidation-reduction indicator). Store at room temperature (22–25°C).
    (a) Reduced state: colorless
    (b) Oxidized state: pink
   (4) Completed medium (2), pH 7.0 ± 0.2

Casein/meat peptone	20.0 g
Yeast extract	10.0 g
L-Cysteine·HCl·H_2O	0.5 g

Resazurin solution	4.0 mL
VPI salt solution	40.0 mL
Vitamin K_1–hemin solution (**optional**)	10.0 mL
Deionized water	1000.0 mL

(*Note:* Growth factors (yeast extract, vitamin K_1-hemin solution) are required by many anaerobes. Cysteine reduces and maintains a low E_h.)

  b. Carbohydrates

  (1) **5 g/L** PY broth

adonitol	erythrose	ribose
amygdalin	glycogen	trehalose
arabinose	melezitose	
dextrin	melibiose	

  (2) **10.0 g/L** PY broth

cellobiose	inulin	rhamnose
dulcitol	lactose	salicin
fructose	maltose	sorbitol
galactose	mannitol	sucrose
glucose	mannose	xylose
inositol	raffinose	

  (3) **8.0 mL/L** PY broth: glycerol

  c. Dispense: screw-cap PRAS tubes: 7.0 mL/tube (15 × 90 mm); store in refrigerator (4–10°C). Shelf life is approximately 6–8 weeks with carbohydrates.
  d. Autoclave: 121°C, 15 lb, 15 min
  e. Fermentation (A/F): pH 5.6 or less, colorless

2. **Thioglycolate (THIO) medium without indicator, without dextrose (thioglycolate fermentation medium)**
  a. Ingredients, pH 7.2 ± 0.2

Casein peptone	20.0 g
L-Cystine	0.4 g

(May substitute L-cysteine for L-cystine, same concentration.)

Sodium chloride, NaCl	2.5 g
Dipotassium phosphate, K_2HPO_4	1.5 g
Sodium thioglycolate, $HSCH_2COONa$	0.6 g
Sodium sulfite, Na_2SO_3	0.2 g
Phenol red	0.018 g
or methylene blue	0.002 g
Agar	0.5 g
Deionized water	1000.0 mL
Single carbohydrate or carbohydrate disks (as desired), 0.5–1.0%	5.0–10.0 g

Sodium thioglycolate ($HSCH_2CH-(NH_2)COOH$) and cystine ($HOOCCH(NH_2)CH_2SSCH_2CH(NH_2)COOH$) or cysteine ($HSCH_2CH_2-(NH_2)COOH$) are reducing agents. They react with and remove (tie up) molecular oxygen from the environment and prevent accumulation of peroxides (e.g., H_2O_2), which may be lethal to some microorganisms. Sulfhydryl groups (-SH) in compounds inactivate arsenic, mercury, and other heavy metal compounds and thus maintain a low redox (E_h) potential and ensure anaerobiosis (32).

Agar helps initiate anaerobic growth and growth from small inocula. It also eliminates the need for seals, as it retards dispersion of CO_2 and diffusion of O_2 and reducing substances. The low concentration reduces convection currents within the medium to enhance anaerobic condition in the **lower portion** of tubed medium.

Methylene blue is an oxidation-reduction indicator; as oxidation increases, more oxygen is absorbed than the reducing agent can remove, and the medium changes from clear to blue-green.

    b. Dispense: screw-cap tubes; 10.0 mL/tube (16 × 125 mm)
    c. Autoclave: **118–121°C, 12–15** lb, 15 min; cool in an **upright position** and tighten down caps.
    d. Storage
       (1) **Un**sealed: room temperature (22–25°C) in the dark
       (2) Sealed: refrigerator, 4–10°C
       (3) Shelf life: approximately 6 months unless more than one third of the upper fluid column becomes oxidized. *Caution:* check the upper portion of **each** tubed medium prior to inoculation. If **more** than one third of the fluid column is oxidized—indicated by a pink or blue-green color depending on the pH indicator used—**discard the tube**. If one third or less is pink or blue-green, boil it in a water bath (100°C) with cap off, **without agitation,** for 10 min to drive off absorbed oxygen. Cool to room temperature **before** use. **Do not boil** (reheat) more than once; frequent boiling results in the development of toxic products.
    e. Inoculation: direct (e.g., swab). It is **not** necessary to prereduce media before use for anaerobic cultivation (12).
    f. Incubation: 35°C, 48 h or longer
    g. Fermentation (A/F)
       (1) With phenol red: yellow color, pH 6.8
       (2) With methylene blue: reduced state, colorless
       (3) Uninoculated (either indicator): light beige

3. **Carbohydrate fermentation broth (CHO medium base)** (10, 11, 33)
    a. Basal medium, pH 7.0±0.2

Casein peptone	15.0 g
Yeast extract	7.0 g
L-Cystine	0.25 g
Sodium chloride, NaCl	2.5 g
Ascorbic acid	0.1 g
Sodium thioglycolate	0.5 g
Bromthymol blue (BTB)	0.01 g
Agar	0.75 g
Deionized water	900.0 mL

(*Note:* Yeast extract and ascorbic acid enhance growth of oxygen-sensitive and fastidious anaerobes (11). Cystine and thioglycolate reduce and maintain a low E_h.)

    b. Additives
       (1) Carbohydrates: filter-sterilized 6.0% solutions of desired carbohydrate; 100.0 mL added to sterile, cooled (50°C) basal medium; final concentration, 6%
       (2) Starch solution: 2.5%; add 100.0 mL to cooled basal medium
    c. Dispense: 7.0 mL/screw-cap tubes (15 × 90 mm or 15 × 125) (2, 10)
    d. Prereduce media in an anaerobic atmosphere (chamber) with caps loosened, and store with caps screwed down in refrigerator (4–10°C).
    e. Inoculation: stab depth of medium with bacteriological loop.

f. Incubation: anaerobically, 35°C, 48 h or longer
g. pH indicator: bromthymol blue (BTB)
    (1) Acid: yellow, pH 6.0
    (2) Alkaline: deep Prussian blue, pH 7.6
    (3) Uninoculated medium: green, pH 7.0 (neutral)
h. Fermentation (F/A): yellow

4. Quality control microorganisms for anaerobic media

   a. Glucose (dextrose) (A/F)
      Positive controls:
      Bacteroides fragilis ATCC 25285
      Clostridium perfringens ATCC 12919
      Clostridium bifermentans ATCC 638
      Escherichia coli ATCC 25922
      Negative controls:
      Bacteroides melaninogenicus ATCC 25611
      Clostridium cochlearium ATCC 17787
      Uninoculated

   b. Lactose (A/F)
      Positive controls:
      Bacteroides fragilis ATCC 25285
      Bacteroides melaninogenicus ATCC 25611
      Clostridium perfringens ATCC 12919
      Negative controls:
      Bacteroides vulgatus ATCC 8482
      Clostridium bifermentans ATCC 0638
      Uninoculated

B. **Carbohydrate fermentation broth for streptococci** (34)
   1. Purpose: to test for fermentation of fastidious *Streptococcus* spp.
   2. Basal medium, pH 7.4 ± 0.2

Beef heart infusion broth	25.0 g
Bromcresol purple (1.6% in 95% ethanol)	1.0 mL
Deionized water	900.0 mL

   3. Carbohydrates; most frequently used, especially for the oral streptococci
      a. Selection: inulin, lactose, mannitol, raffinose, sorbitol, trehalose
      b. Filter sterilized, 10.0 g/100.0 mL deionized water added to basal medium; final concentration, 1.0%
   4. pH indicator: bromcresol purple
      a. Acid: yellow, pH 5.2
      b. Alkaline: purple, pH 6.8
      c. Uninoculated medium: deep purple, pH 7.4
   5. Dispense: 3.0 mL/screw-cap tubes (13 × 100 mm)
   6. Autoclave: 121°C, 15 lb, 10 min
   7. Quality control microorganisms
      a. *Streptococcus mutans* ATCC 25175: positive (A;) for all six sugars listed in IV.B.3.a above.
      b. *Streptococcus sanguis* ATCC 10556: inulin V (variable), lactose +, mannitol −, raffinose V, sorbitol −, trehalose V
   8. Incubation: 35°C, up to 7 days
   9. Fermentation (A/F): acid, yellow

Medium contains the large amounts of protein required by streptococci for optimal growth. Streptococci **do not** produce significant quantities of alkaline by-products from protein degradation, and acid neutralization does not occur; however, do not use with Gram-negative bacteria.

C. **Carbohydrate fermentation medium for staphylococci and Gram-negative enterics**
   1. Purple broth base (PBB); pH 6.8 (2, 16, 19)

Pancreatic digest of gelatin, USP	10.0 g
Sodium chloride, NaCl	5.0 g
Bromcresol purple	0.02 g
Deionized water	1000.0 mL

   2. Carbohydrates, filter sterilized, added to basal medium to a final concentration of 1.0%, or carbohydrate disks
   3. pH indicator: bromcresol purple (see VIII.B.4)
   4. Dispense: 15–20 mL/plate (Petri dish) (100 × 20 mm)
   5. Inoculation
      a. Divide plate into four quadrants.
      b. **Light** inocula; with inoculating needle make **two** 0.5- to 1.0-cm streaks on one quadrant, two streaks per single isolate to be tested.
   6. Quality control: glucose fermentation (A/F)

Escherichia coli	ATCC 25922 AG
Staphylococcus aureus subsp. *aureus*	ATCC 25923 A
Neisseria meningitidis	ATCC 13090 A

   7. Incubation: aerobically (**no** CO_2), 35°C, 24–72 h (may require up to 7 days)
      a. Strong acid reaction may be detected as early as 12–24 h (2)
      b. Moderate acid production usually within 48–72 h (20)
   8. Interpretation: color change from purple to yellow surrounding bacterial colonies (growth) (2)
      a. Positive (A/F): moderate to strong acid-yellow color extends out from culture streaks into surrounding medium within 72 h.
      b. Weak (±): distinct yellow color under streak but **not** extending within 72 h
      c. Negative (−): **no** acid production or very faint yellow color under streak

IX. PRECAUTIONS

A. **General**
   1. Carbohydrates are collectively termed "sugars." However, many are actually polyhydric alcohols (9). The name of a true sugar usually ends with "ose," while alcohols end with "ol"; thus lact**ose** and malt**ose** are examples of sugars, and ducit**ol** and mannit**ol** are alcohols. A few exceptions exist such as the sugar salicin (a glycoside).
   2. The concentration of carbohydrates incorporated into phenol red broth base is usually 1.0%, with the exception of salicin (0.5%). One may use 0.5% concentrations for **all** carbohydrates; however, 1.0% concentrations are recommended since they reduce the possibility of reversion (9).
   3. Orr and Taylor (23) concluded that some types of peptone are unsuitable for the preparation of carbohydrate medium. In their studies, *S. flexneri* type 6, Newcastle, and Manchester biotypes **failed** to produce both acid and gas in certain batches of peptone (23). The basic constituent is casein peptone, which **must** be free of any carbohydrates that may be fermented (26). If commercially prepared dehydrated medium is not available, controls should be run on batches of peptone to determine their suitability for carbohydrate medium made from scratch.

4. Cook and Knox (8) recommend that carbohydrate medium be free of nitrate, which may interfere with gas production.
5. Herrmann (13) recommends avoiding the addition of yeast extract, serum, or ascitic fluid to carbohydrate medium. However, addition of ascitic fluid is recommended to determine the fermentation profile of *Neisseria* spp. (3). The addition of yeast extract is optional; Difco incorporates it and BBL does not, yet both media give identical results.
6. Carbohydrate medium, when hot or upon removal from the autoclave, has a light orange color. This changes to orange-red upon cooling.
7. Caution must be used when interpreting carbohydrate tests, as the color denoting fermentation varies with the pH indicator used in the medium (Table 5.2).

Table 5.2. pH Indicators for Carbohydrate Media

pH Indicator	Acid (Fermentation)	Alkaline (Negative)
Andrade's	Pinkish red	Yellow, colorless
Bromcresol purple (BCP)	Yellow	Purple
Bromthymol blue (BTB)	Yellow	Deep Prussian blue
Phenol red	Yellow	Pinkish red

8. Incorporation of some carbohydrates into the base medium may result in an acid condition. If this occurs, add 0.1 N NaOH drop by drop until the desired orange-red color is obtained (10). Avoid adding excess NaOH and obtaining a deep red color (10); such media may be too alkaline for true fermentation within the usual incubation period.
9. When testing a large battery of carbohydrates (e.g., 15–20 sugars), it may be necessary to use 2–3 separate culture inocula. In this case, always flame the needle or loop before reentering the growth culture. If a swab is used, a new one is needed for each reentry of a growth culture. These precautions avoid any possibility of contaminating the growth culture, which may be needed for further tests or for subculturing.
10. All carbohydrates **must** be properly labeled **immediately** after preparation. **All** carbohydrates look alike, and they should be set up in a rack in a certain order, depending upon the laboratory's worksheet. A microbiologist usually does not label each carbohydrate but follows a certain order **consistently** in a bacteriology laboratory. However, if one is in doubt about the order, label each carbohydrate tube used **as it is set in the rack**. If the identity of a particular sugar is not certain when you are reading results, **repeat** the test.
11. Carbohydrate fermentations are often recorded as positive (+) or negative (−). Acidity is preferred to record fermentation, denoted by an A. A ± usually means a delayed reaction (orange color) and should be reincubated. If visible gas is also observed, fermentation is recorded as AG or Ⓐ; Ⓐ to denote both acidity and gas production. Fermentation may also be denoted by the letter F.
12. Carbohydrate medium is slightly alkaline (pH 7.4). Some carbohydrates are degraded into simpler sugars when subjected to heat at an alkaline pH (3). Glucose in the presence of phosphates is gradually destroyed by autoclaving (29). Autoclaving at 15-lb pressure hydrolyzes maltose and glucose, and gradual destruction of glucose produces acidity (29). McDade and Weaver (21) recommend using a phosphate-reduced medium (0.08% KH_2PO_4) with phenol red pH indicator at a concentration of 0.0072%, which gives a pH of 7.5–7.6. They recommend using these concentrations to test the *Enterobacteriaceae*, a richer medium to test *Streptococcus* spp., and one lacking a buffer (at a low pH, 7.3) for *Neisseria* spp.
13. Visible acidity (fermentation) is reached at different pH readings depending on the pH

indicator used. Bromthymol blue (BTB) exhibits acid production when the pH falls to 6.0 or below, while bromcresol purple (BCP) does not change color until the pH falls to about 5.0 (9). Andrade's indicator is pink at about pH 5.5 (9).

14. Many anaerobes decolorize indicators; to avoid this possibility indicator may be added **after** completion of incubation (9).
15. Gas production may be from protein degradation and thus **not** indicate carbohydrate use (9).
16. Acids produced by nonfermenters are considerably weaker than the mixed acids derived from fermentative bacteria; thus the pH of fermentation media in which a nonfermenter is growing may not become low enough to convert the pH indicator (19). The initial clue is a lack of acid produced in either KIA or triple sugar iron (TSI) agar with an alkaline (red)/alkaline (red) butt (deep) (19).
17. Microbiologists who use prepackaged commercial kits and bypass inoculation of the unknown to KIA or TSI may not know whether to select a fermentative or oxidative system (19). It is recommended that the oxidation/fermentation of all unknown isolates of Gram-negative bacilli be assessed by inoculation to KIA or TSI (19).

B. **Broth medium:** When using a carbohydrate broth medium, a Durham insert is usually placed in an **inverted** position **only** in the glucose tube. If an organism is capable of producing gas in glucose, gas will also be produced in all other carbohydrates used. However, if the organism tested is known not to ferment glucose, it is advisable to add Durham inserts to a few other carbohydrates being tested in the battery. All *Enterobacteriaceae* are glucose fermenters by definition; thus only glucose need be tested for gas production by use of a Durham insert.

Often a microbiologist, especially when working with a member of the *Enterobacteriaceae,* observes no gas production in KIA or TSI. This does not always mean the organism does not produce gas. Always test for gas production when using carbohydrates. Any sign of gas, even a single small bubble, is evidence of gas production. Often so much gas is produced that the medium in the Durham insert is completely replaced by gas, giving it an empty appearance.

Before carbohydrates are autoclaved, place a Durham insert in the glucose and/or other carbohydrate tubes in an **inverted** position. **Do not** attempt to get medium into the Durham insert; usually the tube floats on top of the medium; however, on autoclaving, the medium will be forced up into the inverted Durham insert. If a Durham insert is not inverted, gas production **cannot** be determined.

C. **Semisolid medium**
1. When using semisolid carbohydrate medium, stab the medium with an inoculating needle in the center of the tube to within 1/4 inch from the bottom of the tube. Stab gently and **do not** use an inoculating loop. Rough stabbing or using a loop may mechanically split the medium and give a false appearance of gas production.
2. No Durham insert is required with semisolid carbohydrate medium because gas production is denoted by splitting of the medium, the presence of gas bubbles, or separation of the medium from the sides or bottom of the tube. If a large amount of gas is produced (e.g., as seen with the *Klebsiella-Enterobacter* groups), the medium may be completely blown up into the cap (closure) of the tube. If this occurs, handle the culture cautiously when subculturing to avoid self-contamination or contamination of the culture.
3. After autoclaving, semisolid carbohydrate medium **must** be cooled in an upright position.

D. **With Andrade's pH indicator**
1. Immediately after autoclaving, hot medium is pink; the color disappears upon cooling (9).
2. Media with Andrade's indicator is sterilized at 115°C for 20 min (9).

3. Medium **not** nutritionally rich; is **not** suitable for testing fastidious aerobic bacteria (e.g., streptococci); it is used for enterics.
4. The amount of NaOH used depends on the dye content of different lots of acid fuchsin (33).
5. Andrade's indicator improves somewhat with aging and should be prepared 6 months ahead of anticipated use (33).

E. **With serum: unheated** serum contains an enzyme capable of hydrolyzing maltose to glucose. When using serum to enrich a maltose medium, the serum should be heated for 1 h at 60°C to inactivate the enzyme **before** it is added to the medium.

F. **Streptococci fermentation medium: do not** use for fermentation studies of Gram-negative bacteria and others that produce alkaline products from protein degradation. These products neutralize acid production and mask positive results (false-negative result).

G. **Staphylococci fermentation medium: do not** incubate under CO_2.

H. **Thioglycolate medium**
1. **Do not** heat tubes more than once to drive off absorbed oxygen; frequent boiling results in the development of toxic products. However, it is recommended that **all THIO** media be boiled once prior to its use to enhance the recovery rate.
2. **Do not** shake tubes or invert tubes when boiling.
3. Bring media to room temperature (20–25°C) **prior** to inoculation.
4. Store all media in the dark; light has a deteriorating effect on resazurin indicator.
5. Fluid THIO (Brewer) (5) **should not** be used for fermentation tests because it contains much yeast extract, which is high in carbohydrate.

I. **PY broth with carbohydrates**
1. The pH of arabinose, ribose, and xylose may decrease during incubation, even when carbohydrate is **not** fermented. Therefore, an adjustment **must** be made in interpreting results; report acid as a pH below 5.7 (27).
2. **Do not** use media if it is pink. The E_h indicator is pink in the oxidized state; oxygen has entered tube(s).

REFERENCES

1. Andrade E. Influence of glycerin in differentiating certain bacteria. J Med Res 1906;14:551–556.
2. Balows A, Hausler WJ Jr, Herrmann KL, et al. Manual of Clinical Microbiology, ed 5. Washington, DC: American Society for Microbiology, 1991:232, 1234–1235, 1246–1247.
3. Baron EJ, Finegold SM. Bailey and Scott's Diagnostic Microbiology, ed 8. St Louis: CV Mosby, 1990:A5–A6.
4. BBL. BBL Quality Control and Product Information Manual for Tubed Media. Cockeysville, MD: BBL Microbiology Systems, 1987, T21890, Rev 0.0.
5. Brewer JH. Clear liquid mediums for the "aerobic" cultivation of anaerobes. JAMA 1940;115(8):598–600.
6. Burrows W, Lewert RM, Rippon JW. Textbook of Microbiology. The Pathogenic Microorganisms, ed 19. Philadelphia: WB Saunders, 1968:118–121, 135–138.
7. Cantarow A, Schepartz B. Biochemistry, ed 3. Philadelphia: WB Saunders, 1962:1.
8. Cook GT, Knox R. Some effects of nitrates in bacteriological media. J Clin Pathol 1950;3(4):356–358.
9. Cowan ST. Cowan & Steel's Manual for the Identification of Medical Bacteria, ed 2. Cambridge: Cambridge University Press, 1974:11–12, 30–32, 137, 146.
10. Coykendall AL. Classification and identification of the viridans streptococci. Clin Microbiol Rev 1989;2:315–328.
11. Dowell VR Jr, Lombard GL, Thompson FS, Armfield AY. Media for Isolation, Characterization, and Identification of Obligately Anaerobic Bacteria, USDHEW. Atlanta, GA: Centers for Disease Control, 1977:22.
12. Harrow B, Mazur A. Textbook of Biochemistry, ed 9. Philadelphia: WB Saunders, 1966:199–201, 211.
13. Herrmann W. Beitroge zur frageder Vergarung von saccharose und laktose durch erreger der typhus-paratyphus-enteritis-gruppe. Zentralbl Bakteriol Hyg I Abt Orig 1944;151(7):427–435.
14. Holdeman LV, Cato EP, Moore WEC, eds. Anaerobic Laboratory Manual, ed 4. Blacksburg, VA: Virginia Polytechnic Institute Anaerobic Laboratory, 1977.
15. Holman WL. Value of a cooked meat medium for routine and special bacteriology. J Bacteriol 1919;4(2):149–155.

16. Hugh R, Leifson E. The taxonomic significance of fermentative versus oxidative metabolism of carbohydrates by various gram negative bacteria. J Bacteriol 1953;66(1):24–26.
17. Juhlin I. A new fermentation medium for *N. gonorrhoeae*. HAP medium. Influence of different constituents on growth and indicator colour. Acta Pathol Microbiol Scand 1963;58(1):51–71.
18. Kloos WE, Tornabene TG, Schleifer KH. Isolation and characterization of micrococci from human skin, including two new species: *Micrococcus lylae* and *Micrococcus kristinae*. Int J Syst Bacteriol 1974;24(1):79–101.
19. Koneman EW, Allen SD, Janda WM, et al. Color Atlas and Textbook of Diagnostic Microbiology, ed 4. Philadelphia: JB Lippincott, 1994:114, 194.
20. Krieg NR, Holt JG, eds. Bergey's Manual of Systemic Bacteriology, vol 1. Baltimore: Williams & Wilkins, 1984:493, 495.
21. McDade JJ, Weaver RH. Rapid methods for the detection of carbohydrate fermentation. J Bacteriol 1959;77(1):65–69.
22. Oginsky EL, Umbreit WW. An Introduction to Bacterial Physiology, ed 2. San Francisco: WH Freeman, 1959:236.
23. Orr JO, Ewing J, Taylor J. Variations in the fermentative reactions of antigenically identical strains of Bact. newcastle. Mon Bull Emerg Public Health Lab Serv 1945;4:130–133.
24. Oser BL, ed. Hawk's Physiological Chemistry, ed 14. New York: McGraw-Hill, 1965:60–61.
25. Pelczar MJ Jr, Reid RD. Microbiology, ed 2. New York: McGraw-Hill, 1965:139–141.
26. Powers DA, McCuen PJ, eds. Manual of BBL Products and Laboratory Procedures, ed 6. Cockeysville, MD: BBL Microbiology Systems, 1988:220.
27. Scott TJ. Microbiological Media, A Manual of Products and Procedures. Fiskeville, RI: Scott Laboratories, 1981:616.
28. Smith DT, Conant NF, Willett HP. Zinsser's Microbiology, ed 14. New York: Appleton-Century-Crofts, 1968:112–113.
29. Smith ML. CLXXIII. The effect of heat on sugar solutions used for culture media. Biochem J 1932;26:1467–1472.
30. Sneath PHA, Mair NS, Sharpe ME, Holt JG, eds. Bergey's Manual of Systemic Bacteriology, vol 2. Baltimore: Williams & Wilkins, 1986:1049.
31. Stanier RY, Doudoroff M, Adelberg EA. The Microbial World, ed 2. Englewood Cliffs, NJ: Prentice-Hall, 1963:252, 259, 262–263.
32. The Merck Index, ed 7. Rahway, NJ: Merck and Company, 1960:161, 762.
33. Washington JA. Laboratory Procedures in Clinical Microbiology, ed 2. New York: Springer-Verlag, 1985:774, 801–802.

6 Catalase-Peroxidase Tests

I. PRINCIPLE

To test for the presence of the enzymes catalase and/or peroxidase

II. PURPOSE

(Also see Chapters 43–45)
A. **Catalase test; 3% H_2O_2**
   1. Primarily used to differentiate between genera
      a. *Streptococcus* (−) from *Micrococcus* (+) and/or *Staphylococcus* (V+)
      b. *Bacillus* (+) from *Clostridium* (V−)
      c. *Listeria monocytogenes* (+), *Kurthia* spp. (+), *Corynebacterium* (+) from from other microorganisms that may be similar morphologically: *Erysipelothrix* (−), *Lactobacillus* spp. (V−), *Enterococcus* spp. (−), and group B *Streptococcus* (−) (51). Old *Corynebacterium pyogenes* (catalase −) is now reclassified in the genus *Arcanobacterium* as *A. pyogenes* (82).
      d. *Kingella denitrificans* (−), *Neisseria elongata* subsp. *elongate* (−), and *N. elongata* subsp. *nitroreducens* (−) from other *Neisseria* spp. (+) and *Moraxella catarrhalis* (+) (formerly *Branhamella catarrhalis*) (51)
      e. *Xenorhabdus* spp. (−) from other *Enterobacteriaceae*
   2. To aid in species differentiation
      a. **Gram-positive organisms**
         (1) *Aerococcus urinae* (+) from *Aerococcus viridans* (−)
         (2) Aerotolerant *Clostridium histolyticum*, *C. carnis*, and *C. tertium* (all −) from aerobic bacilli (e.g., lactobacilli)
         (3) *Pediococcus acidilactici* (+) and *P. pentosaceus* (+) from other *Pediococcus* spp. (−)
         (4) *Staphylococcus aureus* subsp. *anaerobius* (−; usually only grows anaerobically) and *S. saccharolytica* (−) from other *Staphylococcus* spp. (+)
      b. **Gram-negative organisms**
         (1) *Campylobacter fetus*, *C. hyointestinalis*, *C. jejuni*, and *C. coli* (all +) from *C. spurorum*, *C. concisus*, and *C. mucosalis* (all −) (53)
         (2) *N. elongata* subsp. *elongata* (−) *N. elongata* subsp. *nitroreducens* (−), and *N. mucosa* (−) from other *Neisseria* spp. including *N. elongata* subsp. *glycolytica* (+) (53)
         (3) *Moraxella bovis* (variable) and *Kingella* spp. (−) from other *Moraxella* spp. (+)
         (4) *Prevotella ovlora* (+) from other frequently isolated *Prevotella* spp. (−)
B. **Superoxol (30% catalase) test**: screening test that tentatively differentiates *Neisseria gonorrhoeae* (+) from *N. meningitidis* and *Neisseria lactamica* (both − or weak and delayed +) cultivated on Thayer-Martin (TM) growth agar (76)
C. **Catalase/peroxidase tests**
   1. To differentiate known strains of *Legionella pneumophila* (catalase −, peroxidase +) from other *Legionella* spp. (catalase +, peroxidase −) (71, 72)

2. To differentiate pathogenic *Leptospira interrogans* (catalase strongly + peroxidase weakly − or −) from nonpathogenic *Leptospira biflexa* (catalase weakly + or −, peroxidase strongly +) (15)

III. BIOCHEMISTRY INVOLVED

General

When reduced flavoproteins or reduced iron-sulfur proteins unite with oxygen and oxidases present in the respiratory chain of all bacteria, two toxic compounds are formed: hydrogen peroxide (H_2O_2) and the superoxide radical O_2^- (32).

$$FADH_2 \rightleftharpoons FAD + 2H^+ + 2\bar{e}$$
Flavoprotein — Reduced flavoprotein

$$O_2 + 2\bar{e} + 2H^+ \xrightarrow{oxidase} H_2O_2 \quad (33)$$

or

$$FADH_2 \rightleftharpoons FAD + 2H + 2\bar{e}$$
Flavoprotein — Reduced flavoprotein

$$2O_2 + 2\bar{e} + 2H^+ \xrightarrow{oxidase} 2O_2^- + 2H^+ \quad (33)$$

H_2O_2 is an oxidative end product of the aerobic breakdown of sugars. Reduced flavoprotein reacts directly with gaseous oxygen via electron reduction to form H_2O_2 (34, 67), **not** by direct action between hydrogen and molecular oxygen (34). Catalases, peroxidases, and superoxide dismutase (SOD) catalytically scavenge intermediates of oxygen-reduction (28). SOD catalytically scavenges the superoxide anion (O_2^-); catalase, H_2O_2 (79). Both enzymes are essential to the biologic defense against oxygen toxicity (79).

Catalases: $$2H_2O_2 \xrightarrow{catalase} 2H_2O + O_2 \uparrow \quad (28, 48)$$

Peroxidases: $$H_2O_2 + RH_2 \xrightarrow{peroxidases^*} 2H_2O + R \quad (28)$$

Superoxide dismutase: $$O_2^- + O_2^- + 2H^+ \xrightarrow{SOD} H_2O_2 + O_2 \uparrow \quad (28, 74)$$
$$\downarrow catalase$$
$$H_2O + O_2 \uparrow$$

* Variety of reductants available to cell.

Catalase and SOD are present in most cytochrome-containing aerobic and facultatively anaerobic (aerotolerant) respiring bacteria (20, 27, 31, 34); the **main exceptions** are *Streptococcus* spp., which lack catalase. Obligate (strict) anaerobes **lack both enzymes; most** anaerobic bacteria (e.g., *Clostridium* spp.) possess peroxidase in lieu of catalase.

There are catalases that are heme proteins (74), and others are found in microorganisms incapable of heme synthesis; they may be flavoproteins (46). There are heme-containing peroxidases (77) that can use a wide variety of electron donors to reduce H_2O_2 (e.g., two bacterial peroxidases, a ferrocytochrome c peroxidase (a heme protein as is found in *Pseudomonas fluorescens*

(57)) and a reduced nicotinamide adenine dinucleotide (NADH) peroxidase, a flavoprotein (as is found in *Enterococcus faecalis* (formerly *Streptococcus faecalis*) (21)).

The principal enzymes that reduce O_2 to O_2^- and/or H_2O_2 are flavoprotein oxidases (7). Flavoprotein NADH oxidases account for most O_2 uptake and H_2O_2 production by streptococci, lactobacilli, and other bacteria that lack cytochromes (22, 83, 84). These bacteria contain both NADH oxidases that can produce O_2^- and H_2O_2 or H_2 and NADH peroxidases that can reduce H_2O_2 to H_2 (73).

$$NADH + H^+ + H_2O_2 \xrightarrow[\text{peroxidase}]{\text{NADH}} NAD^+ + 2H_2O$$

Reduction of cytochrome c can also eliminate O_2^-.

$$O_2^- + \text{Cyto-c}(Fe^{3+}) \longrightarrow O_2 + \text{Cyto-c}(Fe^{2+})$$
(73)

Many lactic acid bacteria are aerotolerant and contain SOD but **lack** true catalase. However, peroxidases are present that oxidize organic compounds (e.g., alcohol, aldehydes) **or** NADH with H_2O_2 (31). According to Molland (63), many anaerobes also contain catalase. In some bacteria catalase is an inducible enzyme that is synthesized in response to O_2, H_2O_2, or some other substance formed when H_2O_2 is present (40). According to Pruitt and Tenovuo (73) the term *catalase* should be reserved for enzymes that yield 0.5 mol O_2 per mol H_2O_2 and preferably for a hemoprotein enzyme having the specific properties of catalase.

Burrows et al. (8) report evidence that some bacteria may possess a non-iron-containing catalase enzyme. Studies by Dacre (17) show a strong and weak catalase activity among lactobacilli. Whittenbury (90) detected two types of catalase among the lactic acid bacteria: (*a*) the classical catalase that decomposes hydrogen peroxide and is insensitive to acid conditions and (*b*) a pseudocatalase that lacks the heme prosthetic group and is sensitive to acid pH. Whittenbury (90) suggests that the lactic acid bacteria may possess a rudimentary respiratory system whereby, when provided a source of iron porphyrins, some organisms may produce a heme protein. Johnston and Delwiche (46) also demonstrated both types of catalase among the lactic acid organisms.

Catalase/Peroxidase

Both catalases and peroxidases are considered "hydroperoxidases" (9). Peroxidases are plant enzymes but are also found in milk and leukocytes; catalases (hydrogen-peroxide: hydrogen-peroxide oxidoreductases, EC 1.11.1.6) are present in animals and plants (37). The active center of catalase is a class of heme proteins called cytochromes. The heme of catalase is a high-spin porphyrin iron complex of protoporphyrin IX (10). Protoporphyrin is alternative nomenclature for catalase heme group; defines its chemical properties (28) (Fig. 6.1).

Protoporphyrin IX
I II III IV = pyrroles

A cytochrome consists of one or more heme prosthetic groups bound by an apoprotein heme composed of porphyrin (four pyrrole rings joined by =CH- bridges) plus a central iron atom that on reduction accepts a single electron (e.g., $Fe^{3+} \leftrightarrow Fe^{2+}$). Iron generally forms an octahedral coordination complex with six ligands; four of these are N atoms of the pyrroles that hold the iron within the plane of the porphyrin ring and the other two are suitable atoms in adjacent amino acid residues (e.g., histidyl-N, methionyl-S) (47). Meso carbon atoms are methinyl carbons (four) that link pyrrole rings; each methinyl or meso carbon bears a hydrogen atom (10). It is a tetramer with each protein unit containing an iron (III) porphyrin; **only one** of these reacts in the catalytic process (10). The four iron atoms in the heme protein are in the oxidized state (Fe^{3+}). In catalases, the heme group itself is the organic radical (1); in cytochrome c peroxidase and other peroxidases, the radical is situated on an amino acid side chain or a sulfur atom (43).

Catalytic Reaction

H_2O_2, if allowed to accumulate, is toxic to bacteria and results in their death. Catalase either decomposes H_2O_2 or oxidizes secondary substrates (9, 26, 81), but it has no action against other peroxides (26). H_2O_2 is decomposed via the action of two enzymes: (*a*) catalase (hydrogen peroxide oxidoreductase) and (*b*) either a peroxidase, NADH, reduced nicotinamide adenine dinucleotide phosphate (NADPH), cytochrome c, or glutathione (20). Catalytic decomposition of H_2O_2 involves reduction of trivalent iron (Fe^{3+}) in catalase by H_2O_2 to its reduced form (Fe^{2+}) and reoxidation of the latter by oxygen (87). Catalase can function in two distinct modes: in catabolism of H_2O_2 (**catalytic reaction**) or **peroxidative oxidation** of small substrates such as ethyl alcohol (ethanol), methyl alcohol (methanol), or elementary mercury ($Hg°$) (80).

Catalytic / Peroxidatic Reactions: (10, 11, 27, 33, 48, 49, 50, 52, 79, 80)

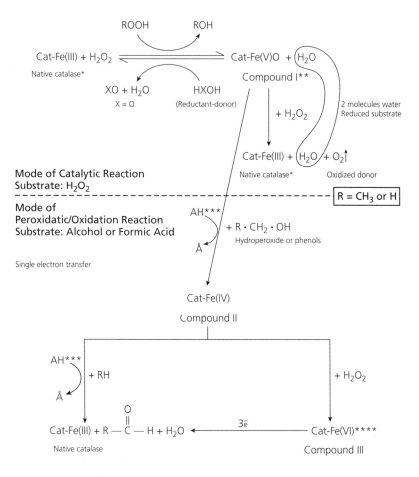

*   Ferricatalase – oxidation state of Fe – neutral pH
** Unstable – common intermediate in reduction of peroxides
*** Electron donor – reductant
**** Tetraperoxide derivative – ferryl state (fero-oxy state) (52)

Dominant pathways exist between ferricatalase and compound I (27, 64). H_2O_2, a powerful oxidizing agent, is a stable molecule that can accumulate in high concentration (73). Catalase catalyzes the dismutation of H_2O_2 (78) from a reduced state to an oxidized state, compound I, and back to a reduced state, native catalase. The compound I structure is **not** an enzyme-substrate (E • S) complex of peroxidase and H_2O_2 (73). Catalase compound I **must** transfer two electrons in a single step, and the iron of native catalase **cannot** be reduced by ordinary reducing agents (80). Compound I is a common intermediate in reduction of peroxides (27); rates are pH independent. The optimal pH for catalase activity is 7.0 (27, 38).

Peroxidative Reaction—Mode of Catalase Action

Compounds I, II, and III are enzyme peroxide derivatives. Neither II nor III occurs in the catalytic reaction; they are **in**active (10). Peroxidases generally differ from catalases in that no organic substrate will convert compound I **directly** to native enzyme (10). Compound I radical is more reactive than compound II (10). Catalase can be **in**activated by a high concentration of substrate, presumably by conversion to a tetraperoxide derivative (10), compound III. Compound III is **non**reactive to most reductants (10).

Catalase compound I can react with a limited number of hydrogen donors such as ethanol or methanol and oxidize them by using the oxygen from a single H_2O_2 molecule in a two-electron oxidation step (80). Oxidation occurs with two distinct one-electron transfers: reduction of compound I to compound II and oxidation of AH_2 to AH (the reduced and oxidized forms of suitable electron (e^-) donors) (73).

A wide variety of organic compounds can serve as AH_2 (73). Besides H_2O_2, substrates for catalase include several alcohols (e.g., ethanol), hydrated formaldehyde ($H_2C(OH)_2$), nitrous acid (HNO_2), and formic acid (HCOOH) (9, 34). Also, nonspecific substrates such as aromatic amines, phenols, and aromatic acids may be used (34). Catalase can use H_2O_2 to oxidize methyl (CH_3OH) and ethyl (C_2H_5OH) alcohols to their corresponding aldehydes (67).

Superoxide Radical (O_2^-)

A compound more toxic than H_2O_2 is produced from oxygen in biologic systems, the superoxide radical, written as either $O_2^-\cdot$ or O_2^-. It is formed by univalent reduction of oxygen with reduced flavins, quinones, or other electron carriers (31); transfer of one electron ($\bar{e}$) from a reduced substance to O_2 is a normal biologic reduction of molecular oxygen (28).

$$\bar{e} + O_2 \longrightarrow O_2^-$$

The anion O_2^- is stable in a strong base, but spontaneous dismutation is rapid at biologically relevant pH (73). The anion can act as an oxidizing agent or a reducing agent and serves as both in the dismutation reaction (73).

Superoxide dismutase (SOD) (superoxide:superoxide oxidoreductase, EC 1.15.1.1.) rapidly converts the free radical form of oxygen, superoxide anion (O_2^-), into molecular oxygen and H_2O_2 (65). SOD protects microorganisms from the deleterious actions of the O_2^- radical by catalyzing its dismutation to H_2O_2 and O_2 (28).

$$O_2^- + O_2^- + 2H^+ \xrightarrow{\text{SOD}} H_2O_2 + O_2$$

Escherichia coli and **all** aerobic and aerotolerant microorganisms contain the enzyme SOD, which converts O_2^- to H_2O_2 and O_2. Obligate anaerobes **do not** contain SOD (28). Synergistic interactions exist between catalase and SOD; in any reaction mixture generating both O_2^- and H_2O_2, the effectiveness of catalase is enhanced by SOD, which prevents conversion of active catalase into relatively **in**active compounds II and III (52). Hydrogen peroxide is formed whenever reduced flavoproteins or reduced iron-sulfur proteins come together with oxygen and oxidases that are present in **all** microorganisms (31).

Superoxide **inhibits** catalase in two distinct ways (52): (*a*) a rapid inhibition that can be prevented and reversed by SOD or (*b*) slow inhibition that can be prevented but **not reversed** by SOD and can be both prevented and reversed by ethanol (52), a two-step reaction. There are three distinct types of SOD that all catalyze the same reaction (28): FeSOD contains iron, MnSOD contains manganese, and Cu/ZnSOD contains both copper and zinc.

Only iron (Fe)-protein SOD and mangano-(Mn)-protein SOD are found in bacteria. Gram-negative bacteria (e.g., *E. coli*) contain both FeSOD and MnSOD (31, 46). Gram-positive bacteria most frequently contain only MnSOD (46); however, *S. aureus* subsp. *aureus* contains both Fe and Mn SODs. In FeSOD and MnSOD, trivalent and bivalent states of the metals are involved in the catalytic cycle (28). The chemical identity of these SODs is not yet established (28).

Cu/Zn and FeSODs can be **in**activated by H_2O_2 (2, 5, 6, 41, 42). This is the basis of the reverse synergism in which catalase prevents inactivation of SOD. According to studies by Kono and Fridovich (52), catalase and SOD clearly constitute a mutually protective set of enzymes. Cooperative interaction of SOD and catalase is distinct from the protection derived from prevention of OH production by iron-catalyzed interaction of O_2^- with H_2O_2 (19, 35, 52, 60).

IV. REAGENTS

A. **Hydrogen peroxide, 30% (Superoxol)**
   1. Store in a dark bottle. Avoid any undue exposure to light.
   2. Keep refrigerated at all times when not in use.
B. **M/15 Phosphate buffer, pH 7.0**
   1. Ingredients; two selections
      a. Formula 1
         (1) Ingredients

Potassium dihydrogen phosphate, KH_2PO_4, anhydrous	1.361 g
Disodium hydrogen phosphate, Na_2HPO_3, anhydrous	1.420 g
Distilled water	1000.0 mL

         (2) Add the salts to a small volume of distilled water (boiled and cooled before use) in a 1-L volumetric flask.
         (3) Dissolve by agitation and bring to 1000 mL with boiled distilled water.
      b. Formula 2 (51)
         (1) Solution 1: disodium hydrogen phosphate, anhydrous, 9.47 g/L
         (2) Solution 2: potassium dihydrogen phosphate, anhydrous, 9.07 g/L
         (3) Mix 61.1 mL of solution 1 with 38.9 mL of solution 2; confirm pH with meter (51).
C. **Tween 80, 10%**
   1. This strong detergent solution helps to disperse the hydrophobic, tightly clumped mycobacteria from large aggregates into individual bacilli to maximize detection of catalase (51).
   2. Commercial product available: Tween 80 (Polysorbate 80)
   3. Method of preparation
      a. Add 1.0 mL of concentrated Tween 80 to a small volume of distilled water in a 10-mL volumetric flask.
      b. Dissolve by agitation and bring to 10 mL with distilled water.
      c. Autoclave: 121°C, 10 min; swirl afterward to disperse the solution.
      d. Store in refrigerator (4–10°C); shelf life at least 6 months.

   Tween 80, a polyoxyethylene derivative of sorbitan monooleate, is a surfactant.

D. **Storage:** Store all reagents in a refrigerator (4°C) when not in use. The stability of the phosphate buffer varies; thus it should be checked periodically and discarded when it shows a negative or weak reaction with a known positive organism.

V. QUALITY CONTROL MICROORGANISMS

Hydrogen peroxide (Superoxol) is very unstable and **should** undergo a quality control check **daily** or immediately **prior to** its use. Positive and negative controls should be run simultaneously (4). Vigorous bubbling or foaming occurs (indicating a positive reaction) when a drop of hydrogen peroxide is placed on a blood agar plate, because of the catalase in red blood cells. A chocolate agar plate may be used for a negative control, since the blood cells have been destroyed (85).

A. **Routine catalase tests**

Staphylococcus aureus subsp. *aureus* ATCC 12600, strongly positive (+)
Streptococcus pyogenes ATCC 12344, negative (−)

B. ***Mycobacterium* catalase tests**
  1. Semiquantitative test
     a. Positive (+); > 45 mm
        Mycobacterium kansasii ATCC 12478, strongly +
        Mycobacterium tuberculosis H37Rv, ATCC 25618, weakly +
  2. Negative (−); < 45 mm
     Mycobacterium avium complex ATCC 25291
     Uninoculated
  3. Catalase heat test
     a. Positive (+)
        Mycobacterium kansasii ATCC 12478, strongly +
     b. Negative (−)
        Mycobacterium tuberculosis ATCC 25177
        Mycobacterium bovis ATCC 19210
        Uninoculated

C. **Whole-cell peroxidase-catalase test**
  1. Catalase strongly positive (+), peroxidase negative (−): *Legionella bozemanii* (now *Fluoribacter bozemanae*) ATCC 33217
  2. Catalase negative (−), peroxidase positive (+): *Legionella pneumophilia* subsp. *pneumophilia* ATCC 33152

VI. PROCEDURES

A. Routine catalase tests, room temperature (22–25°C)
  1. **Slide method, recommended procedure**
     a. With an inoculating needle, pick the **center** of an 18- to 24-h pure colony and place on a clean, glass slide.
     b. The test **cannot** be applied if blood agar is introduced into the H_2O_2.
     c. Place a drop of **30%** H_2O_2 on the organism on the slide with a dropper or Pasteur pipette.
        (1) **Do not** reverse the order of procedure as false-positive results may occur.
        (2) **Do not** mix with inoculating needle or loop. Mixing the culture and H_2O_2 is **not** necessary.
     d. Observe for **immediate** bubbling (gas liberation) and record the result.
     e. Discard slide into a disinfectant.
  2. **Tube method**
     a. Add 1.0 mL of **3%** H_2O_2 directly to an 18- to 24-h **heavily** inoculated **pure** agar slant culture.
     b. Do **not** use a blood agar culture medium.
     c. Observe for immediate bubbling (gas liberation) and record the result.
B. **Catalase tests for *Mycobacterium* differentiation**

(*Note:* Perform procedures under the strictest aseptic conditions, always under a bacteriological hood.)

  1. Three procedures
     a. **Spot test (drop method)** (3, 51)

(1) This screening procedure gives a broad indication of the amount of catalase present; particularly used to determine significant isoniazid resistance in strains of *M. tuberculosis,* which usually reflects prior contact with this drug (3).

(2) Inoculum: a single colony of mycobacterial growth on an egg- or agar-based medium (slant or plate); only use colonies from media without drugs (3).

(3) Add 1–2 drops of **freshly** prepared 1:1 Tween–30% peroxide solution to colony and interpret results.

b. **Semiquantitative test (SQ)** (4, 51, 54, 55).

(1) Purpose: to differentiate strains that are strongly positive from those with a small amount of catalase. It is particularly helpful in identification of isoniazid-resistant *M. tuberculosi* (−) (51). Two subgroups of *M. kansasii* can be separated by the amount of catalase they produce; one produces less than 45 mm, and strains more commonly associated with disease produce a column exceeding 45 mm (3).

(2) Use an inoculum from an egg-based medium **only**; e.g., Middlebrook 7H9 broth culture incubated at 35°C for 5–7 days (4).

(3) Test medium: Löwenstein-Jensen deep (5 mL) tube.
   (a) Inoculate **surface** with 0.1 mL of broth culture; inoculate quality control tubes simultaneously.
   (b) Use a marking pencil to mark the equivalent of a 45-mm column on each tube.
   (c) Leave tubes **upright** in an autoclavable rack.
   (d) Incubate, 37°C, caps loosened, 2 weeks

(4) After incubation, place the rack of tubes in an autoclavable, waterproof tray lined with disinfectant-soaked paper towels. **This is necessary to avoid self-contamination, because columns of bubbles produced may overflow.**

(5) Add 1 mL of **freshly** prepared Tween–30% peroxide solution to each **upright** tube.

(6) After 5 min at room temperature (22–25°C), measure the height of the column of bubbles. This test measures the activity of enzyme by the height of column of bubbles of O_2 formed by the action of **un**treated enzyme produced (4).

c. **Heat-stable catalase (68°C catalase)**

(1) Differentiates *Mycobacterium* spp. under controlled pH and temperature conditions (4, 51, 54) and measures the activity of catalase after heating (54). This test in conjunction with the niacin test is valuable for the recognition of tubercle bacilli (3).

(2) To each **sterile** screw-cap tube (16 × 125 mm), add
   (a) 0.5 mL of M/15 phosphate buffer
   (b) Several loopfuls of *Mycobacterium* growth from an actively growing slant culture, 3–4 weeks old; egg-based medium **only** (52)
   (c) Inoculate quality control microorganisms simultaneously.

(3) Incubate with caps screwed down loosely, in a 68°C water bath or constant-temperature block for **exactly 20 min.** The temperature **must** be strictly monitored during the entire incubation period (4).

(4) Cool to room temperature (22–25°C).

(5) Just before use, prepare a 1:1 mixture of sterile 10% Tween 80 and 30% H_2O_2.

(6) To cooled suspension, add 0.5 mL of the Tween 80–peroxide solution. **Do not shake tube because the Tween 80 in the mixture can give a false impression of bubbles** (51). Interpret results.

All *Mycobacterium* spp. show routine catalase activity at room temperature except some isoniazid-resistant strains (4, 54); e.g., *M. tuberculosis, M. gastri,* and some nonpathogenic, isoniazid-resistant strains of M. kansasii (3). Strains resistant to isoniazid may either lose their catalase activity or exhibit decreased activity (4).

C. **Whole-cell peroxidase-catalase test**
  1. Procedure of Pine, Hoffman, Malcolm, Benson, and Gorman (71)
  2. Purpose: **rapid** adjunct to hippuric acid hydrolysis (hippurate test) for phenotypic description of L. pneumophila subsp. pneumophilia (71)
     a. Rapid catalase and/or peroxidase test
     b. Differentiation of known strains of L. pneumophila subsp. pneumophilia (catalase −, peroxidase +) from other Legionella spp. (catalase +, peroxidase −)
     c. Differentiation of pathogenic Leptospira interrogans (catalase strongly +, peroxidase weak + or −) from nonpathogenic Leptospira biflexa (catalase weak + or −, peroxidase strongly +) (15)
  3. Principle: catalase, peroxidase, and SOD **all** deal with destruction of potentially toxic reduced forms of oxygen (28). All Legionella spp. contain SOD, but peroxidase and catalase are **not** uniformly distributed among Legionella spp.
  4. Procedures
     a. Catalase test is performed in the standard manner with 3% H_2O_2 and read after **10 min.**
     b. Peroxidase test (91)
        (1) Reagent: 1% solution of o-dianisidine in methanol; store in an amber bottle
           (a) H^+ donor
           (b) Dye measures color development.
        (2) Substrate, H_2O_2
           (a) Stock solution: 1.0 mL 30% H_2O_2 (Superoxol) diluted to 100.0 mL with distilled water
           (b) Working solution: 1.0 mL of stock H_2O_2 diluted to 100.0 mL with 0.01 M potassium diphosphate buffer (KH_2PO_4), pH 6.0, prepared **fresh daily.**
        (3) Ethylenediamine tetraacetic acid (EDTA) tetrasodium salt (EDTANa$_4$), $C_{10}H_{12}N_2Na_4O_8$, pH 4.6 is the **optimal** additive. This chelating agent causes cells to stain a strong purple to brown color, and more color and bubbles are formed than with phosphate buffer alone (71).
        (4) Procedure (71)
           (a) To a test tube (6 × 50 mm), add in sequence
              0.1 mL K_2HPO_4 buffer
              0.2 mL EDTA
              0.005 mL o-dianisidine
              0.1 mL cells in a water suspension (absorbance at 660 nm + 1 cm, > 1.0), mixed with plastic stick
              0.1 mL 3% H_2O_2
              mix
              0.1 mL mineral oil layered over surface of mixture
           (b) Press reaction tubes into white clay in **upright position.**
           (c) Incubate at room temperature (22–25°C) for **60** min. Interpret results.

VII. RESULTS

> **See Figure 6.1 (Appendix 1) for colored photographic results**

VIII. INTERPRETATION

A. **Routine catalase test (slide or tube)**
   1. Positive (+): immediate bubbling, easily observed; O_2 formed
   2. Negative (−): **no** bubbling; no O_2 formed
B. **Catalase tests for mycobacteria**
   1. **Spot test (drop method):** positive (+), evolution of bubbles around colonies within 4–5 sec. Some colonies may be positive and others negative (3).
      a. Rapid: strongly positive (+)
      b. Slow: weakly positive (+^{w})
   2. **Semiquantitative test:** measure height of column of bubbles (see Table 6.1 for results with specific mycobacteria).

      > 45–50 mm: strongly positive (+)
      20–50 mm: weakly positive (+^{w}) to positive (+)
      < 20 mm: negative (−)

Table 6.1. Catalase Reactions of the Most Commonly Isolated *Mycobacterium* spp. from Clinical Specimens

Mycobacterium sp.	SQ[a]	68°C[b]
M. asiaticum	>45 mm	+
M. chelonae	>45 mm	V[c]
M. flavescens	>45 mm	+
M. fortuitum	>45 mm	+
M. gordonae	>45 mm	+
M. kansasii	>45 mm	+
M. nonchromogenicum	>45 mm	+
M. phlei	>45 mm	+
M scrofulaceum	>45 mm	+
M. simiae	>45 mm	+
M. smegmatis	>45 mm	+
M. szulgai	>45 mm	+
M. terrae	>45 mm	+
M. triviale	>45 mm	+
M. vaccae	>45 mm	+
M. xenopi	>45 mm	V[c]
M. avium complex	<45 mm	V[c]
M. bovis	<45 mm	−
M. gastri	<45 mm	−
M. haemophilum	<45 mm	−
M. malmoense	<45 mm	V[c]
M. marinum	<45 mm	−
M. tuberculosis	<45 mm	−
M. ulcerans	<45 mm	+

Data from reference 51.
[a]Semiquantitative catalase test.
[b]Heat-stable catalase test.
[c]Variable.

   3. **Heat-stable catalase (68°C):** observe for immediate bubbling (gas liberation). Negative tubes should be held for 20 min before reporting as negative; check carefully, as a few bubbles indicate a positive result (4) (see Table 6.2).
C. **Whole-cell peroxidase-catalase test** (71) (Table 6.2)
   1. **Catalase activity,** after **10 min**
      a. Catalase positive (+)

(1) Continuous vigorous stream of small bubbles rapidly penetrate the oil barrier and form a **temporary** head or foam on surface.
(2) Color **remains** absolutely white.
(3) *Legionella* spp. other than *L. pneumophila*
  b. Catalase-like activity of peroxidase (e.g., formation of molecular oxygen from H_2O_2) **does not** form steady stream of bubbles. Few bubbles are produced that cling to sides of the tube and gradually increase in size until they float to surface of **water** layers.
2. **Peroxidase-positive activity, after 60 min**
   a. Light green to gray color gradually turns to brown or purple-brown; color is observed throughout the tube.
   b. Oxidation of *o*-dianisidine with concomitant reduction of H_2O_2 to H_2O.

Table 6.2. Catalase–Peroxidase–Superoxide Dismutase Reactions of *Legionella* spp. Most Commonly Isolated from Humans

Legionella sp.	Catalase[a]	Peroxidase[b]	SOD[c]
L. pneumophilia	−	+	+
L. dumoffii (42)	+	+	+
L. jordanis	+	−	+
L. longbeachae	+	−	+
L. oakridgensis	+	−	+
L. wadsworthii	+	−	+
L. gormanii[d] (31)	−	+	+
L. bozemanii[e]	+	−	+
L. micdadei[f]	+	−	+

Data from references 44, 45, 70, 72.
[a]When positive, strongly catalase positive.
[b]Hydroperoxidase I (HP I) and II (HPII).
[c]Superoxide dismutase.
[d]*L. gormanii* now *Fluoribacter gormanii*.
[e]*L. bozemanii* now *Fluoribacter bozemanae*.
[f]*L. micdadei* now *Tatlockia micdadei*.

IX. RAPID TESTS

A. **Rapid supplemental catalase test for the *Enterobacteriaceae***
  1. Procedure of Chester and Moskowitz (12); supplement for API 20E
  2. Rapid semiquantitative slide test primarily to differentiate between genera of the *Enterobacteriaceae*, especially
     a. *Serratia* (+) from *Enterobacter* (−)
     b. *Yersinia* (+) from *Escherichia* (−) and *Shigella* (−)
  3. Procedure
     a. Isolate 18- to 24-h colonies grown on 5% sheep blood agar (SBA) or MacConkey (MAC) agar.
     b. With bacteriological **loop**, place a single colony onto a glass and add one drop of **3%** H_2O_2; note time required for bubbles to appear.
  4. Interpretation
     a. Immediate positive
        (1) Instant appearance of bubbles
        (2) Possible genera (12, 85)

        Cedecea   *Providencia*
        Hafnia   *Serratia*

    Morganella   *Yersinia*
    Proteus

 b. Delayed positive
  (1) Any delay of bubbling **no matter how slight**
  (2) Possible genera (12, 85)

    Citrobacter   *Kluyvera*
    Edwardsiella *Salmonella*
    Enterobacter *Shigella*
    Escherichia   *Tatumella*
    Klebsiella

5. Quality control; 3% H_2O_2 tested **daily** against

  Immediate reaction, *Proteus vulgaris* ATCC 13315
  Delayed reaction, *Escherichia coli*   ATCC 25922
  Negative reaction, *Streptococcus pyogenes* ATCC 19615

  The slight, delayed bubbling from peroxidase in erythrocytes (RBCs) and leukocytes (WBCs) in sheep blood agar **does not** interfere with semiquantitative catalase interpretation.

B. **Superoxol catalase test for *Neisseria*** (56, 76)

1. Procedure of Saginur, Clecner, Portnoy, and Mendelson (76)
2. Purpose: **direct** screening test for **presumptive** differentiation of *N. gonorrhoeae* colonies from other *Neisseria* spp. when cultivated on Thayer-Martin (TM) growth agar; it compares favorably with the coagglutination test (76).
3. Reagent: Superoxol; 30% H_2O_2. *Neisseria* spp. produce abundant catalase as exhibited with 3% H_2O_2, but species can be differentiated with 30% H_2O_2.
4. Procedure: add one drop of Superoxol directly onto a suspected colony on a **TM** agar plate.
5. Interpretation on TM medium
 a. *N. gonorrhoeae:* immediate ($<$ 1 sec) rapid, brisk, abundant bubbling
 b. *N. meningitidis:* delayed or weak bubbling

A negative Superoxol test precludes an isolate being *N. gonorrhoeae,* but an organism that grows on TM and is Superoxol positive is likely to be *N. gonorrhoeae;* further biochemical tests **must** be performed for confirmation (76).

X. ALTERNATIVE TESTS

A. **Capillary tube technique**
1. Method of Fung and Petrishko (30)
2. Capillary tubes (commercial): outer diameter, 1 mm; length, 67 mm.
3. Place tubes in a 50 mL beaker.
 a. Add 10 mL of **3%** H_2O_2.
 b. H_2O_2 is drawn into tubes by capillary action to a height of approximately 20 mm.
4. Touch **center** of colony to be tested with an H_2O_2-filled capillary tube.
 a. 18- to 24-h growth on nutrient or blood agar plates
 b. May be a pure or mixed culture as long as colonies are well isolated
5. Observe for immediate effervescence (bubbling) within 10 sec.
6. Record results, semiquantitative scale

 0, no bubbles
 +, few bubbles
 ++, many bubbles
 +++, gas forcing H_2O_2 to tip of the capillary tube

B. **Coverslip technique**
   1. Method of Taylor and Achanzar (85)
   2. Primarily used to aid identification of the *Enterobacteriaceae*
   3. Growth from an 18- to 24-h plate medium
   4. Two methods
      a. To an isolated colony add 1 drop of 0.5% H_2O_2 and a coverslip.
      b. To a glass microscope slide
         (1) When above method gives a weak or delayed reaction
         (2) Add
            (a) Bacteria: **center** of a single colony **picked with an inoculating needle**
            (b) **One drop of 0.5%** H_2O_2 and a coverslip
   5. Observe for immediate bubbling using either method.
      a. Frosted appearance of bubbles elaborated under coverslip indicates the speed of reaction.
      b. Interpret by absence or presence of **trapped** bubbles.

Studies by Taylor and Achanzar (85) using **3.0%** H_2O_2 showed vigorous catalase activity with *Serratia, Proteus,* and *Providencia* organisms; moderate activity with *Salmonella* (74.2%); and rare moderate activity with *Escherichia, Enterobacter,* and *Klebsiella* organisms. *Escherichia* (70.4%), and *Shigella* (65.2%) spp. were usually nonreactive, most *Enterobacter* spp. (67.6%) were usually weakly reactive, and *Klebsiella* strains were divided between nonreactive (48.1%) and weakly reactive (49.4%) (85). However, at an H_2O_2 concentration of **0.5%,** they found that only *Pseudomonas aeruginosa* and *Serratia* organisms were catalase positive, and this positive activity could be used particularly to aid in identifying nonpigmented strains. The only other organisms that are positive at this concentration are the staphylococci.

Positive activity using 0.5 or 3.0% H_2O_2 can be graded as negative (−), weak or delayed (+), moderate (++), or vigorous (+++). When using a 0.5% solution, Taylor and Achanzar (85) recommend not using a coverslip unless reactions are weak or doubtful.

C. **Color reaction streak test**
   1. Method of Hanker and Rabin (36)
   2. Used for catalase-positive microorganisms; primarily to differentiate staphylococci and streptococci
   3. Reagent (Polysciences, see Appendix 11).
      a. Stock solutions
         (1) Dopamine: 20 mg/mL in 0.2 M phosphate buffer, pH 8.0.
         (2) *p*-Phenylenediamine dihydrochloride: 1 mg/mL in 0.2 M phosphate buffer, pH 8.0.
      b. Working reagent

Dopamine	1.0 mL
p-Phenylenediamine dihydrochloride	1.0 mL
H_2O_2 (3%)	2.0 mL
Dimethyl sulfoxide	1.0 mL

   4. Streak **pure** bacterial colony onto chemically clean glass microscopic slide and allow to **air dry.**
   5. Add **1 drop** of working reagent; an enzymatic color reaction happens within seconds.
   6. A catalase-positive reaction is denoted by formation of a highly purple color on the smear; the colored oxidation product lasts for days so the result may be rechecked, if necessary.
   7. Chemistry of reagent action: peroxidases and catalases catalyze the same type of general reaction (59).

$$H_2O_2 + \left.\begin{array}{l} H_2X \\ 2X^n \end{array}\right\} \longrightarrow 2H_2O + \left.\begin{array}{l} X \\ 2X^{n+1} \end{array}\right\}$$

n = positive charge

Catalase differs from peroxidase in using H_2O_2 as an oxidant and a second molecule as an electron donor, or coreductant (9, 59). Peroxidase can catalyze the same reaction, but the general reaction is preferred in which H_2X or X^{nn} can be a phenol or hydroxylamine (9, 59). With the streak test, a peroxidatic (peroxidase-like) oxidation of dopamine–p-phenylenediamine reagent occurs. Catalase mediates the oxidation of certain phenols and aromatic amines by H_2O_2 with liberation of oxygen, and the H_2O_2 is reduced at the expense of several substances that act as electron acceptors (9, 36, 37, 59). A complex process, but overall reaction (9, 36, 37) is

$$H_2O_2 + H_2A \xrightarrow[\text{catalase}]{\text{peroxidase}} 2H_2O + A$$

Aromatic amine and phenol (colorless)   Colored compound (purple)

XII. PRECAUTIONS

A. General

1. Many organisms are fastidious and require certain enrichments such as blood for growth. Therefore, if colonies are tiny and growing on blood agar medium, it is often difficult to pick the center of a colony and obtain enough growth to perform the slide procedure without introducing blood agar into the hydrogen peroxide. Erythrocytes contain catalase/peroxidase, and their presence will give a false-positive result (4, 16, 51).

   To avoid this problem, either use chocolate agar plates for isolation and testing, since the red cells have been destroyed (lysed), or streak a pie plate for **maximum** growth before determining catalase activity. For the pie plate procedure use a single blood agar plate for four separate determinations.

   Mark a blood agar plate into four quadrants (below) on the bottom half of the plate that contains the medium. **Prior to** inoculation, label **each** pie area appropriately to avoid any mixup in the catalase test or its interpretation.

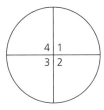

   Pick a single, well-isolated, **pure** colony and streak **one** quadrant for maximum growth. Incubate at 37°C for 18–24 h. This procedure should provide sufficient growth of a **pure** culture for catalase testing. The catalase test must be performed with a **heavy** inoculum.

   Also, few clinical specimens produce a pure bacterial culture on the initial isolation media; thus, if colonies are small and not well isolated, they may contain mixed cell types of catalase-reacting organisms and produce false-positive or doubtful results.

2. In performing the slide test **do not** reverse the order of procedure (addition of H_2O_2 to slide before organism) as the platinum in the inoculation needle may produce a false-positive result. Nichrome wire does not cause bubbling.
3. Growth for catalase testing **must** be from an 18- to 24-h culture. Older colonies may lose their catalase activity and yield a false-negative result (4).
4. Superoxol (30% H_2O_2) is an extremely caustic solution so avoid exposure to skin, because painful burns may occur. If H_2O_2 does get on the skin, **immediately** flood the area with 70% ethanol, **not** water, to neutralize the action. It is a good habit to keep a bottle of 70% ethanol on hand near the hydrogen peroxide to avoid any delay in its use when spillage or accidents occur.
5. H_2O_2 must be fairly fresh because it is unstable and breaks down easily on exposure to light. The solution **must** be kept refrigerated at all times when not in use, and it is advisable to perform a quality control check just prior to its use. Cowan (16) states that the rate of H_2O_2 decomposition **increases** as the temperature increases, because of dissolved oxygen; a false-positive result may occur. This may be avoided by gently shaking a small volume of H_2O_2 reagent **immediately before** its use (16).
6. There are no universal standards for the concentration of H_2O_2 used in catalase testing nor gradations for vigor and speed of catalase activity (85). The concentration and method of reporting are arbitrary and vary from laboratory to laboratory, often even between two microbiologists in the same laboratory. Thus, when investigating a new modified procedure or performing an established procedure, be sure to use the concentration stated. Be consistent in your laboratory concerning both concentration and reporting, by setting up standards.
7. Duke and Jarvis (23) have shown that routine catalase testing is hazardous because of release of bacteria-laden aerosols by liberated oxygen. Use of the color reaction streak test eliminates exposure to a possible aerosol of pathogenic bacteria (36). Also, routine testing must be observed immediately during the procedure because **no record** exists after effervescence subsides (23), but the streak test results can be rechecked for days (36).
8. Catalase is **in**activated by sunlight under aerobic conditions (62).
9. When **an**aerobes are tested, cultures should be exposed to air 30 min **before** addition of H_2O_2 (87). Most aerotolerant anaerobes lack catalase but contain SOD; obligate anaerobes lack **both** enzymes (31).

B. **Rapid supplemental catalase test**
1. **Do not** use cotton swabs or wooden applicator sticks; they obscure the reaction (33).
2. Test **must** be restricted to isolates grown on sheep blood agar and MacConkey agar. Some *Enterobacteriaceae* species in the intermediate reaction category give a delayed reaction and some isolates of delayed species give intermediate reactions when grown on Muller-Hinton (M-H) agar (33).

C. **Mycobacterial catalases**
1. Middlebrook (61) reported that acquisition of isoniazid resistance by *M. tuberculosis* is accompanied by a **loss** of catalase and a **loss** of virulence.
2. The incubation temperature of the heat-stable test **must** be strictly monitored during the entire 20 min incubation period (4).
3. In the heat-stable catalase test, tubes **must not be** shaken in any way, as Tween 80 will bubble by itself; shaking may yield a possible false-positive result (4).
4. Discard any Tween-peroxidase mixture left over; it is **un**stable and should not be reused (51).
5. For heat-stable catalase testing, it is recommended that the inoculum be taken from egg-based medium **only** (51).

D. **Specific microorganisms**
1. Be aware that catalase-negative isolates **may** exist; they are rare but not uncommon.

Funada et al. (29) isolated the first anaerobic, catalase-negative variant of *E. coli* from an acute leukemia patient; its poor growth in air is suspected to be susceptibility to H_2O_2. A few catalase-negative strains of *S. aureus* have been isolated, both from an animal source (24) and a human source (58, 86). A single case investigated by Tu and Palutke (86) was coagulase positive but differed from others (24, 58) in being negative for anaerobic fermentation of mannitol, although all other biochemical test results were typical. The authors tested the isolate by the modified benzidine test (18) and found it did contain a cytochrome system; on further testing it was found to be a penicillinase-producing strain.
2. Dacre (17) reported that catalase activity of the lactobacilli increases when they are cultivated on medium with a low glucose concentration.
3. Studies by Hassan and Fridovich (39) showed production of two catalases by *E. coli*; one **inducible**, with formation repressed by glucose, and the other **constitutive.** These observations were confirmed by Claiborne and Fridovich (13) and Claiborne et al. (14). The enzymes use H_2O_2 as an electron acceptor in oxidative metabolism and are classified as hydroperoxides (hydroperoxidase I (HP I) and hydroperoxidase II (HP II)) (14). Enzymatically, HP I is a peroxidase that demonstrates catalytic activity.
4. Catalase is produced by 80–90% of the *Bacteroides fragilis* group; the only other **an**aerobes that produce catalase are *Eubacterium lentum, Peptococcus, Propionibacterium,* and *Veillonella* (87). *B. fragilis* is catalase positive **only** if there is sufficient hemin in the growth medium; catalase formation is repressed by fermentable carbohydrates in the medium (33). Gregory et al. (33) recommend use of chopped meat broth as the growth medium when testing for catalase.
5. *Streptococcus* species produce peroxidase rather than catalase to degrade H_2O_2.
6. Some *Enterococcus* spp. produce a "pseudocatalase" and react weakly with H_2O_2, particularly *E. faecalis* on primary isolation; however, the strength of the reaction may diminish after a few serial subcultures (51).

E. ***Legionella* whole-cell testing**
   1. **General**
      a. Cell suspensions are made in water; at an absorbance $=1.0$ at 660 nm they give a positive peroxidase reaction. At a lower absorbance they give a weak or negative color reaction. An absorbance above 1.0–1.5 can be used, but at these densities cells form large amounts of bubbles in the presence of **peroxidase only,** which may be falsely interpreted as a catalase-positive result (71).
      b. The test result **does not** describe the **internal** enzyme composition of cells. Strains that exhibit both hippurate-positive and peroxidase-positive reactions, should be confirmed to be *L. pneumophila* by immunofluorescence (71).
      c. Catalase and peroxidase formation is repressed in cells grown on media with glucose as the primary substrate (14). Formation of HP I is repressed by glucose (13), and formation of HP II is repressed by both **an**aerobic conditions and glucose (14).
      d. Addition of toluene inhibits both catalytic and peroxidative reactions (71).
      e. When testing whole-cell catalase or peroxidase activities, use cells stored no longer than 3–5 days, even though enzymatic activities are stable and reliable up to 2 weeks (71).
   2. **Catalase activity**
      a. The media used to cultivate *Legionella* spp. can greatly affect catalase production (32, 39, 92); however, a problem exists because few available media support growth of *Legionella* spp. *Legionella* spp. require complex media for growth, which **must** contain either starch or charcoal plus cysteine and added iron (25, 66, 68, 69). Keto acids (e.g., ketoglutaric acid), added Fe^{2+}, and cysteine together stimulate growth of *Legionella* in the absence of light (70). Iron and cysteine are required for growth (25), but the addition of these substances alone **does not** promote growth (88); addition of charcoal strongly stimulates growth in yeast extract media that contains Fe^{3+} and cysteine (71, 75). (For further information on *Legionella* growth requirements, see reference 72.)

Studies by Pine et al. (71) showed that *Legionella* exhibited greatest catalase activity when grown on BCYE (ACES-buffered charcoal–yeast extract agar); however, **catalase-negative** *Legionella* strains have the **lowest** catalase activity when grown on BCYE and the highest activity on blood agar (BA). *L. pneumophila* is catalase positive (89); however, cells grown on complex organic agar media (e.g., BCYE) or in chemically defined broth exhibit either **extremely** weak or no catalase activity (72). *L. pneumophila* catalase activity is very slight or short-lived (15–60 sec) (71) compared with the strong, continued release (minutes) of oxygen (bubbles) by other *Legionella* species (71, 72).

 b. The optimal concentration of H_2O_2 to demonstrate catalase activity is 3%; increasing the concentration **does not** increase reactivity or give any evidence of inhibition. However, a 0.3% concentration definitely reduces the rate and amount of gas evolved (71).

3. **Peroxidase activity**
   a. **No** direct association of peroxidase with pathogenicity exists (72).
   b. The whole-cell peroxidase test **does not** reflect the true hydroperoxidase composition of the cells, and the test can be seriously affected by the medium upon which the cells are grown (71).
   c. The peroxidase color formation reaction is totally inhibited in the **presence** of a strong catalase reaction (71), and conversely, in the **absence** of catalase, a peroxidase with strong catalytic activity may give both a positive catalase and a positive peroxidase result.
   d. Rapid loss of the peroxidative activity of *L. dumoffii* is reversed by addition of fresh H_2O_2, suggesting that the inhibition of peroxidative activity is due to depletion of H_2O_2 by catalase (73).
   e. *L. pneumophila* strains have only a single hydroperoxidase, which has both catalytic and peroxidative activity (73).

REFERENCES

1. Araiso T, Miyoshi K, Yamazaki I. Mechanism of electron transfer from sulfite to horseradish peroxidase-hydroperoxide compounds. Biochemistry 1976;15(14):3059–3063.
2. Asada K, Yoshikawa K, Takahashi M, et al. Superoxide dismutase from a blue- green alga, *Plectonema boryanum*. J Biol Chem 1975;250(8):2801–2807.
3. Balows A, Hausler WJ Jr, Herrmann KL, et al. Manual of Clinical Microbiology, ed 5. Washington, DC: American Society for Microbiology, 1991:319.
4. Baron EJ, Finegold SM. Bailey & Scott's Diagnostic Microbiology, ed 8. Philadelphia: CV Mosby, 1990:615, 624, 627.
5. Beauchamp CO, Fridovich I. Isozymes of superoxide dismutase from wheat germ. Biochim Biophys Acta 1973;317:50–64.
6. Bray RC, Cockle SA, Fielden EM, et al. Reduction and inactivation of superoxide dismutase by hydrogen peroxide. Biochem J 1974;139(1):43–48.
7. Bright HJ, Porter DJT. Flavoprotein oxidases. In: Boyer PD, ed. The Enzymes, vol 12, part B. New York: Academic Press, 1975:421–505.
8. Burrows W, Lewert RM, Rippon JW. Textbook of Microbiology. The Pathogenic Microorganisms, ed 19. Philadelphia: WB Saunders, 1968:111.
9. Cantarow A, Schepartz B. Biochemistry, ed 3. Philadelphia: WB Saunders, 1962:134, 136, 388–389.
10. Castro CI. Mechanisms of reaction of hemeproteins with oxygen and hydrogen peroxide in the oxidation of organic substrates. Pharmacol Ther 1980;10:171–189.
11. Chance B, Sies H, Boveris A. Hydroperoxide metabolism in mammalian organs. Physiol Rev 1979;59(3):527–605.
12. Chester B, Moskowitz LB. Rapid catalase supplemental test for identification of members of the family *Enterobacteriaceae*. J Clin Microbiol 1987;25(2):439–441.
13. Claiborne A, Fridovich I. Purification of the o-dianisidine peroxidase from *Escherichia coli* B. J Biol Chem 1979;254(10):4245–4252.
14. Claiborne A, Malinowski DP, Fridovich I. Purification and characterization of hydroperoxidase II of *Escherichia coli* B. J Biol Chem 1979;254(22):11664–11667.
15. Corin RE, Boggs E, Cox CD. Enzymatic degradation of H_2O_2 by *Leptospira*. Infect Immun 1978;22(3):672–675.
16. Cowan ST. Cowan & Steel's Manual for the Identification of Medical Bacteria, ed 2. Cambridge: Cambridge University Press, 1974:171.
17. Dacre JC. Catalase production by lactobacilli. Nature 1956;178:700.
18. Deibel RH, Evans JB. Modified benzidine test for the detection of cytochrome containing respiratory systems in microorganisms. J Bacteriol 1960;79(3):356–360.

19. DiGuiseppi J, Fridovich I. Ethylene from 2-keto-4-thiomethyl butyric acid: The Haber-Weiss reaction. Arch Biochem Biophys 1980;205(2): 323–329.
20. Doelle HW. Bacterial Metabolism. New York: Academic Press, 1969:240 and 345.
21. Dolin MI. The *Streptococcus faecalis* oxidases for reduced diphosphopyridine nucleotide. III. Isolation and properties of a flavin peroxidase for reduced diphosphopyridine. J Biol Chem 1957; 225(1):557–573.
22. Dolin MI. Cytochrome-independent electron transport enzymes of bacteria. In: Gunsalus IC, Stanier RY, eds. The Bacteria, vol 2. New York: Academic Press, 1961:425–457.
23. Duke PB, Jarvis JD. The catalase test. A cautionary tale. J Med Lab Technol 1972;29(2):203–204.
24. Everall PH, Stacey PM. Catalase negative *Staphylococcus aureus*. J Med Lab Technol 1956;13: 489–490.
25. Feeley JC, Gorman GW, Weaver RE, et al. Primary isolation media for Legionnaires disease bacterium. J Clin Microbiol 1978;8(3):320–325.
26. Fieser LF, Fieser M. Organic Chemistry, ed 3. New York: Reinhold, 1956:467.
27. Fita I, Rossmann MG. The active center of catalase. J Mol Biol 1985;185.21–37.
28. Fridovich I. The biology of oxygen radicals. Science 1978;201:875–880.
29. Funada H, Hattori K-I, Kosakai N. Catalase-negative *Escherichia coli* isolated from blood. J Clin Microbiol 1978;7(5):474–478.
30. Fung DYC, Petrishko DT. Capillary tube catalase test. Appl Microbiol 1973;26(4):631–632.
31. Gottschalk G. Bacterial Metabolism, ed 2. New York: Springer-Verlag, 1986:34–35, 208–209, and 223.
32. Gregory EM, Kowalski JB, Holdeman LV. Production and some properties of catalase and superoxide dismutase from the anaerobe *Bacteroides distasonis*. J Bacteriol 1977;129(3):1298–1302.
33. Gregory EM, Veltri BJ, Wagner DL, Wilkins TD. Carbohydrate repression of catalase synthesis in *Bacteroides fragilis*. J Bacteriol 1977;129(1):534–535.
34. Gunsalus IC, Stanier RY. The Bacteria, vol II. New York: Academic Press, 1961:342, 427.
35. Halliwell B. Superoxide-dependent formation of hydroxyl radicals in the presence of nonchelates. Is it a mechanism for hydroxyl radical production in biochemical systems? FEBS Lett 1978; 92(2):321–326.
36. Hanker JS, Rabin AN. Color reaction streak test for catalase-positive microorganisms. J Clin Microbiol 1975;2(5):463–464.
37. Harper HA, Rodwell VW, Mayes PA. Review of Physiological Chemistry, ed 16. Los Altos, CA: Lange Medical Publications, 1977:229, 483.
38. Harrow B, Mazur A. Textbook of Biochemistry, ed 9. Philadelphia: WB Saunders, 1966:104.
39. Hassan HM, Fridovich I. Regulation of the synthesis of catalase and peroxidase of *Escherichia coli*. J Biol Chem 1978;253(18):6445–6450.
40. Hassan HM, Fridovich I. Superoxide, hydrogen peroxide, and oxygen tolerance of oxygen-sensitive mutants of *Escherichia coli*. Rev Infect Dis 1979;1:357–367.
41. Hodgson EK, Fridovich I. The interaction of bovine erythrocyte superoxide dismutase with hydrogen peroxide: Inactivation of the enzyme. Biochemistry 1975;14(24):5294–5299.
42. Hodgson EK, Fridovich I. The interaction of bovine erythrocyte superoxide dismutase with hydrogen peroxide: Chemiluminescence and peroxidation. Biochemistry 1975;14(24):5299–5303.
43. Hoffman BM, Roberts JE, Kang CH, Margoliash E. Electron paramagnetic and electron nuclear double resonance of the hydrogen peroxide compound of cytochrome c peroxidase. J Biol Chem 1981;256(13):6556–6564.
44. Hoffman PS, Pine L. Respiratory physiology and cytochrome content of *Legionella pneumophilia*. Curr Microbiol 1982;7(6):351–356.
45. Hoffman PS, Pine L, Bell S. Production of superoxide and hydrogen peroxide in medium used to culture *Legionella pneumophila*: Catalytic decomposition by charcoal. Appl Environ Microbiol 1983;45(3):784–791.
46. Johnston MA, Delwiche EA. Distribution and characteristics of the catalases of *Lactobacillaceae*. J Bacteriol 1965;90(2):347–351.
47. Jones CW. Aspects of Microbiology. Bacterial Respiration and Photosynthesis. Washington, DC: American Society for Microbiology, 1982: 17–18.
48. Keilin D, Hartree EF. Coupled oxidation of alcohol. Proc R Soc Ser B 1935;119:141–159.
49. Keilin D, Hartree EF. Properties of catalase. Catalysis of coupled oxidation of alcohols. Biochem J 1945;39:293–301.
50. Keilin D, Hartree EF. Catalase, peroxidase and metmyoglobin as catalysts of coupled peroxidatic reactions. Biochem J 1955;60:310–325.
51. Koneman EW, Allen SD, Janda WM, et al. Color Atlas and Textbook of Diagnostic Microbiology, ed 4. Philadelphia: JB Lippincott, 1992:38, 314–315, 391, 413, 444, 484, 745–746.
52. Kono Y, Fridovich I. Superoxide radical inhibits catalase. J Biol Chem 1982;257(10):5751–5754.
53. Krieg NR, Holt JG, eds. Bergey's Manual of Systematic Bacteriology, vol 1. Baltimore: Williams & Wilkins, 1984:113, 117, 296.
54. Kubica GP, Jones WD Jr, Abbott VD, et al. Differential identification of mycobacteria. I. Tests on catalase activity. Am Rev Respir Dis 1966;94(3):400–405.
55. Kubica GP, Pool GL. Studies on the catalase activity of acid fast bacilli. I. An attempt to subgroup these organisms on the basis of their catalase activity at different temperatures and pH. Am Rev Respir Dis 1960;81:387–391.
56. Lawton WD, Gaafar HA. Update on the labora-

tory diagnosis of gonorrhea Abstr Annu Meet Am Soc Microbiol C(H) 1979;57:355.
57. Lenhoff HM, Kaplan NO. A cytochrome peroxidase from *Pseudomonas fluorescens*. J Biol Chem 1956;220(2):967–982.
58. Lucas PR, Seeley HW. A catalase negative *Micrococcus pyogenes* var *aureus*. J Bacteriol 1955;69(2):231.
59. Mahler HR, Cordes EH. Biological Chemistry. New York: Harper & Row, 1966:590, 592.
60. McCord JM, Day ED. Superoxide-dependent production of hydroxyl radical catalyzed by iron-EDTA complex. FEBS Lett 1978;86(1):139–142.
61. Middlebrook G. Isoniazid resistance and catalase activity of tubercle bacilli. A preliminary report. Am Rev Tuberc 1954;69(3):471–472.
62. Mitchell RL, Anderson IC. Catalase photoactivation. Science 1965;150(10):74.
63. Molland J. Monograph. Acta Pathol Microbiol Scand (Suppl) 1947;66:(1)9–165.
64. Morrison M, Schonbaum GR. Peroxidase—catalyzed halogenation. Annu Rev Biochem 1976;45:861–888.
65. Oberley LW. Superoxide Dismutase. Vol III. Pathological State. Boca Raton, FL: CRC Press, 1985.
66. Orrison LH, Cherry WB, Tyndall RL, et al. *Legionella oakridgensis*: Unusual new species isolated from cooling tower water. Appl Environ Microbiol 1983;45(2):536–545.
67. Oser BL, ed. Hawk's Physiological Chemistry, ed 14. New York: McGraw-Hill, 1965:423–424.
68. Pasculle AW, Feeley JC, Gibson RJ, et al. Pittsburgh pneumonia agent: Direct isolation from human lung tissue. J Infect Dis 1980;141(6):727–732.
69. Pine L, George JR, Reeves MW, Harrell WK. Physiology: Characteristics of the Legionnaires' disease bacterium in semisynthetic and chemically defined liquid media. In: Jones GL, Hebert GA, eds. Legionnaires, the Disease, the Bacterium, and Methodology, ed 2. Atlanta, GA: Centers for Disease Control, 1979:27–40.
70. Pine L, Hoffman PS, Malcolm GB, Benson RF, Franzus MJ. Role of keto acids and reduced-oxygen-scavenging enzymes in the growth of *Legionella* species. J Clin Microbiol 1986;23(1):33–42.
71. Pine L, Hoffman PS, Malcolm GB, Benson RF, Gorman GW. Whole-cell peroxidase test for identification of *Legionella pneumophila*. J Clin Microbiol 1984;19(2):286–290.
72. Pine L, Hoffman PS, Malcolm GB, Benson RF, Keen MG. Determination of catalase, peroxidase, and superoxide dismutase within the genus *Legionella*. J Clin Microbiol 1984;20(3):421–429.
73. Pruitt KM, Tenovuo JO. The Lactoperoxidase System. New York: Marcel Dekker, 1985:33, 184, 189.
74. Rapoport SM, Muller M. Catalase and glutathione peroxidase. In: Yoskikawa H, Rapoport SM, eds. Cellular and Molecular Biology of Erythrocytes. Baltimore: University Park Press, 1974:167.
75. Ristroph JD, Hedlund KW, Allen RG. Liquid medium for growth of *Legionella pneumophila*. J Clin Microbiol 1980;11(1):19–21.
76. Saginur R, Clecner B, Portnoy J, Mendelson J. Superoxol (catalase) test for identification of *Neisseria gonorrhoeae*. J Clin Microbiol 1982;15(3):475–477.
77. Saunders BC, Holmes-Siedle AG, Stark BP. Peroxidase. Washington, DC: Butterworth, 1964.
78. Schonbaum GR, Chance B. Catalase In: Boyer PD, ed. The Enzymes, vol 13. New York: Academic Press, 1976:363–408.
79. Shimizu N, Kobayashi K, Hayashi K. The reaction of superoxide radical with catalase. Mechanism of the inhibition of catalase by superoxide radical. J Biol Chem 1984;259(7):4414–4418.
80. Sichak SP, Dounce AL. Analysis of the peroxidatic mode of action of catalase. Arch Biochem Biophys 1986;249(2):286–295.
81. Smith DT, Conant NF, Willett HP. Zinsser's Microbiology, ed 14. New York: Appleton-Century-Crofts, 1968:107.
82. Sneath PHA, Mair NS, Sharpe ME, Holt JG, eds. Bergey's Manual of Systematic Bacteriology, vol 2. Baltimore: Williams & Wilkins, 1986:1275.
83. Strittmatter CF. Electron transport to oxygen in lactobacilli. J Biol Chem 1959;234(4):2789–2793.
84. Strittmatter CF. Flavin-linked oxidative enzymes of *Lactobacillus casei*. J Biol Chem 1959;234(4):2794–2800.
85. Taylor WI, Achanzar D. Catalase test as an aid to the identification of *Enterobacteriaceae*. Appl Microbiol 1972;24(1):58–61.
86. Tu KK, Palutke WA. Isolation and characterization of a catalase-negative strain of *Staphylococcus aureus*. J Clin Microbiol 1976;3(1):77–78.
87. Washington JA. Laboratory Procedures in Clinical Microbiology, ed 2. New York: Springer-Verlag, 1985:134, 338.
88. Wayne LG, Diaz GA. Identification of mycobacteria by specific precipitation of catalase with absorbed sera. J Clin Microbiol 1985;21(5):721–725.
89. Weaver RE. Cultural and staining characteristics. In: Jones GL, Hebert GA, eds. Legionnaires, the Disease, the Bacterium, and Methodology. Atlanta, GA: Centers for Disease Control, 1978:17–21.
90. Whittenbury R. Two types of catalase-like activity in lactic acid bacteria. Nature 1960;187:433–434.
91. Worthington Enzyme Manual. Freehold, NJ: Worthington Biochemical Corporation, 1972:43–44, 66–70.
92. Yoshpe-Purer Y, Henis Y. Factors affecting catalase level and sensitivity to hydrogen peroxide in *Escherichia coli*. Appl Environ Microbiol 1976;32(4):465–469.

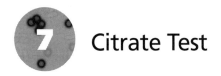

7 Citrate Test

I. PRINCIPLE

To determine if an organism is capable of utilizing citrate as the sole source of carbon for metabolism and growth with resulting alkalinity

II. PURPOSE

(Also see Chapters 43–45)

Citrate is part of the indole–methyl red–Voges-Proskauer–citrate (IMViC) group of tests for identification of the *Enterobacteriaceae,* related Gram-negative microorganisms, and **non**fermentative bacteria.

A. To help differentiate between genera, primarily among the *Enterobacteriaceae*
   1. *Escherichia coli* (usually −) and *Shigella* spp. (−) from most other frequently encountered *Enterobacteriaceae* (Table 7.1)

Table 7.1. Simmons Citrate Reactions among Genera of Family *Enterobacteriaceae*

Arsenophonus	NR	*Obesumbacterium*	−
Budvicia	−	*Pantoea*	+
Buttiauxella	+	*Plesiomonas*	−
Cedecea	+	*Pragia*	V+
Citrobacter	V	*Proteus*	V
Edwardsiella	−	*Providencia*	V
Enterobacter	V+	*Rhanella*	+
Escherichia	−	*Salmonella*	V
Ewingella	+	*Sarratia*	V+
Hafnia	−	*Shigella*	−
Klebsiella	V+	*Tatumella*	−
Kluyvera	V+	*Xenorhabdus*	V
Lecleric	V+	*Yersinia*	V−
Moellerella	V+	*Yokenella*	+
Morganella	V−		

   2. *Edwardsiella* (−) from *Salmonella* (usually +)
   3. *Serratia proteamaculans* (formerly *Serratia liquefaciens*) (+) from *Yersinia pseudotuberculosis* (−) and *Yersinia enterocolitica* (usually −); *Serratia proteamaculans* subsp. *proteamaculans* (formerly *Serratia liquefaciens*) is a collection of several DNA hybridization groups that include *S. proteamaculans* and *Serratia grimesii* (16).
   4. *Klebsiella-Enterobacter* groups (usually +) from *E. coli* (usually −)
   5. *Proteus rettgeri* (formerly *Providencia rettgeri*) (+) from *Morganella morganii* biogroups 1 and 2 (−)

6. *Yokenella regensburgei* (formerly *Koserella trabulsii*) (+) from *Hafnia alvei* (−) (16).
B. To aid in species differentiation
 1. *Leminorella grimontii* (+) from *Leminorella richardii* (−) (16)
 2. *Acidovorax delafieldii* (+) from *A. facilis* (−) and *A. temperans* (−)

III. BIOCHEMISTRY INVOLVED

Energy can be supplied to some bacteria in the absence of fermentation or lactic acid production (15, 20) by the use of citrate as the sole source of carbon. Normally, citrate metabolism involves a condensation of acetyl with coenzyme A and oxalacetate (15) to enter the Krebs' cycle. Citrate metabolism by most bacteria is rapid via the tricarboxylic acid cycle or the citrate fermentation pathway (20). Organisms possessing a transport or permease permit citrate to enter the cell (25). In bacteria, cleavage of citrate involves an enzyme system without coenzyme A involvement, citritase (citrate oxaloacetate-lyase) (25) or citrate desmolase (15). Citratase requires a divalent cation for its activity, magnesium or manganese (23). The initial breakdown of citrate was originally thought to yield oxalacetate (the salt of oxalacetic acid) and acetate (the salt of acetic acid) (15), now known to be intermediates in citrate metabolism (15).

$$\text{Citrate} \longrightarrow \text{Oxalacetate} + \text{acetate} \longrightarrow \text{Pyruvate} + CO_2$$

The products of citrate metabolism depend upon the pH of the medium (12, 15). At a high pH (alkaline), more acetate and formate are produced, and production of lactate and CO_2 decreases (12, 15). Above pH 7.0 there is no production of lactate and the products are (12, 15)

$$\text{Citrate} \longrightarrow CO_2 + \text{formic acid} + 2 \text{ acetic acid}$$

At acid pH, acetylmethylcarbinol (acetoin) and lactate are the major products of citrate metabolism (12, 15). Regardless of the end products produced, the first step in citrate fermentation produces pyruvate. Degradation of pyruvate then depends upon the pH of the medium (5, 14).

$$\text{Citrate} \longrightarrow \text{Oxalacetate} + \text{acetate}$$
$$\text{Oxalacetate} \longrightarrow \text{Pyruvate} + CO_2$$

Alkaline pH

$$\text{Pyruvate} \longrightarrow \text{Acetate} + \text{formate}$$

Acid pH

$$2 \text{ Pyruvate} \longrightarrow \text{Acetate} + CO_2 + \text{lactate}$$
$$2 \text{ Pyruvate} \longrightarrow \text{Acetoin} + 2CO_2$$

The medium for citrate fermentation also contains inorganic ammonium salts. An organism that can use citrate as its sole carbon source also uses the ammonium salts as its sole nitrogen source (16). Ammonium salts (e.g., ammonium phosphate) are broken down to ammonia (NH_3), which increases alkalinity. Bacteria extract nitrogen from ammonium salts with production of ammonia (NH^+) leading to alkalization of medium and conversion of NH_3^{2+} to ammonium hydroxide (NH_4OH) (16).

Deffner and Franke (9, 10) showed that citrate use by *Enterobacter aerogenes* yielded the following products:

$$4\ \text{Citrate} \longrightarrow 7\ \text{Acetate} + 5\,CO_2 + \text{formate} + \text{succinate}$$

Use of organic acids and their salts for a carbon source produces alkaline carbonates and bicarbonates on further degradation (2, 22).

IV. MEDIA EMPLOYED

A. **Simmons citrate medium** (3, 11, 13, 22)
   1. Ingredients, pH 6.9 ± 0.2

Magnesium sulfate, $MgSO_4 \cdot 7H_2O$	0.2 g
Monoammonium phosphate or ammonium dihydrogen phosphate, $NH_4H_2PO_4$	1.0 g
Dipotassium phosphate, K_2HPO_4	1.0 g
Sodium citrate, $Na_3C_6H_5O_7 \cdot 2H_2O$	2.0 g
Sodium chloride, NaCl	5.0 g
Agar	15.0–20.0 g
Bromthymol blue (BTB)	0.08 g
Deionized water	1000.0 mL

      (*Note:* the ammonium salts are the sole source of nitrogen; sodium citrate, an anion, is the sole source of carbon (17).)

   2. pH indicator: bromthymol blue (BTB)
      a. Acid: pH 6.0, yellow color (not observed)
      b. Alkaline: pH 7.6, deep Prussian blue color
      c. Uninoculated medium: pH 6.9, green color
   3. Method of preparation
      a. Weigh amount accurately as directed on the label.
      b. Rehydrate with distilled or demineralized water.
      c. Heat **gently** into solution.
      d. Place approximately 4.0–5.0 mL in each tube (**long slant, short butt**).
   4. Method of sterilization: autoclave, 121°C, 15 lb, 15 min
   5. Allow medium to solidify in a **slanted** position.
   6. Cool before use and refrigerate for storage (4–10°C). Shelf life is approximately 6–8 weeks.
   7. Inoculation
      a. Growth from an 18- to 24-h **pure** culture on Kligler's iron agar (KIA) or other suitable culture; broth suspension is **not** recommended.
      b. Bring media to room temperature prior to inoculation.
      c. **Light** inoculum (4, 22); an inoculating needle (straight wire) is recommended (2).
      d. **Fishtail** (serpentine manner) **slant only.**
   8. Incubation: caps loosened (reaction requires oxygen), 35°C; 24–48 h. Longer incubation (up to 4 days) may be required (13).

Simmons citrate medium is a synthetic modification of the original Koser's medium (17), with the addition of 1.5% agar and a pH indicator, bromthymol blue (21, 22). Either sodium or potassium citrate may be incorporated into the medium for the carbon source (21).

B. **Christensen's citrate sulfide medium** (6, 11, 13)
   1. Ingredients, pH 6.7 ± 0.2

Yeast extract	0.5 g
Glucose (dextrose)	0.2 g
Sodium citrate, $Na_3C_6H_5O_7 \cdot 2H_2O$	3.0 g
Cysteine · HCl	0.1 g
Iron (III) ammonium citrate (50/50) (optional)	0.4 g
Ferric citrate, $C_6H_5O_7$	
Ammonium citrate, $(NH_4)_2HC_6H_5O_7$	
Monopotassium phosphate, KH_2PO_4	1.0 g
Sodium chloride, NaCl	5.0 g
Sodium thiosulfate, $Na_2S_2O_3 \cdot 5H_2O$ (optional)	0.08 g
Phenol red	0.012 g
Agar	15.0 g
Deionized water	1000.0 mL

(*Note:* Iron (III) is the new terminology for ferric ion (Fe^{3+}). Iron (III) ammonium citrate (50/50) is an H_2S indicator)

   2. Christensen's citrate sulfide medium tests for citrate use in the presence of organic nitrogen, cysteine monohydrochloride (13). If hydrogen sulfide production is not being determined, the ferric ammonium citrate and sodium thiosulfate may be eliminated from the medium since they do not affect citrate use (13).
   3. pH indicator: phenol red
      a. Acid: pH 6.8, yellow color
      b. Alkaline: pH 8.4, pink-red color
      c. Uninoculated medium: pH 6.7; cream to tan color (buff)
   4. Preparation, sterilization, storage, inoculation, and incubation as with Simmons citrate medium.

C. **Christensen citrate agar, modified**
   1. Formulation of Costin (8)
   2. Changes
      a. **No** H_2S indicators (iron (III) ammonium citrate or sodium thiosulfate)
      b. L-Cysteinium chloride, 0.1 g, replaces cysteine · HCl.
   3. Preparation, sterilization, storage, inoculation, and incubation as with Simmons citrate medium.

V. QUALITY CONTROL MICROORGANISMS

Positive controls:

Proteus rettgeri	ATCC 13315
Klebsiella pneumoniae subsp. *pneumoniae*	ATCC 13883
Enterobacter cloacae	ATCC 13047
Salmonella choleraesuis subsp. *choleraesuis*	ATCC 13312, ATCC 13314

Negative controls:

Escherichia coli	ATCC 11752 (may exhibit a trace of growth, but no color change)
Shigella flexneri	ATCC 12022
Morganella morganii biogroup 1	ATCC 25830
Uninoculated	

VI. RESULTS

> See Figure 7.1 (Appendix 1) for colored photographic results

VII. INTERPRETATION

A. Simmons citrate medium
  1. Positive (+): growth with an intense blue color on the slant
  2. Negative (−): no growth and no change in color (green)
B. Christensen's citrate medium and modified form
  1. Positive (+): pink-red color on the slant
  2. Negative (−): no color change (buff)

VIII. RAPID TEST: CITRATE BLOOD TEST

A. Method of Cordaro and Sellers (7)
B. Principle: To test the ability of an organism to use citrate in citrated blood to form a clot
C. Media
  1. Inoculum diluent
     a. Ingredients
        (1) Dehydrated brain-heart infusion broth (HIB)   12.5 g/L
        (2) Calcium chloride ($CaCl_2$)   100.0 mg
        (3) Sodium chloride (NaCl)   2.5 g
     b. Preparation
        (1) Dispense into screw-cap bottles (120 mL volume); 85.0 mL broth/bottle.
        (2) Method of sterilization: autoclave 121°C, 15 lb, 15 min
     c. Refrigerate for storage (4–10°C).
  2. Test medium
     a. To one bottle of HIB **aseptically** add 15.0 mL of outdated **citrated** blood bank blood.
     b. Mix and **aseptically** pipette 1.0-mL aliquots into small, **sterile** test tubes. Set up only the number of tubes required for one batch of tests.
     c. The remaining broth-blood mixture is good for 1–2 months when refrigerated.
D. Inoculum
  1. Growth from an 18-h **pure** culture, triple sugar iron agar (TSI)
  2. **Heavy** inoculum, 1 loopful
E. Incubation: 35°C, 1–3.5 h
  1. May require longer incubation, up to 6.5 h
  2. Examine tubes **hourly.**
F. Interpretation
  1. Positive (+): presence of a firm clot
  2. Negative (−): no clot formation; medium remains homogeneous

Formation of a clot in the citrate blood test indicates citrate use (7). According to Cordaro and Sellers (7), a nutritive inoculum medium is essential, but **do not** use saline or media that contains glucose (which delays the clotting time). A small amount of saline (2.5 g) is incorporated into the medium to prevent red blood cell lysis (7). Whole blood is preferred over plasma because it has a faster clotting time and does not require centrifugation.

IX. PRECAUTIONS

A. The color intensity in a citrate-positive result may vary because of differences in lots of commercial pH indicators (22).
B. Using a large inoculum to streak the slant may result in a light yellow to tan color on the slant, without affecting the color of the underlying medium (22). This color, however, **does not** denote a positive result. A too heavy inoculum may also give a false-positive result (4, 16). Preformed organic compounds within the cell walls of dying bacteria may release carbon and nitrogen to produce a false-positive result (16).
C. When inoculating a battery of media with the same culture, either flame the inoculating needle or loop before streaking the citrate medium or inoculate it first. Any carryover of glucose or other nutrients/substrates (e.g., proteins) onto the citrate medium can give a false-positive result (2); media **must** lack any protein or carbohydrates as a possible C source (16). Vaughn et al. (24) showed that if a readily metabolized substance such as peptone, glucose, or acetate is introduced onto the citrate slant, the citrate will be metabolized. Matsen and Sherris (18) and Branson (4) recommend diluting the inoculum in saline before inoculating citrate medium to avoid carrying over other carbon sources.
D. After a 24-h incubation, a citrate-positive organism may show slight alkalinity, barely visible on the slant. If the interpretation is in doubt, compare the tube with an uninoculated citrate tube. Some citrate-positive organisms require incubation for 48 h or longer for a pH change to occur.
E. If results are equivocal (±; e.g., *Providencia* spp.), inoculate a **new** slant and incubate at room temperature (22–25°C) for 7 days (1, 13).
F. H_2S production is indicated in the butt of Christensen's medium as a black discoloration; however, the results of H_2S production **may not** agree with those obtained on KIA and/or TSI.
G. The reaction requires oxygen, so caps must be loosened during incubation.
H. Prepared Simmons citrate medium may be slightly opalescent and may have a slight precipitate (11).
I. A test result may be read as positive even though no color change is evident if there is visible colonial growth along the inoculation streak (16). This is possible because growth is visible only when organisms have entered the log phase of growth, which is possible only if C and N have been assimilated. With incubation for an additional 24 h, color change usually develops (16).
J. To prevent delay in initiation of growth and medium reaction, the inoculum **should not** be taken from a suspension of the organism in liquid or broth. Some *E. coli* strains may give a positive result after 2–3 days incubation because of growth supported by broth (19); this could result in *E. coli* being misidentified as *Citrobacter koseri* (formerly *Citrobacter diversus*).

REFERENCES

1. Balows A, Hausler WJ Jr, Herrmann KL, et al., eds. Manual of Clinical Microbiology, ed 5. Washington, DC: American Society for Microbiology, 1991:1239–1240.
2. Baron EJ, Finegold SM. Bailey & Scott's Diagnostic Microbiology, ed 8. St. Louis: CV Mosby, 1990:366, 376.
3. BBL Quality Control and Product Information Manual for Tubed Media. Cockeysville, MD: Becton-Dickinson Microbiology Systems (BBL), 1987. T21026- Rev 0.0
4. Branson D. Methods in Clinical Bacteriology. Springfield, IL: Charles C Thomas, 1972:15–16.
5. Campbell JJR, Bellamy WD, Gunsalus IC. Organic acids as substrates for streptococci. J Bacteriol 1943;46(6):573.
6. Christensen WB. Hydrogen sulfide production and citrate utilization in the differentiation of enteric pathogens and coliform bacteria. Res Bull Weld County Health Dept (Greeley, CO) 1949;1:3–16.
7. Cordaro JT, Sellers W. Blood coagulation test for citrate utilization. Appl Microbiol 1968;16(1):168–169.
8. Costin ID. Bemerkungen zur Praxis der biochemischen identifizierung der Darmbakterien

in der Routinearbeit. Zentralb Bakteriol Parasitkde I Ref 1965;198(5):385–463.
9. Deffner M. Anaerobic fermentation of citric acid by bacteria. Ann Chem (Leipzig) 1938;536:44.
10. Deffner M, Franke W. Degradation of citric acid by bacteria. Ann Chem (Leipzig) 1939;541:85.
11. Difco Manual, ed 10. Detroit: Difco Laboratories, 1984:219–220 864–865.
12. Doelle HW. Bacterial Metabolism. New York: Academic Press, 1969:335.
13. Ewing WH. Edwards and Ewing's Identification of *Enterobacteriaceae*, ed 4. New York: Elsevier, 1986:517.
14. Gunsalus IC, Campbell JJR. Diversion of the lactic acid fermentation with oxidized substrate. J Bacteriol 1944;48(4):455–461.
15. Gunsalus IC, Stanier RY. The Bacteria, vol II. New York: Academic Press, 1961:130–131.
16. Koneman EW, Allen EW, Janda WM, et al. Color Atlas and Textbook of Diagnostic Microbiology, ed 4. Philadelphia: JB Lippincott, 1983: 121–123, 143, 146, 151, 177.
17. Koser SA. Utilization of the salts of organic acids by the Colon-Aerogenes group. J Bacteriol 1932; 8(5):493–520.
18. Matsen JM, Sherris JC. Comparative study of the efficacy of seven paper reagent strips and conventional biochemical tests in identifying gram-negative organisms. Appl Microbiol 1969;18(3): 452–457.
19. Oberhofer TR. Manual of Practical Medical Microbiology and Parasitology. New York: John Wiley & Sons, 1985:144.
20. Oehr P, Willecke K. Citrate-Mg^{2+} transport in *Bacillus subtilis* studies with 2-fluoro-L-erythro-citrate as a substrate. J Biol Chem 1974;249(7): 2037–2042.
21. Ruchhoft CC, Kallas JG, Chinn B, Coulter EW. Coli-Aerogenes differentiation in water analysis. II. The biochemical differential tests and their interpretation. J Bacteriol 1931;22(1): 125–181.
22. Simmons JS. A culture medium for differentiating organisms of the typhoid-colon aerogenes groups and for isolation of certain fungi. J Infect Dis 1926;39:209–214.
23. Sokatch JR. Bacterial Physiology and Metabolism. New York: Academic Press, 1969:133–141.
24. Vaughn RH, Osborne JT, Wedding GT, et al. The utilization of citrate by *Escherichia coli*. J Bacteriol 1950;60(2):119–127.
25. Washington JA. Laboratory Procedures in Clinical Microbiology, ed 2. New York: Springer-Verlag, 1985.194.

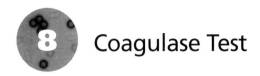

8. Coagulase Test

I. PRINCIPLE

To test the ability of an organism to clot plasma by the action of the enzyme coagulase (staphylocoagulase)

II. PURPOSE

(Also see Chapter 43)

A. The coagulase test is used specifically to differentiate species within the genus *Staphylococcus*.
   1. *S. aureus* subsp. *anaerobius*, *S. aureus* subsp. *aureus*, *S. schleiferi* subsp. *coagulans* are all positive for staphylocoagulase (free coagulase, tube test).
   2. *S. aureus* subsp. *aureus*, *S. lugdunensis* and *S. schleiferi* subsp. *schleiferi* are all positive for clumping factor (bound coagulase, slide test). *S. intermedius* is variable for bound coagulase.
   3. Other human or animal *Staphylococcus* spp. are coagulase positive by the slide or tube procedure or both; however, they are infrequently encountered (Table 8.1).
B. *Peptostreptococcus indolicus* (+) from other *Peptostreptococcus* spp. (−) that may cause human infections
C. Differentiation of *Erysipelothrix rhusiopathiae* (+) from *Listeria* (−) and *Corynebacterium* spp. (−) (82)

Table 8.1. Coagulase-Positive *Staphylococcus* Species

Organism	Coagulase Slide	Coagulase Tube	Heat-Stable Endonuclease
S. aureus subsp. *anaerobius*	−	+[a]	+
S. aureus subsp. *aureus*	+	+	+
S. lugdunensis[b,c]	+	−	−
S. schleiferi subsp. *coagulans*	+	−	+
S. schleiferi subsp. *schleiferi*[b]	+	−	+
S. hyicus[d]	−	V[a]	+
S. intermedius[d]	V	+[a]	+
S. delphini[d]	−	+[a]	−

Data from references 10, 18, 33, 37, 38, 41, 42, 46, 84.
[a]Strains deficient in clumping factor (slide negative) will usually produce free coagulase (tube positive).
[b]Human isolates (33); human plasma is recommended for testing (4).
[c]Latex agglutination is less reliable for detection of clumping factor or fibrinogen (4).
[d]Animal isolates (5, 83). *S. intermedius* and *S. hyicus* are rarely isolated from humans (5). Separation (42):

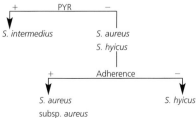

PYR, L-Pyrrolidonyl-β-naphthylamide hydrolysis test.

A positive coagulase result is usually the final diagnostic criterion for the identification of *S. aureus* subsp. *aureus*, and it is frequently used to indicate virulence or pathogenicity. Rarely, an *S. aureus* subsp. *aureus* strain is coagulase negative.

III. BIOCHEMISTRY INVOLVED

Staphylocoagulase (coagulase), the enzyme produced by *S. aureus*, is relatively heat stable, being resistant to temperatures up to 60°C for 30 min (12, 75). This protein is excreted extracellularly by human strains of *S. aureus* (12, 86), and is easily inactivated by proteolytic enzymes (proteases) (65).

The chemical structure of staphylocoagulase is unknown (61, 75); however, there are many hypotheses about the mechanism of coagulase action. Coagulase acts on some constituent of serum to produce a clot or thrombus (78). In vitro, coagulase increases the rate of plasma clotting resulting in formation of a fibrin clot (61).

$$\text{Plasma} \xrightarrow[\text{coagulase}]{\text{bacterium}} \text{Fibrin clot}$$

The normal mechanism of clotting is shown in the following diagram (61).

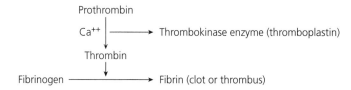

Oginsky and Umbreit (61) state that evidence suggests that coagulase may induce an alternate activating mechanism, either as an enzyme or an activator of a plasma component, to convert fibrinogen to fibrin. Smith et al. (75) suggest that coagulase is a prothrombin-like substance that reacts with normal plasma factors to form a thrombinlike substance that in turn activates fibrinogen to form fibrin.

Burrows et al. (12) state that plasma clotting occurs in two steps: (*a*) a reaction between the bacterial enzyme, a **procoagulase**, with a factor or activator present in plasma to form **coagulase**, and (*b*) the actual plasma clotting activated by coagulase. According to Burrows et al. (12), the actual bacterial factor is procoagulase and the plasma factor is a globulin fraction similar but not identical to prothrombin. Duthrie (25) shows evidence that the enzyme coagulase, which Burrows et al. (12) say is really procoagulase, is present in two forms: bound coagulase (bound to the cell) and free coagulase.

Bound Coagulase

Bound coagulase is detected by the **slide procedure**, the plasma clumping test (12, 25). It is **not** present in culture filtrates (11, 23, 25) but is found on surface of cell walls (46). Bound coagulase, or clumping factor (CF), is responsible for absorbing fibrinogen and altering it so that it precipitates on the staphylococci and causes them to clump (60), resulting in rapid cell agglutination (46). Clumping factor converts fibrinogen to fibrin **directly**, with no involvement of plasma factors, and it is not inhibited by antibodies to free coagulase (23, 64).

Free Coagulase

The **tube coagulase test** detects both free and bound coagulase, with the only distinction between them being antigenic (25). Extracellular free coagulase reacts with a substance in plasma (serum factor) that Dubos and Hirsch (23) and Drummond and Tager (22) called coagulase-reacting factor or CRF, a thermostable, thrombinlike substance (64). CRF is an activator, a modified or derived thrombin molecule (84). Extracellular free coagulase reacts with CRF to form a coagulase-CRF complex, a substance similar but not identical to thrombin. This complex acts **in**directly to convert fibrinogen to fibrin (46). During clotting, similar peptides are released from fibrinogen and the coagulase-CRF complex (22). The main difference is that coagulase-reacting CRF does not require calcium ions to form a clot (11, 73) and is insensitive to heparin (73).

CRF + free coagulase ⟶ Coagulase-CRF complex

Coagulase reacting factor

Coagulase-CRF complex + fibrinogen ⟶ Fibrin clot

Studies by Soulier et al. (76), Tager (80), and Zajdel et al., (94), however, showed that staphylocoagulase and prothrombin possess no enzymatic activity, but their interaction results in the formation of a stable complex with specific proteolytic activity, called staphylothrombin. Staphylocoagulase does not possess proteolytic activation (95); it reacts specifically with prothrombin in a stoichiometric process (definite proportions) (86) that activates prothrombin (95) and converts fibrinogen to a fibrin clot in a manner resembling the action of physiologically formed thrombin (43, 44, 68, 76, 80, 81, 86, 94).

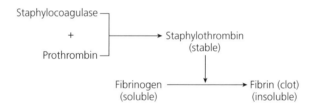

Clotting ability does not depend on calcium ions (9, 11). The staphylocoagulase concentration influences the rate of plasma clotting; the higher the concentration, the faster a clot will be formed. A high concentration causes instantaneous clotting of plasma (39).

The function of coagulase in vivo is still undetermined. For years it was believed that coagulase caused formation of a fibrin layer (wall) around a staphylococcal lesion, thereby possibly providing a deposit of fibrin on the surface of individual staphylococci, creating a barrier against antimicrobial drugs and the phagocytic action of leukocytes (23, 45, 61). Studies by Rogers and Tompsett (71) failed to support the theory that phagocytes cannot engulf *S. aureus* subsp. *aureus* organisms when a fibrin barrier is present. Dubos and Hirsch (23) suggest that the fibrin barrier may localize staphylococcal lesions.

Ekstedt (27), Ekstedt and Nungester (28), and Yotis and Ekstedt (91) showed that coagulase production neutralizes or inhibits the antibacterial activity of normal serum against *S. aureus* subsp. *aureus,* which is normally bactericidal (27). Coagulase-producing *S. aureus* subsp. *aureus* organisms can grow in normal serum; coagulase-negative *Staphylococcus* cannot (28). Ehrenkranz et al. (26) found that human serum may exert a bacteriostatic activity against some coagulase-negative or coagulase-positive strains. The mechanism is undetermined, but Yotis and Ekstedt (91) found that it is not related to the bacterial respiratory mechanism.

Coagulase activity is independent of other staphylococcal toxins that may be produced by *S. aureus* subsp. *aureus* (12). However, Cowan (15) states that all coagulase-positive *S. aureus* subsp. *aureus* strains produce either α or β hemolysins or both. Burrows et al. (12) state that α or δ hemolysins, also indications of virulent strains, are associated with coagulase activity. Young and Leitner (92) found no correlation between hemolysin production and coagulase. Weckman and Catlin (85) correlated coagulase production with deoxyribonuclease formation.

Staphylocoagulase is antigenic (13, 56, 75); Rammelkamp et al. (66), Duthrie (24), and Zen-Yoji et al. (96) recognize seven distinct antigenic staphylocoagulases. However, Miale et al. (56) recognize only four antigenic types (A, B, C, and D), collectively termed isocoagulases. Smith et al. (75) state that there are two distinct types, I and II, with some *S. aureus* subsp. *aureus* producing one or the other and some producing both. A positive coagulase slide reaction resembles specific agglutination and often has been called nonspecific agglutination (13).

In vitro plasma coagulation by *S. aureus* subsp. *aureus* is due to the production of an enzyme concerned with the normal clotting mechanism. Other genera can coagulate plasma, not enzymatically, but by destroying the plasma anticoagulant (7, 32, 39, 54, 63).

IV. REAGENTS EMPLOYED

A. **Plasma or fibrinogen**
  1. Plasma
     a. Recommended: human or rabbit
     b. Alternatives: horse, sheep, or bovine
     c. **Sterile**
     d. Fresh or lyophilized (dehydrated)
  2. Fibrinogen: **sterile** and fresh
B. Commercial lyophilized products are available.
C. Methods of preparation
  1. Commercial plasma
     a. Reconstitute only the amount required for daily use. Storing rehydrated vials is not recommended (65).
     b. With a **sterile** pipette, rehydrate with distilled water according to directions on the label.
        (1) Various company products may differ slightly.
        (2) Vials are prepared containing 1.0, 2.5, 3.0, 15.0, and 25.0 mL.
  2. Fresh plasma from whole blood (16)
     a. Allow red cells to settle out or centrifuge a bag of whole blood.
     b. **Aseptically** remove supernatant (plasma) containing anticoagulant into a **sterile** container. Avoid drawing off red cells.
  3. Fresh fibrinogen (13)
     a. **Aseptically** remove anticoagulant-containing plasma from whole blood.
     b. Precipitate fibrinogen from fresh citrated plasma
        (1) Mix equal volumes of plasma and a saturated salt solution.
        (2) Allow fibrinogen to precipitate.
        (3) Centrifuge.
     c. Make up precipitated fibrinogen to 5 times its volume with **sterile** distilled water.
     d. Store in a **sterile** container.
     e. Fibrinogen is effective for either the slide or the tube coagulase procedure even when diluted up to 1:160.

Before using either citrated plasma or citrated fibrinogen, addition of heparin is recommended to eliminate a false-positive delayed coagulase reaction by organisms capable of using citrate and thus causing plasma to clot (7, 32, 39, 54, 67, 89). Wood (89) suggests adding 5 units of heparin per milliliter of citrated plasma to inhibit coagulation by citrate-using organisms, thereby making the test more specific for *Staphylococcus* spp.

The coagulability of plasma may be checked by its recalcification. Add 1 drop of a 5% calcium chloride solution ($CaCl_2$) to 0.5 mL of plasma (1:2 dilution), and a clot should form (39).

D. Storage: Store unopened dehydrated commercial vials of plasma in a refrigerator (4°C) when not in use, to preserve their stability (65). Keeping reconstituted plasma more than the day of use is not recommended; however, if necessary, it may be refrigerated for a few days and used if there is no evidence of contamination (65). If reconstituted plasma must be stored, freezing (−20°C) is preferred over refrigeration (65).

Fresh plasma or fibrinogen **must** be either refrigerated (4°C) or frozen (−20°C). Many recommend that plasma not be frozen if it is to be used for coagulase testing (16); however, the coagulability of plasma is not affected by freezing, and it is usable as long as a quality control check is performed **prior** to its general use. The stability of all reagents, plasma (either fresh, dehydrated, or frozen), and fibrinogen varies, and each batch or lot should be checked and discarded when it yields a negative or weak reaction with a known positive organism. If commercial plasma does not react properly in a quality control check, the entire lot may be returned to the company for replacement.

The plasma factor among animal species varies, which accounts for its differences in clotting behavior. Most coagulases clot human, pig, rabbit, and horse plasma but not rat, chicken, guinea pig, bovine, or sheep plasma (12, 62). Orth et al. (62) found the highest CRF concentration in human plasma, with decreasing concentrations in pig, rabbit, and horse, and the lowest in bovine, chicken, and sheep. Plasma used for coagulase testing must (a) contain sufficient CRF and fibrinogen, (b) be fairly free of fibrinolytic activity, and (c) be reasonably free of inhibitors (81).

Fibrinolysis occurs when the plasminogen-plasmin (profibrinolysin-fibrinolysin) system is activated by the staphylokinase (Sf) enzyme and staphylococcal Müller factor (MF), resulting in formation of plasmin (fibrinolysin) and lysis of the fibrin clot (40, 62). Orth et al. (62) observed fibrinolysis when rabbit, human, sheep, and horse plasma was used in the coagulase **agar** method. Plasmin activity was strongest in rabbit plasma and decreased with human, sheep, and horse. Bovine, chicken, and pig plasma had the weakest activity (62). The presence of a fibrin clot denotes the absence or weakness of plasmin activity.

Cowan (16) reported that sheep or bovine plasma is clotted by coagulase but gives fewer positive results. Chapman (14) states that rabbit plasma is preferred over human because the clot is firmer and coagulation is faster. Morton and Cohn (57) recommend **not using** human plasma when inoculating a tube test from a solid medium, but either rabbit or human is acceptable when testing a culture grown in a broth. Needham et al. (59) recommend using only rabbit plasma, regardless of the type of medium used to grow the inoculum.

Needham et al. (59) explain their preference for rabbit plasma by suggesting that *S. aureus* subsp. *aureus* loses its ability to produce coagulase when inoculated from a **solid medium** because of inhibition by antibodies in human plasma. Streitfeld et al. (78) showed growth of *S. aureus* but coagulase inhibition due to α-globulin, and Ehrenkranz et al. (26) demonstrated bacteriostatic action in human sera against strains of *Staphylococcus*, which was eliminated by using diluted human plasma inoculated from a possible staphylococcal broth culture.

Yearsly and Carter (90) found that diabetic plasma showed slightly more coagulase activity than normal human plasma as long as the diabetic was not under insulin control.

Dehydrated rabbit plasma with citrate or ethylenediaminetetraacetate (EDTA, or sequestric acid) is recommended for identification of *S. aureus, S. intermedius,* and *S. hyicus;* human plasma is better for *S. lugdunensis* and *S. schleiferi* (47). Plasma from blood samples undergoing biochemical testing may be used if sodium fluoride is not used as the anticoagulant (16). Cowan (16) also recommended not using plasma samples that contain the anticoagulant EDTA. However, most laboratories recommend EDTA, since it is not used by bacteria and it eliminates false-positive coagulation of plasma by citrate-using bacteria (11). Staphylocoagulase will clot plasma regardless of which anticoagulant (oxalate, citrate, or heparin) is present (39). Clotting occurs up to a plasma dilution of 1:100, limited mainly by the amount of fibrinogen present (39). Oxalated or citrated plasma may be used for staphylocoagulase detection, since calcium is not a factor (12).

V. QUALITY CONTROL MICROORGANISMS

(*Note:* Both plasma and fibrinogen, if used, must be tested with known positive and negative cultures before being put into general use.)

A. Positive (+): *Staphylococcus aureus* subsp. *aureus* ATCC 12600
B. Negative (−): *Staphylococcus epidermidis* ATCC 14990

VI. PROCEDURES

A. **Slide test (plasma clumping test):** rapid and relatively specific for detection of bound coagulase (5, 8, 12, 13, 16, 63) with most *S. aureus* subsp. *aureus* strains
   1. Place a **sterile** drop of either distilled water or physiologic saline (0.85% NaCl) on a clear, clean glass slide.
   2. **Gently** emulsify a **heavy** suspension of *Staphylococcus* organism (from an 18- to 24-h **pure** broth culture or a loopful of a single, **pure** isolated colony on plate medium) in the drop of saline (or water).
   3. **Gently** mix a small loopful of pretested **fresh human plasma** in the suspension of staphylococci; the mixture **must** be homogeneous (i.e., smooth).
   4. Set up positive and negative control organisms on the same slide to be tested simultaneously.
   5. Observe for **immediate** formation of macroscopic precipitate in the form of white clumps.
      a. A positive coagulase result usually occurs within 5–20 **sec.**
      b. The result is considered negative if coagulation does not occur within 3–4 **min.**

The slide coagulase test is only a **presumptive** procedure (16), and all negative or delayed results (over 20 sec) **must** be confirmed by the tube test (13, 16, 88), since the results of the slide test do not precisely parallel those of the tube (12, 63).

This procedure is used to screen a large number of possible *S. aureus* subsp. *aureus* cultures, but it is reliable only when performed by an experienced microbiologist who is aware that a heavy inoculum of organism must be used along with a small amount of plasma (13, 88). The rate of coagulation (clumping) depends on the ratio of organisms and plasma concentration; diluting plasma before use decreases the speed of a positive reaction (13). An equal concentration of plasma (undiluted) and organism usually results in immediate clumping (within 5–6 sec) of staphylococci (13).

A suspected colony must be mixed in distilled water or physiologic saline **prior** to the addition of plasma. Any precipitation or clumping that occurs in this mixture is due to autoagglutination by the organism, not by coagulase (13).

B. **Tube test;** detection of **bound** and **free** coagulase (15, 65)
   1. **Sterile** glass tube (13 × 100 mm)
      a. Add 0.5 mL of pretested, **undiluted,** human or rabbit plasma.
      b. Add 0.5 mL of an 18- to 24-h **pure** broth culture of *Staphylococcus* organism or a **large** loopful of a pure colony from an agar plate.
   2. **Rotate tube gently** to suspend the bacteria. **Do not shake.**
   3. Incubation: 37°C water bath, 4 h; observe every 30 min for clotting.
      a. When checking **do not shake or agitate the tube. Gently** slant the tube to observe for a clot.

b. If no clot is visible after 4 h, leave the tube in the water bath or place in a 35°C incubator overnight (24 h).
c. Gillespie (35) and Cowan (15) recommend that the overnight incubation (24 h) be at room temperature (22°C).

Baron and Finegold (5) recommend using a 1:4 dilution of plasma with a broth culture and a 1:5 dilution when adding a single colony to plasma. Cowan (15) suggests using undiluted plasma with a broth culture but diluting plasma 1:2 when suspending a single colony. Harper and Conway (39) recommend a 1:2 dilution, and Gilllspie (35) a 1:10 dilution of plasma. Fisk (31) and Williams and Harper (88) report that the clot forms best when culture and plasma are mixed in equal proportions, with the plasma undiluted. However, staphylocoagulase produces a clot in plasma diluted up to 1:100 (39).

VII. RESULTS

> See Figure 8.1 (Appendix 1) for colored photographic results

VIII. INTERPRETATION

A. **Slide procedure**
  1. Positive (+) (13)
     a. **Marked** clumping within **5–20 sec**
     b. *S. aureus,* virulent strain
  2. Delayed positive (13)
     a. Any clumping or granulation after **20 sec** and up to **1 min**
     b. *S. aureus,* virulent strain
  3. Doubtful (13, 16, 88)
     a. Any granulation after **1 min**
     b. **Repeat;** if result is identical, **confirm by tube** test before reporting result.
  4. Negative (−)
     a. No change; suspension remains homogeneous
     b. **Confirm by tube test** before reporting result.
     c. *S. epidermidis, S. saprophyticus* (5) or other organism
B. **Tube procedure** (5, 88)
  1. Positive (+)
     a. Clot or distinct fibrin threads formed
        (1) Complete: clot throughout tube
        (2) Partial: clot does not extend throughout fluid column. Any clotting is considered positive (see Precautions, XI.E.6, for discussion on clot formation).
     b. *S. aureus,* virulent strain
  2. Negative (−)
     a. No clot formation, suspension remains homogeneous (same as uninoculated)
     b. *S. epidermidis S. saprophyticus* (5) or other organism

IX. ALTERNATIVE TESTS

A. **Pour-plate coagulase test**
  1. Method of Parisi, Baldwin, and Sottile (63)
     a. Detects coagulase production
     b. Primary ingredients

(1) Brain heart infusion agar (BHI) or YETS agar (Trypticase soy broth and 0.3% yeast extract).
            (2) Plasma: **preferred**, swine (pig) (62, 63); alternate, rabbit
        2. Correlation with standard **tube** test is excellent (48). Parisi et al. (63) recommend **not** using human plasma for the pour-plate technique.
    B. **Tube coagulase-thermonuclease test**
        1. Method of Barry, Lachica, and Atchison (6)
            a. Detects
                (1) Free coagulase
                (2) Thermonuclease (heat-stable nuclease)
            b. Primary ingredients
                (1) Brain heart infusion broth (BHI)
                    (a) Inoculum diluent
                    (b) Preincubation medium, **an absolute requirement**
                (2) EDTA-coagulase plasma
                (3) Toluidine blue deoxyribonucleic acid (DNA) agar (TDA) technique
        2. Correlation with standard **tube** test: Barry et al. (6) recommend performing both tests simultaneously as quality control check.
        3. See Chapter 10, Deoxyribonuclease (DNase) and Thermonuclease (Tnase) Tests.
    C. **Coagulase-mannitol agar plate test (C-M)**
        1. Method of Esber and Faulconer (29)
        2. Detects
            a. Both bound and free coagulase
            b. Mannitol fermentation
        3. Primary ingredients
            a. Human blood plasma, 7.0%
            b. Mannitol, 1.0%

X. COMMERCIAL SLIDE COAGULASE TESTS

A. **Latex agglutination tests** (46) are rapid, definitive tests for identification **without** need for further tests on clumping factor–negative isolates (5).
    1. Advantages (47)
        a. Methods and interpretations are standardized
        b. Often higher specificity and sensitivity than conventional slide test for identification of *S. aureus* subsp. *aureus,* but less reliable for identification of *S. lugdunensis*
    2. Principal ingredients
        a. Latex beads coated with plasma
        b. Fibrinogen bound to latex
    3. Detects cell surface antigens; all based on characteristics of coagulase-positive strains.
        a. Clumping factor
        b. Protein A, a staphylococcal cell-wall protein able to bind IgA molecules by Fc region; coagulase-negative staphylococci (CONS) lack protein A (11).
    4. Commercial systems
        a. Larsson and Sjoquist's procedure; latex beads coated with chicken anti–protein A antibodies (53)
        b. Kits (see Chapter 42, Multitests, *Staphylococcus* Identification II.U.1)

XI. PRECAUTIONS

A. **General**
    1. The most virulent strains of *S. aureus* possess coagulase; coagulase production is con-

sidered synonymous with invasive pathogenic potential (45). Ehrenkranz et al. (26), Morton and Cohn (57), and Wegrzynowicz et al. (86) recommend **not** using the presence or absence of staphylocoagulase as a criterion for virulence; the clinical symptoms are of greater significance in determining pathogenicity (26, 57). S. aureus and coagulase-negative mutants produce lesions of the same character, and the correlation of coagulase with virulence is often only coincidental (17).
  2. *S. aureus* strains that are resistant to methicillin are deficient in clumping factor (19, 51). Oberhofer (60) and Koneman et al. (46) recommend confirming negative-reacting methicillin-resistant strains by the tube test or thermonuclease test.
  3. Including an autoagglutination control decreases the number of false-positive results (clot) (5).
B. **Culture**
  1. Weak or negative coagulase activity may occur if mutant strains are present, if a broth culture of suspected organism is too old (must be an 18- to 24-h culture), or if growth is scant (65).
  2. Storing agar cultures (regardless of temperature or other conditions of storage) results in significant loss of clumping factor activity, which is often **not** restored after subculture.
C. **Plasma**
  1. In the coagulase test, plasma is the source of prothrombin (CRF) and fibrinogen, and the procedure is based on the **assumption** that clot formation is **solely** due to staphylocoagulase (79). However, plasma proenzymes (prothrombin and plasminogen) may be activated by proteases (1–3, 20, 72, 86, 87), which hydrolyze peptide bonds of proteins to yield polypeptides (40). Proenzymes are catalytic inactive forms of enzymes that undergo limited proteolysis (conformational changes) and are converted to active enzyme (thrombin and plasmin) by either proteolytic enzymes or H^+ ions (40). Staphylococci produce several extracellular proteases that **cannot** form staphylothrombin but can cause a pseudocoagulase (86). These proteases, under certain conditions, stimulate the clotting effect of staphylocoagulase and the lytic effect of staphylokinase in **rabbit** plasma in the **absence of staphylocoagulase**; they activate prothrombin and/or plasminogen by limited proteolysis (86). Which protease causes clotting/fibrinolysis is currently unknown; Wegrzynowicz et al. (86) consider it more likely that interactions of several staphylococcal proteases are involved. Arvidson (1, 2), Arvidson et al. (3), Drapeau (20), and Rydén et al. (72) have isolated several proteases that exhibit properties different from proteases from single strains of *S. aureus* subsp. *aureus*; these proteases possess narrower and broader substrate specificity (1, 72).

  Proteases such as trypsin and papain in low concentration in plasma can digest prothrombin and/or plasminogen (49, 55, 74). *Bacteroides melaninogenicus* (86, 87) proteases temporarily convert prothrombin and/or plasminogen to thrombin and/or plasmin (86).

  Dilution of **fresh** rabbit plasma may increase the effect of proteases because of simultaneous dilution of natural inhibitors (86). Therefore, to determine **true** staphylocoagulase activity and to avoid possible false-positive (clot) and false-negative (lysis) results, **addition** of protease inhibitors to the test plasma is recommended to block protease action (86). Inhibitors are inactive against true staphylocoagulase or its substrate, but they block proteases.

  To a 0.05-mL aliquot of an **incubated** staphylococcal culture grown in heart infusion broth (HIB), add 0.5 mL of either (*a*) **sterile** fresh rabbit citrated plasma diluted 1:5 with **sterile** saline, (*b*) plasma containing in 1 mL, 100 U of aprotinin (Trasylol, Bayer; see Appendix 11) and 50 U of hirudin (Reanal), or (*c*) plasma containing in 1 mL, 100 U of aprotinin and 20 U of heparin. Wegrzynowicz et al. (87) found that a mixture of aprotinin and hirudin inhibits nonspecific clotting more strongly than aprotinin and heparin. Differences are due to the fact that commercial hirudin contains basic enzymatic activity plus some inhibitors of various proteases (34).

Hirudin inhibits thrombin (i.e., is an antithrombin). It is a scarce and extremely expensive substance extracted from the salivary glands of leeches. Aprotinin, a polypeptide, is a protease and plasmin inhibitor from animal organs.

Staphylothrombin is **resistant** to natural thrombin inhibitors such as heparin, hirudin, and antithrombin III (48, 76) but **sensitive** to specific antibodies, EDTA, and diisopropylfluorophosphate (an inhibitor of serine proteases) (1, 21, 72).

2. Fresh plasma is **un**stable and may coagulate or form particles that produce turbidity or a deposit, making it difficult to interpret a weak-positive coagulase result (16).
3. Plasma used for coagulase testing should **not** be filtered (15, 16); filtering removes blood clotting agents (39).
4. If using plasma from outdated human blood bank blood or freshly drawn blood from hospitalized patients, be aware that inhibitors may be present. If variable amounts of coagulase-reactive factor and antistaphylococcal antibodies are present, **do not use** (46). Test the usual quality control organisms (a strong positive and a negative) **plus** a weakly positive organism (5, 57). If only such blood is available, the problem can be alleviated by diluting the plasma and taking the inoculum from a broth culture (57). Human plasma **must** be checked before use, since it may contain antibiotic or antibodies to staphylococci, as well as hepatitis antigen (60).
5. Sperber and Tatini (77) found that 55 non–*S. aureus* strains produced 3+ and 2+ clots with Difco rabbit plasma but were nonclotting with BBL plasma. Variations in clotting and type of plasma were also demonstrated by Yrios (93). Therefore, it is **absolutely necessary** that positive and negative controls be set up each day plasma is used and better yet, with each batch of test organisms.
6. Rabbit plasma is superior for tube test because reactions are faster (60). Rabbit plasma with EDTA is recommended for both slide and tube procedures (46).
7. Plasma stored in a refrigerator may be sufficiently cold to delay coagulation, especially in the slide test. It is advisable to allow plasma to come to room temperature (22–25°C) before use (16).
8. Storage of rehydrated plasma is **not** recommended (65).

D. **Slide test**
1. The slide test is only a **presumptive** procedure (12), and all negative or delayed results (over 20 sec) must be confirmed by the tube test (8, 12, 59). Some strains of *S. aureus* (10–15, 47) may be negative by the slide test (5); they lack the clumping factor (5).
2. Balows et al. (4) consider it **absolutely necessary** to use **fresh, human plasma** rather than commercial dehydrated plasma for the slide test.
3. In the slide procedure, any granulation or clumping in the organism-distilled water (or saline) suspension **prior** to addition of plasma is most likely due to autoagglutination by the organism, **not** coagulase activity (13). Cadness-Graves et al. (13) reported three autoagglutinable strains. The bacterial suspension **must** be observed for autoagglutination, since failure to detect it will give a false-positive slide coagulase test result.
4. Cadness-Graves et al. (13) recommend confirming a positive slide coagulase result by a Gram stain, checking for typical *Staphylococcus* morphology (Gram-positive cocci in grapelike clusters). Branson (10) recommends checking morphology by staining the positive slide with crystal violet.
5. If the colony does not emulsify (mix) smoothly, the test cannot be interpreted (10).
6. **Do not** use growth from an inhibitory medium containing salt (e.g., mannitol salt agar (10)); high salt causes some strains to autoagglutinate (10, 46).
7. The most frequent cause of false-negative results (lysis) is insufficient suspension of organism on the slide. A **heavy** inoculum is a must (60).
8. False-positive results (clot) occur when the reaction time exceeds 10 sec (47).

E. **Tube test**
   1. When performing the tube test **do not shake or agitate the tube** when checking for clot formation. A doubtful or false-negative (lysis) result may occur due to clot breakdown early in the coagulation stage (88); the clot will not reform with additional incubation.
   2. If plasma is inactivated or if a 1:10,000 solution of the preservative merthiolate is added, there will be interference with the tube test but not with the slide procedure (12).
   3. Some *S. aureus* subsp. *aureus* strains produce a high concentration of fibrinolysin resulting in the absence of a clot because of early lysis or a small clot early in incubation which soon lyses (16, 62, 93) and yields a false-negative result. This is particularly possible with use of rabbit plasma (62). Therefore, the tube should be observed every 30 min for clot formation, particularly during the first hour of incubation (95).
   4. Some *S. aureus* subsp. *aureus* strains produce so little staphylocoagulase that clotting activity is observed only after a 24-h incubation (16, 95).
   5. Coagulase activity is generally considered specific for *S. aureus*. However, other organisms can coagulate citrated plasma. The ability to coagulate citrated plasma is widely distributed among bacteria. Bayliss and Hall (7) and Fredericq (32) reported such activity by *Serratia marcescens*. Krech (50) reported a cell-free filtrate of *Escherichia coli* capable of clotting plasma, and Billaudelle (8) reported clotting ability in some strains of *Bordetella pertussis*. Other Gram-negative organisms found capable of clotting plasma are *Actinomyces* (32), *Klebsiella-Enterobacter* (36), and *Pseudomonas aeruginosa* (12, 54).

      It is generally agreed (7, 12, 30, 39, 54, 58, 63, 70) that these organisms do not produce coagulase but that they break down the anticoagulant citrate, releasing calcium ions that in turn activate the normal mechanisms of blood clotting, the conversion of prothrombin to thrombin (7). Paper chromatography studies by Bayliss and Hall (7) show that positive coagulase tests with organisms other than *S. aureus* coincide with the absence of citrate from the test citrated plasma.

      Coagulation does not occur if plasma has been filtered or inactivated by heparin (39). Also, clot formation is lacking if there is a high concentration of citrate or if the calcium ions are tied up by the anticoagulant oxalate (a nonmetabolizable salt) (39). The anticoagulant EDTA is not broken down by citrate-using bacteria; EDTA chelates divalent ions and is the recommended anticoagulant for the coagulase test (60). If citrated plasma is diluted more than 1:8, a clot will not form, since the clotting elements are too dilute to act (39). Most Gram-negative citrate-destroying organisms usually require 18 h or longer to form a clot; catabolism depends on the concentration of citrate present and the organism's rate of growth (39). Staphylocoagulase clots plasma regardless of the anticoagulant used: oxalate, citrate, EDTA, or heparin.

      Evans et al. (30) reported that group D *Enterococcus* spp. can clot citrated plasma, mainly as a delayed reaction (24 h), but not plasma containing other anticoagulants. Bayliss and Hall (7), Lotter and Horstmann (54), and Young and Leitner (92) also reported clotting activity by *Enterococcus faecalis*. This clot formation, according to Evans et al. (30), is due to citrate use, not to production of coagulase; only the citrate-positive group D enterococci can form a clot in rabbit plasma. However, Wood (89) attributes coagulation of rabbit plasma by group D enterococci not to citrate use but to an agent released by the organism, probably an enzyme. According to Wood (89), this enzyme activity is the same as that of staphylocoagulase; however, its action on human or horse plasma does not parallel its activity on rabbit plasma. This action might be due to variance in inhibitor activation by plasmas of different species (89). Wood (89) also states that the clotting ability of group D *Enterococcus* spp. characterizes strains, not species, and adding 5 units of heparin per mL of citrated plasma inhibits enterococcal coagulation.

      Often group D *Enterococcus* spp. are mistaken for *Staphylococcus* since many can tolerate a high salt concentration. Some can ferment mannitol, thereby possibly exhibiting growth and fermentation on mannitol salt agar, which is usually considered selective for the identification of *Staphylococcus* spp. However, the staphylococcal colonies on mannitol salt agar (MSA) are large compared with those of enterococci (small or pinpoint colonies with slight mannitol fermentation). If in doubt, do a catalase test prior to testing for coagulase activity; *Staphylococcus* spp. are catalase positive, all *Enterococcus* spp. are catalase negative. Evans et al. (30) recommend that if a coagulase result in citrated plasma is delayed (3–24 h for a clot to form), one should suspect that the organism is not *S. aureus*. They also recommend using an anticoagulant other than citrate.

Burrows et al. (12), Smith et al. (75), and Bayliss and Hall (7) reported that *Bacillus subtilis*, a Gram-positive bacillus, can clot citrated or oxalated plasma, human or rabbit, because of a metabolic product. Rammell (67) reported that citrate inhibits the growth of *S. aureus*. The use of heparinized plasma prevents false-positive reactions by citrate-using organisms.

6. Balows et al. (4) state that a positive tube coagulase reaction result is indicated by the presence of either a partial clot (loose clot suspended in plasma) or a complete clot (solid, immovable when the tube is inverted). A flocculent and/or fibrous precipitate is **not** a true clot and should be recorded as a negative result (4).

However, if the coagulase test is the only procedure performed for *S. aureus* subsp. *aureus* differentiation and identification, Zarzour and Belle (95), Rayman et al. (69), and Yrios (93) recommend using degree of clotting: 3+ or 4+ clot, **conclusive;** 2+ or below, **not conclusive.** Sperber and Tatini (77) consider **only** a positive reaction conclusive. When the degree of clotting is **not** conclusive, other tests such as mannitol fermentation and thermonuclease are necessary; Zarzour and Belle (95) suggest performing the thermonuclease test on **all** clinical isolates yielding a 2+ or 1+ clot, to confirm and identify any weak or doubtful coagulase strains of *S. aureus* subsp. *aureus*.

7. Some strains of coagulase-positive staphylococci may be positive at 2–4 h and then revert (10). A tube showing a negative result after 4 h at 35°C should be held at room temperature (22–25°C) and read again at 18–24 h because some strains produce fibrinolysin on prolonged incubation at 35°C, which causes dissolution of the clot (46).

S. aureus subsp. *aureus* strains encountered by Landau and Kaplan (52) that failed to produce coagulase at 36°C did so at room temperature (22–25°C). Strains that were always negative at 37°C (after 24 h) and were positive at room temperature were called "cold coagulases" (52). These authors recommend retesting an otherwise typical *S. aureus* subsp. *aureus* colony that gives a negative coagulase result and reading the results after overnight incubation at room temperature. A typical *S. aureus* colony has a golden pigment, is hemolytic, ferments mannitol, is DNase positive, and has an antimicrobial susceptibility pattern consistent with that of *S. aureus* subsp. *aureus* (52).

Studies suggest that a higher temperature inhibits production of enzyme rather than affecting enzyme activity; Landau and Kaplan (52) recommend two temperature procedures for isolates that remain coagulase negative after incubation for 3–6 h at 36°C. If incubation exceeds 4 h, Kloos and Lambe (47) recommend considering the following points:

   a. Staphylokinase produced by some strains may lyse a clot after prolonged incubation, resulting in a false-negative result. False-negative results occur when *S. aureus* subsp. *aureus* produce so much staphylokinase that it lysis fibrin clots. Lysis due to staphylokinase production activates the formation of fibrinolysin and converts plasminogen to plasmin; it is generally more of a problem with human plasma than with rabbit plasma (60).
   b. Use of **un**sterile plasma (some are not sterile) may yield either a false-positive or a false-negative result.
   c. Inoculum from an agar-grown colony may not be pure; a contaminant may produce false results after prolonged incubation.

8. Veterinary clinical laboratories should note that some strains of *S. intermedius* and most

coagulase-positive strains of *S. hyicus* require more than 4 h for a positive coagulase result; these species may require incubation for 12–24 h (47).

F. **Coagulase mannitol agar:** *E. coli* also ferments mannitol and may be weakly coagulase positive; however, colony morphology visualized by a Gram stain will rule out a Gram-negative bacillus (65).

REFERENCES

1. Arvidson S. Studies on extracellular proteolytic enzymes from *Staphylococcus aureus*. II. Isolation and characterization of an EDTA-sensitive protease. Biochim Biophys Acta 1973;302:149–157.
2. Arvidson S. Hydrolysis of casein by three extracellular proteolytic enzymes from *Staphylococcus aureus*, strain V 8. Acta Pathol Microbiol Scand Sect B 1973;81(5):538–544.
3. Arvidson S, Holme T, Lindholm B. Studies on extracellular proteolytic enzymes from *Staphylococcus aureus*. I. Purification and characterization of one neutral and one alkaline protease. Biochem Biophys Acta 1973;302:135–148.
4. Balows A, Hausler WJ Jr, Herrmann KL, et al., eds. Manual of Clinical Microbiology, ed 5, Washington, DC: American Society for Microbiology, 1991:229.
5. Baron EJ, Finegold SM. Bailey & Scott's Diagnostic Microbiology, ed 8. Philadelphia: CV Mosby, 1990:105, 325.
6. Barry AL, Lachica RVF, Atchison FW. Identification of *Staphylococcus aureus* by simultaneous use of the coagulase and thermonuclease tests. Appl Microbiol 1973;25(3):496–497.
7. Bayliss BG, Hall ER. Plasma coagulation by organisms other than *Staphylococcus aureus*. J Bacteriol 1965;89(1):101–105.
8. Billaudelle H. Studien an *Haemophilus pertussis* (Bordet-Gengou). II. Die Koagulase bei *Haemophilus pertussis*. Acta Pathol Microbiol Scand 1955;37(1):5–13.
9. Blazevic DJ, Ederer GM. Principles of Biochemical Tests in Diagnostic Microbiology. New York: John Wiley & Sons, 1975:19–21.
10. Branson D. Methods in Clinical Bacteriology. Springfield, IL: Charles C Thomas, 1972:16–18.
11. Branson D. Coagulase-negative staphylococci and *Aerococcus*. REMEL Microbiol Newsletter 1984;2(3).
12. Burrows W, Lewert RM, Rippon JW. Textbook of Microbiology. The Pathogenic Microorganisms, vol I, ed 19. Philadelphia: WB Saunders, 1968:272–273.
13. Cadness-Graves B, Williams R, Harper GJ, Milles AA. Slide-test for coagulase-positive staphylococci. Lancet 1943;1:736–737.
14. Chapman GH. The comparative value of human plasma and human whole blood for testing the coagulating power of staphylococci. J Bacteriol 1944;47(2):211.
15. Cowan ST. The classification of staphylococci by precipitation and biological reactions. J Pathol Bacteriol 1938;46(1):31–45.
16. Cowan ST. Cowan & Steel's Manual for the Identification of Medical Bacteria, ed 2. Cambridge: Cambridge University Press, 1974:10, 32–33, 171–172.
17. Cassell GH. Staphylococci. In: McGhee JR, Michalek SM, Cassell GH, eds. Dental Microbiology. Philadelphia: Harper & Row, 1982:404–408.
18. Devriese LA, Hájek V, Oeding P, et al. *Staphylococcus hyicus* (Sompolinsky, 1953) com. nov. and *Staphylococcus hyicus* subsp. *chromogenes* subsp. nov. Int J Syst Bacteriol 1978;28:482–490.
19. Dickson JIS, Marples RR. Coagulase production by strains of *Staphylococcus aureus* of differing resistance characters: A comparison of two traditional methods with a latex agglutination system detecting both clumping factor and protein A. J Clin Pathol 1986;39(4):371–375.
20. Drapeau GR. Protease from *Staphylococcus aureus*. Methods Enzymol 1976;45:469–475.
21. Drummond MC, Tager M. Enzymatic activities associated with clotting of fibrinogen by staphylocoagulase and coagulase-reacting factor and their inhibition by diisopropylfluorophosphate. J Bacteriol 1962;3(5):975–980.
22. Drummond MC, Tager M. Fibrinogen clotting and fibrino-peptide formation by staphylocoagulase and the coagulase-reacting factor. J Bacteriol 1963;85(3):628–635.
23. Dubos RJ, Hirsch JG, eds. Bacterial and Mycotic Infections of Man, ed 4. Philadelphia: JB Lippincott, 1965:419–426.
24. Duthrie ES. Variation in the antigenic composition of staphylococcal coagulase. J Gen Microbiol 1952;7(4):320–326.
25. Duthrie ES. Evidence of two forms of staphylococcal coagulase. J Gen Microbiol 1954;10(3):427–436.
26. Ehrenkranz NJ, Elliott DF, Zarco R. Serum bacteriostasis of *Staphylococcus aureus*. Infect Immun 1971;3(5):664–670.
27. Ekstedt RD. Further studies on the antibacterial activity of human serum on *Micrococcus pyogenes* and its inhibition by coagulase. J Bacteriol 1956;72(2):157–161.
28. Ekstedt RD, Nungester WJ. Coagulase in reversing antibacterial activity of normal human serum on *Micrococcus pyogenes*. Proc Soc Exp Biol Med 1955;89(1):90–94.
29. Esber RJ, Faulconer RJ. A medium for initial visual demonstration of production of coagulase and

29. fermentation of mannitol by pathogenic staphylococci. Am J Clin Pathol 1959;32(2):192–194 (reprinted from Tech Bull Reg Med Tech 1959; 29(7):108–110).
30. Evans JB, Buettner LG, Niven CF Jr. Occurrence of streptococci that give a false-positive coagulase test. J Bacteriol 1952;64(4):433–434.
31. Fisk A. The technique of the coagulase test for staphylococci. Br J Exp Pathol 1940;21:311–314.
32. Fredericq P. 1. Sur la coagulation du plasma oxalaté par les cultures de *B. prodigiosus*. 2. Sur la coagulation du plasma oxalaté par les cultures d'actinomyces. C R Soc Biol 1946a;140:1132, 1946b;140:1166.
33. Freney J, Brun Y, Bes M, et al. *Staphylococcus lugdunensis* sp. nov. and *Staphylococcus schleiferi* sp. nov., two species from human clinical specimens. Int J Syst Bacteriol 1988;38:168–172.
34. Fritz H, Oppitz KH, Geeebhardt M, et al. Über das Vorkommen eines Trypsin-Plasmin-Inhibitors in Hirudin. Hoppe-Seyler's Z Physiol Chem 1969; 350:91–92.
35. Gillespie EH. The routine use of coagulase test for staphylococci [Abstract]. Mon Bull Hyg 1943;18: 681.
36. Graber CD, Boltjes BH, Morillo M. Comparison of the slide and coagulase-mannitol agar methods for adducing staphylocoagulase. Am J Med Technol 1968;34(4):211–214.
37. Hájek V. *Staphylococcus intermedius*, a new species isolated from animals. Int J Syst Bacteriol 1976; 26:401–408.
38. Hájek V, Devriese LA, Mordarski M, et al. Elevation of *Staphylococcus hyicus* subsp *chromogenes* (Devriese et al., 1978) to species status: *Staphylococcus chromogenes* (Devriese et al., 1978) comb. nov. Syst Appl Microbiol 1986;8:169–173.
39. Harper EM, Conway NS. Clotting of human citrated plasma by gram-negative organisms. J Pathol Bacteriol 1948;60(2):247–251.
40. Harper HA, Rodwell VW, Mayes PA. Review of Physiological Chemistry, ed 16. Los Altos, CA: Lange Medical Publications, 1977:37, 84, 563.
41. Hébert GA. Hemolysins and other characteristics that help differentiate and biotype *Staphylococcus lugdunensis* and *Staphylococcus schleiferi*. J Clin Microbiol 1990;28(11):2425–2431.
42. Hébert GA, Crowder CG, Hancock GA, et al. Characteristics of coagulase-negative staphylococci that help differentiate these species and other members of the family *Micrococcaceae*. J Clin Microbiol 1988;26(10):1939–1949.
43. Hemker H, Bas BM, Muller AD. Activation of a proenzyme by a stoichiometric reaction with another protein. The reaction between prothrombin and staphylocoagulase. Biochim Biophys Acta 1975;379:180–184.
44. Hendrix H, Lindhout T, Mertens K, et al. Activation of human prothrombin by stoichiometric levels of staphylocoagulase. J Biol Chem 1983;258:3637–3644.
45. Jawetz E, Melnick JL, Adelberg EA. Review of Medical Microbiology, ed 17. Los Altos, CA: Appleton & Lange, 1987:162, 219.
46. Koneman EW, Allen SD, Janda WM, et al. Color Atlas and Textbook of Diagnostic Microbiology, ed 4. Philadelphia: JB Lippincott, 1992:39, 414–415, 419.
47. Kloos WE, Lambe DW Jr. *Staphylococcus*. In: Balows A, Hausler WJ Jr, Herrmann KL, et al., eds. Manual of Clinical Microbiology, ed 5. Washington, DC: American Society for Microbiology, 1991:222–237.
48. Kopeć M, Wegrzynowicz A, Budzyński Z, et al., Formation and properties of fibrin clots resulting from staphylocoagulase (SC) action. Thromb Diath Haemorrh 1967;18:475–486.
49. Kowalski E, Latao Z, Niewiarowski S. Untersuchungen über die Aktivierung des Plasminogens und die Inaktivierung des Plasmins. Folia Haematol (Leipzig) 1957;75(2):225–241.
50. Krech U. Untersuchungen über die Koagulation von menschlichem und tierischem Plasma durch *Bacterium coli*. Z Immun Forsch 1952; 109:206–209.
51. Lally R, Woolfrey B. Clumping factor defective MRSA. Eur J Clin Microbiol 1984;3:151–152.
52. Landau W, Kaplan RL. Room temperature coagulase production by *Staphylococcus aureus* strains. Clin Microbiol Newslett 1980;2(15):10.
53. Larsson A, Sjöquist J. Novel latex agglutination method with chicken anti-protein A for detection of *Staphylococcus aureus* infections. J Clin Microbiol 1989;27(12):2856–2857.
54. Lotter LP, Horstman BSM. Comparison of a tube method and a plate method for detecting coagulase production. Am J Clin Pathol 1967; 48(1):153–155.
55. Mammen EF. Physiology and biochemistry of blood coagulation. In: Bang NV, Beller FK, Deutsch E, eds. Thrombosis and Bleeding Disorders. Stuttgart: Thieme, 1971:1–56.
56. Miale JB, Winningham AR, Kent JW. Staphylococcal isocoagulase. Nature 1963;197:392.
57. Morton HE, Cohn J. Coagulase and deoxyribonuclease activities of staphylococci isolated from clinical sources. Appl Microbiol 1972;23 (4):725–733.
58. Mushin R, Kerr VJ. Clotting of citrate plasma and citrate utilization by intestinal gram-negative bacilli. J Gen Microbiol 1954;10(3):445–451.
59. Needham GM, Ferris V, Spink WW. The correlation of the rapid slide method with the tube method for differentiating coagulase-positive from coagulase-negative strains of staphylococci. Am J Clin Pathol 1945;15(Tech Suppl 9):83–85.
60. Oberhofer TR. Manual of Practical Medical Microbiology and Parasitology. New York: John Wiley & Sons, 1985:144–147.
61. Oginsky EL, Umbreit WW. An Introduction to Bacterial Physiology, ed 2. San Francisco: WH Freeman, 1959:425–426.
62. Orth DS, Chung LR, Anderson AW. Compari-

62. son of animal sera for suitability in coagulase testing. Appl Microbiol 1971;21(3):420–425.
63. Parisi JT, Baldwin JN, Sottile M. Pour-plate method for the detection of coagulase production by *Staphylococcus aureus*. Appl Microbiol 1973;25(4):558–561.
64. Parker MT. Staphylococcus and Micrococcus; The Anaerobic Gram-Positive Cocci. In: Wilson G, Miles A, Parker MT, eds. Topley and Wilson's Principles of Bacteriology, Virology and Immunology, vol 2, ed 7. Baltimore: Williams & Wilkins, 1983:225, 228.
65. Powers DA, McCuen PJ. Manual of BBL Products and Laboratory Procedures, ed 6. Cockeysville, MD: Becton Dickinson Microbiology Systems, 1988:136–137, 342.
66. Rammelkamp CH Jr, Hezebicks MM, Dingle JH. Specific coagulases of *Staphylococcus aureus*. J Exp Med 1950;91(3):295–307.
67. Rammell CG. Inhibition by citrate of the growth of coagulase-positive staphylococci. J Bacteriol 1965;84(5):1123–1124.
68. Raus J, Love DN. Comparison of the affinities to bovine and human prothrombin of the staphylocoagulases from *Staphylococcus intermedius* and *Staphylococcus aureus* of animal origin. J Clin Microbiol 1991;29(3):570–572.
69. Rayman MK, Park CE, Philpott J, Todd ECD. Reassessment of the coagulase and thermostable nuclease tests as means of identifying *Staphylococcus aureus*. Appl Microbiol 1975;29(4):451–454.
70. Rita G. Sulla natura del fenomeno della coagulazione del plasma citrate ad opera di alcuni ceppi di *B. typhi*. Boll Soc Ital Biol Sper 1945; 20:227–230.
71. Rogers DE, Tompsett R. The survival of staphylococci within human leukocytes. J Exp Med 1952;95(2):209–230.
72. Rydén AC, Rydén L, Philipson L. Isolation and properties of a staphylococcal protease, preferentially cleaving glutamoyl-peptide bonds. Eur J Biochem 1974;44:105–114.
73. Sanders E. Inhibition of coagulase reaction of pathogenic staphylococci by heparin in vitro. II. Use of sterile, cell-free preparations of coagulase. J Bacteriol 1963;86(6):1350–1351.
74. Schultze HE, Schwick G. Über den Mechanismus der Thrombinbildung im isolierten System. Hoppe-Seyler's Z Physiol Chem 1951;289:26–43.
75. Smith DT, Conant NF, Willett HP. Zinsser's Microbiology, ed 14. New York: Appleton-Century-Crofts, 1968:323–333.
76. Soulier JP, Prou O, Halle L. Further studies on thrombin-coagulase. Thromb Diath Haemorrh 1970;23:37–49.
77. Sperber WH, Tatini SR. Interpretation of the tube coagulase test for identification of *Staphylococcus aureus*. Appl Microbiol 1975;29(4):502–505.
78. Streitfeld MM, Sallman B, Shoelson SM. Staphylocoagulase inhibition by pooled human gamma-globulin. Nature (London) 1959;184: 1665–1666.
79. Subcommittee on Taxonomy of Staphylococci and Micrococci. Recommendations. Int Bull Bacteriol Nomen Taxon 1975;15:109–110.
80. Tager M. Current views on the mechanism of coagulase action in blood clotting. Ann NY Acad Sci 1974;236:277–289.
81. Tager M, Drummond MC. Section II. An analysis of the *Staphylococcus*: Extracellular products. Staphylocoagulase. Ann NY Acad Sci 1965;128: 92–111.
82. Tesh MJ, Wood RL. Detection of coagulase activity in *Erysipelothrix rhusiopathiae*. J Clin Microbiol 1988;26(5):1058–1060.
83. Varaldo PE, Kilpper-Bälz R, Biavasco F, et al. *Staphylococcus delphine* sp. nov., a coagulase-positive species isolated from dolphins. Int J Syst Bacteriol 1988;38:436–439.
84. Washington JA. Laboratory Procedures in Clinical Microbiology, ed 2. New York: Springer-Verlag, 1985:135.
85. Weckman BG, Catlin BW. Deoxyribonuclease activity of micrococci from clinical sources. J Bacteriol 1957;73(6):747–753.
86. Wegrzynowicz Z, Heczko PB, Jeljaszewicz J, et al. Pseudocoagulase activity of staphylococci. J Clin Microbiol 1979;9(1):15–19.
87. Wegrzynowicz Z, Ko HL, Pulverer G, Jeljaszewicz J. The nature of clotting and fibrinolytic activities of *Bacteroides melaninogenicus*. Zentralbl Bakteriol Abt 1 Orig A 1978;240:106–111.
88. Williams REO, Harper GJ. Determination of coagulase and alpha-haemolysin production by staphylococci. Br J Exp Pathol 1946;27(2):72–81.
89. Wood M. The clotting of rabbit plasma by group D streptococci. J Gen Microbiol 1959;21(2): 385–388.
90. Yearsley KG, Carter PB. Diabetic plasma in the determination of coagulase activity of staphylococci. Am J Med Technol 1966;32(6):369–372.
91. Yotis WW, Ekstedt RD. Studies of staphylococci. I. Effect of serum coagulase on the metabolism of coagulase positive and coagulase negative strains. J Bacteriol 1959;78(4):567–574.
92. Young CS, Lettner JE. The isolation of coagulase positive enterococci from clinical material. Am J Med Technol 1964;30(3):199–203.
93. Yrios JW. Comparison of rabbit and pig plasma in the tube coagulase test. J Clin Microbiol 1977;5(2):221–224.
94. Zajdel M, Wegrzynowicz Z, Sawecka J, Mechanism of action of staphylocoagulase. Zentralbl Bakteriol Parasitenkd Infektionskr Hyg Abt 1 Suppl 1976;5:549–575.
95. Zarzour JY, Beele EA. Evaluation of three test procedures for identification of *Staphylococcus aureus* from clinical sources. J Clin Microbiol 1978;7(2):133–136.
96. Zen-Yoji H, Tetrayama T, Benoki M, Kuwahara W. Studies on staphylococcal coagulase. I. Antigenic difference of coagulase and distribution of the anticoagulase in human sera. Jpn J Microbiol 1961;5(2):237–247.

Decarboxylase Tests (Lysine-Ornithine-Arginine) and Dihydrolase Test (Arginine)

I. PRINCIPLE

To measure the enzymatic ability of an organism to decarboxylate an amino acid to form an amine with resulting alkalinity

II. PURPOSE

(Also see Chapters 43–45)
(*Note:* The decarboxylase tests are used primarily to determine bacterial groups among the *Enterobacteriaceae*. They test for lysine, ornithine, and arginine decarboxylases.)

A. **Lysine decarboxylase**
   1. To aid in differentiation between genera
      a. *Edwardsiella* (+) and *Salmonella* (usually +) from *Citrobacter* spp. (−)
      b. *Escherichia coli* (+) from *Shigella* spp. (−)
   2. To aid in species differentiation
      a. *Enterobacter aerogenes* (+), *Enterobacter gergoviae* (+), *Hafnia alvei* (+), and *Hafnia alvei* biogroup 1 (+) from other *Enterobacter* spp. (−) and *Pantoea agglomerans* (−) (formerly *Enterobacter agglomerans*)
      b. *Pseudomonas cepacia* (+) and *Pseudomonas pseudoalcaligenes* (variable, usually +) from other *Pseudomonas* spp. (−)
      c. *Klebsiella pneumoniae* subsp. *rhinoscleromatis* (−) and *K. pneumoniae* subsp. *ozaenae* (variable) from other *Klebsiella* spp. (+) (27)
      d. *Burkholderia cepacia* (+) from *B. gladioli* (−), *B. mallei* (−), and *B. pseudomallei* (−)
B. **Ornithine decarboxylase**
   1. To aid in differentiation between genera
      a. *Enterobacter* (V, usually +) from *Klebsiella* (−)
      b. *Morganella morganii* biogroups 1 and 2 (+) from *Providencia* spp. (−)
   2. To aid in species differentiation
      a. *Salmonella typhi* (−) and *Salmonella choleraesuis* serovar *gallinarum* (−, 24 h) (30) from other *Salmonella* spp. (+)
      b. *Shigella sonnei* (+) from other *Shigella* spp. (−)
      c. *Proteus mirabilis* (+) from other *Proteus* spp. (−)
      d. *Aeromonas veronii* (+) from other *Aeromonas* spp. (−) most frequently isolated
C. **Arginine dihydrolase**; to aid in species differentiation
   1. *Lactococcus garviae* (+), *L. lactis* subsp. *hordniae* (+), and *L. lactis* subsp. *lactis* (+) from other *Lactococcus* spp. (V, usually −)
   2. *Aeromonas salmonicida* subsp. *smithia* (V, usually −) and *A. veronii* (−) from other *Aeromonas* species (+) most frequently isolated
   3. *Burkholderia mallei* (+) and *B. pseudomallei* (+) from *B. cepacia* (−) and *B. gladioli* (−)

4. *Capnocytophaga canimorsus* (+) and *C. cynodegmi* (+) from *C. gingivalis* (−), *C. ochracea* (−), and *C. sputigena* (−)
5. *Haemophilus paracumiculus* (+) from other *Haemophilus* spp. (−)
6. *Mobiluncus mulieris* (−) from *M. curtisii* subsp. *curtisii* (+) and *M. curtisii* subsp. *holmesii* (+)
7. *Pediococcus acidilactici* (+) and *P. pentosaceus* (+) from other *Pediococcus* spp.

III. BIOCHEMISTRY INVOLVED

Decarboxylation is the process in which bacteria that possess specific decarboxylase enzymes attack amino acids at their carboxyl end (COOH) to yield an amine or a diamine and carbon dioxide (36).

$$R-CH-NH_2-COOH \longrightarrow R-CH_2-NH_2 + CO_2$$
Amino acid → Amine + Carbon dioxide

There are numerous decarboxylase enzymes, each specific for a given substrate. In a clinical bacteriology laboratory the three important decarboxylases used for bacterial identification are lysine, ornithine, and arginine. These decarboxylases are adaptive, or induced, enzymes. They are formed only when an organism is cultivated in an acid environment in the presence of a specific substrate, and the products of decarboxylation shift the pH to the alkaline range (36).

Decarboxylation is restricted to amino acids that possess at least one chemically active group other than an amine (NH_2) or a carboxyl group (COOH) (19), and the breakdown of amino acids occurs anaerobically (29). Decarboxylation is irreversible, is nonoxidative, and usually requires a common coenzyme, pyridoxal phosphate (8), which further enhances decarboxylase activity (27).

The amino acid L-lysine is decarboxylated to yield cadaverine (a diamine) and carbon dioxide by the action of the specific enzyme lysine decarboxylase (9, 29).

L-Lysine →(Lysine decarboxylase, $-CO_2$)→ Cadaverine (diamine) + CO_2

The amino acid L-ornithine is decarboxylated by the enzyme ornithine decarboxylase to yield the diamine putrescine and carbon dioxide (29).

L-Ornithine →(Ornithine decarboxylase, $-CO_2$)→ Putrescine (diamine) + CO_2

Both cadaverine and putrescine are stable when produced under anaerobic conditions (29). The bacterium to be studied is cultivated anaerobically by overlaying the surface of the medium with either paraffin or mineral oil. By sealing the tubes, all unbound oxygen is consumed by the organism during the initial growth phase, and the pH of the medium during decarboxylation rises (to alkalinity) as carbon dioxide is produced (29). Since the pH can be controlled, it is possible to incorporate a pH indicator, either bromcresol purple or cresol red, into the medium containing the amino acid.

The amino acid L-arginine is catabolized (degraded) via two systems, which may occur either simultaneously or separately (29). These two pathways are the arginine dihydrolase system and the arginine decarboxylase system.

Arginine Decarboxylase System (21, 22, 29)

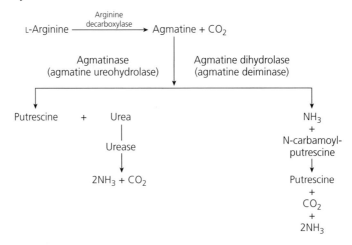

In the decarboxylase system, L-arginine undergoes decarboxylation to yield agmatine, a larger molecule than putrescine, which cannot be considered the final product in the catabolism of arginine by living bacteria (29). Further breakdown of agmatine occurs by one of two pathways. The catalytic action of the enzyme agmatinase splits agmatine into two compounds, putrescine and urea. If the enzyme urease is present, urea is further catabolized to yield two molecules of ammonia (NH_3) and carbon dioxide (CO_2). Møller (29) found that putrescine does not undergo further breakdown to any demonstrable degree.

Møller also demonstrated that all strains of *Enterobacteriaceae* produce agmatinase and thus exhibit a strong catabolism of agmatine, yielding putrescine and urea, or putrescine and 2 NH_3 and CO_2 molecules if urease is also present (29). Agmatine is catabolized by agmatine dehydrolase to putrescine, CO_2, and NH_3 via an intermediate compound, N-carbamoylputrescine (29).

In the dihydrolase system, L-arginine breakdown was shown by Knivett (26), Slade and Slamp (35), and Oginsky and Gehrig (32, 33) to occur in a two-step process: first a breakdown of L-arginine to L-citrulline, followed by a citrulline-splitting system. The overall reaction results in formation of L-ornithine, CO_2, and NH_3 from the substrate L-arginine.

Arginine Dihydrolase System (21, 22, 29)

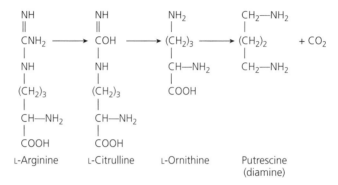

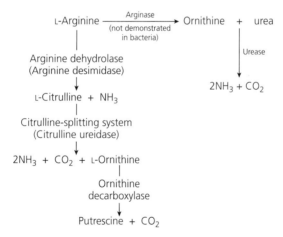

The first step involves hydrolytic removal of NH_2 from arginine by the action of an arginine dihydrolase, arginine desimidase (29) (or L-arginine iminohydrolase (2)), to yield citrulline, ammonia, and inorganic phosphate (Pi) (2, 37). The second step involves a citrulline-splitting system whereby citrulline undergoes phosphorolytic cleavage in the presence of H_3PO_4 and the enzyme ornithine carbamoyltransferase (2) (or citrulline ureidase (29)) to yield ornithine and carbamoyl phosphate (2, 37).

Carbamoyl phosphate under the catalytic action of carbamate kinase and adenosine diphosphate (ADP) yields NH_3, CO_2, and adenosine triphosphate (ATP) (2, 37). The breakdown of L-arginine to L-citrulline is an energy-yielding reaction that provides a major source of ATP for an organism (2, 13, 24, 37). This catabolism is used mostly by anaerobes for ATP synthesis in the carbamate kinase reaction (22). In most cases, arginine deaminase occurs together with carbamate kinase, composing the arginine dihydrolase system (24).

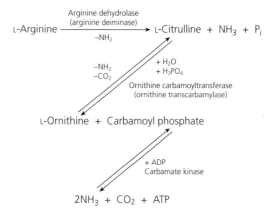

(Redrawn from Kakimoto, T., Shibatani, T., Nishimura, N., and Chibata, I. Enzymatic production of L-citrulline by *Pseudomonas putida,* Appl. Microbiol., 1971, *22,* 992, with permission of the American Society for Microbiology, Washington, D.C.)

If an organism can break down L-arginine to L-ornithine by the dihydrolase system, under the catalytic action of ornithine decarboxylase, L-ornithine is further degraded to putrescine and carbon dioxide. However, determining the presence of an ornithine decarboxylase requires a separate test using only the amino acid substrate L-ornithine. It is impossible to determine both arginine and ornithine degradation in a single test.

If urease is not produced by the organism being studied, the formation of ammonia (NH_3) indicates that the dihydrolase system was used in the breakdown process (29). The formation of ammonia can be determined directly with Nessler's reagent (29).

A rapid, strong pH indicator shift to alkalinity indicates that L-arginine catabolism was due to the arginine dihydrolase system (29). A weaker and slower pH shift with no formation of ammonia occurs when L-arginine is degraded only by the arginine decarboxylase system (29). However, the time factor is not a reliable way to determine which pathway was used.

IV. MEDIA EMPLOYED

(*Note:* Møller's name has been Anglicized to Moeller in most texts, but the author will adhere to the original spelling.)

A. Møller's decarboxylase base (29)
1. Ingredients; pH 6.0 ± 0.2

Peptone (pepsin)	5.0 g
Beef extract	5.0 g
Bromcresol purple (BCP)	0.1 g
Cresol red	0.005 g
Pyridoxal phosphate	0.005 g
Glucose (dextrose)	0.5 g
Deionized water	1000 mL

2. pH indicators
   a. Bromcresol purple (BCP)
      (1) Acid: yellow color, pH 5.2
      (2) Alkaline: purple color, pH 6.8

b. Cresol red (alkaline)
     (1) Alkaline: yellow color, pH 7.2
     (2) Alkaline: red color, pH 8.3
  c. Uninoculated medium: pH 6.0, deep brilliant purple color
3. Method of preparation
  a. Weigh amount accurately as directed on the label.
  b. Rehydrate with distilled or demineralized water.
  c. Heat **gently** into solution.
  d. Add 10 g (1% concentration) of desired amino acid.
     (1) 1% L-(+)-lysine dihydrochloride
     (2) 1% L-(+)-ornithine dihydrochloride
     (3) 1% L-(+)-arginine monohydrochloride

If a DL-isomer (racemic) mixture of an amino acid is used, a 2% concentration (20 g/L) is optimal, since microbial enzymes are apparently only active against the L-(+) forms of amino acids (29).

It is not necessary to adjust the pH when using L-arginine and L-lysine. However, with L-ornithine, adjustment is necessary **before** sterilization, since it is so highly acidic. For a liter of medium containing 1% L-ornithine, adjusting the pH to 6.0 usually requires the addition of approximately 4.6 mL of a 10 N solution of sodium hydroxide (16). A small amount of floccular precipitate may be observed in the ornithine medium, but it does not interfere with its use (16).

Møller's medium is more acidic than most culture media. A low pH is necessary because decarboxylase enzymes are not optimally active until the pH of the medium is below 5.5 (27). A drop from pH 6.0 to 5.5 results from growing bacteria that use the small amount of glucose in the medium to produce mixed acids (27).

  e. Dispense approximately 3.0–4.0 mL per screw-cap tube (16) (13 × 100 mm)
4. Method of sterilization: autoclave, 121°C, 15 lb, 10 min
5. Cool, tighten screw-caps, and refrigerate for storage (4–10°C).
6. Inoculation
  a. Growth from an 18- to 24-h **pure** culture: Kligler's iron agar (KIA) (25, 29)
  b. **Light** inoculum (16)
  c. A control tube **without** an amino acid should be inoculated with each battery of amino acids under investigation (16): (*a*) C, control; (*b*) L, lysine; (*c*) A, arginine; (*d*) O, ornithine.
  d. Overlay **all** tubes including the control with 2–3 mL of either **sterile** paraffin or **sterile** mineral oil. Under these conditions, the oxygen in the medium is consumed by the microorganism; this controls the pH (29). Mineral oil overlay ensures that fermentation of glucose takes place (vs. oxidation) and prevents oxidative degradation of peptone, which results in alkalization at the surface of the medium and eventually diffusing throughout the medium (38). (See Chapter 33, Oxidation-Fermentation Test, Section IV.G.4 for preparation and sterilization of sealants.)
7. Incubation: 35°C, 24 h–4 days (17); examine daily. Prolonged incubation (6–10 days or longer) may be required to demonstrate weak reactions due to poor decarboxylase activity (29).

Møller's decarboxylase medium may be used without glucose; however, Møller (29) found that a 0.05% concentration of glucose and a pH of 6.0 gave better growth and more reliable results when a pH indicator is incorporated into the medium. Pyridoxal phosphate, a synthetic product of codecarboxylase, is effective in activating denatured decarboxylase enzyme (19). Addition of pyridoxal phosphate enhances decarboxylase activity but is not required for microorganisms that exhibit strong decarboxylase activity (29).

B. **Falkow's lysine decarboxylase broth** (17)
   1. Ingredients, pH 6.8 ± 0.2

Peptone or Gelysate (BBL) pancreatic digest of gelatin	5.0 g
Yeast extract	3.0 g
Dextrose (glucose)	1.0 g
L-Lysine	5.0 g
Bromcresol purple (BCP)	0.02 g
Deionized water	1000.0 mL

   2. pH indicator: bromcresol purple (BCP)
      a. Acid: yellow color, pH 5.2
      b. Alkaline: purple color, pH 6.8
      c. Uninoculated medium: pH 6.8; deep brilliant purple color
   3. Method of preparation
      a. Weigh amount accurately as directed on the label.
      b. Rehydrate with distilled or demineralized water.
      c. Heat **gently** into solution.
      d. Dispense approximately 4.0–5.0 mL per screw-cap tube (16 × 125 mm).
   4. Method of sterilization: autoclave, 121°C, 15 lb, 15 min
   5. Cool, tighten caps, and refrigerate for storage (4–10°C).
   6. Inoculation
      a. Growth from an 18- to 24-h **pure** culture (KIA)
      b. **Light** inoculum
      c. Run a control tube containing no amino acid with each organism being investigated for lysine degradation (25).
      d. It is **recommended** that all tubes, including the control, be overlaid with 2–3 mL of either **sterile** paraffin or **sterile** mineral oil.
   7. Incubation
      a. 35°C
      b. No less than 24 h (17); prolonged incubation up to 4 days may be required.

Falkow lysine broth is a modification of Møller's decarboxylase medium, but this medium uses only a 0.5% concentration of lysine. Also, oil seals are not necessary (17), but the caps must be screwed down tightly on the tubes during incubation. Falkow medium depends only on a shift in the pH indicator (17, 27), and neither an anaerobic nor acid environment is required. However, medium **cannot** be used to detect lysine decarboxylation in certain members of the *Klebsiella-Enterobacter-Serratia-Hafnia* group because they produce acetylmethylcarbinol (Voges-Proskauer (VP) positive), which interferes with the final alkaline pH shift and leads to false-negative results (27).

All *Enterobacteriaceae* cause an initial fermentation of glucose-producing acid that causes a change in the pH indicator from purple to yellow within the first 10 to 12 h of incubation. In response to the acidity, organisms that produce lysine decarboxylase form an amine (cadaverine), causing the pH indicator to revert to alkalinity (purple).

Falkow lysine broth may be used to study arginine and ornithine decarboxylase activity. To the basic formula add a 0.5% concentration (5 g/L) of the L-amino acid desired. If a DL-mixture is used, increase the concentration to 1%.

V. REAGENTS EMPLOYED

A. **10 N Sodium hydroxide (40%)**
   1. Ingredients

NaOH, carbonate free, R. G. (reagent grade)	40.0 g
Distilled water	100.0 mL

2. Method of preparation
   a. **Rapidly** weigh the sodium hydroxide and dissolve in less than 100 mL of distilled water in a beaker. This reagent is highly hygroscopic.
   b. Place beaker in a circulating cold water bath to control the temperature.
   c. Cool and transfer the NaOH solution to a 100-mL volumetric flask and bring to 100 mL with distilled water.
   d. Store in a polyethylene- or paraffin-lined glass reagent bottle.
   e. Label correctly.

   Sodium hydroxide is extremely caustic, so avoid exposure to skin, as painful burns may occur.

3. Method of use to adjust the pH of decarboxylase medium containing L-ornithine
   a. Møller's decarboxylase medium containing 1% L-ornithine (16)
      (1) Add approximately 4.6 mL/L.
      (2) Adjust pH to 6.0.
   b. Falkow decarboxylase medium containing 0.5% L-ornithine
      (1) Add approximately 2.1 mL/L.
      (2) Adjust pH to 6.8.

B. **Nessler's reagent**
   1. Method of preparation (12)
      a. Dissolve 5.0 g of potassium iodide (KI) in 5.0 mL of distilled water; distilled water **must** be ammonia (NH_3) free.
      b. Add cold **saturated** mercuric chloride ($HgCl_2$) solution until a slight precipitate remains after shaking.
      c. Add 40 mL of 9 N NaOH.
      d. Dilute with distilled water to 100 mL.
      e. Allow to stand 24 h before use. A slight amount of precipitate will settle to the bottom; **do not** disturb when using.
      f. Store in a paraffin-lined glass bottle or a dark bottle. Avoid exposure to light.
   2. Method of use to detect NH_3 production in L-arginine breakdown (25)
      a. Remove a loopful from a 4-day L-arginine culture and place into 0.5 mL of ammonia-free distilled water.
      b. Add 1 drop of Nessler's reagent.
      c. Run the same check on the control.
   3. Interpretation: a brown color indicates that arginine degradation (in the absence of urease) occurred by the arginine dihydrolase system (12).

VI. QUALITY CONTROL MICROORGANISMS

A. **Lysine**
   1. Positive (+): *Klebsiella pneumoniae* subsp. *pneumoniae* ATCC 10031
   2. Negative (−): *Enterobacter cloacae* ATCC 13047
   3. Uninoculated
B. **Arginine**
   1. Positive (+): *Enterobacter cloacae* ATCC 13047
   2. Negative (−): *Klebsiella pneumoniae* subsp. *pneumoniae* ATCC 10031
   3. Uninoculated
C. **Ornithine**
   1. Positive (+): *Enterobacter cloacae* ATCC 13047
   2. Negative (−): *Klebsiella pneumoniae* subsp. *pneumoniae* ATCC 10031
   3. Uninoculated

(*Note:* One **must** include an uninoculated, amino acid–free substrate control tube with each individual test, to be used as color controls. Also, with Møller's medium this ensures that the initial drop in pH has occurred, showing acidification (27). Alternative controls are listed in Table 9.1.

Table 9.1. Possible Control Microorganisms

Selection	ATCC	Arginine	Lysine	Ornithine
Proteus vulgaris	9484	−	−	−
Klebsiella pneumoniae subsp. *pneumoniae*	10031	−	+[a]	−
Morganella morganii bio group 1	25830	−	−	+
Salmonella typhi	6539	+	+	−
Enterobacter cloacae	13047	+	−	+
Enterobacter aerogenes	13048	−	+	+
Salmonella typhimurium	14028	+	+	+

[a]May be variable at times.

VII. RESULTS

> See Figure 9.1 (Appendix 1) for colored photographic results

VIII. INTERPRETATION

(*Note:* Any amino acid gives the same color results; e.g., lysine decarboxylase.)

A. Positive (+): turbid purple to a faded yellow-purple color (cadaverine produced)
B. Negative (−): bright, clear yellow color (only glucose fermented)
C. Uninoculated control tube (no amino acid substrate): remains yellow (**only** glucose fermented)

IX. ALTERNATIVE TESTS

A. **Lysine-iron agar (LIA)** (14, 34)
   1. Solid medium of Edwards and Fife (14); based on Falkow's formula (17)
   2. Detects whether *Enterobacteriaceae* decarboxylate or deaminate lysine
      a. Basic preliminary screening medium to detect fecal pathogens; aid in identification of *Salmonella* spp., most which are H_2S positive and lysine positive (27)
      b. **Not** a substitute for Møller's medium (3)
   3. Medium ingredients, pH 6.7 ± 0.2
      a. L-lysine, 0.1%
      b. Glucose, 0.1%
      c. H_2S indicators (see Chapter 15, Hydrogen Sulfide Tests for biochemistry of reaction)
         (1) Ferric ammonium citrate
         (2) Sodium thiosulfate
      d. pH indicator: bromcresol purple (see IV.A.2.a for color reactions)
   4. Dispense 4-mL amounts (13 × 100 mm test tubes); **deep butt** (for anaerobiosis)/**short slant**
      a. With inoculating **needle**, streak slant and **stab** butt **twice**.
      b. Loosen cap; 18- to 24-h incubation at 35°C
   5. Controls

Citrobacter freundii, Alk/A, H$_2$S,   ATCC 8454
Salmonella choleraesuis subsp. *arizonae*,   ALK/ALK, H$_2$S, ATCC 13314
Proteus vulgaris,   ALK/A ATCC 9484

6. Interpretation
   a. Lysine **decarboxylation**; biochemistry and precautions same as with Møller's or Falkow's media
      (1) Positive (+): purple slant/**purple butt** (alkaline), with or without H$_2$S
         (a) Purple (alkaline) slant due to aerobic **deamination** of **peptone**
         (b) Butt reaction may be masked by H$_2$S black color; H$_2$S is **only** produced in an alkaline (purple) environment. Reaction takes place anaerobically in the butt (3).
      (2) Negative (−): purple slant/**yellow butt** (acid); fermentation of glucose **only**
   b. **Lysine deamination**
      (1) **Red slant/yellow butt**
         (a) Slant reaction is characteristic of *Proteus* and *Providencia* spp. (6).
         (b) Butt reaction is due to fermentation of glucose.
      (2) H$_2$S-producing *Proteus* spp. **do not** blacken this medium (3).
      (3) Slant reaction with *M. morganii* biogroup 2 may be variable after a 24-h incubation (3).

Edwards and Fife (14) found that when pH indicator was omitted, *Proteus* and *Providencia* spp. produced an orange color throughout the medium because of deamination of lysine; this orange-colored product combines with the pH indicator bromcresol purple to produce a distinct red color on the slant (aerobiosis). However, it is not known which compound formed is responsible for development of the red color.

Lysine deamination (24)

1. 1 mol L-Lysine

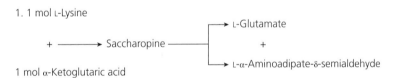

2.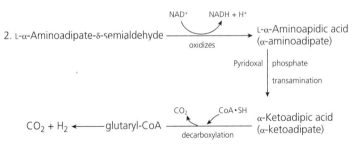

L-lysine was formerly thought to be catabolized via pipecolic acid, a cyclic imino acid (23), but it now appears to be degraded via saccharopine (29).

B. **Ninhydrin broth**
   1. Procedure of Carlquist (10)
   2. Sensitive detection of lysine decarboxylation; compound reacts directly with amines (27).
      a. Most commonly used to detect weak decarboxylase activity of many nonfermenting, Gram-negative bacteria and certain anaerobic bacteria (14, 27).
      b. Differentiates between anaerogenic, nonmotile *E. coli/Shigella* and *Citrobacter/Salmonella* (15)

c. Confirmatory test for pseudomonads; recognition of *Stenotrophomonas maltophila* (formerly *Pseudomonas maltophilia*)
3. Principle
   a. Cadaverine extracted with chloroform (soluble in chloroform) reacts with ninhydrin to produce a pink-purple color.
   b. See Chapter 14, Hippurate Hydrolysis Test, for the biochemistry of ninhydrin
4. Medium
   a. Ingredients, pH 7.2 ± 0.2 (**no** pH indicator)

Pancreatic digest of casein (Casitone)	15.0 g
Potassium phosphate K_2HPO_4	3.0 g
Glucose (dextrose)	1.0 g
Deionized water	1000.0 mL

   b. See Section IV.A.4–8 for method of preparation, sterilization, inoculation, and incubation.
5. Reagents
   a. Ninhydrin, 0.1% (1,2,3-triketohydrindene); 0.1 g/100 mL of chloroform
   b. **4 N** NaOH; 20 mL of 10 N (40%) NaOH brought to 50 mL with distilled water
6. Test procedure
   a. Add 1 mL of 4 N NaOH to **incubated** culture and mix.
   b. Add 2 mL of chloroform; **shake vigorously**.
   c. Centrifuge **lightly** for a few minutes until the chloroform separates into a distinct **clear** layer **below** a layer of denatured protein.
   d. **Aseptically,** by pipette, **carefully** remove 0.5 mL of **clear** chloroform extract to small test tube (13 × 100 mm); **avoid any carryover of alkaline emulsion.**
      (1) Add 0.5 mL of 0.1% ninhydrin.
      (2) Observe reaction at **room temperature** for 4 min.
7. Interpretation
   a. Positive (+): deep purple color
   b. Negative (−): no color change

X. RAPID TESTS

A. **Lysine decarboxylase**
   1. **Spot plate test**
      a. Semimicro method of Gerlach, Steiner, and Weaver (20)
      b. Results within 6–24 h of incubation
      c. Amino acid substrate solution, total volume 100 mL
         (1) Lysine, 1.0% in 0.004 M potassium acid phthalate buffer (pH 5.7)
         (2) Pyridoxal phosphate, 1–2 mg
         (3) Bromphenol red indicator, 0.0016%
         (4) Chloroform (preservative), several drops. Store in the refrigerator (4–10°C) (good for several months).
      d. Procedure
         (1) Control well **only**
            (a) Buffer
            (b) Indicator
         (2) Test well(s)
            (a) 4 drops of amino acid solution
            (b) A **single** drop (capillary pipette) of cell suspension
               1. Growth from a 6-h agar slant

2. **Sterile** swab of growth in 0.5 mL of 0.004 M potassium acid phthalate buffer (adjusted to pH 5.7)
   (3) Cover plate with Saran Wrap
   (4) Incubation: 35°C, 24 h; read at 6 h and 24 h
   (5) Interpretation
       (a) Positive (+): rose-red color
       (b) Negative (−): no color change, remains yellow
2. **Method of Brooker, Lund, and Blazevic** (8)
   a. Results within 4 h of incubation
   b. Medium and preparation
      (1) Ingredients

Peptone	0.5 g
Yeast extract	0.3 g
Deionized water	100.0 mL

      (2) Warm **gently** to dissolve into solution then add

L-lysine monohydrochloride, 1.0%	1.0 g
Alcoholic bromthymol blue	0.5 g

      (3) Adjust pH to 5.0–5.2.
   c. Dispensing and sterilization (choice)
      (1) Dispense 1.0-mL aliquots into borosilicate tubes and cap; autoclave, 121°C, 15 lb, 15 min
      (2) Filter with Millipore filter and **aseptically** dispense 1.0-mL aliquots into borosilicate tubes and cap.
   d. Procedure
      (1) Inoculation: 1 **heavy** loopful
      (2) Overlay with 1.0 mL of **sterile** mineral oil or melted paraffin.
      (3) Incubation
          (a) Choice
              1. 37°C water bath (recommended) (8)
                 a. Better heat exchange
                 b. Positive results obtained in shorter time
              2. 35°C dry air incubator
          (b) Read at 1, 2, 3, and 4 h
   e. Interpretation
      (1) Positive (+): green or blue color (pH 6.1)
      (2) Negative (−): yellow color

A heavy inoculum (10^6 cells or more) is essential; if an inoculum from a sheep blood agar (SBA) or MacConkey's agar (MAC) plate is too light, false-negative results may occur at the end of 4 h of incubation (5). Results are interpreted within a **4-h limit**; incubation may be safely extended to a maximum of 8 h but no longer. At 24 h, lysine-negative *Citrobacter* strains may become falsely positive (7).

B. **Ornithine decarboxylase:** method of Fay and Barry (18)
   1. Results within 2–4 h of incubation
   2. Identification of **non**fermenters; more sensitive than Møller's medium (31)
   3. Modified decarboxylase medium
      a. **No** glucose
      b. pH decreased to 5.5
      c. Medium and preparation

(1) Ingredients

Peptone	5.0 g
Yeast extract	3.0 g
Bromcresol purple 0.2% (w/v) in 50.0% (v/v) ethanol	5.0 mL
Deionized water to bring to	1000.0 mL

   (2) Warm **gently** to dissolve, **then add** 10.0 g of L-ornithine hydrochloride (Difco).
   (3) Adjust to pH 5.5 with concentrated hydrochloric acid (HCl) or sodium hydroxide (NaOH).
 4. Sterilization: autoclave, 121°C, 15 lb, 15 min
 5. Procedure
    a. On day of testing **aseptically** dispense 1.0-mL aliquots into **sterile** tubes (12 × 75 mm).
    b. Inoculation: single colony from an 18- to 24-h culture (SBA or MAC)
    c. Overlay tubes with at least 0.5 mL of **sterile** mineral oil.
    d. Incubation: 37°C heating block, 2–4 h
 6. Interpretation
    a. Positive (+): dark purple color
    b. Negative (−): yellow color
 7. Correlation with Møller's standard test is 100% (18).

Occasionally, *E. coli* may reduce the indicator to a light gray color; if this occurs add a drop of bromcresol indicator directly to the tube and reinterpret (18). Also, some ornithine-positive strains of *E. coli* and *Proteus* may exhibit only a slight purple color at the end of 4 h; confirm a positive result by incubating an additional 30–60 min (18).

C. **Arginine dihydrolase:** use thin-layer chromatography (TLC) (39)
D. **Gas chromatography** method of Lambert and Moss (28)
   1. Analysis by gas-liquid chromatography (GLC) for detection of
      (1) Putrescine from ornithine decarboxylation
      (2) Cadaverine from lysine decarboxylation
   2. Results within 3–5 h
   3. Procedure: see reference 29

XI. PRECAUTIONS

A. **General**
   1. After incubation, a decarboxylase test may show two layers of different colors, yellow and purple. Shake the tube gently **before** attempting an interpretation.
   2. Often a positive decarboxylase test result is difficult to read because of an indistinct yellowish purple color. If this occurs, always compare it with an uninoculated tube. Any trace of purple denotes a positive result if the tube has been incubated at least 24 h. In some cases a color is indistinct or lost after prolonged incubation (several days) because of destruction of the pH indicator (29); addition of bromcresol purple to the tube proves this is the cause. This discoloration or indistinct reading occurs frequently with *P. mirabilis* and *P. vulgaris* (29).
   3. Label all decarboxylase tubes **prior to** inoculation. A mixup of the various amino acid tubes will give an invalid bacterial identification. An accepted labeling is C, control; A, arginine; L, lysine; O, ornithine.
   4. The **un**inoculated control tube containing no amino acid should remain yellow after 18–24 h of incubation, denoting that only glucose was fermented. A positive uninoculated control (purple) result invalidates all the amino acid decarboxylase tests and no interpretation can be made.

5. Metabolizing bacteria may catabolize amino acids in another manner, and the amines formed may be further degraded. These possibilities occur particularly with the breakdown of L-arginine. L-Arginine catabolism can occur simultaneously by different pathways: the decarboxylase and/or the dihydrolase system (29).
6. Bromcresol purple pH indicator in the medium gives more-distinct changes in pH reactions, but an earlier pH shift in the controls appears earlier than those in the decarboxylase test system (29).
7. When using Falkow's or Møller's decarboxylase tests **do not** attempt to interpret results until the tubes have been incubated at least 18–24 h. Earlier interpretations may give a false-negative result. Within the first 10–12 h of incubation, glucose is fermented, which results in a yellow color (acid pH). The decarboxylase activity is only observed after glucose is fermented.
8. *S. choleraesuis* serovar *gallinarum* gives a delayed positive ornithine decarboxylase reaction that requires 5–6 days of incubation. This delayed reaction is due to a slight permeability for ornithine in the living bacterium and is a rare exception (29).
9. Many *E. coli* strains, including those that ferment adonitol, exhibit a delayed reaction for ornithine decarboxylase activity (29).
10. Since decarboxylase media contain peptones, it is necessary to exclude air by sealing to prevent a false-positive alkaline reaction due to oxidation and deamination of peptones, which starts at the surface of the media (4, 6). Acid is not oxidized anaerobically, so no peptone deamination occurs; an alkaline reaction is thus caused by amino acid decarboxylation (6). Anaerobiosis may also be obtained by adding agar to the medium, making it either solid or semisolid. If tubes are **not** sealed, reactions are **not valid** after a 24-h incubation; the control tube may also be alkaline, which makes test results invalid and impossible to interpret.
11. Gale (19), states six conditions **required** for formation of active bacterial amino acid decarboxylases: (*a*) the organism must possess the potential to elaborate a specific decarboxylase enzyme; (*b*) growth must occur in a specific amino acid substrate; (*c*) the enzyme must synthesize a codecarboxylase enzyme or it must be added to the medium; (*d*) the medium must be acidic; (*e*) the organism must be incubated at optimal temperature for decarboxylase production; and (*f*) formation will occur only at the end of active cell division.
12. Specific decarboxylase activity is greatly enhanced at pH 5 or below and greatly decreased or completely depressed at pH 8.0 or above (19).
13. Many nonfermenters display weak decarboxylase activity and may produce **in**sufficient amines to convert the pH indicator system (27). This may be overcome by (*a*) using small quantities of substrate (e.g., 1–2 mL), (*b*) using a heavy inoculum of pregrown organisms in which a high concentration of enzymes has accumulated, and (*c*) increasing sensitivity by overlaying medium with 4 mm of petrolatum (Vaseline) (27).
14. Ornithine is highly acidic; during medium preparation, it may be necessary to adjust the pH with 1 N NaOH **before** sterilization (30).
15. **Non**fermenting bacteria that are arginine positive must be accompanied by a negative lysine and negative ornithine result. A positive lysine combination or an arginine-ornithine combination indicates that the medium is contaminated (31).
16. The reactions of **non**fermenters are slow compared with those of the *Enterobacteriaceae;* often a 48-h incubation is required (31).
17. A small amount of floccular precipitate in ornithine tubes does not interfere with their use.
18. Negative uninoculated controls **must** be used to ensure that an initial drop in pH has occurred (27).
19. Formation of lysine decarboxylase is enhanced in media containing additional organic nitrogen (11).
20. Some amino acids inhibit lysine decarboxylase production (11). Pyridoxine aids lysine

production; *E. coli* converts it to pyridoxal phosphate, the coenzyme that functions with lysine decarboxylase (11).

B. **Møller's decarboxylase medium**
   1. According to Balows et al. (1), numerous versions of Møller's procedure exist that vary in (*a*) the kind of peptone used, (*b*) the amount of beef extract used, (*c*) the amount of bromcresol purple indicator used, (*d*) the volume of media, (*e*) the size of tubes and inocula, and (*f*) the type of overlay. Møller's procedure was developed for the *Enterobacteriaceae* and may not be suitable for other groups of bacteria (1).
   2. Møller's decarboxylase medium requires a low pH, anaerobic conditions, and strict controls. The Falkow decarboxylase medium simply depends on a change in the pH indicator (17).

C. **Falkow's lysine decarboxylase medium**
   1. Falkow lysine decarboxylase activity produces a distinct pH shift to purple in 24 h. The lysine decarboxylase activity in *Salmonella* is used to differentiate this group from *Citrobacter* spp. However, *S. choleraesuis* serovar *paratyphi* A gives a negative reaction (yellow) in 24 h and represents an exception to the reaction discussed for the test.
   2. Falkow's medium is **not satisfactory** for determining the lysine decarboxylase activity of certain members of the *Klebsiella-Enterobacter-Serratia-Hafnia* group (12, 15, 27). They produce acetylmethylcarbinol (VP positive) (29), which interferes with the final alkaline pH shift and yields false-negative results (27). Since the results may be equivocal, Falkow's method is **not** recommended for identification of these microorganisms (12, 15, 27).

D. **LIA:** Lysine-iron agar (LIA) is **not** a substitute for Møller's test medium (3).

E. **Ninhydrin broth procedure**
   1. The ninhydrin test is **not** used for *Enterobacter* (17).
   2. Ninhydrin is **destroyed** if any of the alkaline emulsion (NaOH layer) is carried over with the chloroform layer; remove an aliquot of chloroform layer **carefully**.
   3. It is necessary to centrifuge and extract cadaverine from lysine in the ninhydrin test. Lysine will also give a purple (positive) color with ninhydrin reagent (10).
   4. Time and temperature are important for accurate ninhydrin test results; a higher temperature (above room temperature) or longer time (more than 4 min) may give a false-positive result (6).
   5. There is **no** pH indicator in Carlquist's ninhydrin broth.

F. **Rapid decarboxylase medium of Fay and Barry** (17): original formulation omitted glucose; however, decarboxylation is favored by the absence of glucose. A small amount (0.1 g/L) was introduced; this does not affect the reactions of nonfermenters but does permit use of the same medium to test fermenters (31).

REFERENCES

1. Balows A, Hausler WJ Jr, Herrmann KL, et al. Manual of Clincal Microbiology, ed 5. Washington, DC: American Society for Microbiology, 1991:1243.
2. Barile MF, Schimke RT, Riggs DB. Presence of arginine dihydrolase pathway in *Mycoplasma*. J Bacteriol 1966;91(1):189–192.
3. Baron EJ, Finegold SM. Bailey & Scott's Diagnostic Microbiology, ed 8. Philadelphia: CV Mosby, 1990:A–17.
4. Blazevic DJ, Ederer GM. Principles of Biochemical Tests in Diagnostic Microbiology. New York: John Wiley & Sons, 1975:29–35.
5. Borchardt KA. Simplified method for identification of enteric and other gram-negative bacteria using reagent-impregnated strips. Am J Clin Pathol 1968;49(5):748–750.
6. Branson D. Methods in Clinical Bacteriology. Springfield, IL: Charles C Thomas, 1972:29–32.
7. Brooker DC, Lund ME, Blazevic DJ. Rapid test for lysine decarboxylase activity in *Enterobacteriaceae*. Appl Microbiol 1973;26(4):622–623.
8. Burrows W, Lewert RM, Rippon JW. Textbook of Microbiology. The Pathogenic Microorganisms, vol 1, ed 19. Philadelphia: WB Saunders, 1968:143.
9. Cantarow A, Schepartz B. Biochemistry, ed 3. Philadelphia: WB Saunders, 1962:284–286.

10. Carlquist PR. A biochemical test for separating paracolon groups. J Bacteriol 1956;71(3):339–341.
11. Cascieri T Jr, Mallette MF. Stimulation of lysine decarboxylase production in Escherichia coli by amino acids and peptides. Appl Microbiol 1973;26(6):975–981.
12. Cowan ST. Cowan & Steel's Manual for the Identification of Medical Bacteria, ed 2. Cambridge: Cambridge University Press, 1974:167, 169.
13. Doelle HW. Bacterial Metabolism. New York: Academic Press, 1969:405.
14. Edwards PR, Fife MA. Lysine-iron agar in the detection of Arizona cultures. Appl Microbiol 1961;9(6):478–480.
15. Ewing WH. Enterobacteriaceae. Biochemical Methods for Group Differentiation. US Public Health Service Publ no. 734, 1962.
16. Ewing WH. Edwards and Ewing's Identification of Enterobacteriaceae, ed 4. New York: Elsevier, 1986:518.
17. Falkow S. Activity of lysine decarboxylase as an aid in the identification of salmonellae and shigellae. Am J Clin Pathol 1958;29(6):598–600.
18. Fay GD, Barry AL. Rapid ornithine decarboxylase test for the identification of Enterobacteriaceae. Appl Microbiol 1972;23(4):710–713.
19. Gale EF. The bacterial amino acid decarboxylases. Adv Enzymol 1946;6:1–32.
20. Gerlach EH, Steiner S, Weaver RH. A rapid test for lysine decarboxylase production by Enterobacteriaceae cultures. Am J Med Technol 1967;33(5):372–374.
21. Goldschmidt MC, Lockhart BM, Perry K. Rapid methods for determining decarboxylase activity: Ornithine and lysine decarboxylases. Appl Microbiol 1971;22(3):344–349.
22. Gottschalk G. Bacterial Metabolism, ed 2. New York: Springer-Verlag, 1986:147.
23. Harper HA, Rodwell VW, Mayes PA. Review of Physiological Chemistry, ed 16. Los Altos, CA: Lange Medical Publications, 1977:350–351, 353.
24. Kakimoto T, Shibatani T, Nishimura N, Chibata I. Enzymatic production of L-citrulline by Pseudomonas putida. Appl Microbiol 1971;22(6):992–999.
25. Kauffmann F, Moller V. On amino acid decarboxylases of Salmonella types and on the KCN test. Acta Pathol Microbiol Scand 1955;36(2):173–178.
26. Knivett VA. Citrulline as an intermediate in the breakdown of arginine by Streptococcus faecalis [Abstract]. Biochem J 1952;50:30–31.
27. Koneman EW, Allen SD, Janda WM, et al. Color Atlas and Textbook of Diagnostic Microbiology, ed 4. Philadelphia: JB Lippincott, 1992:123–124, 133, 140, 147, 198, 452.
28. Lambert MAS, Moss CW. Use of gas chromatography for detecting ornithine and lysine decarboxylase activity in bacteria. Appl Microbiol 1973;26(4):517–520.
29. Møller V. Simplified tests for some amino acid decarboxylases and for the arginine dihydrolase system. Acta Pathol Microbiol Scand 1955;36(2):158–172.
30. Oberhofer TR. Manual of Practical Medical Microbiology and Parasitology. New York: John Wiley & Sons, 1985:150–151.
31. Oberhofer TR. Manual of Nonfermenting Gram-Negative Bacteria. New York: John Wiley & Sons, 1985:27–29.
32. Oginsky EL, Gehrig RF. The arginine-dehydrolase system of Streptococcus faecalis. I. Identification of citrulline as an intermediate. J Biol Chem 1952;198(2):791–797.
33. Oginsky EL, Gehrig RF. The arginine-dehydrolase of Streptococcus faecalis. III. The decomposition of citrulline. J Biol Chem 1953;204(2):721–729.
34. Power DA, McCuen PJ. Manual of BBL Products and Laboratory Procedures, ed 6. Cockeysville, MD: Becton Dickinson Microbiology Systems, 1988:180–181.
35. Slade HD, Slamp WC. The formation of arginine dehydrolase by streptococci and some properties of the enzyme system. J Bacteriol 1952;64(4):455–466.
36. Smith DT, Conant NF, Willett HP. Zinsser's Microbiology, ed 14. New York: Appleton-Century-Crofts, 1968:118–119.
37. Sokatch JR. Bacterial Physiology and Metabolism. New York: Academic Press, 1969:169–170.
38. Washington JA. Laboratory Procedures in Clinical Microbiology, ed 2. New York: Springer-Verlag, 1985:196–197.
39. Williams GA, Blazevic DJ, Ederer GM. Detection of arginine dihydrolase in nonfermentative gram-negative bacteria by use of thin-layer chromatography. Appl Microbiol 1971;22(6):1135–1137.

10 Deoxyribonuclease (DNase) and Thermonuclease (TNase) Tests

I. PRINCIPLE

A. To determine the ability of an organism to produce enzyme deoxyribonuclease (DNase) capable of depolymerizing deoxyribonucleic acid (DNA) (9, 10, 42)

B. To determine thermonuclease (TNase) stability characteristic of *Staphylococcus aureus* subsp. *aureus* DNase subjected to heating

II. PURPOSE

(Also see Chapters 43–45)

A. **Presence of DNase**
  1. Used primarily as a supplemental test to identify potential pathogenic staphylococci (23, 26, 96). Helps identify possible *Staphylococcus aureus* subsp. *aureus* strains that fail to give a definite positive coagulase test reaction (18, 41, 76, 86, 96); *S. aureus* subsp. *aureus* (+), *S. epidermidis* (usually −) (41, 96, 100)
  2. Aid in differentiating between closely related genera of the *Klebsiella-Enterobacter-Serratia* division of *Enterobacteriaceae: Serratia* spp. (+) **except** *Serratia proteamaculans* subsp. *proteamaculans* (formerly *Serratia liquefaciens*) (V, variable; usually (+)) and *Serratia fonticola* (−) (43) from *Klebsiella-Enterobacter* spp. (−) (7, 22, 63, 79)

(Note: *S. proteamaculans* is a collection of several DNA hybridization groups that includes *proteamaculans* and *grimesii* (43), and *S. fonticola* (−), probably not a true member of the *Serratia* genus (3, 43), conforms to definition of family *Enterobacteriaceae*; does not conform to present definition of genus *Serratia* (46).)

  3. Differentiate and distinguish *Moraxella catarrhalis* (formerly *Branhamella catarrhalis*) (+) and *Kingella denitrificans* (formerly TM-1 group) (V) (32, 86) from *Neisseria* spp. (−). *M. catarrhalis* and *K. denitrificans* are easily separated by catalase reaction; *K. denitrificans* (−), *M. catarrhalis* (+). DNase test agar–toluidine blue O (DTA-TBO) procedures especially enhance recovery from mixed bacterial populations (85). DTA-TBO suppresses growth of upper respiratory flora and permits rapid differentiation between *M. catarrhalis* and *Neisseria* spp. (85).
  4. Differentiate *Plesiomonas shigelloides* (−) from *Aeromonas* spp. (+) (43, 46).
  5. Differentiate *Campylobacter jejuni* (V), *Campylobacter coli* (V, usually (+), *C. coli* 16% (+) (4) to 75% (+) (78)), *Campylobacter lari* (+), and *Helicobacter pylori* (+) (formerly *Campylobacter pylori* (34)) from other *Campylobacter* spp. (−) (29). Lior and Patel (60) recommend DTA-TBO procedure over DNase test agar–methyl green (DTA-MG) for Lior's (59) biotyping scheme for campylobacters.
  6. Differentiate between less commonly encountered microorganisms
     a. *Sphingobacterium spiritivorum* (+) (formerly *Flavobacterium spiritivorum*, CDC IIk-3) from other yellow-pigmented pseudomonads *Sphinx multivorum* (−) (formerly *Flavo-bacterium multivorum*, CDC IIk-2) (43), *Sphingomonas paucimobilis* (formerly *Pseudo-monas paucimobilis*), CDC IIk-1) (−), *Chryseomonas luteola* (−)

(formerly *Chromobacterium typhiflavum*, *Pseudomonas luteola*, *Pseudomonas polytricha*, and CDC Ve-1) (33, 43), and *Flavimonas oryzihabitans* (−) (formerly CDC Ve-2) (43)
   b. Differentiate RNA group V *Stenotrophomonas maltophila* (formerly *Xanthomonas maltophilia* and *Pseudomonas maltophilia*) (+) and RNA group IV, *Shewanella putrefaciens* (+) (formerly *Pseudomonas putrefaciens* (61)) from *Brevundimonas vesicularis* (formerly *Pseudomonas diminuta*) (V, usually (−), and *Brevundimonas paucimobilis* (formerly *Pseudomonas vesicularis*) (−) (43)
   c. Differentiate *M. catarrhalis* (+) from other *Moraxella* spp. (−) most frequently isolated
7. Determine the immunologic response to group A streptococcal infections (94), a serologic procedure that is not discussed further in this text

Group A *Streptococcus pyogenes* is DNase positive in four antigenic variants: A, B, C, and D (93). Most strains produce two or more types; type B is most common (93).

B. **Thermonuclease test**: determine and confirm the presence of *S. aureus* subsp. *aureus* DNase from that produced by *S. epidermidis* or other micrococci

(*Note:* Not all methods presently in use to determine hydrolysis of DNase are applicable in a clinical laboratory (9).)

III. BIOCHEMISTRY INVOLVED

Nucleic Acid

DNA (desoxy- or deoxyribonucleic acid), deoxypentosenucleic acid (12), is a member of the family of polymers called nucleic acids. It is a long-chain polynucleotide composed of repeating purine and pyrimidine mononucleotide monomeric units called deoxyribonucleotides bound to one another by phosphodiester bridges (9, 30, 31, 35, 83). The deoxy- prefix means "lacking in an oxygen atom found in a closed structural relative" (35). Nucleic acids are organic nitrogen-containing molecules.

Nucleotide units consist of repeating units of a pentose sugar and phosphate with a nitrogenous base attached to each deoxyribose–phosphoric acid (phosphate) residue (31, 83).

The 5-carbon sugar is D-2-deoxyribose in furanose form to which phosphoric acid is esterified (attached) at position 3′ and/or 5′ (9, 12, 31). The phosphoric acid unit on one nucleotide splits out water and joins with an alcohol unit (–OH) of the next nucleotide to form an internucleotide phosphate ester (–O–) linkage (bridge, bond) between two molecules (12, 35); thus, deoxyribonucleotides are phosphoric acid esters of nucleosides (9).

D-2-Deoxyribose
2-Deoxy-β-D-ribofuranose
β-D-Deoxyribose (29)

Phosphoric acid (phosphate)

The "backbones" of nucleic acids are the alternating sugar-phosphate units and, from the sugar moiety, various heterocyclic nitrogenous amines (bases) are projected in repeating sequences (35, 74). There are four amines of two types: two purine bases, adenine and guanine, and two pyrimidine bases, thymine and cytosine.

Pyrimidines (32)

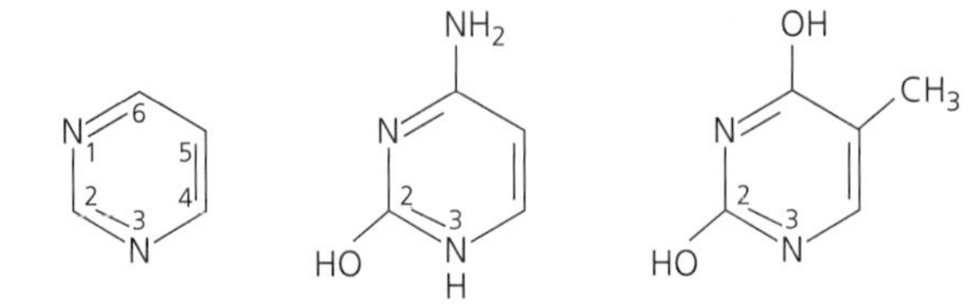

General structure

Cystosine (C)
(2-oxy-4-amino-pyrimidine)

Thymine (T)
(2,4-dioxy-5-methyl-pyrimidine)

Purines (32)

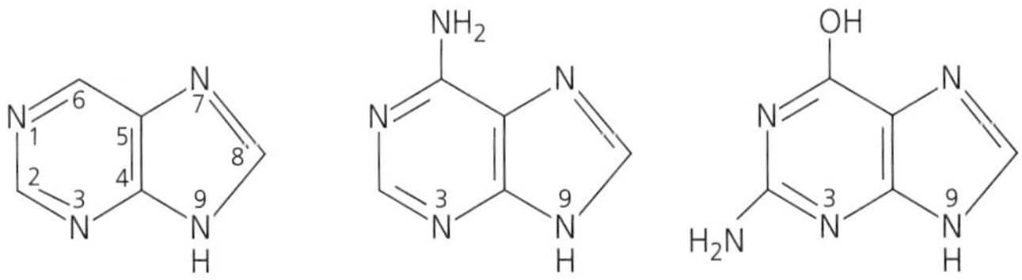

General structure

Adenine (A)
(6-aminopurine)

Guanine (G)
(2-amino-6-oxypurine)

In polynucleotides, nucleotide residues are held together by phosphodiester linkages between the 3'-carbon of one deoxyribose residue and the 5'-carbon of the adjacent deoxyribose residue (31). Deoxyribose is attached to the 9'- and 3'-carbon of purines and pyrimidines, respectively, in β-glucosidic linkage (12).

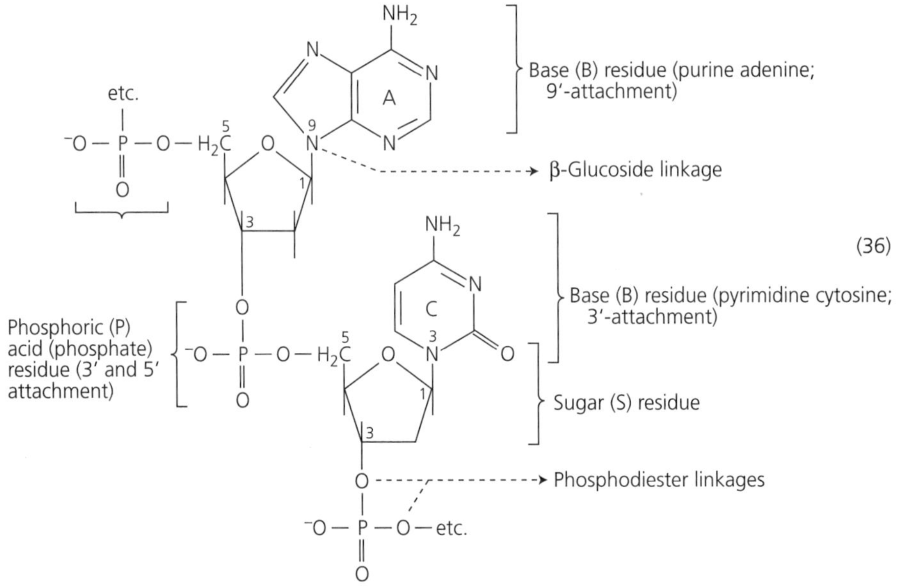

(36)

Base (B) residue (purine adenine; 9'-attachment)

β-Glucoside linkage

Base (B) residue (pyrimidine cytosine; 3'-attachment)

Phosphoric (P) acid (phosphate) residue (3' and 5' attachment)

Sugar (S) residue

Phosphodiester linkages

Two general types of DNA exist: in animal tissue and yeast adenine and thymine predominate, and in bacteria and some insect viruses there is an excess of guanine and cytosine (12). Some bacteria such as *Escherichia coli* have equimolar proportions of the four major bases (12).

DNA is a double helix with two coiled intertwined chains of a backbone of sugar-phosphate complexes with bases located between chains forming a ladderlike structure (19, 35). Purine-pyrimidine base combinations on one chain are linked to those in the other chain by hydrogen bonds (19, 35, 74); a thymine (T) on one chain fits the adenine (A) exactly opposite it on the second chain, and the guanine (G) on one chain pairs with cytosine (C) (71), resulting in molar equivalence of the bases (19, 30, 35).

Monomeric units of DNA (adenylate, guanylate, cytidylate, and thymidylate; A, G, C, T) constitute a single strand of DNA held together in polymeric form by 3′,5′-phosphodiester bridges (30). Hydrogen-bonded purines and pyrimidines occur in definite pairs. Three hydrogen bonds hold G to C; A and T are held together by two hydrogen bonds; thus G:C is the stronger of the two pairs (30). However, in general, hydrogen bonds are very weak and are easily broken (35).

DNA exists in nature as a double-stranded molecule (30). The two strands are antiparallel; one strand runs in the 5′ to 3′ direction, the other 3′ to 5′ (30). This gives the DNA polymer polarity; one end has a 5′-hydroxyl or phosphate terminus; the other a 3′-phosphate or hydroxyl moiety (30). However, in bacteria the two ends of DNA molecule are joined to create a closed circle with no termini; polarity is not destroyed, but **all** 3′ and 5′ free hydroxyl and phosphoryl groups are eliminated (30).

DNA can be hydrolyzed enzymatically to inorganic phosphate and nucleotides (12, 31). The major nucleotides and nucleosides of DNA (9, 12, 83) are shown in Table 10.1.

(Redrawn from Holum, J. R. *Elements of General and Biological Chemistry,* 4th ed., 1975, p. 512, with permission of John Wiley and Sons, Inc., New York.)

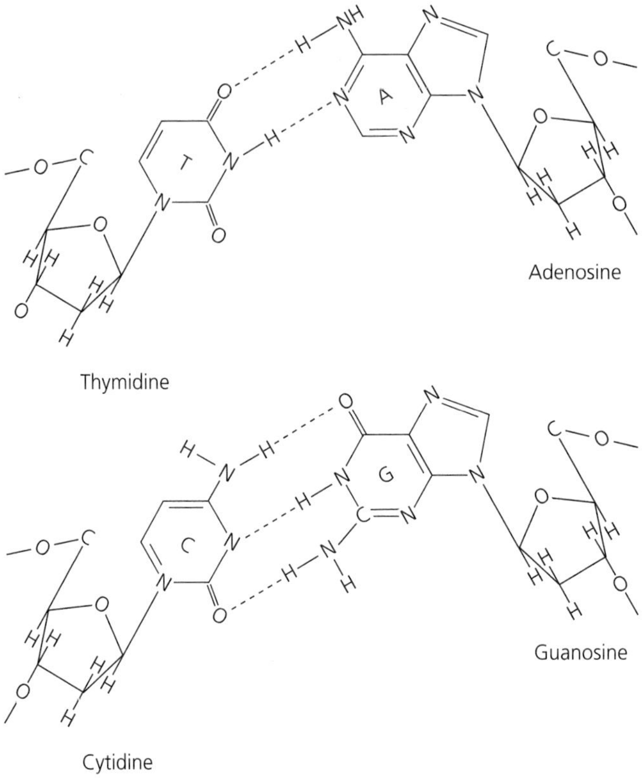

Adenosine

Thymidine

Guanosine

Cytidine

(Redrawn from Harper, H. A., Rodwell, V. W., and Mayes, P. A. *Review of Physiological Chemistry,* 16th ed., 1977, p. 134, wih permission of Lange Medical Publications, Los Altos, Calif.)

$$DNA \xrightarrow[H_2O]{Enzyme} Nucleotides \xrightarrow[H_2O]{Enzyme} Nucleosides + P_i$$

(base-sugar-phosphate complex) (B-S-P)
(base-sugar-complex) (B-S)
Inorganic phosphorus (phosphate)

Table 10.1. Major Nucleotides and Nucleosides of DNA

Base	Deoxyribonucleotides (B–S–P)	Deoxyribonucleosides (B–S)
Adenine (A)	Adenosine-5′-phosphate (AMP, 5′-AMP) (adenosine-5′-monophosophate) (deoxyadenylic(5′) acid) (deoxyadenosine-5′-phosphate)	Adenosine
Guanine (G)	Guanosine-5′-phosphate (GMP, 5′-GMP) (guanosine-5′-monophosphate) (deoxyguanylic(5′)acid) (deoxyguanosine-5′-phosphate)	Guanosine
Cytosine (C)	Cytidine-5′-phosphate (CMP, 5′-CMP) (cytosine-5′-monophosphate) (deoxycytidylic(5′)acid) (deoxycytidine-5′-phosphate)	Cytidine
Thymine (T)	Thymidine-5′-phosphate (TMP, 5′-TMP) (thymidine-5′-monophosphate) (deoxythymidylic (5′) acid) (deoxythymidine-5′-phosphate)	Thymidine

DNase enzymes

Nuclease enzymes capable of degrading nucleic acids are classified as either (*a*) **endonucleases**, which cleave an internal phosphodiester bond, producing 3′-hydroxyl and 5′-phosphoryl or 5′-hydroxyl and 3′-phosphoryl termini, or (*b*) **exonucleases**, which hydrolyze (cleave) a nucleotide only when it is present at a terminus of a molecule (30). Some nucleases cleave both strands; others cleave only one (30). The physical and chemical properties of DNA differ from those of oligonucleotides or mononucleotides, and these differences are used to detect hydrolysis of DNA by DNase (9). DNase can catalyze the depolymerization of DNA (i.e., break the linkage of polymers to form smaller monomer units of nucleic acid DNA) (70).

DNase is an extracellular endonuclease (30) that is specific for hydrolysis (degradation) of DNA (9, 30). Most bacterial DNases require divalent cations for their activity (70, 94), which are usually provided by peptones in growth/test medium (9). The pH range for enzyme activity is 5.5–8.5 (70, 94), and optimal pH is 7.2. Various DNases may be differentiated from each other antigenically (65, 95) or by differences in response to specific inhibitors (6, 13, 45).

On hydrolysis, approximately one fourth of the internal nucleotide phosphodiester and hydrogen bonds holding complementary sequences of DNA nucleotides together are cleaved, yielding a mixture of oligonucleotides (chains of several deoxyribonucleotides). Oligonucleotides possess a 3′-hydroxyl and 3′-phosphoryl and/or 5′-phosphoryl or 5′-hydroxyl terminus (31). Partial degradation (depolymerization) by DNase action, heating, or pH extremes denatures DNA, with corresponding changes in physical properties; these include decreased viscosity of the DNA solution and increased absorption of ultraviolet light at 260 mμ (31, 96). The effect of DNase is the formation of deoxyribonucleotides having higher percentages of purines than the DNA substrate (31).

DNases are present in extracts of a variety of microorganisms (79); however, extracellular DNases are reported in a few bacterial species such as *S. aureus* subsp. *aureus* (16), group A streptococci (94), *Corynebacterium diphtheriae* (66), *Serratia marcescens* (20, 42), *Pseudomonas aeruginosa* (42), *Bacillus* spp. (42), and *Vibrio* spp. (63).

Staphylococcal DNase

Both *S. aureus* subsp. *aureus* and *S. epidermidis* produce extracellular DNase (1, 77, 100); however, *S. aureus* subsp. *aureus* has more DNase activity (96, 100), and the DNase test depends on a **quantitative** discrimination (100). The DNase test is used primarily to determine potential pathogenic staphylococci (23, 26, 96) (e.g., *S. aureus* subsp. *aureus*).

S. aureus subsp. *aureus* DNase, ribonucleate (deoxyribonucleate) 3′-nucleotidohydrolase (deoxyribonuclease) (100), differs from other DNases in that it requires calcium (Ca^{2+}) as a cation activator (i.e., cofactor) (24, 52, 96), it has a higher optimal pH of 8.6–9.0 (96), it degrades DNA more extensively (96), it is remarkably heat stable, and its activity correlates somewhat with that of coagulase (8, 18, 96).

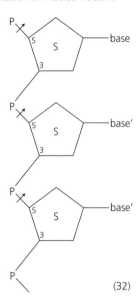

(32)

DNA hydrolysis by micrococcal nuclease produces primarily mono- and dinucleotide fragments (70) by specifically cleaving bonds between the 5'-carbon of the sugar-phosphate (S–P) residue attached on the other end to the 3'-carbon of an adjacent S–P residue (31); its products terminate in 3'-phosphate groups (24, 70). Oligonucleotides containing adenylic or thymidylic acid residues are cleaved preferentially (70), and DNase is more active on denatured than on native DNA (70).

Certain related saprophytic staphylococci may produce DNase (e.g., *S. epidermidis*) (69); however, the thermostability of the nuclease produced by all *S. aureus* subsp. *aureus* strains appears to be a constant and unique property (5, 52, 55, 76, 86, 90, 98, 99), and no DNase from another source has been reported to possess this characteristic (52). Lachica et al. (55) found that production of thermostable nuclease appears to be as accurate as coagulase production as an indicator of *S. aureus* subsp. *aureus*; no *S. epidermidis* strains showed thermostable nuclease activity (99). The DNase of *S. aureus* subsp. *aureus* can withstand boiling (100°C) for 15 min (16).

Serratia DNase

The DNase test shows potential as an aid in identification of *Serratia* spp., especially the nonpigmented strains, which are the most commonly isolated (14, 21, 22, 36). These nonpigmented strains are biochemically and morphologically similar to other *Enterobacteriaceae*, especially *Klebsiella-Enterobacter* spp. Rothberg and Swartz (79) and Elston and Elston (22) showed that DNase activity is absent in *Klebsiella-Enterobacter* spp. All species of *Serratia* produce DNase except *S. fonticola* (43).

Serratia extracellular DNase is a nonspecific phosphodiesterase (20, 63, 79), and the major products of hydrolysis are di-, tri-, and tetranucleotides terminating in a 5'-phosphate (70). DNase is predominantly endonucleolytic, and less than 2% of the degradation products are mononucleotides; DNase can degrade native and denatured DNA substrates, both single- and double-stranded DNA, at similar rates (70). Enzyme production increases during cell growth (log phase), peaks just after the stationary phase, and declines steadily thereafter (70).

S. marcescens nuclease requires magnesium (Mg^{2+}) or manganese (Mn^{3+}) ions for activation; its pH range is 7.0–10.0, with the optimum at 8.5. It is heat labile; heating to 44°C or above reduces enzymatic activity, and all activity stops after heating for 40 min (70). Concentrations of calcium or sodium ions (e.g., CaCl$_2$ or NaCl) above 10^{-4} M inhibit *Serratia* DNase, and it is completely inactivated by 0.1 M EDTA (70).

Differences between *S. aureus* subsp. *aureus* and *S. marcescens* DNase (70) are shown in Table 10.2.

Table 10.2. Differences between *S. aureus* subsp. *aureus* and *Senatia marcescens* DNase

	S. aureus subsp. *aureus*	*S. marcescens*
Ions required for activation	Ca^{2+}	Mg^{2+} or Mn^{3+}
pH range	8.6–9.0	7.0–10.0
Optimal pH		8.5
Heating, 44°C or above	Thermostable (heat resistant)	Thermolabile (heat sensitive)
Preferred DNA substrate type	Denatured	Native and denatured; single or double strands
Major products formed	Mono- and dinucleotides	Di-, tri- and tetranucleotides
Product terminus	3'-phosphate	5'-phosphate

Data from reference 70.

Streptococcal DNase

Streptococcal extracellular DNases (42, 83) A, B, C, and D are serologically distinct enzymes that degrade the same substrate (DNA) (83). Nuclease B elicits antibodies that are a useful index of streptococcal infection. All group A streptococci produce DNase as well as those in some other Lancefield groups (94). The DNase of group A streptococci yields products with a chain length of 3–10 deoxyribonucleotide units along with mononucleotides (94). Streptococcal DNases require magnesium (Mg^{2+}) ions for activation (83). Extracellular nucleases are produced primarily by the same species that produce the proteose gelatinases (3).

IV. MEDIUM EMPLOYED: STANDARD DNASE TEST AGAR (DTA)

A. Acid-DNase test procedure of Jeffries, Holtman, and Guse (42); precipitation test
B. Ingredients, pH 7.3 ± 0.2

Deoxyribonucleic acid (DNA), 0.2%	2.0 g
Pancreatic digest of casein, USP	15.0 g
Palmic digest of soybean meal, USP	5.0 g
Sodium chloride, NaCl	5.0 g
Agar, 1.5%	15.0 g
Deionized water	1000.0 mL

C. DNA: Sigma Chemical Co. (87) (see Appendix 11)
D. Commercial products (3) (see Appendix 11)
   1. Thermal agar
   2. Thermonuclease agar; REMEL
E. Method of preparation
   1. Weigh out amounts accurately as directed on the label. Various company products may differ slightly.
   2. Rehydrate with distilled or demineralized water.
   3. Heat **gently** into solution to avoid formation of insoluble protein threads (48).
F. Method of sterilization: autoclave; 121°C, 15 lb, 15 min
G. Place flask of sterilized medium into a 50°C water bath to cool down but **not solidify** medium.
   1. Periodically during cooling, remove flask(s) from water bath and place against forearm.

2. If cool to touch, medium should be right temperature to pour.
3. **Never** place an **unsterile** thermometer into flask to check temperature.
H. Pour into disposable **presterilized** plastic (or glass) Petri dishes (15 × 100 mm).
   1. Open commercially packaged dishes carefully at one end and save bags for storage.
   2. Flame mouth of flask and pour approximately **12–15 mL/plate.**
   3. If air bubbles appear in poured plates, pass a Bunsen flame **quickly** over agar **before** it sets (solidifies).
   4. Allow agar to set with plates in an **upright** position with lids slightly ajar (cracked) to get rid of excess moisture.
I. Incubation; sterility check
   1. **Inverted** position (lid on bottom); 35°C, 18–24 h
   2. Discard all plates showing **any** contamination or poorly mixed areas of medium.
J. Storage
   1. Refrigeration, 4–10°C
   2. **Inverted** position
   3. It is preferable to store in bags to minimize water loss (original bags are saved from IV.H.1 above).
K. Inoculation (18, 42, 79)
   1. Growth from an 18- to 24-h **pure** culture; brain-heart infusion (BHI) broth, heart infusion agar (HIA) slants, sheep blood agar (SBA) plate, Kligler's iron agar (KIA), or other suitable culture.
   2. Can inoculate from 4 to as many as 8 test organisms per single plate
   3. Two methods; both use inoculating **needle**
      a. Band (i.e., line) streak inoculations
         (1) **Heavy** inocula (63)
         (2) At least 1½–1 inch long
         (3) From rim to center of plate
      b. Spot inoculations
         (1) **Heavy** inocula
         (2) Diameter of ⅛ to ¼ inch
L. Incubation (18, 42, 79): 35°C; 18–24 h or period and temperature suitable for organisms being tested
   1. Continue incubation to 36 h, if necessary, until good growth.
   2. Incubate at least 24 h before reporting as negative result.
M. Add 1 N HCl reagent **directly** to **incubated** plate(s) **before** attempting to interpret; allow plate(s) to remain **upright** (lid on top) to avoid spilling the reagent, as it takes a few minutes to be absorbed into the medium.

The composition of culture medium, amount of aeration, pH, temperature, and incubation period are important factors in DNase activity in culturing and testing the micrococci (96). Weckman and Catlin (96) found that BHI produced the highest DNase activity levels in micrococci, while activities in cultures from Trypticase soy broth (TSB), tryptose phosphate broth, or heart infusion (HI) were increased by supplementation with yeast extract. Activity increases even more when cultures are shaken (aerated) at room temperature for 40–72 h. Jeffries et al. (42), showed that organisms are more exacting about pH for enzyme production than about temperature. Zierdt and Golde (100) recommend adding niacin and thiamine (5 µg/mL) to standard DTA plates, which markedly increases the number of positive reactions. Blood may be added to DTA medium for cultivation of more fastidious organisms (e.g., streptococci).

For DTA prepared from scratch, commercial DNA substrate is available in various purity grades: the highest grade and most polymerized is derived from calf thymus (Sigma Chemical Co.), the intermediate grade is not as highly polymerized, and the crude DNA is derived from herring sperm (100) (see Appendix 11). Zierdt and Golde (100) showed that purified DNA gave 100% positive reactions with larger zones with atypical staphylococcal strains and that crude DNA was too insensitive for nuclease production. The lower the purity of DNA used, the less sensitive the test for nuclease production becomes. However, Zierdt and Golde (100) found that lower-grade DNA discriminated better between *S. aureus* subsp. *aureus* and *S. epidermidis* because the small amount of DNase produced by *S. epidermidis* is not detected, and hence, DNase production indicates *S. aureus* subsp. *aureus*. The storage life of DNA solution is 3 months at $-10°C$ if tubes are tightly capped (28).

V. ALTERNATIVE ADDITIONS TO DTA MEDIUM

A. **Mannitol**
   1. Incorporation of 1% mannitol and pH indicator before sterilization (15)
   2. pH indicator: either bromthymol blue or phenol red
      a. Alkaline: red (phenol red); Prussian blue (bromthymol blue)
      b. Acid: yellow; phenol red and bromthymol blue
   3. Permits mannitol use, indicated by yellow zones around colonies
   4. **Subsequent addition of acid** can then be used to detect DNase production on the **same plate.**

(*Note:* Various dye indicator systems are incorporated directly into medium thus **eliminating the need to use a reagent** (e.g., 1 N HCl) to demonstrate specific DNase-producing bacteria (84).)

The advantages of DTA-TBO and DTA-MG media are that plate colonies may be examined at a glance without the use of an additional reagent; therefore, if colony growth is insufficient in a normal incubation period or there are questionable zones of DNase activity, plates may be reincubated and reexamined, and colonies may be subcultured, if necessary, since organisms are still viable (84).

B. **DNase test agar medium–toluidine blue O modifications (DTA-TBO, TBO-DTA, DTB)**
   1. Procedures of Waller, Hodel, and Nuti (91); modification of procedures of Schreier (80) and Jeffries et al. (42)

(*Note:* There are two procedures; be aware that the concentration of TBO varies according to procedure used.)

   a. **TBO flooding**
      (1) According to studies by Waller et al. (91), flooding technique produces much more delineated zones of DNase activity than does DNA precipitation DNase test with 1.0 N HCl.
      (2) TBO final concentration: **0.05%** (91)
      (3) Flood colony growth with 5–6 mL of TBO solution.
      (4) Let stand 3–5 min and decant.
      (5) Read at 5-min intervals up to 30 min.
   b. **Incorporation of TBO into DNase test medium**
      (1) Incorporating TBO into DTA demonstrates DNase production more clearly than the HCl–DNA precipitation DNase test (91).
      (2) Add TBO to DTA medium before sterilization.
      (3) TBO optimal final concentration, 0.005%; acceptable range 0.0025–0.0075% (91)
   2. **Procedure of Lior and Patel (60) for *Campylobacter* spp.;** recommended as a replacement for DTA-MG used in Lior's (59) biotyping scheme for campylobacters.
      a. Tris buffer
         (1) 0.05 M; pH 9.0

(2) Prepared according to manufacturer's directions from TRIZMA-9.0; Sigma Chemical Co; (see Appendix 11)

b. Medium

DNA	0.3 g
Calcium chloride, 0.01 M	1.0 mL
Sodium chloride, NaCl	10.0 g
Agar, 6.5%	6.5 g
Tris buffer (see above)	1000.0 mL

c. Heat to boiling (100°C) 25 min or until agar and DNA are completely dissolved.
d. Cool to 50°C.
e. Add 2.5 mL of a 3% solution of TBO in distilled water (certified stain; Fisher Scientific Co.); final pH, 8.7
f. Mix well and dispense; sterilization **not** required
   (1) Flasks or bottles for storage; stable up to 3 months at room temperature (22–25°C)
   (2) 25 mL aliquots/Petri dish (90 mm)
g. Incubation 24–48 h; best results at **43°C**, 48 h

TBO allows growth and DNase production by **both Gram-positive and Gram-negative** bacteria; provides better delineation of DNase activity (91)

3. **Procedure of Soto-Hernandez, Nunley, Holtsclaw-Berk, and Berk** (85)
   a. Selective and differential medium used for rapid primary isolation of *M. catarrhalis* (+) (formerly *B. catarrhalis*) from *Neisseria* spp. (−) in mixed cultures; suppresses growth of other upper respiratory tract flora. Used in routine sputum culture when Gram-stained smear shows inflammatory cells and Gram-negative diplococci.
   b. Medium; DNase test agar, 42 g/L, pH 7.26 ± 0.2, to which is added

Vancomycin	10 μg/mL
Trimethoprim	8 μg/mL
Amphotericin B	2 μg/mL

   c. Inoculation: **heavy** inoculum; up to 8 inocula/plate
   d. Incubation: 35°C, 5% CO_2, 48 h
   e. Flood (overlay) colonies with 1 drop of a buffered 0.04% TBO solution.
      (1) TBO, Fisher; actual dye content 57%; conversion factor (CF) 100 divided by actual dye content used to prepare concentration of solution.
      (2) Tris hydrochloride buffer, 0.20 M, pH 7.8
      (3) Filter mixture with a 0.2-μm pore-sized filter.
   f. Results within 15 min
      (1) Positive (+)
         (a) Dye around colony forms a magenta halo, stable 2–4 h
         (b) Indicates interaction of dye with both agar and hydrolyzed DNA
      (2) Negative (−)
         (a) Medium remains a deep royal blue color
         (b) A drop of buffered TBO in an area of plate where there are **no** colonies provides a color contrast.

TBO is a dye (80) that exhibits metachromasia, a property whereby dye will not stain true because of complexes formed with some substances that change the absorption spectrum from that of the original dye (17, 68)). True, or orthochromatic, staining of TBO is royal blue; metachromatic coloring is pink-red-violet (58). When TBO complexes with **un**hydrolyzed DNA, a royal blue color results; however, when DNA is hydrolyzed and TBO complexes with oligonucleotides or mononucleotides that change the dye structure, the resulting absorption spectrum shifts to a different wave length of light, yielding a bright pink color that is the metachromatic, or staining, pattern of TBO (9, 68, 91). TBO may inhibit Gram-positive bacteria, and staphylococci may not grow on this medium (9).

Commercial TBO dye preparations contain actual dye contents varying from 60 to 95% (91). The dye content, as stated on commercial labels, **must be adjusted** so that dye solutions and media contain the desired percentage of dye rather than the percentage supplied by the manufacturer (91). A conversion factor **must** be included to account for true dye content:

CF (conversion factor) = 100 ÷ % dye in commercial preparation

Powder required (in g) ÷ 100 mL dye in water or agar = % dye required × CF

C. **Methyl green–DNase test agar (DTA-MG)**
1. Smith, Hancock and Rhoden (84) modification of Jeffries et al. (42) procedure
2. Stock solution
   a. Methyl green (MG) dye (Fisher, Difco; see Appendix 11)
   b. Prepare a 0.5% concentration in distilled or demineralized water; 0.5 g/100 mL.
   c. Extract repeatedly with approximately equal volumes of chloroform.
      (1) Usually 6–7 extractions
      (2) Continue until chloroform layer is colorless.
   d. Sterilize by filtration.
   e. Store in glass-stoppered reagent bottle at 4°C.
3. Working solution
   a. Add 1 mL of MG **stock** dye solution to each 100 mL of **sterile** melted DTA medium; 10 mL/L.
   b. Final optimal concentration of dye, 0.005%
4. Supports growth of both **Gram-positive** and **Gram-negative** bacteria.

MG requires a highly polymerized DNA substrate (54). It combines with polymerized DNA to form a stable, green complex at pH 7.5 (48–50). As hydrolysis progresses at pH 7.5, MG is released; when not combined at this pH, MG fades and becomes colorless (48, 50). Fading is not instantaneous; it takes 4–6 h (48, 50). According to Smith et al. (83), incorporation of MG into DTA medium yields an improved, highly sensitive medium that may be used for primary isolation of *S. aureus* subsp. *aureus* and group A *S. pyogenes* as well as the *Enterobacteriaceae*.

VI. REAGENT EMPLOYED: 1 N HYDROCHLORIC ACID (HCL) (42, 74)

A. Method of preparation, 1 N (N/1) concentration (42)
1. To a 1-L volumetric flask, add approximately 250 mL of distilled or demineralized water.
2. **Do not pipette concentrated HCl by mouth. Use a bulb (Pro) pipette.** Add 90 mL of concentrated HCl to the flask, allowing the acid to run down the side of **tilted** flask **slowly** with **gentle** swirling of flask to mix well.
3. Discard the pipette in an appropriate container.
4. Bring the volume up to 1 L with distilled or demineralized water.
5. Concentrated HCl is extremely caustic, and any splatters may cause burns. If acid contacts any skin, flood area **immediately** with running cold water.
6. Store in glass-stoppered reagent bottle in small aliquots; e.g., 100 mL.

B. Method of use
1. Procedure of Jeffries, Holtman, and Guze (42)
2. Flood **incubated** DTA plate with 1 N HCl.

C. Chemistry of reagent action: in a positive test result, oligonucleotides liberated by hydrolysis dissolve in acid; the size of the clear zone is related to the amount of exocellular enzyme produced (42). Adjacent to the clear zone a white cloudy (hazy) area is **always** present because of reaction of HCl with DNA salts in medium (23). Unhydrolyzed DNA is insoluble in acid, and the acid precipitates the salts in the medium, causing it to become cloudy (42).

VII. QUALITY CONTROL MICROORGANISMS

A. **DNase test agar**
 1. Positive (+)
    Staphylococcus aureus subsp. *aureus* ATCC 25923
    Streptococcus pyogenes ATCC 19615
 2. Negative (−)
    Staphylococcus epidermidis ATCC 12228
B. **DTA-TBO/DTA-MG**
 1. Positive (+)
    Serratia marcescens ATCC 13880
 2. Negative (−)
    Klebsiella pneumoniae subsp. *pneumoniae* ATCC 33495

VIII. INTERPRETATION

A. **Standard acid–DTA medium** (42)
 1. Positive (+)
    a. **Clearing** zone immediately surrounding bacterial colony (inoculum: streak or spot)
    b. Adjacent to clear zone a white, cloudy area; precipitated salts in medium
    c. DNA hydrolyzed (depolymerized)
    d. Size of zone related to amount of DNase produced
 2. Negative (−)
    a. No clearing around colonies
    b. **Cloudy precipitate** around colony and throughout medium (23) due to precipitated salts in medium
    c. DNA **not** hydrolyzed
B. **Standard acid-mannitol-DTA medium**
 1. Mannitol use
    a. Fermentation (F): yellow zones surround colonies; acid production
    b. Nonfermentation (NF): medium remains unchanged, reddish orange color
 2. DNA hydrolysis (+): same as standard acid procedure (see Section VIII.A above)
C. **DTA-TBO** (9, 10, 17, 80)
 1. Positive (+)
    a. Bright **rose-pink** zone around bacterial streak (or spot) inoculum; royal blue background
    b. DNase production
 2. Negative (−)
    a. **No change** in color of medium
    b. Medium remains same as uninoculated, clear royal blue
D. **DTA-MG** (10, 84)
 1. Positive (+)
    a. Distinct **clear** zone around bacterial streak (or spot) in otherwise green agar
    b. Clear zones **best observed against a white background**
 2. Negative (−)
    a. **No change** in color of medium
    b. Medium remains same as uninoculated, a green color

IX. THERMONUCLEASE TESTS

(*Note:* TNase activity is used for rapid detection of *S. aureus* subsp. *aureus* in foods (25, 44, 56, 73) and in blood cultures (5, 25, 62, 66, 75, 76).

A. **TNase test for blood cultures** (62, 75)
   1. Procedure of Madison and Baselski (62)
   2. Purpose: rapid differentiation of *S. aureus* subsp. *aureus* (+) from *Micrococcaceae* spp. in blood cultures
   3. Controls: **must** be from blood culture bottles containing blood and a known-positive *S. aureus* subsp. *aureus* strain and a known-negative staphylococcus strain (e.g., *S. epidermidis*). Controls and test specimens are processed simultaneously. Control test bottles may be used for up to 1 week and kept at room temperature (22–25°C).
   4. Specimens: **only** those bottles that show **Gram-positive** cocci in **cluster** on a **direct** Gram stain
   5. Procedure
      a. **Aseptically,** with a **sterile** capillary pipette, remove 2–3 mL of the blood broth, including erythrocytes (RBCs) and place into a **sterile** screw-cap tube.
      b. Place in boiling (100°C) water bath, 15 min.
      c. Cool to room temperature (22–25°C).
   6. Medium: DTA-TBO test plate (15 × 100 mm)
      a. With **sterile** capillary pipette, cut up to 12 wells/plate; 6-mm diameter.
      b. With **sterile** pipette, add 2–3 drops of **cooled** broth to each well. Plates may be used on successive days as long as a positive and negative control are used.
   7. Quality controls: same as for acid-DNase test agar procedure
   8. Interpretation
      a. Positive (+)
         (1) Pink zone of clearing at edge of well with a darker blue ring at outer periphery of zone
         (2) TNase activity; **presumptive** *S. aureus* subsp. *aureus*
         (3) Report: "indicating *S. aureus* subsp. *aureus*"
      b. Negative (−)
         (1) Medium has no change; no TNase activity
         (2) Report: "Gram-positive cocci in clusters; **not** *S. aureus* subsp. *aureus*"

Madison and Baselski (62) showed that *S. aureus* subsp. *aureus* TNase activity should be detectable in blood cultures when Gram stain shows Gram-positive cocci in clusters. Identification in aerobic and anaerobic blood culture bottles has occurred as early as 12 h after receipt of samples in the laboratory (62). Studies and confirmations (5, 66, 76, 82) have shown 100% agreement between direct TNase on blood cultures and subsequent tube coagulase tests by standard procedures.

S. epidermidis is the most frequently encountered coagulase-negative staphylococcus in blood cultures (64, 81); this species has not been identified as one that may give a positive TNase result (27).

B. **Simplified thermonuclease (STN) test**
   1. Procedure of Lachica for foods (51)
   2. *S. aureus* subsp. *aureus* selective isolation plate media; several choices
      a. Baird-Parker medium
      b. Tellurite–polymyxin–egg yolk agar
      c. Tellurite-glycine agar
      d. Egg yolk–sodium azide agar

3. Selective plate media with growing colonies **preheated**
   a. 60°C oven, 2 h
   b. Inactivates nucleases produced by non–*S. aureus* bacteria
4. Preheated plates overlaid with 10 mL of melted DTA-TBO and incubated at 35°C, 3 h
5. *S. aureus* subsp. *aureus*: bright pink halos around colonies; halo diameter varies among strains

C. **Metachromatic agar–diffusion microslide technique (MAD)**
   1. Screening procedure of Lachica, Hoeprich, and Franti (54)
   2. Quantitative assay for **staphylococcal TNase** in heterogeneous systems; e.g., broth and milk
   3. MAD reagent (enzyme solution)
      a. Well-buffered agar (pH 9.0) containing DNA, TBO (indicator), and iron agar no. 2
      b. Prepared as described by Lachica et al. (53), on plastic immunoplates (2.5 × 7.5 cm)
      c. Extremely stable; slides may be dried and preserved.
   4. Procedure
      a. Pipette 3.0 mL of molten reagent onto immunoplate; depth 1.6 mm
      b. Allow to harden and cut wells 2–3 mm in diameter; up to 10–20 equidistant wells per plate
      c. Fill wells with overnight broth culture suspensions (e.g., BHI) of staphylococci to be tested, steamed at 100°C, 15 min, 2–3 loopfuls
      d. Cover to minimize dessication (drying).
      e. Incubation: 35°C, 3 h
   5. Positive reaction
      a. Pink halo (hydrolysis zone) surrounding well; DNase production
      b. Quantitative determination by measuring zone diameter. Zone diameter is related to, and significantly affected by, the concentration of reagent and time and temperature of incubation. Concentrations as low as 0.05 µg/mL and as high as 2.0 µg/mL can be determined after 3 h at 35°C (54).

Advantages of the MAD technique are that highly polymerized DNA is not required and quantitatively reproducible results can be obtained with impure, opaque systems that contain high concentrations of protein (54).

D. **Acridine orange–deoxyribonucleate agar (ADA) overlays**
   1. Procedure of Lachica and Deibel (52)
   2. ADA overlay mixture; two choices (see Appendix 11 for commercial products)
      a. Ingredients, pH 9.0 ± 0.2

Acridine orange (Eastman Organic Chemicals)	1.0 mg
Sodium deoxynucleate (Sigma Chemical Co.)	15.0 mg
Dipotassium phosphate, K_2HPO_4	0.5 g
Agar (1%)	1.0 g
Deionized water	100.0 mL

      b. Stock solution 0.4% acridine orange (AO) (Matheson, Coleman, and Bell or Eastman Organic Chemicals); 1 mL stock solution to each 100 mL of DTA (69)
      c. Autoclave, 121°C, 15 lb, 15 min and cool to 50°C
      d. Stable 4 weeks in screw-cap bottles; better results when subjected to several melting cycles
   3. Two procedures
      a. Colony (semisolid) overlay

(1) Detects **only** DNase activity
(2) Growth medium
   (a) DTA plates; see standard acid medium of Jeffries et al. (42), section IV
   (b) Streak for isolation.
(3) **Before** incubation, flood plate with 8–10 mL of ADA mixture.
   b. Disk-broth overlay
   (1) Detects **DNase** activity of various organisms and **TNase** resistance of *Staphylococcus*
   (2) Growth medium: overnight BHI broth culture
   (3) Test base agar: DTA fortified with 1.5% Tryptone, 0.5% dipotassium phosphate (K_2HPO4), and 2.0% agar
   (4) Testing
      (a) Add 1 drop of each broth culture to be tested onto a paper disk (1.27 cm diameter).
      (b) If testing **confirmed staphylococci, heat** remaining broth to boiling (100°C) in a water bath for 15 min.
         1. Cool and add 1 drop each culture to another set of disks in Petri dish, labeled accordingly.
         2. Determines heat resistance of staphylococcal DNase
      (c) Place disks onto surface of fortified base agar and overlay with 10 mL of ADA mixture; testing DNase activity
4. Incubation; either procedure
   a. 35°C; **upright** (lid on top)
   b. 1–5 h; or at temperature favorable for DNase activity of test organisms (controls)

Serratia marcescens	ATCC 13880, 3–4 h
Pseudomonas aeruginosa	ATCC 10145, 3–4 h
Staphylococcus aureus subsp. *aureus*	ATCC 25924, 2–4 h
Bacillus subtilis	ATCC 6051, 2–5 h

5. Observe plates in a dark room under ultraviolet light
6. Interpretation (Table 10.3)

Table 10.3. ADA Results of *S. aureus* subsp. *aureus* and *Serratia marcescens*

	Unheated	Heated
S. aureus subsp. *aureus*	+	+
S. marcescens	+	−

   a. **Colony or un**heated broth culture (disk) overlays
      (1) Positive (+)
         (a) **Nonfluorescing clear** halos around colonies or disks
         (b) DNase-producing organisms
      (2) Negative (−)
         (a) **Fluorescence; light-green** color in medium
         (b) Intact DNA; absence of DNase
   b. **Heated** broth culture (disk) overlay
      (1) Positive (+)
         (a) **Nonfluorescing clear** halos around disks; DNase-producing *S. aureus* subsp. *aureus*
         (b) **Heat-resistant** DNase–producing *S. aureus;* DNase from no other source has been reported to possess this characteristic (16).

(2) Negative (−): non-DNase-producers **or** thermo**labile** DNase–producing organisms

Both procedures avoid direct addition of the ADA mixture to the growth medium, which eliminates the possibility of mutagenic effects or curing of episomes (52). Episomes are a class of bacterial genetic elements that exist as either chromosomal segments or freely replicating extrachromosomal fragments; they contain DNA (11) and can be eliminated by treatment with acridine dyes (88).

Acridine orange (Trad) (basic orange), a basic dye that imparts an orange-yellow color with green fluorescence, is used as a fluorochrome for nucleic acids (58). Acridine orange reacts strongly with nucleic acids; at low concentration, monovalent, green fluorescent cation prevails (58). *Fluorescence* is absorption of one wavelength and emission of another (71).

X. ALTERNATIVE TEST PROCEDURES

A. **Rapid well–agar diffusion method**
   1. Procedure of Hänninen (29)
   2. Purpose: detection of DNase production by *C. jejuni, C. coli, C. lari* (formerly *C. laridis* (44)), and *H. pylori* (formerly *C. pylori*)
   3. Cell suspension of test organism(s)
      a. **Heavy** suspension made in Tris buffer, pH 7.3. Campylobacters are poor producers of DNase (29).
      b. Growth media; choices
         (1) *C. jejuni* and *C. coli:* Brucella blood agar plates
         (2) *H. pylori:* brain-heart infusion (BHI)
   4. Polymyxin B pretreatment
      a. A polycationic antibiotic that improves sensitivity when added to a suspension of test organism **before** inoculation into agar test wells
      b. Enhances leakage of cell-bound DNase
   5. Medium: DTA
   6. Inocula
      a. 50 µL (2 mg/mL) added to 0.5 mL of a **heavy** bacterial suspension in Tris buffer. Hold at 4°C, 15 min.
      b. Two wells/test organism; with and without pretreatment
   7. Controls
      a. Two known *Campylobacter* spp.; positive and negative
      b. One well with just Tris buffer and polymyxin B
   8. Incubation: aerobically, 35°C; examine at 4, 8, 20, and 40 h
   9. Results
      a. Positive (+): strong pink zone with distinctive edges around wells
      b. Negative (−): colorless or lightly pinkish, narrow zones with irregular edges

According to Hänninen (29), the agar diffusion method is more reliable for DNase detection with *H. pylori* strains that do not grow well on DTA. Pretreatment with polymyxin B shortened detection time for visible results in 8 h with *C. jejuni* and *C. coli* (29). Results confirmed after 20–24 h when pink zones were larger than those of **un**treated cells; however, pretreatment did not increase width of pink zones with *H. pylori* (29), suggesting the presence of cell-associated DNase and extracellular DNase in *C. jejuni* and *C. coli. H. pylori* has only extracellular DNase, since pretreatment with polymyxin did not increase width of pink zones.

B. **Turbidimetric assay staphylococcal nuclease test**
   1. Procedure of Erickson and Deibel (24)
   2. Modification of Houck's spectrophotometric procedure for turbidimetric estimation of RNA and DNase (37, 38)

3. Tube assay of DNase and differentiation between heat-stable and heat-labile nuclease activity
4. DNA-containing broth growth culture is denatured by heat and the turbidity formed upon acidification is read in a spectrophotometer; directly related to the amount of unhydrolyzed nucleic acid present
5. Assay based on relation between turbidity and amount of precipitable DNA present
6. Decreased turbidity indicates DNA hydrolysis.

C. **Rapid indirect determination of DNase activity**
   1. Procedure of Wolf, Horwitz, Mandeville, Vaquez, and von der Muehll (97)
   2. Substitutes 5-bromo-4-chloro-3-indoyl-thymidine-3-phosphate for DNA substrate
      a. Substituted substrate has phosphate bonds similar to those of DNA, which are cleaved by DNase.
      b. Localizes endonuclease phosphodiesterases
      c. Substrate cleaved at site of attachment of indolyl ring to thymidine-3-phosphate
      d. Test solution
         (1) Very expensive
         (2) 2.0 mL of sodium acetate buffer, pH 5.2, 0.1 M in 2 mg of indolyl phosphate substrate
   3. Inoculated and incubated: 35°C; reaction within 4 h; intensified after 18–24 h
   4. Positive (+): blue-green-indigo throughout incubated solution and on bacterial growth at bottom of test tube
   5. Indigogenic reaction (97)

Indolyl phosphate (colorless) → Indolyl + Phosphoric acid (via DNase, phosphodiesterase, H_2O; produces H_3PO_4)

Indolyl-2 molecules + O_2 → Insoluble blue-green indigo deposited at site of enzyme + $2H_2O$

D. **Acidometric DNase test**
   1. Included on API Quad Ferm + Strip (see Appendix 11)
   2. Identification of *Neisseria*; 2-h carbohydrate degradation method (39)
E. **Lombard-Dowell DNA agar** (39); quadrant in Presumpto Quadrant Plate #2 (43)

XI. PRECAUTIONS

A. **General**
   1. Most bacterial DNases require divalent cations for their activity.
   2. Quantitative procedures of DNase activity are laborious, involved, and (in some cases) affected by purity of enzyme and substrate preparations (94).
   3. Detection of nucleases is most sensitive at room temperature (22–25°C) (3)

B. ***S. aureus* subsp. *aureus* identification**
   1. DNase activity is used primarily to determine or confirm potential pathogenic *S. aureus* subsp. *aureus* strains (23, 26, 41, 96) and to differentiate *S. aureus* subsp. *aureus* from *S. epidermidis*. The correlation between *S. aureus* subsp. *aureus* coagulase and DNase production varies among investigators (8, 18, 23, 41, 69, 96, 99, 100). Jeffries (41) showed 91.3% correlation between coagulase and DNase production, most disagreement stemmed from production of DNase by coagulase-negative strains along with a few strains that were coagulase positive, but DNase negative. Morton and Cohn (69) found that 98% of coagulase-positive *S. aureus* subsp. *aureus* cultures and 13.5% of coagulase-negative *S. epidermidis* produced DNase; these findings were also obtained by Zarzaur and Belle (99). *S. aureus* subsp. *aureus* may lose its ability to coagulate plasma through mutations but still be pathogenic (23). Morton and Cohn (69) showed that DNase production correlated better with coagulase production than did fermentation of mannitol.

      The DNase test **cannot** be relied on as the only criterion for identification of *S. aureus* subsp. *aureus* (40, 99), but when strains give doubtful clot reactions (1+ or 2+ in coagulase test) a positive DNase result confirms *S. aureus* subsp. *aureus* (99). Morton and Cohn (69) state that coagulase and DNase may be useful for identifying *S. aureus* subsp. *aureus*, but these properties **should not** be taken to indicate pathogenicity nor their absence, nonpathogenicity. There is no reliable in vitro test to determine the potential pathogenicity of staphylococci for man. Total reliance on DNase production to detect coagulase-positive *S. aureus* subsp. *aureus* may result in some staphylococci being missed (84, 100). DNase testing should be a supplemental test to help identify positive *S. aureus* subsp. *aureus* strains that do not give a definite (4+) coagulase test reaction (76, 86).

      Classification of pathogenic *Staphylococcus* species depends on colony characteristics, pigmentation, catalase test, and both slide and tube coagulase tests (40). Some *S. epidermidis* produce DNase as do *S. pyogenes* and occasionally other β-hemolytic streptococci (94).
   2. Spot inoculations are necessary because some *S. aureus* subsp. *aureus* strains **do not** grow well on the media, and growth is not required for detection of DNase activity (43).
C. ***Serratia* spp. identification**
   DNase testing shows potential in identifying *Serratia* spp., especially nonpigmented strains (22) from closely related nonpigmented members of the *Klebsiella-Enterobacter-Serratia* (K-E-S) group of *Enterobacteriaceae* (7, 79). Most isolated *Serratia* spp. are nonpigmented (14, 21, 36), which creates difficulty biochemically and morphologically with other members of the K-E-S division. Elston and Elston (22) recommend DNase as a differential test in enteric bacteriology. However, since *Hafnia alvei* enzyme systems characteristically switch in many instances when incubation temperatures of 25°C and 37°C are used, plates should be incubated at both temperatures for 24 h (91). Martin and Ewing (63) recommend caution and do not rely on the results of the DNase test alone when identifying *Enterobacteriaceae* and other Gram-negative bacteria. All *Serratia* spp. except *S. fonticola* are DNase positive (51).
D. **Other organisms positive/variable for DNase production are**
   Achromobacter spp. (22, 42)
   Aeromonas hydrophilia (51)
   Bacillus spp. (22, 42, 51)
   Bordetella bronchiseptica (7)
   Clostridium septicum (22)
   Corynebacterium diphtheriae (67)
   Escherichia coli (22)

Pasteurella pestis (22)
Proteus mirabilis (7)
Proteus vulgaris (7)
Pseudomonas aeruginosa (22, 42, 87)
Streptococcus spp. (42, 92)
Vibrio spp. (63)

E. **Standard acid–DTA test procedure**
1. The agar–DNase test, because of its lengthy incubation (18–24 h), elicits a positive reaction from relatively small amounts of nuclease, and at the same time, there is a possibility of DNA breakdown due to enzymes other than DNase or metabolic products such as organic acids (100).
2. The HCl-flooding technique is limited by interference with proteins (54).
3. The semisynthetic medium of Jeffries et al. (42) **cannot** grow many fastidious organisms; often results with micrococci are unsatisfactory.
4. Heavy inocula are recommended, and such inocula **do not** encourage development of well-isolated colonies (42).
5. The HCl reagent is **bactericidal** for either isolated colonies or a heavier, more confluent growth. Once HCl is applied, the test **must** be read and **cannot** be continued by reincubation (42).
6. **Do not pipette concentrated HCl by mouth. Use a syringe or bulb (Pro) pipette.** Add concentrated acid to the volumetric flask, running the acid down the side of the flask slowly with gentle swirling of flask to mix well. **Never** add water directly to an acid; always add **acid to water** because concentrated HCl is extremely caustic and any splatters may cause burns. If acid does contact any skin, wash the area **immediately** with cold running tap water.
7. Jeffries et al. (42) found that the standard test with HCl containing serum in a concentration of 2 mL/100 mL or above became turbid on addition of HCl, obscuring the zone of nucleic acid hydrolysis.
8. When preparing DTA medium, **gently** mix to avoid forming insoluble protein threads; DNA tends to precipitate as fibers (48).
9. The standard DTA-acid procedure is **unsatisfactory** for testing pyocyanin-producing strains of *Pseudomonas;* extracellular pyocyanin is red-brown when acidified; it overlaps growth areas and may obscure clear zones indicating DNase production (87). In this case, perform DNase testing on DTA-TBO (87).

F. **DTA-TBO and DTA-MG**
1. Many bovine strains, reference strains, and type strains of newly described and recognized *Staphylococcus* spp. **do not** grow on DTA-MG or DTA-TBO. TBO and MG dyes are **not** recommended for detection of staphylococci of bovine origin or for use with many newly defined staphylococci species (57).
2. Reaction of metachromatic color changes stable for 2–4 h, after which dye slowly diffuses into agar and loses its well-demarcated borders.
3. Strict attention **must** be paid to dye content of commercially available TBO dye powders; TBO concentrations **must** reflect actual dye concentrations. Calculations **must** include a conversion factor that accounts for the true dye content of commercial powders (91). Two factors in addition to dye concentration affect results of TBO flooding procedures (91): (*a*) length of time dye is in contact with agar and (*b*) length of time between decanting dye solution and reading DNase activity result. A 0.05% TBO solution is superior to 0.01% (80) TBO as a flooding agent for detecting DNase activity of colonies grown on DNase agar (91).
4. Smith et al. (84) recommend performing appropriate biochemical tests to confirm the identity of all DNase-producing staphylococci and streptococci selected from DTA-MG.
5. DTA-MG rarely, if ever, fails to identify DNase-producing group A *S. pyogenes* (84, 94),

but it may give an occasional false positive result (84); some strains of other Lancefield groups of streptococci may also produce DNase (94).
6. A positive DTA-MG reaction indicated by a clear zone around colonies in otherwise green agar is best observed by holding plate against a white background in indirect light (59, 84).
7. DTA-MG is technically difficult to prepare, and Black et al. (7) showed that DNase production is less clearly shown than with either the HCl-DTA or DTA-TBO procedures.
8. Of all methods for DNase activity, only those using MG are applicable to **impure** systems (54).
9. Lior (59) showed that increasing the concentration of MG in medium from 0.005 to 0.006% provided a better contrast and reduced questionable, narrow, hazy zones that are difficult to interpret.
10. By observing both colony size and zone of DNase activity and by performing a Gram stain, highly accurate **presumptive** identification can be made; Gram-negative enteric organisms are not readily confused with staphylococci or group A streptococci because of differences in colony size and consistency (84).
11. MG methods require highly purified DNA substrate (50).
12. According to Lior (59), MG is toxic for at least some *Campylobacter* strains

G. **DTA with acridine orange**
1. Care should be exercised, as certain selective media (e.g., DTA-AO) may inhibit either nuclease activity or its production (52).
2. **Do not** use lids on plates during DTA-AO heating phase; unsatisfactory results may occur because of water loss or excessive condensation that may distort the agar surface (52).
3. The surface-plating DTA-AO procedure should be used for quantitative studies instead of pour plates; surface plating gives a stronger reaction (52).
4. Cross contamination may occur during DTA-AO overlay; isolates should be pure before proceeding with ADA overlaying (52).

H. **Metachromatic agar-diffusion (MAD) technique:** with the MAD procedure (54), concentration, temperature, and time significantly affect staphylococcal assay; these three factors must be standardized.

I. **TNase**
1. Thermal stability (heat resistance) is unique to the nuclease of *S. aureus* subsp. *aureus* (55); it is characteristic of all *S. aureus* subsp. *aureus* strains (76, 86, 98, 99). Zarzaur and Belle (99) recommend performing the TNase test on all clinical isolates yielding 2+ or 1+ clot in the coagulase test to confirm and identify any weak coagulase producers or doubtful *S. aureus* subsp. *aureus* strains.

   Various investigators (5, 86, 99) have shown that the nuclease produced by *S. aureus* subsp. *aureus* is uniquely and consistently **thermostable,** whereas nucleases produced by coagulase-negative staphylococci are thermolabile when tested by the method of Lachica et al. (53).
2. Vogel and Johnson medium and *Staphylococcus* 110 medium cannot be used in STN test; TNase is produced with 110 medium, but activity is inhibited (51).
3. Some strains of *S. epidermidis*, *S. simulans*, and *S. carnosus* can demonstrate weak TNase activity (2).
4. *Enterococcus* spp. may produce TNase (72).
5. Differentiation of thermophilic campylobacters into species and into biotypes provides valuable markers for epidemiologic investigations (59).

J. **Well–agar diffusion method:** agar diffusion method is more reliable for DNase detection of *H. pylori* strains that **do not** grow well in DNase test medium (29).

REFERENCES

1. Baird-Parker AC. The classification of staphylococci and micrococci from world-wide sources. J Gen Microbiol 1965;38(3):363–387.
2. Balows A, Hausler WJ Jr, Herrmann KL, et al. Manual of Clinical Microbiology, ed 5. Washington, DC: American Society for Microbiology, 1991:229–230.
3. Baron EJ, Finegold SM. Bailey & Scott's Diagnostic Microbiology, ed 8. Philadelphia: CV Mosby, 1990:111, 366, 382.
4. Barrett TJ, Patton CM, Morris GK. Differentiation of *Campylobacter* species using phenotypic characterization. Lab Med 1988;19(2):96–102.
5. Barry AL, Lachica RVF, Atchison FW. Identification of *Staphylococcus aureus* by simultaneous use of tube coagulase and thermostable nuclease tests. Appl Microbiol 1973;25(3):496–497.
6. Bernheimer AW, Ruffier NK. Elaboration of deoxyribonuclease by streptococci in the resting state and inhibition of the enzyme by a substance extractable from the cocci. J Exp Med 1951;93(4):399–413.
7. Black WA, Hodgson R, McKechnie A. Evaluation of three methods using deoxyribonuclease production as a screening test for *Serratia marcescens*. J Clin Pathol 1971;24(4):313–316.
8. Blair EB, Emerson JS, Tull AH. A new medium, salt mannitol plasma agar, for the isolation of *Staphylococcus aureus*. Am J Clin Pathol 1967;47(1):30–39.
9. Blazevic DJ, Ederer GM. Principles of Biochemical Tests in Diagnostic Microbiology. New York: John Wiley & Sons, 1975:37–40.
10. Branson D. Methods in Clinical Bacteriology. Springfield, IL: Charles C Thomas, 1972:18–19.
11. Campbell AM. Episomes. Adv Genet 1962;11:101–145.
12. Cantarow A, Schepartz B. Biochemistry, ed 3. Philadelphia: WB Saunders, 1962:99, 105–109.
13. Catlin BW. Extracellular deoxyribonucleic acid of bacteria and a deoxyribonuclease inhibitor. Science 1956;124:441–442.
14. Clayton E, von Graevenitz A. Nonpigmented *Serratia marcescens*. JAMA 1966;197(13)1059–1064.
15. Coobe ER. The rapid recognition of *Staphylococcus aureus*: Deoxyribonuclease and coagulase tests in correlation with sensitivities and other properties. Ulster Med J 1968;37:146.
16. Cunningham L, Catlin BW, Privat de Garilhe MP. A deoxyribonuclease *Micrococcus pyogenes*. J Am Chem Soc 1956;78(16):4642–4645.
17. Davidsohn I, Henry JB. Todd-Stanford Clinical Diagnosis by Laboratory Methods, ed 14. Philadelphia: WB Saunders, 1969:94.
18. DiSalvo JW. Desoxyribonuclease and coagulase activity of micrococci. Med Tech Bull US Armed Forces Med J 1958;9(5):191–196.
19. Dubos RJ, Hirsch JG, eds. Bacterial and Mycotic Infections of Man, ed 4. Philadelphia: JB Lippincott, 1965:75.
20. Eaves GN, Jeffries CD. Isolation and properties of an exocellular nuclease of *Serratia marcescens*. J Bacteriol 1963;85(2):273–278.
21. Elston HR. A bacteriological study of non-chromogenic variants of *Serratia marcescens*. J Clin Pathol 1965;18(5):618–621.
22. Elston HR, Elston JH. Further use of deoxyribonuclease in a screening test for *Serratia*. J Clin Pathol 1968;21(2):210–212.
23. Elston HR, Fitch DM. Determination of potential pathogenicity of staphylococci. Am J Clin Pathol 1964;42(4):346–348.
24. Erickson A, Deibel RH. Turbidimetric assay of staphylococcal nuclease. Appl Microbiol 1973;25(3):337–341.
25. Erickson A, Deibel RH. Production and heat stability of staphylococcal nuclease. Appl Microbiol 1973;25(3):332–336.
26. Fusillo MH, Weiss DL. Qualitative estimation of staphylococcal deoxyribonuclease. J Bacteriol 1959;78(4):520–522.
27. Gramoli JL, Wilkinson BJ. Characterization and identification of coagulase-negative, heat-stable deoxyribonuclease-positive staphylococci. J Gen Microbiol 1978;105:275–285.
28. Greenwood JR, Pickett MJ. Deoxyribonuclease: Detection with a three-hour test. J Clin Microbiol 1976;4(5):453–454.
29. Hänninen M-L. Rapid method for the detection of DNase of campylobacters. J Clin Microbiol 1989;27(9):2118–2119.
30. Harper HA, Rodwell VW, Mayes PA. Review of Physiological Chemistry, ed 16. Los Altos, CA: Lange Medical Publications, 1977:131–133, 411, 430.
31. Harrow B, Mazur A. Textbook of Biochemistry, ed 9. Philadelphia: WB Saunders, 1966:130, 134, 136, 141, 142, 144, 149, 152.
32. Hollis DG, Wiggins GL, Weaver RE. An unclassified gram-negative rod isolated from the pharynx on Thayer-Martin medium (selective agar). Appl Microbiol 1972;24:772–777.
33. Holmes B, Steigerwalt AG, Weaver RE, Brenner DJ. *Chryseomonas luteola* comb. nov. and *Flavimonas oryzihabitans* gen. nov. comb. nov. *Pseudomonas*-like species from human clinical specimens and formerly known respectively, as groups Ve-1 and Ve-1. Int J Syst Bacteriol 1987;37:245–250.
34. Holt JG, Bruns MA, Caldwell BJ, Pease CD. Stedman's Bergey's Bacteria Words. Baltimore: Williams & Wilkins, 1992:63.
35. Holum JR. Elements of General and Biological Chemistry, ed 4. New York: John Wiley & Sons, 1975:507–508, 510.
36. Hotz RM, Dowell VR Jr. Extended study of *Ser-*

ratia in a diagnostic bacteriology laboratory. Can J Microbiol 1966;12:99–103.
37. Houck JC. The microdetermination of ribonuclease. Arch Biochem Biophys 1958;73(2):384–390.
38. Houck JC. The turbidimetric determination of deoxyribonuclease activity. Arch Biochem Biophys 1959;82(1):135–144.
39. Janda WM, Zigler KL, Bradna JJ. API Quad-FERM + with Rapid DNase for identification of *Neisseria* spp. and *Branhamella catarrhalis*. J Clin Microbiol 1987;25(2):203–206.
40. Jarvis JD, Wynne CD. A short survey of the reliability of deoxyribonuclease as an adjunct in the determination of staphylococcal pathogenicity. J Med Lab Technol 1969;26:131–133.
41. Jeffries CD. Comparison of six physiologic characteristics of staphylococci from laboratory specimens. Am J Clin Pathol 1961;36(2):114–118.
42. Jeffries CD, Holtman F, Guse DG. Rapid method for determining the activity of microorganisms on nucleic acids. J Bacteriol 1957;73(4):590–591.
43. Koneman EW, Allen SD, Janda WM, et al. Color Atlas and Textbook of Diagnostic Microbiology, ed 4. Philadelphia: JB Lippincott, 1992:140, 143, 202–204, 207–208, 252, 271, 416, 546.
44. Koupal A, Deibel RH. Rapid qualitative method for detecting staphylococcal nuclease in food. Appl Environ Microbiol 1978;35(2):1193–1197.
45. Kozloff LM. Origin and fate of bacteriophage material. Cold Spring Harbor Symp Quant Biol 1953;18:209–220.
46. Krieg NR, Holt JG, eds. Bergey's Manual of Systematic Bacteriology, vol 1. Baltimore: Williams & Wilkins, 1984:484, 550.
47. Kurnick NB. Discussion of article by Michaelis L. The nature of the interaction of nucleic acids and nuclei with basic dye stuffs. Cold Spring Harbor Symp Quant Biol 1947;12:141–142.
48. Kurnick NB. The determination of desoxyribonuclease activity by methyl green; application to serum. Arch Biochem Biophys 1950;29(1):41–53.
49. Kurnick NB. Methyl green pyronin. Basis of selective staining of nucleic acids. J Gen Microbiol 1950;33(2):243–264.
50. Kurnick NB, Foster M. Methyl green. III. Reaction with desoxyribonucleic acid, stoichiometry, and behavior of the reaction product. J Gen Physiol 1950;34(2):147–159.
51. Lachica RVF. Simplified thermonuclease test for rapid identification of *Staphylococcus aureus* recovered on agar medium. Appl Environ Microbiol 1976;32(4):633–634.
52. Lachica RVF, Deibel RH. Detection of nuclease activity in semisolid and broth cultures. Appl Microbiol 1969;18(2):174–176.
53. Lachica RVF, Genigeorgis C, Hoeprich PD. Metachromatic agar-diffusion methods for detecting staphylococcal nuclease activity. Appl Microbiol 1971;21(4):585–587.
54. Lachica RVF, Hoeprich PD, Franti CE. Convenient assay for staphylococcal nuclease by the metachromatic well-agar-diffusion technique. Appl Microbiol 1972;24(6):920–923.
55. Lachica RVF, Hoeprich PD, Genigeorgis C. Nuclease production and lysostaphin susceptibility of *Staphylococcus aureus* and other catalase-positive cocci. Appl Microbiol 1971;21(5):823–826.
56. Lachica RVF, Hoeprich PD, Genigeorgis C. Metachromatic agar-diffusion microslide technique for detecting staphylococcal nuclease in foods. Appl Microbiol 1972;23:168–169.
57. Langlois BE, Harmon RJ, Akers K, Aaron DK. Comparison of methods for determining DNase and phosphatase activities of staphylococci. J Clin Microbiol 1989;27(5):1127–1129.
58. Lillie RD. HJ Conn's Biological Stains, ed 9. Baltimore: Williams & Wilkins, 1977:356–357.
59. Lior H. New, extended biotyping scheme for *Campylobacter jejuni, Campylobacter coli,* and *Campylobacter laridis.* J Clin Microbiol 1984;20 (4):636–640.
60. Lior H, Patel A. Improved toluidine blue-DNA agar for detection of DNA hydrolysis by campylobacters. J Clin Microbiol 1987;25(10):2030–2031.
61. MacDonell MT, Colwell RR. Phylogeny of the *Vibrionaceae,* and recommendation for two new genera, *Listonella* and *Shewanella.* Int J Syst Bacteriol 1985;6:171–182.
62. Madison BM, Baselski VS. Rapid identification of *Staphylococcus aureus* in blood cultures by thermonuclease testing. J Clin Microbiol 1983; 18(3):722–724.
63. Marsik EJ, Brake S. Species identification and susceptibility to 17 antibiotics of coagulase-negative staphylococci isolated from clinical specimens. J Clin Microbiol 1982;15(4):640–645.
64. Martin WJ, Ewing WH. The deoxyribonuclease test as applied to certain gram-negative bacteria. Can J Microbiol 1967;13(5):616–618.
65. McCarty M. The inhibition of streptococcal desoxyribonuclease by rabbit and human antisera. J Exp Med 1949;90(6):543–554.
66. Menzies RE. Comparison of coagulase, deoxyribonuclease, and heat-stable nuclease for identification of *Staphylococcus aureus.* J Clin Pathol 1977;30:606–608.
67. Messinova OV, Yusupova DV, Shamsutdinov NS. Deoxyribonuclease activity of *Corynebacterium* and its relation to virulence. Fed Proc 1963;22:T1033–T1035.
68. Michaelis L, Granick S. Metachromasy of basic dyestuffs. J Am Chem Soc 1945;67:1212–1219.
69. Morton HE, Cohn J. Coagulase and deoxyribonuclease activities of staphylococci isolated from clinical sources. Appl Microbiol 1972;23 (4):725–733.
70. Nestle M, Roberts WK. An extracellular nuclease from *Serratia marcescens.* I. Purification and some properties of the enzyme. II. Specificity of

the enzyme. J Biol Chem 1969;244(19):5213–5218, 5219–5225.
71. Nussenbaum S. Organic Chemistry. Boston: Allyn & Bacon, 1963:455, 602.
72. Park CE, de Melo Serrano A, Landgraf M, et al. A survey of microorganisms for thermonuclease production. Can J Microbiol 1980;26:532–535.
73. Park CE, El Derea HB, Rayman MK. Evaluation of staphylococcal thermonuclease (TNase) assay as a means of screening foods for growth of staphylococci and possible enterotoxin production. Can J Microbiol 1978;24(2):1135–1139.
74. Pelczar MJ Jr, Reid RD. Microbiology, ed 2. New York: McGraw-Hill, 1965:155.
75. Ratner HB, Stratton CW. Thermonuclease test for same-day identification of *Staphylococcus aureus* in blood cultures. J Clin Microbiol 1985;21(6):995–996.
76. Rayman MK, Park CE, Philpott J, Todd ECD. Reassessment of the coagulase and thermostable nuclease tests as means of identifying *Staphylococcus aureus*. Appl Microbiol 1975;29(4):451–454.
77. Raymond EA, Traub WH. Identification of staphylococci isolated from clinical material. Appl Microbiol 1970;19(6):919–922.
78. Roop II RM, Smibert RM, Johnson JL, Krieg NR. Differential characteristics of catalase-positive campylobacters correlated with DNA homology groups. Can J Microbiol 1984;30(7):938–951.
79. Rothberg NW, Swartz MN. Extracellular deoxyribonucleases in members of the family Enterobacteriaceae. J Bacteriol 1965;90(1):294–295.
80. Schreier JB. Modification of deoxyribonuclease test medium for rapid identification of *Serratia marcescens*. Am J Clin Pathol 1969;51(6):711–716.
81. Sewell CM, Clarridge JE, Young EJ, Guthrie RK. Clinical significance of coagulase-negative staphylococci. J Clin Microbiol 1982;16(2):236–239.
82. Shanholtzer CJ, Peterson LR. Clinical laboratory evaluation of the thermonuclease test. Am J Clin Pathol 1982;77(5):587–591.
83. Smith DT, Conant NF, Willett HP. Zinsser's Microbiology, ed 14. New York: Appleton-Century-Crofts, 1968:123, 431.
84. Smith PB, Hancock GA, Rhoden DL. Improved medium for detecting deoxyribonuclease-producing bacteria. Appl Microbiol 1969;18(6):991–993.
85. Soto-Hernandez JL, Nunley D, Holtsclaw-Berk S, Berk SL. Selective medium with DNase test agar and a modified toluidine blue O technique for primary isolation of *Branhamella catarrhalis* in sputum. J Clin Microbiol 1988;26(3):405–408.
86. Southamer AH, de Haan PG, Bulten EJ. Kinetics of F-curing by acridine orange in relation to the number of F-particles in *Escherichia coli*. Genet Res 1962;4(2):305–317.
87. Sperber WH, Tatini SR. Interpretation of the tube coagulase test for identification of *Staphylococcus aureus*. Appl Microbiol 1975;29(4):502–505.
88. Streitfeld MM, Hoffmann EM, Janklow HM. Evaluation of extracellular deoxyribonuclease activity in *Pseudomonas*. J Bacteriol 1962;84(1):77–80.
89. Valu JA. Use of the deoxyribonuclease test as an aid in the differentiation of *Paracolobactrum (Hafnia)* from *Serratia*. J Bacteriol 1966;91(1):467–468.
90. Victor R, Lachica F, Weiss KF, Deibel RH. Relationships among coagulase, enterotoxin, and heat-stable deoxyribonuclease production by *Staphylococcus aureus*. Appl Microbiol 1969;18(1):126–127.
91. Waller JR, Hodel SL, Nuti RN. Improvement of two toluidine blue O-mediated techniques for DNase detection. J Clin Microbiol 1985;21(2):195–199.
92. Wannamaker LW. The differentiation of three distinct deoxyribonucleases of group A streptococci. J Exp Med 1958;107(6):797–812.
93. Wannamaker LW. Characterization of a fourth desoxyribonuclease of group A streptococci. Fed Proc 1962;21:231.
94. Wannamaker LW. Streptococcal deoxyribonuclease. In: Uhr JW, ed. The Streptococcus, Rheumatic Fever, Glomerulonephritis. Baltimore: Williams & Wilkins, 1964:140–165.
95. Warrack GH, Bidwell E, Oakley CL. The beta-toxin (deoxyribonuclease) of *Cl. septicum*. J Pathol Bacteriol 1951;63(2):293–302.
96. Weckman BG, Catlin BW. Deoxyribonuclease activity of micrococci from clinical sources. J Bacteriol 1957;73(6):747–753.
97. Wolf PL, Horwitz J, Mandeville R, et al. A new and unique method for detecting bacterial deoxyribonuclease in the clinical laboratory. Tech Bull Reg Med Technol 1969;39(4):83–86.
98. Yrios JW. Comparison of rabbit and pig plasma in the tube coagulase test. J Clin Microbiol 1977;5(2):221–224.
99. Zarzour JY, Beele EA. Evaluation of three test procedures for identification of *Staphylococcus aureus* from clinical sources. J Clin Microbiol 1978;7(2):133–136.
100. Zierdt CH, Golde DW. Deoxyribonuclease-positive *Staphylococcus epidermidis* strains. Appl Microbiol 1970;20(1):54–57.

11 β-Galactosidase (ONPG and PNPG) Tests

I. PRINCIPLE

To demonstrate the presence or absence of the enzyme β-galactosidase by use of the organic compound *o*-nitrophenyl-β-D-galactopyranoside (ONPG) or *p*-nitrophenyl-β-D-galactoside (PNPG)

II. PURPOSE

(Also see Chapters 43–45)

A. **ONPG**
  1. To rapidly differentiate lactose-delayed organisms from lactose-negative organisms: help distinguish some strains of *Citrobacter* spp. (+) and *Salmonella bongori* (+), *Salmonella choleraesuis* subsp. *arizonae* (+), and *S. choleraesuis* subsp. *diazonae* (+) from most other *Salmonella* spp. (V⁻) (15)
  2. To aid in species differentiation of *Burkholderia cepacia* (formerly *Pseudomonas cepacia*) (V) and *Stenotrophomonas maltophilia* (formerly *Xanthomonas maltophilia*) and *Pseudomonas maltophilia*) (+) (13, 28) from other *Pseudomonas* species (−) (1)
  3. To aid in species differentiation of *Neisseria lactamica* (+) from other fastidious *Neisseria.* spp. (−) (2). ONPG test on *Neisseria* should be restricted to identifying only species that will grow on selective media; e.g., *N. gonorrhoeae*, *N. meningitis,* and *N. lactamica* (1)
  4. To differentiate *Klebsiella pneumoniae* subsp. *rhinoscleromatis* (−) from *Klebsiella pneumoniae* subsp. *pneumoniae* (+) and *Klebsiella pneumoniae* subsp. *ozaenae* (V)
  5. To differentiate *Corynebacterium bovis* (+) from other *Corynebacterium* spp. (−) (14)
  6. To differentiate *Norcardia* (+), *Nocardiopsis* (+), and *Streptomyces* (+) from other aerobic *Actinomyces* (−) (2)
  7. To differentiate *Flavimonas oryzihabitans* (formerly *Pseudomonas oryzihabitans*–taxonomy uncertain) (−) (1, 13)) from *Chryseomonas luteola* (formerly *Pseudomonas luteola* (+) (12, 13)
  8. To differentiate between four H₂S-producing enterics: *Budvicia aquatica* (+) from *Leminorella grimontii* (−), *Leminorella richardii* (−), and *Pragia fontium* (−)
  9. To differentiate oxidase-positive, fermentative, Gram-negative bacilli, *Chromobacterium violaceum* (−) from *Aeromonas hydrophilia* (+), *Plesiomonas shigelloides* (+), and *Vibrio cholerae* (+)
  10. To differentiate *Capnocytophaga gingivalis* (+) from *C. canimorsus*, (−), *C. cynodegmi* (−), *C. ochracea* (−), and *C. sputigena* (−)
  11. To differentiate *Deincoccus radiopugnans* (+) from other most frequently isolated *D. proteolyticus* (−), *D. radiodurans* (−), and *D. radiophilus* (−)
  12. To differentiate *Shigella sonnei* (+) from other *Shigella* spp. (−)
B. **PNPG**: to differentiate among certain species of *Mycobacterium* (see Section IX.D)

III. BIOCHEMISTRY INVOLVED

Bacterial enzymes are classified as either constitutive or adaptive. An adaptive, or induced, enzyme is one produced by a bacterium only when its specific substrate is present; a constitutive enzyme is produced in either the absence or presence of the substrate (4, 17). The process of substrate mediated enzyme synthesis is called **enzyme induction,** and the compound turning on enzyme synthesis is called an **inducer** (10). β-Galactosidase is an inducible enzyme that acts specifically on simple galactosides (5). Formation of an induced enzyme is controlled genetically; however, an induced enzyme may decrease in cells after several generations if the inducer is removed (11). Also, gene mutation can cause an induced enzyme to become constitutive; the mechanism of formation is the same (11). Cohen and Monod (6) reported that in mutants, β-galactose inhibits formation of constitutive β-galactosidase.

A glycoside is an acetal compound $\left(RCH{<}{}^{OR^1}_{OR^1}\right)$ formed from a carbohydrate that exists in one of two forms: α or β. In the β form the hydroxyl group (OH) at carbon number 1 is above the ring plane, or to the left in the straight-chain structural formula of a carbohydrate; in the α form it is below the plane, or to the right in a straight chain.

α form   β form

In the disaccharide lactose, two monosaccharides, glucose and galactose, are linked through hydroxyl groups by a glycosidic link.

Glucose residue   Galactose residue

$$\text{Galactose residue} \quad \text{Glucose residue}$$

β-Glycosidic linkage
β-Lactose
(4-*o*-(β-D-galactopyranosyl)-D-glucopyranose)

β-Galactosidase is sometimes referred to as lactase (5, 9, 16, 17, 24) because it cleaves lactose. However, it can also hydrolyze other galactosides (24); this hydrolysis usually is not catalyzed by a specific lactase (5). Lactose is a natural galactosidase that when catalyzed by a β-D-galactosidase, yields β-D-galactose and D-glucose; the bond is split between carbon 1 of galactose and oxygen (27).

Active lactose-fermenting organisms possess two genetically distinct induced enzymes: β-galactoside permease and β-D-galactosidase (6, 7, 17, 23). The occurrence of β-galactosidase and β-galactoside permease is controlled by two different genes, and both enzymes are required for lactose fermentation (20). Bacteria that possess both ferment lactose rapidly (20).

Before lactose can be metabolized by an organism, it must penetrate the cell wall. β-Galactoside permease located on the cell membrane is concerned with the transport of lactose. Transport of all nutrients is controlled by specific protein permeases (6, 18); β-galactoside permease is specific for galactose (27) or galactosides. β-Glucosidases are widely distributed in bacteria and fungi. In bacteria, phospho-β-D-glucosidases phosphorylate substrates during active transport by specific permease systems (25, 26). β-Galactoside permease can be induced by the presence of lactose in the medium or by other galactosides such as melibiose, methyl-α-D-galactoside, or propyl-α-D-galactoside; however, conditions for protein synthesis must exist (23).

Mechanism of Permease Action

β-D-Galactosidase is an intracellular enzyme concerned with the hydrolysis of lactose and other β-galactosides (6, 7, 17, 23); lactose is hydrolyzed to galactose and glucose. Three enzymes are synthesized when lactose is added to growth medium: (*a*) lactose permease, (*b*) β-galactosidase, and (*c*) β-acetyltransferase (10).

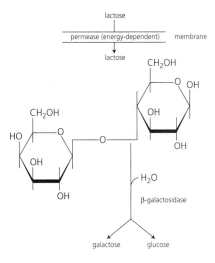

Conversion of lactose to galactose and glucose.

(Redrawn from Gottschalk, G. Bacterial Metabolism, 2nd ed. New York: Springer-Verlag, 1986 with permission.)

Lactose permease catalyzes an energy-dependent transport of lactose into the cell, and β-glactosidase hydrolyzes lactose into glucose and galactose (10). β-Galactoside acetyltransferase acetylates lactose to glucose and galactose with acetyl–coenzyme A (CoA); its biologic function is probably that of a detoxification enzyme (10). Nonmetabolizable structural analogs of lactose are acetylated and excreted (10). Glucose formed from lactose is phosphorylated to glucose-6-phosphate by hexokinase.

β-Galactosidase is required by *Escherichia coli* during growth on lactose, but **not** if glucose serves as a substrate (10). The inducer is not lactose directly, but allolactose (α-D-galactosyl-β-1,6-D-glucose), a compound derived from lactose (α-D-galactosyl-β-1,4-D-glucose) by β-galactosidase (10). The breakdown of lactose requires the permease, β-galactosidase, and the enzymes that convert galactose into glucose-6-phosphate (10). The galactose formed from lactose induces synthesis of three enzymes: (*a*) galactokinase, (*b*) glucose:galactose-1-phosphouridylyl-transferase, and (*c*) uridine diphosphate (UDP)-glucose epimerase; these three enzymes further metabolize galactose to glucose-1- phosphate, which is fed into the Embden-Meyerhof-Parnas and subsequent pathways (10).

Some organisms are active lactose fermenters, others are delayed or slow fermenters, and some cannot ferment lactose under any condition. The active coliform lactose fermenters produce both β-galactoside permease and β-galactosidase and thus rapidly (within 18–24 h) catabolize lactose to carbon dioxide and hydrogen (CO_2 + H_2) through the intermediates galactose and glucose.

Non–lactose fermenters lack both enzymes, and lactose can neither enter the cell nor be degraded. However, Lowe (18) states that cells unable to ferment lactose may exhibit one of two phenotypes: (*a*) lack β-galactosidase but have permease (G^-P^+) and thus accumulate galactosides but cannot metabolize them or (*b*) possess β-galactosidase but lose the permease (G^+P^-).

Slow or delayed lactose fermenters are ONPG-positive organisms that do not possess a specific lactose permease but do possess β-galactosidase. Delayed lactose fermenters, or so-called late lactose fermenters, lack the β-galactoside permease (17). Delayed fermenters can potentially ferment lactose, since they produce the necessary intracellular enzyme. When a 1% concentration of lactose is used, these organisms over time (48 h to several days or weeks) produce some mutant cells that possess the permease (17, 18) along with non-lactose-fermenting cells (18), and "late lactose fermentation" will be observed. Lowe and Evans (19) found that delayed fermenters were impermeable to a 1% concentration of lactose. However, increasing the lactose concentration (up to 10%) decreases the fermentation time in some bacterial strains (17, 19). Lowe (18) states that evidence suggests that delayed or "late" fermenters can metabolize lactose by virtue of possessing β-galactosidase. Thus, the time for lactose fermentation to occur is longer when the organism lacks the permease enzyme when inoculated into a 1% lactose medium than it is when both enzymes are present. The time depends on the rate of development of mutant cells and the rate of diffusion of the substrate into the cell.

The ability to ferment lactose can be predicted by demonstrating the presence or absence of β-galactosidase activity when ONPG is used (4, 5).

$$\text{Bacterium} + \underset{\text{(colorless)}}{\text{ONPG}} \xrightarrow[\text{β-galactosidase}]{\text{hydrolyzed}} \underset{\text{(yellow)}}{o\text{-Nitrophenol}} + \text{galactose}$$

o-Nitrophenyl-β-D-galactopyranose (ONPG) $\xrightarrow[\text{β-galactosidase}]{\text{hydrolyzed} \\ H_2O}$ Galactose + o-Nitrophenol (ONP)

If actively metabolizing galactosidase-positive cells are present, the colorless ONPG reagent is hydrolyzed to liberate a yellow chromogenic compound, o-nitrophenol (ONP); a positive β-galactosidase reaction is based on detection of ONP (16–18). Released ONP undergoes a tautomeric change at alkaline pH, producing a yellow color (16); the acid tautomer is practically colorless (20). Since ONP is a weak acid that is almost colorless under acidic conditions, one must determine β-galactosidase activity in a well-buffered solution (16). ONP can be detected or measured at a low concentration (16).

IV. REAGENTS EMPLOYED

A. **Sodium phosphate buffer, 0.01 M**, pH 7.0 (17, 18)
   1. Add 6.9 g of Na_2HPO_4 to 45 mL of distilled water in a 50-mL volumetric flask.
   2. Dissolve by warming to 37°C.
   3. **Slowly** add approximately 7.5 mL of 5 N sodium hydroxide (NaOH) (or 3.0 g) while adjusting the pH to 7.0.
   4. Bring the volume to 50.0 mL with distilled water.
   5. Label correctly.

Sodium hydroxide is extremely caustic; avoid exposure to the skin, as painful burns may occur.

B. ***o*-Nitrophenyl-β-D-galactopyranoside (*o*-nitrophenyl-β-D-galactoside)**
   1. May substitute *p*-nitrophenyl-β-D-galactoside for the ortho (o) compound (11)
   2. Commercial product available (see Appendix 11)
      a. Sigma Chemical Company
      b. Calbiochem
   3. Method of preparation
      a. Add 80.0 mg of ONPG reagent to 15.0 mL of distilled water in a flask.
      b. Warm flask to 37°C to dissolve crystals. **Do not overheat**.

c. Add 5.0 mL of phosphate buffer and adjust to pH 7.0.
d. Store in a dark glass bottle. Avoid undue exposure to light.
e. Label correctly.

The ONPG solution must be colorless to determine β-galactosidase activity.

C. Toluene, analytical grade
D. Physiologic saline (0.85% NaCl)
E. Storage: store all reagents in a refrigerator (4°C) when not in use. Their stability varies; thus they should be given a periodic quality control check and discarded when they demonstrate a negative or weak reaction with a known-positive organism. The ONPG solution should be placed in a 37°C water bath prior to its use, to redissolve the phosphate that crystallizes out on storage (17).

V. QUALITY CONTROL MICROORGANISMS

A. ONPG positive (+)

Escherichia coli	ATCC 25922
Salmonella choleraesuis subsp. *arizonae*	ATCC 13314
Neisseria lactamica	ATCC 23970

B. ONPG negative (−)

Proteus mirabilis	ATCC 29245
Neisseria meningitis	ATCC 13077

(Note: System restricted to identification of only those species that grow on selective media (1).)

VI. PROCEDURES

A. **Method 1**
  1. Broth growth culture: appropriate to organism
     a. Inoculate **heavily** with organism to be tested (1 loopful) (17, 18).
     b. Incubation: 37°C; 18–24 h
  2. Method of use
     a. After incubation, centrifuge, and discard supernatant into a disinfectant.
     b. To the sediment of cells, add 0.25 mL of normal saline (0.85%).
     c. Add 1 drop of toluene and shake tube (17).
     d. Place tube in a 37°C water bath for 5–10 min.
     e. Add 0.25 mL of ONPG solution to cell suspension.
     f. Reincubate: 37°C water bath; 20 min–24 h.
        (1) Read tube at end of 20 min.
        (2) If negative (no color change), continue incubation and read at 1, 2, 3, and 24 h or until a color change occurs within a 24-h period.

ONPG test is performed with toluene-treated cell suspensions in a physiologic saline solution (20). Toluene helps release enzyme from bacterial cells. β-Galactosidase activity is greatly increased when bacteria are subjected to lytic treatment and by the presence of sodium (Na) ions (16).

B. **Method 2**
  1. Growth medium: ONPG broth (18)
     a. ONPG solution
        (1) Ingredients

ONPG	6.0 g
Sodium phosphate buffer, pH 7.5, 0.01 M	1000.0 mL

(2) Method of preparation
  (a) Dissolve at room temperature (25°C).
  (b) Sterilization: filtration
    1. Millipore membrane filter method
    2. Membranes, 0.45-μ pore diameter
b. Peptone water, 1% (7, 18)
  (1) Ingredients

Peptone	10.0 g
Sodium chloride, NaCl	5.0 g
Distilled water	1000.0 mL

  (2) Method of preparation
    (a) Place ingredients in a flask and dissolve by heating.
    (b) Adjust pH to 8.0–8.4.
    (c) Boil 10 min.
    (d) Filter.
    (e) Readjust pH to 7.2 to 7.4.
  (3) Method of sterilization: autoclave; 115°C, 20 min
2. Method of use (7, 18)
  a. **Aseptically,** add 1 part **sterile** ONPG solution (250 mL) to 3 parts **sterile** 1% peptone water (750 mL) in a **sterile** flask. To eliminate use of an additional sterile flask, add 250 mL (1 part) of prepared ONPG solution directly to 750 mL (3 parts) of peptone water.
  b. Dispense approximately 2.5 mL of ONPG broth per **sterile** tube. Tubed medium is stable for a month when refrigerated (4°C) (7).
  c. Inoculate a tube of ONPG–peptone water broth **heavily** (1 loopful) (17).
  d. Incubation
    (1) 37°C water bath or incubator
    (2) 20 min–24 h
      (a) Read tube after 20 min
      (b) If negative (no color change), continue incubation and read at 1, 2, 3, and 24 h, or until a color change occurs within a 24-h period.

Le Minor and Hamida (17) recommend using toluene to enhance the liberation of β-galactosidase. However, Lowe (18) states that toluene is not essential for enzyme liberation if the organism is incubated overnight in an ONPG broth suspension. A positive β-galactosidase test result is based on an observable color change; therefore, the total volume is not critical.

VII. RESULTS

> See Figure 11.1 (Appendix 1) for colored photographic results

VIII. INTERPRETATION

A. Positive result
  1. Yellow color within 20 min to 24 h
  2. Organism contains lactose-fermenting enzymes; classified as a lactose fermenter
B. Negative result: colorless after 24 h

If a heavy inoculum is used, a rapid positive reaction will occur within a 20 min–3 h incubation period; a yellow color at 20 min is a strong positive reaction (17, 18). The yellow color produced is stable and will not fade if a positive reaction is not observed immediately.

IX. RAPID TESTS

A. **Key ONPG test tablets**
  1. Manufacturer: Key Scientific Products Company; follow manufacturer's directions.
  2. Results: within 6 h or less; an organism with strong β-galactosidase activity may produce a positive result within a few minutes after inoculation of medium (15).
  3. Correlation with standard test (3)
     a. Occasional false negative result due to insufficient inoculum
     b. Heavy inoculum required from triple sugar iron agar (TSI)/Kligler's iron agar (KIA)
B. **ONPG filter disks**
  1. Manufacturers: REMEL; follow manufacturer's directions
  2. Store: 2–8°C
C. **PNPG test for *Mycobacterium* spp.** (8)
  1. Procedure of David and Jahan (8)
  2. *Mycobacterium* enzymes **not** phospho-β-D-glucosidases
  3. Identifies and differentiates mycobacteria by ability to hydrolyze PNPG enzymatically to a yellow *p*-nitrophenol (PNP)
     a. *Mycobacterium tuberculosis* (+) from *M. bovis,* including Calmette-Guerin bacillus (BCG) strains (−)
     b. Runyon group II
        (1) *Mycobacterium scrofulaceum* (−) from other group II species (+)
        (2) Can be a rapid substitution for prolonged Tween 80 degradation test
  4. Substrate: 0.5 mL of colorless 2 M solution of PNPG (Sigma Chemical Co.; see Appendix 11) in 0.05 M Tris (hydroxymethylaminomethane) buffer, pH 7.0. Store at 4°C.
  5. Procedure
     a. To 0.5 mL of substrate, add 1 spadeful of bacterial cells (2–5 mg net weight) scraped from slant surface of 3-week-old Lowenstein-Jensen medium.
     b. Controls
        (1) Positive (+): *Mycobacterium fortuitum* ATCC 6841
        (2) Negative control: substrate solution **only; un**inoculated
     c. Incubation: 37°C, 3 h
  6. Interpretation: if test organism is chromogenic (yellow), centrifuge before interpreting results.
     a. Positive reaction
        (1) Development of a distinct yellow color; enzymatic hydrolysis of PNPG
        (2) Release of PNP
     b. Negative reaction: solution remains colorless
     c. Control
        (1) Liberation of PNP is a function of incubation time.
        (2) If allowed to remain overnight, spontaneous hydrolysis occurs in controls containing no cells.

X. PRECAUTIONS

A. **General**
  1. A **heavy** inoculum (1 loopful) is necessary with either method, to obtain a high concentration of enzyme (if present) and to increase the speed of a positive reaction (17).

2. **Prior** to use, ONPG solution or broth **must** be placed in a 37°C water bath to redissolve the phosphate that crystallizes out during storage (17).
3. If ONPG solution is not properly buffered, false-negative or false-positive results may occur. A false-negative (colorless) result may occur if the solution is acid. Liberated ONP is a weak acid and its acid, benzenoid tautomer, is almost colorless (16). Therefore, determination of released ONP **must** be made under one of two conditions: (a) in a well-buffered solution, pH 7.0–7.5, in which a fixed proportion is dissociated to produce a yellow color, or (b) at a strongly alkaline pH, 10.0 or higher, in which a negligible portion remains undissociated and colorless (16).

   A false-positive result (yellow) may occur if the solution is not properly buffered, because of stimulation of apparent galactosidase activity by sodium ions (16, 17). Rubidium (Rb) and substituted ammonium ions such as ethanolammonium and ethylenediammonium inhibit galactosidase activity (16). Lederberg (16) suggests that these ions compete with each other and possibly with the hydrogen ion, since inhibition by rubidium ions is reversed by sodium or potassium ions. He reported that divalent ions such as chloride, sulfate, nitrate, acetate, and phosphate had no effect on enzyme activity.

   Lederberg (16) also found that storing bacterial cells in M/10 buffer can activate galactosidase activity; storage under refrigeration in distilled water has no effect. Caution must be exercised to preserve cell suspensions in their original condition (16).
4. Prepared ONPG solution **must** be colorless **prior to** its use for determination of enzyme activity. In the ONPG broth, peptone itself may impart a slight yellow color to the cell-broth suspension, although it is present at only a 1% concentration. A positive reaction may vary in the intensity of the yellow color; therefore, when using an ONPG broth-cell suspension, a negative control should be run simultaneously.
5. The test **cannot** be used with yellow-pigmented (chromogenic) bacteria such as flavobacteria, unless they are centrifuged **before** interpreting results or a second tube containing inoculum **only** is used to differentiate a tube reaction from a pigment effect (21).
6. Glucose inhibits β-galactosidase activity, and cells grown on glucose show activity slower than those grown with lactose (16).
7. ONPG test **is not** a substitute for the determination of lactose fermentation because **only** the enzyme β-galactosidase is measured (15, 20); also perform conventional lactose fermentation tests (20).
8. Inoculum **must** be recovered from a lactose-containing medium because of the inducible nature of the enzyme (21).
9. **Do not** report a negative result before 24 h incubation.
10. Inoculum from either KIA or TSI agar produces optimal results in the ONPG test (15).

B. **Disk test:** a large volume of fluid should not be added to disk to prevent dilution of color intensity (21).

C. **PNPG test**
1. The substrate tends to be **un**stable during storage. Prepare solution weekly and store at 4°C or frozen at $-70°C$. Each aliquot should be examined for spontaneous hydrolysis before use.
2. Do not allow overnight incubation. After prolonged incubation, the substrate often hydrolyzes spontaneously in controls without added cells (22).

REFERENCES

1. Balows A, Hausler WJ Jr, Herrmann KL, et al. Manual of Clinical Microbiology, ed 5. Washington, DC: American Society for Microbiology, 1991:266, 437–438, 1267.
2. Baron EJ, Finegold SM. Bailey & Scott's Diagnostic Microbiology, ed 8. Philadelphia: CV Mosby, 1990:360, 472–473.
3. Belliveau RR, Grayson JW, Butler TJ. A rapid,

simple method of identifying *Enterobacteriaceae*. Am J Clin Pathol 1968;50(1):126–128.
4. Burrows W, Moulder JW. Textbook of Microbiology, vol II, ed 19. Philadelphia: WB Saunders, 1968:115.
5. Cantarow A, Schepartz B. Biochemistry, ed 3. Philadelphia: WB Saunders, 1962:241–242.
6. Cohen GN, Monod J. Bacterial permeases. Bacteriol Rev 1957;21(3):169–194.
7. Cowan ST. Cowan & Steel's Manual for the Identification of Medical Bacteria, ed 2. Cambridge: Cambridge University Press, 1974:39, 177.
8. David HL, Jahan MT. β-Glucosidase activity in mycobacteria. J Clin Microbiol 1977;5(3):383–384.
9. Fieser LF, Fieser M. Organic Chemistry, ed 3. New York: Reinhold, 1956:461.
10. Gottschalk G. Bacterial Metabolism, ed 2. New York: Springer-Verlag, 1986:97–98, 178–179.
11. Harrow B, Mazur A. Textbook of Biochemistry, ed 9. Philadelphia: WB Saunders, 1966:381.
12. Holmes B, Steigerwalt AG, Weaver RE, Brenner DJ. *Chryseomonas luteola* comb. nov. and *Flavimonas oryzihabitans* gen. nov. comb. nov., *Pseudomonas*-like species from human clinical specimens and formerly known respectively, as groups Ve-1 and Ve-2. Int J Syst Bacteriol 1987; 37:245–250.
13. Holt JG, Bruns MA, Caldwell BJ, Pease CD. Stedman's Bergey's Bacteria Words. Baltimore: Williams & Wilkins, 1992:74, 117, 349.
14. Jackman PJH, Pitcher DG, Pelcynska S, Borman P. Classification of corynebacteria associated with endocarditis (group JK) as *Corynebacterium jeikeium* sp. nov. Syst Appl Microbiol 1987;9:83.
15. Koneman EW, Allen SD, Janda WM, et al. Color Atlas and Textbook of Diagnostic Microbiology, ed 4. Philadelphia: JB Lippincott, 1992:380–382.
16. Lederberg J. The beta-D-galactosidase of *Escherichia coli*, strain K-12. J Bacteriol 1950; 60(4):381–392.
17. Le Minor L, Hamida FB. Advantages de la recherche de la β-galactosidase sur celle de la fermentation du lactose en milieu complexe dans le diagnostic bactériologique, en particulier des *Enterobacteriaceae*. Ann Inst Pasteur 1962; 102:267–277.
18. Lowe GH. The rapid detection of lactose fermentation in paracolon organisms by the demonstration of β-galactosidase. J Med Lab Technol 1962;19:21–25.
19. Lowe GH, Evans JH. A simple medium for the rapid detection of salmonella- like paracolon organisms. J Clin Pathol 1957;10(4):318–321.
20. Lubin AH, Ewing WH. Studies on the beta-D-galactosidase activities of *Enterobacteriaceae*. Public Health Lab 1964;22:83–101.
21. Oberhofer TR. Manual of Nonfermenting Gram-Negative Bacteria. New York: John Wiley & Sons, 1985:7–9.
22. Oberhofer TR. Manual of Practical Medical Microbiology and Parasitology. New York: John Wiley & Sons, 1985:368–369.
23. Oginsky EL, Umbreit WW. An Introduction to Bacterial Physiology, ed 2. San Francisco: WH Freeman, 1959:393.
24. Oser BL, ed. Hawk's Physiological Chemistry, ed 14. New York: McGraw-Hill, 1965:395 and 404.
25. Schaefler SA, Malamy A. Taxonomic investigation on expressed and cryptic phospho-β-glucosidases in *Enterobacteriaceae*. J Bacteriol 1969;99(2):422–433.
26. Schaefler S, Malamy A, Green I. Phospho-β-glucosidases and β-glucoside permeases in *Streptococcus, Bacillus,* and *Staphylococcus*. J Bacteriol 1969;99(2):434–440.
27. Sokatch JR. Bacterial Physiology and Metabolism. New York: Academic Press, 1969:62, 67.
28. Swings J, De Vos P, Van den Mooter M, De Lay J. Transfer of *Pseudomonas maltophilia* Hugh 1981 to the genus *Xanthomonas* as *Xanthomonas maltophilia* (Hugh 1981) comb. nov. Int J Syst Bacteriol 1983;33:409–413.

12 Gelatin Liquefaction Tests

I. PRINCIPLE

To determine the ability of an organism to produce proteolytic-type enzymes (gelatinases) that liquefy/hydrolyze gelatin or show characteristic changes due to degradation products

II. PURPOSE

(Also see Chapters 43–45)

Gelatinase production is used as a taxonomic aid for identification and classification of both fermentative (e.g., *Enterobacteriaceae*) and nonfermentative bacteria, mainly to identify pure cultures.

A. To aid in differentiation between genera
   1. Among the *Enterobacteriaceae* only the following can liquefy gelatin:
      a. *Arsenophonus nasoniae* (+)
      b. *Erwinia amylovora* (+)
      c. *Pantoea agglomerans* (+)
      d. *Photorhabdus* (*Xenorhabdus*) *luminescens* (variable, V)
      e. *Proteus myxofaciens* (+), *Proteus mirabilis* (+), *Proteus vulgaris* (+), and *Proteus penneri* (V)
      f. At 22°C, *Serratia* spp. (usually +)
      g. *Xenorhabdus* spp. (V) at 25°C
      h. *Yersinia ruckeri* (V; negative at 35°C and 25°C; positive at 30°C after 14 days) at 22°C
   2. *Staphylococcus aureus* subsp. *aureus* (+) from *Staphylococcus epidermidis* (+, slow) and *Micrococcus* spp. (+); *Stomatococcus mucilaginosus* (+) (25) (formerly *Micrococcus mucilaginosus* (23))
   3. *Listeria monocytogenes* (−) from
      a. *Arcanobacterium pyogenes* (formerly *Actinomyces pyogenes*, *Corynebacterium pyogenes*) ((+) after 24 h) (11, 12, 31, 39)
      b. *Corynebacterium striatum* (V; negative at 35°C and 25°C; positive at 30°C after 14 days), *C. pseudotuberculosis* (V, usually +) (41), and *C. ulcerans* (V; no liquefaction or weak at 37°C, liquefaction at 25°C) (1)
      c. *Cellulomonas turbata* (formerly *Oerskovia turbata*, CDC groups A-3 and A-4 (42)) (+) and *Cellulomonas cellulans* (formerly *Oerskovia xanthineolytica*, and CDC A-1 and A-2 groups (+) (42)) (1) (positive at 22°C)
B. To aid in species differentiation
   1. *S. aureus* (+) from *S. epidermidis* (+, slow)
   2. Anaerobic lecithinase-positive *Clostridium* spp.; *C. baratii* (−) from other lecithinase-positive clostridia (+)
   3. Definitive test for distinguishing *Pseudomonas fluorescens* biovars I, II, III (+) from *P. putida* biovars A and B (−) (5, 43)
   4. *Nocardia brasiliensis* (+) from *N. asteroides* (−), *N. farcinia* (−), *N. nova* (−), *N. otidiscaviarum* (−), and *N. transvalensis* (−)

5. *Propionibacterium acnes* (strong +) and *P. avidium* (strong +) from other *Propionibacterium* spp. (−) most frequently isolated
6. *Prevotella heparinolytica* (−) and *P. oulora* (−) from other *Prevotella* spp. (+) most frequently isolated
7. *Selenomonas acidaminovorans* (+) from other *Selenomonas* spp. (−) most frequently isolated
8. *Acidovorax facilis* (+) from *A. delafieldii* (−) and *A. temperans* (−)
9. *Acinetobacter haemolyticus* (V, usually positive) from other *Acinetobacter* spp. (−)
10. *Alcaligenes latus* (+) from *A. faecalis* (−)
11. *Eubacterium combesii* (+) from other *Eubacterium* spp. (V, usually negative) that may cause human infections
12. *Capnocytophaga sputigena* (+) from *C. canimorsus* (−), *C. cynodegmi* (−), *C. gingivalis* (−), and *C. ochracea* (−)
13. Differentiate *Nocardia* and *Streptomyces* (2) (see BCYE$_\alpha$ gelatin medium)

III. BIOCHEMISTRY INVOLVED

Gelatin, a protein derivative of animal collagen, is incorporated into various media to determine an organism's ability to produce proteolytic-type enzymes (proteinases), detected by digestion or liquefaction of the gelatin. Enzymes capable of gelatinolysis are termed **gelatinases.** These proteolytic enzymes are often important in the virulence factor of some microorganism (2).

Naturally occurring proteins are too large to enter a bacterial cell; thus, for a cell to use proteins, they must first be catabolized into smaller components. Exocellular gelatinases are secreted by certain bacteria to break down proteins, and this ability aids bacterial identification.

Catabolism of proteins by gelatinases is a two-step process; the end result is a mixture of individual amino acids.

$$\text{Protein} + \text{H}_2\text{O} \xrightarrow[\text{proteinases}]{\text{gelatinases}} \text{Polypeptides} \qquad (1)$$

$$\text{Polypeptides} + \text{H}_2\text{O} \xrightarrow[\text{peptidases}]{\text{gelatinases}} \text{Individual amino acids (AA)} \qquad (2)$$

Gelatin is hydrolyzed by gelatinase into its constituent amino acids with a loss of its gelling characteristics. There are basically five media/methods for detection of gelatin degradation by microorganisms:

Liquid basal medium; liquefaction (2, 10, 13, 19, 27, 32)
Nutrient agar medium; hydrolysis (13, 37, 40, 43)
Charcoal-gelatin strips; hydrolysis (21, 35)
X-ray film; degradation of gelatin (5, 38)
Gelatin agar; alkalization (21, 35)

IV. MEDIA EMPLOYED

A. **Kohn gelatin medium** (24, 28); **highly recommended**
   1. Denatured gelatin–charcoal disks
      a. Ingredients

Nutrient gelatin	15.0 g
Inactivated, finely powdered charcoal	3.0–5.0 g
Cold tap or distilled water	100.0 mL

b. Method of preparation (24)
   (1) Sprinkle the nutrient gelatin across the surface of the water. Wait a few minutes for the mixture to soak well and produce a homogeneous suspension.
   (2) Bring the gelatin mixture to a boil.
   (3) Add powdered charcoal.
   (4) Shake thoroughly and cool to 48°C in a water bath.
   (5) Pour into a large **glass** Petri dish or other suitable flat glass container with the bottom previously smeared with a thin line of Vaspar (wax) or Vaseline to a depth of 3 mm.
      (a) Pour mixture at a cool temperature to allow quick setting to avoid formation of charcoal sediment.
      (b) A lined container prevents the gelatin-charcoal mixture from sticking to the glass and permits easy removal.
   (6) Allow mixture to set until hard.
   (7) **Gently,** lift out the gelatin-charcoal sheet intact and place in 10% formalin for 24 h.

Calcium carbonate ($CaCO_3$)	1.0 g
Sodium chloride (NaCl)	0.9 g
Formaldehyde, 40%	10.0 mL
Deionized water	90.0 mL

   (8) Cut gelatin-charcoal disks, 1 cm in diameter.
   (9) Wrap gelatin disks in gauze and place under running tap water for 24 h.
   (10) Place disks in screw-cap tubes (1 per tube) and cover with a small amount of water. Loosen caps.
c. Method of sterilization (24): two methods
   (1) Flowing steam, 30 min
   (2) Repeated heating, 3 times
      (a) Water bath, 90–100°C
      (b) 20 min each time
d. After sterilization
   (1) **Aseptically** decant water.
   (2) Add 3.0–4.0 mL of sterile Trypticase soy broth (TSB) or other suitable **sterile** liquid growth medium per tube.
   (3) Incubate 24 h for sterility; check before use.
e. Cool before use, tighten caps, and refrigerate for storage (4–10°C).
2. Inoculation
   a. Growth from an 18- to 24-h pure culture: Kligler's iron agar (KIA)/triple sugar iron agar (TSI), or other suitable culture
   b. **Heavy** suspension
3. Set up control tube (uninoculated) to run with tube of bacterium being tested. Label **control.**
4. Incubation
   a. Broth test and control tubes simultaneously
   b. Routine work: 35–37°C (24, 28)
   c. 18–24 h or longer

The Kohn gelatin test depends on the presence of a preformed or induced gelatinase that liquefies gelatin, thus releasing charcoal particles (13). Inoculation of the medium with a heavy inoculum of the bacterium being tested is recommended because liquefaction time is determined by the amount of preformed enzyme present (28).

The gelatin-charcoal acts only as a substrate for determining gelatinase activity, **not** as a nutrient (24). This substrate contains many minute charcoal particles bound by a small amount of gelatin that upon even slight liquefaction, releases easily detectable charcoal particles (24). Hence, released charcoal particles indicate gelatin liquefaction (24).

The Kohn charcoal-formalin-denatured gelatin procedure is rapid because of the heat stability of the formalin-denatured gelatin (28). Proteins are usually denatured when subjected to heat, but gelatin is an exception (16). With Kohn gelatin, liquefaction may occur at 37°C, and only a slight amount of gelatin need be liquefied to release charcoal particles, denoting a positive result. Gelatin liquefaction may be detected within 24 h, compared with 7 days or longer with the more common procedure, the nutrient gelatin stab incubated at 22°C.

Kohn (24) recommends **not** autoclaving his medium, since this tends to soften the gelatin. Also, false-positive results do not occur if the Kohn culture medium is mechanically shaken; in fact, shaking is recommended when interpreting the results (24).

B. **Nutrient gelatin stab medium**, pH 6.8 (3, 13, 14)
   1. Ingredients

Beef extract, veal extract, or infusion broth	3.0 g
Peptone	5.0 g
Gelatin, 12%	120.0 g
Deionized water	1000.0 mL

      Sodium thiosulfate, 0.05%, may be added for cultivation of certain clostridia in an anaerobic environment (2).

   2. Methods of preparation
      a. Individual ingredients
         (1) First add only gelatin to deionized water and let stand 15–30 min.
         (2) Heat to 50°C to dissolve gelatin.
         (3) Add beef extract and peptone and again heat to 50°C to dissolve all constituents.
         (4) **Do not** overheat.
         (5) Adjust pH to 6.8–7.0 (3, 13, 14).
      b. Dehydrated commercial medium
         (1) Weigh out amount accurately as directed on the label.
         (2) Rehydrate with deionized water.
         (3) Heat **gently** into solution.
         (4) Dispense approximately 4.0–5.0 mL per screw-cap tube; "**deeps**" (i.e., allow medium to solidify in upright position, **do not slant**).
         (5) Loosen caps.
   3. Method of sterilization: autoclave, 121°C, 15 lb, 15 min
   4. Cool in an upright position, tighten caps, and refrigerate for storage (4–10°C).
   5. Inoculation
      a. Keep gelatin tubes in the refrigerator until just before inoculation; medium should be solidified.
      b. Inoculating needle
         (1) Growth from an 18- to 24-h pure culture: KIA or other suitable culture
         (2) **Heavy** inoculum
         (3) Stab medium to a depth of ½ to 1 inch.
   6. Set up a control tube (uninoculated) to be run along with bacterium being tested. Label **control.**
   7. Incubation
      a. Both test and control tubes simultaneously
      b. 22–25°C or 35°C
      c. 24 h–14 days
         (1) Observe for growth (turbidity) and liquefaction.

(a) At the end of each 24 h, place both tubes (test bacterium and control) in a refrigerator or ice bath long enough (approximately 2 h) (13) to determine whether digestion of gelatin (liquefaction) has occurred.
(b) Make the transfer from incubator to refrigerator **without shaking** the tubes.
(2) Check tubes daily up to 2 weeks (13) unless liquefaction occurs sooner.
(a) Occasionally, prolonged incubation (30 days to 6 weeks) may be required.
(b) For routine testing, liquefaction results are determined at the end of 2 weeks incubation at 35°C.

Nutrient gelatin stab medium is **not** suitable for **routine** testing of gelatinase activity since many species require prolonged incubation before liquefaction is evident (13, 28). In routine diagnostic procedures for identifying bacteria, the duration of incubation should be a reasonable time.

C. **Nutrient gelatin plate medium** (33)
  1. Measurement of products of gelatinase degradation; evident by changes in composition of gelatin in place of gelatin liquefaction
     a. Low concentration of gelatin (4%) acts as a solidifying agent **and** a binding agent; prevents mixing of degradation products with **un**changed gelatin
     b. Zonal changes observed directly **without** the need to chill medium or use a protein precipitant
  2. Ingredients: add 40 g of gelatin (4%) to 1 L of Trypticase soy agar (TSA), pH 7.2
  3. Method of sterilization: autoclave; 121°C, 15 lb, 15–20 min
  4. Dispense 12–15 mL per Petri dish (plate) (15 × 100 mm); dry plates **overnight at room temperature** (22–25°C).
  5. Inoculation: band or spot inoculate
  6. Incubation:
     a. Routine: 35°C, 18–24 h
     b. Selected pseudomonads: room temperature (22–25°C), 18–24 h

D. **Thioglycolate gelatin medium**, pH 7.0 (6)
  1. Supports growth of strict (obligate) anaerobes, aerobes, and facultative organisms; many fastidious microorganisms
  2. Ingredients

Casitone	15.5 g
Yeast extract	5.0 g
Dextrose (glucose)	2.0 g
Sodium chloride (NaCl)	2.5 g
l-Cystine	0.25 g
Sodium sulfite (NaSO$_2$)	0.1 g
Thioglycolic acid	0.3 mL
Agar	0.75 g
Gelatin	50.0 g
Deionized water	1000.0 mL

     Pancreatic digest of casein, 20.0 g, may be substituted for Casitone and yeast extract.
  3. Commercial products available: Thioglycollate Broth w/5% gelatin, Thiogel (BBL), Supplemented Thio.
  4. Method of preparation
     a. Weigh out amount accurately as directed on the label.
     b. Rehydrate with **cold** distilled or deionized water.
     c. Place in a 50°C water bath to wet all ingredients.
     d. Heat **gently** into solution.
     e. Dispense approximately 8.0 mL per screw-cap tube (16 × 125 mm).

f. Loosen caps.
5. Method of sterilization: autoclave; 121°C, 15 lb, 15 min
6. Cool in an **upright** position, tighten caps, and store at room temperature (22°C); just before use, boil 2 min (recommended) then cool to room temperature **without agitation** (3).
7. Inoculation
   a. Growth from an 18- to 24-h pure culture: KIA or other suitable culture
   b. **Heavy** suspension
8. Set up a control tube (uninoculated) to be run along with bacterium being tested. Label **control.**
9. Incubation
   a. Both test and control tubes simultaneously; caps tightened
   b. 22–25°C or 35°C
   c. 24 h to 14 days
      (1) Observe for growth (turbidity) and test for liquefaction at the end of each 24 h by placing both test and control tubes in a refrigerator or an ice bath long enough to determine whether gelatin liquefaction has occurred.
         (a) Interpret as soon as uninoculated control tube solidifies; usually anywhere from 5 min to 1 h.
         (b) Remove tubes to room temperature (22–25°C) and invert.
      (2) Check tubes daily up to 2 weeks unless liquefaction occurs sooner. Occasionally, prolonged incubation (30 days) may be required.
   d. **No** increased CO_2

Thioglycolate gelatin medium may also be prepared by simply adding a 5.0% concentration of gelatin to dehydrated thioglycolate medium (3). This medium permits determination of gelatin liquefaction regardless of bacterial oxygen requirements; thus no special incubation procedures are required (e.g., anaerobiosis). Sodium thioglycolate and cystine are reducing agents that remove molecular oxygen (by binding) and thus prevent accumulation of peroxides that are lethal (toxic) to certain microorganisms.

Among bacteria, gelatinase activity varies with incubation temperature; the amount of enzyme produced differs from genus to genus (28). Staphylococci produce more gelatinase when incubated at 20°C than at 37°C (28). Gorini (20) showed that the greatest gelatinase activity occurred when a culture was incubated for growth at 26°C rather than 37°C.

V. QUALITY CONTROL MICROORGANISMS

A. **Nutrient gelatin media**
   1. **Facultative** microorganisms
      a. Growth **and** liquefaction (G/L)
         Proteus vulgaris   ATCC 8427
         Serratia proteamaculans subsp. *proteamaculans*   ATCC 19323
      b. Growth, no liquefaction (G/NL)
         Escherichia coli ATCC 25922
   2. **Anaerobic** microorganisms
      a. Growth and liquefaction (G/L)
         Bacteroides fragilis ATCC 25285
      b. Growth, no liquefaction (G/NL)
         Clostridium perfringens ATCC 12924
B. **Thiogel**
   1. Growth, moderate to heavy; liquefaction (G/L)

Staphylococcus aureus subsp. *aureus* ATCC 25923
Bacteroides fragilis ATCC 25285

2. Growth, heavy; no liquefaction (G/NL)

    Clostridium tetani ATCC 19406

Use a 10^{-1} dilution of an 18- to 24-h culture grown in Trypticase soy broth (TSB) of *S. aureus* subsp. *aureus* and a 10^{-1} dilution of a 3- to 5-day-old culture grown on cooked meat for *Clostridium* and *Bacteroides* spp.

VI. RESULTS

> See Figure 12.1 (Appendix 1) for colored photographic results

VII. INTERPRETATION

A. **Kohn gelatin-charcoal medium**
   1. Liquefaction (L); test microorganism
      a. Free particles of charcoal settle to the bottom of the tube.
      b. Shake tube **gently** to resuspend particles, observed as "cloudy visible black cloud" (24).
   2. No liquefaction (NL); test microorganism
      a. Gelatin-charcoal mixture intact
      b. **No** free charcoal particles in medium
      c. Reincubate for additional time.
   3. Control tube
      a. Gelatin-charcoal mixture intact
      b. **No** free charcoal particles in medium
B. **Nutrient gelatin stab medium or thioglycolate medium. Caution:** cool medium incubated at 35°C **before** interpreting results.
   1. Liquefaction (L); test microorganism: medium liquefied. Liquefaction of gelatin starts at the surface of the medium and flows, extent depends on degree of liquefaction.
   2. No liquefaction (NL); test microorganism
      a. Medium remains solid.
      b. Reincubate for additional time.
   3. Control tube: Medium remains solid; a firm gel because of resolidification of unliquefied gelatin
C. **Nutrient gelatin plate medium** (33)
   1. Liquefaction (L): zonal clouding around growth
      a. Rest of medium remains clear.
      b. Strong positive result has milky-white precipitation; zone 3–6 mm wide
   2. No liquefaction (NL): **no** zonal changes; medium remains clear.

Pickett et al. (36) showed that hydrolysis of gelatin in a plate medium has several advantages: (*a*) it detects extracellular proteins, (*b*) medium is solid at both 30° and 35°C, and (*c*) it may also give earlier positive results.

VIII. ALTERNATIVE TESTS

A. **Mercuric chloride procedure of Frazier** (4, 17)
   1. Principle: detection of a change in composition of gelatin rather than its liquefaction (4)

2. Media: two choices
   a. Nutrient broth containing 12% gelatin (17)
   b. Nutrient agar or brain-heart infusion agar (BHIA) containing 0.4% gelatin (6)
3. Heat **gently** to dissolve; avoid sticking and scorching of gelatin.
4. Autoclave: 121°C, 15 lb, **12 min**
5. Dispense: two choices
   a. Petri plates (15 × 100 mm)
      (1) Approximately 12–15 mL per plate
      (2) Store **inverted** (lid down)
   b. Test tubes (13 × 100 mm)
      (1) 3.0 mL per tube
      (2) Cool in upright position ("**deeps**")
6. Storage: refrigeration (4–10°C); warm to room temperature **just prior to use**
7. Developer: acid mercuric chloride, a protein precipitant, precipitates (binds to) **un**digested gelatin in medium (25)
   a. Ingredients

Mercuric chloride (HgCl$_2$)	15.0 g
Concentrated HCl	20.0 mL
Deionized water	100.0 mL

   b. Add HCl to about 50 mL of water.
   c. Add HgCl$_2$ and shake **gently** until completely dissolved.
8. Inoculation: **heavy**
   a. Plates: spot inoculate; can inoculate 2–4 test organisms per plate
   b. Tube: stab upper ¼ to ½ of medium several times (Fig. 12.2)

   (e.g.,).

9. Incubation
   a. 28°C (4), 30°C (2)
   b. 24 h (4) to 3 days (2, 4)
   c. **No** increased CO$_2$
10. **Add** reagent (developer)
    a. Several drops to each tube or on each plate/spot inocula
    b. Allow reagent to penetrate agar medium for 10–20 min **before** interpreting results.
11. Interpretation
    a. Positive result
       (1) Plate: clearing around colony
       (2) Tubed medium
          (a) Upper ¼ of medium **below** reagent layer clear
          (b) Lower medium cloudy
       (3) Gelatin hydrolyzed
    b. Negative result
       (1) Plate: **no** clearing; cloudy precipitate
       (2) Tubed medium: entire medium **below** reagent layer is cloudy
       (3) **Non**hydrolyzed gelatin; undigested gelatin coagulates, producing a cloudy precipitate

B. **X-ray film method** (5, 36, 38, 45)
   1. Principle: visible removal of gelatin coating from exposed x-ray film
   2. Film (commercial, Eastman x-ray film, type AA; see Appendix 11)

a. Exposed but **not** developed
b. Strips approximately 1¼ inches and narrow enough to fit inside test tubes. Strips do not have to be sterilized (34); however, if desired, place strips in a Petri dish and sterilize by ethylene oxide treatment (33).
3. Procedure
   a. Add 0.5 mL of **sterile** saline or **sterile** distilled water to test tubes (13 × 100 mm). Alternative: 1.0 mL of THIO without glucose, without indicator
   b. Inoculate **heavily** with a loopful of 18- to 24-h bacterial growth.
   c. Insert exposed x-ray strip into saline (or water) suspension and cap tube. **Do not** press strips to side of tube.
   d. Incubate: 37°C water bath and observe at 1, 2, 3, 4, and 24 h for removal of the green gelatin emulsion from the strip; incubate 48 h before reporting as negative. Include a saline blank.
4. Interpretation
   a. Positive: green gelatin emulsion comes off immersed portion of film leaving a transparent (clear) blue film strip.
   b. Negative: strip remains green; greenish emulsion remains on immersed portion of film.

(*Note:* Test may be adapted to a well containing 50 μl of organism suspension in Minitek plate (BBL) (45).)

IX. ALTERNATIVE GELATIN-CONTAINING MEDIA

A. **Chapman Stone agar**
   1. Formulation of Chapman (8); modification of Chapman's *Staphylococcus* agar 110 (7)
   2. Purpose
      a. Isolation of pathogenic staphylococci from clinical specimens
      b. Especially recommended for suspected food poisoning studies
      c. Determination of gelatinase production and mannitol fermentation
   3. Gelatinase activity: positive Stone reaction indicated by a clear zone around colonies
B. **Gelatin metronidazole cadmium (GMC) medium**
   1. Formulation of Korman and Loesche (26)
   2. Purpose: isolation and **presumptive** identification of microaerophilic oral *Actinomyces viscosus* and *A. naeslundii* from dental plaque flora (26)
C. **Lombard-Dowell (LD) gelatin agar**
   1. Formulation of Whaley, Dowell, Wanderlinder, and Lombard (46) (see Chapter 42, Multitest Systems)
   2. Purpose: determination of gelatinase activity; mainly *Clostridium* spp.
D. ***Staphylococcus* agar 110 (Staph-110, S-110) (Stone gelatin agar)**
   1. Formulation of Chapman (7–9)
   2. Purpose
      a. Isolation of *Staphylococcus*
      b. Differentiation of *S. aureus* subsup. *aureus* from *S. epidermidis*
      c. Recommended for studies of food-poisoning outbreaks
E. **Peptone yeast (PY) gelatin medium**
   1. Formulation of VPI Anaerobic Laboratory (22)
   2. Purpose: study of gelatinase activity in anaerobic microorganisms
F. **BCYE$_\alpha$ (buffered charcoal yeast extract) agar with added α-ketoglutarate (1)**
   1. Purpose: identification of *Legionella micdadei*, *L. nautarum*, and *L. feelei* (NL) from other *Legionella* spp. (L) (1, 4)
   2. Gelatin substituted for agar
      a. Dispense 2.0 mL per small capped tube
      b. Preincubate medium 35°C for 72 h.

      c. Inoculate **heavily.**
      d. Check daily at 35°C for 7 days.
      e. Store: 4°C; shelf life 2 months.
  G. **Dilute gelatin medium** (2)
    1. Purpose: differentiation of *Nocardia* and *Streptomyces*
    2. Ingredients; pH 7.0
      a. Gelatin, 4%; 4.0 g/L of deionized water
      b. Autoclave 121°C, 15 lb, 5 min
      c. Dispense 5.0 mL/tube.
    3. Inoculate small fragment of growth from a Sabouraud dextrose agar slant.
    4. Incubate: room temperature (22–25°C), 21–25 days
    5. Interpretation
      a. *N. asteroides:* **no** growth (NG) or very sparse, thin, flaky growth
      b. *N. brasiliensis:* good growth (G); round compact colonies
      c. *Streptomyces* spp.: poor to good growth (G); stringy or flaky
  H. **Gelatin agar (GA) plate method**
    1. Formulation of Syed (44)
    2. Purpose
      a. Rapid agar medium for detection of gelatinase activity of human dental plaque flora
      b. Study of aerobic, anaerobic, and facultative microorganisms of clinical significance
    3. Medium: many salts plus menadione (vitamin K_3), which enhances growth of *Prevotella melaninogenicus* (formerly *Bacteroides melaninogenicus*), and reducing agents, cysteine · Cl and dithiothreitol (Cleland's reagent)
  I. **Aerobic low peptone (ALP) basal medium (1, 21, 35)**
    1. Procedure of Greenwood (21)
    2. Purpose: gelatin liquefaction by nonfermenting Gram-negative bacteria. According to Pickett et al. (36), alkalization of gelatin in ALP basal medium is the test procedure of choice for gelatin liquefaction by fluorescent pseudomonads; in studies 20 of 24 *P. fluorescens* strains exhibited liquefaction within 7 days.
    3. Basal medium ingredients, pH 6.5

Casitone (Difco)	0.5 g
Yeast extract (Difco)	0.5 g
Diammonium phosphate, $(NH_4)_2HPO_4$	1.0 g
Potassium chloride, KCl	0.2 g
Magnesium sulfate heptahydrate, $MgSO_4 \cdot 7H_2O$	0.2 g
Phenol red pH indicator	0.02 g
Agar	15.0 g
Demineralized water	1000 mL

    4. Basal medium supplemented with 0.02% glucose for gelatin determination
    5. Gelatin substrate; final concentration 1%
      a. Substrates sterilized in screw-cap tubes over a slight excess of chloroform
      b. Add to basal medium **before** slanting.
    6. Dispense 3 mL per screw-cap tube (13 × 100 mm).
    7. Autoclave 121°C, 15 min, 15 lbs; **slants**
    8. Inoculation: **heavy,** from an infusion broth culture

X. PRECAUTIONS

A. **General**
    1. Gelatin varies in gelling ability (7). Always run a control tube (uninoculated) in parallel with the organism being tested; a single control is sufficient if several organisms are tested simultaneously only **if** all tubes are inoculated at the same time.

2. Gelatin is solid when incubated at 20°C or below and liquid at a temperature of 35°C or above. Gelatin changes from a gel (solid) to a liquid at about 28°C. Therefore, if gelatin tubes are incubated at 35°C or above, they **must** be placed in a refrigerator or ice bath and cooled before liquefaction may be determined.
3. **Do not** shake gelatin tubes while warm, since growth and liquefaction of gelatin frequently occur only on the surface layer (18). If the gelatin is shaken and allowed to be mixed with the warm fluid of the medium, a microbiologist might overlook a positive result and thus report a false-negative result.
4. The rate of liquefaction depends on the age of the gelatin medium; the viscosity of autoclaved gelatin increases with storage at room temperature (22°C) (30).
5. Lautrop (28) found that some bacteria (e.g., *Salmonella, Serratia, Staphylococcus*) produce a calcium-requiring gelatinase; he recommends incorporating 0.01 M $CaCl_2$ into the suspending medium.
6. Gelatin liquefaction sensitivity is **increased** at lower concentrations; 4% gelatin forms a gel at 5°C that is retained at 21°C (36).
7. Most fastidious bacteria grow in infusion broth, but some **will not grow** in nutrient or peptone broth (1).
8. Gelatin **must** be free of fermentable carbohydrates.
9. At 30–35°C incubation, gelatin is a fluid; therefore, slants are **not** applicable (36).

B. **Kohn gelatin-charcoal medium**
1. After preparation of gelatin-charcoal disks, it is **essential** to wash them well in running water for 24 h to remove all traces of formalin. Any remaining formalin on the disks may inhibit gelatinase activity (28).
2. Kohn found that peptone broth was superior to nutrient broth as a liquid medium for gelatin liquefaction. According to Kohn, nutrient broth has "a definitely inhibitory effect and the results are somewhat delayed" (24).
3. Ewing (15) recommended adding 0.1 mL of toluene per tube of Kohn's medium to accelerate bacterial strains that liquefy gelatin slowly. Toluene decreases the time for liquefaction, with 1–3 days and even up to 6–7 days gained in obtaining a positive result (28). Toluene is a lipid solvent that increases the release of intracellular enzymes by increasing cell wall permeability (28). However, Lautrop (28) states that the toluene effect varies; it may increase or inhibit liquefaction, depending on the incubation temperature. Lautrop (28) suggests the possibility of two gelatinase enzymes: one produced only at 20°C that is heat and toluene sensitive; the second produced at both 20 and 37°C, which is heat stable and unaffected by toluene. The growth temperature influences the amount and type of enzyme produced (28). Toluene's usefulness applies mainly to slow gelatin liquefiers. However, since some bacterial strains are inhibited by toluene, Lautrop (28) recommends that if toluene is used, two tubes per organism being tested should be incubated simultaneously, one without the addition of toluene.

C. **Nutrient gelatin stab medium**
1. The type of gelatin liquefaction (e.g., fir tree, inverted fir tree) does **not** have great importance in routine diagnostic work. Simply record as liquefaction (positive) or no liquefaction (negative) of gelatin (13).
2. Mesophilic bacteria may grow slowly, if at all, when incubated at 22–25°C. To avoid this problem, incubate tubes at 35°C and cool before interpreting results (13).
3. According to Cowan (13), some bacteria do not grow in nutrient gelatin medium.
4. A gelatin concentration of 12–15% **may** inhibit growth (6).
5. Hydrolyzing gelatin is two-step process, to polypeptides and then to individual amino acids. A positive reaction starts at the surface of the medium and the flow depends upon the degree of liquefaction.
6. Liquefaction by **non**fermentative Gram-negative bacteria may be delayed; hold test 7

days (34). Some species produce gelatinase faster, and some solely at room temperature rather than at 35°C; if such organisms (e.g., *P. fluorescens*) are suspected, inoculate a second tube of nutrient gelatin and incubate at room temperature (34).
7. Thiogel should be used to determine gelatin liquefaction by fastidious species and obligate anaerobes (3).

D. **Mercuric chloride procedure**
1. The acidic mercuric chloride procedure **does not** detect rate of liquefaction and **cannot** be used for many organisms such as *Klebsiella* (4).
2. If medium **immediately** becomes opaque and white around area of bacterial growth, gelatin has been precipitated, **not** hydrolyzed, by test organism.

E. **X-ray film method**
1. Cut film strips 1 × 1½ inches. If strips are too narrow they will cling to the side of the tubes and may not be fully immersed; if too wide, they will **not** adhere to side and will fall to bottom of the tube (33).
2. Overnight incubation is **not** recommended (possible false-positive results). On 18- to 24-h incubation, some batches of buffered saline and/or broth may randomly strip gelatin from film in the **un**inoculated control (33).
3. Photographic strips are recommended for general use by many investigators (5, 29, 38). However, Pickett et al. (36) found that photographic strips fail to detect weak proteolysis; they recommend confirming negative test results by a more sensitive test medium such as 4% gelatin broth or alkalization of ALP gelatin.

F. **ALP medium:** alkalization of gelatin is **not** applicable to *Acinetobacter* and *Alcaligenes* spp. (36).

REFERENCES

1. Balows A, Hausler WJ Jr, Herrmann KL, et al. Manual of Clinical Microbiology, ed 5. Washington, DC: American Society for Microbiology, 1991:279, 443, 450, 1248.
2. Baron EJ, Finegold SM. Bailey & Scott's Diagnostic Microbiology, ed 8. Philadelphia: CV Mosby, 1990:382, A-14.
3. Becton Dickinson. Manual of BBL Products and Laboratory Procedures, ed 6. Cockeysville, MD: Becton Dickinson Microbiology Systems, 1988: 215–216.
4. Blazevic DJ, Ederer GM. Principles of Biochemical Tests in Diagnostic Microbiology. New York: John Wiley & Sons, 1975:46.
5. Blazevic DJ, Koepcke MH, Matsen JM. Incidence and identification of *Pseudomonas fluorescens* and *Pseudomonas putida* in the clinical laboratory. Appl Microbiol 1973;25(1):107–110.
6. Branson D. Methods in Clinical Bacteriology. Springfield, IL: Charles C Thomas, 1972:21–22.
7. Chapman GH. A single culture medium for selective isolation of plasma-coagulating staphylococci and for improved testing of chromogenesis, plasma coagulation, mannitol fermentation, and the Stone reaction. J Bacteriol 1946;51(3):409.
8. Chapman GH. An improved Stone medium for the isolation and testing for food-poisoning staphylococci. Food Res 1948;13:100–105.
9. Chapman GH. A simple method for making multiple tests of a microorganism. J Bacteriol 1952;63(1):147.
10. Clark WA, Hollis DG, Weaver RE, Riley P. Identification of unusual pathogenic gram-negative aerobic and facultatively anaerobic bacteria. Atlanta: Centers for Disease Control, 1984.
11. Collins MD, Farrow JAE, Phillips BA, Kandler O. Validation of the publication of new names and new combinations previously effectively published outside the IJSB. List no. 14. Int J Syst Bacteriol 1984;34(2):270–271.
12. Collins MD, Jones D. Reclassification of *Corynebacterium pyogenes* (Glage) in the genus *Actinomyces* as *Actinomyces pyogenes* comb. nov. J Gen Microbiol 1982;128:901–903.
13. Cowan ST. Cowan & Steel's Manual for the Identification of Medical Bacteria, ed 2. London: Cambridge University Press, 1974:24, 34–35, 156, 173.
14. Difco Manual, ed 10. Detroit: Difco Laboratories, 1984:624–625.
15. Ewing WH. Edwards and Ewing's Identification of Enterobacteriaceae, ed 4. New York: Elsevier, 1986:245–246.
16. Fieser LF, Fieser M. Organic Chemistry, ed 3. New York: Reinhold, 1956:417, 450.
17. Frazier WC. A method for the detection of changes in gelatin due to bacteria. J Infect Dis 1926;39:302–309.
18. Frobisher M. Fundamentals of Microbiology, ed 6. Philadelphia: WB Saunders, 1957:239.
19. Gilardi GL. *Pseudomonas* and related genera. In: Balows A, Hausler WJ Jr, Herrmann KL, et al.,

19. eds. Manual of Clinical Microbiology, ed 5. Washington, DC: American Society for Microbiology, 1991:429–441.
20. Gorini L. Le rôle du calcium dans l'activité et la stabilité de quelques proteinases bactériennes. Biochim Biophys Acta 1951;6:237–255.
21. Greenwood JR. Methods of isolation and identification of glucose-nonfermenting gram-negative rods. In: Gilardi GL, ed. Nonfermentative Gram-Negative Rods. Laboratory Identification and Clinical Aspects. New York: Marcel Dekker, 1985:1–16.
22. Holdeman LV, Cato EP, Moore WEC, eds. Anaerobic Laboratory Manual, ed 4. Blacksburg, VA: Virginia Polytechnic Institute Anaerobic Laboratory (VPI), 1977.
23. Holt JG, Bruns MA, Caldwell BJ, Rease CD. Stedman's Bergey's Bacteria Words. Baltimore, Williams & Wilkins, 1992:10, 28, 167, 233, 295.
24. Kohn J. A preliminary report of a new gelatin liquefaction method. J Clin Pathol 1953;6(3):249.
25. Koneman EW, Allen SD, Janda WM, et al. Color Atlas and Textbook of Diagnostic Microbiology, ed 4. Phildelphia: JB Lippincott, 1992:144, 422, 546.
26. Korman KS, Loesche WJ. New medium for isolation of *Actinomyces viscosus* and *Actinomyces naeslundii* from dental plaque. J Clin Microbiol 1978;7(6):514–518.
27. Lampe AS. A variant of the test for gelatin liquefaction in non-fermentative gram-negative rods. Antonie van Leeuwenhoek 1982;48:207–208.
28. Lautrop H. A modified Kohn's test for the demonstration of bacterial gelatin liquefaction. Acta Pathol Microbiol Scand 1956;39(5):357–369.
29. Le Minor L, Piechaud M. Note technique. Une méthode rapide de recherche de la protéolyse de la gélatine. Ann Inst Pasteur 1963;105:792–794.
30. Levine M, Carpenter DC. Gelatin liquefaction by bacteria. J Bacteriol 1923;8(4):297–306.
31. MacLean PD, Liebow AA, Rosenberg AA. A haemolytic corynebacteria resembling *Corynebacterium ovis* and *Corynebacterium pyogenes* in man. J Infect Dis 1946;79:69–90.
32. Nash P, Krenz MM. Culture media. In: Balows A, Hausler WJ Jr, Herrmann KL, et al., eds. Manual of Clinical Microbiology, ed 5. Washington, DC: American Society for Microbiology, 1985:1226–1288.
33. Oberhofer TR. Manual of Practical Medical Microbiology and Parasitology. New York: John Wiley & Sons, 1985:166–169.
34. Oberhofer TR. Manual of Nonfermenting Gram-Negative Bacteria. New York: John Wiley & Sons, 1985:45, 53.
35. Pickett MJ, Greenwood JR. Identification of oxidase-positive, glucose-negative, motile species of nonfermentative bacilli. J Clin Microbiol 1986;23(5):920–923.
36. Pickett MJ, Greenwood JR, Harvey SM. Tests for detecting degradation of gelatin: Comparison of five methods. J Clin Microbiol 1991;29(10):2322–2325.
37. Pitt TL, Dey D. A method for the detection of gelatinase production by bacteria. J Appl Bacteriol 1970;33:687–691.
38. Porres JM, Harris D. Rapid gelatin liquefaction test. Am J Clin Pathol 1974;62(3):428–430.
39. Reddy CA, Cornell CP, Fraga AM. Transfer of *Corynebacterium pyogenes* (Glage) Eberson to the genus *Actinomyces pyogenes* (Glage) comb. nov. Int J Syst Bacteriol 1982;32(4):419–429.
40. Smith HL Jr, Goodner K. Detection of bacterial gelatinases by gelatin agar plate methods. J Bacteriol 1958;76(6):662–665.
41. Sneath PHA, Mair NS, Sharpe ME, Holt JG, eds. Bergey's Manual of Systematic Bacteriology, vol 2. Baltimore, Williams & Wilkins, 1986:1268.
42. Sottnek FO, Brown JM, Weaver RE, Carroll GF. Recognition of *Oerskovia* species in the clinical laboratory: Characterization of 35 isolates. Int J Syst Bacteriol 1977;27:263–270.
43. Stanier RY, Palleroni NJ, Doudoroff M. The aerobic pseudomonads: A taxonomic study. J Gen Microbiol 1966;43(2):159–271.
44. Syed SA. A new medium for the detection of gelatin-hydrolyzing activity of human dental plaque flora. J Clin Microbiol 1976;3(2):200–202.
45. Washington JA. Laboratory Procedures in Clinical Microbiology, ed 2. New York: Springer-Verlag, 1985:355–356.
46. Whaley DN, Dowell VR Jr, Wanderlinder LM, Lombard GL. Gelatin agar medium for detecting gelatinase production by anaerobic bacteria. J Clin Microbiol 1982;16(2):224–229.

13 Gluconate Oxidation Test

I. PRINCIPLE

To determine the ability of an organism to oxidize gluconate (gluconic acid), its sole carbon source, to the reducing compound 2-ketogluconate, which in turn reduces copper sulfate

II. PURPOSE

(Also see Chapters 44 and 45)

A. To aid in differentiation between genera: *Pseudomonas aeruginosa* (+) from *Alcaligenes faecalis* (−).
B. Primarily to aid in species differentiation of the fluorescent pseudomonads from other **non-fermentative bacilli (NFB)**: *P. aeruginosa* (+), *P. fluorescens* (V, variable, usually +), *P. putida* (V, usually +), *P. aureofaciens* (V), and *P. chlororaphis* (+). Often included in battery of tests to identify oxidase-positive NFB.

III. BIOCHEMISTRY INVOLVED

The substrate, potassium gluconate, is a potassium salt of gluconic acid. Gluconate oxidation was originally used by Haynes (5) to differentiate the pseudomonads, but other organisms, mainly those among the *Enterobacteriaceae,* are now known to possess this ability. Gluconate is one of the oxidation products formed from glucose by aerobic microorganisms that metabolize carbohydrates by the Entner-Doudoroff pathway.

Bacteria metabolize carbohydrates by either fermentation or oxidation. In fermentation, glucose catabolism involves initial phosphorylation, then a splitting into two triose molecules. However, when glucose is metabolized **oxidatively** to gluconic acid, **no initial phosphorylation occurs,** and only organisms capable of oxidative metabolism can use potassium gluconate as their sole carbon source (6, 10, 11). These oxidative organisms are obligate aerobes. Sebek and Randles (11) attribute the lack of phosphorylation in the initial stage of oxidation to the inability of adenosine triphosphate (ATP) to penetrate the bacterial cell.

$$\begin{array}{c}
\boxed{\text{CHO}} \longrightarrow \text{Aldehyde group} \\
\text{H}-\underset{1}{\text{C}}-\text{OH} \\
\text{HO}-\underset{2}{\text{C}}-\text{H} \\
\text{HO}-\underset{3}{\text{C}}-\text{OH} \\
\text{H}-\underset{4}{\text{C}}-\text{OH} \\
\underset{5}{\text{CH}_2\text{OH}}
\end{array} \xrightarrow[\text{no phosphorylation}]{\text{oxidation}} \begin{array}{c}
\boxed{\text{COOH}} \longrightarrow \text{Carboxyl group} \\
\text{H}-\underset{2}{\text{C}}-\text{OH} \\
\text{HO}-\underset{3}{\text{C}}-\text{H} \\
\text{H}-\underset{4}{\text{C}}-\text{OH} \\
\text{H}-\underset{5}{\text{C}}-\text{OH} \\
\underset{6}{\text{CH}_2\text{OH}}
\end{array}$$

Glucose   Gluconic acid (gluconate)

In oxidation, glucose is **not** split into two trioses; the aldehyde group is directly oxidized to a carboxyl group, forming gluconic acid. Aldose sugars such as glucose and galactose are

polyhydric aldehydes in which each molecule contains an aldehyde group (CHO or H–C=O).
When only the aldehyde groups are oxidized to carboxyl groups (–COOH or $\overset{\overset{O}{\|}}{C}$–OH), the series of compounds derived are called "aldonic acids," of which gluconic acid is one (9, 13).

Gluconic acid can be further degraded to 2-ketogluconic acid (2-ketogluconate), the key intermediate in the gluconate test, which may accumulate or be slowly metabolized further (11). Structurally, 2-ketogluconic acid differs from gluconic acid by a carbonyl at C2 (3).

Oxidative Metabolism of Glucose (2, 6, 10)

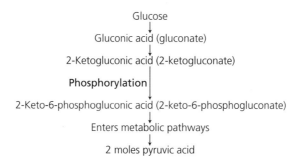

Gluconic acid and gluconate are **not** reducing compounds, but some bacteria can oxidize gluconate via the oxidative metabolic pathway into intermediates such as 2-ketogluconate, which has reducing properties (5, 10).

IV. MEDIA EMPLOYED

A. **Gluconate peptone broth**
   1. Modification of Haynes medium (5, 12)
   2. Ingredients, pH 7.0 ± 0.2

Casein peptone	1.5 g
Yeast extract	1.0 g
Dipotassium phosphate, K_2HPO_4	1.0 g
Potassium gluconate, $KC_6H_{11}O_7$	40.0 g
Deionized water	1000.0 mL

      Potassium gluconate may be replaced by 37.25 g of sodium gluconate (4).
   3. Method of preparation
      a. Heat **gently** into solution.
      b. Filter (Millipore).
      c. Dispense approximately 2.0 mL per screw-cap (snap-cap) tube (13 × 100 mm).
   4. Method of sterilization: autoclave; 115°C, 15 lb, 15 min
   5. Finished uninoculated medium appearance: clear, yellowish liquid, tubed medium
   6. Cool before use and refrigerate for storage (4–10°C); shelf life approximately 6–8 weeks at 2–8°C
   7. Inoculation
      a. **Heavy** inoculum (1)
      b. Growth from an 18- to 24-h **pure** culture: Kligler's iron agar (KIA)/triple sugar iron agar (TSI)
   8. Incubation: 35°C; 48 h (4, 5)
   9. Add Benedict's reagent or a Clinitest tablet **directly** to the **incubated** tube **before** attempting to interpret.

The potassium salt of gluconate is routinely used because it gives a clear solution and is readily available (5). A 4% solution (wt/wt) is used because at the end of the 48-h incubation this amount permits *P. aeruginosa* to accumulate at least 50% of potassium 2-ketogluconate (5).

B. **Key gluconate substrate test tablet**
   1. Manufacturer: Key Scientific Products
   2. Procedure: follow manufacturer's directions

V. REAGENTS EMPLOYED: TWO CHOICES

A. **Benedict's qualitative solution**
   1. Ingredients (4)

Copper sulfate, $CuSO_4 \cdot 5 H_2O$	1.73 g
Sodium carbonate, anhydrous, Na_2CO_3	10.0 g
Sodium citrate, $C_3H_4OH(COO)_3Na_3$	17.3 g
Deionized water	100.0 mL

   2. Method of preparation (4)
      a. Solution 1: dissolve sodium citrate and carbonate in 60.0 mL of deionized water.
      b. Solution 2: dissolve copper sulfate in 20.0 mL of distilled water.
      c. Add solution 2 to solution 1 with constant stirring.
      d. Adjust volume to 100 mL with deionized water.
   3. Storage: store in a warm location; this reagent is highly susceptible to crystallization when cold (4).
   4. Chemistry of reagent action: the carbohydrate intermediate 2-ketogluconate, if present, reduces soluble cupric hydroxide (copper sulfate) when heated to an insoluble cuprous oxide, which precipitates (9).

$$Cu{<}^{OH}_{OH} + \text{2-Ketogluconate} \xrightarrow[\text{reduction}]{\text{heat}} Cu_2\downarrow + 2H_2O + O$$

| Cupric hydroxide $2\ Cu(OH)_2$ (blue color) | Reducing agent | Cuprous oxide (yellow to orange-red colored precipitate) (characteristic odor of decaying cabbage) (5) |

B. **Clinitest tablets**
   1. Manufacturer: Ames
   2. Add **one-half** Clinitest tablet **directly** to **incubated** gluconate tube.
   3. Storage: Clinitest tablets are stable indefinitely when stored **unopened** at room temperature; however, they are hygroscopic and highly susceptible to humidity. They are also destroyed at temperatures above 120°F. Tablets that show any dark blue discoloration should be discarded. Since their stability varies each week tablets should be given a quality control check and discarded when demonstrating a negative or weak reaction with a known positive organism.
   4. Chemistry of reagent action (7): the Clinitest tablet contains copper sulfate, sodium carbonate, a small amount of citric acid, and sodium hydroxide (NaOH). The sodium carbonate and citric acid provide effervescence to speed up dissolving of the tablet, while sodium hydroxide provides the alkalinity necessary for reduction. The self-heating system is generated by both sodium hydroxide and the reaction between sodium hydroxide and citric acid.

$$2\ Cu^{++} + \text{2-Ketogluconate} \xrightarrow[\substack{\text{NaOH} \\ \text{reduction}}]{\text{heat}} Cu_2O\downarrow + \text{oxidized compound}$$

Cupric ions   Reducing   Cuprous oxide
(blue color)   agent   (yellow to orange-red
                                                     precipitate)

VI. QUALITY CONTROL MICROORGANISMS

Either reagent **must** be tested **with known** positive and negative cultures before being put into general use.

A. Positive (+)

Klebsiella pneumoniae subsp. *pneumoniae*	ATCC 13883
Pseudomonas aeruginosa	ATCC 10145
Citrobacter freundii	ATCC 8090

B. Negative (−)

Escherichia coli	ATCC 11775
Uninoculated	

VII. INTERPRETATION—EITHER REAGENT

A. Add Benedict's solution or a Clinitest tablet **directly** to **incubated** tubes **before** attempting to interpret.
1. **Benedict's solution**
   a. Add 1.0 mL **directly** to each gluconate tube.
   b. Mix well and place in a boiling water bath (100°C), 10 min.
2. **Clinitest tablet:** add one-half tablet to each tube; wait 5 sec after boiling has stopped, then shake tube **gently** before interpreting color (7).

B. Positive (+)
1. A yellow to orange to orange-red precipitate. The color produced depends on the amount of reducing substance accumulated; the greater the amount, the more orange to orange-red the color becomes. However, any reducing activity, with colors ranging from slight green (1+) to deep orange (4+) indicates oxidation (8).
2. Presence of a reducing substance, 2-ketogluconate. 2-Ketogluconate reduces copper sulfate (blue color) when heated to an insoluble cuprous oxide (Cu_2O), which is precipitated out.

C. Negative (−)
1. **No** color change; medium remains blue or bluish green after addition of Benedict's solution or a Clinitest tablet.
2. No reducing substance present.

VIII. PRECAUTIONS

A. **Clinitest tablet**
1. **Do not** use the commercial impregnated **Clinistix** dip stick test because it is specific for glucose, a reducing sugar (1, 7).
2. Clinitest tablets are stable indefinitely when stored **un**opened at room temperature (22–25°C); however, they are hygroscopic and highly susceptible to humidity. They are also destroyed at temperatures above 120°F. Tablets that show any dark blue discoloration should be discarded.

B. **Key gluconate substrate tablet** (Key Scientific Products): Pease et al. (10) found the tablet

to be more accurate than gluconate broth. In their tests, 93% of fluorescein-producing pseudo-monads were positive for gluconate. They found too many false-positive and false-negative results with the broth medium (10).
C. Test specific for fluorescent pseudomonads; other microorganisms such as *Achromobacter* and *Pseudomonas cepacia* occasionally give a false-positive test result (8).
D. Oberhofer (8) recommends recording reactions in degrees of positivity rather than just positive and negative; weak reactions are useful for characterizing microorganisms.

REFERENCES

1. Branson D. Methods in Clinical Bacteriology. Springfield IL: Charles C Thomas, 1972:23.
2. Burrows W, Lewert RM, Rippon JW. Textbook of Microbiology. The Pathogenic Microorganisms, ed 19. Philadelphia, WB Saunders, 1968: 118–121.
3. Cohen SS. Glucokinase and the oxidative path of glucose-6-phosphate utilization. J Biol Chem 1951;189(2):617–628.
4. Cowan ST. Cowan & Steel's Manual for the Identification of Medical Bacteria, ed 2. Cambridge: Cambridge University Press, 1974:116, 146.
5. Haynes WC. *Pseudomonas aeruginosa*—its characterization and identification. J Gen Microbiol 1951;5(5):939–950.
6. Hugh R, Leifson E. The taxonomic significance of fermentative versus oxidative metabolism of carbohydrates by various gram negative bacteria. J Bacteriol 1953;66(1):24–26.
7. Kark RM, Lawrence JR, Pollak VE, et al. A Primer of Urinalysis, ed 2. New York: Hoeber Medical Division, Harper & Row, 1963:36–38.
8. Oberhofer TR. Manual of Practical Medical Microbiology and Parasitology. New York: John Wiley & Sons, 1985:172–173.
9. Oser BL, ed. Hawk's Physiological Chemistry, ed 14. New York: McGraw-Hill, 1965:80–81, 89.
10. Pease M, Malcolm J, Chernaik R, Dunlop S. An approach to the problem of differentiating pseudomonads in the clinical laboratory. Am J Med Technol 1968;34(1):51–57.
11. Sebek OK, Randles CI. The oxidative dissimilation of mannitol and sorbitol by *Pseudomonas fluorescens*. J Bacteriol 1952;63(6):693–700.
12. Shaw C, Clarke PH. Biochemical classification of *Proteus* and *Providence* cultures. J Gen Microbiol 1955;13(1):155–161.
13. Stanier RY, Doudoroff M, Adelberg EA. The Microbial World, ed 2. Englewood Cliffs, NJ: Prentice-Hall, 1963:269.

14 Hippurate Hydrolysis Test

I. PRINCIPLE

A. To determine the enzymatic ability of an organism to hydrolyze sodium hippurate (hippuric acid) to benzoic acid and glycine by the action of the enzyme hippurate hydrolase (hippuricase).
B. Enzymatic activity is determined by testing for either end product, benzoic acid or glycine.

II. PURPOSE

(Also see Chapters 43 and 45)

A. Along with a combination of other tests aids in differentiation of bovine β-hemolytic group B *Streptococcus* (*S. agalactiae*) (+) from human β-hemolytic *Streptococcus* spp. (usually −) (2, 6, 7) and **presumptive** identification of group B *Streptococcus*
B. Differentiates β-hemolytic group B *Streptococcus* from β-hemolytic groups A and nonenterococcal D and the β-hemolytic *Enterococcus* spp.
C. Hippurate hydrolysis testing is critical for differentiation of *Campylobacter jejuni* subsp. *jejuni* (+) and subsp. *doylei* (+) (36) from *C. coli* (−), *C. lari* (−) and other *Campylobacter* spp. (−) (30, 38, 42, 47, 55, 56, 60). *C. jejuni* is the only campylobacter to hydrolyze hippurate (38). Differentiation of *C. coli* from *C. jejuni* relies almost entirely on hippurate hydrolysis (50). An occasional strain of *C. jejuni* is hippurate negative (28, 30, 55).
D. Additional diagnostic aid along with other biochemical tests (gelatin liquefaction and β-lactamase) in the identification of *Legionella pneumophila* (+) and *L. feeleii* (V, variable) from other *Legionella* and *Legionella*-like species (−) (29, 38).
E. Additional diagnostic aid along with other biochemical tests (starch hydrolysis, α- and β-glucosides) in the identification of *Gardnerella vaginalis* (+) (4, 24, 41).
F. Aids in differentiation of
   1. *Actinobacillus lignieresii* (+) from *Actinobacillus equuli* (−)
   2. *Brevibacterium iodinum* (−) from most frequently isolated *B. casei* (+), *B. epidermidis* (+), and *B. linens*
   3. *Listeria grayi* (−) from *L. innocua* (+), *L. ivanovii* (+), and *L. monocytogenes* (+)
   4. *Mobiluncus mulieris* (−) from *M. curtisii* subsp. *curtisii* (+), and *M. curtisii* subsp. *holmesii* (+)
   5. Aerobic, sporeforming *Bacillus* spp. (52)

The test should **not** be applied indiscriminately to all groups of streptococci; it is only useful in relation to β-hemolytic streptococci of human or bovine origin and should be used only with them (2).

III. BIOCHEMISTRY INVOLVED

Hippuric acid (N-benzoyl glycine, benzoylaminoacetic acid, $C_6H_5CONHCH_2COONa$) is a benzoyl acid derivative of glycine; an aromatic ring compound benzoyl ($C_6H_5CO^-$) conjugated with amino acid glycine (NH_2CH_2COOH). Hippuric acid is an aryl-substituted carboxylic acid with a carboxyl group (–COOH) attached directly to the aromatic (benzene) ring;

the hydroxyl portion (–OH) of the carboxyl group is removed (RC—) and replaced in this case by an amide (–NH$_2$).

Benzoyl radical + Glycine ⇌ Hippuric acid + H$^+$OH$^-$

(Carbonyl group; Amino group labeled on Hippuric acid structure)

Hippuric acid is acidic because it can donate a hydrogen ion to a more basic solution. Also, as an amide it is readily hydrolyzed (48) with chemical splitting by the addition of water and a catalytic action of the specific enzyme hippurate hydrolase.

Hippuric acid (benzoylglycine) + H$_2$O ⇌ (hippurate hydrolase / hydrolysis) Benzoic acid + Glycine (glycocoll) (5, 31)

A salt of hippurate (C$_6$H$_5$CONHCH$_2$COO$^-$Na$^+$) is used in test medium, forming sodium benzoate (C$_6$H$_5$COO$^-$Na$^+$) and sodium glycinate (NH$_2$CH$_2$COO$^-$Na$^+$) on hydrolysis. Acid end products of hippuric hydrolysis, benzoic acid and glycine, are insoluble in water; their salts are soluble (48). Salt formation depends on acid strength (or degree of ionization); if the acid is RCOOH, its ionization (an equilibrium process) is (48)

$$RCOOH \rightleftharpoons RCOO^- + H^+$$
Undissociated carboxylic acid — carboxylate ion

Carboxylic acids react stoichiometrically (equivalent for equivalent) with bases to form salts that are 100% dissociated in solution (26). Sodium salts are usually water soluble and produce alkaline aqueous solutions; because they are salts of strong bases and weak acids they are hydrolyzed (27). The substrate sodium hippurate pH shift to alkalinity is probably due to the amino acid product, glycine (12).

Benzoic acid (benzene carboxylic acid, phenylformic acid, dracylic acid) is a volatile weak acid (6). It is a monocarboxylic acid of the aromatic series related to benzene (C$_6$H$_5^-$), a benzene derivative (1). Glycine (glycocoll) is a monoaminomonocarboxylic acid (15); its functional group is the amine group (–NH$_2$) (48).

Hippuricase promotes hydrolysis at the peptide linkage of hippuric acid; evidence suggests that combination of the enzyme with substrate takes place through glycine (or amino acid portion) (17). The amide linkage between an α amino acid and a carboxyl group is called a **peptide linkage** (48).

Peptide link

Glycine-alpha(α) carbon, carbon next to functional group (—NH or amino acid)

Hippurate hydrolysis may be determined by detecting either end product (16). Benzoic acid in the medium can be demonstrated by addition of either an acidified ferric chloride ($FeCl_3$) solution or an inorganic acid; the $FeCl_3$ procedure is the more sensitive of the two methods (2). The end product glycine is detected by the ninhydrin method (16).

The enzyme earlier called **histozyme** (39), a name replaced by the widely used term **hippuricase** (39), has been designated **hippurate hydrolase** (N- benzoylamino acid amidohydrolase, aminocylase) (52, 54); it splits the benzoyl derivative of natural L-amino acids (39). Hydrolases are a class of enzymes that catalyze hydrolytic reactions without coenzymes. Hippuric acid–splitting enzymes are widely distributed in nature, but the biologic significance of hippurate hydrolase is unclear. The specificity of these enzymes for substrates other than hippuric acid may differ from species to species (19). It has not been purified, and its biochemical characteristics are poorly defined (19).

Hippurate hydrolase (hippuricase), a constitutive enzyme (33), is heat labile and antigenic and requires a pH of 7.1–9.0 for optimum activity (19). Ferrieri et al. (19) showed that treatment with the proteolytic enzyme trypsin resulted in complete loss of hippurate hydrolase activity. They also showed that hippurate hydrolase is largely intracellular and not cell wall associated, but there may be a slight tendency for membrane association. Their studies confirmed the association of hippurate hydrolase activity with group B streptococci, ruling out release of enzyme extracellularly into medium. Studies confirm that filtrates are not capable of hippurate hydrolysis; however, washed cells, either dead or alive, reacted with the substrate in a manner similar to whole-cell broth cultures (19). According to studies by Hwang and Ederer (34), group B streptococci appear to possess inherent enzyme systems.

As hippuric acid is split into benzoic acid and glycine, the amino nitrogen content of the medium should increase, unless glycine is used by bacteria (2). A large increase in amino nitrogen constitutes another test for hydrolysis (2).

IV. REAGENT EMPLOYED: ACIDIC FERRIC CHLORIDE

A. Formulations; two choices
  1. Formulation 1

     Ferric chloride, aqueous, $FeCl_3 \cdot 6H_2O$, 12%   12.0 g
     Concentrated hydrochloric acid, HCl (37%)   5.4 mL
     Deionized water to bring to 94.6 mL

  2. Formulation 2 (3)
     a. Aqueous HCl, 2%: 5.4 mL/94.6 mL deionized water
     b. Ferric chloride, 12.0 g/100 mL 2% aqueous HCl
B. Method of preparation
  1. Add approximately 75 mL of distilled or deionized water to a 100-mL volumetric flask.

2. With transfer pipette (TC, to contain), add 2.5 mL of HCl to the flask, running the acid down the sides of the flask.
3. Add 12.0 g of ferric chloride.
4. Dissolve by warming the flask **gently,** swirling contents to mix well.
5. Bring the volume up to 100 mL with distilled or deionized water.
6. Solution appears orange.

C. Reagent quality control
1. Must be performed **before** adding reagent to any test organism(s).
2. Negative control (NC) tube 1.
   a. Contains 0.8 mL of **incubated** broth culture
   b. Add 0.2 mL of a 12% $FeCl_3$ reagent.
   c. **Immediately** shake tube **gently**.
   d. Let stand 10–15 min before interpreting results with occasional shaking (18).
      (1) If negative
         (a) **Clearing** of initial precipitate within 15 min (18) or precipitate redissolves on shaking
         (b) Ferric ion is **in excess**.
         (c) Proceed to determine results on test organism(s) (see V, Medium Employed, part N).
      (2) If positive
         (a) Initial precipitate **does not** redissolve or clear within 10–15 min on shaking (18).
         (b) Ferric ion **not** in excess
         (c) Titrate $FeCl_3$ to determine optimal amount of reagent required to be in excess (step 3).
3. Titration of $FeCl_3$ reagent (13)
   a. To 1.0-mL aliquots in negative control (NC) tubes 3, 4, 5, and 6 rapidly add 0.2, 0.3, 0.4, and 0.5 mL of $FeCl_3$, respectively.
   b. **Immediately** shake **gently**.
   c. Let stand 10–15 min **before** interpreting results with occasional shaking (18).
   d. The **smallest amount** of acidic $FeCl_3$ reagent that gives a clear solution indicates ferric (Fe^{3+}) ion is in excess; this quantity is used for test organism(s).
   e. **Proceed to determine results on test organism(s) (part E).**
4. Positive control (PC)
   a. Heavy precipitate remaining after 10–15 min with occasional shaking (18)
   b. Hippurate hydrolyzed

D. Method of use—test organism(s)
1. Add appropriate amount of acidic 12% $FeCl_3$ reagent as determined by quality control of reagent (part C) to all incubated tubes.
2. Shake tubes **gently**.
3. Let stand 10–15 min before interpreting results with occasional shaking (18).

Recent terminology for iron-containing compounds is iron (III) for ferric (Fe^{3+}) ion and iron (II) for ferrous (Fe^{2+}) ion (40). The ferric chloride test depends on the relative solubilities of benzoate and hippurate of a Fe^{3+} (iron (III)) salt; complexes of ferric benzoate and ferric hippurate differ in stability (52, 59). The final concentration of iron is critical and must be measured in both broth culture fluid and reagent (13, 59); if a definite amount of $FeCl_3$ reagent is added to a fixed quantity of medium, the reaction is balanced. Protein (glycine), residual hippurate, and benzoate are precipitated by the reagent; however, the protein and hippurate precipitates are more soluble and will redissolve after shaking or in an excess of ferric chloride, while benzoate remains an insoluble precipitate (2, 13, 14, 25, 33). Ferric chloride is very sensitive, reacting with even traces of benzoic acid (52). Acidified ferric chloride, like hydrochloric acid, redissolves the iron phosphate formed in the medium (2) besides entering into the color reaction.

E. Storage: store reagent in a refrigerator (4°C) when not in use. Ferric chloride should be placed in dark bottles to avoid exposure to light. Its stability varies; therefore, it should be given a quality control check weekly and discarded when demonstrating a negative or weak reaction with a known positive organism.
F. Chemistry of reagent action: ferric chloride in solution gives color with a number of organic derivatives: phenols, enols, hydroxamic acids, and some carboxylic acids (57). Wesp and Brode (61) showed that the requirements for color reaction with $FeCl_3$-phenol solutions are (a) Fe^{3+} ions (iron (III)), (b) a mildly acidic –OH or –SH group such as occurs in phenols, and (c) a solvent capable of coordination. The reagent consists of a hydrated ferric ion, $FeCl_3 \cdot 6H_2O$, in which water is held in combination with the ferric (iron (III)) ion; this is often referred to as water of crystallization, or water of hydration (indicated by the chemical dot (·) in formula) (40). It may also be written as $Fe(H_2O)_6^{3+}3Cl$. The ferric chloride solution exists as a solvated (hydrated) molecule or dissociated molecule to give solvated ions.

Addition of phenol (C_6H_5OH) displaces the solvent and produces an anionic (negative) iron-phenol complex; when in water, water serves as a proton acceptor so that it is a phenoxide (phenolate) ($C_6H_5O^-$) ion, which can displace a molecule of solvent (H_2O) from the solvated ferric ion (57). The reagent solvent plays a part in color formation (57). The hydrated ferric ion, $Fe(H_2O)_6^{3+}$, is pale violet but loses protons very rapidly (53). Ferric salts in solution are yellow or brown because of formation of hydroxide complexes, and solutions containing the chloride ion are more intensely yellow or brown because of formation of ferric chloride complexes (53); a free hydroxyl group (OH) is needed on an aromatic ring to produce the color reaction.

Phenolic carboxylic acids compete for the solvated ferric ion or molecule of ferric chloride (57). Basic salts have a replaceable OH; they contain −OH ions that can combine with a proton (40). Sodium benzoate is a base insoluble in water, but the carboxylate ion ($RCOO^-$) is a good proton acceptor especially with hydrochloric acid (HCl), a proton (positive) donor (32). The use of an aqueous ferric chloride acidified with a strong acid (HCl) provides the necessary proton; strong acids readily give up protons (40).

Coordination is a condition in which a pair of electrons or more are shared by at least two atoms. Atoms with unshared electrons such as oxygen (O) can act as ligands for metallic ions (46). A **ligand** is a molecule that supplies necessary electrons to form coordinate covalent bonds with metallic ions. Ferric (Fe^{3+}, iron (III)) or ferrous (Fe^{2+}, iron (II)) ions have a high affinity for oxygen and are tightly bound; metallic ions are bound more tightly as the pH rises (46).

Overall Reaction

The color complex is a negative (anionic) ion (57, 61); its color is due to formation of complex coordinated ions of type $Fe(OR)_6^{\equiv}$, where OR is ionized phenol (46). The color may be destroyed by the addition of acids or bases (61).

All three compounds, glycinate, residual hippurate, and benzoate, are precipitated by reagent; however, ferric glycinate and ferric hippurate precipitates are more readily soluble and will redissolve after shaking or in an excess of ferric chloride (2, 13, 19, 25, 34, 43), leaving ferric benzoate as sole precipitate (33). Ferric benzoate separates from water as either a liquid layer or, in this case, an insoluble precipitate (48) that is permanent (2, 13, 14, 25, 34). The hydronium ion (H_3O^+) is found in all water solutions of acids.

Overall Reaction

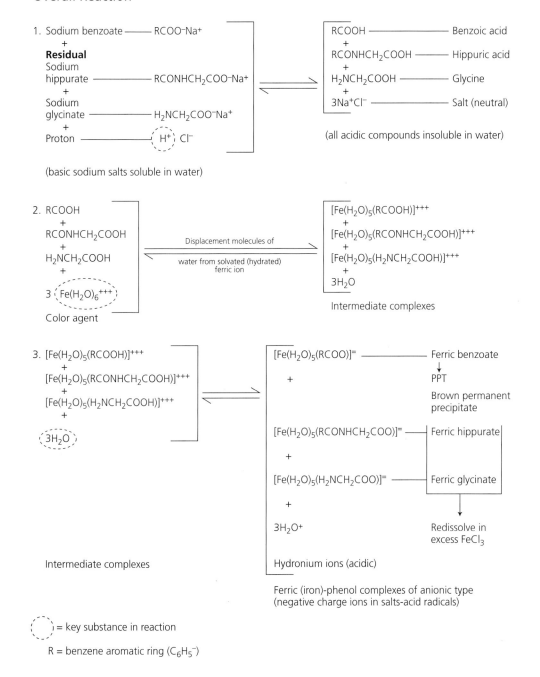

= key substance in reaction

R = benzene aromatic ring ($C_6H_5^-$)

V. MEDIUM EMPLOYED: HIPPURATE (SODIUM) BROTH

A. Ayers and Rupp broth (2); procedure modified by Facklam et al. (18)
B. Benzoic acid detection
C. Ingredients
    1. Basal medium: two choices
        a. Routine: (heart) infusion broth (HIB), pH 7.4 ± 0.2
        b. Growing larger volumes of test organisms: Todd-Hewitt broth (THB); pH 7.8 ± 0.2 (19)

2. Formulation 1

HIB **or** THB	1000 mL
Sodium hippurate (N-benzoylglycine, benzoylaminoacetic acid; $C_6H_5CONHCH^2COONa$), 1%	10.0 g

3. Formulation 2

Beef heart, infusion from	500.0 g
Casein/yeast (50/50) peptone	10.0 g
Sodium chloride, NaCl	5.0 g
Sodium hippurate	10.0 g
Deionized water	1000.0 mL

D. Method of preparation
  1. Weigh out amount accurately as directed on the label. Various company products may vary slightly.
  2. Rehydrate with distilled or deionized water.
  3. Dissolve 10.0 g of sodium hippurate in broth.
  4. Heat **gently** into solution.
  5. Dispense approximately 5.0 mL per screw-cap tube (15 × 125 mm) (18); loosen caps.
E. Method of sterilization: autoclave; 121°C, 15 lb, 15 min
F. Cool and tighten caps **firmly**.
G. **Before use** or **storage**, mark level of medium in each tube with a wax pencil to check later for possible evaporation.
H. Refrigerate for storage (4–10°C)
I. Inoculation
  1. Tube(s) labeled 1, 2, 3, etc.: test organism(s)
     a. Growth from an 18- to 24-h pure culture of confirmed β-hemolytic *Streptococcus*
     b. **Heavy** inoculum; 1–2 drops (18)
     c. To save time, Facklam et al. (18) suggest inoculating with 1–2 isolated colonies from original isolation plate.
  2. Tube labeled PC: positive control
  3. Tube labeled NC: negative control
J. Incubation–all tubes: 35°C; 48 h (2); 42–66 h (18, 34)
K. **Before** adding reagent, **if necessary,** bring medium level to pencil mark with **sterile** distilled water. The concentration of sodium hippurate **must** be exactly 1%.
L. If culture is densely turbid (cloudy), centrifuge to sediment growth and use clear supernatant fluid for test (18).
M. **Aseptically,** transfer a specific aliquot of culture (or its supernatant) to small test tubes (Wassermann or Kahn).
  1. Test organism(s): 0.8 mL
  2. Five negative controls (NC) per batch organisms being tested in one setup
     a. NC 1: 0.8 mL
     b. NCs 2–5: 1.0 mL
N. Add ferric chloride reagent.
  1. Test for the proper amount of reagent to add (see Section V.C) **before adding reagent to other tubes**.
  2. The appropriate amount of reagent must be added to **all** incubated tubes **before** attempting an interpretation.

Hydrolysis of hippuric is faster in dextrose broth (e.g., Todd-Hewitt) medium during first 24 h of incubation, but after that the results are practically identical (2). The presence of dextrose or beef broth does not interfere with hydrolysis, and 48-h incubation is sufficient (2). The influence of hydrogen ion concentration (pH) on enzyme action (e.g., development of acidity in medium due to benzoic acid production) does not interfere with the hydrolysis of hippurate and need not be considered in connection with tests for this reaction (2). Ayers and Rupp (2) also showed that if a medium is suitable for good growth of a *Streptococcus* capable of splitting hippurate, its composition or reaction has no effect on the hydrolysis. Beef infusion (peptone) medium requires a longer time to become clear when hippurate has not been hydrolyzed (2). The disadvantage of (heart) infusion broth is the prolonged incubation period of 42–66 h (6).

VI. QUALITY CONTROL MICROORGANISMS

A. Positive (+)

Streptococcus agalactiae	ATCC 27956
Campylobacter jejuni	ATCC 33560

B. Negative (−)

Streptococcus salivarius	ATCC 13419
Campylobacter coli	ATCC 33559
Uninoculated	

VII. RESULTS

> See Figures 14.1 and 14.2 (Appendix 1) for photographic results

VIII. INTERPRETATION

A. Positive (+)
  1. Brown, flocculant, insoluble precipitate (ppt) persisting on shaking **after** 10 min (2, 18, 19, 21, 25)
     a. Heavy; well marked when one fifth or more of hippurate has been split (2)
     b. Cloudy (turbid) when less than one fifth of hippurate split (2)
  2. Permanent precipitate ferric benzoate complex (38)
  3. Hippurate hydrolyzed (19); report "presumptive group B *Streptococcus* by hippurate hydrolysis" (38).
B. Negative (−)
  1. Precipitate, if any, dissolves on shaking.
     a. Initial precipitate clears **within** 10 min (18). If solution clears within 10 min, reaction is nonspecific because of interaction with **un**hydrolyzed hippurate or with the protein in the medium (38).
     b. There may be slight turbidity (cloudiness) or opalescence; clear amber (orange) color (2, 19).
  2. Hippurate **not** hydrolyzed.

IX. RAPID TESTS: DETECTION OF GLYCINE END PRODUCT

A. **Procedure of Hwang and Ederer** (34)
  1. Substrate
     a. 1% Aqueous sodium hippurate solution

Sodium hippurate	1.0 g
Distilled or deionized water	100.0 mL

b. Dispense approximately 0.4 mL per **sterile** tube; may use screw-cap tubes (15 × 125 mm). For convenience, tubes may be prepared ahead of time and stored at −20°C (3).
c. Tighten down caps or cork **tightly**.
d. Storage: refrigeration; **freeze;** −20°C. Thaw before use. Hippurate solution deteriorates within 7 days at 4°C and **must** remain frozen when not in use (49).
2. Ninhydrin solution
   a. Ninhydrin, 3.5 g in 100 mL of a 1:1 mixture of acetone and butanol (butyl alcohol) (4)
   b. Mix acetone and butanol together and then add ninhydrin (4).
   c. Store in a **tightly sealed** brown bottle at room temperature (22–25°C); shelf life maximum of 6 months.
3. Inoculation
   a. **Heavy** inoculum; a large loopful of **pure** culture β-hemolytic *Streptococcus* spp.
   b. Growth from tryptic soy agar (TSB) with 5% sheep blood or other suitable medium such as 5% sheep blood agar (SBA)
   c. Emulsify inoculum into test medium; the suspension should be cloudy.
4. Incubation
   a. Heating block (temperature block) or water bath; 37°C; 2 h
   b. With a pipette, add 0.2 mL (5 drops) of ninhydrin reagent; add ninhydrin **slowly** down the side of tube **to form an overlay**.
   c. **Do not shake tubes**.
   d. Continue incubation in heating block or water bath 10 min.
   e. Remove from heat; **do not incubate longer than 30 min** as false positives could result.
   f. **Immediately** record results.
5. Interpretation
   a. Positive (+)
      (1) Deep purple-blue (crystal violet) color within 10 min **after** addition of ninhydrin reagent
      (2) Hippurate hydrolyzed
   b. Negative (−)
      (1) No color change; the medium remains colorless or occasionally has a faint tinge of purple.
      (2) Hippurate not hydrolyzed

Test results correlated well with those from the test of Facklam et al. (18). Ninhydrin can be used because the substrate contains only aqueous sodium hippurate, which does not react with ninhydrin, and because only one of the products, glycine, is an amino acid (34).

6. Chemistry of reagent reaction: ninhydrin, $C_6H_4(CO)_3 \cdot H_2O$ (51), is a strong oxidizing agent (4, 33) that evokes oxidative deamination of O-amino group (43); the α-carbon is the carbon next to the functional group.

$$(R \;\text{—}\; \underset{H}{\overset{NH_2}{C}} \;\text{—}\; COOH).$$

Testing with ninhydrin for the presence of end product glycine, involves a two-step process initially in which an amino group is removed: (*a*) hydrogen is removed, yielding an imino acid, and eventually combines with oxygen (from ninhydrin) to form water and (*b*) the imino acid is hydrolyzed to a keto acid and ammonia. The ammonia does not accumulate but is transformed (48) in sequential steps, producing color.

Ninhydrin is positive for all free groups, whether in amino acids, peptides, or proteins (11). In the case of a free amino acid that possesses a free carboxyl group (COOH) adjacent to the amino group, further reaction causes decarboxylation of the imino acid to carbon dioxide and the next lower aldehyde, ammonia, and color reaction (11). The decarboxylating ninhydrin reaction is positive for peptides and proteins (11). One of the products of hydrolysis, serine, can be deaminated by ninhydrin, which is reduced to a purple product in the process (20).

The ninhydrin reaction is based on (a) measurement of CO_2, (b) determination of NH_3 present, and (c) color change (51). In hippurate hydrolysis only color development is used to denote a positive reaction, although the other means of determination can be used to identify glycine. An aldehyde, NH_3, CO_2, and reduced ninhydrin are released during oxidation. NH_3 reacts with residual ninhydrin and reduced ninhydrin, hydrindantin, to form a purple reaction product (33).

Reaction Steps (11, 26, 43, 48)

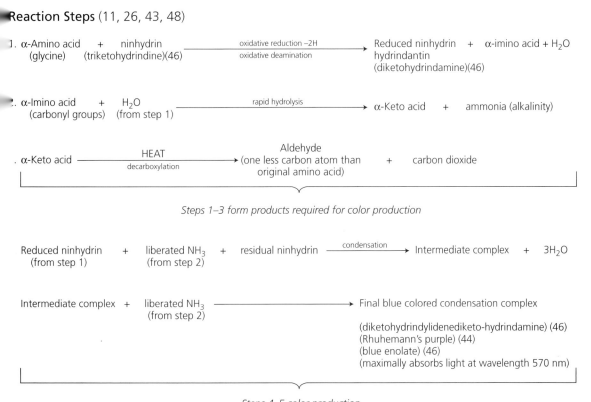

Overall Reaction

[Reaction scheme showing ninhydrin reaction with α-amino acid]

- Free carboxyl group
- Free amino group

R—CH—COOH → *[R—CH—COOH] →(rapid hydrolysis)→ R—C—COOH →(HEAT, decarboxylation)→ R—CHO
  | | ‖
  NH_2 NH   O

α-Amino acid   α-Imino acid   α-Keto acid   Aldehyde

oxidative deamination / oxidative reduction → H_2O

Ninhydrin → Partially reduced form ninhydrin-hydrindantin + Ammonia + Residual ninhydrin

condensation → $3H_2O$

Final color complex (deep purple-blue color) ←(NH_3)— Intermediate color complex

*[R—C—COOH] not actually isolated as an intermediate.
   ‖
   NH

(Redrawn and modified from Harper, H. A., Rodwell, V. W., and Mayes, R. A. *Review of Physiological Chemistry*, 16th ed., 1977, p. 26, with permission of Lange Medical Publications, Los Altos, Calif.)

Gas liquid chromatography (GLC) (37) is more reproducible than conventional tube methods for determination of hippurate hydrolysis in *Campylobacter* spp. (47). According to Morris et al. (47), tubes are satisfactory for routine use; however, GLC method is recommended when tube tests give questionable results.

Thin layer chromatography (TLC) may be used to evaluate hippurate hydrolase activity (52) or to confirm doubtful results of glycine liberation (59). The advantage of TLC is its ability to determine the products glycine or benzoic acid semiquantitatively (52, 59).

B. **Hippurate disk** (41, 46, 56)
   1. Manufacturer: REMEL (see Appendix 11); follow manufacturer's directions.
   2. Test to distinguish *C. jejuni* (+) from *C. coli* (−) and *C. laridis* (−).
   3. Results within 3 h
   4. Positive results based on presence of a blue color irrespective of its intensity (10). Sensitivity 95% and specificity 94%
C. **MA hippurate hydrolysis test;** test using reagents rhodamine B and uranium acetate as color developers. Not a routine procedure (see 2nd edition for procedure).

X. PRECAUTIONS

A. **General**
   1. If either $FeCl_3$ or ninhydrin reagents are used, positive and negative controls **must** be run along with the test organisms; if uninoculated medium is used for a negative control, the tube **must be incubated** (6) along with the test organisms to simulate the same environment.
   2. Bovine group B *S. agalactiae,* a common cause of bovine mastitis (19), is found in udders of cows and hence in milk from such animals (2). Group B streptococci are normally present in the vagina of the female genital tract (7) but have been isolated from various body sites and fluids (19), e.g., in normal throats of humans (2, 7). Group B streptococci are frequently incriminated in severe infections (34) and are significant human pathogens (7, 45, 63) causing maternal septicemia and meningitis and pneumonia in neonates and infants (34). Braunstein et al. (7) showed that the organism was a potential urinary tract pathogen, the cause of skin infections, and (almost exclusively in females) pharyngitis. Bovine strains split hippurate, but none of the human types possess this ability, and hippurate hydrolysis assists in properly placing the bovine culture found in normal throats (2).
   3. Hippurate hydrolysis is used for identification within the genus *Streptococcus;* however, this enzymatic ability is also found among some species of other genera:

   Aerococcus viridans, 100% positive hydrolysis (18)
   Bacillus spp. (14)
   Beneckea spp. (5)
   Corynebacterium spp. (8)
   Enterobacteriaceae (59)
   Listeria spp. (4, 18)
   Mycobacterium and *Nocardia* (22, 23)
   Pediococcus spp. (62)
   Pseudomonas spp. (35)
   Staphylococcus spp., usually positive; may vary among strains (35)
   Streptomyces spp. (64)

   Among these genera the **only** ones of concern when performing hippurate hydrolysis are the catalase-negative Gram-positive cocci: *Streptococcus, Enterococcus, Aerococcus, Leuconostoc, Lactococcus, Pediococcus,* and *Gemella;* other genera are catalase-positive and/or Gram-positive or Gram-negative bacilli except *Staphylococcus* spp. which are Gram-positive, catalase-positive cocci. *Aerococcus* spp. are Gram-positive cocci arranged in tetrads that produce large zones of α-hemolysis on sheep blood agar (SBA); *Pediococcus* spp. are plant saprophytes (9) and are not likely to be involved in human infections.
   4. The test should **not** be applied indiscriminately to all groups of streptococci; it is useful only in relation to β-hemolytic streptococci of human or bovine origin (2). When β-hemolysis is the criterion for performing hippurate hydrolysis, one is concerned pri-

marily with differentiating group B β-hemolytic streptococci from groups A and D β-hemolytic streptococci and group D enterococci.

A β-hemolytic organism **must** be identified as a member of the genus *Streptococcus* **before** being tested for hippurate hydrolysis by first performing the catalase test and doing a Gram morphology. All *Streptococcus* spp. are catalase-negative, Gram-positive cocci arranged in chains, pairs, or singly.

Hippurate hydrolysis is used to **aid** in the identification of group B streptococci (18). Hwang and Ederer (34) consider this test the best means of identifying β-hemolytic group B streptococci. No single test should be relied upon for **presumptive** identification of group B human or bovine organisms; many microbiologists (7, 18) recommend using positive hippurate reaction **in combination with other tests.** Serologic testing is the **only** way to confirm group B identification.

Facklam et al. (18) recommend clinical diagnosis and culture source along with hydrolysis. Braunstein et al. (7) recommend preliminary group B identification by correlating the source with colony morphology on sheep blood agar followed by two confirmatory tests: (*a*) bacitracin disks to rule out group A β-streptococci, and (*b*) hippurate hydrolysis to verify the presence of group B organisms. Susceptibility to bacitracin is used to distinguish group A from non–group A, β-hemolytic streptococci along with immunofluorescent studies (61) and to differentiate group A, β-hemolytic group from β-hemolytic streptococci not group A (7, 18). Group B organisms are often confused with group A organisms, especially if they are grown from throat cultures (7). Probably, *S. agalactiae* in throat cultures is occasionally assigned incorrectly to group D (assumed insignificant) or group A (different significance) when incomplete studies are done (7). Group B streptococci are also often confused with other bacteria, especially those in group D, if growth in *Streptococcus faecalis* (SF) broth is the sole criterion (7).

β-Hemolytic streptococci that hydrolyze hippurate are in either group B or group D; they can be differentiated by bile esculin hydrolysis (18, 34) (group B, negative; group D, 99% positive (18)) for **presumptive** identification of this organism (34). Facklam et al. (18) showed that no group A streptococci hydrolyzed hippurate, 96% of group B hydrolyzed hippurate, and 6.9% of group D enterococci hydrolyzed hippurate. Both human and bovine streptococci exhibit β-hemolysis (clear zone), but the human type shows larger hemolytic zones around colonies on blood agar plates after 24 h incubation (2); group B zones are relatively narrow (small) and hazy (7).

5. Hippurate hydrolysis is **not** limited to β-hemolytic types (2); some α types from cow udder **do not** produce hydrolysis, while hydrolyzing is a common property among α and γ lactic-type streptococci (2). Nonhemolytic group B streptococci have been isolated from humans. Many *Enterococcus* spp. can hydrolyze hippurate (7, 9, 18, 58), and Facklam et al. (18) showed that a small percentage (6.9%) of group D enterococci are β-hemolytic, with no one species hydrolyzing more often than another and no correlation of hemolysis with hippurate hydrolysis among these strains. Other streptococci that may hydrolyze hippurate and are α- or γ-hemolytic are *S. acidominimus* and *S. uberis*, viridans streptococci that are rarely found in specimens from human infections (7, 18). Another species not β-hemolytic that is isolated from humans and variable for hydrolysis is *S. dysgalactiae* (Table 14.1).

Table 14.1. *Streptococcus/Enterococcus/Lactococcus* Positive/Variable for Hippurate Hydrolysis

	Lancefield Group	Hemolysis, 5% Sheep Blood Agar	Hippurate Hydrolysis
S. agalactiae[a]	B	α, β, γ	+
S. dysgalactiae	C	α, γ	V−
S. bovis	D	α, γ	V
E. faecalis[b]	D	α, β, γ	+
L. lactis[c]	N	α, γ	V
S. acidominimus[d]	Non-groupable	α	+
S. uberis	Non-groupable	α, γ	V

Data from reference 9.
V, variable; V−, variable, usually −.
[a]Glycerol fermentation (aerobically) +; arginine hydrolysis +.
[b]Formerly *Streptococcus faecalis*.
[c]Formerly *Streptococcus lactis* (55).
[d]Glycerol fermentation −, arginine hydrolysis −, slow hippurate hydrolysis.

6. Hippurate solution deteriorates in 7 days at 4°C and **must** remain frozen when not in use (49).
7. Since the concentration of sodium hippurate broth affects test results, hippurate media should be tightly sealed to prevent evaporation during storage (33).

B. **Ferric chloride procedure**
1. This test requires adding reagents to cultures, which rules out repeated tests on the same culture (59) unless aliquots are **aseptically** removed for testing.
2. If the culture is densely turbid, centrifuge to sediment growth and use clear supernatant fluid for testing (18); heavy turbidity could result in a false-positive precipitate that would not clear in the allotted 10–15 min.
3. When beef infusion (peptone) medium is used, a longer time is required for the medium to clear when hippurate has **not** been hydrolyzed (2).
4. After addition of $FeCl_3$ reagent, tubes must be shaken before interpreting results, because both shaking and excess $FeCl_3$ help **redissolve** soluble hippurate and glycinate precipitates to give negative results. Failure to shake the tubes could give false-positive results if hippurate is not hydrolyzed.
5. The ferric chloride procedure requires an extended period of incubation, centrifugation, and determination of a somewhat equivocal end point (16); this is a long process when rapid results are desired. Appropriate amount of ferric chloride needed to reach an excess of ferric ions varies with the amount of hippurate medium being tested and the concentration of sodium hippurate in the medium (33). A delicate balance exists between volume ratio of $FeCl_3$ reagent and cell-free supernatant needed to obtain accurate results; adequate positive and negative controls **must** be used to ensure an excess of ferric ions during testing (33).
6. If the medium contains phosphates it is necessary to use an acidic (HCl) $FeCl_3$ solution to redissolve the iron phosphate formed (2), which could result in a false-positive precipitate.
7. Beef infusion peptone medium requires using a **12%** concentration of **acidic** $FeCl_3$ solution, **no less** (2).
8. To control the constancy of constituents of the medium with added hippurate, tubes **must be tightly sealed after sterilization** to prevent evaporation of water from broth (6); considerable error occurs if the hippurate concentration has varied appreciably for any reason (21). If evaporation occurs and hippurate concentration is below 1% before reagent is added, a false-positive reaction may occur. Therefore, **before use or storage,**

mark the level of medium in **each tube,** and **before** reagent is added, bring the level to mark, if necessary, with distilled water. Tightly capped tubes and a proper fluid level before use balance the quantity of medium spent and the amount of reagent to give a more carefully controlled test (6).

9. The test depends on relative solubilities of ferric benzoate and ferric hippurate; the final iron concentration is critical and titration of broth culture fluid and reagent is required (13) **before** any reagent is added to the test organism(s).
10. Place the reagent solution in brown stoppered bottles and store in a dark place to avoid exposure to light. Excessive light causes deterioration, and false-negative results may occur. Perform quality control checks weekly, and discard if solution is negative or weakly reactive with a known positive control.
11. The colored precipitate may be destroyed by addition of acids or bases (61).
12. Concentrated HCl is extremely caustic, so when preparing acidified reagent avoid exposure to skin, as painful burns may occur. If the acid does contact skin, **immediately** flood the area with water. **Do not pipette acid by mouth;** use a Pro pipette and always run the concentrated acid slowly down the side of the flask when adding to water, and discard pipette in appropriate container.

C. **Ninhydrin procedure**
1. **Do not** incubate the tubes in heating block longer than 30 min, as false positive results could occur (34).
2. The procedure is limited by **not** having growth capabilities and in requiring a nonprotein milieu (environment) (16). Since most growth media contain protein and free amino acids, ninhydrin **cannot** be used to test for hippurate hydrolysis in protein-containing growth media (34). **Test** must contain **only** hippurate, since ninhydrin might react with any free amino acids in growth medium or other broths (4).
3. Reaction time longer than 10 min will give **un**wanted positive results with group D streptococci or enterococci. However, 6.5% salt and bile esculin tests and, in most instances, hemolysis, will preclude misidentification of these microorganisms as group B streptococci (48).

REFERENCES

1. Allinger NL, Cava MP, DeJongh DC, et al. Organic Chemistry, ed 2. New York: McGraw-Hill, 1936:236.
2. Ayers SH, Rupp P. Differentiation of hemolytic streptococci from human and bovine sources by the hydrolysis of sodium hippurate. J Infect Dis 1922;30:388–399.
3. Balows A, Hausler WJ Jr, Herrmann KL, et al. Manual of Clinical Microbiology, ed 5. Washington, DC: American Society for Microbiology, 1991:305.
4. Baron EJ, Finegold SM. Bailey & Scott's Diagnostic Microbiology, ed 8. Philadelphia: CV Mosby, 1990:109, 112.
5. Baumann P, Baumann L, Mandel M. Taxonomy of marine bacteria: The genus *Beneckea*. J Bacteriol 1971;107(1):268–294.
6. Blazevic DJ, Ederer GM. Principles of Biochemical Tests in Diagnostic Microbiology. New York: John Wiley & Sons, 1975:53–58.
7. Braunstein H, Tucker EB, Gibson CB. Identification and significance of *Streptococcus agalactiae* (Lancefield group B). Am J Clin Pathol 1969;51(2):207–213.
8. Brooks RF, Hucker GJ. A study of certain members of the genus *Corynebacterium*. J Bacteriol 1944;48(3):295–312.
9. Buchanan RE, Gibbons NE, eds. Bergey's Manual of Determinative Bacteriology, ed 8. Baltimore: Williams & Wilkins, 1974.
10. Cacho JB, Aguirre PM, Hernanz A, Velasco AC. Evaluation of a disk method for detection of hippurate hydrolysis by *Campylobacter* spp. J Clin Microbiol 1989;27(2):359–360.
11. Cantarow A, Schepartz B. Biochemistry, ed 3. Philadelphia: WB Saunders, 1962:90–91.
12. Cowan ST. Biochemical test for bacterial characterization. I. Hippurate test. Int Bull Bacteriol Nomencl Taxon 1955;5(3):97–104.
13. Cowan ST. Cowan & Steel's Manual for the Identification of Medical Bacteria, ed 2. Cambridge: Cambridge University Press, 1974:36,174.
14. Davis GHG. The classification of lactobacilli from the human mouth. J Gen Microbiol 1955;13(3):481–493.
15. Desha LJ. Organic Chemistry. New York: McGraw-Hill, 1936:416–418, 423, 548–549.
16. Edberg SC, Samuels S. Rapid colorimetric test

for the determination of hippurate hydrolysis of group B *Streptococcus*. J Clin Microbiol 1976;3(1):49–50.
17. Ellis S, Walker BS. The action of hippuricase on ring substituted derivatives of hippuric acid. J Biol Chem 1942;142(1):291–298.
18. Facklam RR, Padula JF, Thacker LG, et al. Presumptive identification of group A, B, and D streptococci. Appl Micro biol 1974;27(1):107–113.
19. Ferrieri P, Wannamaker LW, Nelson J. Localization and characterization of the hippuricase activity of group B streptococci. Infect Immun 1973;7(5):747–752.
20. Finegold SM, Baron EJ. Bailey and Scott's Diagnostic Microbiology, ed 7. St. Louis: CV Mosby, 1986:377–378.
21. Gilbert I, Frobisher M Jr. The hydrolysis of sodium hippurate by various bacteria. Bull John Hopkins Hosp 1930;47:55–60.
22. Gordon RE. Some strains in search of a genus: *Corynebacterium, Mycobacterium, Nocardia* or what? J Gen Microbiol 1966;43(3):329–343.
23. Gordon RE, Hoan AC. A piecemeal description of *Streptomyces griseus* (Krainsky) Waksam and Henriei. J Gen Microbiol 1968;50(2):223–233.
24. Greenwood JR, Pickett MJ. Transfer of *Haemophilus vaginalis* Gardner and Dukes to a new genus *Gardnerella: G. vaginalis* (Gardner and Dukes) comb. nov. Int J Syst Bacteriol 1980;30(1):170–178.
25. Hajna AA, Damon SR. Differentiation of A. *aerogenes* and A. *cloacae* on basis of hydrolysis of sodium hippurate. Am J Epidemiol 1934;19:545–548.
26. Harper HA, Rodwell VW, Mayes PA. Review of Physiological Chemistry, ed 16. Los Altos, CA: Lange Medical Publications, 1977:10, 25–26.
27. Hart H, Schuetz RD. A Short Course in Organic Chemistry, ed 2. Boston: Houghton Mifflin, 1959:175–176.
28. Harvey SM, Greenwood JR. Relationships among catalase-positive camylobacters determined by deoxyribonucleic acid-deoxyribonucleic acid hybridization. Int J Syst Bacteriol 1983;33(2):275–284.
29. Hébert GA. Hippurate hydrolysis by *Legionella pneumophila*. J Clin Microbiol 1981;13(1):240–242.
30. Hébert GA, Edmonds P, Brenner DJ. DNA relatedness among strains of *Campylobacter jejuni* and *Campylobacter coli* with divergent serogroup and hippurate reactions. J Clin Microbiol 1984;20(1):138–140.
31. Henry RJ. Clinical Chemistry: Principles and Technics. New York: Hoeber Medical Division, Harper & Row, 1968:540.
32. Holum JR. Elements of General and Biological Chemistry, ed 4. New York: John Wiley & Sons, 1975:294.
33. Howard BJ, Klaas J II, Rubin SJ, et al. Clinical and Pathogenic Microbiology. St. Louis: CV Mosby, 1987:874.
34. Hwang M, Ederer GM. Rapid hippurate hydrolysis method for presumptive identification of group B streptococci. J Clin Microbiol 1975;1(1):114–115.
35. Kameda Y, Kuramotat T, Matsui K, Ebara T. Studies on acylase activity and microorganisms. XXV. Purification and properties of benzoylamino acid amidohydrolase in KT 801 (*Pseudomonas* sp.). Chem Pharm Bull (Tokyo) 1968;16(6):1023–1029.
36. Kasper G, Dickgiesser N. Isolation from gastric epithelium of *Campylobacter*-like bacteria that are distinct from *Campylobacter pyloridis*.Lancet 1985;1:111–112.
37. Kodaka H, Lombard GL, Dowell VR Jr. Gas-liquid chromatography technique for detection of hippurate hydrolysis and conversion of fumarate to succinate by microorganisms. J Clin Microbiol 1982;16(5):962–964.
38. Koneman EW, Allen SD, Janda WM, et al. Color Atlas and Textbook of Diagnostic Microbiology, ed 4. Philadelphia: JB Lippincott, 1992:250–251, 343, 362, 449.
39. Lethardt F. Hippuricase (histozyme). In: Summer JB, Myrback K, eds. The Enzymes: Chemistry and Mechanisms of Action, vol 1. New York: Academic Press, 1951:951–955.
40. Lewis JR. College Chemistry, ed 9. New York: Barnes & Noble, 1971:60–63, 109, 297.
41. Lien EA, Hillier SL. Evaluation of the enhanced rapid identification method for *Gardnerella vaginalis*. J Clin Microbiol 1989;27(3):566–567.
42. Luechtefeld NW, Wang W-LL. Hippurate hydrolysis by and triphenyltetrazolium tolerance of *Campylobacter fetus*. J Clin Microbiol 1982;15(1):137–140.
43. Mahler HR, Cordes EH. Biological Chemistry. New York: Harper & Row, 1966:54.
44. Mallette FM, Clagett CO, Phillips AT, McCarl RL. Introductory Biochemistry. Baltimore: Williams & Wilkins, 1971:388–389.
45. McCracken GH. Group B streptococci: The new challenge in neonatal infections. J Pediatr 1973;82(4):703–706.
46. McGilvery RW. Biochemistry. Philadelphia: WB Saunders, 1970:147–149, 700–701.
47. Morris GK, El Sherbeeny MR, Patton CM, et al. Comparison of four hippurate hydrolysis methods for identification of thermophilic *Campylobacter* spp. J Clin Microbiol 1985;22(5):714–718.
48. Nussenbaum S. Organic Chemistry. Boston: Allyn & Bacon, 1963:296–297, 334, 346–347, 395–397, 431–432, 441, 445, 454, 575, 597.
49. Oberhofer TR. Manual of Practical Medical Microbiology and Parasitology. New York: John Wiley & Sons, 1985:187.
50. On SLW, Holmes B. Assessment of enzyme detection tests useful in identification of campylobacteria. J Clin Microbiol 1992;30(3):746–749.
51. Oser BL, ed. Hawk's Physiological Chemistry, ed 14. New York: McGraw-Hill, 1965:139.

52. Ottow JCG. Detection of hippurate hydrolase among *Bacillus* species by thin layer chromatography and other methods. J Appl Bacteriol 1974;37(1):15–30.
53. Pauling L. General Chemistry, ed 2. San Francisco: WH Freeman, 1953:542.
54. Rischka W, Roehr M. Induced biosynthesis of hippurate hydrolysis in *Streptococcus durans*. Zentralb Bakteriol Parasitenk Infektionskr Hyg Abt 2 1972;127(3):222–226.
55. Roop II RM, Smibert RM, Johnson JL, Krieg NR. Differential characteristics of catalase-positive campylobacters correlated with DNA homology groups. Can J Microbiol 1984;30(7):938–951.
56. Skirrow MB, Benjamin J. Differentiation of enteropathogenic *Campylobacter*. J Clin Pathol 1980;33(11):1122.
57. Soloway S, Wilen SH. Improved ferric chloride test for phenols. Anal Chem 1952;24(6):979–983.
58. Swift HF. The streptococci. In: Dubos R. Bacterial and Mycotic Infections of Man. Philadelphia: JB Lippincott, 1948:237–294.
59. Thirst ML. Hippurate hydrolysis in *Klebsiella-Cloaca* classification. J Gen Microbiol 1957;17(2):390–395.
60. Walder M, Sandstedt K, Ursing J. Phenotypic characteristics of thermotolerant *Campylobacter* from humans and animal sources. Curr Microbiol 1983;9:291–296.
61. Wesp EF, Brode WR. The absorption spectra of ferric compounds. I. The ferric chloride-phenol reaction. J Am Chem Soc 1934;56(5):1037–1042.
62. Whittenbury R. A study of some pediococci and their relationship to *Aerococcus viridans* and the enterococci. J Gen Microbiol 1965;40(1):97–106.
63. Wilkinson HW, Facklam RR, Wortham EC. Distribution by serological type of group B streptococci isolated from a variety of clinical material over a five-year period (with special reference to neonatal sepsis meningitis). Infect Immun 1973;8(2):228–235.
64. Ziegler P, Kutzner HJ. Hippurate hydrolysis as a taxonomic criterion in the genus *Streptomyces* (order *Actinomycetales*). Z Allg Mikrobiol 1973;13(3):265–272.

15 Hydrogen Sulfide Test

I. PRINCIPLE

To determine whether hydrogen sulfide (H_2S) gas has been liberated enzymatically from sulfur-bearing amino acids to produce a visible, black color reaction in the presence of an H_2S indicator system

II. PURPOSE

(Also see Chapters 43 and 45)

A. To aid in species differentiation
  1. *Proteus mirabilis* (+), *P. penneri* (+), and *P. vulgaris* (+) from other *Proteus* spp.(−)
  2. Triple sugar iron agar (TSI): *Erysipelothrix rhusiopathiae* (+) (2) from *Corynebacterium* spp. (−) and *Listeria monocytogenes* (−)
  3. TSI: *Campylobacter coli* (+), *C. concisus* (+), *C. hyointestinalis* (+), *C. mucosalis* (+), *C. sputorum* biovar *bubulus* (+), and *C. sputorum* biovar *sputorum* (variable, usually positive; V$^+$) (25)
  4. *Microbacterium arborescens* (+) and *M. laevaniformis* (+) from *M. imperiale* (−) and *M. lacticum* (−)
  5. *Sphingomonas paucimobilis* (+) from *S. parapaucimobilis* (−)
  6. *Selenomonas ruminatium* (+) from other *Selenomonas spp.* (−) most frequently isolated
  7. *Vagococcus salmoninarum* (+) from *V. fluvialis* (−)
  8. *Aeromonas hydrophila* (+), *A. salmonicida* subsp. *masoucida* (+), and *A. salmonicida* subsp. *smithia* (+) from other *Aeromonas* spp. (−) most frequently isolated
B. To aid in identifying
  1. Enterobacteriaceae: *Budvicia aquatica* (V, usually +); *Citrobacter freundii* (V, usually +); *Edwardsiella tarda* (+); *Salmonella* (usually +); *Proteus mirabilis, P. penneri,* and *P. vulgatis* (V, usually +); *Leminorella* spp. (+); *Morganella morganii* biogroup 2 (V); and *Pragia fontium* (V, usually +)
  2. *Shewanella putrefaciens* (+) (27) (formerly *Alteromans putrefaciens*); **only** nonfermenter that produces H_2S on Kligler's iron agar (KIA)/TSI (25)
  3. TSI: *Arcobacter nitrofigilis* (+) (formerly *Campylobacter nitrofigilis*) (48)
  4. *Wolinella succinogenes* (+)

III. BIOCHEMISTRY INVOLVED

The proteolysis of proteins yields individual amino acids; certain heterotrophic bacteria can enzymatically liberate sulfur from the various sulfur-containing (-SH) amino acids, producing H_2S gas (33). Peptone, cysteine, cystine, methionine, and thiosulfate are all sources of sulfur, but different species use different sulfur-containing compounds or amino acids to produce H_2S (7). The enzymes responsible for this activity are cysteine desulfhydrase (14, 31, 36) (formerly called cysteinase (14)), and thiosulfate reductase (31).

The sulfur (-SH)-containing amino acids are (18)

$$\underset{\text{Methionine}}{\underset{|}{\overset{|}{\underset{S-CH_3}{\underset{|}{\overset{|}{\underset{(CH_2)_2}{H_2N-CH\cdot COOH}}}}}}} \qquad \underset{\text{Cystine}}{\overset{H_2N-CH\cdot COOH}{\underset{CH_2-S\cdot S-CH_2}{|}}\overset{H_2N-CH\cdot COOH}{|}}$$

Cystine $\xrightarrow{+2H}$ A reduction product of cystine (5,14)

$$\underset{\text{Cysteine}}{\underset{|}{\overset{|}{\underset{CH_2\cdot SH}{H_2N-CH\cdot COOH}}}}$$

An H_2S-producing organism cultivated in an organic medium such as peptone reduces sulfur by hydrogenation, producing H_2S gas (8, 13).

Anaerobic catabolism of cysteine yields H_2S, pyruvic acid, and ammonia (18, 33).

$$\underset{\text{Cysteine}}{\underset{|}{\overset{|}{\underset{COOH}{\underset{|}{\overset{|}{\underset{CH\cdot NH_2}{CH_2\cdot SH}}}}}}} + H_2O \xrightarrow{\text{Cysteine desulfurase}} \underset{\substack{\text{Pyruvic} \\ \text{acid}}}{\underset{|}{\overset{|}{\underset{COOH}{\underset{|}{\overset{|}{\underset{C=O}{CH_3}}}}}}} + \underset{\substack{\text{Hydrogen} \\ \text{sulfide} \\ \text{gas}}}{H_2S\uparrow} + \underset{\text{Ammonia}}{NH_3}$$

Many peptone iron-containing media are on the market to detect H_2S production among the *Enterobacteriaceae*. The sulfide indicators vary among these media: peptonized iron, ferrous sulfate, ferrous or ferric ammonium sulfate, ferric citrate, sodium thiosulfate, bismuth sulfite, or lead acetate; however, the principle is the same. In one such medium, KIA, the H_2S indicators are a salt, ferric ammonium citrate, and another chemical, sodium thiosulfate. Both indicators **must** be present, since the end result is a two-step procedure.

Step 1

Thiosulfate is an intermediate in the reduction of sulfate to H_2S by sulfate-reducing bacteria (24). The bacterium reacts with sodium thiosulfate in a reduction reaction that yields a sulfite and a sulfate (11). An acid pH and a source of H^+ ions **must** exist in the KIA butt for thiosulfate reduction to occur. Two carbohydrates are present to provide this acidity and increase in H^+ ions (25). This is an anaerobic respiration process in which the sulfur atom serves as the electron acceptor for the oxidation of organic substrates (38). Thiosulfate ($S_2O_3^{2-}$) replaces sulfate as an electron acceptor and is an organism's source of sulfur (11).

$$4H^+ + 4e + \underset{\text{Thiosulfate}}{3S_2O_3^{2-}} \xrightarrow{\substack{\text{thiosulfate} \\ \text{reductase}}} \underset{\text{Sulfite}}{2SO_3^{2-}} + \underset{\substack{\text{Hydrogen} \\ \text{sulfide gas}}}{2H_2S\uparrow}$$

H_2S is a colorless gas; therefore, a second indicator is necessary to visualize H_2S production.

Step 2

The colorless gas H_2S reacts with a heavy iron salt, ferric ammonium citrate, to produce an **insoluble black precipitate**, heavy metal ferrous sulfide. Ferric ammonium citrate is recommended over ferric citrate because it is more soluble. Ferrous sulfate may be substituted for the ferric salt. H₂S production is detected when the gas comes in contact with certain metals, lead, iron, or bismuth, and forms sulfides of these metals.

$$\text{Hydrogen sulfide gas} + \text{ferric ions} \longrightarrow \text{Ferrous sulfide} \downarrow \text{ (black precipitate)}$$

Overall Reaction

$$\text{Bacterium (acid environment)} + \text{sodium thiosulfate} \longrightarrow H_2S \text{ gas} \uparrow \quad (1)$$

$$H_2S + \text{ferric ions} \longrightarrow \text{Ferrous sulfide} \downarrow \text{ (insoluble black precipitate)} \quad (2)$$

H₂S gas, therefore, can be produced either by reduction of an inorganic sulfur source such as thiosulfate ($-S_2O_3$) or reduction of organic sulfur supplied by the R_1-SH functional group of the amino acid cysteine, which is present in peptone (32).

Lead acetate, $Pb(C_2H_3O_2)_2 \cdot 3H_2O$ (PbAc), the salt of the metal, is also an indicator of H₂S production. Upon contact with PbAc, H₂S produces lead sulfide, a black precipitate, in a visible black color reaction. PbAc is extremely sensitive and can detect small quantities of H₂S; a concentration of at least 0.2 mM is required for sulfide detection in a peptone medium (50).

$$Pb(C_2H_3O_2)_2 \cdot 3H_2O + H_2S \longrightarrow PbS\downarrow + H_2O + Ac^-$$

Lead acetate — Hydrogen sulfide gas — Lead sulfide (black precipitate) — Acetate

The ability of an organism to produce H₂S is a consistent characteristic, and an H₂S producer usually produces gas ($CO_2 + H_2$) in carbohydrate media. In determining H₂S production four factors must be considered (7, 25): (a) the type and availability of the sulfur source; (b) the sensitivity of the test for H₂S detection; (c) growth of organism in a basal medium; (d) the presence of the H₂S-producing enzyme system in the organism being tested. Many means of detecting H₂S production exist, but the PbAc procedures are the most sensitive for detecting minute amounts of H₂S in bacteria other than the *Enterobacteriaceae*.

IV. MEDIA EMPLOYED

(Also see Table 15.1)

Table 15.1. Most Commonly Used[a] H$_2$S-Detecting Media

Medium	Purpose	Sulfur Source(s)	H$_2$S Indicator(s)
Bile esculin agar (BEA)	Isol/diff gp d *Streptococcus/ Enterococcus*	Peptone	Ferric ammonium citrate
Bismuth sulfite agar (BSA)	Selective isol *Salmonella*	Peptone & sulfite[b]	Ferrous sulfate
Citrate sulfide agar[c]	Aid diff between genera	Sodium thiosulfate[d]	Ferric ammonium citrate
Deoxycholate citrate agar (DCA)	Isol Gram-neg enterics	Peptone	Ferric citrate
Hektoen enteric (HE) agar	Selective isol/ diff *Salmonella/ Shigella*	Sodium thiosulfate	Ferric ammonium citrate
Kligler iron agar (KIA)	Aid id Gram-neg enterics	Sodium thiosulfate	Ferrous sulfate or ferric ammonium citrate
Lead acetate (PbAc) strips	Bacteria that exhibit small amts of H$_2$S	Sodium thiosulfate	Lead acetate
Lysine iron agar (LIA)	Aid id Gram-neg enterics	Sodium thiosulfate	Ferric ammonium citrate
Peptone iron agar	Aid id Gram-neg enterics	Sodium thiosulfate	Ferric ammonium citrate
Salmonella-Shigella agar (SS)	Selective isol *Salmonella/ Shigella*	Sodium thiosulfate	Ferric citrate
Sulfide-indole-motility (SIM)	Aid id Gram-neg enterics	Sodium thiosulfate	Peptonized iron, ferrous ammonium sulfate
Thiosulfate citrate-bile sucrose agar (TCBS)	Selective isol/ diff vibrios	Peptone, sodium thiosulfate	Ferric citrate
Triple sugar iron agar (TSI)	Aid id Gram-neg enterics	Sodium thiosulfate	Ferrous sulfate, ferrous ammonium sulfate
Xylose lysine desoxy-cholate agar (XLD)	Isol/diff *Salmonella/ Shigella*	Sodium thiosulfate	Ferric ammonium citrate

Data from references 2 and 25.

[a]H$_2$S-detecting media **not** routinely used are Tergitol 7 (T7) agar/broth, Tinsdale agar, *Vibrio parahaemolyticus* (VP) agar, Lombard-Dowell esculin agar, motility sulfide medium, cooked (choppped) meat (CM) medium, Rimler-Shotts (RS) medium, oleandomycin-polymyxin-sulphadiazine-perfringens agar (OPSP), and Önöz *Salmonella* agar.

[b]In the presence of glucose fermentation, sulfite (e.g., bismuth sulfite) is reduced with production of iron sulfide.

[c]Christensen's citrate medium **only**; optional additives.

[d]Sodium thiosulfate is an inorganic compound added to a medium as a supplement.

A. Most commonly used commercial media containing sulfur amino acids
   1. **H$_2$S detection of the *Enterobacteriaceae***
      a. **Kligler's iron agar (KIA)** (see Chapter 18, Kligler Iron Agar)
      b. **Triple sugar iron agar (TSI)** (see Chapter 18, Kligler Iron Agar/Triple Sugar Iron Agar)
      c. **Bismuth sulfite agar (BSA)**
         (1) Formulation of Wilson and Blair (49); modified by Hajna (16) and Hajna and Damon (17)
         (2) Ingredients, pH 7.5 ± 0.2

Casein/meat (50/50) peptone	10.0 g
Beef (meat) extract	5.0 g
Glucose (dextrose)	5.0 g
Disodium phosphate, Na$_2$HPO$_4 \cdot$ 12H$_2$O	4.0 g
Ferrous sulfate, FeSO$_4 \cdot$ 7H$_2$O	0.3 g

Bismuth sulfite, $Bi_2(SO_3)_3$	8.0 g
Brilliant green	0.025 g
Agar	20.0 g
Deionized water	1000.0 mL

d. **Deoxycholate (sodium deoxycholate) agars** (Table 15.2)

(*Note:* Desoxy-; alternate spelling)

(1) **Deoxycholate agar (DC)**

Casein/meat (50/50) peptone	10.0 g
Lactose	10.0 g
Sodium chloride, NaCl	5.0 g
Dipotassium phosphate, $K_2HPO_4 \cdot 12H_2O$	2.0 g
Ferric citrate, $FeC_6H_5O_7 \cdot 5H_2O$, (or ferric ammonium sulfate, $FeNH_4(SO_4)_2 \cdot 12H_2O$)	1.0 g
Sodium citrate, $Na_3C_6H_5O_7 \cdot 2H_2O$	1.0 g
Sodium deoxycholate, $C_{24}H_{40}O_4Na$	1.0 g
Agar	15.0 g
Neutral red	0.033 g (33 mg)

(Best added as an aqueous 1% solution; add 3.0 mL/L (26))

Deionized water	1000.0 mL

(*Note:* If medium is to be used as streak plates for enteric pathogens, ferric citrate may be omitted; however, then it is best to continue to add 0.1% sodium citrate to clear medium.)

(2) **Deoxycholate citrate agar (DC agar):** Leifson's (26) modification; higher concentration of sodium citrate and sodium deoxycholate
(3) **Deoxycholate lactose agar (DCL):** formulation of Leifson (26); decreased concentration of sodium deoxycholate
(4) **Deoxycholate citrate-lactose-sucrose agar (DCLS):** formulation of Leifson (26)
(5) **Deoxycholate citrate-lactose-sucrose agar (DCLS):** formulation of Hajna and Damon (17)

Table 15.2. Primary Differences Between Various Deoxycholate Base Agars

Ingredient	Concentration (g/L)				
	D	DC	DCL	DCLS	DCLS
Lactose	10.0	10.0	10.0	5.0	7.5
Sucrose				5.0	7.5
Na citrate	1.0	20.0[a]	2.0	6–10.5[a]	10.0[a]
Na deoxycholate	1.0	5.0	0.5[b]	2.5–3.0	10.0
Na thiosulfate				5.0	7.5
pH indicator	NR	NR	NR	NR	BCP
Final pH	7.3	7.3–7.5	7.1	7.2–7.5	7.2

NR, neutral red; BCP, bromcresol purple.
[a]Increased concentration for isolation of enteric pathogens, *Salmonella* and *Shigella* spp.
[b]Decreased concentration for enumeration of coliforms.

e. **Hektoen enteric agar (HE agar, HEA)**
   (1) Modification of King and Metzger (20–22); formulation according to APHA (37) specifications
   (2) Ingredients; pH 7.5–7.6 ± 0.2

Meat peptone	12.0 g
Yeast extract	3.0 g
Lactose	12.0 g
Sucrose	12.0 g
Salicin	2.0 g
Bile salts	9.0 g
Ferric ammonium citrate	1.5 g
(50/50 mixture ferric citrate, $FeC_6H_5O_7 \cdot 5H_2O$ and ammonium citrate, $(NH_4)_3C_6H_5O_7$)	
Sodium thiosulfate, $Na_2S_2O_3 \cdot 5H_2O$	5.0 g
Sodium chloride, NaCl	5.0 g
Acid fuchsin	0.19 g
Bromthymol blue (BTB)	0.065 g
Agar	14.0 g
Deionized water	1000.0 mL

f. **Lysine iron agar (LIA)**
   (1) Formulation of Edwards and Fife (12)
   (2) **Not** a substitute for Møller's decarboxylase medium (2) nor does it replace or substitute for KIA or TSI
   (3) Ingredients, pH 6.7 ± 0.2

Gelatin peptone	5.0 g
Yeast extract	3.0 g
Glucose (dextrose)	1.0 g
l-Lysine · HCl	10.0 g
Ferric ammonium citrate	0.5 g
Sodium thiosulfate, $Na_2S_2O_3 \cdot 5H_2O$	0.04 g
Bromcresol purple (BCP)	0.02 g
Agar	15.0 g
Deionized water	1000.0 mL

g. **Peptone iron agar (PIA)**; semisolid medium; pH 6.7 ± 0.2 (10)

Peptone	20.0 g
Ferric ammonium citrate	0.5 g
Sodium thiosulfate, $Na_2S_2O_3 \cdot 5H_2O$	0.08 g
Dipotassium phosphate, K_2HPO_4	1.0 g
Agar	15.0 g
Deionized water	1000.0 mL

h. **Sulfide-indole-motility agar (SIM)**; semisolid medium
   (1) Aids in identifying the *Enterobacteriaceae,* especially *Salmonella* and *Shigella,* on basis of sulfide production, indole formation, and motility; following presumptive evidence on differential tubed media (e.g., KIA/TSI).
   (2) Ingredients, pH 7.3 ± 0.2

Casein peptone	20.0 g
Meat peptone	6.1 g
Ferrous ammonium sulfate, $FeNH_4(SO_4)_2 \cdot 12H_2O$ (or peptonized iron 0.2 g)	0.2 g

Sodium thiosulfate, $Na_2S_2O_3 \cdot 5H_2O$	0.2 g
Agar	3.5 g
Deionized water	1000.0 mL

(*Note:* the casein peptone contains tryptophan, necessary for indole production.)

  i. ***Salmonella-Shigella* agar (SS)**
   (1) Modification of deoxycholate-citrate agar of Leifson (26)
   (2) Ingredients, pH 7.0 ± 0.2

Casein/meat (50/50) peptone	5.0 g
Beef (meat) extract	5.0 g
Lactose	10.0 g
Sodium citrate, $C_3H_4OH(COO)_3Na_3$	8.5 g
Bile salts mixture	8.5 g
Sodium thiosulfate, $Na_2S_2O_3 \cdot 5H_2O$	8.5 g
Ferric citrate, $FeC_6H_5O_7 \cdot 5H_2O$	1.0 g
Neutral red	0.025 g
Brilliant green	0.00033 g (0.33 mg)
Deionized water	1000.0 mL

  j. **Xylose lysine desoxycholate (XLD) agar**
   (1) Isolation and identification of enteric pathogens; especially supports growth of more fastidious *Shigella* and *Providencia* spp. (40–45)
   (2) Ingredients, pH 7.5 ± 0.2

Yeast extract	3.0 g
Xylose	3.5 g
L-Lysine · HCl	5.0 g
Lactose	7.5 g
Sucrose (saccharose)	7.5 g
Sodium chloride, NaCl	5.0 g
Sodium deoxycholate, $C_{24}H_{40}O_4Na$	2.5 g
Sodium thiosulfate, $Na_2S_2O_3 \cdot 5H_2O$	6.8 g
Ferric ammonium citrate	0.8 g
Phenol red	0.08 g
Agar	13.5 g
Deionized water	1000.0 mL

2. ***Streptococcus/Enterococcus* spp.: bile esculin agar (BEA)** (see Chapter 2)
3. **Aids in differentiating genera: Christensen's citrate sulfide agar** (6), pH 6.7 ± 0.2

Yeast extract	0.5 g
Glucose (dextrose)	0.2 g
Sodium citrate, $Na_3C_6H_5O_7 \cdot 2H_2O$	3.0 g
Cysteine · HCl	0.1 g
Ferric ammonium citrate	0.4 g
Monopotassium phosphate, KH_2PO_4	1.0 g
Sodium chloride, NaCl	5.0 g
Sodium thiosulfate, $Na_2S_2O_3 \cdot 5H_2O$	0.08 g
Phenol red	0.012 g
Agar	15.0 g
Deionized water	1000.0 mL

4. **Isolation/differentiation of vibrios: thiosulfate-citrate-bile salts-sucrose (TCBS) agar (*Vibrio* selective agar)**
   a. Formulation of Nakanishi (30); modified by Kobayashi, Enomoto, Sakazaki, and Kuwahara (23)

(2) Ingredients, pH 8.6 ± 0.2

Casein/meat (50/50) peptone	10.0 g
Yeast extract	5.0 g
Sucrose	20.0 g
Sodium citrate, $Na_3C_6H_5O_7 \cdot 2H_2O$	10.0 g
Sodium thiosulfate, $Na_2S_2O_3 \cdot 5H_2O$	10.0 g
Bile salts	8.0 g
(or sodium cholate, 3.0 g and	
Oxgall dehydrated, 5.0 g (34))	
Sodium chloride, NaCl	10.0 g
Ferric citrate, $FeC_6H_5O_7 \cdot 5H_2O$	1.0 g
Thymol blue	0.04 g
Bromthymol blue (BTB)	0.04 g
Agar	15.0 g
Deionized water	1000.0 mL

5. Method of preparation: **any of the above media**
   a. Weigh out amount accurately as directed on the label. Various company products may differ slightly.
   b. Rehydrate with distilled or deionized water.
   c. Heat **gently** into solution.
   d. Dispense media **prior** to sterilization.
      (1) Tubes: 4–5 mL/tube (13 × 100 mm): KIA, TSI, BEA, citrate sulfide, LIA, PIA
      (2) Tubes: 8 mL/tube (16 × 125 mm): SIM
      (3) Plate medium: BEA; sterilize flask of medium **before** pouring.
   e. Method of sterilization for all **tubed** media and BEA flask: autoclave; 121°C, 15 lb, 15 min. **Do not autoclave the following media:** BSA, deoxycholate agars, Hektoen agar, SS agar, TCBS, and XLD agars (see IX. Precautions).
   f. Cool tubed media.
      (1) **Slanted** position with **deep butts:** KIA, TSI, LIA
      (2) **Slanted** position with **long slants/short butt:** BEA and citrate sulfide agar
      (3) Vertical position (upright): semisolid media PIA and SIM
   g. Water bath, 37°C: **all** plate media
      (1) Cool flask of medium to 45–50°C.
      (2) **Aseptically** pour 15–20 mL per **sterile** Petri dish.
      (3) Cool in an upright position (lid up).
      (4) Crack lid (slightly ajar) to dry surface.
      (5) Use same day as poured.
   h. Method of inoculation
      (1) **Pure** culture, single colony
      (2) Pick center of colony with an **inoculating needle**.
      (3) **Slanted** tubed media
         (a) Fishtail slant
         (b) Stab butt
            1. To within 1/4 inch from the bottom
            2. Withdraw needle following line of entrance
         (c) Order may be reversed if preferred.
      (2) **Vertical** (PIA, SIM), stab butt
         (a) To within 1/4 to 1/2 inch from the bottom
         (b) Withdraw needle following initial line of inoculation.
   d. Plate media; streak for isolation (4-quadrant method). (See Chapter 31 for procedure.)
6. Incubation

a. 35°C
b. All tubed media, 18–24 h
c. Plate media
   (1) Invert (lid down)
   (2) Up to 48 h before reporting as negative
B. **PbAc strip test**, primarily for H_2S detection by bacteria other than *Enterobacteriaceae*; nonenteric organisms that may produce small amounts of H_2S
1. Reagent strips
   a. Reagent: **hot, saturated,** 5% aqueous solution of PbAc
   b. Commercial H_2S test strips available
   c. Preparation of PbAc paper strips
      (1) Cut white filter paper into strips approximately 1/2 inch wide and 2 inches long.
      (2) Soak strips in **hot** PbAc solution and place (with forceps) in large **glass** Petri dish or widemouthed screw-cap jar.
      (3) Air dry or place in oven at 50–60°C.
      (4) Seal Petri dish with autoclave tape; close jar loosely.
   d. Method of sterilization: autoclave; 121°C, 15 lb, 15 min
   e. Cool and dry, then tighten caps.
   f. Label container with date autoclaved. Resterilize after 3 weeks to maintain sterility.
2. Media employed
   a. **Routine H_2S detection**; 3 choices
      (1) Nutrient broth, pH 6.9 ± 0.2

Peptone or protease peptone	5.0 g
Beef extract	3.0 g
Deionized water	1000.0 mL

      (2) Thiopeptone broth, pH 6.8 ± 0.2

Thiotone peptone	5.0 g
Beef extract	3.0 g
Deionized water	1000.0 mL

      (3) Trypticase soy broth (TSB), pH 7.3 ± 0.2

Trypticase peptone	17.0 g
Peptone (soy bean)	3.0 g
Sodium chloride, NaCl	5.0 g
Dipotassium phosphate, K_2HPO_4	2.5 g
Dextrose (glucose)	2.5 g
Deionized water	1000.0 mL

      (4) Method of preparation: any of the above media
         (a) Weigh out amount accurately as directed on label. Various company products may differ slightly.
         (b) Rehydrate with distilled or deionized water.
         (c) Heat **gently** into solution.
         (d) Dispense approximately 4.0–5.0 mL per tube, except Thiotone peptone (Thiopeptone), 0.8 mL per tube (75 × 10 mm) (29).
      (5) Method of sterilization of all media: autoclave; 121°C, 15 lb, 15 min
      (6) Cool to 45°C in a water bath
   b. *Brucella* spp. H_2S detection: serum glucose agar slants (19) or Tryptose agar slants (1)
      (1) Ingredients, **nutrient base**

Peptone	10.0 g
Beef extract	5.0 g

Sodium chloride, NaCl	5.0 g
Agar	20.0 g
Deionized water	1000.0 mL

(2) Preparation of nutrient base (see Section IV.B.2.a.(iv)–(vi).)
(3) **Aseptically,** add sterile enrichments to cooled base medium.

Horse serum	50.0 mL
Glucose, 20% aqueous solution	50.0 mL
Nutrient base	1000.0 mL

(4) Mix thoroughly.
(5) **Aseptically,** dispense approximately 5.0 mL per **sterile** tube.
(6) Cool in a **slanted position** and refrigerate for storage (4–10°C).

The genus *Brucella* requires additional enrichments with sulfhydryl bonds (−SH) for H_2S detection.

3. Procedures
   a. **Macroprocedure**
      (1) Method of ZoBell and Feltham (50)
      (2) Media: several choices
         Trypticase soy broth (TSB)
         Nutrient broth
         Serum glucose agar slants, *Brucella* spp. only
      (3) Inoculation
         (a) Growth from an 18- to 24-h **pure** culture: KIA or other suitable culture
         (b) **Heavy** inoculum
      (4) **Aseptically** suspend a **sterile** PbAc strip **above** broth level.
         (a) Place strip in tube.
            1. Along one side
            2. About 10 mm above broth level
            3. **Do not** immerse strip in broth.
         (b) Secure strip.
            1. Fold one end of strip over lip of tube.
            2. Replace closure (cap) to hold strip in place.
      (5) Incubation
         (a) *Brucella* spp.
            1. 35°C
            2. Increased CO_2 tension (10%)
            3. **Change** PbAc strip **daily** up to 7 days of incubation.
            4. Record results **daily**.
         (b) All other organisms
            1. 30°C (optimal) to 35°C (47)
            2. Read after 12 and 24 h.
               a. A positive result may occur within the first 12 h of incubation
               b. If negative at the end of 24 h, reincubate.
            3. Hold up to 6 days before reporting as negative.
               a. Read daily.
               b. **Do not** change strips. Use the same strip for the entire 6 days.

Tittsler (47) found that with certain bacteria, more H_2S was detected when cultures were incubated at 30°C. H_2S detection with PbAc paper strips is more advantageous than actually incorporating PbAc into the medium, since it obviates possible toxic effects of the metallic salt

(7). Also, it is easier to detect H$_2$S on PbAc strips than to observe a color reaction in the medium; the strip detects as little as 0.01 mmol of sulfide liberated from peptone (50).

A heavy inoculum of test organism is essential because the amount of H$_2$S produced and the time to detection depends on the concentration of the suspension (8). When a heavy inoculum is used, a positive reaction may develop as soon as 15–30 min after incubation and usually in 1–2 h with most organisms (8).

  b. **Microprocedure**
    (1) Method of Morse and Weaver (29)
    (2) Medium: Thiopeptone broth. If prepared just **prior** to use there is no need to sterilize either tubes or medium (29).
    (3) Inoculation (29)
      (a) Warm tubes in a 37°C water bath.
      (b) Growth from a **6-h** logarithmic-phase, **pure** culture grown on an enriched medium (e.g., infusion agar slant)
      (c) Transfer inoculum with a swab.
        1. Swab does not have to be sterile.
        2. Swab half the surface of the slant; **heavy** inoculum.
      (d) Swirl swab **gently** in medium; discard swab in disinfectant.
    (4) **Aseptically,** suspend a sterile PbAc strip about 10 mm above broth level; secure strip by folding a 1 cm section over the mouth of the tube. **Do not** immerse strip in broth.
    (5) Incubation: 35°C; read results at 15-min intervals up to a final period of 45 min.

According to Morse and Weaver (29), their microprocedure gives results comparable to those obtained by macromethods; however, a longer incubation increases the sensitivity, and many organisms exhibit H$_2$S production not observed by macrotechniques. Thiopeptone (BBL-Thiotone Peptone) is especially rich in sulfur. The time for H$_2$S detection increases if the culture used for inoculation is not in the logarithmic growth phase (29). According to Morse and Weaver (29), H$_2$S production variances among organisms "differ quantitatively rather than qualitatively."

V. QUALITY CONTROL MICROORGANISMS

A. **H$_2$S detection primarily of the *Enterobacteriaceae***
  1. Positive (+)

    Salmonella choleraesuis subsp. *arizonae*   ATCC 13314

  2. Negative (−)

    Shigella flexneri   ATCC 12022
    Escherichia coli   ATCC 25922

B. **SIM**

Organism	ATCC	H$_2$S	Indole	Motility
Salmonella typhimurium	13311	+	−	+
Shigella flexneri	9199	−	−	−
Escherichia coli	25922	−	+	+

C. **Bile esculin agar (BEA)**
  1. Positive (+): *Enterococcus faecalis*   ATCC 29212
  2. Negative (−): *Streptococcus pyogenes*   ATCC 19615

D. **Thiosulfate-citrate-bile-sucrose (TCBS) agar**
  1. Positive (+): *Enterococcus faecalis*   ATCC 29212
  2. Negative (−): *Vibrio parahaemolyticus*   ATCC 17802

E. **Lysine iron agar (LIA)**
   1. Positive (+)

Salmonella choleraesuis subsp. *arizonae*	ATCC 13314
Citrobacter freundii	ATCC 8454

   2. Negative (−): *Proteus vulgaris*   ATCC 9484

VI. RESULTS

> See Figure 15.1 (Appendix 1) for colored photographic results

VII. INTERPRETATION

A. **Sulfur-containing amino acid media**
   1. Tubed media: KIA, TSI, BEA, LIA, citrate sulfide, SIM, PIA
      a. Positive (+): **any** blackening of medium
         (1) Along line of inoculation. Blackening first seen where acid fermentation is **maximum** along inoculation line (25)
         (2) Throughout entire butt
      b. Negative (−): **no** blackening
   2. Plate media, BSA, deoxycholate Agar, Hektoen, SS, TCBS, XLD
      a. Positive (+): black colonies surrounded by a brownish black zone in the medium
         (1) Zone diameter may be several times the size of the colony.
         (2) Zone area may exhibit a metallic sheen.
      b. Negative (−): no blackening and no metallic sheen

B. **PbAc strip**
   1. Routine H_2S detection
      a. Positive (+)
         (1) Brownish black coloration of paper strip; may have a sheen
         (2) Record degree of blackening; trace (T) to 4+
      b. Negative (−)
         (1) No change, no coloration of strip
         (2) Check reaction by removing strip and adding a few drops of 2 N HCl (170 mL of HCl brought to 1 L with distilled water) to culture.
            (a) Acid releases dissolved H_2S, if present.
            (b) Replace strip and again observe after a few minutes
   2. *Brucella* spp. H_2S detection (9)
      a. The time H_2S is produced is significant only with *Brucella* spp.
      b. Record daily results: examples
         (1) "H_2S produced on the first 2 days."
         (2) "H_2S produced from the 1st to 5th day"
      c. Results
         (1) Positive (+): brownish black coloration of paper strip; may have a sheen
         (2) Negative (−): no change, no coloration of strip

The amount of blackening of a PbAc strip may be measured in millimeters making the test a quantitative procedure (50).

VIII. RAPID TEST

BBL's H_2S/Indole Disks: Follow manufacturer's directions

IX. PRECAUTIONS

A. **Sulfur-containing amino acid media**
   1. **General**
      a. The following conditions must obtain to detect H_2S production: (*a*) medium must contain a source of sulfur (-SH); e.g., amino acids, cysteine and methionine, (*b*) an H_2S indicator must be present, (*c*) medium must support growth of microorganism being tested, and (*d*) bacteria present must possess an H_2S-producing enzyme system (25). Differences among the various H_2S-detection media are due to alterations in one or more of these four conditions; H_2S production by a specific organism in one medium may **not** be detected in another (25). One must know the exact test system to interpret results.
      b. Controls **should** be run on peptone used in H_2S medium to determine if the sulfur content suffices for H_2S detection. If the peptone is deficient for rapid H_2S detection, cysteine may be added to enrich the concentration of sulfhydryl bonds (-SH).
      c. According to Tittsler (47), some H_2S inhibition occurs when the test is incubated at 34°C, and inhibition increases as the temperature increases to 40°C. Tittsler ran experiments with *Salmonella pullorum* and found the optimal incubation temperature range for maximum H_2S production was 30–34°C.
      d. Ferrous sulfate H_2S detector is somewhat less sensitive than other ferric or ferrous salts; therefore, there may be discrepancies in H_2S readings between KIA/TSI and other H_2S-detection media (25).
      e. Most bacteria use sulfate as principal sulfur source; however, sulfate **must** be reduced, since sulfur in most sulfur-containing compounds is at the oxidation level of H_2S (15).
   2. **KIA/TSI**
      a. H_2S production may be evident on KIA, but negative on TSI because of the sucrose present only in TSI (4). Bulmash and Fulton (4) showed that sucrose use may suppress the enzyme mechanisms responsible for H_2S production, masking the iron sulfide indicator in the medium. Padron and Dockstader (32) state that not all H_2S-producing *Salmonella* spp. are positive on TSI, nor does this medium give clear-cut separations of other H_2S-producing members of the *Enterobacteriaceae*.
      b. KIA more sensitive than TSI because sucrose is believed to suppress enzyme mechanisms responsible for H_2S production (25).
      c. KIA/TSI media lack inhibitors, and all but the most fastidious bacteria will grow, with the exception of obligate anaerobes (25). Therefore, these media can only be used when test bacteria are selected from a single colony recovered on primary or selective agar plates (25).
   3. **Bismuth sulfite agar**
      a. Dehydrated BSA quickly deteriorates when exposed to the atmosphere; deterioration indicated by aggregation into solid, nonfriable mass with development of a brown color. On rehydration, medium remains brown instead of normal green and loses selective and differential properties (46).
      b. BSA **should not** be stored in the refrigerator (4°C) for longer than 2 days; after 3 days of storage the medium becomes green and loses selectivity, so that smaller numbers of *Salmonella* are recovered (28). Preferably, medium should be used on day prepared and **not** stored.
      c. Do **not** allow sunlight to shine on BSA plates; a reaction sets in that destroys the usefulness of the medium (39).

d. Only colonies of *S. typhi* growing close to surface or on the surface exhibit a decided black metallic sheen.
   e. Specimens preserved in glycerol **must** first be diluted with water to reduce glycerol content, since *S. typhi* is inhibited in as much as 2% glycerol (10).
   f. Typical *S. typhi* colonies usually develop within 24 h; however, all plates should be incubated for 48 h to allow growth of all typhoid strains (10).
   g. **Do not autoclave**; heating longer than necessary to just dissolve ingredients destroys its selectivity (10).
4. **Deoxycholate citrate agars:** boil medium only until it melts; excessive heating at any time increases inhibition. **Do not autoclave.** Citrate and iron (Fe) combination has a strong hydrolyzing effect on agar if the medium is heated, producing a soft, nonelastic agar; if autoclaved it becomes soft and almost impossible to streak (26).
5. **Hektoen enteric (HE) agar (HEA):** do not autoclave medium; excessive heat may alter ingredients. Sterilization is not necessary; the medium is highly inhibitory to Gram-positive microorganisms.
6. **Lysine iron agar (LIA)**
   a. H_2S-producing *Proteus* spp. **do not** blacken this medium (2). Ferrous sulfide (FeS) may not be seen with microorganisms that **do not** produce lysine decarboxylase since acid in butt may suppress its formation; however, this is no problem if medium is used in conjunction with KIA or TSI medium.
   b. All organisms inoculated on LIA **must** be glucose fermenters.
7. **Sulfide-indole-motility (SIM) medium**
   a. Hydrogen sulfide reactions are intensified by motile culture (10).
   b. An H_2S-producing organism may exhibit blackening on SIM medium (positive) but none on TSI medium (negative) (3).
   c. SIM medium is more sensitive than KIA because of its semisolid consistency, lack of carbohydrates to suppress H_2S formation, and the use of peptonized iron as an indicator (25).
8. **Xylose lysine agars**
   a. Incubation period exceeding 48 h may yield false-positive results; however, 48-h incubation increases production of black centers due to H_2S production.
   b. *Salmonella* serovar *paratyphi* A, *S. choleraesuis*, *Salmonella* serovar *pullorum,* and *Salmonella* serovar *gallinarum* may form red colonies without H_2S, thus resembling *Shigella* spp.
   c. Some *Proteus* spp. may develop black centers on XLD and rarely on XLBG medium.
   d. H_2S **only produced** when alkaline conditions exist; e.g., *Salmonella, Citrobacter,* and *Proteus* usually H_2S-negative on XLD medium because of acid reaction from carbohydrate fermentation(s).
9. **Christensen's citrate sulfide agar:** H_2S production is observed in butt as a black discoloration; however, the results of H_2S production may **not** agree with those obtained on KIA/TSI.

B. **Lead Acetate Strip**
1. Some workers treat PbAc strips with glycerol to enhance hydroscopicity. ZoBell and Feltham (50) state that this practice has no real usefulness in increasing H_2S detection.
2. PbAc strip procedures are 10 times more sensitive than procedures that incorporate the metal in the medium (50); the PbAc result may be positive when butt reaction in KIA/TSI is negative or only weakly positive.
3. PbAc is toxic to bacterial growth, exhibiting a bacteriostatic action that inhibits liberation of H_2S from peptone (50); therefore, **do not** allow the PbAc strips to touch the broth medium.
4. When testing for H_2S production among the *Brucella* spp., it is **essential** to change PbAc strips daily. The time period of production is significant also (9).

5. Studies by Rodler et al. (35) with *Escherichia coli* showed that the black color obtained with PbAc was due to the interaction of indicator with mercaptans produced from cystine. They recommend using only H_2S indicators such as iron salts, which **do not** react with mercaptans (35).
6. PbAc strips are extremely sensitive and should be used whenever bacteria exhibit only trace amounts of H_2S on routine H_2S detection media (25).
7. Disadvantage of PbAc is that it may also inhibit growth of many fastidious bacteria, specifically those that may require a more sensitive H_2S-detector system (25).
8. The extreme sensitivity of PbAc strips makes it possible to drape the impregnated filter paper strip under cap of a KIA or TSI tube **without** incorporating it directly into the medium (25).

REFERENCES

1. Balows A, Hausler WJ Jr, Herrmann KL, et al. Manual of Clinical Microbiology, ed 5. Washington, DC: American Society for Microbiology, 1991:459.
2. Baron EJ, Finegold SM. Bailey & Scott's Diagnostic Microbiology, ed 8. Philadelphia: CV Mosby, 1990:83–85, 116.
3. Branson D. Methods in Clinical Bacteriology. Springfield, IL: Charles C Thomas, 1972:24–25.
4. Bulmash JM, Fulton M. Discrepant tests for hydrogen sulfide. J Bacteriol 1964;88(2):1813.
5. Cantarow A, Schepartz B. Biochemistry, ed 3. Philadelphia: WB Saunders, 1962:286.
6. Christensen WB. Hydrogen sulfide production and citrate utilization in the differentiation of enteric pathogens and coliform bacteria. Res Bull Weld County Health Dept (Greeley, Colo) 1949;1:3–16.
7. Clarke PH. Hydrogen sulphide production by bacteria. J Gen Microbiol 1953;8(3):397–407.
8. Clarke PH, Cowan ST. Biochemical methods for bacteriology. J Gen Microbiol 1952;6(2):187–197.
9. Cowan ST. Cowan & Steel's Manual for the Identification of Medical Bacteria, ed 2. Cambridge: Cambridge University Press, 1974:36, 167, 174.
10. Difco Manual, ed 10. Detroit: Difco Laboratories, 1984:132–136, 654.
11. Doelle HW. Bacterial Metabolism. New York: Academic Press, 1969:99–100, 224.
12. Edwards PR, Fife MA. Lysine-iron agar in the detection of *Arizona* cultures. Appl Microbiol 1961;9(6):478–480.
13. Fieser LF, Fieser M. Organic Chemistry, ed 3. New York: Reinhold, 1956:155.
14. Fromageot C. Desulfhydrases. In: Summer JB, Myrback K, eds. The Enzymes, Chemistry and Mechanism of Action, vol 1, part 2. New York: Academic Press, 1951:1237.
15. Gottschalk G. Bacterial Metabolism, ed 2. New York: Springer-Verlag, 1986:42.
16. Hajna AA. Preparation and application of Wilson and Blair's bismuth sulfite agar medium. Public Health Lab 1951;9:48–50.
17. Hajna AA, Damon SR. New enrichment and plating medium for the isolation of *Salmonella* and *Shigella* organisms. Appl Microbiol 1956; 4(6):341–345.
18. Harrow B, Mazur A. Textbook of Biochemistry, ed 9. Philadelphia: WB Saunders, 1966:21, 419.
19. Jones LM, Morgan WJB. A preliminary report on a selective medium for the culture of *Brucella*, including fastidious types. Bull WHO 1958;19(1): 200–203.
20. King S, Metzger WI. A new medium for the isolation of *Salmonella* and *Shigella* species. Bacteriol Proc 1967:77.
21. King S, Metzger WI. A new plating medium for the isolation of enteric pathogens. I. Hektoen enteric agar. Appl Microbiol 1968;16(4):577–578.
22. King S, Metzger WI. A new plating medium for the isolation of enteric pathogens. II. Comparison of Hektoen agar with SS and EMB agar. Appl Microbiol 1968;16(4):579–581.
23. Kobayashi T, Enomoto S, Sakazaki R, Kuwahara S. A new selective isolation medium for the vibrio group: On a modified Nakanishi medium (TCBS agar medium). Jpn J Bacteriol 1963; 18:387–392.
24. Kobayashi K, Tachibana S, Ishimoto M. Intermediary formation of trithionate in sulfite reduction by a sulfate-reducing bacterium. J Biochem 1969;65:155–157.
25. Koneman EW, Allen SD, Janda WM, et al. Color Atlas and Textbook of Diagnostic Microbiology, ed 4. Philadelphia: JB Lippincott, 1992:113–114, 124, 125, 212, 213, 251, 337, 568.
26. Leifson E. New culture media based on sodium desoxycholate for the isolation of intestinal pathogens and for the enumeration of colon bacilli in milk and water. J Pathol Bacteriol 1935;40(3):581–599.
27. MacDonell MT, Colwell RR. Phylogeny of the *Vibrionaceae,* and recommendation for two new genera *Listonella* and *Shewanella*. Int J Syst Bacteriol 1985;6:171–182.
28. McCoy JM, Spain GE. Bismuth sulphite media in the isolation of salmonellae. In: Shapton DA,

Gould GW, eds. Isolation Methods for Microbiologists. New York: Academic Press, 1969: 20.
29. Morse ML, Weaver RH. Rapid microtechnics for identification of cultures. III. Hydrogen sulfide production. Am J Clin Pathol 1950;20(3):481–484.
30. Nakanishi Y. An isolation agar medium for cholerae and enteropathogenic halophilic vibrios. Mod Media 1963;9:246.
31. On SLW, Holmes B. Assessment of enzyme detection tests useful in identification of campylobacteria. J Clin Microbiol 1992;30(3):746–749.
32. Padron AP, Dockstader WB. Selective medium for hydrogen sulfide production by salmonellae. Appl Microbiol 1972;23(6):1107–1112.
33. Pelczar MJ Jr, Reid RD. Microbiology, ed 2. New York: McGraw-Hill, 1965:573.
34. Power DA, McCuen PJ. Manual of BBL Products and Laboratory Procedures, ed 6. Cockeysville, MD: Becton Dickinson Microbiology Systems, 1988:246.
35. Rodler M, Vadon V, Pekar K. Untersuchung des H_2S-Bildungsvermogens verschiedener Bakterien. Zentralbl Bakteriol 1968;206(1):117–122.
36. Smythe CV. Desulfhydrases and dehydrases. In: Colowick SP, Kaplan NO, eds. Methods in Enzymology, vol 2. New York: Academic Press, 1955:315.
37. Speck ML, ed. Compendium of Methods for the Microbiological Examination of Foods. Washington, DC: American Public Health Association, 1976.
38. Stanier RY, Doudoroff M, Adelberg EA. The Microbial World, ed 2. Englewood Cliffs, NJ: Prentice-Hall, 1963:272.
39. Stewart JA. Methods of Media Preparation for the Biological Sciences. Springfield, IL: Charles C Thomas, 1974.
40. Taylor WI. Isolation of Shigellae. I. Xylose lysine agars: New media for isolation of enteric pathogens. Am J Clin Pathol 1965;44(4):471–475.
41. Taylor WI, Harris B. Isolation of shigellae. II. Comparison of plating media and enrichment broths. Am J Clin Pathol 1965;44(4):476–479.
42. Taylor WI, Harris B. Isolation of shigellae. III. Comparison of new and traditional media with stool specimens. Am J Clin Pathol 1967;48(3):350–355.
43. Taylor WI, Schelhart D. Isolation of shigellae. IV. Comparison of plating media with stools. Am J Clin Pathol 1967;48(3):356–362.
44. Taylor WI, Schelhart D. Isolation of shigellae. V. Comparison of enrichment broths with stools. Appl Microbiol 1968;16(9):1383–1386.
45. Taylor WI, Schelhart D. Isolation of shigellae. VII. Comparison of Gram-negative broth with Rappaport's enrichment broth. Appl Microbiol 1969;18(3):393–395.
46. The Oxoid Manual, ed 4. Basingstoke Hampshire, England: Oxoid Limited, 1980.
47. Tittsler RP. The effect of temperature upon the production of hydrogen sulphide by *Salmonella pullorum*. J Bacteriol 1931;21:111–118.
48. Vandamme P, Falsen E, Rossau R, Hoste B, et al. Revision of *Campylobacter, Helicobacter,* and *Wolinella* taxonomy: Emendation of generic descriptions and proposal of *Arcobacter* gen. nov. Int J Syst Bacteriol 1991;41:88–103.
49. Wilson WJ, Blair MM. A combination of bismuth and sodium sulphite affording an enrichment and selective medium for the typhoid-paratyphoid groups of bacteria. J Pathol Bacteriol 1926;29(3):310–311.
50. ZoBell CE, Feltham CB. A comparison of lead, bismuth, and iron as detectors of hydrogen sulphide produced by bacteria. J Bacteriol 1934;28:169–176.

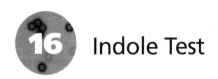# 16 Indole Test

I. PRINCIPLE

To determine the ability of an organism to split indole from tryptophan

II. PURPOSE

(Also see Chapters 43–45)

A. To aid in differentiation between genera
   1. Separation of *Escherichia coli* (+) from members of the *Klebsiella* (variable, usually negative; V⁻)-*Enterobacter* (V⁻)-*Hafnia* (−)-*Serratia* (V⁻) and one species of *Pantoea*, *P. agglomerans* (−) (formerly *Enterobacter agglomerans*) (30)
   2. *Cardiobacterium hominis* (+ᵂᵉᵃᵏ) (formerly CDC group II D) from *Eikenella corrodens* (−), *Kingella* spp. (−), and *Suttonella indologenes* (−) (formerly *Kingella indologenes*) (30)
B. To aid in species differentiation along with other biochemical tests
   1. *Paenibacillus alvei* (formerly *Bacillus alvei*) (+) from other *Bacillus* spp. (usually −)
   2. *Escherichia coli* (+), *E. hermanii* (+), and *E. fergusonii* (+) from *E. vulneris* (−) and *E. blattae* (−) (30)
   3. *Citrobacter freundii* (−) from *C. koseri* (formerly *C. diversus*) (+), and *C. amalonaticus* and biogroup 1 (+)
   4. *Klebsiella oxytoca* (+) and *K. ornithinolytica* (+) from other *Klebsiella* spp. (V⁻) (30)
   5. *Proteus vulgaris* (+), *P. inconstans* (+), *P. rettgeri* (+) from other *Proteus* species (−) (30)
   6. *Pasteurella dagmatis* (+), *P. dagmatis* subsp. *septica* (V⁺), *Pasteurella multocida* (+), *P. multocida* subsp *gallicida* (+), and *P. multocida* subsp. *multocida* (+), *P. pneumotropica* (+) from *P. haemolytica* (−) and *Actinobacillus ureae* (formerly *Pasteurella ureae*) (−) (30)
   7. *Paenibacillus alvei* (+) from most frequently isolated species *P. macerans* (−), and *P. polymgxa* (−)
   8. *Peptostreptococcus asaccharolyticus* (+) and *P. indolicus* (+) from other *Peptostreptococcus* spp. (−) that may cause human infections
   9. *Propionibacterium acnes* (+) from most frequently isolated *Propionibacterium* spp. (−)
C. Spot indole test
   1. Along with other tests (urease and ornithine) subdivides *Haemophilus influenzae* and *Haemophilus parainfluenzae* into biotypes (30, 51) *H. influenzae* biotypes I, II, V, and VII are indole positive; III, IV, VI, and VIII are indole negative. *H. parainfluenzae* biotypes IV, VI, VII, and VIII are indole positive; I, II, and III are indole negative. Other *Haemophilus* spp. are indole negative except *H. paracuniculus* (+). According to Welch and Ahlin (51) spot indole test alone can provide **presumptive** identification of *H. influenzae* in respiratory tract specimens, since indole-positive biotype II strains represent 40–70% of *H. influenzae* strains found in respiratory specimens.
   2. Along with sialidase, α- and β-glucosidase, and α-fructosidase, differentiates between the black-pigmented anaerobes (formerly *Bacteroides* genus): *Porphyromonas asaccharolyticus* (+), *P. endodontalis* (+), *P. gingivalis* (+), and *Prevotella intermedia* (+) from

Prevotella corporis (−), *P. denticola* (−), *P. loescheii* (−), *P. melaninogenica* (−), and *Porphyromonas levii* (formerly *Bacteroides levii*) (−) (38).

III. BIOCHEMISTRY INVOLVED

Tryptophan is an amino acid that can be oxidized by certain bacteria to form three major indolic metabolites: indole, skatole (methyl indole), and indoleacetic acid (IAA, indoleacetate) (8, 22, 54). Various intracellular enzymes involved are collectively called "tryptophanase," a general term used to denote the **complete** system of enzymes that mediate production of indole (22) by hydrolytic activity on substrate tryptophan (23, 53). The major intermediate in tryptophan degradation is indolepyruvic acid, from which indole can be formed through deamination, and skatole through decarboxylation of IAA (22). Tryptophan degradation in vitro (54) is shown below.

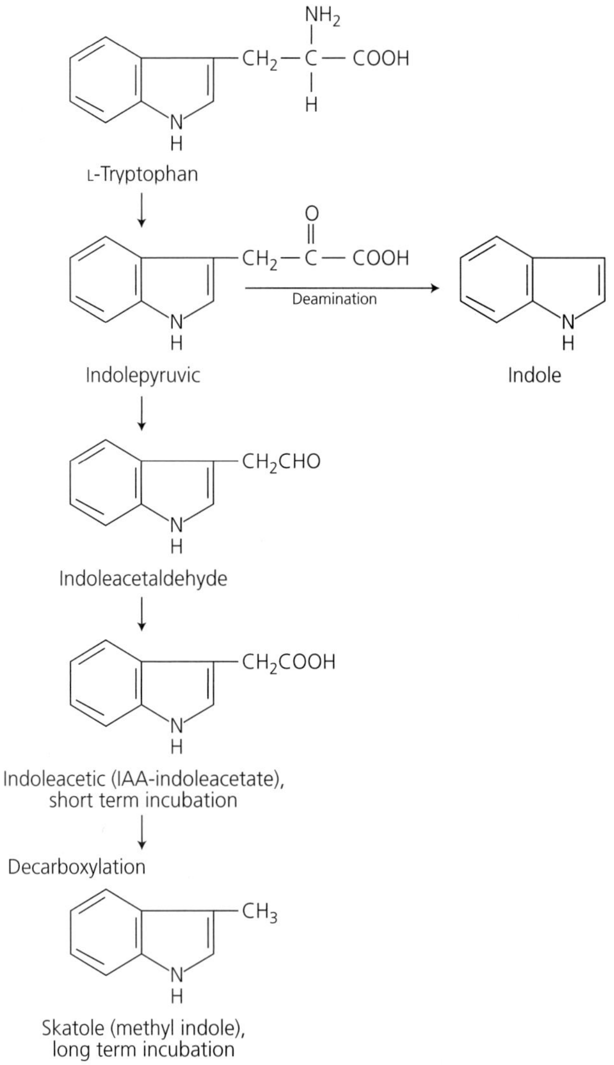

L-Tryptophan

↓

Indolepyruvic —Deamination→ Indole

↓

Indoleacetaldehyde

↓

Indoleacetic (IAA-indoleacetate), short term incubation

↓ Decarboxylation

Skatole (methyl indole), long term incubation

Chief indolic metabolites produced. (Redrawn in abbreviated form from Yokoyama, M. T., and Carlson, J. R. (1974) Appl. Microbiol., 27, 546, with permission of the American Society for Microbiology.)

Tryptophanase catalyzes the deamination reaction (12), attacking the tryptophan molecule only in its side chain and leaving the aromatic ring intact as indole (9).

$$\text{L-Tryptophan} \xrightarrow[\text{H}_2\text{O}]{\text{Tryptophanase Deamination}} \text{Indole} + CH_3-\overset{O}{\underset{\|}{C}}-COOH + NH_3$$

(L-Tryptophan → Indole + Pyruvic acid + Ammonia)

Deamination and hydrolysis take place with addition of a molecule of water in the presence of tryptophanase and the coenzyme pyridoxal phosphate (9). In deamination, the amine (NH_2) portion of the amino acid is removed, with release of a molecule of ammonia. Two types of deamination exist: oxidative and reductive. Oxidative deamination removes the NH_2 group from an amino acid and adds a double bond to the deaminated product (an unsaturated compound) and forms NH_3 and energy (9).

$$R-\underset{NH_2}{\underset{|}{C}}-COOH \xrightarrow[\tfrac{1}{2}O_2]{\text{Oxidative deamination}} R-\underset{O}{\overset{\|}{C}}-COOH + NH_3 + \text{Energy}$$

(Amino acid → Keto acid)

Tryptophan deamination is reductive; the NH_2 is removed and released as NH_3 and energy, which is used by the bacterium. Degradation of tryptophan releases indole, pyruvic acid, ammonia, and energy. The pyruvic acid can be further metabolized either via the glycolytic cycle or by entering the Krebs' cycle to release CO_2, H_2O, and a large yield of energy. The NH_3 can be used to synthesize new amino acids by using the energy present for the anabolic reaction. Indole split from the tryptophan molecule can be detected by a reagent that involves a chemical combination producing a distinct color. The presence or absence of indole formation is used for bacterial identification.

IV. MEDIA EMPLOYED

A. **Tryptophan or peptone broth**
  1. Ingredients
     a. Basal medium: most commercial peptone, pancreatic digest of casein broth (Tryptone) or enzymatic casein hydrolysate contains sufficient tryptophan for determination of indole (4).

Casein peptone (a protein fraction)	10.0 g
Sodium chloride, NaCl	5.0 g
Deionized water	1000.0 mL

     b. Tryptophan: variable, 1% concentration may be incorporated into peptone broth.
  2. Method of preparation
     a. Weigh out amount accurately as directed on the label. Various company products may vary slightly.
     b. Rehydrate with distilled or deionized water.
     c. Heat **gently** into solution.
     d. Dispense approximately 4.0 mL per tube.
  3. Method of sterilization: autoclave; 121°C, 15 lb, 15 min
  4. Cool before use and refrigerate for storage (4–10°C).
  5. Inoculation

a. **Light** inoculum (16)
   b. Growth from an 18- to 24-h **pure** culture: Kligler's iron agar (KIA)
6. Incubation: 35°C; 24 to 48 h
7. Add Kovacs' or Ehrlich's reagent **directly** to the incubated tube **before** attempting an interpretation.
B. **Casein medium**
  1. A pancreatic digest of casein solution may be prepared if commercial medium is unavailable.
     a. Ingredients

Pancreatic digest of casein	2.0 g
Sodium chloride, NaCl	0.5 g
Deionized water	100.0 mL

     b. Method of preparation
        (1) Dissolve by moderate heating.
        (2) Dispense 4.0 mL amounts into tubes.
     c. Method of sterilization: autoclave; 121°C, 15 lb, 15 min
     d. Proceed as with a commercial type of medium.
  2. Casein contains 1.2 g of tryptophan per 100 g (10)

V. REAGENTS USED

(*Note:* Choice between Ehrlich or Kovacs' reagent is a laboratory's preference; however, the Ehrlich reagent is more sensitive and is preferred when testing nonfermentative bacilli or anaerobes with minimal indole production (30)).

A. **Ehrlich's indole test** (2, 44).
  1. Ingredients; a light-colored solution stable at room temperature (22–25°C) when stored in a brown glass bottle

p-Dimethylaminobenzaldehyde (DMAB)	1.0 g
Ethyl alcohol (absolute)	95.0 mL
HCl (concentrated)	20.0 mL

  2. Method of use
     a. Add 1.0 mL of ether (4, 52) or xylene (4) to a 24- or 48-h incubated broth tube; these solvents extract and concentrate indole. **Do not** exceed the recommended amount of solvent; even minimal dilution may lower the concentration of indole below sensitivity.
     b. Shake well.
     c. Wait for the ether to rise to the surface of the medium.
     d. **Gently** add 0.5 mL of Ehrlich's reagent to the tube, tilting the tube so that the reagent runs down its side.
B. **Kovacs' indole test** (4, 7, 31)
  1. Ingredients: pale solution; store in a brown glass bottle.

Pure amyl or isoamyl alcohol (butyl alcohol may be substituted)	150.0 mL
p-Dimethylaminobenzaldehyde (DMAB)	10.0 g
HCl (concentrated)	50.0 mL

  2. Method of preparation
     a. Dissolve the aldehyde in the alcohol; may require **gentle** heating to put into solution.
     b. **Slowly** add the acid to the aldehyde-alcohol mixture.
  3. Method of use
     a. Add 5 drops of Kovacs' reagent directly to a 24- or 48-h incubated tube.
     b. Shake the tube **gently.**

Gadebusch and Gabriel (20) reported that substitution of isoamyl alcohol makes Kovacs' reagent more stable. With either reagent, dissolving the aldehyde in solvent may require **gentle** heating in a 50–60°C water bath. When performing the indole test, Ewing and Davis (17) recommend Kovacs' reagent; Ehrlich's reagent is used with nonfermenters such as *Flavobacterium* (28) and with anaerobes (24). Reagents are **not** dyes or stains, but upon hydrolysis, they yield substances that are converted simultaneously or subsequently into insoluble azo dyes (32).

C. With either reagent, if a 24-h incubated tube is tested for indole production, it is recommended that a 2.0 mL portion be removed aseptically for the test.
   1. A positive reaction after 24 h denotes a completed test.
   2. If the 24-h culture is negative, it should be incubated an additional 24 h and then retested.
D. Quality control: either reagent **must** be tested with known positive and negative cultures before being put into general use.
E. Storage: store both reagents in a refrigerator (4°C) when not in use. Their stability varies; therefore, each week they should be given a quality control check and discarded when demonstrating a negative or weak reaction with a known positive organism.
F. Chemistry of reagent action: indole, if present, combines with the color in the alcohol layer (10). This reaction occurs by a condensation process formed by an acid splitting of the protein (19). The reaction will occur without heat if the reagent is prepared with concentrated HCl.

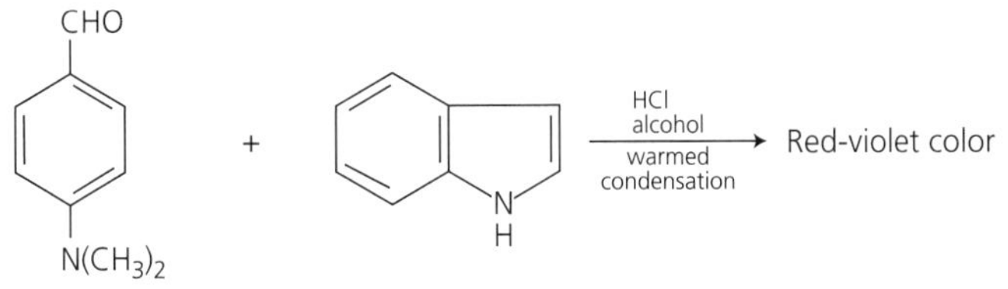

p-Dimethylamino-benzaldehyde (DMAB, DMABA) + Indole $\xrightarrow[\text{warmed condensation}]{\text{HCl alcohol}}$ Red-violet color

Indole is volatile, whereas α-methyl indole is not, and either heat or acid demonstrates volatile indole (6). The color reaction is based on the pyrrole structure present in indole.

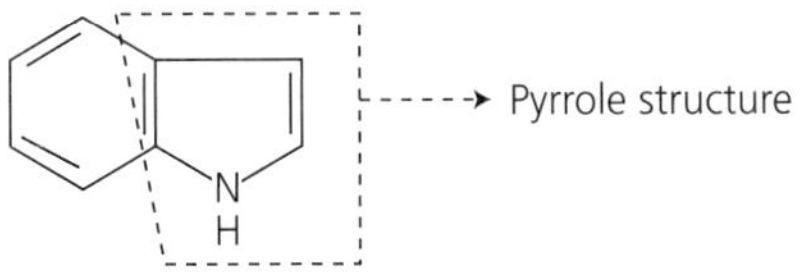

Indole → Pyrrole structure

The pyrrole structure can react in its tautomeric forms (when in solution, some of the molecules rearrange so that two forms are present) (40).

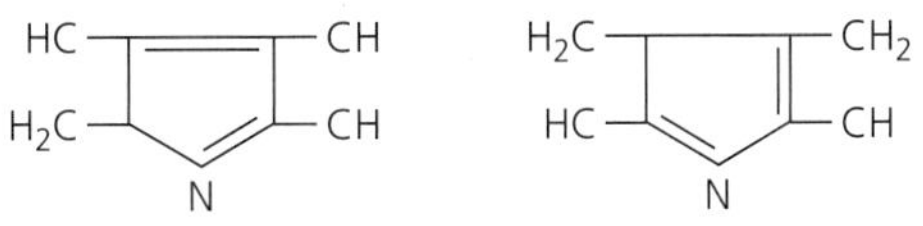

Pyrrole Tautomeric forms

The CH$_2$ groups in either pyrrole form permit condensation with the aldehyde in a two-step procedure (19).

A quinone or a quinoidal-type structure is an important color-producing compound (40) Reaction steps 1 and 2 occur immediately with DMAB in concentrated HCl (19). The derivatives of pyrrole show the same condensation reactions provided they have an intact CH group at the α or β position relative to the cyclic NH group (19). The alcoholic layer extracts and concentrates the red color complex. This complex is soluble in ethyl ether, ethyl alcohol, isoamyl alcohol, amyl alcohol, or butyl alcohol.

VI. QUALITY CONTROL MICROORGANISMS

A. **Routine**
　1. Positive (+)
　　　Escherichia coli　　　　　　ATCC 25922
　2. Negative (−)
　　　Enterobacter cloacae　　　　ATCC 23355
　　　Pseudomonas aeruginosa　　ATCC 27853

B. **Indole-nitrite medium**

Strain	ATCC	Indole	Nitrate
Pasteurella multocida	6529	+	+
Clostridium perfringens	13124	−	+
Clostridium sordellii	9714	+	−

C. **Motility-indole-ornithine (MIO) medium**

Strain	ATCC	Motility	Indole	Ornithine
Escherichia coli	25922	+	+	+
Enterobacter aerogenes	13048	+	−	+
Klebsiella pneumoniae subsp. pneumoniae	13883	−	−	−

VII. RESULTS

> See Figure 16.1 (Appendix 1) for colored photographic results

VIII. INTERPRETATION—EITHER REAGENT

A. Positive (+): **within seconds**, a red (bright fuchsia) ring at the interface of the medium in the lower portion, alcoholic phase, layers above the medium.
B. Negative (−): no color development at the alcohol layer or a cloudy ring; takes the color of the Kovacs' or Ehrlich's reagent (yellow).
C. Variable (±): an orange color at the surface of the medium due to skatole, a methylated compound that may be a precursor to indole formation (23).

IX. RAPID TESTS

A. **Indole spot test**
  1. Method of Vracko and Sherris (49)
  2. Presumptive characterization of E. coli, rapid speciation of swarming Proteus from primary isolation plates (2)
  3. Reagents; selection
     a. Kovacs': p-dimethylaminobenzaldehyde (DMAB)
        (1) Manufacturer: Eastman Organic Chemicals (see Appendix 11)
        (2) 5% solution in acidified amyl alcohol (3.0 mL of amyl alcohol in 1.0 mL of concentrated HCl)
     b. p-Dimethylaminobenzaldehyde (DMAB)
        (1) 1.0% solution in 10% (v/v) concentrated HCl
        (2) Prepare fresh every **4 months.**
        (3) Detects 6–12 µg of indole per mL (34)
        (4) Most stable and most economic reagent
     c. p-Dimethylaminocinnamaldehyde (DMACA, PACA)
        (1) Vinyl analog of DMAB (34, 49)
        (2) Manufacturer: Aldrich Chemical Company, (see Appendix 12)
        (3) 1.0% solution in 1% (v/v) concentrated HCl
        (4) Prepare fresh every **2 months**
        (5) Detects 3 µg of indole per mL (34)
        (6) Most sensitive reagent
  4. Inoculum: 18- to 24-h **pure** culture, sheep blood agar (SBA); preferred if available: Trypticase soy blood agar, 5.0% sheep blood (33, 47)
  5. Procedure
     a. No. 1 Whatman filter paper (9.0 cm)
        (1) Place in Petri dish cover.
        (2) Moisten with 1.0–1.5 mL of Kovacs' reagent (or other reagent listed above).
     b. Smear inoculum (cell paste) onto moistened filter paper. Many tests may be performed on a single filter paper.
  6. Interpretation
     a. Positive (+) (47)
        (1) Kovacs' reagent
           (a) Brown to reddish brown to red color
           (b) 1–3 min

(2) DMAB
    (a) Pink to red color
    (b) 1–3 min
(3) DMACA
    (a) Blue or green color
    (b) Within a few seconds

B. **Indole spot test for anaerobic bacteria** (4, 47)
  1. Use the same procedure as spot test of Vracko and Sherris (49) with the **exception** of reagent; use 1% DMACA in 10% (v/v) concentrated HCl; store in a dark bottle.
  2. Interpretation
     a. Positive (+): **immediate** formation of a blue color around growth
     b. Negative (−): no color change or a pinkish color
     c. **Late color development should be ignored.**

C. **Indole microtechnique**
  1. Method of Arnold and Weaver (1)
  2. Media: two choices
     a. Broth 1

        | Tryptone | 1% |
        | Beef extract | 0.3% |

     b. Broth 2

        | Tryptophan | 0.03% |
        | Peptone | 0.1% |
        | Dipotassium phosphate, K_2HPO_4 | 0.5% |

     c. Optimal pH for indole production, 7.4–7.8
     d. Dispense 1.0-mL broth aliquots into small test tubes (10 × 75 mm).
        (1) Sterility not necessary (1)
        (2) Caps **not** necessary
  3. Reagent: Kovacs' reagent
     a. Must be fresh
     b. Best solvent: isoamyl alcohol
  4. Procedure
     a. **Preheat** broth tubes; **absolute requirement**
        (1) Water bath, 37°C
        (2) Shortens time required for indole production (1)
     b. **Heavy inoculum** (1)
        (1) Preferred: from tryptone agar or broth
        (2) Alternate: any tryptophan medium or synthetic medium that contains tryptophan
     c. Add 4 drops of **fresh** Kovacs' reagent.
  5. Incubation, preferred: water bath, 37°C, 6 min–2 h
  6. Interpretation
     a. Positive (+): pink to red color in alcohol layer
     b. Negative (−): no color change; medium remains light yellow.

X. MULTITESTS

A. **Indole-nitrite medium (Trypticase nitrate broth)**
  1. Supports growth of aerobes and facultative and obligate anaerobes.
  2. Differentiates by ability to reduce nitrate and/or produce indole
  3. Ingredients, pH 7.2 ± 0.2

     | Casein peptone | 20.0 g |
     | Glucose (dextrose) | 1.0 g |

Disodium phosphate, Na$_2$HPO$_4$ 2.0 g
Potassium nitrate, KNO$_3$ 1.0 g
Agar   1.0 g
Deionized water   1000.0 mL

4. Dispense 5 mL/tube (13 × 100 mm).
5. Sterilization: 118–121°C, 15 lb, 15 min
6. Inoculum: 18- to 24-h **pure** culture; e.g., blood agar
7. Interpretation
    a. Indole: either reagent, Kovacs' or Ehrlich's; same as routine tests
    b. Nitrate: see Chapter 30, Nitrate Reduction Test.

B. **Motility-indole-lysine (MIL)/with sulfide (MILS)**
1. One-tube test of Reller and Mirrett (45)
2. Identification of *Enterobacteriaceae* from fecal specimens (14)
3. Procedure: see Chapter 28, Motility Test

C. **Motility-indole-ornithine (MIO) medium**
1. Formulation of Ederer and Clarke (13) and Oberhofer and Hajkowski (41)
2. Differentiation of the *Enterobacteriaceae* (see Chapter 28, Motility Test)

D. **Sulfide-indole-motility (SIM) medium:** see Chapter 15, Hydrogen Sulfide Test

XI. PRECAUTIONS

A. **General**
1. When a peptone broth is used instead of a tryptophan broth for the indole test, the medium itself should be tested with a known indole-producing organism. This determines if the peptone is suitable for indole production and also checks for the optimal incubation period required (48). Different lots and commercial varieties of peptone media are on the market, and some are unsuitable for indole production because they contain too little tryptophan.
2. Peptone medium containing glucose **must not** be used for indole detection. Indole formation occurs only with organisms capable of fermenting carbohydrates. Organisms that use carbohydrates oxidatively **cannot** produce indole (26). The high acidity produced by glucose fermentation may prevent growth of the organism (5) or inhibit the enzyme (15). Addition of tryptophan stimulates indole production, while glucose inhibits its production (11, 18, 54).
3. Some organisms form indole but break it down as rapidly as it is produced; therefore, a false-negative reaction may occur (44). This occurs mainly among some *Clostridium* spp. (44).
4. The optimal pH for tryptophanase activity is slightly alkaline (pH 7.4–7.8); a decrease in pH (toward acidity) decreases indole production (50) and may give a false-negative or weakly positive result.
5. Cultures to be tested for indole production **must** be incubated aerobically. Decreased oxygen tension decreases indole production (18, 22).
6. The ability of an organism to produce indole interferes with antimicrobial activity by either chemical or genetic means (29). Klein et al. (29) showed that with *Klebsiella*, indole-producing strains are prevalent in clinical specimens, and these organisms are more susceptible to action of antibiotics than non–indole producers. Martin et al. (36) reported similar findings.
7. According to Müller (39), indole positivity is lost upon prolonged incubation; however, studies by Pickett (42) showed no loss after 96 h incubation.
8. Differentiation between *C. hominis, Kingella* spp., *E. corrodens,* and *S. indologenes* requires a **heavy** inoculation in tryptone broth, incubation for 48 h, and extraction with xylene or chloroform using Ehrlich's reagent (30).

9. *Comamonas acidovorans* (formerly *Pseudomonas acidovorans*) produces a distinct "pumpkin orange" indole reaction because of formation of anthranilic acid rather than indole from tryptophan (35).
10. Minor modifications may be required in testing for indole production by certain weakly positive **non**fermenters; an enriched medium is required, such as heart infusion broth (30).
11. According to Maslow et al. (37), differentiating *Klebsiella* spp. solely on the basis of tryptophanase activity may be unreliable; differentiation is clonal (37). The tryptophanase operon from *Klebsiella* spp. has not been formally analyzed (37).

B. **Ehrlich's and Kovacs' reagents**
1. Kovacs' and Ehrlich's reagents are not specific for indole. α-Methylindole (indoleacetic acid) will also be produced from tryptophan and will react with reagent to yield a red color. Isenberg and Sundheim (27) found that indole reagent will react with 17 different indole compounds to yield a red color; however, by using a solvent (e.g., xylene, ether, or chloroform) to first extract indole, the red color obtained in solvent layer **only occurs** with indole and skatole (5-methyl indole).

$$\text{Indole} + \text{skatole (5 methyl indole)} + \text{test reagent} \longrightarrow \text{Pink color}$$

2. Care **must** be taken to add only a small amount of extractant; even minimal dilution may lower the concentration of indole below sensitivity of detection by either reagent (30).
3. Because indole is soluble in organic compounds, xylene or chloroform should be added to the test medium before addition of Ehrlich's reagent (30); the extraction step is less critical with Kovacs' reagent because amyl alcohol is used for the diluent (30).
4. Using Kovacs's reagent **without** shaking the tube is the method of choice (42).
5. Hemo-De (PMP Medical Industries) and Shandon (Shandon Inc.) are terpene-based solvents and less toxic extractants; these xylene substitutes may be used although they are less effective. In doubtful cases xylene should be used (21). Because of blocking action, use of indole-nitrate cannot be recommended (21). Hemo-De is a satisfactory xylene substitute in the Happold and Hoyle (22) modification of Ehrlich's indole test.
6. Kovacs' reagent should be fresh; however, it can be kept **several days** in a refrigerator (4–10°C). If it is allowed to stand at room temperature any length of time, the color changes from pale yellow to brown and it becomes **less** sensitive (1).

Both reagents should be stored in brown bottles with glass stoppers.

C. **Spot indole test**
1. Weakly false positive reactions may occur with the spot test if the inoculum is a mixed culture of indole-positive and -negative organisms. A pure culture must be obtained. Use a single, well-isolated colony for testing. Also, the inoculum **must** be cultivated on a medium that enhances indole production, a Tryptone or tryptophan medium. Since indole produced by adjacent colonies may diffuse into the medium and produce false-positive results, test colonies should be separated by at least 5 mm (25).

   MacConkey (MAC) or eosin–methylene blue agar (EMB) are **not** acceptable since they contain pH indicators, which could result in color carryover onto the acid-moistened filter paper and false-positive interpretations (25); blood agar plates are preferred (30). Spot indole test is also better performed on colonies growing on blood agar since pigmentation of lactose-positive colonies on MAC will make interpretation of color reaction difficult (30). However, the medium must contain enough tryptophan to initiate indole positivity (3); 1-day incubated blood agar plates may give false-negative results (42).

2. Spot indole reagent may not be sensitive enough for weakly indole-positive bacteria such as *C. hominis* and *Suttonella indologenes* (30).
3. PACA is more sensitive than Kovacs' reagent (30).
4. Certain strains of *Proteus vulgaris, Providencia* and *Aeromonas* will give a false-negative result with the indole spot test (6).

D. **Indole-nitrite medium**
   1. Medium can be used for nitrite tests with members of the *Enterobacteriaceae*, but is **not** recommended for indole testing of organisms that reduce nitrate to nitrite, which prevents detection of indole (46). Nitrites present in medium may block detection of indole (46).
   2. If medium is more than 2 days old, just before use, boil tubed medium for 2 min and cool **without** agitation (43).

REFERENCES

1. Arnold WM, Weaver RH. Quick microtechniques for the identification of cultures. I. Indole production. J Lab Clin Med 1948;33(10):1334–1337.
2. Bale MJ, McLaws SM, Matsen JM. The spot indole test for identification of swarming *Proteus.* Am J Clin Pathol 1985;83:87–90.
3. Balows A, Hausler WJ Jr, Herrmann KL, et al. Manual of Clinical Microbiology, ed 5, Washington, DC: American Society for Microbiology, 1991:1295.
4. Baron EJ, Finegold SM. Bailey & Scott's Diagnostic Microbiology, ed 8. Philadelphia: CV Mosby, 1990:378, 394.
5. Berman N, Rettger LF. 1. Bacterial nutrition: Further studies on the utilization of protein and non-protein nitrogen. 2. The influence of carbohydrate on the nitrogen metabolism of bacteria. J Bacteriol 1918;2(4):367–388, 389–402.
6. Blazevic DJ, Ederer GM. Principles of Biochemical Tests in Diagnostic Microbiology. New York: John Wiley & Sons, 1975:63–67.
7. Böhme A. Die Anwendung der Ehrlichschen Indolreaktion für bakteriologische Zwecke. Zentralbl Bakteriol Parasitenkd Infektionskr Hyg Abt 1 Orig 1905;40:129–133.
8. Branson D. Methods in Clinical Bacteriology. Springfield, IL: Charles C Thomas, 1972:25–27.
9. Burrows W, Moulder JW. Textbook of Microbiology. The Pathogenic Microorganisms, vol I, ed 19. Philadelphia: WB Saunders, 1968:144.
10. Cantarow A, Schepartz B. Biochemistry, ed 3. Philadelphia: WB Saunders, 1962:81, 135.
11. Clarke PH, Cowan ST. Biochemical methods for bacteriology. J Gen Microbiol 1952;6(2):187–197.
12. Doelle HW. Bacterial Metabolism. New York: Academic Press, 1969:410.
13. Ederer GM, Clark M. Motility-indole-ornithine medium. Appl Microbiol 1970;20(5):849–850.
14. Ederer GM, Lund ME, Balazevic DJ, et al. Motility-indole-lysine-sulfide medium. J Clin Microbiol 1975;2(3):266–267.
15. Epps HMR, Gale EF. The influence of the presence of glucose during growth on the enzymatic activities of *Escherichia coli:* Comparison of the effect with that produced by fermentation acids. Biochem J 1942;36:619–623.
16. Ewing WH. Edwards and Ewing's Identification of Enterobacteriaceae, ed 4. New York: Elsevier, 1986:521.
17. Ewing WH, Davis BR. Media and Tests for Differentiation of *Enterobacteriaceae*. Atlanta: Centers for Disease Control, 1970.
18. Fay GD, Barry AL. Methods for detecting indole production by gram-negative nonsporeforming anaerobes. Appl Microbiol 1974;27(3):562–565.
19. Feigl F. Spot Tests in Organic Analysis, ed 7. New York: Elsevier, 1966:372, 381–382.
20. Gadebusch HH, Gabriel S. Modified stable Kovacs' reagent for detection of indol. Am J Clin Pathol 1956;26(11):1373–1375.
21. Gubash SM, Bennett EE. Use of terpene-based solvents (Hemo-De, Histoclear, and Shandon and BDH xylene substitutes) in place of xylene in the Ehrlich indole test. J Clin Microbiol 1989;27(9):2136–2137.
22. Happold FC, Hoyle L. CCXXVII. The coli-tryptophan-indole reaction. I. Enzyme preparations and their action on tryptophan and some indole derivatives. Biochem J 1935;29:1918–1926.
23. Harrow B, Mazur A. Textbook of Biochemistry, ed 9. Philadelphia: WB Saunders, 1966:412.
24. Holdeman LV, Moore WEC. Anaerobe Laboratory Manual. Blacksburg, VA: Virginia Polytechnic Institute and State University, 1972.
25. Howard BJ, Klaas J II, Rubin SJ, et al. Clinical and Pathogenic Microbiology. St. Louis: CV Mosby, 1987:876.
26. Hugh R, Leifson E. The taxonomic significance of fermentative versus oxidative metabolism of carbohydrates by various gram negative bacteria. J Bacteriol 1953;66(1):24–26.
27. Isenberg HD, Sundheim LH. Indole reactions in bacteria. J Bacteriol 1958;75(6):682–690.
28. King EO. The Identification of Unusual Patho-

genic Gram Negative Bacteria. Atlanta: Centers for Disease Control, 1967.
29. Klein D, Spindler JA, Matsen JM. Relationships of indole production and antibiotic susceptibility in the *Klebsiella* bacillus. J Clin Microbiol 1975;2(5):425–429.
30. Koneman EW, Allen SD, Janda WM, et al. Color Atlas and Textbook of Diagnostic Microbiology, ed 4. Philadelphia: JB Lippincott, 1992:39, 121, 133, 140, 145, 174, 175, 197, 293, 310, 311, 325, 341.
31. Kovács N. Eine vereinfachte Methode zum Nachweis der Indolbildung durch Bakterien. Z Immunitaetsforsch 1928;55:311–315.
32. Lillie RD. HJ Conn's Biological Stains, ed 9. Baltimore: Williams & Wilkins, 1977:217.
33. Lovrekovich L. Detection of indole produced by bacteria on blood agar plates. Am J Med Technol 1972;38(4):130.
34. Lowrance BL, Reich P, Traub WH. Evaluation of two spot-indole reagents. Appl Microbiol 1969;17(6):923–924.
35. Marraro RV, Mitchell JL, Payet CR. A chromogenic characteristic of an aerobic pseudomonad species in 2% tryptone (indole) broth. J Am Med Technol 1977;39:13–19.
36. Martin WJ, Yu PKW, Washington JA II. Epidemiologic significance of *Klebsiella pneumoniae*: A 3-month study. Mayo Clin Proc 1971;46:785–793.
37. Maslow JN, Brecher SM, Adams KS, et al. Relationship between indole production and differentiation of *Klebsiella* species: Indole-positive and -negative isolates of *Klebsiella* determined to be clonal. J Clin Microbiol 1993;31(8):2000–2003.
38. Mincla BJ, Braham P, Rabe LK, Hillier SL. Rapid presumptive identification of black-pigmented gram-negative anaerobic bacteria by using 4-methylumbelliferone derivatives. J Clin Microbiol 1991;29(9):1955–1958.
39. Müller HE. Production and degradation of indole by gram-negative bacteria. Zentralbl Bakteriol Mikrobiol Hyg Ser A 1986;261:1–11.
40. Nussenbaum S. Organic Chemistry. Boston, Allyn & Bacon, 1963:297, 349.
41. Oberhofer TR, Hajkowski R. Evaluation of non-lactose-fermenting members of the Klebsiella-Enterobacter-Serratia division. I. Biochemical characteristics. Am J Clin Pathol 1970;54(11):720–725.
42. Pickett MJ. Methods for identification of flavobacteria. J Clin Microbiol 1989;27(10):2309–2315.
43. Power DA, McCuen PJ. Manual of BBL Products and Laboratory Procedures, ed 6. Cockeysville, MD: Becton Dickinson Microbiology Systems, 1988:168, 200.
44. Reed RW. Nitrate, nitrite, and indole reactions of gas gangrene anaerobes. J Bacteriol 1942;44(4):425–432.
45. Reller LB, Mirrett S. Motility-indole-lysine medium for presumptive identification of enteric pathogens of *Enterobacteriaceae*. J Clin Microbiol 1975;2(3):247–252.
46. Smith RF, Rogers RR, Bettge CL. Inhibition of the indole test reaction by sodium nitrite. Appl Microbiol 1972;23(2):423–424.
47. Sutter VL, Carter WT. Evaluation of media and reagents for indole-spot test in anaerobic bacteriology. Am J Clin Pathol 1972;58(3):335–338.
48. Tilley FW. Influence of peptone on indol formation by *Bacillus coli*. Am J Public Health 1921;11(9):834–836.
49. Vracko R, Sherris JC. Indole-spot test in bacteriology. Am J Clin Pathol 1963;39(4):429–432.
50. Weaver DK, Lee EKH, Leahy MS. Comparison of reagent-impregnated paper strips and conventional methods for identification of *Enterobacteriaceae*. Am J Clin Pathol 1968;49(4):494–499.
51. Welch DF, Ahlin PA, Matsen JM. Differentiation of *Haemophilus* spp. in respiratory isolate cultures by an indole spot test. J Clin Microbiol 1982;15(2):216–219.
52. Wilson TM, Davidson LSP. Ehrlich's aldehyde test for urobilinogen. Br Med J 1949;1(2312):884–887.
53. Wood WA, Gunsalus IC, Umbreit WW. Function of pyridoxal phosphate: Resolution and susceptibility of the tryptophanase enzyme of *Escherichia coli*. J Biol Chem 1947;170(1):313–322.
54. Yokoyama MT, Carlson JR. Dissimilation of tryptophan and related indolic compounds by ruminal microorganisms in vitro. Appl Microbiol 1974;27(3):540–548.

17 Indoxyl Substrate Hydrolysis Tests

I. PRINCIPLE

To determine the ability of specific bacterial esterases to hydrolyze specific indoxyl substrates to an indigo dye with a resultant dark blue color

II. PURPOSE

(Also see Chapter 43)

A. **Indoxyl acetate (IA) hydrolysis:** rapid and selective differential test to distinguish between a limited number of *Campylobacter* spp. and former *Campylobacter,* and related genera *Helicobacter* and *Wolinella* spp. (1): *C. jejuni* (+), *C. coli* (+), *C. upsaliensis* (+), *Arcobacter cryaerophila* (+), *Helicobacter fennelliae* (+), and *H. cinaedi* (variable, V), usually −) from other *Campylobacter* spp. (−) (6, 11, 15), *Campylobacter*- like organisms (CLOs) −, *Helicobacter pylori* −, and *Wolinella succinogenes* − (15)
   1. Distinguish *Helicobacter cinaedi* − (formerly in genus *Campylobacter*) from *Campylobacter upsaliensis* (+) (6), especially *C. upsaliensis* variants (+) that fail to grow at 42°C (14)
   2. Distinguish *Campylobacter lardi* (−) (formerly *C. laridis*) from *C. jejuni* (+) and *C. coli* (+) (8, 15)
   3. Distinguish *Helicobacter cinaedi* (−) from *Campylobacter fennelliae* (+) (15)
   4. Distinguish *Helicobacter pylori* (−) from *H. mustelae* (+) (15)
   5. Distinguish *Wolinella succinogenes* (−) from *W. recta* (+) and *W. curva* (+) (15)
B. **Indoxyl sulfate (IS) hydrolysis:** identification of *Providencia stuartii* (+) and *Klebsiella pneumoniae* (+) (3)
C. **Indoxyl butyrate (IB) hydrolysis (tributyrin hydrolysis)**
   1. Rapid differentiation of former *Branhamella* species, *Moraxella catarrhalis* (+), *M. caviae* (+), and *M. ovis* (+) from other oxidase-positive, Gram-negative cocci − (2)
   2. Other bacteria that may be positive for hydrolysis are *Pseudomonas aeruginosa* (+) and *Staphylococcus aureus* (V, usually +) (2).
D. **Indoxyl-β-D-glucuronide (IBDG) hydrolysis:** direct screen and rapid identification of *Escherichia coli* in urine and environmental samples and replica plate technology (4, 9, 18)

III. BIOCHEMISTRY INVOLVED

Indoxyl is a product of putrefactive decomposition of tryptophan in the intestines of humans via bacterial action (13). It is a heterocyclic 5-member ring fused to a benzene ring.

Bacterial hydrolases release indoxyl from acetate, sulfate, butyrate, and β-D-glucuronide (15). In the presence of air (O_2) and alkali, indoxyl hydrolyzes spontaneously to form indigo white, and in an acid environment, then indigo (3). Indigo white and indigo (indigo blue) produce a dark blue color indicating that the indoxyl compound was metabolized.

Indoxyl Substrate Hydrolysis (3, 5, 10, 15)

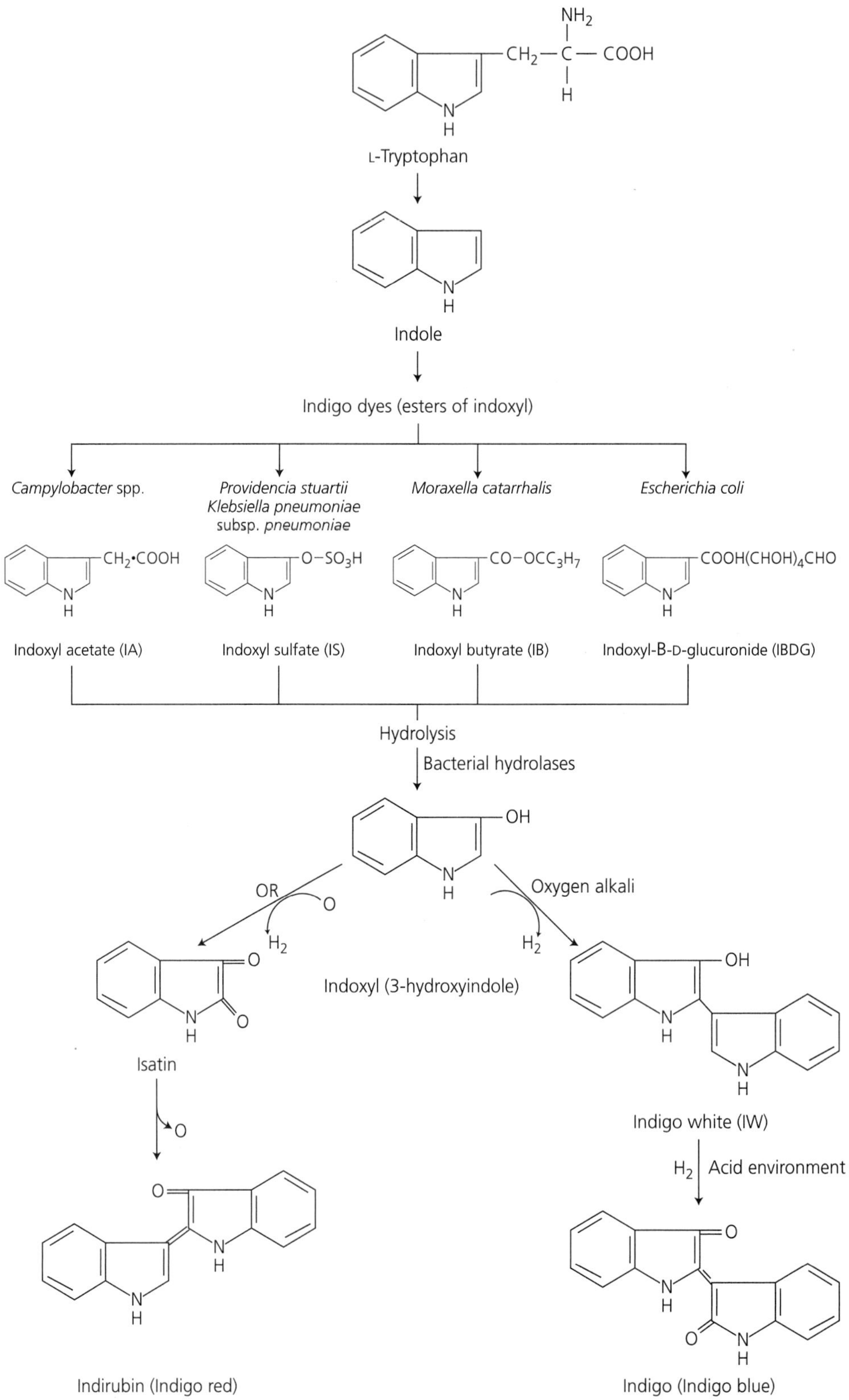

L-Tryptophan

↓

Indole

↓

Indigo dyes (esters of indoxyl)

Campylobacter spp.	Providencia stuartii, Klebsiella pneumoniae subsp. pneumoniae	Moraxella catarrhalis	Escherichia coli
Indoxyl acetate (IA)	Indoxyl sulfate (IS)	Indoxyl butyrate (IB)	Indoxyl-B-D-glucuronide (IBDG)

Hydrolysis
Bacterial hydrolases

↓

Indoxyl (3-hydroxyindole)

— OR / O, H_2 → Isatin → Indirubin (Indigo red)

— Oxygen alkali, H_2 → Indigo white (IW) → H_2 | Acid environment → Indigo (Indigo blue)

Exact chromophore is uncertain; ketones (C=O) in a closed ring occur often in dyes. Indigo is regarded as having chromophore properties (10).

Dealler et al. (3) showed that all bacteria that had indoxyl sulfatase activity also had indoxyl phosphatase activity, suggesting that the same enzyme hydrolyzes the two substrate. Optimal pH is 5.1 for both activities (3).

Esterases break ester linkages between substrate groups and carrier molecules (2). Loss of substrate moiety releases indoxyl, which reacts spontaneously to produce indigo blue and indirubin (6). The color compounds indigo white, indigo, and indirubin (indigo red) are visible at very low concentrations, which makes tests sensitive and rapid.

IV. PROCEDURES/RESULTS

A. **Indoxyl acetate (IA) hydrolysis (IAH)**
  1. Method of Mills and Gherna (11)
  2. Reagent
     a. Indoxyl acetate: Sigma Chemical Co. (see Appendix 11)
     b. Solution: 10% (wt/vol) indoxyl acetate in acetone; 1 g indoxyl in 10 mL acetone
  3. Differential disk preparation
     a. Disks: 0.64 cm (0.25 in.) diameter
        (1) Commercially available
            (a) American Type Culture Collection (ATCC), Manassas, VA (see Appendix 11)
            (b) Centers for Disease Control (CDC)
     b. Impregnation of disk(s); two methods
        (1) Method 1: place **sterile** disk(s) on a dry surface and add 0.5 mL (50 µL) per disk. Air dry away from direct light.
        (2) Method 2
            (a) Place 100 **sterile** blank concentration disks in dark bottle containing 0.25 g of indoxyl acetate dissolved in 2.5 mL of acetone.
            (b) Spread saturated disks on **glass** Petri dish and air dry away from direct light.
     c. Shelf life is 6–8 months if stored in a tightly capped amber bottle, protected from light, under a desiccant (silica gel), at 4°C (refrigerator) (6). On and Holmes (12) showed that disks impregnated with 25 µL of substrate were more reliable than those with 50 µL. Mills and Gherna (11) showed that all strains that hydrolyzed indoxyl acetate did so regardless of culture medium used.
  4. Inocula
     a. **Pure** cultures of organisms being tested; inocula from heart infusion agar supplemented with 5% defibrinated rabbit blood (HIA-RB) incubated at 36°C, in 5% CO_2 for 18–24 h.
     b. **Heavy** inocula (6)
  5. Procedures; three choices
     a. **Method 1**
        (1) Colonies of *Campylobacter* spp. smeared onto a disk
        (2) Moisten each disk with a drop of **sterile** distilled water
        (3) Results at room temperature (22–25°C) (11)
            (a) Positive (+)
                1. Dark blue color **5–10 min;** weakly positive (+ʷ) a paler blue color in 10–30 min (15)
                2. Hydrolysis
            (b) Negative −: no color change within 20 min; no hydrolysis
     b. **Method 2 (tube)**

(1) Suspend colonies in 0.3 mL of **sterile** distilled water; 13 × 100 mm glass tube.
(2) Add disk to suspension.
(3) Results at room temperature (22–25°C)
  (a) Positive (+)
    1. Dark blue color within 10–15 min (11); weakly positive (+^{w}) is pale blue in 10–45 min
    2. Hydrolysis
  (b) Negative −: no color change; no hydrolysis
  c. **Method 3** (6)
    (1) Disks impregnated with indoxyl acetate; 0.25 g dissolved in 2.5 mL acetone
    (2) Place disk on glass microscopic slide and moisten with 1–2 drops **sterile** distilled water.
    (3) Smear colonies onto disk.
    (4) Results at room temperature (22–25°C)
      (a) Positive (+): blueness within 1 min; color intensifies on prolonged standing up to 20 min
      (b) Negative (−): no color change within 20 min
B. **Indoxyl sulfate (IS) hydrolysis**
  1. Determined on purple bag syndrome (PUBS) in which urinary catheter bag of a patient turns purple over a period of hours or days following catheterization (1, 17). Chemical identity unknown, but suggested to be a mixture of indigo and indirubin, although indirubin not specifically identified (16)
  2. Plates of blood agar base supplemented with 7.9 mM indoxyl sulfate (3); Sigma Chemical Co.
  3. Four-quadrant streaking of test organism for maximum isolation
  4. Incubation: 35°C, 48 h
  5. Positive (+): colonies a deep blue color; hydrolysis
C. **Indoxyl butyrate (IB) hydrolysis**
  1. Indoxyl butyrate strips
    a. Butylase Lab M. Co., Bury, England
    b. Store in sealed plastic at 4°C with desiccant; shelf life 4 months (2)
  2. Inocula
    a. Growth medium: chocolate agar, nutrient agar, or blood agar plate
    b. **Pure** culture
    c. Incubation: 35°C, 14–18 h, 5% CO_2
  3. Procedure
    a. Smear enough **pure** culture onto filter paper strip to be visible.
    b. Moisten strip with 10 μL of water at room temperature (22–25°C). Studies showed no difference between wetting with tap water, sterile distilled water, Tris buffer (pH 7.5), or 0.9% saline (2). Leave at room temperature.
    c. Positive (+): blue-green color at inoculum site within 2.5 min (2)
D. **Indoxyl β-D-glucuronide (IBDG) hydrolysis** (4)
  1. Differentiation of lactose fermenters, nonlactose fermenters, and IBDG-positive *E. coli* (4); immediate visualization and detection of *E. coli* on primary plates
  2. MacConkey (MAC) agar supplemented with 0.8 g IBDG/L (MAC-IBDG agar)
  3. With calibrated loop, inoculate plate with 0.01 mL of urine; streak four-quadrant method with loop.
  4. Incubate 35°C, 18 h
  5. Positive (+)
    a. Deep blue-black colonies
    b. *E. coli*

V. QUALITY CONTROL MICROORGANISMS

(*Note:* Do a quality control check when disks are first prepared and monthly thereafter.)

A. **Indoxyl acetate**
   1. Positive (+): *Campylobacter jejuni* ATCC 29428
   2. Negative −: drop of water to disk
B. **Indoxyl sulfate**
   1. Positive (+): *Providencia stuartii* ATCC 29914
   2. Negative −: *Escherichia coli* ATCC 25922
C. **Indoxyl butyrate**
   1. Positive (+): *Moraxella catarrhalis* ATCC 11020
   2. Negative −: *Neisseria lactamica* ATCC 23970
D. **Indoxyl-β-D-glucuronide**
   1. Positive (+): *Escherichia coli* ATCC 25922
   2. Negative −: *Klebsiella pneumoniae* subsp. *pneumoniae* ATCC 10031

VI. PRECAUTIONS

A. **Indoxyl acetate**
   1. Freshly prepared disks are white. On prolonged storage (up to 1 year), disks become discolored (pale purple) (6). Discard any discolored disks.
B. **Indoxyl butyrate**
   1. If cold container is opened and closed frequently, strips may have a slight pink discoloration caused by condensation of water (2).
   2. Dealler et al. (2) showed that positive results with *Acinetobacter lwoffii*, an oxidase-negative organism, and *Moraxella lacunata*, an uncommon Gram-negative coccobacillus that forms clear colonies, cause no problems in identification of *M. catarrhalis* on strip.
C. **Indoxyl-β-D-glucuronide**
   1. β-Glucuronidase activity is confined to genera *Escherichia*, *Shigella*, and *Salmonella* (7), which should be differentiated easily by ability to ferment lactose. *Shigella* and *Salmonella* spp. are rarely found in urine and may also be differentiated by ONPG and spot indole tests (7).
   2. Delisle and Ley (4) showed that *E. coli* 0157:H7 did not hydrolyze IBDG.

REFERENCES

1. Barlow GB, Dickson JAS. Purple urine bags. Lancet 1978;i:220–221.
2. Dealler SF, Abbott M, Croughan MJ, Hawkey PM. Identification of *Branhamella catarrhalis* in 2.5 min with an indoxyl butyrate strip test. J Clin Microbiol 1989;27(6):1390–1391.
3. Dealler SF, Hawkey PM, Millar MR. Enzymatic degradation of urinary indoxyl sulfate by *Providencia stuartii* and *Klebsiella pneumoniae* causes the purple bag syndrome. J Clin Microbiol 1988;26(10):2152–2156.
4. Delisle GJ, Ley A. Rapid detection of *Escherichia coli* in urine samples by a new chromogenic β-glucuronidase assay. J Clin Microbiol 1989;27(4):778–779.
5. Guibault GG, Kramer DN. Resorufin butyrate and indoxyl acetate as fluorigenic substrates for cholinesterase. Anal Chem 1965;37:120–123.
6. Hodge DS, Borczyk A, Wat L-L. Evaluation of the indoxyl acetate hydrolysis test for the differentiation of campylobacters. J Clin Microbiol 1990;28(6):1482–1483.
7. Killian M, Bulow P. Rapid diagnosis of *Enterobacteriaceae*. I. Detection of bacterial glycosidases. Acta Pathol Microbiol Scand Sect B 1976;84(5):245–251.
8. Koneman EW, Allen SD, Janda WM, et al. Color Atlas and Textbook of Diagnostic Microbiology, ed 4. Philadelphia: JB Lippincott, 1992:443.
9. Ley AN, Bowers RJ, Wolfe S. Indoxyl-beta-D-glucuronide, a novel chromogenic reagent for the specific detection and enumeration of *Escherichia coli* in environmental samples. Can J Clin Microbiol 1988;34:690–693.
10. Lillie RD. HJ Conn's Biological Stains, ed 9. Baltimore: Williams & Wilkins, 1977:451–452.

11. Mills CK, Gherna RL. Hydrolysis of indoxyl acetate by *Campylobacter* species. J Clin Microbiol 1987;25(8):1560–1561.
12. On SLW, Holmes B. Assessment of enzyme detection tests useful in identification of campylobacteria. J Clin Microbiol 1992;30(3):746–749.
13. Oser BL, ed. Hawk's Physiological Chemistry, ed 14. New York: McGraw-Hill, 1965:851.
14. Patton CM, Shaffer N, Edmonds P, et al. Human disease associated with *Campylobacter upsaliensis* (catalase-negative or weakly positive *Campylobacter* species) in the United States. J Clin Microbiol 1989;27(1):66–73.
15. Popovic-Uroic T, Patton CM, Nicholson MA, Kiehlbauch JA. Evaluation of the indoxyl acetate hydrolysis test for rapid differentiation of *Campylobacter, Helicobacter,* and *Wolinella* species. J Clin Microbiol 1990;28(10):2335–2339.
16. Sapira JD, Somani S, Shapiro AP, et al. Some observations concerning mammalian indoxyl metabolism and its relationship to the formation of urinary indigo pigments. Metabolism 1971;20:474–486.
17. Stott A, Khan M, Roberts C, Galpin IJ. Purple urine bag syndrome. Ann Clin Biochem 1987;24:185–188.
18. Watkins WD, Rippey SR, Clavet CR, et al. Novel compound for identifying *Escherichia coli*. Appl Environ Microbiol 1988;54:1874–1875.

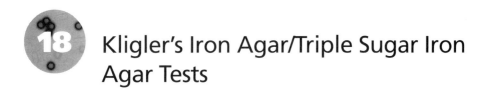

18 Kligler's Iron Agar/Triple Sugar Iron Agar Tests

I. PRINCIPLE

To determine the ability of an organism to attack a specific carbohydrate(s) incorporated in a basal growth medium, with or without the production of gas, along with the determination of possible hydrogen sulfide (H_2S) production

II. PURPOSE

(Also see Chapter 45)

(*Note:* An asterisk in front of an organism's name indicates variable reactions. Organisms in boldface are those most frequently encountered in the specific KIA/TSI reaction listed. For more detail about a particular microorganism (e.g., former classification, human or environmental organism) see tables in Chapter 45 on identification schemas for *Enterobacteriaceae* and intestinal bacteria.)

A. H_2S production and/or fermentation patterns are generally characteristic of specific bacterial groups, genera, or species, especially among the *Enterobacteriaceae* (5, 9).
  1. Acid/acid, with/without gas
     a. KIA/TSI

         Butvicia aquatica
         Buttiauxella agrestis*
         **Cedecea davisae*
         **Cedecea lapageri*
         **Cedecea neteri*
         ***Citrobacter* spp.**
         Enteric group 64
         Enterobacter aerogenes
         **Enterobacter amnigenus* biogroups 1 & 2
         **Enterobacter asburiae*
         Enterobacter cloacae
         **Enterobacter dissolvens*
         **Enterobacter gergoviae*
         Enterobacter intermedius
         Enterobacter nimipressuralis
         Enterobacter sakazakii
         Escherichia coli
         ***Escherichia coli* inactive**
         **Escherichia hermannii*
         Escherichia vulneris
         Ewingella americana
         Klebsiella ornithinolytica
         Klebsiella oxytoca

Klebsiella planticola
   ***Klebsiella pneumoniae** subsp. ozaenae*
   Klebsiella pneumoniae subsp. *pneumoniae*
   Klebsiella terrigena
   Kluyvera spp.
   Leclerica adecarboxylata
   Moellerella wisconsensis
   Pantoea agglomerans
   Plesiomonas shigelloides biogroups 1 & 2
   Rahnella aquatilis
   **Serratia ficaria*
   Serratia fonticola
   Serratia odorifera biogroups 1 & 2
   **Serratia plymuthica*
   Serratia rubidaea
   **Yersinia bercovieri*
   **Yersinia frederiksenii*
   Yersinia intermedia
   **Yersinia mollaretii*

 b. **TSI only**

   Arsenophonus nasoniae
   **Cedecea* species 3
   Cedecea species 5
   Edwardsiella hoshinae
   Edwardsiella tarda biogroup 1
   Enteric group 68
   Enterobacter hormaechae
   **Klebsiella pneumoniae* subsp. *rhinoscleromatis*
   **Pantoea dispersa*
   Proteus inconstans
   Proteus myxofaciens
   Proteus penneri
   Proteus rettgeri
   **Providencia rustigianii*
   Providencia stuartii
   Serratia entomophila
   Serratia grimesii
   Serratia marcescens
   Serratia proteamaculans
   Tatumella ptyseos
   **Yersinia aldovae*
   Yersinia enterocolitica
   Yersinia rohdei

2. **Acid/acid, H$_2$S**
   a. **KIA/TSI**

      **Budvicia aquatica*
      Citrobacter freundii
      Salmonella choleraesuis** subsp. **arizonae
      **Salmonella choleraesuis* subsp. *diarizonae*
      Salmonella indica

b. **TSI only**
   *Proteus mirabilis
   *Proteus penneri
   *Proteus vulgaris
3. **Alkaline/acid, with/without gas**
   a. **KIA only**
      *Arsenophonus nasoniae
      *Cedecea davisae
      *Cedecea neteri
      Cedecea subsp. 5
      *Citrobacter amalonaticus biogroup 1
      Edwardsiella hoshinae
      Edwardsiella tarda biogroup 1
      Enteric group 68
      Enterobacter ammigenus biogroup 1
      Enterobacter asburiae
      *Enterobacter dissolvens
      *Enterobacter gergoviae
      Enterobacter hormaechae
      Pantoea agglomerans
      Pantoea dispersa
      Proteus inconstans
      Proteus myxofaciens
      *Proteus penneri
      Proteus rettgeri
      Serratia entomophila
      *Serratia ficaria
      Serratia grimesii
      Serratia marcescens
      Serratia plymuthica
      Serratia proteamaculans
      Tatumella ptyseos
      *Yersinia bercovieri
      Yersinia enterocolitica
      *Yersinia frederiksenii
      *Yersinia intermedia
      *Yersinia mollaretii
      Yersinia rohdei
   b. **KIA/TSI**
      *Budvicia aquatica
      *Cedecea lapagei
      *Cedecea species 3
      ****Citrobacter amalonaticus**
      ****Citrobacter freundii**
      ****Citrobacter koseri**
      Edwardsiella ictaluri
      Enteric group 63
      *Enterobacter aerogenes
      Enterobacter amnigenus biogroup 2
      Enterobacter cancerogenus

Escherichia blattae
Escherichia coli inactive
Escherichia fergusonii
Escherichia hermannii
Escherichia vulneris
Ewingella americana
Hafnia alvei
Hafnia alvei biogroup 1
Klebsiella pneumoniae subsp. *ozaenae*
Klebsiella pneumoniae subsp. *rhinoscleromatis*
Kluyvera cryocrescens
Morganella morganii
***Morganella morganii* biogroups 1 & 2**
  Obesumbacterium proteus
Pragia fontinum
Providencia spp.
Salmonella choleraesuis serovar. *choleraesuis*
Salmonella choleraesuis serovar. *paratyphi* A
  Shigella spp.
Yersinia aldovae
  Yersinia kristensenii
Yersinia pestis
  Yersinia pseudotuberculosis
  Yersinia ruckeri
  Yokenella regensburgei
  Xenorhabdus spp.

4. **Alkaline/acid, gas, H$_2$S**
   a. **KIA only**

      Proteus penneri
      Proteus vulgaris

   b. **KIA/TSI**

      Budvicia aquatica
      Citrobacter freundii
      Edwardsiella tarda
      Leminorella spp.
      Morganella morganii biogroup 2 (rare)
      Pragia fontinum
      Proteus mirabilis
      ***Salmonella* spp.**

5. **Alkaline/alkaline or alkaline/no change: KIA and TSI**

      Acinetobacter baumanni
      Acinetobacter calcoaceticus
      Acinetobacter lwoffii
      Alcaligenes faecalis
      Alcaligenes latus
      Alcaligenes piechaudii
      Alcaligenes xylosoxidans
      Pseudomonas aeruginosa

6. To aid in genus speciation

a. *Yersinia enterocolitica* (TSI, acid/acid) from *Y. pestis* (TSI, alkaline/acid) and *Y. pseudotuberculosis* (TSI, alkaline/acid)
   b. *Edwardsiella tarda* (H_2S +) from other *Edwardsiella* spp. (H_2S −)
   c. *Proteus inconstans, P. myxofaciens,* and *P. rettgeri* (all H_2S −), and *P. penneri* (H_2S variable) from *P. mirabilis* (H_2S +) and *P. vulgaris* (H_2S +)
B. Aid in identification of bacteria other than the *Enterobacteriaceae*
   1. *Shewanella putrefaciens* (H_2S +) (formerly *Pseudomonas putrefaciens*) from *S. hanedai* (H_2S −) and *S. benthica* (H_2S −) (1, 9)
   2. Aerotolerant former campylobacters, *Arcobacter nitrofigilis* (H_2S +) from *A. butzleri* (H_2S −) and *A. cryaerophilus* (H_2S −) (9)
   3. Differentiation of *Erysipelothrix rhusiopathiae* (H_2S +) from other nonenteric Gram-negative bacilli (H_2S −) (9)

III. BIOCHEMISTRY INVOLVED

Kligler's iron agar (KIA) and triple sugar iron agar (TSI) are tubed differential media that serve a dual purpose: (*a*) determination of carbohydrate fermentations, and (*b*) determination of H_2S production. An organism can use various substrates incorporated into the medium; the pattern of substrates metabolized is used to differentiate among various groups, genera, or species, primarily among the *Enterobacteriaceae*.

KIA contains two carbohydrates: **1.0%** lactose and **0.1%** glucose. TSI may be substituted for KIA; the primary **difference** is the addition of a third carbohydrate, sucrose, at **1.0%** concentration. The biochemistry is basically the same as that in KIA. Thus only KIA is discussed in detail. In KIA, some organisms can ferment **both** carbohydrates, others ferment **only** glucose; still others can ferment **neither** lactose nor glucose. Carbohydrate fermentation may occur with or without gas production (CO_2 + H_2).

Fermentation occurs both aerobically (on the slant) and anaerobically (in the butt). On the slant the monosaccharide glucose is initially catabolized via the Embden-Meyerhof-Parnas anaerobic pathway used by both aerobes and anaerobes to yield the key intermediate pyruvic acid. Pyruvic acid is then further degraded to completion via the Krebs' cycle by either aerobes or facultative anaerobes to yield CO_2, H_2O, and energy.

Both pathways, the Embden-Meyerhof-Parnas and the Krebs' cycle, involve sequential steps that produce many intermediates, each step mediated by specific enzymes. Lactose is a disaccharide composed of two monosaccharide units: glucose and galactose.

$$\text{Lactose} \xrightarrow{\beta \text{ Galactosidase}} \text{Glucose} + \text{galactose}$$

$$\text{Glucose or galactose} \xrightarrow[\text{aerobic}]{\text{Krebs' cycle}} CO_2 + H_2O + \text{energy}$$

In the KIA butt (deep), anaerobic conditions exist so that glucose is metabolized via the Embden-Meyerhof-Parnas pathway to ATP and pyruvic acid, which is converted further to various **stable** end products: lactic acid and/or other organic acids, aldehydes, alcohols, CO_2, H_2, and energy.

$$\text{Glucose} \xrightarrow[\text{anaerobic}]{\text{Embden-Meyerhof-Parnas pathway}} \begin{cases} \text{organic acids} \\ \text{aldehydes} \\ \text{alcohols} \\ CO_2 + H_2 \\ \text{energy} \end{cases}$$

KIA reactions are used **primarily** to identify members of the *Enterobacteriaceae* (the enterics), which are by definition catalase-positive, Gram-negative bacilli, **all** of which ferment glucose to acid. Also, many nonenteric Gram-negative intestinal bacilli exist whose identification or separation from the *Enterobacteriaceae* is aided by their KIA reactions. Three basic fermentation patterns are observed on KIA medium: (*a*) glucose fermentation **only**, (*b*) fermentation of both glucose and lactose, and (*c*) failure to ferment glucose or lactose.

For identification purposes **all** KIA tubes **must** be interpreted for carbohydrate fermentation at the end of 18–24 h of incubation. Earlier or delayed interpretations may yield invalid fermentation patterns that will result in mistakes in grouping organisms among the *Enterobacteriaceae* or in identifying genus and/or species.

Fermentation of Glucose Only (Alkaline/Acid)

The first KIA pattern after 18–24 h of incubation is an alkaline slant and an acid butt (alkaline/acid). This reaction is observed with organisms capable of fermenting **only** glucose; they are non–lactose fermenters.

The slant is alkaline (red), indicating aerobic degradation of glucose. After 18–24 h of incubation the low glucose concentration (0.1%) is depleted, and the organism starts to use the peptones in the medium for its growth nutrients. Catabolism of peptone releases ammonia (NH_3) yielding an alkaline pH with phenol red, the pH indicator incorporated in the medium.

However, the butt of KIA has a yellow color because of the anaerobic degradation of glucose. The glucose here is also degraded after 18–24 h of incubation; however, acid end products are formed yielding an acid pH (yellow color); the acid reaction is maintained in the butt because of a lower oxygen tension.

If a glucose-fermenting organism on KIA were read earlier (e.g., 12 h or less), the slant would be acid, since in this short time the glucose has not yet been depleted completely and would give a false reaction. A microbiologist would interpret the organism as capable of fermenting both carbohydrates present, glucose and lactose. Likewise, if the KIA tube is not read until after incubation for 48 h or longer, the slant and butt may both be alkaline (red), indicating that neither carbohydrate was fermented. The acidity normally present in the butt is due to production of stable acid products; eventually, however, these products are oxidized, and the organism shifts to using peptones for its nutrients, resulting in an alkaline pH throughout the KIA tube (both slant and butt).

Fermentation of Lactose and Glucose (Acid/Acid)

Some organisms can ferment both lactose and glucose for their nutrients, resulting in a KIA reaction of an acid slant and an acid butt (acid/acid) after 18–24 h of incubation. The lactose concentration (1.0%) is 10 times that of glucose. In 18–24 h, the lactose (present in a greater amount) has not been depleted, and an acid condition still exists. If the same KIA tube were read after 48 h or longer, the slant would eventually turn alkaline because of depletion of lactose and use of peptones.

Neither Lactose nor Glucose Fermented (Alkaline/Alkaline; Alkaline/No Change)

Certain bacteria, mainly the Gram-negative nonenteric bacilli, cannot ferment either glucose or lactose. These bacteria are present in the intestinal tract along with members of the *Enterobacteriaceae,* and it is necessary to definitely identify them as nonenterics. Since these bacteria cannot derive their nutrients from the carbohydrates, they rely on the peptone in the medium. These nonenterics can use peptone either aerobically or anaerobically, resulting in two possible KIA reactions. An organism that yields a KIA with an alkaline slant and alkaline butt degrades peptone both aerobically and anaerobically. A reaction of an alkaline slant and no change in the butt is the result of an organism that can only catabolize peptone aerobically; hence, only the slant exhibits a color change (red). When peptones are degraded producing an alkaline pH due to the release of ammonia (NH_3), the medium is imparted with a deep red color.

$$\text{Peptones} \xrightarrow[\text{anaerobically}]{\text{aerobically}} \text{Ammonia } (NH_3)$$

Therefore, a KIA reaction can be interpreted in four ways depending on the bacteria being tested:

1. Alkaline/acid: **only** glucose attacked
2. Acid/acid: glucose **and** lactose attacked
3. Alkaline/alkaline: **neither** glucose **nor** lactose attacked; peptones used
4. Alkaline/no change: **neither** glucose **nor** lactose attacked; peptones used

A KIA tube is observed to determine if the bacteria present can ferment lactose and/or glucose and also, if gas (CO_2 and O_2) is produced as an end product of carbohydrate metabolism. A gas producer is termed **aerogenic** and is evident by splitting of the medium, a single gas bubble, complete displacement of the medium from the bottom of the tube leaving a clear area, or a slight indentation of the medium from the side of the tube. Non–gas producing organisms are termed **anaerogenic**.

H_2S Formation

Another system for differentiation is afforded by H_2S indicators in the medium; a salt, ferric ammonium citrate, and another chemical, sodium thiosulfate. Both indicators **must** be present, since the end result is a two-step procedure.

Step 1

$$\text{Bacterium (acid environment)} + \text{sodium thiosulfate} \longrightarrow H_2S \text{ gas} \uparrow$$

H_2S is a colorless gas; thus a second indicator is necessary to visualize H_2S production.

Step 2

$$H_2S + \text{ferric ions} \longrightarrow \text{Ferrous sulfide} \downarrow \text{(insoluble black precipitate)}$$

(See Chapter 15, Hydrogen Sulfide Test, for a more detailed explanation of the biochemistry of H_2S production.) The black precipitate of ferrous sulfide indicating H_2S production may mask the acid condition produced in the KIA butt; therefore, if H_2S is produced, an acid condition exists **even if not observable.** Tittsler (15) notes a parallel between an organism's ability to produce H_2S and the gases CO_2 and H_2 from carbohydrate fermentations. Not all monosaccharides are degraded by all bacterial species; their fermentation patterns and H_2S production differ, aiding in group, genus, or species identification. Fermentation is an anaerobic process, and bacterial fermenters are usually facultative anaerobes (6).

When reading a KIA after 18–24 h of incubation, look for (a) fermentation of lactose and/or glucose, (b) production of CO_2 and H_2 from carbohydrate metabolism, and (c) H_2S production.

IV. MEDIA EMPLOYED

A. **Kligler's iron agar (KIA)**
   1. Formulation of Kligler (7, 8); a combination of Kligler's lead acetate medium and Russell's double sugar agar (13)
   2. Ingredients, pH 7.4 ± 0.2

Beef (meat) extract	3.0 g
Yeast extract	3.0 g
Peptone	15.0 g
Proteose peptone	5.0 g
Lactose	10.0 g
Glucose (dextrose)	1.0 g
Ferrous sulfate, $FeSO_4 \cdot 7H_2O$	0.2 g
or Ferric ammonium citrate (50/50)	0.5 g
Ferric citrate, $FeC_6H_5O_7$	
Ammonium citrate, $[(NH_4)_3C_6H_5O_7]$	
Sodium chloride, NaCl	5.0 g
Sodium thiosulfate, $Na_2S_2O_3 \cdot 5H_2O$	0.3 g
Phenol red	0.024 g
Agar	12.0 g
Deionized water	1000.0 mL

(*Note:* ferrous, Fe^{2+} or iron (II); ferric, Fe^{3+} or iron (III))

B. **Triple sugar iron agar (TSI)**
  1. Formulation of Krumwiede and Kohn (triple sugar medium) (10); Russell double sugar medium (13) modified by addition of sucrose. Sulkin and Willett (14) made a further modification by adding H_2S indicators; final formulation is a modification by Hajna (4).

  Grouping the *Enterobacteriaceae* by TSI reactions varies slightly from that by KIA, since some non–lactose fermenters can ferment sucrose, which results in a different slant reaction (Table 16.1). For example, *Proteus vulgaris* is alkaline/acid on KIA but is usually acid/acid on TSI.

  2. Addition of sucrose aids in screening for *Salmonella* and *Shigella,* since only rare strains use either lactose or sucrose.
  3. Ingredients: same as KIA with the following **additions:**
     a. Sucrose, 10.0 g/L (1%).
     b. H_2S indicators: ferrous ammonium sulfate, $FeNH_4(SO_4)_2 \cdot 12H_2O$ or ferrous sulfate, $FeSO_4 \cdot 7H_2O$

  Both KIA and TSI contain four protein derivatives: beef extract, yeast extract, peptone, and proteose peptone; these ingredients make both media nutritionally rich (9).

Table 18.1. KIA/TSI Reactions and Colors

Reaction	KIA	TSI
Alk/A (red/yellow)	Glucose only fermented Peptones used	Glucose only fermented Peptones used
A/A (yellow/yellow)	Glucose fermented Lactose fermented	Glucose fermented Lactose +/or sucrose fermented
Alk/Alk (red/red)	Neither glucose nor lactose fermented; peptones used	Neither glucose, lactose, nor sucrose, fermented; peptones used

C. Carbohydrates
  1. KIA

     Lactose, 1.0%
     Glucose (dextrose), 0.1%

  2. TSI

Lactose, 1.0%
Sucrose, 1.0%
Glucose (dextrose), 0.1%
- D. pH indicator: phenol red
    1. Alkaline: red
    2. Acid: yellow
    3. Uninoculated medium: pH 7.4; reddish orange
- E. H_2S indicators
    1. Sodium thiosulfate
    2. Ferric ammonium citrate, ferric ammonium sulfate, ferrous ammonium sulfate or ferrous sulfate
- F. Method of preparation
    1. Weigh out amount accurately as directed on the label. Various company products may differ slightly.
    2. Rehydrate with distilled or deionized water.
    3. Heat **gently** into solution.
    4. Dispense approximately 5.0 mL per tube.
    5. Autoclave; 121°C, 15 lb, 15 min
    6. Cool in a **slanted** position with **deep butts** ("deeps")
- G. Method of inoculation
    1. **Pure** culture, single colony
    2. Pick center of colony with an inoculating needle.
    3. Slanted tubed medium: fishtail slant; stab butt. Order may be reversed if preferred.
- H. Incubation: 35°C; 18–24 h, **no earlier or later**

V. QUALITY CONTROL MICROORGANISMS FOR KIA/TSI

Organism	ATCC	Slant	Butt	H_2S
Escherichia coli	25922	Acid	Acid, gas	−
Shigella flexneri	12022	Alk	Acid	−
Edwardsiella tarda	15947	Alk	Acid	+
Pseudomonas aeruginosa	27853	Alk	Alk	−

VI. RESULTS

> See Figures 18.1–18.8 (Appendix 1) for colored photographic results

VII. INTERPRETATION

- A. **Carbohydrate** use
    1. Fermentation of **only** glucose
        a. Slant
            (1) Alkaline reaction
            (2) Red color
        b. Butt
            (1) Acid reaction
            (2) Yellow color
                (a) If H_2S gas is also produced, the black precipitate may mask the acidity.
                (b) An acid condition exists in the butt and is recorded as such.

2. Fermentation of **both** glucose and lactose
   a. Slant
      (1) Acid reaction
      (2) Yellow color
   b. Butt
      (1) Acid reaction
      (2) Yellow color
         (a) *Citrobacter freundii* produces H_2S besides fermenting both carbohydrates.
         (b) However, an acid condition exists in the butt and is recorded as such if unobservable.
3. **Neither** glucose **nor** lactose fermented (nonenterics)
   a. Slant
      (1) Alkaline reaction
      (2) Red color
   b. Butt
      (1) Aerobic organism
         (a) No growth
         (b) No change in color
            1. Color same as uninoculated tube
            2. Reddish orange color
            3. If unsure compare with an uninoculated tube
      (2) Facultative organism
         (a) Alkaline reaction
         (b) Red color
4. **Neither** glucose **nor** lactose fermented; fairly common
   a. Slant
      (1) **Growth only**
      (2) No change in color; same as uninoculated tube (reddish orange color)
   b. Butt
      (1) **Growth only**
      (2) No change in color; same as an uninoculated tube (reddish orange color)
B. **Gas production**
   1. Aerogenic
      a. Gas production: CO_2 and H_2
      b. Evident by one of the following:
         (1) A **single** gas bubble
         (2) Bubbles in the medium
         (3) Splitting of medium
         (4) Complete displacement of the medium from the bottom of the tube, leaving a clear area
         (5) Slight indentation of medium from the side of the tube
   2. Anaerogenic: **no** gas production
C. **H_2S production:** a black precipitate (ferrous sulfide) is evidenced by
   1. A black color spread throughout the entire butt, masking the acidity; **may** even be slight evidence on the slant
   2. A black ring near the top of the butt area
   3. A black precipitate scattered throughout the butt but not entirely masking the acidity present

Any combination of the above reactions **may** be observed in interpreting a KIA result. **Always** observe for all three characteristics: (*a*) carbohydrate fermentations, (*b*) gas production (CO_2 and H_2), and (*c*) H_2S production. Record all observations.

VIII. PRECAUTIONS

TSI may be substituted for KIA. The primary **difference** is the addition of a third carbohydrate, 1% sucrose. However, the principle, purpose, and biochemistry are basically the same as those for KIA. These precautions pertain to both media.

A. A KIA tube **must** be read and interpreted within an 18- to 24-h incubation period. If read earlier (e.g., 12 h), a false-positive result of acid/acid may occur or the carbohydrate fermented may not have yet produced enough acid to change the pH indicator (phenol red) incorporated in the medium. A KIA tube read **after** 24 h may give a false alkaline/alkaline result because the organism used peptones, resulting in an alkaline pH.
B. An H_2S-producing organism may produce so much black precipitate (ferrous sulfide) that the acidity produced in the butt is completely masked. However, if H_2S is produced, an acid condition **does exist** in the butt even if not observable and should be so recorded.
C. KIA results are **always** written in a standard manner. First the slant reaction then the butt reaction, separated by a slash mark (i.e., slant reaction/butt reaction). The slant reaction involves the presence or absence of acidity (carbohydrate fermentation). When interpreting the butt reaction observe for (a) absence or presence of acidity (carbohydrate fermentation) or use of peptones, (b) presence of CO_2 and H_2 gases, and (c) the presence of a black precipitate indicating H_2S production. H_2S is a gas, but since it is colorless, the second H_2S indicator is necessary to detect its presence. The ferric ammonium citrate reacts with H_2S **gas** to yield the black precipitate ferrous sulfide observed in the butt. Thus, when recording H_2S production **do not** use the word *gas*; the symbol H_2S implies that the gas was produced.

The various KIA reactions that may be observed may be written out completely or may be abbreviated with abbreviations that are standard throughout all bacteriology laboratories. Acidity may be denoted by the letter *A*; alkalinity, the abbreviation *Alk* or the symbol *K*. The gases CO_2 and H_2 may be denoted by the word *gas*, the symbol *G*, or by circling the butt reaction. H_2S is denoted only by H_2S.

The various ways of recording the different KIA reactions are listed below; remember that the **slant reaction is first, the butt reaction second**.
1. Acid/acid: A/A
2. Acid/acid, gas

    A/A, gas
    A/A, G
    A/Ⓐ

3. Alkaline/acid

    Alk/A
    K/A

4. Alkaline/acid, gas

    Alk/A, gas   K/A, gas
    Alk/A, G   K/A, G
    Alk/Ⓐ   K/Ⓐ

5. Alkaline/acid, gas, H_2S

    Alk/A, gas, H_2S K/A, gas, H_2S
    Alk/A, G, H_2S K/A, G, H_2S
    Alk/Ⓐ, H_2S K/Ⓐ, H_2S

6. Alkaline/acid, H_2S

Alk/A, H$_2$S

K/A, H$_2$S

7. Acid/acid, H$_2$S   A/A, H$_2$S
8. Alkaline/alkaline

    Alk/alk

    K/K

9. Alkaline/no change

    Alk/NC

    K/NC

10. No change/no change: NC/NC

The symbol K, denoting alkalinity, is acceptable and is frequently used in laboratories or reference books. Before using this symbol make sure it is acceptable in your particular bacteriology laboratory.

D. KIA contains **no** inhibitor; therefore, any organism may grow on this medium; it permits growth of the most fastidious species **excluding** obligate (strict) anaerobes. KIA tubed differential medium is used to identify all members of the *Enterobacteriaceae* (enterics) and the nonenteric Gram-negative intestinal bacilli. Hence, before inoculating a KIA tube with an unknown organism **be sure** it is a catalase-positive, Gram-negative bacillus. If other organisms are inoculated onto KIA, a variety of reactions may be observed, and some will fit no pattern for enteric groupings (e.g., acid/alkaline, acid/no change). Medium **can only** be used to test a single colony recovered on primary or selective plates.

A **pure** culture is essential for inoculating a KIA tube. Always pick the center of a well-isolated colony on solid plate medium with an **inoculating needle**. If KIA is inoculated with a mixed culture, irregular observations may occur after incubation; following biochemical testing mixed reactions are usual, which makes it impossible to fit the organism accurately into a particular pattern for group, genus, or species identification.

Even if an organisms is a glucose fermenter and is suspected of being an enteric, a cytochrome oxidase test should be performed to exclude organisms belonging to other genera of fermenting bacteria such as *Aeromonas, Plesiomonas, Vibrio,* and *Pasteurella,* which are oxidase positive (9).

E. After the results of a KIA tube are recorded, refrigerate it to inoculate biochemicals for genus or genus and species identification or confirmation. Set the KIA tube in a rack along with tubes of biochemical test media to be inoculated. The KIA tube is incubated along with the biochemicals to maintain **continuity** of the specimen, since the KIA tube **should** have been labeled appropriately to identify the specimen. Usually biochemicals inoculated from a KIA tube are not labeled; hence, the KIA tube is placed in the first position in the rack, followed by the order for biochemical testing in your laboratory. This also maintains continuity when inoculating the various biochemical tubes. After incubation of the rack of biochemicals **do not** attempt to interpret the KIA tube again. The reaction has already been interpreted and recorded. A change in reaction is of no significance.

F. KIA will detect two types of gases: (*a*) CO$_2$ and H$_2$, which are end products of carbohydrate metabolism, and (*b*) H$_2$S. H$_2$S is colorless and it yields a black precipitate when it comes in contact with the salt ferric ammonium citrate or ferrous sulfate. Therefore, **only** the gases CO$_2$ and H$_2$ are recorded using the word *gas;* H$_2$S is used alone to denote hydrogen sulfide gas. **Do not** use the word *gas* to denote H$_2$S production.

Often an organism that produces CO$_2$ and H$_2$ **does not** exhibit any evidence of these gases in the KIA butt: bubbles, splitting of the medium, a slight indentation of the medium from the side of the tube, or a displacement of the medium from the bottom of the tube leaving a clear space. If gas is not observed with an organism normally producing gas, do not be disturbed. If gas is formed it will be detected in various carbohydrate tests (mainly glucose) using a Durham insert or semisolid medium.

If an organism can produce H_2S gas, its detection depends on the presence of **both** H_2S indicators: sodium thiosulfate and either ferric ammonium citrate or ferrous sulfate. If one is absent, H_2S **cannot** be detected.

G. Salmonella typhi usually produces a ring of H2S near the surface of the butt. However, this characteristic is not sufficient for identification purposes. Biochemical tests and serologic typing must be performed for definite identification and confirmation. Other H2S-producing organisms may at times produce a false-appearing ring of H2S because only a small amount of H2S is formed in the 18- to 24-h incubation period. Do not rely on the presence of a ring of H2S for definite identification of S. typhi.

H. **Do not** use an inoculating loop to inoculate a KIA tube. Stabbing the butt causes mechanical splitting that gives a false appearance of gas production (CO_2 and H_2).

I. **Do not** fail to stab the KIA butt during inoculation; failure to do so makes the result invalid. The order for inoculating a KIA tube: (*a*) fishtail slant, stab butt or (*b*) stab butt, fishtail slant is of no significance as long as both are inoculated. The order used depends on the microbiologist's preference.

J. BBL (12) recommends preparing KIA tubes the day they are to be used for greater accuracy; If not feasible then the medium should be melted and resolidified just before use.

K. The H_2S indicators in KIA medium are not as sensitive as lead acetate strips for detecting H_2S production. H_2S determination using KIA medium should be limited to members of the *Enterobacteriaceae;* other organisms require the **more sensitive** lead acetate strip procedure to detect H_2S formation.

L. Some organisms, mainly the *Klebsiella-Enterobacter* groups, produce so much gas (CO_2 and H_2) that the medium may be completely displaced by gas and be blown up into the closure (cap) of the tube. If this occurs handle the culture with great caution when subculturing, to avoid contamination of the culture or self-contamination.

M. The amount of H_2S produced by certain organisms varies. Some produce so much gas that the butt is completely blackened by the ferrous sulfide precipitate, others produce a moderate amount making the butt black but leaving the acidity visible, while still others produce only minute amounts in the 18- to 24-h incubation period. However, **any trace** of **blackening** in the butt indicates H_2S production and should be recorded as such. Occasionally *Proteus rettgeri* (formerly *Providencia rettgeri*) or *Morganella morganii* exhibits a darkening of the KIA butt, but this should **not** be interpreted as H_2S production.

N. Occasionally a KIA result of no change/no change is observed after incubation. **Do not** be hasty in discarding the tube. Check the tube carefully to see if there is **growth.** If there is **no growth,** possibly the microbiologist failed to inoculate the tube; look for a stab line in the butt and streak marks on the slant. Certain bacteria grow on KIA but exhibit no action on the carbohydrates present within 24 h nor a change in the pH indicator toward alkalinity. If growth is present, record the KIA reaction as NC/NC and proceed to the inoculation of biochemical tubes for identification after performing a Gram stain to confirm the presence of a Gram-negative bacillus.

O. Occasionally a KIA tube exhibits an **acid** reaction on the slant but **no change** in the butt. This could result from (*a*) inoculation with a Gram-positive organism that can only use lactose aerobically or (*b*) failure of the microbiologist to stab the butt. If this occurs, check the butt for a stab line, recheck the colony morphology on the plate medium used for KIA inoculation, and perform a Gram stain and a catalase test on the growth present on the slant.

P. *Klebsiella-Enterobacter* groups usually cause a rapid reversion of the slant within an 18- to 24-h incubation. Normally these groups exhibit a KIA reaction of A/A, gas. Report the KIA reaction **exactly** as observed; e.g., with reversion alkaline/acid, gas. If you suspect reversion due to colony morphology, you may write *reversion* in parentheses after the KIA reaction: alkaline/acid, gas (reversion). If reversion does occur, it usually starts at the top of the slant, with a reversion to alkalinity. This should create no problem if the colony morphology on solid media and the KIA slant are checked. These organisms usually are **extremely mucoid** both on plate media and the KIA slant, and they usually produce an abundance of gas that displaces the medium near or into the tube closure. Biochemical tests should still be performed for identification of the groups, genus, or genus and species present.

Q. **Do not** use screw-cap tubes for KIA/TSI media nor tightly stoppered or capped tubes during incubation. Enhancing the alkaline condition on the slant requires free exchange of air through the use of **loose** caps on tubes. If caps are too tight, an acid condition may involve the slant solely because of glucose fermentation.

R. In preparing medium, the slant and butt must be equal in length, approximately 1.5 inches, or 3 cm, to preserve the two-chamber effect (9).

S. Microbiologists who use packaged commercial kits and bypass inoculation of unknown to KIA/TSI may **not** know whether to select a fermentative or oxidative system; oxidation/fermentation (OF) of **all** unknown isolates of Gram-negative bacilli should be assessed by inoculation onto KIA or TSI.

T. Acids produced by nonfermenters are considerably weaker than mixed acids derived from fermentative bacteria, thus pH in fermentation media in which a nonfermenter is growing may **not** drop enough to affect the pH indicator; initial indication is a lack of acid production in either KIA/TSI with alkaline (red) slant and alkaline butt (red deep).

U. H_2S production may be evident on KIA but negative on TSI because sucrose is present **only** in TSI. Studies by Bulmash and Fulton (3) showed that sucrose use may suppress the enzyme mechanisms responsible for H_2S production. Padron and Dockstader (11) state that not all H_2S-producing *Salmonella* spp. are positive on TSI, nor does this medium give clear-cut separations of other H_2S- producing members of the *Enterobacteriaceae*.

V. Controls **should** be run on peptone used in H_2S medium to determine whether the sulfur content suffices for H_2S production. If the peptone is deficient for rapid H_2S detection, cysteine may be added to enrich the concentration of sulfhydryl bonds ($-SH$).

W. An H_2S-producing organism may exhibit blackening on sulfide-indole-motility (SIM) medium (positive) but none on TSI medium (negative) (2).

X. According to Tittsler (15), some H_2S inhibition occurs when the test is incubated at 34°C, and inhibition increases as the temperature increases to 40°C. In experiments with *Salmonella pullorum* Tittsler (15) found that the optimal incubation temperature for maximum H_2S production was 30–34°C.

Y. Sucrose is added to TSI to eliminate certain sucrose-fermenting, non-lactose-fermenting bacteria (e.g., *Proteus* and *Citrobacter* spp.) (15).

REFERENCES

1. Balows A, Hausler WJ Jr, Herrmann KL, et al. Manual of Clinical Microbiology, ed 5, Washington, DC: American Society for Microbiology, 1991:439.
2. Branson D. Methods in Clinical Bacteriology. Springfield, IL: Charles C Thomas, 1972:24–25.
3. Bulmash JM, Fulton M. Discrepant tests for hydrogen sulfide. J Bacteriol 1964;88(2):1813.
4. Hajna AA. Triple-sugar iron agar medium for the identification of the intestinal group of bacteria. J Bacteriol 1945;49(5):516–517.
5. Howard BJ, Klaas J II, Rubin SJ, et al. Clinical and Pathogenic Microbiology. St. Louis: CV Mosby, 1987:299–301.
6. Hugh R, Leifson E. The taxonomic significance of fermentative versus oxidative metabolism of carbohydrates by various gram negative bacteria. J Bacteriol 1953;66(1):24–26.
7. Kligler IJ. A simple medium for the differentiation of members of the typhoid-paratyphoid group. Am J Public Health 1917;7(12):1042–1044.
8. Kligler IJ. Modifications of culture media used in

the isolation and differentiation of typhoid, dysentery, and allied bacilli. J Exp Med 1918; 28(3):319–322.
9. Koneman EW, Allen SD, Janda WM, et al. Color Atlas and Textbook of Diagnostic Microbiology, ed 4. Philadelphia: JB Lippincott, 1992: 113, 114, 127–131, 154–158, 212, 251, 483.
10. Krumwiede C Jr, Kohn LA. A triple-sugar modification of the Russell double sugar medium. J Med Res 1917;37:225–227.
11. Padron AP, Dockstader WB. Selective medium for hydrogen sulfide production by salmonellae. Appl Microbiol 1972;23(6):1107–1112.
12. Power DA, McCuen PJ. Manual of BBL Products and Laboratory Procedures, ed 6. Cockeysville, MD: Becton Dickinson Microbiology Systems, 1988:171.
13. Russell FF. The isolation of typhoid bacilli from urine and feces with the description of a new double sugar tube medium. J Med Res 1911;25:217–229.
14. Sulkin SE, Willett JC. A triple sugar-ferrous sulfate medium for use in identification of enteric organisms. J Lab Clin Med 1940;25(6):649–653.
15. Tittsler RP. The effect of temperature upon the production of hydrogen sulphide by *Salmonella pullorum*. J Bacteriol 1931;21:111–118.

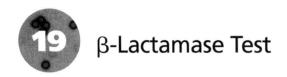

19 β-Lactamase Test

I. PRINCIPLE

To determine the susceptibility of specific microorganisms to penicillinase-susceptible penicillins or cephalosporinase-susceptible cephalosporins as determined by their ability to elaborate a β-lactamase enzyme that hydrolyzes the β-lactam ring to produce penicilloic acid or cephalosporoic acid

II. PURPOSE

(Also see Chapters 43 and 44)

β-Lactamases are found in a variety of Gram-positive and Gram-negative bacteria (42). Significance of enzymes produced by many enteric bacteria *(Enterobacteriaceae)* is less clear, and these bacteria **should not** be tested for β-lactamase (42); little value is due to diversity of enzymes with different substrate specificities that may be produced within the species, or even by a single strain (98).

A. *Haemophilus influenzae/Haemophilus parainfluenzae* (39, 94)
   1. β-Lactamase testing should be performed on all clinically significant *Haemophilus* species; any isolate considered a pathogen (42).
   2. TEM-1 β-lactamase (plasmid-mediated) can be detected by any variety of in vitro β-lactamase assays (94, 100).
B. *Neisseria gonorrhoeae* (4)
   1. β-Lactamase test should be performed for all clinically significant *N. gonorrhoeae;* any isolate considered a pathogen (42).
   2. Penicillin-resistant β-lactamase-producing strains are encountered with increased frequency and **must** be detected **before** antibiotic therapy is begun (42).
C. *Moraxella (Branhamella) catarrhalis* (57)
   1. All clinically revelant isolates should be routinely tested for β-lactamase production (70).
   2. Nitrocefin test **cannot** differentiate BRO-1 type (Ravisio-type) strains from BRO-2 type (1908-type); **all** β-lactamase-producing strains should be interpreted and reported as resistant to penicillin (70).
   3. Nitrocefin assay has lowest rate of false-negative results and is method of choice (19, 21, 23, 24, 32, 45).
D. *Enterococcus faecalis:* nitrocefin chromogenic assay is method of choice (68)
E. **Certain *Bacteroides/Prevotella* species** (63)
   1. Presumptive identification of members of *Bacteroides fragilis* group and other β-lactamase-producing former *Bacteroides* species: *Prevotella melaninogenicus* and *Prevotella oralis*
   2. *B. fragilis* group β-lactamase detected primarily by chromogenic Nitrocefin assay method
   3. *P. melaninogenicus* detected by both chromogenic and starch-iodine tests (11)
F. ***Staphylococcus aureus* subsp. *aureus*** (74, 109): chromogenic Nitrocefin test preferred (1, 24, 41)

G. **Legionella species**: *L. cincinnatiensis* (−), *L. feelei* (−), *L. micdadei* (−), and *L. maceachernii* (−); *L. bozemanii* (V, variable) and *L. longbeachae* (V) from other *Legionella* species (+) (92)

H. **β-Lactamase has been reported in *Clostridium* and *Fusobacterium* spp.** (58).

III. BIOCHEMISTRY INVOLVED

Plasmids/Resistance

Plasmids are extrachromosomal DNA particles, circular pieces of DNA that act independently of chromosomes (42). Gene coding (information) for production of β-lactamase usually resides on plasmids (episomes) that carry genes that determine and control resistance to antibiotics (103). At times they are physically distinct from the bacterial chromosome, and some bacteria can transfer them from one bacterium to another (107), which explains diffusion of the resistance (52). Other mechanisms of resistance are emerging; in addition to production of inactivating enzyme is the "intrinsic resistance" (52).

Linking resistant genes from multiple antibiotics on a plasmid permits bulk transfer of resistance that characterizes many newly resistant organisms. Plasmid DNA is easily transferred from one strain to another, one species to another, even one genus to another (42). However, some antibiotic resistance is chromosome mediated (107).

The most common mechanism of transferring resistant genes to other bacteria is via a **transposon** (transposable genetic element); which carries portion of plasmids and a piece of chromosome from one bacterium to another by **conjugal transfer** (conjugative transposon or "jumping gene") (42). Usually, resistance depends entirely or partly on β-lactamases (55).

Plasmid genes are responsible for acquired resistance, which is either mutational or acquired (92). Acquired resistance to many penicillins is by production of β-lactamases. Transposal gene coding for one plasmid-determined β-lactamase is the TEM β-lactamase found in *H. influenzae* and *N. gonorrhoeae* (92). Plasmid-mediated β-lactamases are principally TEM and SHV types.

β-Lactamases

More than 50 different β-lactamases or penicillinases are known (35). β-Lactamases (penicillinases) are modifying enzymes (drug-inactivating enzymes) found in all types of bacteria, Gram positive and Gram negative. They are heterogeneous bacterial enzymes; penicillin-destroying enzymes that cleave (i.e., open) the β-lactam ring of penicillins and cephalosporins to **in**activate the antibiotic (35, 42). However, β-lactamases produced by different resistant bacterial strains are **not** all identical (52).

β-Lactamase-producing organisms can reduce the efficiency of β-lactam antibiotics in eradicating infection at various body sites (12). These organisms not only protect themselves from penicillin but can also protect penicillin-susceptible organisms that may be present at the site of the infection (13).

β-Lactamases may be **induced** or **constitutive**. An inducible enzyme is produced only when an organism is exposed to a β-lactam antibiotic (60); enzyme produced only in presence of (i.e., exposure to) a challenge substrate of a β-lactam antimicrobial agent, after which production of enzyme is turned on (42). An induced cell that contains the gene for resistance has a control mechanism that enables it to refrain from synthesizing an enzyme (e.g., β-lactamase) when there is no need for it (e.g., in absence of antibiotic) (52). However, in the presence of antibiotic, mechanism called **induction** is evoked, and the cell synthesizes the inactivating enzyme (52). Antibiotic does **not** cause resistance; it only induces the expression of resistance potentially present in cell (52). Constitutive enzyme is expressed continuously whether an inciting challenge is present or not (42).

β-Lactamase is only **one** of several factors contributing to resistance to penicillin and cephalosporins by Gram-negative bacteria; other factors include (a) the outer membrane of Gram-negative bacteria, which constitutes a hydrophobic barrier layer, and (b) crypticity, which refers to interaction of cell-bound β-lactamase and barrier function of cell envelope (98).

Most β-lactamases in Gram-positive bacteria have enhanced affinity for penicillins rather than cephalosporins (penicillinases) (42). In Gram-negative bacteria, chromosomal enzymes have a greater specificity for cephalosporins than for penicillins (cephalosporinases).

Some enzymes are secreted into extracellular environment where they exert their antibacterial action; e.g., β-lactamases of Gram-positive cocci such as staphylococci are secreted (42). Most Gram-negative enzymes are cell bound and exert their effects only if antibiotic enters the cell (42).

Bacterial resistance to antimicrobial agents is thought to be due to (a) a defect, enzyme inactivation of antibiotic by β-lactamases of Gram-positive and Gram-negative bacteria, and (b) alteration of binding proteins for a variety of β-lactam antibiotics, for both Gram-positive and Gram-negative bacteria (42); alteration in penicillin-binding proteins (peptidoglycantranspeptidases) that are essential to activity of β-lactam antibiotics (42, 55). Binding proteins can attach to a particular antibiotic. Several different proteins of the inner membrane, called penicillin-binding proteins, can specifically bind β-lactams (52). Different β-lactams vary in their binding affinity (52).

β-Lactams

β-Lactam group includes two of the most important families of antibiotics: penicillins and cephalosporins. Bacteria can have high affinity for any β-lactam drug of any class (42). All penicillins and all cephalosporins are β-lactam drugs that selectively inhibit bacterial cell wall synthesis (35) by inserting antibiotic into the peptidoglycan structure (42). Cell wall is composed of peptidoglycan, a macromolecule, (mucopeptide or glycopeptide or murein) and other polymers (polysaccharides, lipoproteins, etc.) that vary in different types of bacteria (52).

Inhibitors of peptidoglycan synthesis are classified into three groups according to process with which they interfere; β-lactams inhibit cross-linking and are bactericidal (cause irreversible damage) (52). All β-lactams have similar but not identical mechanisms of action: preventing or interrupting peptidoglycan maturation by inhibiting cross-linking (42, 52).

The following model for the mechanism of the irreversible effects of β-lactams (cell lysis) is indirectly related to their interference with their primary targets (PBPs) (52):

1. Inhibition of activity of one or more enzymes in peptidoglycan synthesis (PBPs), thus inhibiting bacterial growth.
2. A "signal" (unknown) is generated that triggers release of teichoic acids into the medium.
3. Loss of teichoic acids activates one or more peptidoglycan-hydrolyzing activities.
4. They sever covalent bonds of cell wall, exposing cell membrane.
5. Osmotic lysis of cell wall ensues.

Penicillins

Narrow-spectrum **penicillin** antibiotics are mainly active against Gram-positive and some Gram-negative cocci, with little action against Gram-negative bacilli. Penicillin G and penicillin V are examples of narrow-spectrum antibiotics (92). Penicillinase-resistant penicillins have narrow spectra but are active against penicillinase-producing staphylococci.

Penicillins inhibit cell wall synthesis; they attach to penicillin-binding proteins adjacent to the cytoplasmic membrane and block the transpeptidation reaction that links peptidoglycan molecules by pentapeptide bridges to provide structural strength to the cell wall (92). Different β-lactam antibiotics may have predominant effect on different combinations of penicillin-binding enzymes (92).

Synthetic penicillins (e.g., methicillin, oxacillin, nafcillin) are resistant to penicillinases produced by staphylococci.

β-Lactam Action

β-lactam drugs are cyclic amides; examples of heterocyclic compounds. **Penicillin G,** the most widely used natural penicillin, is the prototype penicillin. All penicillins share the same basic structure: 6-aminopenicillanic acid (6APA); a two-ringed nucleus composed of a five-atom thiazolidine ring attached to an unstable four-atom β-lactam ring (106) that carries a free amino group (35, 74) on an acyl side chain. Properties of penicillin depend on the side chain on the 6-β carbon atom. An acidic radical attached to an amino group can be split off by bacterial and other amidases (35).

Different radicals (R) attached to aminopenicillanic acid determine the essential pharmacologic properties of resultant drugs.

Representative Penicillins (35, 92)

"R" radical–follow structures can be substituted at R to produce a new penicillin

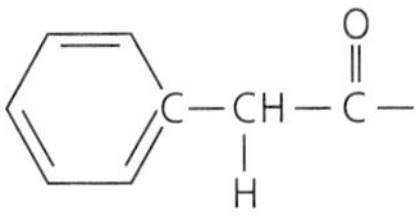

Penicillin G (benzylpenicillin) Destroyed by β-lactamese

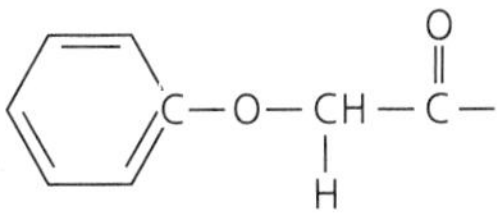

Penicillin V (phenoxymethyl penicillin)

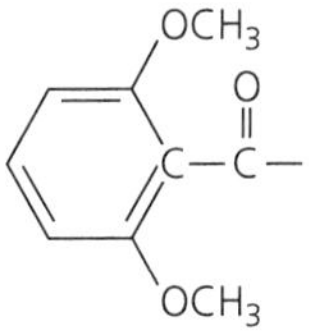

Methicillin (dimethoxyphenyl penicillin)

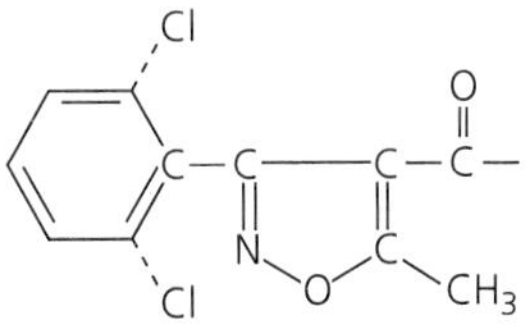

Oxacillin; cloxacillin (one Cl in structure; dicloxacillin (2 Cl's in structure); flucloxacillin (one Cl and one F in structure) (iso oxazoyl penicillins)

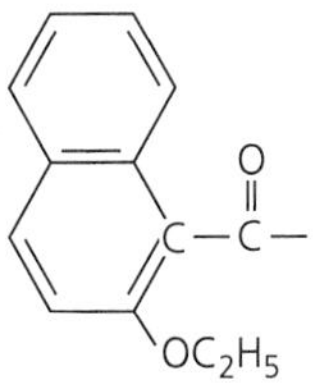

Nafcillin (ethoxynaphthamido penicillin)

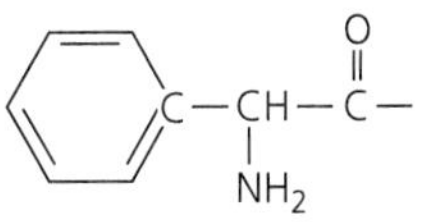

Ampicillin (α-aminobenzylpenicillin) Destroyed by β-lactamase

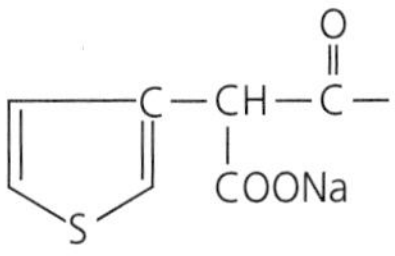

Ticaicillin

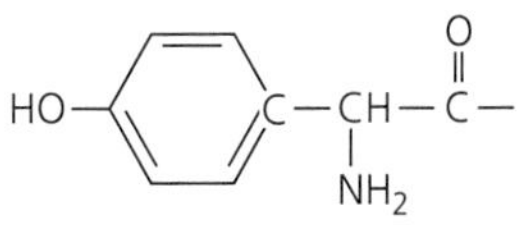

Amoxicillin

Under hydrolysis, β-lactamase (penicillinase) opens the β-lactam ring to yield penicilloic acid, which is **devoid of antibacterial activity** (15) but carries an antigenic determinant of the penicillins and acts as a sensitizing hapten when attached to carrier proteins (35). The β-lactam ring can be opened enzymatically or chemically. The side chain of the β-lactam ring confers the antibacterial activity. Cleavage of the β-lactam ring often decreases the pH (15); penicilloic acid is more acid than penicillin, hence acidic pH and a color change.

Hydrolysis of Penicillin by Acylase and β-Lactamase (15, 35, 92, 106)

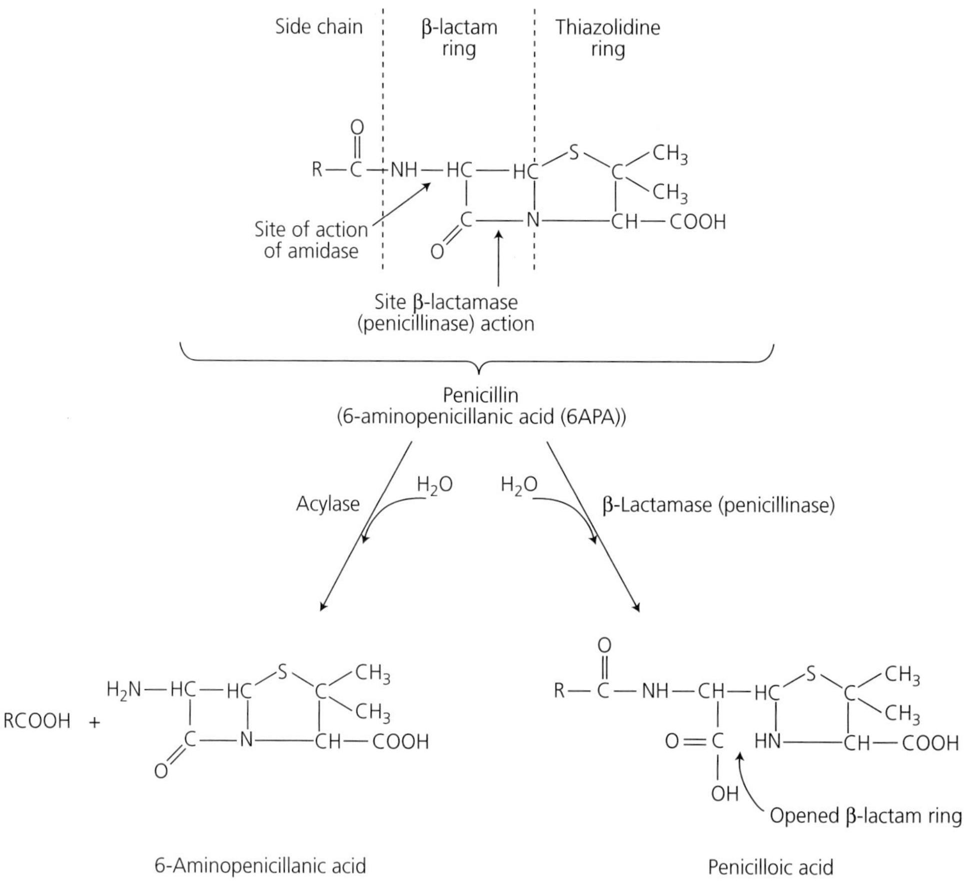

6-Aminopenicillanic acid

Penicilloic acid

Cephalosporins

All cephalosporins originate from cephalosporin C; active against penicillin-resistant *S. aureus* subsp. *aureus*, but more active against Gram-negative bacteria (52) (for examples of cephalosporins see the following figure).

Representative Cephalosporins (22, 52, 77, 92)

	R_1	R_2	Name
First Generation	thiophene-2-yl-CH₂—	—OCOCH₃	Cephalothin
	thiophene-2-yl-CH₂—	phenyl	Cephaloridine
	phenyl-S—CH₂—	—OCO—CH₃	Cephapirin
	N≡C—CH₂—	—OCO—CH₃	Cephacetrile
	tetrazol-1-yl-CH₂—	—S—(1,3,4-thiadiazol-2-yl)—CH₃	Cefazolin
2nd and 3rd Generation	phenyl-CH(OH)—	—S—(tetrazolyl, N—CH₃)	Cefamandole
	(tetrahydrofuran-2-yl)—C(=N—OCH₃)—	—O—CO—NH₂	Cefuroxime
	(2-amino-thiazol-4-yl)—C(=N—OCH₃)—	—O—CO—CH₃	Cefotaxime
	HO—C₆H₄—CH(NHCO—piperazinyl—N—C₂H₅)—	—S—(triazolyl, N—CH₃)	Cefoperazone

Cephalosporins resemble penicillins, but differ from them in that the central nucleus is 7-aminocephalosporanic acid and the five-atom thiazolidine ring is replaced by a six-atom dihydrothiazine ring and a second (R_2) radical group at position 3.

Hydrolysis of Cephalosporin by Acylase and β-Lactamase (15, 92)

Mechanism of action is comparable to that of penicillin, including attachment to receptors and inhibition of final transpeptidation of bacterial cell wall peptidoglycan (35). Most common β-lactamases have a serine-based mechanism as seen in staphylococcal penicillinase, the TEM and SHV types and the class I enzymes of Gram-negative bacteria; **all** operate with this mechanism (55):

1. Free hydroxyl of β-lactam ring residue first associates noncovalently with antibiotic.
2. It forms covalent acyl ester with opened β-lactam ring.
3. Ester hydrolysis ensues.

Microbial acylases, produced by many organisms, cleave acyl side chains of susceptible penicillins and cephalosporins (102).

β-Lactamases hydrolyze amide bonds of β-lactam ring of sensitive penicillins and cephalosporins; they play an important role in microbial resistance to β-lactam antibiotics (15). The microbial assay methods are based on loss of antibacterial activity after hydrolysis of the β-lactam ring (97). However, β-lactamases **do not** act exclusively on penicillin or cephalosporin; many show a predominance of either penicillinase or cephalosporinase activity (75, 97, 98).

Staphylococcus β-Lactamase

Only one class of enzymes is produced by resistant strains (1, 41). Staphylococci have three different β-lactamases (42); they may be inducible or constitutive and they are borne on plasmids (42) and secreted into periplasmic space (42, 60).

β-lactamases are **not** active against penicillin-resistant penicillins or cephalosporins (42). Studies (6, 9, 26, 27, 46–51, 72, 85) have shown oxacillin, methicillin, nafcillin, and cephalothin to be only partially resistant to hydrolysis by staphylococcal β-lactamase, and increased production could cause increased resistance (60). Methicillin is the least active penicillinase-resistant penicillin (7). Penicillin resistance is associated with cell wall or penicillin-binding protein (PDP) alterations, **not** β-lactamase production (92). Multiresistance is usually plasmid determined and acquired by **transduction** (92).

Growth medium composition can greatly affect how much enzyme is extracellular (60). Coles and Gross (17) reported that inorganic phosphate liberated cell-bound enzyme. Kim and Chipley (40) reported that 5 or 10% salt (NaCl) optimally stimulated both constitutive and induced synthesis of β-lactamase. Release of β-lactamase in staphylococci is **not** due to cell damage; high salt concentration also favored release of β-lactamase (40).

Neisseria gonorrhoeae β-Lactamase

Penicillinase-producing *N. gonorrhoeae* are widely distributed (42). In 1976, strains producing plasmid-mediated β-lactamase were reported in the United States (78). Currently, penicillinase-producing *N. gonorrhoeae* (PPNG) are endemic in certain regions of the United States (70). Only one class of enzymes is produced by resistant strains (4). PPNG produce plasmid-coded TEM-type β-lactamases identical to those of members of the *Enterobacteriaceae* and ampicillin-resistant *H. influenzae* (92). In 1983 an outbreak due to chromosomally mediated resistant *N. gonorrhoeae* (CMRNG) was reported (33). Unlike PPNG, CMRNG cannot be detected by chromogenic, iodometric, or acidometric tests (14, 30, 68, 74).

Moraxella catarrhalis β-Lactamase

First reported in 1977 (57), most clinical isolates of *M. catarrhalis* produce a β-lactamase (2, 23, 56, 61, 95) in small amounts that remains strongly cell associated (24, 32, 36, 45). It is constitutive and chromosomally mediated (20, 23, 32).

β-Lactamases of *M. catarrhalis* are of one of two types: Ravasio type and 1908 type (41, 67). The BRO-1 type (or Ravisio type) is the most common and is constitutive, Nitrocefin positive, and inhibited by clavulanic acid and sulbactam (20, 31). BRO-2 type (or 1908-type) is produced in lesser amounts but is Nitrocefin positive.

M. catarrhalis produces significantly more activity against Nitrocefin than against either penicillin or ampicillin (32, 96). Nitrocefin test is the procedure of choice for susceptibility to penicillin and ampicillin (19, 20, 23, 24, 43, 71, 82, 105); chromogenic assays yield the fewest false-negative results. Enzyme is more active against penicillin than cephalosporin (20, 23, 32) and is inhibited by clavulanate (23, 31, 32).

Enterococcus faecalis β-Lactamase

Penicillin-resistant enterococci, first discovered in the early 1980s (65) resulted from plasmid-mediated β-lactamase (70). β-Lactamase-producing strains appear to make an enzyme similar to the plasma-mediated enzyme found in *Staphylococcus aureus* subsp. *aureus*. This plasmid is self-transferable, so potential exists for spread (62, 65, 66, 76, 89, 93). β-Lactamase enterococcal plasmids are heterogenous. Constitutive cell-bound enzyme is readily detected by the Nitrocefin test (62, 64, 76, 77).

Haemophilus influenzae β-Lactamase

Only one class of enzyme is produced by most resistant strains: TEM-1 type β-lactamase (94, 100) and less commonly, ROB-1 (68). Ampicillin-resistant strains produce potent β-lactamase that is plasma-mediated and identical to that found in other Gram-negative bacteria (92). Some 20–40% of *H. influenzae* type b produce β-lactamase (22); however, any isolate considered a pathogen should be tested. β-Lactamase of *H. influenzae* is readily detected by acidometric (30), iodometric (14), and chromogenic tests (70, 74).

Bacteroides fragilis Group/*Prevotella* β-Lactamase

Bacteroides/Prevotella produce a variety of enzymes with different substrate specificities: *Prevotella melaninogenicus* and *P. oralis* are specific for penicillins (penicillinase) (88) and *B. fragilis* group for cephalosporins (18). *B. fragilis* group, *P. melaninogenica* and *P. oralis* are the most resistant of the anaerobes (8). Resistance primarily to β-lactam drugs is mediated by β-lactamase against cephalosporinases, they also have a significant ability to hydrolyze penicillins (8).

Inhibitors

Most β-lactamase inhibitors are β-lactam compounds that compete with β-lactam antibiotics for the enzyme (106).

Clavulanic acid, a natural product of *Streptomyces clavuligerus* (69, 80), inhibits activity of staphylococcal β-lactamase, most plasmid-mediated β-lactamases of Gram-negative bacilli (7), and some chromosomal enzymes (e.g., those from *B. fragilis* group with little intrinsic bacterial activity).

Sulbactam is a semisynthetic 6-desaminopenicillin sulfone with weak antibacterial activity (5, 28) and little intrinsic bacterial activity. It effectively inhibits certain plasmid and chromosomally mediated β-lactamases (7) and is active against many β-lactamases of Gram-negative and Gram-positive bacteria. It is less active than clavulanic acid and considered less able to penetrate cells than clavulanic acid.

Tazobactam is active against plasmid-mediated β-lactamases of Gram-negative bacteria. No significant differences exist between clavulanate and tazobactam except for their spectra of activity. Tazobactam is superior to sulbactam.

β-Lactamase Inhibitors (106)

Clavulanic acid

Sulbactum

These compounds are irreversible inhibitors (28, 80, 81, 83) that form irreversible acyl enzyme complex with β-lactamase, leading to loss of enzyme activity (7). These compounds by themselves, generally do not inhibit bacteria (60).

IV. RAPID ASSAY METHODS

(*Note:* Microbiological assay methods are based on loss of antibacterial activity after hydrolysis of β-lactam ring (97).)

Since β-lactam antibiotics inhibit or compete for β-lactamase, the rate of color formation is inversely proportional to concentration of antibiotic (7).

A. **Nitrocefin-chromogenic cephalosporin test** (63, 74, 104)
   1. Principle: In the presence of β-lactamase and the opening of the β-lactam ring, conjugation of the dinitrostyryl group at position 3 with the dihydrothiazine ring increases, with a change in color from yellow to red (104). Electron shift in a chromogenic cephalosporin (104)
   2. Most sensitive of the three methods
   3. Reagent solutions
      a. Phosphate buffer, pH 7.0

Monopotassium phosphate, 1/15 M, KH_2PO_4	39.2 mL
Disodium phosphate, 1/15M, $Na_2HPO_4 \cdot 12H_2O$	60.8 mL

      b. Working solution

Nitrocefin powder or PADAC	5.0 mg
Dimethyl sulfoxide (DMSO), $(CH_3)_2SO$	0.5 mL
Phosphate buffer, 0.1 mol/L, pH 7.0	9.5 mL

Nitrocefin is chromogenic cephalosporin 87/312 (Glaxo, LTD, Greenford, Middlesex, England). Commercial Nitrocefin-impregnated disks are available as Cefinase from BBL. Nitrocefin has the widest spectrum of susceptibility and sensitivity of commercially available β-lactams. It is not known to react with other microbial enzymes and is effective for detection of **all** known β-lactamases including staphylococcal penicillinases (63, 74, 94).

   c. Dissolve Nitrocefin in dimethyl sulfoxide and dilute to 10.0 mL with phosphate buffer; final concentration 500 μg/mL
   d. Dispense 0.2 mL-aliquots; small test tubes (13 × 100 mm)
   e. Store at −20°C.

An alternate chromogenic cephalosporin is PADAC, pyridine-2-azo-dimethylaniline cephalosporin (70) (Calbiochem-Behring), developed by Schindler and Huber (90). PADAC, a chromophore-3-substituted cephalosporin, changes from yellow to purple (bromcresol purple pH indicator) on action of β-lactamase (90). PADAC exhibits little antimicrobial activity against Gram-negative bacteria, but good activity against *S. aureus,* comparable to Nitrocefin (36). Available as dipsticks (Behringwerke, Germany) or powder and disks (Calbiochem-Behring).

Pyridine-2-Azo-Dimethylaniline Cephalosporin (37)

4. Procedure; two choices
   a. Method 1
      (1) Saturate a Whatman no. 1 filter paper disk (7-cm diameter) with Nitrocefin.
      (2) Place disk in a closed Petri dish to avoid drying out.
      (3) Smear a small loopful or heavy suspension of a **pure** colony of suspected organism onto impregnated disk.
   b. Method 2
      (1) Add 2 drops of Nitrocefin/well of microdilution plate.
      (2) Inoculate each test well with test organism(s).
      (3) Seal plate with strips of cellophane tape to prevent evaporation.
5. Incubation; room temperature (22–25°C): most reactions occur within 30 sec, but take final reading of disk after 15 min at room temperature (22–25°C) or 1 h at 37°C (15, 34); reaction may take up to 6 h (7).
6. Interpretation
   a. Positive (+): presence of β-lactamase
      (1) Nitrocefin: red color that deepens to deep burgundy within 10–30 min. Weak reaction exhibits a dark orange coloration.
      (2) PADAC: purple color
   b. Negative (−)
      (1) Either Nitrocefin or PADAC: color remains yellow.
      (2) Absence of β-lactamase

(3) Test negative results after induction with methicillin; loopful 18- to 24-h growth around methicillin disk (5 μg) (34) or cefoxitin (108).

B. **Iodometric slide test** (86, 104)
  1. Principle: Starch and iodine react in solution to produce a purple color. β-Lactamase causes the β-lactam ring to open with production of penicilloic acid, which reacts with iodine, making it **un**available to react with starch. The presence of β-lactamase is indicated by decolorization of (or failure to form) the starch-iodine complex (73). Intact (active) penicillin does **not** bind iodine, whereas penicilloic acid does (54). Penicilloic acid acts as a reducing agent to reduce iodine in the complex (15).
  2. Test is less sensitive than chromogenic Nitrocefin assay, and it requires a large test sample.
  3. Reagents
      a. Starch solution
          (1) 0.4%: dissolve 0.4 g starch in 100 mL of deionized water
          (2) Autoclave, 121°C, 15 lb, 15 min, and store in the refrigerator (4–10°C).
      b. Iodine solution; two choices
          (1) Selection 1
              (a) Phosphate buffer, 0.1 mol/L, pH 6.4: 60 mL of pH 6 buffer and 40 mL of pH 7 buffer
              (b) Ingredients

Potassium iodide (KI)	1.5 g
Iodine (I) crystals	0.3 g
Phosphate buffer, 0.1 mol/L	100.0 mL

          (2) Selection 2: Gram's iodine (solution used for Gram stain technique)

Potassium iodide (KI)	2.0 g
Iodine crystals (I)	1.0 g
Deionized water	100.0 mL

      c. Penicillin solution
          (1) To a 10^6-unit vial of penicillin, add 1.0 mL of sterile water.
          (2) Withdraw entire volume and freeze 0.15 mL aliquots in small (1-dram) vials.
  4. Procedures (14)
      a. Procedure 1
          (1) Add 1.1 mL of iodine solution to a vial of penicillin solution.
          (2) On flamed side of a glass slide, emulsify organism to be tested in a drop of the penicillin-iodine solution; make a **heavy** suspension.
          (3) Add 1 drop of starch solution.
      b. Procedure 2
          (1) Penicillin-starch impregnated disks
              (a) Immerse penicillin-starch disks in a solution of Gram's iodine until they become uniformly deep purple.
              (b) Drain excess liquid and place on paper towels until they lose their shine.
          (2) Place impregnated disk onto a primary chocolate agar plate of isolated colonies of suspected organism; ensure contact with agar surface for 10 min.
          (3) Remove disk that contains adherent imprint of colonies on underside of filter paper. Place in Petri disk to observe for clearing of purple color.
  5. Interpretation: initially, solution of all samples will turn purple.
      a. Positive (+)
          (1) Solution: clearing of purple color to white within 5 min; read at 1, 10, and 30 min. The entire mixture does not have to clear; clearing of definite clumps or areas is sufficient to denote a positive result.

(2) Disk: clearing of purple color within 1 min in immediate vicinity of suspected gonococcal isolates.
   b. Negative (−): no clearing of solution; mixture remains purple, denoting formation of a starch-iodine complex; disk remains purple.
C. **Acidometric test** (42, 101, 104)
   1. Principle: Penicilloic acid, produced by opening the β-lactam ring, is more acidic than penicillin. Alteration (decrease) to acid pH is detected by using phenol red in the presence of a new carboxyl group.
   2. Test is less sensitive than Nitrocefin chromogenic method.
   3. Reagent: phenol red pH indicator
      a. 0.5% solution
      b. Dilute 2.0 mL of 0.5% phenol red with 16.6 mL of deionized water.
   4. Procedure: to a vial containing 20 million units (10^6) of penicillin G, (buffered potassium penicillin G, USP) add
      a. Phenol red solution, 2.0 mL
      b. NaOH, 1 mol/L, dropwise (0.5 mL) until solution **just turns** purple-violet, pH 8.5

A high concentration of penicillin G is used to detect strains of *Staphylococcus aureus* subsp. *aureus* that are low penicillinase producers (72).

   c. Store aliquots at −20°C for up to 1 week. Thawed tubes may be kept at 4°C for entire working day; longer storage periods are not advisable because of possible hydrolysis of penicillin.

As penicillin is hydrolyzed, in the presence or absence of penicillinase, the color of the solution changes from violet or deep red (basic form of phenol red) to yellow (acid form); solution color adequately indicates suitability of solutions for use after storage.

   5. Procedures; selections
      a. Method 1
         (1) Dip one end of a capillary tube (blue tip coagulation capillary tube, 0.5–0.9 mm diameter) into phenol red solution; fill tube to a height of 1 cm by capillary action.
         (2) Scrape **filled end** of capillary tube across a pure colony of bacteria to be tested; a plug should form in the end of the tube. Take care that no air is trapped between bacteria and solution. Formed plug must be in contact with solution.
         (3) Incubate at room temperature (22–25°C) for 1 h in vertical position, with bottom of tube containing plug of bacteria **not** in contact with solid surface.
      b. Method 2
         (1) β-Lactam disks or strips impregnated with penicillin and pH indicator, bromcresol purple; commercially available
         (2) Disk/strip rehydrated with a single drop of **sterile** 0.85% physiologic saline (NaCL) (pH 7.0); follow manufacturer's directions.
         (3) Transfer 3–5 isolated colonies onto surface of disk/strip by use of wooden sticks.
         (4) Incubate at room temperature (22–25°C), 1, 10, and 30 min.
   6. Interpretation
      a. Positive (+): either method, yellow color (acidity); production of β-lactamase (penicillinase) and thus resistant to penicillin
      b. Negative (−)
         (1) Phenol red: color remains yellow.
         (2) Bromcresol purple: color remains violet-purple.

V. QUALITY CONTROL MICROORGANISMS

Moraxella catarrhalis   ATCC 43617, 43618, 43628
Neisseria gonorrhoeae   ATCC 49226
Staphylococcus aureus subsp. *aureus*   ATCC 25923, 29213

VI. PRECAUTIONS

A. **General**
1. Interpretation of β-lactam assays must take into consideration the following: *(a)* sensitivity of test for different classes of β-lactamase enzymes, *(b)* types of β-lactamases produced by different taxonomic groups of organisms, and *(c)* substrate specificities of different β-lactamases (79).
2. β-Lactamase test should be performed for all clinically significant *H. influenzae* and *N. gonorrhoeae* isolates. Penicillin-resistant β-lactamase-producing strains are encountered with increased frequency and **must** be detected **before** antibiotic therapy is begun (42).
3. Control strains **must** be included with each battery of tests.
4. Although microbial β-lactamases **do not** act exclusively on penicillins or cephalosporins, many show a predominance of either penicillinase or cephalosporinase activity (75, 97, 98); therefore, chemical or microbial methods that use either a penicillin alone or a cephalosporin alone can give **false-negative** results for β-lactamase activity (3, 25, 29, 38, 53, 59, 87).
5. Significance of enzymes produced by many enteric (*Enterobacteriaceae*) bacteria is less clear, and these bacteria **should not** be tested for β-lactamase (42).

B. **Nitrocefin-chromogenic cephalosporin** test
1. Test **must** be used when testing *Moraxella catarrhalis* (42).
2. Incubation with human sera can cause color change with Nitrocefin (74); therefore, Nitrocefin is **not** suitable for detecting β-lactamase in the presence of certain body fluids (15). PADAC is not adversely influenced (non- enzyme-related color change) by protein content of specimens (37).
    O'Callaghan et al. (74) showed **false-positive** results with Nitrocefin when reagent was added to broth cultures that were highly alkaline (pH 10.0) or that contained serum, albumin, thiols, cysteine, glutathione, mercaptoethanol, or dimercaprol and recommended caution when testing colonies obtained from media containing any of these substances.
3. PADAC color changes occur more slowly than those with Nitrocefin (37).
4. PADAC poor antimicrobial agent against Gram-negative species (37).

C. **Iodometric slide** test
1. Once iodine and penicillin solutions are mixed, they **must** be used within 1 h to avoid false-positive results (104).
2. Test is less sensitive than chromogenic method and requires a large test sample.

D. **Acidometric** test
1. Test less sensitive than chromogenic method (42).
2. Test may be unable to detect β-lactamase present in small amounts and tightly bound to the cell as β-lactamase produced by *Staphylococcus saprophyticus;* for these organisms, Nitrocefin solution is best (7).
3. Cleavage of acyl side chain from β-lactam antibiotics often decreases pH and reduces antibiotic activity; thus, acidometric methods **may not** differentiate β-lactamase activity from acylase activity (99).
4. Store aliquots at $-20°C$ for up to 1 week. Thawed tubes may be kept at 4°C for entire

working day; longer storage periods are not advisable because of possible hydrolysis of penicillin.

E. **Staphylococcus**
   1. Previous studies have shown that staphylococcal β-lactamase, when present in sufficient quantities for sufficient duration, **slowly** hydrolyzes penicillinase-resistant penicillins (PRPs) and cephalosporins (6, 9, 26, 27, 46–51, 72, 85). Some *S. aureus* subsp. *aureus* produce large quantities of β-lactamase, which can slowly inactivate so-called PRPs (60). Additional sodium chloride is needed to promote growth and subsequent detection of heteroresistant staphylococci, but this salt may at the same time promote production and release of β-lactamase (60).
   2. Although the vast majority of penicillin-resistant staphylococci owe their resistance to their ability to produce penicillinase (16), some strains are resistant for other reasons (91).
   3. Always run a test that depends upon inhibition of growth to be sure you are not dealing with a rare methicillin-resistant strain.
   4. β-Lactamase induced by exposure to penicillins is **not** active against cephalosporins or penicillinase-resistant penicillins such as methicillin and nafcillin unless large amounts are produced (42).
   5. Generally β-lactamases produced by *S. aureus* subsp. *aureus* inactivate penicillin only, **not** cephalosporins (52).

F. **Neisseria gonorrhoeae**
   1. In 1983, an outbreak of gonorrhoeae occurred due to chromosomally mediated resistant *N. gonorrhoeae* (CMRNG) (33). Unlike PPNG, CMRNG **cannot** be detected by screening for β-lactamase (33).
   2. All clinical isolates of *N. gonorrhoeae* in areas where therapy other than ceftriaxone is being used should be screened for resistance to penicillin (70). Koneman et al. (42) recommend testing all clinically significant isolates.
   3. Some strains are resistant to penicillin by nonenzymatic means (84), and susceptibility tests should also be performed **if** treatment fails (42).

G. **Haemophilus influenzae**
   1. When performing β-lactamase tests, it is extremely important to test more than one colony (about 10 colonies) from culture plate, since both β-lactamase-positive and β-lactamase-negative strains can be simultaneously recovered from same specimen (44).
   2. β-Lactamase **should** be tested for on any isolate considered pathogenic (42).
   3. Occasional reports of β-lactamase nonproducing strains should be tested against ampicillin by a diffusion or dilution susceptibility test (10). β-Lactamase-negative strains are **not** necessarily ampicillin susceptible, since at least a small percentage of *H. influenzae* strains are resistant to ampicillin via a mechanism other than production of TEM-1 β-lactamase (68).

H. **Moraxella catarrhalis**
   1. Nitrocefin test **cannot** differentiate RBO-1 type (Ravasio-type) strains from BRO-2 type (1908-type); all β-lactamase-producing strains should be interpreted and reported as resistant to penicillin (70).
   2. Chromogenic assay has lowest rate of false-negative results.
   3. β-Lactamase of *M. catarrhalis* is produced in small amounts and remains strongly cell associated (32, 45); conventional β-lactamase assays to detect activity among clinical isolates could lead to **false-negative** results (24, 36). Studies showed 36% false-negative results with iodometric test, 31% with PADAC, and most accurate (4%) with Nitrocefin (24). Not all β-lactamase strains of *M. catarrhalis* are equally reactive in individual β-lactamase assays (24). In length of time to detect positive results, sensitivity of tube Nitrocefin equals that of disk; Nitrocefin > disk PADAC > disk acidometric > broth acidometric > iodometric test (24).

I. *Enterococcus faecalis*
   1. Certain isolates of β-lactamase-producing enterococci are **not** reliably detected by routine susceptibility testing (7).
   2. *E. faecalis* is moderately sensitive to penicillins and almost totally insensitive to most cephalosporins (52).

REFERENCES

1. Adam AP, Barry AL, Benner EJ. A simple, rapid test to differentiate penicillin-susceptible from penicillin-resistant *Staphylococcus aureus*. J Infect Dis 1970;122:544–546.
2. Alvarez S, Jones M, Holtsclaw-Berk S, et al. In vitro susceptibilities and beta-lactamase production of 53 clinical isolates of *Branhamella catarrhalis*. Antimicrob Agents Chemother 1985; 27:646–647.
3. Anhalt JP, Nelson R. Failure of PADAC test strips to detect staphylococcal beta-lactamase. Antimicrob Agents Chemother 1982;21:993–999.
4. Ashford WA, Golash RG, Hemming VG. Penicillinase-producing *Neisseria gonorrhoeae*. Lancet 1976;2:657–658.
5. Aswapokee N, Neu HC. A sulfone beta-lactam compound which acts as a beta-lactamase inhibitor. J Antibiot 1978;31:1238–1244.
6. Ayliffe GAJ, Barber M. Inactivation of benzylpenicillin and methicillin by hospital staphylococci. Br Med J 1963;2:202–205.
7. Balows A, Hausler WJ Jr, Herrmann KL, et al. Manual of Clinical Microbiology, ed 5. Washington, DC: American Society for Microbiology, 1991:613, 1070, 1194–1195, 1160.
8. Baron EJ, Finegold SM. Bailey & Scott's Diagnostic Microbiology, ed 8. Philadelphia: CV Mosby, 1990:533.
9. Basker MJ, Edmondson RA, Sutherland R. Comparative stabilities of penicillins and cephalosporins to staphylococcal beta-lactamase and activities against *Staphylococcus aureus*. J Antimicrob Chemother 1980;6:333–341.
10. Bell SM, Plowman D. Mechanisms of ampicillin resistance in *Haemophilus influenzae* from respiratory tract. Lancet 1980;1:279–280.
11. Bourqault A-M, Rosenblatt JE. Characterization of anaerobic gram-negative bacilli by using rapid slide tests for β-lactamase production. J Clin Microbiol 1979;9(6):654–656.
12. Brook I. Microbiological rapid methods useful in the office laboratory, part I. Am Clin Products Rev 1987;Aug:34–36.
13. Brook I, Calhoun L, Yocum P. Beta lactamase-producing isolates of *Bacteroides* species from children. Antimicrob Agents Chemother 1980; 18:164–166.
14. Catlin BW. Iodometric detection of *Haemophilus influenzae* beta-lactamase. Rapid presumptive test for ampicillin resistance. Antimicrob Agents Chemother 1975;7:265–270.
15. Chen KCS, Knapp JS, Holmes KK. Rapid, inexpensive method for specific detection of microbial β-lactamases by detection of fluorescent end products. J Clin Microbiol 1984;19(6):818–825.
16. Citri N, Pollock MR. The biochemistry and function of β-lactamase (penicillinase). In: Nord FF, ed. Advances in Enzymology, vol 28. New York: Interscience, 1966:237–323.
17. Coles NW, Gross R. Liberation of surface-located penicillinase from *Staphylococcus aureus*. Biochem J 1967;102:742–747.
18. Del Bene VE, Farrar WE. Cephalosporinase activity in *Bacteroides fragilis*. Antimicrob Agents Chemother 1973;3:369–372.
19. Doern GV. *Branhamella catarrhalis:* An emerging human pathogen. Clin Microbiol Newsl 1985; 7:75–78.
20. Doern GV. Antimicrobial resistance among clinical isolates of *Haemophilus influenzae* and *Branhamella catarrhalis*. Clin Microbiol Newsl 1988; 10:185–187.
21. Doern GV, Jones RN. Antimicrobial susceptibility testing of *Haemophilus influenzae, Branhamella catarrhalis,* and *Neisseria gonorrhoeae*. Antimicrob Agents Chemother 1988;32:1747–1753.
22. Doern GV, Jorgensen JH, Thornsberry C, Preston DA. Prevalence of antimicrobial resistance among clinical isolates of *Haemophilus influenzae*. A collaborative study. Diagn Microbiol Infect Dis 1986;4:95–107.
23. Doern GV, Siebers KG, Hallick LM, Morse SA. Antibiotic susceptibility of beta-lactamase-producing strains of *Branhamella (Neisseria) catarrhalis*. Antimicrob Agents Chemother 1980; 17:24–29.
24. Doern GV, Tubert TA. Detection of beta-lactamase activity among clinical isolates of *Branhamella catarrhalis* with six different β-lactamase assays. J Clin Microbiol 1987;25(8):1380–1383.
25. Durkin JP, Dmitrienko GI, Viswanatha T. N-(2-Furyl)acryloyl penicillin: A novel compound for the spectrophotometric assay of beta-lactamase. Int J Antibiot (Tokyo) 1977;30:883–885.
26. Dyke KGH. Penicillinase production and intrinsic resistance to penicillins in *Staphylococcus aureus*. Lancet 1966;1:835–838.
27. Duke KGH. Penicillinase production and intrinsic resistance to penicillins in methicillin-resistant cultures. J Med Microbiol 1969;2:261–278.
28. English AR, Retsema JA, Girard AE, et al. CP-45, 899, a beta-lactamase inhibitor, that extends the antibacterial spectrum of beta-lactams: Initial

28. bacteriological characterization. Antimicrob Agents Chemother 1978;14:414–419.
29. Ericsson H. The effect of beta-lactamases of varying origin on different types of cephalosporins. Scand J Infect Dis Suppl 1978;13: 33–34.
30. Escamilla J. Susceptibility of *Haemophilus influenzae* to ampicillin as determined by use of a modified, one-minute beta-lactamase test. Antimicrob Agents Chemother 1976;9:196–198.
31. Farmer T, Reading C. Beta-lactamases of *Branhamella catarrhalis* and their inhibition by clavulanic acid. Antimicrob Agents Chemother 1982;21:506–508.
32. Farmer T, Reading C. Inhibition of the beta-lactamases of *Branhamella catarrhalis* by clavulanic acid and other inhibitors. Drugs 1986;31(Suppl 3):70–78.
33. Faruki H, Kohmescher RN, McKinney WP, Sparling PF. A community-based outbreak of infection with penicillin-resistant *Neisseria gonorrhoeae* not producing penicillinase (chromosomally mediated resistance). N Engl J Med 1985;313:607–611.
34. Hébert GA, Cooksey RC, Clark NC, et al. Biotyping coagulase-negative staphylococci. J Clin Microbiol 1988;26(10):1950–1956.
35. Jawetz E, Melnick JL, Adelberg EA. Review of Medical Microbiology, ed 17. Los Altos, CA: Appleton & Lange, 1987:13–131, 143–144, 148.
36. Jones RN, Sommers HM. Identification and antimicrobial susceptibility testing of *Branhamella catarrhalis* in the United States laboratories. Drugs 1983–1985;31(Suppl 3):34–39.
37. Jones RN, Wilson HW, Novick WJ Jr. In vitro evaluation of pyridine-2-azo-*p*-dimethylaniline cephalosporin, a new diagnostic chromogenic reagent, and comparison with Nitrocefin, Cephacetrile, and other beta-lactam compounds. J Clin Microbiol 1982;15(4):677–683.
38. Jorgensen JH, Crawford SA, Alexander GA. Pyridinium-2-azo-dimethylaniline chromophore, a new chromogenic cephalosporin for rapid beta-lactamase testing. Antimicrob Agents Chemother 1982;22:162–164.
39. Khan W, Ross S, Rodriquez W, et al. *Haemophilus influenzae* type b resistant to ampicillin. JAMA 1974;299:298–301.
40. Kim TK, Chipley JR. Effect of salts on penicillinase release by *Staphylococcus aureus*. Microbios 1974;10A:55–63.
41. Kirby WMM. Extraction of a higher potent penicillin inactivator from penicillin-resistant staphylococci. Science 1944;99:452–453.
42. Koneman EW, Allen SD, Janda WM, et al. Color Atlas and Textbook of Diagnostic Microbiology, ed 4. Philadelphia: JB Lippincott, 1992:43, 362, 409–411, 611–616, 638–640.
43. Kovatch AL, Wald ER, Michaela RH. Beta-lactamase-producing *Branhamella catarrhalis* causing otitis media in children. J Pediatr 1983;102: 261–264.
44. Krieger PS, Naidu S. Simultaneous recovery of beta-lactamase-negative and beta-lactamase-positive *Haemophilus influenzae* type b from cerebrospinal fluid of neonate. Pediatrics 1980;68:253–254.
45. Labia R, Barthelemy M, Le Bouquennec CB, Hoi-Dang Van AB. Classification of beta-lactamases from *Branhamella catarrhalis* in relationship to penicillinases produced by other bacterial species. Drugs 1986;31(Suppl 3):40–47.
46. Lacey RW. Antibiotic resistance plasmids of *Staphylococcus aureus* and their clinical importance. Bacteriol Rev 1975;39:1–32.
47. Lacey RW. Stability of the isoxazolyl penicillins to staphylococcal β-lactamase. J Antimicrob Chemother 1982;9:239–243.
48. Lacey RW. Treatment of staphylococcal infections. J Antimicrob Chemother 1983;11:3–6.
49. Lacey RW. Mechanisms of resistance to beta-lactam antibiotics. Scand J Infect Dis 1984;42 (Suppl):64–71.
50. Lacey RW, Lewis EL. Further evolution of a strain of *Staphylococcus aureus* in vivo: Evidence for significant inactivation of flucloxacillin by penicillinase. J Med Microbiol 1975;8:337–347.
51. Lacey RW, Stokes A. Susceptibility of the "penicillinase-resistant" penicillins and cephalosporins to penicillinase of *Staphylococcus aureus*. J Clin Pathol 1977;30:35–39.
52. Lancini G, Parenti F. Antibiotics: An Integrated View. New York: Springer-Verlag, 1982:8, 39, 42–49, 81, 106–107, 115, 117.
53. Lee DT, Rosenblatt JE. A comparison of four methods for detecting beta-lactamases in anaerobic bacteria. Diagn Microbiol Infect Dis 1983;1:173–175.
54. Lee W-S, Komarmy L. Iodometric spot test for detection of beta-lactamase in *Haemophilus influenzae*. J Clin Microbiol 1981;13(1):224–225.
55. Livermore DM. Carbapenemases: The next generation of β-lactamases? ASM News 1993;59 (3):129–135.
56. Luman I, Wilson RW, Wallace RJ Jr, Nash DR. Disk diffusion susceptibility of *Branhamella catarrhalis* and relationship of beta-lactam zone size to β-lactamase production. Antimicrob Agents Chemother 1986;30:774–776.
57. Malmvall B-E, Brorsson JE, Johnson J. In vitro sensitivity to penicillin V and beta-lactamase production of *Branhamella catarrhalis*. Antimicrob Agents Chemother 1977;3:374.
58. Marrie TJ, Haldane EV, Swantee CA, Kerr EA. Susceptibility of anaerobic bacteria to nine antimicrobial agents and demonstration of decrease susceptibility of *Clostridium perfringens* to penicillin. Antimicrob Agents Chemother 1981; 19:51–55.
59. Marshall MJ, Ross GW, Chanter KV, Harris AM.

Comparison of the substrate specificities of the beta-lactamases from *Klebsiella aerogenes* 1082 E and *Enterobacter cloacae*. Appl Microbiol 1972; 23:765–769.
60. McDougal LK, Thornsberry C. The role of beta-lactamase in staphylococcal resistance to penicillinase-resistant penicillins and cephalosporins. J Clin Microbiol 1986;23(5):832–839.
61. McLeod DT, Power JT, Calder MA, Seaton A. Bronchopulmonary infection due to *Branhamella catarrhalis*. Br Med J 1983;287:1446–1451.
62. Moellering RC Jr, Korzeniowski OM, Sande MA, Wennersten CB. Species-specific resistance to antimicrobial synergism in *Streptococcus faecalis*. J Infect Dis 1979;140:203–208.
63. Montgomery K, Raymundo L Jr, Drew WL. Chromogenic cephalosporin spot test to detect beta-lactamase in clinically significant bacteria. J Clin Microbiol 1979;9(2):205–207.
64. Murray BE, Church DA, Wanger A, et al. Comparison of two beta-lactamase-producing strains of *Streptococcus faecalis*. Antimicrob Agents Chemother 1986;30:861–864.
65. Murray BE, Mederski-Samoraj BD. Transferable beta-lactamase: A new mechanism for in vitro penicillinase resistance in *Streptococcus faecalis*. J Clin Invest 1983;72:1168–1171.
66. Murray BE, Mederski-Samoraj BD, Foster SK, et al. In vitro studies of plasmid-mediated penicillinase from *Streptococcus faecalis* suggest a staphylococcal origin. J Clin Invest 1986;77:289–293.
67. Nash DR, Wallace RJ, Steingrub VA, Shurin PA. Isoelectric focusing of beta-lactamases from sputum and middle ear isolates of *Branhamella catarrhalis* in the United States. Drugs 1986;31 (Suppl 3):47–53.
68. National Committee for Clinical Laboratory Standards. Approved Standard: M2-A4. Performance Standards for Antimicrobial Disk Susceptibility Tests, ed 4. Villanova, PA: National Committee for Clinical Laboratory Standards, 1990.
69. Neu HC, Fu KP. Clavulanic acid, a novel inhibitor of beta-lactamases. Antimicrob Agents Chemother 1978;14:650–655.
70. Neumann MA, Sahm DF, Thornsberry C, McGowan JE Jr. New development in antimicrobial agent susceptibility testing: A practical guide. Cumitech 6A, Washington, DC: American Society for Microbiology, 1991.
71. Ninane G, Joly J, Kraytman M, Piot P. Bronchopulmonary infection due to beta-lactamase-producing *Branhamella catarrhalis* treated with amoxycillin/clavulanic acid. Lancet 1978;1:257–259.
72. Novick RP, Richmond MH. Nature and interactions of the genetic elements governing penicillinase synthesis in *Staphylococcus aureus*. J Bacteriol 1965;90:467–480.
73. Oberhofer TR, Towle DW. Evaluation of the rapid penicillinase paper strip test for detection of beta-lactamase. J Clin Microbiol 1982;15(2):196–199.
74. O'Callaghan CH, Morris A, Kirby SM, Shingler AH. Novel method for detection of beta-lactamases by using a chromogenic cephalosporin substrate. Antimicrob Agents Chemother 1972; 1(4):283–288.
75. Ogawara H. Antibiotic resistance in pathogenic and producing bacteria, with special reference to beta-lactam antibiotics. Microbiol Rev 1981; 45:591–619.
76. Patterson JE, Masecar BL, Zervos MJ. Characterization and comparison of two penicillinase-producing strains of *Streptococcus (Enterococcus) faecalis*. Antimicrob Agents Chemother 1988; 32:122–124.
77. Patterson JE, Zervos MJ. Susceptibility and bactericidal activity studies of four beta-lactamase-producing enterococci. Antimicrob Agents Chemother 1989;33:251–253.
78. Phillips I. Beta-lactamase-producing penicillin-resistant gonococcus. Lancet 1976;2:656–657.
79. Power DA, McCuen PJ. Manual of BBL Products and Laboratory Procedures, ed 6. Cockeysville, MD: Becton Dickinson Microbiology Systems, 1988:336–337.
80. Reading C, Cole M. Clavulanic acid: A beta-lactamase-inhibiting beta-lactam from *Streptococcus clavuligerus*. Antimicrob Agents Chemother 1977;11:852–857.
81. Reading C, Hepburn P. The inhibition of staphylococcal beta-lactamase by clavulanic acid. Biochem J 1979;179:67–76.
82. Renkonen OV. Antibacterial activity of nine oral antibiotics against *Streptococcus pneumoniae*, *Haemophilus influenzae*, and *Branhamella catarrhalis*. Scand J Infect Dis Suppl 1973;39:106–108.
83. Retsema JA, English AR, Girard AE. CP-45, 899 in combination with penicillin or ampicillin against penicillin-resistant *Staphylococcus*, *Haemophilus influenzae*, and *Bacteroides*. Antimicrob Agents Chemother 1980;17:615–622.
84. Rice RJ, Biddle JW, JeanLouis YA, et al. Chromosomally mediated resistance in *Neisseria gonorrhoeae* in the United States: Results of surveillance and reporting, 1983–1984. J Infect Dis 1986;153:340–345.
85. Richmond MH. Purification and properties of the exopenicillinase from *Staphylococcus aureus*. Biochem J 1963;88:452–459.
86. Rosenblatt JE, Neumann AM. A rapid slide test for penicillinase. Am J Clin Pathol 1978;69:351–354.
87. Ross GW, Chanter KV, Harris AM, et al. Comparison of assay techniques for beta-lactamase activity. Anal Biochem 1973;54:9–16.
88. Salyers AA, Wong J, Wilkins TD. Beta-lactamase activity in strains of *Bacteroides melaninogenicus* and *Bacteroides oralis*. Antimicrob Agents Chemother 1977b;11:142–146.

89. Schaberg DR. Resistant nosocomial enterococcal infections. Infect Dis Newsl 1988;7:73–75.
90. Schindler P, Huber G. Use of PADAC, a novel chromogenic β-lactamase substrate. In: Brodbeck U, ed. Enzyme Inhibitors. Weinheim: Verlag Chemie, 1980:169.
91. Seligman SJ. Penicillinase negative variants of methicillin resistant *Staphylococcus aureus*. Nature (London) 1966;209:994–996.
92. Sherris JC, Ryan KJ, Ray CG, et al., eds. Medical Microbiology. An Introduction to Infectious Diseases. New York: Elsevier, 1984:126–131, 154–155, 214, 221, 234.
93. Shlaes DM. Antibiotic-resistant enterococci. Infect Dis Newsl 1989;8:53–55.
94. Skinner A, Wise R. A comparison of three rapid methods for the detection of beta-lactamase activity in *Haemophilus influenzae*. J Clin Pathol 1977;30:1030–1032.
95. Slevin NJ, Aitken J, Thornley PE. Clinical and microbiologic features of *Branhamella catarrhalis* bronchopulmonary infections. Lancet 1984;1:782–783.
96. Stobberingh EE, van Eck HJ, Houben AW, van Boven CPA. Analysis of the relationship between ampicillin resistance and beta-lactamase production of *Branhamella catarrhalis*. Drugs 1986;31(Suppl 3):23–27.
97. Sykes RB, Bush K. Physiology, biochemistry, and inactivation of β-lactamases. In: Morin RB, Gorman M, eds. Chemistry and Biology of β-Lactam Antibiotics, vol 3. New York: Academic Press, 1982:155–207.
98. Sykes RB, Matthew M. The beta-lactamases of gram-negative bacteria and their role in resistance to beta-lactam antibiotics. J Antimicrob Chemother 1976;2:115–157.
99. Sykes RB, Matthew M; Detection, assay and immunology of β-lactamases. In: Hamilton-Miller JMT, Smith JT, eds. Beta-Lactamases. New York: Academic Press, 1979:17–49.
100. Thornsberry C, Kirven LA. Ampicillin resistance in *Haemophilus influenzae* as determined by a rapid test for beta-lactamase production. Antimicrob Agents Chemother 1974;6:653–654.
101. Tu KK, Jorgensen JH, Stratton CW. A rapid paper-disk test for penicillinase. Am J Clin Pathol 1981;75:557–559.
102. Vandamme EJ. Enzymes involved in beta-lactam antibiotic biosynthesis. Adv Appl Microbiol 1977;21:89–123.
103. Waldvogel FA. *Staphylococcus aureus* (including toxic shock syndrome). In: Mandell GL, Douglas RG, Bennett JE, eds. Principles and Practice of Infectious Diseases, ed 3. New York: Churchill Livingstone, 1990:1489–1510.
104. Washington JA. Laboratory Procedures in Clinical Microbiology, ed 2. New York: Springer-Verlag, 1985:305, 308–310.
105. Wilhelmus KR, Peacock J, Coster DJ. *Branhamella keratitis*. Br J Ophthalmol 1980;64:892–895.
106. Wilson G, Miles A, Parker MT, eds. Topley and Wilson's Principles of Bacteriology, Virology, and Immunology, vol 1, ed 7. Baltimore: Williams & Wilkins, 1983:103, 105, 115, 115.
107. Wistreich GA, Lechtman MD. Microbiology, ed 3. New York: Macmillan, 1980:398–399.
108. Woods GL, Hall GS, Rutherford I, Pratt K, Knapp CC. Antibiogram comparisons: Methicillin-resistant vs methicillin-susceptible coagulase-negative staphylococci. Lab Med 1987;18(11):765–768.
109. Workman RG, Edmund WJ. Activity of penicillinase in *Staphylococcus aureus* as studied by the iodometric method. J Infect Dis 1970;121:433–437.

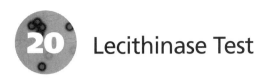

20 Lecithinase Test

I. PRINCIPLE

To determine ability of microorganisms to produce the enzyme lecithinase evidenced by appearance of egg yolk opacity (12, 21) or serum turbidity (20, 22)

II. PURPOSE

(Also see Chapters 43 and 44)

A. Identification of anaerobes: Primarily useful in the identification of *Clostridium* spp.: *C. perfringens* (+), *C. bifermentans* (+), *C. sordellii* (+), *C. baratii* (+), *C. haemolyticum* (+), *C. ghoni* (+), *C. limosum* (+), and *C. novyi* A and B (V, variable, usually +) from other most frequently isolated *Clostridium* spp. (−) with subterminally located spores (1, 12, 13, 16, 20)
B. Aid in identification of *Bacillus* species: Differentiation of *B. anthracis* (+), *B. cereus* (+), *B. mycoides* (+), and *B. licheniformis* (+) from other *Bacillus* spp. (−) (17).
C. Aid in identification of most phage-typable *Staphylococcus aureus* subsp. *aureus* strains (10). Active lecithinase-producing nonfermentative bacteria are hemolytic for human red cells (23).

III. BIOCHEMISTRY INVOLVED

Howard (12) first recognized the value of opalescence in the identification of *Clostridium perfringens* (formerly *C. welchii*); she referred to the test as Nagler reaction. Nagler test is a test for *C. perfringens* antitoxin. MacFarlane and Knight (19) showed that α-toxin of *C. perfringens* is a lecithinase, which they designated lecithinase C (EC 3.1.4.3), responsible for lecithinase reaction of egg yolk agar and hazy zone of hemolysis on blood agar.

Lecithins

Lecithins are classified as phosphoglycerides or phosphatides (phospholipids), a group of compounds that contain fatty acids, phosphoric acid, glycerol, and choline (14). They are glyceryl esters (diglycerides) of two long-chain fatty acid molecules (R and R') linked at their third carbon to choline ester of phosphoric acid (phosphatidic acid, H_3PO_4), which in turn is bound by ester linkage to a nitrogenous base, choline (an amino alcohol); $CH_2(R)CH(R')CH_2OPO(OH)O(CH_2N(OH)(CH_2)_3$ (11, 14, 31).

Lecithinase C

Willis (28) showed actions of four types of lecithinase; however, lecithinase C is the one usually produced by bacteria. Lecithinase C (also referred to as phospholipase C, phosphatidase D, or phosphatidylcholine-phosphotidylhydrolase) is in the general class of enzymes known as phosphodiester hydrolases (16). Lecithinases (or phospholipases) A, B, and D also break down lecithin, but hydrolyze lecithin at different places on molecule with resulting production of substances **other than** phosphorylcholine and diglyceride (16, 27). Lecithinase C hydrolyzes lecithin and other phospholipids such as sphingomyelin, phosphatidylethanolamine, cephalin, and thromboplastin (26).

Phosphatidase D acts on phosphatide lecithin molecules and hydrolyzes specific ester linkages; the phosphorylcholine group is removed from the 3 position to yield a 1,2-diglyceride (α,β-diglyceride) (11).

Hydrolysis of Lecithin (3,11)

$$\text{L-}\alpha\text{-lecithin (phosphatidylcholine)} \xrightarrow[\text{Lecithinase C (phosphatidylcholine cholinephosphohydrolase)}]{\text{Phosphatidase D}} \text{1,2-Diglyceride} + \text{Phosphorylcholine}$$

Egg Yolk Factor

Lecithin is normal component of egg yolk; lecithovitellin (LV) lipoprotein component of egg yolk that can be obtained as a clear yellow liquid by mixing egg yolk with saline (5). When egg yolk–saline mixture is mixed with certain bacterial toxins or lecithinases, liquid becomes opalescent, and flocculation and separation of a thick curd of fat may follow (5).

Lecithinase, or egg yolk factor, acts on the lipoprotein component of egg yolk; hydrolysis of lecithin liberates phosphorus and choline in stages, and precipitation of **in**soluble fat (diglyceride) causes opalescence (23). An opaque halo surrounds colonies growing on egg yolk–containing medium (2).

Willis and Gowland (29) studied the mechanism of opacity production and showed that opalescence was due to a combination of three factors:

1. Fat (diglyceride) produced from lecithin upon its breakdown

2. Free fats from egg yolk emulsion after breakdown of lecithin (which stabilizes egg yolk emulsion)
3. Water-insoluble proteins from egg yolk (vitellin and vitellenin) that precipitate free fats

MacFarlane et al. (20) stated that opalescence caused by α-toxin (lecithinase C) is due to liberation of free fat from either serum or lecithovitellin, with the reaction with lecithovitellin more rapid and more sensitive than that with serum.

IV. MEDIA EMPLOYED

(*Note:* A number of egg yolk agar (EYA) media are available; selection depends on one's laboratory preference and/or microorganisms being tested.)

Any suitable growth medium (e.g., Trypticase soy agar (TSA), brain-heart infusion (BHI) agar, soybean casein digest agar) with 10% egg yolk enrichment may be used for **aerobic** bacteria (23).

A. **Egg yolk emulsion**
   1. Preparation from scratch
      a. Scrub and then soak antibiotic-free hen egg in 95% ethanol (ethyl alcohol), 1 h.
      b. **Aseptically** aspirate or separate egg yolk.
      c. Add 1 egg yolk to 500 mL of agar base.
      d. With **sterile** pipette, stir to smooth suspension.
   2. Commercial egg yolk emulsion is available.
B. **Lecithin-lactose anaerobic agar (anaerobic lecithin-lactose agar)**
   1. Modified formulation of Ellner and O'Donnell (8)
   2. Selective because of inhibitors sodium azide and neomycin sulfate. Inhibits Gram-negative bacteria; aerobic Gram-positive bacilli. Gram-positive cocci are markedly attenuated (suspended). Differentiation by ability to ferment lactose and/or produce lecithinase; primarily for histotoxic *Clostridium* spp.
   3. Ingredients
      a. **Calcium-cysteine solution**

Cysteine · HCl	5.0 g
Calcium chloride, $CaCl_2 \cdot 2H_2O$	0.5 g
Deionized water	100.0 mL
Acidify with glacial acetic acid, CH_3COOH, 99.4%, USP	1 drop

      b. **Lecithin emulsion**

Egg lecithin	3.3 g
Deionized water	100.0 mL
Adjust to pH 7.0 with 0.1 N NaOH	

      c. **Columbia agar base,** pH 7.4 ± 0.2 (24)

Pancreatic digest of casein	12.0 g
Peptic digest animal tissue	5.0 g
Yeast extract	3.0 g
Beef extract	3.0 g
Corn starch	1.0 g
Sodium chloride, NaCl	5.0 g
Agar	13.5 g
Deionized water	1000.0 mL

   4. **Original formulation** (8), pH 6.7 ± 0.2: to 1 L of Columbia agar base (46.6 g/L) add

Lactose	10.0 g
Sodium azide, NaN_3	0.2 g
Bromcresol purple (1.25% alcoholic (ethanol) solution)	2.0 mL

After sterilization cool and add

Neomycin sulfate, **sterile**	0.15 g
Calcium-cysteine solution, **sterile**	10.0 mL
Lecithin emulsion, sterile	20.0 mL

5. **Alternate formulation** (24), pH 6.8 ± 0.2

Pancreatic digest casein	12.65 g
Peptic digest animal tissue	5.5 g
Pancreatic digest heart muscle	3.3 g
Yeast extract	3.85 g
Corn starch	1.1 g
Sodium chloride, NaCl	5.5 g
Lactose	10.0 g
Sodium azide, NaN_3	0.2 g
L-cysteine · HCl	0.5 g
Calcium chloride, $CaCl_2 \cdot 2H_2O$	0.05 g
Agar	15.0 g
Egg lecithin	0.66 g
Bromcresol purple (BCP)	25.0 mg
Deionized water	1000.0 mL

6. **Lecithin-lactose anaerobic agar, modified**
   a. Formulation of Ellner, Granato, and May (7)
   b. Ingredients, pH 7.0 ± 0.2

Casein/meat (50/50) peptone	10.0 g
Casein/yeast (50/50) peptone	10.0 g
Heart peptone	3.0 g
Lactose	10.0 g
Corn starch	1.0 g
Sodium chloride, NaCl	5.0 g
Sodium azide, NaN_3	0.2 g
L-Cysteine · HCl	0.5 g
Palladium chloride, $PdCl_2$	0.33 g
Dithiothreitol	0.1 g
Magnesium sulfate, $MgSO_4 \cdot 7H_2O$	0.01 g
Tris (hydroxymethyl) aminomethane	1.66 g
Tris (hydroxymethyl) aminomethane · HCl	5.75 g
Calcium chloride, $CaCl_2 \cdot 2H_2O$	0.01 g
Lecithin	0.66 g
Bromcresol purple (BCP)	0.025 g
Agar	13.5 g
Deionized water	1000.0 mL
After sterilization, cool and add:	
Neomycin sulfate, **sterile**	0.015 g

(*Note:* $PdCl_2$ (palladous chloride, palladium dichloride) and dithiothreitol, also known as Cleland's reagent, are reducing agents. Tris (hydroxymethyl) aminomethane (THAM; 2-amino-2-hydroxymethyl-1,3- l-1,3-propanediol; tris amine buffer) is $(CH_2OH)_3CNH_2$.)

C. **Lecithin-lipase anaerobic agar (anaerobic lecithin-lipase agar, modified McClung-Toabe agar)**
   1. Modification of McClung and Toabe agar (21)
   2. Purpose: isolation and differentiation of *Clostridium* species by ability to produce lecithinase and/or demonstrate lipase activity; most widely used medium for detection of

lecithinase activity (21); supports good growth of various clostridia and gives more intense zones of opacity than serum media
3. Ingredients, pH 7.6 ± 0.2

Casein peptone	40.0 g
Yeast extract	5.0 g
Glucose (dextrose)	2.0 g
Sodium chloride, NaCl	2.0 g
Monopotassium phosphate, KH_2PO_4	1.0 g
Disodium phosphate, $Na_2HPO_4 \cdot 12H_2O$	5.0 g
Magnesium sulfate, $MgSO_4 \cdot 7H_2O$	0.1 g
Agar	25.0 g
Deionized water	1000.0 mL
After sterilization, cool and add:	
Egg yolk suspension	100.0 mL

D. *Clostridium difficile* agar (cycloserine-cefoxitin-fructose–egg yolk (CCFA) agar)
   1. Formulation of George, Sutter, Citron, and Finegold (9)
   2. Selective because of antimicrobic inhibitors cycloserine and cefoxitin, which inhibit *Bacillus* and *Pseudomonas* spp., most cocci (**except** *Enterococcus faecalis*), most Enterobacteriaceae, clostridia (**except** *C. difficile*), and Gram-negative nonsporulating anaerobic bacilli.
   3. With egg yolk: differentiates by ability to produce lecithinase and lipase
   4. Ingredients, pH 7.2 ± 0.2 (24)

Peptic digest of animal tissue	32.0 g
Fructose	6.0 g
Monopotassium phosphate, KH_2PO_4	1.0 g
Disodium phosphate, Na_2HPO_4	5.0 g
Sodium chloride, NaCl	2.0 g
Magnesium sulfate, $MgSO_4 \cdot 7H_2O$	0.1 g
Neutral red (NR)	0.03 g
Agar	20.0 g
Deionized water	1000.0 mL
After sterilization, cool and add	
Cycloserine (C), **sterile**	500 µg/mL
Cefoxitin (C), **sterile**	16 µg/mL
Egg yolk suspension in saline, 50%, sterile 5.0 mL	

E. CDC modified McClung-Toabe egg yolk agar (1)
   1. Formulation of Lombard, Thompson, and Armfield (6) at Communicable Disease Centers (CDC), Atlanta, GA, USA
   2. **Non**selective enrichment agar used primarily to isolate **most** anaerobic bacteria from clinical specimens
   3. Ingredients, pH 7.4 ± 0.2

Pancreatic digest casein	40.0 g
Yeast extract	5.0 g
D-Glucose (dextrose)	2.0 g
Sodium chloride, NaCl	2.0 g
Sodium phosphate, $Na_2HPO_4 \cdot 12H_2O$	5.0 g
Magnesium sulfate, $MgSO_4 \cdot 7H_2O$, 5% aqueous solution	0.2 mL
Agar	25.0 g
Deionized water	900.0 mL
Egg yolk suspension	100.0 mL

278   Biochemical Tests for Identification of Medical Bacteria

(*Note:* Trypticase soy agar (TSA), 72.0 g/L, may be substituted for the pancreatic digest of casein and yeast extract.)

- F. Method of sterilization
    1. Base: autoclave, 121°, 15 lb, 15 min
    2. Calcium-cysteine solution, lecithin emulsion egg yolk suspension: filtration (Millipore)
- G. Dispense: Petri dishes, 15–20 mL/plate (15 × 100 mm)
- H. Finished/uninoculated medium appearance
    1. Lecithin-lactose anaerobic agar: purple plate medium
    2. Lecithin-lipase anaerobic agar: yellowish plate medium
    3. *C. difficile* agar: orange plate medium
- I. Storage
    1. Media, calcium-cysteine solution, and lecithin emulsion: refrigerator, 2–8°C; plates inverted (lids down)
    2. Shelf life
        a. Lecithin-lactose anaerobic agar: completed medium approximately 2 weeks (8)
        b. Lecithin-lipase anaerobic agars: approximately 2–4 weeks
        c. *C. difficile* agar with cycloserine and cefoxitin: no longer than 5–7 days (30)
        d. CDC agar: approximately 6–8 weeks
- J. Inoculation
    1. Prereduce plates by incubation in GasPak 24 h.
    2. Growth from a **pure** culture
    3. Direct; four-quadrant streaking for maximum isolation
- K. Incubation: anaerobically, 35°C, 48–72 h; plates inverted (lids down)

V. QUALITY CONTROL MICROORGANISMS

Test each new lot of egg yolk agar (EYA) plates (2) (Table 20.1).

Table 20.1. Quality Control Microorganisms

Species	ATCC	Lecithinase	Lactose	Lipase
Clostridium bifermentans	638	+	−	−
Clostridium perfringens	13124	+	A	−
Clostridium difficile	9689	−	−	−
Clostridium septicum	6008	−	A	−
Clostridium sporogenes	3584	−	−	+
Uninoculated				

VI. RESULTS

> See Figures 20.1 and 20.2 in Appendix 1 for colored photographic results

VII. INTERPRETATION

(See Table 20.2)

- A. **Lecithinase activity**
    1. Positive (+): opaque, opalescent (milky white) zone surrounding some colonies; **insoluble** precipitate best seen in transmitted light (1, 17)

2. Negative (−): no opaque zone in medium
B. Lactose fermentation
   1. Positive (A): yellow zone surrounding colonies; acid condition
   2. Negative (−): no color change in medium surrounding colonies
C. Lipase positive (+): iridescent sheen on growth surface (see Chapter 22, Lipase Test)

Table 20.2. *Clostridium* Species: Lecithinase, Lipase, and Lactose Reactions on Egg Yolk Media

Species	Lecithinase	Lactose	Lipase
Lecithinisae, lactose, lipase negative			
C. aminovalericum	−	−	−
C. argentinense[a]	−	−	−
C. cadaveris	−	−	−
C. difficile	−	−	−
C. glycolicum	−	−	−
C. hastiforme	−	−	−
C. histolyticum	−	−	−
C. malenominatum	−	−	−
C. novyi C	−	−	−
C. putrefaciens	−	−	−
C. putrificum	−	−	−
C. symbiosum[b]	−	−	−
Lecithinase positive/lactose positive/lipase negative			
C. perfringens[c]	+	A	−
C. baratii[c,d]	+	A	−
Lecithinase positive/lactose negative/lipase variable			
C. bifermentans[c]	+	−	−
C. ghoni	+	−	+
C. haemolyticum	+	−	−
C. limosum	+	−	−
C. novyi A	+	−	+
C. novyi B	+	−	−
C. sordellii[c]	+	−	−
Lecithinase negative/lactose negative/lipase positive			
C. cochlearium	−	−	+
C. sporogenes	−	−	+
Lecithinase negative/lactose positive/lipase negative			
C. bijerinckii	−	A	−
C. butyricum	−	A	−
C. celatum	−	A	−
C. chauvoei	−	A	−
C. clostridioforme[e]	−	A	−
C. indolis	−	A	−
C. oroticum	−	A	−
C. paraputrificum	−	A	−
C. ramosum	−	A	−
C. sartagoforme	−	A	−
C. septicum	−	A	−
C. sphenoides	−	A	−
C. spiroforme	−	A[w]	−
C. tertium	−	A	−
Lecithinase, lactose, lipase, variable			
C. botulinum	V	−	+
C. carnis	−	V	−
C. fallax	−	V+	−

continued

Table 20.2. (*continued*) *Clostridium* Species: Lecithinase, Lipase, and Lactose Reactions on Egg Yolk Media

Species	Lecithinase	Lactose	Lipase
C. innocuum	−	V	−
C. leptum	−	V	−
C. subterminale	V	−	−
C. symbiosum	−	V	−
C. tetani	−	−	V

V, variable, V +, variable, usually positive; A, acid production; A^w, weak acid production.
[a]Formerly *C. botulinum* G, some nontoxic *C. hastiforme*, and *C. subterminale*.
[b]Formerly *Fusobacterium symbiosum*.
[c]Nagler positive.
[d]Formerly *C. barti, C. perenne, C. paraperfringens*.
[e]Formerly *C. clostridiiforme*.

VIII. PRECAUTIONS

A. **General**
 1. A slight clearing around spot inoculum is a result of proteolysis and **should be ignored** (15).
 2. Reaction can be inhibited by adding certain antitoxic or antilecithinase sera to surface of medium **before** inoculation (5). Eggs should be from chickens **not** receiving antibiotics, to avoid inhibition of growth (26).
 3. When testing **non**fermenters for lecithinase activity, temperature relationship of organism **must** be kept in mind; e.g., *Pseudomonas fluorescens* and *Acinetobacter haemolyticus* grow faster and more strongly at room temperature (22–25°C) than at 35°C; whereas, the reverse is true with *Pseudomonas aeruginosa* and *P. cepacia* (23).
 4. MacFarlane and Knight (19) determined an optimal pH for the enzyme of 7.0–7.6; activity is stimulated by calcium ions.
 5. Lipolytic microorganisms may produce small zones of opacity (4).
 6. Lipase-positive, iridescent, "pearly" layer at edge of growth should be ignored and **not** recorded because activity is inconsistent within species (23).
 7. Clostridia and *Bacillus* species produce large (4–5 mm) zones of opacity extending from edge of growth; nonfermenters produce small (1–2 mm) zones of opacity (23).
 8. Lecithinase factor in clostridia is an α-toxin, best demonstrated when medium is supplemented with magnesium (Mg) ions; e.g., McClung-Toabe EYA containing magnesium used for aerobes and anaerobes (23).

B. *Staphylococcus*
 1. Most strains of *S. aureus* subsp. *aureus* produce an egg yolk reaction, but over one fourth of coagulase-negative staphylococci do also; therefore, opacity is **not** of great value for staphylococci (23).
 2. Addition of egg yolk to *Staphylococcus* 110 medium **does not** distinguish coagulase-negative from coagulase-positive staphylococci (18).

C. **Anaerobic lecithin-lactose agar**
 1. Occasionally an additional 24-h incubation is necessary for clear-cut reactions to occur (8).
 2. Occasionally, Gram-positive cocci grow as pinpoint colonies with **neither** reaction **nor** color change in agar **except** for a yellow color that sometimes occurs around attenuated enterococci colonies (8).

D. *Clostridium difficile* agar (CCFA agar)
 1. Typical Gram stain morphology of *C. difficile* may **not** be evident on this medium; several transfers on blood agar (BA) may be necessary to achieve morphology consistent with *C. difficile*. The two antimicrobics cycloserine and cefoxitin cause marked elongation of cells and loss of spores on Gram stain (9). Usually a single pass on BA will restore characteristic morphology (9).

2. Growth of *C. difficile* may be inhibited by some strains of lactobacilli and enterococci (25). Also presence of *C. difficile* may inhibit some *Bacteroides, Peptococcus,* and *Peptostreptococcus* (25).
3. *C. difficile* is negative for both lecithinase and lipase activity; therefore, the need for egg yolk agar in a selective medium for *C. difficile* isolation has not been established (30).

REFERENCES

1. Balows A, Hausler WJ Jr, Herrmann KL, et al. Manual of Clinical Microbiology, ed 5. Washington, DC: American Society for Microbiology, 1991:431, 498, 500, 1236.
2. Baron EJ, Finegold SM. Bailey & Scott's Diagnostic Microbiology, ed 8. St. Louis: CV Mosby, 1990:494.
3. Blazevic DJ, Ederer GM. Principles of Biochemical Tests in Diagnostic Microbiology. New York: John Wiley & Sons, 1975:69–71.
4. Branson D. Methods in Clinical Bacteriology. Springfield, IL: Charles C Thomas, 1972:28–29.
5. Cowan ST. Cowan & Steel's Manual for the Identification of Medical Bacteria, ed 2. Cambridge: Cambridge University Press, 1974:37.
6. Dowell VR Jr, Lombard GL, Thompson FS, Armfield AY. Media for isolation, characterization and identification of obligately anaerobic bacteria. CDC Laboratory Manual, publ no. CDC-530–009/64745. Atlanta, GA: Centers for Disease Control, reprinted 1987.
7. Ellner PD, Granato PA, May CB. Recovery and identification of anaerobes: A system suitable for the routine clinical laboratory. Appl Microbiol 1973;26(6):904–913.
8. Ellner PD, O'Donnell ED. A selective differential medium for histotoxic clostridia. Am J Clin Pathol 1971;56(2):197–200.
9. George WL, Sutter VL, Citron D, Finegold SM. Selective and differential medium for isolation of *Clostridium difficile*. J Clin Microbiol 1979;9(2):214–219.
10. Graber CD, Boltjes BH, Morillo M. Comparison of the slide and coagulase-mannitol agar methods for adducing staphylocoagulase. Am J Med Technol 1968;34(4):211–214.
11. Harrow B, Mazur A. Textbook of Biochemistry, ed 9. Philadelphia: WB Saunders, 1966:277, 279–280.
12. Hayward NJ. Rapid identification of *Cl. welchii* by the Nagler reaction. Br Med J 1941;1 811–814.
13. Hayward NJ. The rapid identification of *Cl. welchii* by the Nagler tests in plate cultures. J Pathol Bacteriol 1943;55:285–293.
14. Holum JR. Elements of General and Biological Chemistry, ed 4. New York: John Wiley & Sons, 1975:340.
15. Howard BJ, Klaas J II, Rubin SJ, et al. Clinical and Pathogenic Microbiology. St. Louis: CV Mosby, 1987:339, 346.
16. Ispolotovskaya MV. Type A *Clostridium perfringens* toxin. In: Kodis S, Montie TC, Ajl SL, eds. Microbial Toxins, vol 2A. New York: Academic Press, 1971:109–158.
17. Koneman EW, Allen SD, Janda WM, et al. Color Atlas and Textbook of Diagnostic Microbiology, ed 4. Philadelphia: JB Lippincott, 1992:476–477, 546, 592.
18. Koskitalo LD, Milling ME. Lack of correlation between egg yolk reaction in *Staphylococcus* medium 110 supplemented with egg yolk and coagulase activity of staphylococci isolated from cheddar cheese. Can J Microbiol 1969;15:132–133.
19. MacFarlane MG, Knight BCJG. The biochemistry of bacterial toxins. I. The lecithinase activity of *Cl. welchii* toxins. Biochem J 1941;35(8):884–902.
20. MacFarlane RG, Oakley CL, Anderson CC. Haemolysis and the production of opalescence in serum and lecitho-vitellin by the α-toxin of *Clostridium welchii*. J Pathol Bacteriol 1941;52:99–103.
21. McClung LS, Toabe R. The egg yolk plate reaction for the presumptive diagnosis of *Clostridium sporogenes* and certain species of the gangrene and botulinum groups. J Bacteriol 1947;53(2):139–147.
22. Nagler FP. Observations on a reaction between the lethal toxin of *Cl. welchii* (type A) and human serum. Br J Exp Pathol 1939;20(6):473–485.
23. Oberhofer TR. Manual of Nonfermenting Gram-Negative Bacteria. New York: John Wiley & Sons, 1985:73–77.
24. Power DA, McCuen PJ. Manual of BBL Products and Laboratory Procedures, ed 6. Cockeysville, MD: Becton Dickinson Microbiology Systems, 1988:135, 137, 175.
25. Rolfe RD, Helebian S, Finegold SM. Bacterial interference between *Clostridium difficile* and normal fecal flora. J Infect Dis 1981;143(3):470–475.
26. Smith LDS, Holdeman LV. The Pathogenic Anaerobic Bacteria. Springfield, IL: Charles C Thomas, 1968:27.
27. White A, Handler P, Smith EL. Principles of Biochemistry, ed 5. New York: McGraw-Hill, 1973:584–586.
28. Willis AT. Clostridia of Wound Infection. London: Butterworths, 1969.
29. Willis AT, Gowland G. Some observations on the mechanism of the Nagler reaction. J Pathol Bacteriol 1962;83:219–226.
30. Wilson KH, Kennedy MJ, Fekety FR. Use of sodium taurocholate to enhance spore recovery on a medium selective for *Clostridium difficile*. J Clin Microbiol 1982;15(3):443–446.
31. Wistreich GA, Lechtman MD. Microbiology, ed 3. New York: Macmillian, 1980:83.

21 Leucine Aminopeptidase (Leucine Arylamidase) (LAP) Test

I. PRINCIPLE

To detect the presence of the enzyme leucine aminopeptidases (LAP)

II. PURPOSE

Presumptive preliminary characterization of catalase-negative, Gram-positive cocci of streptococci, enterococci, and streptococcus-like genera (4). LAP is often used in conjunction with PYR and other biochemical tests (Table 21.1).

Table 21.1. Characteristics of *Streptococcus*, *Enterococcus*, and *Streptococcus*-like Organisms

Organism	Catalase	Lap	Pyr	Esculin Hydrolysis	Growth 6.5% NaCl	Vancomycin
Beta (β) *Streptococcus*						
S. pneumoniae	−	+	V	V	−	S
S. pyogenes, group A	−	+	+	+	−	S
Other (β) *Streptococcus* spp.	−	−	−	−	−	S
Enterococcus spp., group D	−	+	+	+	V+	S
Aerococcus						
A. viridans	−	−	+	V	+	S
A. urinae	−	+	−	V	+	S
Alloiococcus otitis	+	+	+	−	+[a]	S
Gemella						
G. hemolysans	−	V	+	−	−	S
G. morbillorum	−	+	+[wb]	−	−	S
Globicatella sanguis	−	−	+	V	+	S
Helcococcus kunzii	−	−	+	+	V	S
Lactococcus spp.	−	+	+	+	−	S
Leuconostoc spp.	−	−	−	−	V	R
Nutrionally variant streptococci						
Abiotrophia adiacens	−	+	V	−	−	S
Abiotrophia defectiva	−	+	V	−	−	S
Pediococcus spp.	−	+	−	+	V	R
Tetragenacoccus spp.	−	+	−	NR	NR	S
Vagacoccus spp.	−	+	+	+	+	S

(Data from reference 2.)
NR, no results; +[w], weakly positive; S, susceptible (sensitive); R, resistant.
[a]May take 2–7 days.
[b]Large inoculum **must** be used.

III. ENZYME/SUBSTRATE

Enzyme

Leucine aminopeptidase (LAP) (leucine arylamidase) is an exopeptidase that hydrolyzes a peptide bond adjacent to a free amino group. It is called leucine aminopeptidase because it reacts most rapidly with leucine compounds (6).

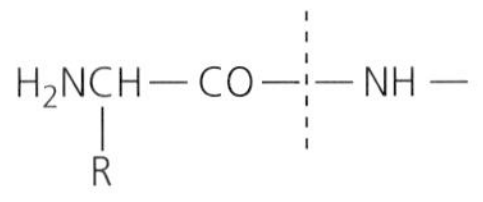

$$H_2NCH-CO-\vdots-NH-$$
$$|$$
$$R$$

Leucine-aminopeptidase

R is leucine or other aliphatic side chain.

Aminopeptidases require a free terminal NH_4 group and depend on metal ions for their activity; breakdown of chain liberates free amino acid (deamination) (1). Deamination initiates breakdown of amino acid; start with removal of water (H_2O). Leucine aminopeptidase is a metal-activated peptidase (Mn^{2+} or Mg^{2+}). Metal ions are tightly bound and are necessary for enzymatic activity. The metal forms a bridge between substrate and enzyme.

IV. REAGENT p–DIMETHYLAMINOCINNAMALDEHYDE (DMACA)

(Note: Same reagent is used for pyrrolidonyl-β-naphthylamide (PYR) test (Chapter 37).)

A. **Properties**
 1. *p*-Dimethylaminocinnamaldehyde (DMACA) is a vinyl analog of *p*-dimethylaminobenzaldehyde (DMABA).
 2. **Not** a dye or stain, but upon hydrolysis it yields a substance that is converted into an **insoluble azo dye** (3).
 3. Acid solution; concentration 1% in 10% concentrated hydrochloric acid (HCl)
 4. Prepare fresh every 2 months.

B. **Chemistry of reagent action**

LAP reagent is an acid solution containing detergent that forms a red Shiff base with free β-naphthylamine. β-Naphthylamines are not reactive because the amino group is involved in amide bond.

1. Step 1

Leucine-β-naphthylamide is hydrolyzed by leucine aminopeptidase, releasing free β-naphthylamine.

2. Step 2

Color results when chromophore azo group -N=N- results from coupling with enzymatically released naphthols or naphthylamine (3).

Step 1

Leucine-β-naphthylamide $\xrightarrow[\text{enzymatic hydrolysis}]{\text{leucine aminopeptidase}}$ Leucine + free β-naphthylamine

Substrate $\qquad\qquad\qquad\qquad\qquad\qquad$ $C_6H_{13}O_2N$ $\quad$ $C_{10}H_7NH_2$
$\qquad\qquad\qquad\qquad\qquad\qquad\qquad\quad$ Colorless $\qquad\;\;$ Colorless

Step 2

β-Naphthylamine + p-Dimethylaminocinnamaldehyde $\xrightarrow[\text{dye coupler}]{\text{diazo}}$ Red color

Substrate $\qquad$ LAP/PYR reagent $\qquad\qquad\qquad\qquad$ Shiff base
Colorless

Diazo compounds combine with aromatic amines or phenols (e.g., β-naphthylamine). Azo group –N=N– (or diazo group if an N is connected to an element other than carbon) yields a colored compound (3).

V. COMMERCIAL TEST SYSTEMS

A. **Disk spot tests**; disks with reagents
   1. Manufacturers; follow manufacturer's directions
      a. LAP disk: REMEL (5)
      b. LAP (LAPNA): Key Scientific
      c. Leucine Minitek: BBL
   2. Procedure (2, 5)
      a. Rehydrate disk; two methods
         (1) Moisten with **sterile** distilled water.
         (2) Place disk on agar surface; e.g., sheep blood agar (SBA).
      b. With a wooden applicator stick or an inoculating loop, **heavily** rub several **pure** colonies from an 18- to 24-h agar plate onto disk. If slow-growing isolate, incubate 2–3 days for sufficient inoculum.
      c. Incubate room temperature (22–25°C) **5 min**
      d. **After** incubation, add **1 drop** of detection reagent to disk; allow **1 min** for color development.
B. **Assay for enzyme included in kit systems** (2)
   1. Manufacturers
      a. API Rapid Strep; bioMérieux
      b. Bacti Card Streptococcus Test; REMEL
         (1) System consists of PYR, LAP, and esculin hydrolysis.
         (2) Card used with vancomycin susceptibility provides preliminary characteristics of *Aerococcus, Enterococcus, Gemella, Globicatella, Lactococcus, Leuconostoc,* and *Pediococcus*.
C. **Storage:** disks and systems, 2–8°C

VI. QUALITY CONTROL MICROORGANISMS

A. Positive (+)

   Enterococcus faecalis $\qquad$ ATCC 29212

B. Negative (−)

   Aerococcus viridans $\qquad$ ATCC 11563

VII. RESULTS

> See Figure 21.1 (Appendix 1) for colored photographic results

VIII. INTERPRETATION

A. Positive (+): red color
B. Weakly positive (+^{w}): pink color
C. Negative (−): no color change; yellow

IX. PRECAUTIONS

A. **General**
   1. DHEW publ no. (NIH) 76–900 lists amino acid β-naphthylamines as known carcinogens. Care must be taken during preparation and storage of LAP substrate.
   2. Preferably, clinical isolates of streptococci should be tested prior to 48-h incubation or subcultured prior to testing.
   3. **Before** performing the LAP test, confirm that organism is a Gram-positive coccus and is catalase negative.
B. **REMEL disks** (5)
   1. Store disks in original container at 2–8°C; do not freeze or overheat. Allow them to come to room temperature before use; do not incubate.
   2. Color development after 1 min **should be disregarded**.
   3. False-negative result may occur if inadequate inoculum is used.
   4. Further biochemical and serologic testing may be necessary for definitive identification.

REFERENCES

1. Doelle HW: Bacterial Metabolism. New York: Academic Press, 1969:403.
2. Koneman EW, Allen SD, Janda WM, et al. Color Atlas and Textbook of Diagnostic Microbiology, ed 5. Philadelphia: JB Lippincott, 1997:606–629.
3. Lillie RD. H. J. Conn's Biological Stains, ed 9. Baltimore: Williams & Wilkins, 1977:200.
4. Murray PR, Baron EJ, Pfaller MA, Tenover FC, Yolken RH. Manual of Clinical Microbiology, ed 6. Washington, DC: American Society for Microbiology, 1995:258.
5. REMEL LAP Disk Technical Information no. 21129. Lenexa, KS: REMEL, 1993.
6. Worthington Biochemical Corporation. Worthington Manual. Freehold, NJ: Worthington Biochemical Corporation, 1972:115.

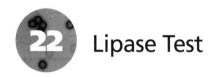

22 Lipase Test

I. PRINCIPLE

To determine the ability of microorganisms to produce the enzyme lipase that catalyzes the hydrolysis of triglycerides and diglycerides to fatty acids and glycerol as evidenced by an oily, iridescent sheen on and surrounding colonies on plate medium

II. PURPOSE

(Also see Chapters 43 through 45)

A. Aid in identification of obligate anaerobic Gram-negative bacilli
   1. *Fusobacterium necrophorum* (+) from other *Fusobacterium* spp. (−) (20)
   2. *Propionibacterium acnes* (V, variable) and *P. granulosum* (V) from *P. avidum* (−) and *P. propionicus* (−) (20)
B. Aid in identification of *Clostridium* species: *C. botulinum* (+), *C. sporogenes* (+), *C. novyi* A (+), *C. ghoni* (+), *C. cochlearium* (+), and *C. leptum* (V, usually −) from other *Clostridium* spp. (−) (also see Chapter 20, Lecithinase Test, Table 20.2)
C. *Pseudomonas aeruginosa* (+) (6, 15) and *Burkholderia cepacia* (formerly *Pseudomonas cepacia*) (+) from other *Pseudomonas* spp. (−) (2, 8, 15, 24, 27, 29, 32, 34)
D. *Ureaplasma urealyticum* (+) from other *Ureaplasma* spp. (−)
E. *Mycoplasma hominis* (+) (30), *Mycoplasma mycoides* (+) (7), and *Acholeplasma laidlawii* (+) (37)
F. *Corynebacterium pseudotuberculosis* (+) and *C. ulcerans* (+)) from other *Corynebacterium* spp. (−) (3)
G. Lipase activity specific among the *Enterobacteriaceae*
   1. *Serratia fonticola* (−) from other *Serratia* spp. (usually +); unique among the *Enterobacteriaceae* in that lipase, gelatinase, and DNase are positive (18, 20, 21)
   2. *Proteus vulgaris* (V, usually +), *P. myxofaciens* (+), and *P. penneri* (V) from *P. inconstans* (−), *Providencia* spp. (−), and *Morganella morganii* biogroups 1 and 2 (−)
   3. *Cedecea* spp. (V, usually +)
H. Other lipase-positive bacteria: *Staphylococcus aureus* subsp. *aureus* (18, 21)

III. BIOCHEMISTRY INVOLVED

Lipids

Lipid is an all-inclusive term to describe a group of fats or derived fats. Lipids are classified into three main groups: (*a*) **simple (neutral) fats** that on hydrolysis yield esters of fatty acids and alcohol, (*b*) **compound fats** that on hydrolysis yield products other than alcohols and fatty acids (e.g., **phospholipids** and **glycolipids**), and (*c*) **derived fats** that are obtained by hydrolysis of simple or compound lipids. **Neutral fats** are esters of glycerol and long-chain fatty acids. The *R* is a carbon chain of fatty acids (alkyl side chains of fatty acids) esterified to glycerol (glycerin), a trihydric (polyhydric) alcohol. **Phospholipids** are complex esters of alcohol, fatty acid, phosphoric acid, and a nitrogenous base. Choline is just one of the alcohols that may be present; others are ethanolamine, serine, and inositol (16). **Glycolipids** are complex lipids containing sphingosine, a fatty acid, and a sugar but **no** phosphoric acid; a sugar moiety other than D-mannose may be galactose, glucose, or an oligosaccharide (16).

$$
\begin{array}{l}
CH_2-O-\overset{O}{\underset{\|}{C}}-R \\
CH-O-\overset{O}{\underset{\|}{C}}-R \\
CH_2-O-\overset{O}{\underset{\|}{C}}-R
\end{array}
\quad \text{Lipid}
$$

$$
\begin{array}{l}
CH_2-O-\overset{O}{\underset{\|}{C}}-R \\
CH-O-\overset{O}{\underset{\|}{C}}-R \\
CH_2-O-\underset{\underset{O^-}{|}}{\overset{O}{\underset{\|}{P}}}-O-CH_2-N^+\!\!\underbrace{\begin{array}{l}-CH_3 \\ -CH_3 \\ -CH_3\end{array}}_{\text{Choline}}
\end{array}
\quad \text{Phospholipid}
$$

Glycolipid, with D-mannose (16)

Bacteria contain considerable lipids as constituents of their membrane systems, especially phospholipids and glycolipids.

Fatty Acids

Fatty acids are carboxylic acids; the precursor of fatty acids is acetyl-coenzyme A (CoA). Most fatty acids in lipids contain 16–18 carbon atoms; they are saturated or have one (seldom more) double bond between carbon atoms in the alkyl chain. The three hydroxyl groups (OH) of glycerol ($C_3H_5(OH)_3$) offer many combinations for fatty acid ester formation. Some **un**saturated fatty acids are also important constituents of phospholipids (e.g., palmitoleate and *cis*-vaccenate in *Escherichia coli* (16).

Glycerides

Glycerides are large molecules with ester groups; e.g., triglycerides, diglycerides, and monoglycerides. The term "fat" usually refers to triglycerides. Triglycerides are a mixture of long-chain fatty acids and glycerol where R, R' and R'' are alkyl side chains of saturated and unsaturated fatty acids. They are the chief component of fats and oils (e.g., in vegetable oils, olive oils, corn oil). Both fats and oils, regardless of their source, are mixtures of different glyceride molecules (19); there are **no chemical** differences between fat and oil.

$$\begin{array}{l} CH_2-O-\overset{O}{\overset{\|}{C}}-R \qquad \text{1 or } \alpha \text{ (saturated)} \\ CH-O-\overset{O}{\overset{\|}{C}}-R' \qquad \text{2 or } \beta \text{ (unsaturated)} \\ CH_2-O-\overset{O}{\overset{\|}{C}}-R'' \qquad \text{3 or } \alpha_1 \text{ (saturated)} \end{array}$$

Triglyceride (fat)

Hydrolysis

The enzyme lipase acts on emulsified esters of glycerides and/or lipids. Triglycerides (triacylglycerols) are hydrolyzed to monoglycerides (monoacylglycerols), glycerol, and a variety of different saturated or unsaturated fatty acids. Lipase is specific for α and α_1 chains of triglycerides.

Hydrolysis of Triglyceride

$$\begin{array}{c} CH_2-O-\overset{O}{\overset{\|}{C}}-R \quad HO|H \\ CH-O-\overset{O}{\overset{\|}{C}}-R' + HO|H \\ CH_2-O-\overset{O}{\overset{\|}{C}}-R'' \quad HO|H \end{array} \xrightarrow{\text{lipase}} \begin{array}{c} CH_2OH \\ | \\ CHOH \\ | \\ CH_2OH \end{array} + HO-\overset{O}{\overset{\|}{C}}-R + HO-\overset{O}{\overset{\|}{C}}-R' + HO-\overset{O}{\overset{\|}{C}}-R''$$

L-Triglyceride   Water   Glycerol   3 Different fatty acids

When hydrolyzed, ester linkages (carbonyl-oxygen bonds) break, and elements of water combine with the fragments (19). When ester linkages in glyceride are hydrolyzed, fatty acids behave as ordinary carboxylic acids (19) and are **in**soluble in water.

Phospholipases

Many lipases are produced constitutively, although their production may be influenced by nutritional and physical conditions of the culture (22). The physical role of extracellular lipases is probably nutritional; some may hydrolyze exogenous triglycerides to provide free fatty acids for use as an energy source (26). They are important catabolic enzymes in phospholipid metabolism; mechanism of their action in infectious process is not well understood (9).

Phospholipase A_1 and A_2 hydrolyze phospholipids to lysophospholipid and fatty acids (11). Phospholipase A_2 is involved in resynthesis of phospholipids via deacylation-reacylation (23) and in the production of prostaglandin precursors (36).

Phospholipase C is a phosphoryl hydrolase that liberates 1,2-diglyceride and phosphorylester (9, 36). Phospholipase C activity has been reported as secreted phosphorylhydrolase in many bacterial species (1, 9). Its secretion may play a role in the physiologic effects of infection, but the function of phospholipases as secreted toxins in perinatal infection is not yet delineated (11). Phospholipase C catalyzes hydrolysis of phosphatidylcholine (a phospholipid in membranes of animal cells) into phosphorylcholine and diglyceride (diacylglycerol) (15).

Hydrolysis of Diglyceride

$$\begin{array}{c} CH_2-O-\overset{O}{\overset{\|}{C}}-R \\ | \\ CH\ -O-\overset{O}{\overset{\|}{C}}-R' \\ | \\ CH_2OH \end{array} + 2H_2O \xrightarrow{\text{lipase}} \begin{array}{c} CH_2OH \\ | \\ CHOH \\ | \\ CH_2OH \end{array} + HO-\overset{O}{\overset{\|}{C}}-R$$

D-α-β-Triglyceride   Glycerol   Fatty acid
(1,2-diglyceride)   (saturated variety)

Egg Yolk

Egg yolk (suspension) is an indicator for lipase (or lecithinase) activity in culture media. Egg yolk is a mixture of lipids, phospholipids, lipoproteins and other complex components; thus, the egg yolk reaction may be caused by a number of enzymes acting on a variety of substrates (26). Free fats in egg yolk are degraded by lipase to glycerol and fatty acid.

Ureaplasma/Mycoplasma/Acholeplasma

Ureaplasma spp. have phospholipases A_1, A_2, and C; however, A_2 activity varies among serovars studied (10). Variation in levels of specific activity or unique enzyme characteristics may account for differences in virulence among *Ureaplasma* serovars (11). Phospholipase C in *U. urealyticum* differs from that in most bacteria in being membrane bound; most bacteria secrete it into culture medium (1, 9). Endogenous phospholipases are localized primarily in the plasma membrane of exponential-phase cells (11); other investigators have made the same observations in *M. hominis* (31), *A. laidlawii* (37), and *M. mycoides* (7). Mycoplasmas adhere to host cells, and their enzyme can interact with cell membrane (25). Phospholipases localized in membrane are important in delineating mechanism of pathogenesis (11); they function as virulence factors in infection (5, 9).

Staphylococcus aureus subsp. *aureus*

Lipase may help spread the organism in cutaneous and subcutaneous tissues (20). *S aureus* subsp. *aureus* produces lipase that may, by hydrolyzing lipids on epithelial surface of humans, enhance colonization of the skin (38). *S. aureus* subsp. *aureus* contains two phospholipases: one hydrolyzes phosphatidyl inositol and lysophosphatidyl inositol; the other hydrolyzes sphingomyelin (13).

IV. MEDIA EMPLOYED

A. *C. botulinum* isolation (inhibitory) (CBI) agar (12, 20)
   1. Formulation of Dezfulian, McCroskey, Hatheway, and Dowell (12); selective medium
      a. Rapid quantitative and qualitative isolation of *C. botulinum* types A, B, and F and *C. argentinense* (formerly *C. botulinum* type G) from human feces; suppresses growth of

other obligate anaerobes and a few *Clostridium* spp. Results comparable to those on egg yolk agar (EYA).
   b. Aids in differentiating *C. botulinum* types A, B, and F (lipase +) from *C. argentinense* and other clostridia that grow on CBI (lipase −).
2. Egg yolk suspension: 50% in physiologic saline (NaCl)
3. Stock solutions
   a. Cycloserine (C, Cyclo): 1%, dissolve in distilled water
   b. Sulfamethoxazole (S, SMX): 1.9%, dissolve in distilled water; just enough 10% NaOH to get into solution
   c. Trimethoprim (T, TMP): 0.1%, dissolve in distilled water; just enough 0.05 N HCl to get into solution
4. Medium, pH 7.4 ± 0.2

Trypticase peptone	40.0 g
Yeast extract	5.0 g
D-Glucose (dextrose)	2.0 g
Disodium phosphate, $Na_2HPO_4 \cdot 12H_2O$	5.0 g
Magnesium sulfate (5% aqueous solution)	0.2 mL
Sodium chloride, NaCl	2.0 g
Agar	20.0 g
Deionized water	900.0 mL
After sterilization, cool, and add	
Egg yolk suspension, **sterile**	100.0 mL
Cycloserine (C), **sterile**	250.0 mg/mL
Sulfamethoxazole (S), **sterile**	76.0 mg/mL
Trimethoprim (T), **sterile**	4.0 mg/mL

B. **Botulinum selective medium (BSM)**
1. Formulation of Mills, Midura, and Arnon (28); modification of *C. botulinum* inhibitory medium (CBI) (12)
2. Rapid, quantitative recovery of lipase-positive *C. botulinum* in infant botulism and food-borne botulism along with a Gram stain and fecal toxin testing
3. Antibiotic stock solutions
   a. Cycloserine: 25 mg/mL in distilled water
   b. Sulfamethoxazole: 15 mg/mL in 0.1N sodium hydroxide (NaOH)
   c. Trimethoprim: 50 mg
      (1) Dissolve in 5 mL of 0.05 N HCl at 55°C.
      (2) Add distilled water to final volume of 50 mL; 1 mg/mL final concentration.
4. Egg yolk suspension: 50% egg yolk in physiologic saline (NaCl; 0.85%)
5. Medium, pH 7.4 ± 0.2

Heart infusion (HI) broth	25.0 g
Agar	20.0 g
Deionized water	1000.0 mL
After **sterilization**, cool and add	
Egg yolk suspension, **sterile**	30.0 mL
Cycloserine, **sterile**	250.0 mg/mL
Sulfamethoxazole, **sterile**	76.0 mg/mL
Trimethoprim, **sterile**	4.0 mg/mL
Thymidine phosphorylase, **sterile**	100 IU

(*Note*: Thymidine phosphorylase suppresses nonbotulinum fecal flora.)

C. See Chapter 20, Lecithinase Test, for additional egg yolk agar (EYA) media that may also be used for lipase test and preparation of egg yolk from scratch. Antibiotics C-S-T may also be added to CDC modified EYA medium.

D. **Lipase salt mannitol (LSM) agar (mannitol salt egg yolk agar, mannitol salt lipase (test) agar)**
   1. Formulation of Gunn, Dunkelberg, and Creitz (17), and O'Brien and Lewis (30)
   2. Primary isolation and identification of *S. aureus* subsp. *aureus* (V^+) from *Staphylococcus epidermidis* ($-$)
   3. Ingredients, pH 7.4 ± 0.2

Casein/meat (50/50) peptone	10.0 g
Beef extract	1.0 g
D-Mannitol	10.0 g
Sodium chloride, NaCl	75.0 g
Phenol red	0.025 g
Deionized water	1000.0 mL
After **sterilization**, cool, and add	
Egg yolk suspension, 2%, **sterile**	20.0 mL

E. Method of sterilization
   1. Basal agar media: autoclave, 121°C, 15 lb, 15 min
   2. Antibiotics (C-S-T), thymidine phosphorylase, and egg yolk suspension: filtration, Millipore)
F. Dispense: Petri dishes; 20 mL/plate (15 × 100 mm)
G. Storage
   1. Refrigerator, 4–10°C; seal tightly in original bags with plates inverted (lids down)
   2. Shelf life: **no longer** than 2 weeks
H. Inoculation
   1. Anaerobes: hold plates in anaerobic glove box 4 h **before use**; if delayed, place in jar flushed with nitrogen.
   2. Direct specimen; four-quadrant streaking for maximum isolation
I. Incubation: aerobic/anaerobic, depending on microorganisms being tested; 35°C; plates inverted (lids down)
   1. Anaerobes: 48 h
   2. Staphylococci: 24–36 h

V. QUALITY CONTROL MICROORGANISMS

Positive (+):
    Clostridium sporogenes   ATCC 3584
    Staphylococcus aureus subsp. *aureus*   ATCC 12600
Negative (−):
    Clostridium perfringens   ATCC 13124
    Staphylococcus epidermidis   ATCC 14990
Uninoculated

VI. RESULTS

> See Figure 22.1 in Appendix 1 for colored photographic results

VII. INTERPRETATION

A. **Botulinum media**
 1. Positive (+)
    a. Iridescent sheen (mother-of-pearl sheen) on surface of colonies and on agar immediately around bacterial growth or either as a surface "oil-on-water" layer that covers colonies and may extend beyond colony edge or as an opaque zone directly beneath the colonies (4).
    b. To best see the "oil-on-water" phenomenon, hold plate at an angle to a light source (4); use reflected light (20).
    c. If questionable results, add a few drops of water and look for a film that floats on top of the water (20).
    d. Clearing of medium indicates proteolysis, **not** a lipase-positive result.
 2. Negative (−): **no** change in appearance of colonies or medium
B. **Lipase salt mannitol (LSM)**
 1. Lipase positive (+)
    a. Opaque zone around yellow colonies; lipovitellin-lipase activity
    b. *S. aureus* subsp. *aureus,* 90.4% (17); according to Gunn et al. (17), LSM correlates with coagulase production on 94.7% of cultures tested.
 2. Lipase negative (−): **no** zone around colonies; *S. epidermidis*

VIII. PRECAUTIONS

A. Phospholipase C production of *P. aeruginosa* is suppressed by inorganic phosphate (6).
B. It may be necessary to reincubate plates up to 2 weeks to detect slow lipase producers (4).
C. **All** clostridia, pigmented *Bacteroides* spp., and fusobacteria should be tested for lipase production (4).
D. Enzyme that hydrolyzes water-soluble Tween 80 **is not** a true lipase (39) but an esterase and should be treated separately. Organisms that have lipases **do not** necessarily split Tween 80 (14, 33).
E. Dezfulian et al. (12) recommend simultaneous use of both selective CBI and nonselective EYA medium for isolation of *C. botulinum* from primary specimen and, if necessary, from enriched culture to avoid missing drug-susceptible strains such as *C. botulinum* type E (35).
F. To best observe opaque zone on LSM, wipe off a colony with a swab; zones may be observed this way that would otherwise be delayed.

REFERENCES

1. Baine WB, Rasheed JK, Mackel DC, et al. Exotoxin activity associated with the Legionnaires disease bacterium. J Clin Microbiol 1979;9(3):453–456.
2. Ballard RW, Palleroni NJ, Doudoroff M, et al. Taxonomy of the aerobic pseudomonads: *Pseudomonas cepacia, P. marginata, P. alliicola, P. caryophylli.* J Gen Microbiol 1970;60:199–214.
3. Barksdale L, Linder R, Sulea IT, Pollice M. Phospholipase D activity of *Corynebacterium pseudotuberculosis (C. ovis)* and *Corynebacterium ulcerans,* a distinctive marker within the genus *Corynebacterium.* J Clin Microbiol 1981;13(2):335–343.
4. Baron EJ, Finegold SM. Bailey & Scott's Diagnostic Microbiology, ed 8. Philadelphia: CV Mosby, 1990:366, 494.
5. Bejar R, Curbelo V, Dairs C, Gluck L. Premature labour. Obstet Gynecol 1981;57:479–482.
6. Berka RM, Gray GL, Vasil ML. Studies of phospholipase C (heat-labile hemolysin) in *Pseudomonas aeruginosa.* Infect Immun 1981;34:1071–1074.
7. Bhandari S, Asnani PJ. Characterization of phospholipase A2 of *Mycoplasma* species. Folia Microbiol 1989;34:294–301.
8. Carson LA, Favero MS, Bond WW, Petersen NJ. Morphological, biochemical, and growth characteristics of *Pseudomonas cepacia* from distilled water. Appl Microbiol 1973;25:476–483.
9. Dennis EA. Phospholipases. In: Boyer PD, ed. The Enzymes. New York: Academic Press, 1983:307–353.
10. De Silva NS, Quinn PA. Endogenous activity of phospholipase A and C in *Ureaplasma urealyticum.* J Clin Microbiol 1986;23(2):354–359.
11. De Silva NS, Quinn PA. Localization of endogenous activity of phospholipases A and C in *Ure-*

aplasma urealyticum. J Clin Microbiol 1991;29 (7):1498–1503.
12. Dezfulian M, McCroskey LM, Hatheway CL, Dowell VR Jr. Selective medium for isolation of *Clostridium botulinum* from human feces. J Clin Microbiol 1981;13(3):526–531.
13. Doery HM, Magnusson BJ, Cheyne IM, Gulasekharam J. A phospholipase in staphylococcal toxin which hydrolyses sphingomyelin. Nature 1963;198:1091–1092.
14. Elston HR, Elston JH. Further use of deoxyribonuclease in a screening test for *Serratia.* J Clin Pathol 1968;21(2):210–212.
15. Esselmann MT, Liu PV. Lecithinase production by gram-negative bacteria. J Bacteriol 1961;81: 939–945.
16. Gottschalk G. Bacterial Metabolism, ed 2. New York: Springer-Verlag, 1986:66, 68.
17. Gunn BA, Dunkelberg WE Jr, Creitz JR. Clinical evaluation of 2%-LSM medium for primary isolation and identification of coagulase-positive staphylococci. Am J Clin Pathol 1972;57(2): 236–240.
18. Holt JG, Krieg NR, Sneath PHA, et al. Bergey's Manual of Determinative Bacteriology, ed 9. Baltimore: Williams & Wilkins, 1994:203.
19. Holum JR. Elements of General and Biological Chemistry, ed 4. New York: John Wiley & Sons, 1975:342, 344–345.
20. Koneman EW, Allen SD, Janda WM, et al. Color Atlas and Textbook of Diagnostic Microbiology, ed 4. Philadelphia: JB Lippincott, 1992:143, 409, 546, 573, 586.
21. Krieg NR, Holt JG, eds. Bergey's Manual of Systematic Bacteriology, vol 1. Baltimore: Williams & Wilkins, 1984:514.
22. Kurioka S, Matsuda M. Phospholipase C assay using *p*-nitrophenylphosphorylcholine together with sorbitol and its application to studying the metal and detergent requirement of the enzyme. Anal Biochem 1975;75:281–289.
23. Lands WEM. Metabolism of glycerolipids. II. The enzymatic acylation of lysolecithin. J Biol Chem 1960;235:2233–2237.
24. Lawrence RC, Fryer TF, Reiter B. The production and characterization of lipases from a micrococcus and a pseudomonad. J Gen Microbiol 1967;48:401–418.
25. Lingwood C, Schramayr S, Quinn PA. The male germ cell specific sulfogalactoglycerolipid is recognized and degraded by mycoplasmas allocated with male infertility. J Cell Physiol 1990;142:170–176.
26. Lonon MK, Woods DE, Straus DC. Production of lipase by clinical isolates of *Pseudomonas cepacia.* J Clin Microbiol 1988;26(5):979–984.
27. McKevitt AI, Woods DE. Characterization of *Pseudomonas cepacia* isolates from patients with cystic fibrosis. J Clin Microbiol 1984;19(2): 291–293.
28. Mills DC, Midura TF, Arnon SS. Improved selective medium for the isolation of lipase-positive *Clostridium botulinum* from feces of human infants. J Clin Microbiol 1985;21(6):947–950.
29. Morris MB, Roberts JB. A group of pseudomonads able to synthesize poly-β-hydroxybutyric acid. Nature (London) 1959;183:1538–1539.
30. O'Brien SM, Lewis JF. Evaluation of a medium for isolation and identification of coagulase positive staphylococci. Am J Med Technol 1967; 33(6):490.
31. Rottem S, Hasin M, Razin S. Differences in susceptibility to phospholipase C of free and membrane-bound phospholipids of *Mycoplasma hominis.* Biochim Biophys Acta 1973;323:520–531.
32. Sinsabaugh HA, Howard GW Jr. Emendation of the description of *Pseudomonas cepacia* Burkholder (synonyms: *Pseudomonas multivorans* Stanier et al., *Pseudomonas kingae* Jonsson: EO-1 group). Int J Syst Bacteriol 1975;25:187–201.
33. Smith RF, Willett NP. Lipolytic activity of human cutaneous bacteria. J Gen Microbiol 1968; 52:441–445.
34. Starr MP, Burkholder WH. Lipolytic activity of phytopathogenic bacteria determined by means of spirit blue agar and its taxonomic significance. Phytopathology 1941;32:598–604.
35. Swenson JM, Thornsberry C, McCroskey LM, et al. Susceptibility of *Clostridium botulinum* to thirteen antimicrobial agents. Antimicrob Agents Chemother 1980;18(1):13–19.
36. Van den Bosch H. Intracellular phospholipases A. Biochim Biophys Acta 1980;604:191–246.
37. Van Golde LMG, McElhaney RN, Deenen LLMV. A membrane-bound lysophospholipase from *Mycoplasma laidlawii* strain B. Biochim Biophys Acta 1971;231:245–249.
38. Willett HP. *Staphylococcus.* In: Joklik WK, Willett HP, eds. Zinsser's Microbiology, ed 16. New York, Appleton-Crofts, 1976:412.
39. Willis ED. Lipases. Adv Lipid Res 1965;3:197–240.

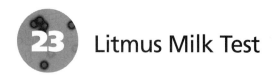

23 Litmus Milk Test

I. PRINCIPLE

To differentiate organisms on the basis of their multiple metabolic reactions in a milk medium

II. PURPOSE

(Also see Chapters 43 and 44)

Differential medium used primarily for study of selective microorganisms, e.g., Gram-negative nonfermenters, clostridia, and the enterococci (16)

A. To aid in species differentiation primarily within the genus *Clostridium* (Table 23.1)

Table 23.1. Reactions of the Most Frequently Isolated *Clostridium* spp. in Litmus Milk

Digestion/clot (DC)[a]
- *C. cadaveris*
- *C. perfringens* (GS)

Clot/digestion (CD)[b]
- *C. haemolyticum*
- *C. septicum*

Clot (C)
- *C. baratii*[c]
- *C. beijerinckii*
- *C. butyricum* (GS)
- *C. celatum* (slight curd)
- *C. chauvoei*
- *C. clostridioforme*[d]
- *C. fallax*
- *C. indolis*
- *C. novyi* A
- *C. oroticum*
- *C. paraputrificum*
- *C. ramosum*
- *C. sartagoforum*
- *C. sphenoides*
- *C. spiroforme*
- *C. symbiosum*[e]
- *C. tertium*

Digestion (D)
- *C. argentinense* (variable)[f]
- *C. bifermentans*
- *C. botulinum*
- *C. ghoni*
- *C. hastiforme*
- *C. histolyticum*
- *C. limosum*
- *C. novyi* B[g]
- *C. putrefaciens*
- *C. putrificum*
- *C. sordellii*
- *C. sporogenes*
- *C. subterminale*[h]

No reaction/negative
- *C. carnis*
- *C. cochlearium*
- *C. difficile*
- *C. glycolicum*
- *C. innocuum*
- *C. leptum*
- *C. malenominatum*
- *C. novyi* C
- *C. tetani*[i]

[a]Digestion priority over clot.
[b]Clot priority over digestion.
[c]Formerly *C. barti*, *C. perenne*, *C. paraperfringens*, *C. perennet*.
[d]Formerly *C. clostriidiforme*.
[e]Formerly *Fusobacterium symbiosum* and *Fusobacterium biacutus*.
[f]Formerly *C. botulinum* G, some nontoxic *C. hastiforme*, and *C. subterminale*.
[g]*C. novyi* B reports variable and long delayed.
[h]Slow.
[i]*C. tetani* reports variable and long delayed.

B. Most *Enterococcus* spp. reduce milk to a white color by using litmus as an electron acceptor (19) in presence of preformed enzyme.
C. *Streptococcus bovis* (growth) from *S. equinus* (no growth).
D. To aid in species differentiation of cutaneous *Propionibacterium acnes* (+) and *P. avidum* (+) from *P. granulosum* (−) (20) (see alternative test procedure)
E. Along with other tests (esculin, slime production, sodium chloride broth reaction, and carbohydrates arabinose, melibiose, raffinose, and trehalose) aids in differentiating *Leuconostoc lactis* (acid/clot) and *L. pseudomesenteroides* (acid/clot) from *L. mesenteroides* (−; occasional exception) and *L. citreum* (−) (1)

III. BIOCHEMISTRY INVOLVED

Litmus milk is a differential medium used to determine several metabolic functions of an organism: (*a*) lactose fermentation, (*b*) caseolysis, and (*c*) casein coagulation (6). Litmus incorporated in milk indicates both pH and E_h (oxidation-reduction); thus the medium can denote several metabolic functions. Milk alone contains the carbohydrate lactose along with three main proteins: casein, lactalbumin, and lactoglobulin (4). Therefore, an organism may exhibit one or several metabolic properties in litmus milk, each specific for a particular species, aiding bacterial identification: (*a*) lactose fermentation, (*b*) litmus reduction, (*c*) clot formation, (*d*) peptonization (digestion), and (*e*) gas formation.

Lactose Fermentation (Acidification)

Litmus as a pH indicator is red in an acid solution (pH 4.5) and blue under alkaline conditions (pH 8.3). Litmus milk exhibits a purplish blue color (pH 6.8) when uninoculated, but if an organism can ferment lactose, producing **mainly** lactic acid, an acid condition results that changes the medium to a pink-red color. Occasionally, butyric acid is the end product of lactose fermentation (3). Certain alkali-forming bacteria **do not** ferment lactose, but act on the nitrogenous substances present in the milk, releasing ammonia (3) and thereby yielding an alkaline pH denoted by a bluish purple color.

$$\text{Lactose} \longrightarrow \text{Glucose} + \text{galactose}$$

$$\text{Glucose} \longrightarrow \text{Pyruvic acid} \longrightarrow \begin{cases} \text{lactic acid} \\ \text{butyric acid} \\ CO_2 + H_2 \end{cases}$$

Reduction of Litmus

Litmus is a pH indicator (acid-base indicator) **and** simultaneously an oxidation-reduction indicator (E_h indicator). Reduction of oxygen levels often accompanies acid formation in depth of tube; the depth of top layer depends on the rate of reduction, not air oxidation (16). Certain organisms can reduce litmus to a leuco (white) base.

Clot Formation and Digestion (Casein Liquefaction/Peptonization)

Proteolytic enzymes (caseases) hydrolyze milk proteins, which coagulates the milk; the main enzyme responsible for clot formation is rennin (3, 9). Formation of a clot in litmus milk medium is caused by **either** precipitation of casein by acid formation **or** conversion of casein to paracasein by rennin. Peptonization may be accompanied by alkalinization, seen as a clear purple layer at the milk surface (16). Casein, a complex phosphoprotein, is the main protein present in milk (4, 17). It is a globular protein that is soluble in either water or an aqueous solution of acids, bases, or salts (8).

Alkalinization

Moderate activity on casein may produce alkaline products (16). Alkalization is seen at the surface of milk as a purple ring because of a basic shift in the pH of litmus in the presence of curd (16).

Formation of an Acid Clot

Precipitation of casein by organic acids from lactose (3) under acid conditions yields a firm, gelatinous clot that **does not** retract from the sides of the tube and is easily dissolved under alkaline conditions. Fresh milk has a pH of 6.6–6.9 due to the presence of acid phosphates. Cantarow and Schepartz (4) state that casein "is probably present as a salt (calcium caseinate) and precipitates on acidification as in souring (lactic acid fermentation)." Acidifying milk to a pH of 4.5 breaks up the complex protein casein to yield a precipitate (17). Lactose fermentation with litmus indicator exhibits a pinkish red color at pH 4.5. Lactose fermentation yields lactic acid and other organic acids as the end products of glycolysis, which in turn combine with the water-soluble salt calcium caseinate to yield caseinogen, which precipitates as an insoluble clot.

$$\text{Lactose} \longrightarrow \text{Lactic acid}$$

$$\text{Lactic acid} + \text{calcium caseinate} \xrightarrow{\text{casease}} \text{Caseinogen} \downarrow$$

(Acid environment)   (Salt of casein) (Soluble)   (Insoluble) precipitate

According to Burrows et al. (3), enzymatic hydrolysis of casein yields a final conversion of the caseinogen precipitate to a clear fluid, a process termed **peptonization.** Peptonization is exhibited by a watery clearing of the medium caused by digestion of the precipitate (clot) and milk proteins by proteolytic enzymes. However, peptonization **only** occurs when the bacteria growing in litmus milk contain casease (3). Peptonization is more often referred to as **digestion.**

Formation of a Curd (Clot)

Another form of a clot is a curd, or the curdling of milk by the conversion of casein to paracasein by the digestive enzymes rennin (rennase), pepsin, or chymotrypsin (chymosin) (4). The best-known enzyme is rennin (rennet) (17), which according to Cantarow and Schepartz (4), is secreted as prorennin and then activated by hydrogen ions (H^+). A dried commercial extract of rennin (rennet) is available.

Rennin curdles milk (a rennet clot) by converting the soluble casein salt (calcium caseinogenate) to an insoluble paracasein (calcium caseinate), which is the curd (4, 8). Curd contains calcium and calcium phosphates. Casein has been regarded as principle protein in milk, but it is actually a colloidal aggregate composed of several identifiable proteins together with phosphorus and calcium (10), a heterogeneous complex called calcium caseinate.

$$\text{Casein} \xrightarrow[\text{Ca}^{++}]{\text{rennin}} \text{Paracasein} \downarrow$$

(Salt calcium caseinogenate) (soluble)   (Calcium caseinate) (insoluble)   curd

According to Oser (17), rennin activity "hydrolyzes one peptide bond per 10,000 in casein." Harrow and Mazur (9) state that rennin's action is probably initial removal of a peptide bond in casein followed by formation of a clot or curd; calcium present as the salt acts as a stabilizing agent. However, Cantarow and Schepartz (4) state that casein is hydrolyzed to soluble paracasein that with calcium is converted to an insoluble casein, calcium paracaseinate, to form a "milk curd."

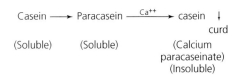

Paracasein precipitates as calcium paracaseinate (4, 17) above pH 4.5. This curd is soft, insoluble, and not dissolved under alkaline conditions; it retracts from the sides of the tube after a few hours, yielding a clear grayish or straw-colored residual fluid called "whey" (4, 5).

In recording clot formation, which enzymatic process was involved is not significant for identification purposes. Simply record the presence or absence of a clot.

Gas Formation/Stormy Fermentation

Gases (CO_2 and H_2) may result from lactose fermentation. Stormy fermentation results when an abundance of gas present breaks up an **acid** clot (acidification and clotting of casein). As milk proteins are coagulated by acid, curd is torn apart by gas production during fermentation. This may occur with certain anaerobic *Clostridium* spp. (*C. perfringens* and *C. butyricum*), and it is of great significance for species identification.

Proteolytic bacteria can hydrolyze milk enzymatically to form a clot (curd) or produce an alkaline reaction (3). Some organisms produce the enzyme lipase, which catabolizes the fats present in milk to yield a yellow transparent clear fluid (3).

One of these metabolic reactions or a variety of combinations may occur with a single bacterial isolate.

Acid, clot, gas, stormy fermentation (ACGS)
Acid only (A)
Acid with gas (AG)
Acid with clot (AC)
Acid, clot, gas (ACG)
Acid, digestion (AD)
Alkaline (Alk)
Clot, digestion (CD)
Clot, gas (CG)
Clot (C)
Digestion (D)
No change, negative (NC/−)
Reduction (Red)

Standard symbols or abbreviations are used to record all metabolic reactions occurring in litmus milk.

Acid, A
Alkaline, Alk or K
Clot, C
Digestion, D
GAs, G

Stormy fermentation, S
Reduction, R or Red
No change, NC, −, or neg

IV. INDICATOR (LITMUS SOLUTION)

(*Note:* Litmus, a vegetable indicator, a nonsynthetic product, or azolitmin, a commercial substance isolated from natural litmus, may be used in milk media.)

A. Ingredients (5)

Litmus, granular	250.0 g
Ethanol (ethyl alcohol) 40%, C_2H_5OH	1000.0 mL

B. Method of preparation of solvent **ethanol, 40%**
   1. Stock: 95% ethanol
   2. Calculations
      a. % required/% stock = x/amount required
      b. 40/95 = x/100 mL
      c. 4000/95 = 42.1 mL of 95% ethanol
   3. Amount desired of a 40% solution
      a. 100 mL = 42.1 mL of 95% ethanol brought to 100 mL with distilled water
      b. 1000 mL = 421.0 mL of 95% ethanol brought to 1000 mL with distilled water
C. Method of preparation: **litmus solution**
   1. Grind litmus to a fine powder.
   2. In a 2-L flask add 500 mL of 40% ethanol and ground litmus.
   3. Boil **1 min.**
   4. **Carefully** decant supernatant (liquid) into another 2-L flask.
   5. Add remaining 500 mL of 40% ethanol to residue in initial flask.
   6. Boil again for **1 min.**
   7. **Carefully** decant supernatant into flask containing the first 500 mL portion of boiled liquid.
   8. Centrifuge supernatant and decant into a 1-L graduated cylinder.
   9. Adjust volume to 1000 mL with 40% ethanol.
   10. Drop by drop, add 1 N HCl (hydrochloric acid) until solution turns **purple**.
D. Control testing of litmus reaction (5)
   1. Boil 10.0 mL of distilled water.
   2. Cool.
   3. Add 1 **drop** of litmus solution and **mix well.**
   4. If properly prepared, the water turns **mauve**.
   5. The concentration of litmus indicator is approximately 2.5% (5).

Litmus (lichen blue) is a natural product whose chemical composition is only partly known; the major coloring matter is a 7-hydroxy-2-phenoxazone derivative with 3,6-substituents (14); it is structurally similar to indophenol (11). Azolitmin **is not** the entire coloring matter of litmus; litmus may contain several constituents (11). The pH range of litmus is 4.8–8.3 (13) and of azolitmin, 5.0–8.0/4.5–8.3 (12, 13).

V. MEDIUM EMPLOYED: LITMUS MILK MEDIUM, pH 6.8 (6)

(*Note:* Fresh clean-skimmed cow's milk or commercial dehydrated skim milk may be used to prepare litmus milk medium (2).)

A. Ingredients: three choices
   1. With litmus; pH 6.8 ± 0.2

a. Formulation 1

Skim milk, dehydrated	100.0 g
Litmus powder	5.0 g
Deionized water	1000.0 mL

b. Formulation 2

Skim milk, dehydrated	100.0 g
Peptone	10.0 g
Sodium thiosulfate, $HSCH_2COONa$	0.5 g
Litmus	5.0 g
Deionized water	1000.0 mL

2. With azolitmin, pH 6.5 ± 0.2

Skim milk, dehydrated powder	100.0 g
Sodium sulfite, $Na_2SO_3 \cdot 7H_2O$	0.5 g
Azolitmin	0.5 g
Deionized water	1000.0 mL

3. Check pH; correct to 6.8 by slight addition of more litmus/azolitmin, checking after each addition.
4. A liquid solution of litmus may be added in place of the powder. If so, rehydrate the skim milk with distilled water and then add sufficient litmus solution (Section IV) to obtain a **purplish blue** color (pH 6.8) (5).

B. pH indicator: litmus
   1. Acid: red color, pH 4.5
   2. Alkaline: blue color, pH 8.3
   3. Uninoculated: pH 6.8; purplish blue color

C. Method of preparation
   1. Weigh out amount accurately as directed on the label.
   2. Rehydrate with distilled or deionized water; heat water to 50°C before using for rehydration.
   3. Heat **gently** into solution.
   4. Mix well to obtain a homogeneous solution.
   5. Dispense approximately 5.0 mL per **screw-cap** tube; loosen caps.

D. Method of sterilization
   1. Autoclave
   2. Usual: 121°C, 15 lb, 15 min
      a. Difco (6) recommends 121°C, 15 lb, 15 min.
      b. BBL (18) recommends 113–115°C, 20 min.
      c. Baron and Finegold (2) recommend 10 lb, 10 min.
      d. Cowan (5) recommends two methods
         (1) Autoclaving: 115°C, 10 min
         (2) Fractional steam (tyndallization) 30 min on 3 consecutive days

During autoclaving litmus milk is reduced to a white base; however, upon **cooling**, oxygen is absorbed and the original purplish blue color returns.

E. Cool before use, tighten caps, and refrigerate for storage (4–10°C).
F. Inoculation
   1. Growth from an 18- to 24-h **pure** culture; Kligler's iron agar (KIA) or other suitable plate medium
   2. If *Clostridium* is suspected add **sterile** iron (e.g., iron powder, nails paper clips, metal filings) to the tube.

G. Incubation
1. Routine: 35°C; 18–24 h; longer periods up to 14 days may be necessary (5); record reactions at various intervals during incubation.
2. Fluorescent pseudomonads: 25°C; examine on days 4 and 7 of incubation (15).
3. Anaerobes: **sterile** mineral oil may be layered over medium (18).

VI. QUALITY CONTROL MICROORGANISMS

AC	*Lactobacillus acidophilus*	ATCC 314
ACGS	*Clostridium perfringens*	ATCC 3624
	Clostridium butyricum	ATCC 859
A	*Escherichia coli*	ATCC 25922
ALK	*Alcaligenes faecalis*	ATCC 8750
RED	*Enterococcus faecalis*	ATCC 29212
D	*Pseudomonas aeruginosa*	ATCC 10145
NC	*Proteus vulgaris*	ATCC 13315
Uninoculated		

VII. RESULTS

> See Figures 23.1 and 23.2 (Appendix 1) for colored photographic results

VIII. INTERPRETATION

A. **Pinkish red** (A)
1. Acid reaction
2. Lactose and/or glucose (dextrose) fermented
3. May have stormy fermentation; strong evolution of gas by certain strains of clostridia
4. As lactose is converted to lactic acid, subsurface first changes to pale pink while upper layer remains pink-purple. As more acid is produced, the top layer becomes light pink and the bottom pink portion fades to white. As still more acid is produced, curdling appears (acid-coagulate) leaving just a narrow band or collar of pink at the top because of decreased oxidation (16). A firm clot may be formed that resists flow when tube is tilted (16).

B. **Purplish blue** (NC/−)
1. **No** fermentation of lactose
2. **No change** of litmus pH indicator; same as uninoculated

C. **Blue (Alk/K)**
1. Alkaline reaction; clear purple layer at surface of milk (16)
2. **No** fermentation of lactose
3. Organism attacks nitrogenous substances in medium; activity on lactalbumin with production of ammonia (NH_3) or basic amines (18).

D. **White (Reduction)**
1. Reduction of litmus throughout tube to a white leuco base when litmus serves as an electron acceptor
2. Action of reductases removes oxygen to form decolorized leucolitmus compound (18).

E. **Clot or curd formation (C)** from milk protein by one of two processes.
1. Precipitation by acid produced from lactose. Clot **does not** retract and is soluble in alkali (5).
2. Conversion of casein to paracasein by rennin (16). Rennet clot is soft and retracts and expresses a clear grayish (straw-colored) fluid called **whey** at top of thoroughly coagu-

lated tube. Whey formation occurs as casein is curdled, and rapidly forming clot is accompanied by separation of a clear, straw-colored liquid (16). Clot is **in** soluble in alkali. Peptonization or digestion of clot may follow (5).
F. **Digestion (D) (Peptonization)**
   1. Milk protein digested
   2. Medium clears
   3. Digestion (dissolution) of curd or milk proteins by proteolytic enzymes. Proteolytic organisms or those that produce alkaline generally **do not** coagulate milk; however, a soft coagulum called rennin curd is formed (16). This is followed by hydrolysis of casein (dissolution of rennin clot) by proteolytic extracellular enzymes, with conversion of milk proteins to soluble compounds (16).
G. **Gas (CO_2 and H_2) (G)**
   1. Bubbles in medium
   2. Clot may be broken up
H. **Stormy fermentation (S):** acid clot is disrupted by an abundance of gas production.

IX. ALTERNATIVE TESTS

A. **Litmus milk agar (LMA)**
   1. Procedure of Webster and McGinley (20)
   2. Presumptive identification of cutaneous *Propionibacterium* spp.; anaerobic, Gram-positive, nonsporeforming species
   3. Medium
      a. Add 1.5% agar to 5% litmus milk medium (BBL) (see Section V for preparation)
      b. Pour into Petri plates to a depth of approximately 14 mm.
   4. Inoculation: up to 5 test organisms per plate; swab area for maximum growth, about 4–5 mm diameter.
   5. Incubation
      a. 35°C, inverted position (lid down)
      b. Anaerobically (GasPak, BBL); **7 days**
   6. Interpretation
      a. Positive (+)
         (1) Clearing zone; zone size 1.5–2.0 cm diameter
         (2) Casein hydrolysis; *P. acnes* or *P. avidum*
         (3) **No** correlation between intraspecific serotype and zone size
      b. Negative (−): no zone of clearing; *P. granulosum*
B. **Rapid caseolysis *Enterococcus* test** (19)
   1. Studies by Schierl and Blazevic (19) showed that 83% of enterococci reduce litmus within 4 h.
   2. Decreased volume of milk with increased inoculum size
      a. Dispense 0.5 mL of medium/tube (13 × 100 mm or 6 × 50 mm); cap tubes.
      b. Inoculum from 18- to 24-h sheep blood agar (SBA) culture; **large** inocula; growth scrapped with bacteriological loop
   3. Incubation: 37°C heating block; read at 1/2 h and then hourly for total of 4 h.
   4. Interpretation
      a. Positive (+): white; reduction
      b. Negative (−): pink; acid production

X. PRECAUTIONS

A. Clot formation is simply recorded as a clot (C). **Do not** attempt to differentiate between a clot or a curd.

B. Litmus milk **must** have a pH of 6.8. If unsure about the proper reactions occurring in the medium, set up controls before putting the medium into general use.
C. Homogenized milk is **un**suitable for preparing litmus milk medium (5). If **skim milk** is not available, place **fresh** milk in a refrigerator (4–10)°C) and let it stand overnight; then siphon off the skim milk layer **avoiding** the cream layer. Steam the skim milk for 1 h, cool to 4–10°C, filter, and measure filtrate (5). To the skim milk add enough litmus **solution** to give purplish blue color (pH 6.8) (5). Dispense into tubes, sterilize, and use as you would use dehydrated skim milk.
D. Litmus is reduced during sterilization to a colorless leuco base; it takes on color as the medium cools and absorbs oxygen. Overheating during sterilization caramelizes milk sugar and should be avoided (5, 16).
E. Reactions observed in litmus milk are **not** sufficient for speciation; additional biochemical and serologic tests **must** be performed.
F. Azolitmin **does not** successfully replace litmus, even though differences in pH range are small; it **does not** represent the entire color matter of litmus (11).
G. Viridans streptococci may reduce litmus milk during prolonged incubation (7); a test for enterococci should **not** be read after 4 h.

REFERENCES

1. Balows A, Hausler WJ Jr, Herrmann KL, Isenberg HD, Shadomy HJ. Manual of Clinical Microbiology, ed 5. Washington, DC: American Society for Microbiology, 1991:254.
2. Baron EJ, Finegold SM. Bailey & Scott's Diagnostic Microbiology, ed 8. Philadelphia: CV Mosby, 1990:A19.
3. Burrows W, Lewert RM, Rippon JW. Textbook of Microbiology. The Pathogenic Microorganisms, ed 19. Philadelphia: WB Saunders, 1968:324.
4. Cantarow A, Schepartz B. Biochemistry, ed 3. Philadelphia: WB Saunders, 1962:273, 792–793.
5. Cowan ST. Cowan & Steel's Manual for the Identification of Medical Bacteria, ed 2. Cambridge: Cambridge University Press, 1974:138, 152, 176.
6. Difco Manual, ed 9. Detroit: Difco Laboratories, 1953:192–193.
7. Facklam RR. Physiological differentiation of viridans streptococci. J Clin Microbiol 1977;5(2):184–201.
8. Fieser LF, Fieser M. Organic Chemistry, ed 3. New York: Reinhold, 1956:417, 461.
9. Harrow B, Mazur A. Textbook of Biochemistry, ed 9. Philadelphia: WB Saunders, 1966:355.
10. Hawley GG. The Condensed Chemical Dictionary, ed 10. New York: Van Nostrand Reinhold, 1981:203.
11. Lillie RD. HJ Conn's Biological Stains, ed 9. Baltimore: Williams & Wilkins, 1977:374, 403–404.
12. Long C. Biochemist's Handbook. Princeton, NJ: Van Nostrand, 1961.
13. Stecher PG, ed. Merck Index, ed 7. Rahway, NJ: Merck and Co. 1960.
14. Musso H, Kramer H. Ober orceinfarbstoffe. X. Lichtabsorption und chromophor des Lackmus. Chem Ber 1959;92:751–753.
15. Oberhofer TR. Manual of Nonfermenting Gram-Negative Bacteria. New York: John Wiley & Sons, 1985:77.
16. Oberhofer TR. Manual of Practical Medical Microbiology and Parasitology. New York: John Wiley & Sons, 1985:199.
17. Oser BL, ed. Hawk's Physiological Chemistry, ed 14. New York: McGraw-Hill, 1965:374.
18. Power DA, McCuen PJ. Manual of BBL Products and Laboratory Procedures, ed 6. Cockeysville, MD: Becton Dickinson Microbiology Systems, 1988:177–178.
19. Schierl EA, Blazevic DJ. Rapid identification of enterococci by reduction of litmus milk. J Clin Microbiol 1981;14(2):227–228.
20. Webster GF, McGinley KJ. Use of litmus milk agar for presumptive identification of cutaneous propionibacteria. J Clin Microbiol 1977;5(6):661–662.

24 Lysostaphin Susceptibility Test

I. PRINCIPLE

To determine the ability of an organism to produce endopeptidase enzyme, lysostaphin, that cleaves glycine-rich pentapeptide cross-bridges in staphylococcal cell-wall peptidoglycan (13, 26), which renders cells susceptible to osmotic lysis (17)

II. PURPOSE

(Also see Chapter 43)
  Rapid screening test to differentiate *Staphylococcus aureus* subsp. *aureus* and other *Staphylococcus* spp. from *Micrococcus* spp. (26); useful in blood cultures
A. Baker (1) found that most S. aureus subsp. aureus isolates tested lysed lysostaphin, but lysis of coagulase-negative staphylococci was inconsistent.
B. Sabath et al. (20) reported diminished lysis of methicillin-resistant *S. aureus* subsp. *aureus* (MRSA); but Seligman (25) reported enhanced lysis of MRSA by lysostaphin. Schleifer and Kloos (16, 23) and Heddaeus et al. (11) found considerable strain-to-strain variation in susceptibility of staphylococci to lysostaphin.
C. Zygmunt et al. (28, 29) found no naturally occurring lysostaphin-resistant strains of *S. aureus* subsp. *aureus* and also found that over 400 strains of multiply-resistant methicillin-susceptible *S. aureus* subsp. *aureus* (MSSA) lysed lysostaphin.

III. BIOCHEMISTRY INVOLVED

Peptidoglycan

Bacterial cell wall (rigid outer layer) owes its strength to a layer composed of a substance called murein, mucopeptide, or **peptidoglycan** (all synonyms) (15). One purpose of the cell wall is to provide osmotic protection.
  Gram-positive bacteria contain peptidoglycan as a major component of their cell wall, some 80–90% (8); other components are teichoic acids. Peptidoglycan is a complex polymer of polysaccharides and highly cross-linked polypeptides (15). Polysaccharides contain three parts: (*a*) a backbone of alternating sequences of amino sugars, *N*-acetyl glucosamine, and *N*-acetylmuramic acid connected by β-1,4-linkages, (*b*) a set of identical tetrapeptide side chains attached to *N*-acetylmuramic acid, and (*c*) a set of identical cross-bridges (8, 15).

A. Segment of Peptidoglycan of *Staphylococcus aureus*

(N-Acetyl-glucosamine) — (N-Acetyl-muramic acid peptide) — (N-Acetyl-glucosamine) — (N-Acetyl-muramic acid peptide)

Peptide side chain (from N-Acetyl-muramic acid):

(α NH)
|
L-Alanine
|
D-Isoglutamine
|
L-Lysine
|
D-Alanine
(α COOH)

B. Schematic Representation of Peptidoglycan Lattice Formed by Cross-linking

Repeating backbone: —GlcNAc—MurNAc—GlcNAc—MurNAc—GlcNAc—

From each MurNAc:
L-ALA
|
D-I-GLU-N
|
L-LYS
|
D-ALA — [GLY]$_5$ — (cross-link to adjacent chain)

(Redrawn from Jawetz E., Melnick J. L., Adelberg, E. A. *Review of Medical Microbiology,* ed 17, p. 16, 1987, with permission of Appleton & Lange, Norwalk, Connecticut.)

Peptide chains cross-linked between parallel polysaccharides form a lattice. Bridges composed of pentaglycine peptide chains (GLY) connect the α- carboxyl of the terminal D-alanine residue of one chain with the amino group of an L-lysine residue of the next chain (15).

$$NH_3CHCOO^- \quad\quad NH_2CHCOO^-$$
$$| \quad\quad\quad\quad\quad\quad |$$
$$CH_3 \quad\quad\quad\quad (CH_2)_3$$
$$\quad\quad\quad\quad\quad\quad\quad |$$
$$\quad\quad\quad\quad\quad\quad CH_2$$
$$\quad\quad\quad\quad\quad\quad\quad |$$
$$\quad\quad\quad\quad\quad\quad\; ^+NH_3$$

Alanine   Lysine

Final rigidity imparted to the cell wall by cross-linkage of adjacent chains is brought about by closure of bridges between some of the peptide units (8) by **transpeptidation** (8). Cross-linkage by transpeptidation occurs outside cytoplasm (8) and is mediated by several enzymes (15).

Lysostaphin specificity appears to be based on its peptidolytic action on pentaglycine cross-linkages peculiar to staphylococcal cell walls (14). Since all peptidoglycan chains are cross-linked, each peptidoglycan layer is a single giant molecule (15).

Gram-positive bacteria vary greatly in the composition of their peptidoglycans (8). Cross-bridging reactions occur in growing, but **not** resting, cells (8). Significant differences exist in tetrapeptide side chains and peptide cross-bridges; they vary from species to species (15). There are also significant differences among various *Staphylococcus* spp.; thus some species are more susceptible to lysostaphin than others (4, 18). *S. aureus* subsp. *aureus*, *S. simulans*, *S. xylosus*, and *S. cohnii* are more susceptible to lysostaphin (18). *S. saprophyticus*, *S. haemolyticus*, *S. hominis* are less susceptible than *S. aureus* subsp. *aureus* because of serine in the interpeptide bridge (19); susceptibility of various strains of staphylococci depends on contents of the interpeptide bridge (19). Cell walls of *Staphylococcus aureus* subsp. *aureus* and *S. epidermidis* differ in relative amounts of glycine and serine in interpeptide bridging pentapeptides (6, 7, 27, 29).

Lysostaphin

Lysostaphin is a mixture of enzymes; peptidases and lysozyme. The most active component is a lytic endopeptidase that cleaves pentapeptide cross-linking bridges of peptidoglycan (3, 14); it cleaves glycine-glycine bridges. Staphylolytic endopeptidase (lysostaphin) cleaves interpeptide pentaglycine bridges (19), and liberation of N-terminal glycine and alanine causes lysis. Staphylococci are sensitive to peptidase but resistant to lysozyme. Lysostaphin lyses staphylococci but is **in**active against most other microorganisms (5, 18, 21). Micrococci **lack** both interpeptide bridges in peptidoglycan and teichoic acids (2).

Growth Media

Composition of growth media is important. Growth of staphylococci in serine-rich medium **increases** serine content of the cell wall (22), which renders cells **more resistant** to lysostaphin (3).

In complex media, source of peptone influences amino acid (AA) concentration (23). Peptone prepared from meat has high glycine and relatively low serine content; peptone prepared from casein is much lower in glycine and relatively high in serine (22). To maximize sensitivity of lysostaphin, bacteria to be tested **should be cultured in meat extract** broths (12). Susceptible interpeptide chain of peptidoglycan depends on the amino acid content of culture medium (12).

Depending on the species and relative amount of glycine present in growth medium, some glycine residues may be substituted with L-serine or L-alanine (2). Cell walls of staphylococci grown in serine-rich media are more resistant to lysostaphin than those of staphylococci grown in glycine-rich medium (23).

IV. REAGENTS

A. **Phosphate buffer, 0.02 M,** pH 7.3 0.2 (12, 26)

Monosodium phosphate, 0.2M, $NaH_2PO_4 \cdot H_2O$	9.5 mL
Disodium phosphate, 0.2 M, $Na_2HPO_4 \cdot 12H_2O$	40.5 mL
Distilled water	100.0 mL

B. **Lysostaphin stock solution** (10×) (12)

(*Note:* Lysostaphin (Sigma) with specific activity of 287 U/mg is used for all lysostaphin procedures.)

1. Method of Hájek (10)
2. Ingredients, pH 7.4 ± 0.2

Lysostaphin (Sigma)	10.0 g
Phosphate buffer	40.0 mL
Sodium chloride, NaCl	0.4 g

3. Final concentration lysostaphin in mixture is 250 μg/mL
4. Dispense 1.0 mL aliquots/test tube (13 × 100 mm).
5. Storage: −20°C until reconstituted in phosphate-buffered solution (14)

C. **Lysostaphin working solution** (25 μg/mL) (12)
   1. Ingredients: to 1.0 mL tube containing 1.0 mL lysostaphin stock solution **add** 9.0 mL of phosphate buffer
   2. Mix thoroughly.
   3. Storage
      a. Refrigerator, 4–10 C, **no longer** than 2 days
      b. −20°C, less than 30 days (26)
      c. −70°C, prolonged periods

V. PROCEDURES

A. **Disk test**
   1. Disk; procedure of Poutrel and Caffin (18)
      a. Impregnate **sterile** 6-mm paper disks with 10 μg/mL of lysostaphin solution with specific activity of 287 U/mL.
      b. Sterilize by filtration; 0.20 μm filter.
      c. Lyophilize; store in dry conditions at 4°C until needed
   2. Inoculate Muller-Hinton (M-H) agar plate with test organisms; 0.5 McFarland turbidity standard (17). Swab a portion of the plate for **heavy** growth; may inoculate up to 4 test organisms per plate.
   3. **Aseptically,** place disk onto each inoculum.
   4. Incubate: 35°C, 24 h; plates **upright (lids up)**
B. **Commercial lysostaphin solution test kit** (REMEL); follow manufacturer's directions (19)
C. **Agar overlays**; two choices
   1. Procedure 1 (12)
      a. P agar; ingredients

Peptone	10.0 g
Yeast extract	5.0 g

Glucose (dextrose)	1.0 g
Sodium chloride, NaCl	5.0 g
Agar	15.0 g
Deionized water	1000.0 mL

       (1) Sterilize: autoclave, 121°C, 15 lb, 15 min
       (2) Dispense 10–20 mL/Petri dish (15 × 100 mm)
    b. Overlay; spot test
       (1) Add 0.1 mL saline suspension (approximately 10^7 colony-forming units/mL) of test organism to tube containing 3 mL fluid, soft P agar.
       (2) Mix and pour on surface of dry, soft P agar plate.
       (3) Place 1 drop **sterile** lysostaphin solution (200 µg/mL) on inoculated agar. Lysostaphin diffuses rapidly into medium (18).
       (4) Incubate 35°C, 24–48 h.
  2. Procedure 2 (12)
    a. Inoculum
       (1) Heart infusion broth (HIB)
       (2) Incubate 35°C no longer than 18–24 h.
    b. Shake culture and add 5 drops to each of two tubes (test and control).
    c. Add 5 drops phosphate buffer to control tube (C).
    d. Add 5 drops lysostaphin to test (T) tube.
    e. 35°C, water bath; examine at 30, 60, and 120 min

VI. QUALITY CONTROL MICROORGANISMS

A. Susceptible (sensitive, sens, S, +)

Staphylococcus aureus subsp. *aureus*	ATCC 25923
Staphylococcus epidermidis	ATCC 14990
Staphylococcus saprophyticus	ATCC 15305

B. Resistant (R, −): *Micrococcus luteus*   ATCC 4698

VII. RESULTS

> See Figure 24.1 (Appendix 1) for colored photographic results

VIII. INTERPRETATION

A. Susceptible (sensitive, sens, S)
  1. Complete growth inhibition around disk or spot inoculum or clearing of solution suspension
  2. *Staphylococcus* spp.
B. Resistant (Res, R)
  1. **No** inhibition of growth around disk or spot inoculum; visible growth or **no** clearing of solution suspension
  2. *Micrococcus* spp.

IX. PRECAUTIONS

A. Media-dependent action of lysostaphin should be considered when lysostaphin susceptibility test is used to distinguish *Staphylococcus* spp. from *Micrococcus* spp. (9). To obtain optimal results, test isolate should be grown on high-glycine, beef peptone–based medium rather than casein-peptone (17). Critical factor is glycine content of medium since glycine is an important part of staphylococcal cell wall and is essential for lysostaphin action (17). Medium made with casein needs supplementation with 0.2–0.3% glycine for lysostaphin test (23).

B. Some strains of *Micrococcus luteus, Kocuria rosea* (formerly *Micrococcus roseus*), *Arthrobacter agilis* (formerly *Micrococcus agilis*) and *Kytococcus sedentarius* (formerly *Micrococcus sedentarius*) demonstrate susceptibility to lysostaphin, presumably because of contaminating levels of endo- β-N-acetylglucosaminidase activity (2). Approximately 10% of *Micrococcus* have been reported either susceptible or weakly susceptible to lysostaphin, and occasional strains of *S. epidermidis, S. haemolyticus, S. warneri, S. capitis,* and *S. hominis* have been found slightly resistant (23, 24).

C. According to Gunn et al. (9), lysostaphin test as a single distinguishing test for staphylococci and micrococci may vary depending on source of isolate, testing method, and criteria used to assess susceptibility. Hájek (10) suggested that 50% or more reduction in turbidity after 2 h incubation be considered positive for susceptibility. However, Gunn et al. (9) showed that using Hájek's interpretation would cause many staphylococci to be misidentified. Gunn et al. (9) found 83% of staphylococci and 4% of micrococci tested susceptible to lysostaphin.

D. In the disk test, the time required to read results is independent of incubation time; diameter of inhibition zones did not differ after 6-, 16-, or 24-h incubation (18).

E. Addition of lysostaphin solution to plate medium **decreases** lysostaphin activity over time; solution **must** be made up when needed or stored in frozen fractions (18).

F. Cross-bridging reactions occur in growing, but **not** resting, cells (8).

G. When problems arise with lysostaphin test for staphylococcal identification, glucose oxidation-fermentation (OF) test and facultative growth in semisolid thioglycolate (THIO) agar should be used (9).

H. Most strains of staphylococci that are resistant to lysostaphin produce acid from glycerol (23). Slightly lysostaphin-resistant or lysostaphin-sensitive micrococci **do not** produce acid from glycerol and are susceptible (sensitive) to lysozyme (23).

REFERENCES

1. Baker JS. Comparison of various methods for differentiation of staphylococci and micrococci. J Clin Microbiol 1984;19(6):875–879.
2. Balows A, Hausler WJ Jr, Herrmann KL, et al. Manual of Clinical Microbiology, ed 5. Washington, DC: American Society for Microbiology, 1991:223.
3. Browder HP, Tavormina PA, Zygmunt WA. Optical configuration of staphylococcal cell wall serine. J Bacteriol 1968;96:1452–1453.
4. Browder HP, Zygmunt WA, Young JR, Tavormina PA. Lysostaphin: Enzymatic mode of action. Biochem Biophys Res Commun 1965; 19:383–389.
5. Cisani G, Varaldo PE, Grazi G, Soro O. High-level potentiation of lysostaphin antistaphylococcal activity by lysozyme. Antimicrob Agents Chemother 1982;21:531–535.
6. Ghuysen JM. Use of bacteriolytic enzymes in determination of wall structure and their role in cell metabolism. Bacteriol Rev 1968;32:425–464.
7. Ghuysen JM, Tipper DJ, Birge CH, Stromiger JL. Structure of the cell wall of *Staphylococcus aureus* strain Copenhagen. VI. The soluble glycopeptide and its sequential degradation by peptidases. Biochemistry 1965;4:2245–2254.
8. Gottschalk G. Bacterial Metabolism, ed 2. New York: Springer-Verlag, 1986:77.
9. Gunn BA, Singleton FL, Peele ER, Colwell RR, Keiser JK, Kapfer CO. Comparison of methods for identifying *Staphylococcus* and *Micrococcus* spp. J Clin Microbiol 1981;14(2):195–200.
10. Hájek V. *Staphylococcus intermedius,* a new species isolated from animals. Int J Syst Bacteriol 1976;26:401–408.
11. Heddaeus H, Heczko PB, Pulverer G. Evaluation of the lysostaphin-susceptibility test for the classification of staphylococci. J Med Microbiol 1979;12:9–15.
12. Howard BJ, Klaas J II, Rubin SJ, et al. Clinical and Pathogenic Microbiology. St. Louis: CV Mosby, 1987:879.
13. Huber MM, Huber TW. Susceptibility of methicillin-resistant *Staphylococcus aureus* to lysostaphin. J Clin Microbiol 1989;27(5):1122–1124.

14. Iverson O, Grov A. Studies and characterization of three enzymes. Eur J Biochem 1973;38:293–306.
15. Jawetz E, Melnick JL, Adelberg EA. Review of Medical Microbiology, ed 17. Los Altos, CA: Appleton & Lange, 1987:14–16, 130.
16. Kloos WE, Schleifer KH. Simplified scheme for routine identification of human staphylococcal species. J Clin Microbiol 1975;1(1):82–88.
17. Koneman EW, Allen SD, Janda WM, et al. Color Atlas and Textbook of Diagnostic Microbiology, ed 4. Philadelphia: JB Lippincott, 1997:550.
18. Poutrel B, Caffin J-P. Lysostaphin disk test for routine presumptive identification of staphylococci. J Clin Microbiol 1981;13(6):1023–1025.
19. Lysostaphin Reagent Set TI no. 21130. Lenexa, KS: REMEL, 1984.
20. Sabath LD, Leaf CD, Gerstein DA, Finland M. Cell walls of methicillin-resistant *Staphylococcus aureus*. Antimicrob Agents Chemother 1969;9:73–77.
21. Schindler CA, Schuhardt VT. Lysostaphin: A new bacteriolytic agent for the *Staphylococcus*. Proc Natl Acad Sci USA 1964;51:414–421.
22. Schleifer KH, Hammes WP, Kandler O. Effect of endogenous and exogenous factors on the primary structures of bacterial peptidoglycan. Adv Microb Physiol 1976;13:245–292.
23. Schleifer KH, Kloos WE. A simple test system for the separation of staphylococci from micrococci. J Clin Microbiol 1975;1(3):337–338.
24. Schleifer KH, Kloos WE. Isolation and characterization of staphylococci from human skin. I. Amended descriptions of *Staphylococcus epidermidis* and *Staphylococcus saprophyticus* and descriptions of three new species: *Staphylococcus cohnii, Staphylococcus haemolyticus,* and *Staphylococcus xylosus*. Int J Syst Bacteriol 1975;25:50–61.
25. Seligman SJ. Autolytic activity in methicillin-resistant *Staphylococcus aureus*. Antimicrob Agents Chemother 1970;10:218–222.
26. Severance PJ, Kauffman CA, Sheagren JN. Rapid identification of *Staphylococcus aureus* by using lysostaphin sensitivity. J Clin Microbiol 1980;11(6):724–727.
27. Tipper DJ. Structure of the cell wall peptidoglycan of *Staphylococcus epidermidis* Texas 26 and *Staphylococcus aureus* Copenhagen. II. Structure of neutral and basic peptides from hydrolysis with *Myxobacter* A1–1 peptidase. Biochemistry 1969;8:2192–2202.
28. Zygmunt WA, Browder HP, Tavormina PA. Lytic action of lysostaphin on susceptible and resistant strains of *Staphylococcus aureus*. Can J Microbiol 1967;13:845–853.
29. Zygmunt WA, Tavormina PA. Lysostaphin: Model for a specific enzymatic approach to infectious disease. Prog Drug Res 1972;16:309–333.

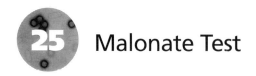

25 Malonate Test

I. PRINCIPLE

To determine an organism's ability to use sodium malonate as the sole source of carbon with resulting alkalinity

II. PURPOSE

(Also see Chapters 43 through 45)

A. To differentiate among *Enterobacteriaceae* species
   1. *Salmonella choleraesuis* subsp. arizonae (+) and *Salmonella choleraesuis* subsp. *diazonae* (+) from other *Salmonella* spp. (−)
   2. *Enterobacter asburiae* (−), *E. cloacae* (V, variable) and *E. sakazakii* (V, usually −) from other *Enterobacter* spp. (+) (10)
   3. *Escherichia blattae* (+), *E. fergusonii* (V), and *E. vulneris* (V, usually +) from other *Escherichia* spp. (usually −) (10)
   4. *Citrobacter amalonaticus* (−) and *C. freundii* (V, usually −) from *C. koseri* (+) (10)
   5. *Klebsiella pneumoniae* subsp. *ozaenae* (−) from other *Klebsiella* spp. (+) (10)
   6. *Edwardsiella hoshinae* (+) from other *Edwardsiella* spp. (−) (10)
   7. *Serratia rubidaea* (+) and *S. fonticola* (V, usually +) from other *Serratia* subspecies (−) (10)
   8. *Salmonella choleraesuis* subsp. *salamae* (+) from other *S. choleraesuis* subspecies. (−) (10)
   9. *Pantoea agglomerans* (+) (formerly *Enterobacter agglomerans*) from *P. dispersa* (−) (10)
   10. *Cedecea davisae* (+), *C. lapagei* (+), and *C. neteri* (+) from *Cedecea* species 3 & 5 (−)
   11. *Erwinia cacticida* (+) and *E. persicinus* (+) from other *Erwinia* spp. (−)
B. To aid in differentiation between genera: *Leclercia adecarboxylata* (+) (formerly *Escherichia adecarboxylata*) from *Escherichia coli* (−) and *Pantoea agglomerans* (V) (formerly *Enterobacter agglomerans*) (11)
C. Other malonate-positive enterics: *Kluyvera* spp. (V, usually +) (11), *Rahnella aquatilis* (+), enteric group 64 (+), *Hafnia alvei*, *Hafnia alvei* biogroup 1 (V), and *Budvicia aquatica* (V)

III. BIOCHEMISTRY INVOLVED

Malonate is an enzyme inhibitor (9, 15, 17). Quastel and Woodridge (17) first demonstrated that malonic acid (malonate) interfered with the oxidation of succinic acid to fumaric acid by inhibiting the catalytic action of the enzyme succinic dehydrogenase. Malonic acid inactivates the enzyme by a process called competitive inhibition. Succinic dehydrogenase transfers hydrogen to a suitable acceptor in the conversion of succinic acid to fumaric acid (2, 8, 9, 15), but this reaction can be inhibited by an organic compound structurally similar to the normal substrate, succinic acid (15). Malonic acid is structurally similar to succinic acid and it competes for sites on the enzyme.

Malonic acid differs chemically from the substrate by being a 3-carbon dicarboxylic acid while succinic acid is a 4-carbon dicarboxylic acid (1, 15).

```
        COOH              COOH
         |                 |
        CH₂              (CH₂)₂
         |                 |
       3*COOH            4*COOH

     Malonic acid       Succinic acid
      (malonate)
```

Malonic acid attaches to the enzyme and ties up the active sites; thus the enzyme cannot combine with its normal substrate, succinic acid, and succinic acid oxidation is blocked (15). An enzyme-substrate complex is necessary for activation of the substrate, and if activation is blocked, no new product (fumaric acid) is formed:

$$E + S \rightleftharpoons ES\ complex \longrightarrow E + P$$

Blocked by malonate

where E is enzyme, S is substrate, and P is product.

The degree of inhibition is inversely related to the ratio of the concentration of the inhibitor to that of the substrate (1, 2). Malonic acid inhibits succinic acid because it is an analog of the normal metabolite, succinic acid, and this metabolic antagonism inhibits growth (1, 2, 17). However, competitive inhibition is reversible (17). If the normal concentration of substrate (succinate) is added to the medium and a hydrogen acceptor is present (17), malonate is released from the enzyme, which is free to catalyze the oxidation of succinic acid to fumaric acid.

Malonate inhibition of succinic dehydrogenase ties up the enzyme stoichiometrically (8), and succinic acid accumulates (8, 13). Depending on the concentration of malonate, it may either retard the rate of oxidation of succinic acid or bring about complete inhibition.

In the Krebs' cycle, each acid compound is acted upon independently by specific enzymes; one molecule is used up and one is formed in a stepwise procedure. If the formation of a single acid (e.g., fumaric acid) is suppressed and it is not replaced, the Krebs' cycle ceases to function (1).

Since much energy for bacterial metabolism is provided by the Krebs' cycle (1), the bacterial cell must then rely on the glyoxylic acid cycle to produce intermediates for further biosynthesis for continual metabolism. By the glyoxylic cycle the bacterial cell regulates the amount of acetyl coenzyme A (acetyl-CoA) introduced into the cycle for its continuation, which is controlled by the activity of the enzyme isocitratase (1). However, increased concentration of succinic acid also inhibits isocitratase, which results in an absence of glyoxylic and acetic acid formation (1).

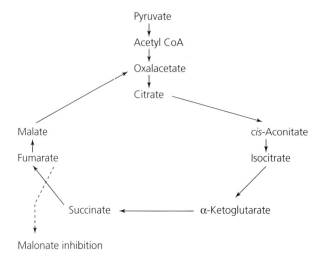

Abbreviated Krebs Cycle

Most bacteria can synthesize a small amount of isocitrate under any condition, but this synthesis is inhibited by addition of succinic acid to culture medium (1).

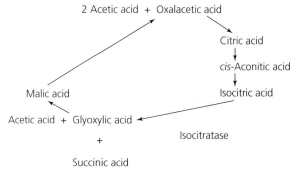

Glyoxylic Acid Cycle (1)

Therefore, accumulation of succinic acid due to inhibition of succinic dehydrogenase interrupts the Krebs' cycle, depriving some organisms of their energy source, and also interferes with the glyoxylic acid cycle, halting production of further intermediates required for the biosynthesis of new compounds necessary for metabolism. The end result is that an organism cannot grow and reproduce unless it can ferment (12) or utilize (18) sodium malonate as its sole source of carbon. If such a reaction is essential for a bacterium's metabolic activity, then the inhibitor malonate exhibits antibacterial activity.

Leifson (12) described the sodium malonate test as a fermentation, while Shaw (18) calls it a utilization. Leifson (12) also showed a correlation between acetylmethylcarbinol (acetoin) production and fermentation of sodium malonate by *Escherichia coli* and the *Klebsiella-Enterobacter* groups. This correlation does not pertain to other members of the *Enterobacteriaceae* (11) (Table 25.1).

Table 25.1. Malonate and Acetoin Results of *Escherichia-Klebsiella-Enterobacter*

	Escherichia coli	*Klebsiella-Enterobacter* Groups
Acetoin (VP)	−	+
Na malonate	−	+

IV. MEDIA EMPLOYED

A. **Malonate broth modified (malonate broth, Ewing)** (4, 6, 12, 16)
  1. Modification from Leifson's original formulation (12) by addition of yeast extract and glucose by Ewing, Davis, and Reavis (7)
  2. Ingredients, pH 6.7 ± 0.2

Yeast extract	1.0 g
Ammonium sulfate, $(NH_4)_2SO_4$	2.0 g
Dipotassium phosphate, K_2HPO_4	0.6 g
Monopotassium phosphate, KH_2PO_4	0.4 g
Sodium chloride, NaCl	2.0 g
Sodium malonate	3.0 g
Glucose (dextrose)	0.25 g
Bromthymol blue (BTB)	0.025 g
Deionized water	1000.0 mL

  3. pH Indicator: bromthymol blue (BTB)
     a. Acid: yellow color, pH 6.0
     b. Alkaline: deep Prussian blue color, pH 7.6
     c. Uninoculated medium: pH 6.7; green color

  The phosphates present in the medium adjust the pH to 6.7 (slight acidity), making the medium green with BTB pH indicator (4, 12, 16)

B. **Malonate broth with phenylalanine**
  1. Medium of Shaw and Clarke (19)
  2. Add DL-phenylalanine, 0.2%; 2.0 g/L to malonate base **before** sterilizing base. If L-phenylalanine is used, use only 1.0 g/L (3).
  3. **After** interpreting malonate results, add directly to tube
     a. N/10 HCl: 5 drops
     b. Ferric chloride solution, 8%: 3–5 drops
     c. See Chapter 34, Phenylalanine Deaminase Test, for interpretation.
C. **Malonate disks:** commercially available from BBL; follow manufacturer's directions
D. Method of preparation; either medium
  1. Weigh out amount accurately as directed on the label. Various company products may differ slightly.
  2. Rehydrate with distilled or deionized water.
  3. Heat **gently** into solution.
  4. Dispense approximately 3.0 mL per screw-cap tube (13 × 100 mm).
E. Method of sterilization: autoclave; 121°C, 15 lb, 15 min
F. Cool before use and refrigerate for storage (4–10°C) for up to 3 months (14).
G. Inoculation
  1. Growth from an 18- to 24-h **pure** culture: Kligler's iron agar (KIA) or other suitable culture
  2. **Light** inoculum
H. Incubation: 35°C; 24–48 h; observe for growth at the end of each period (6).

Both glucose and malonate serve as carbon source (20). However spontaneous alkalization caused by bacterial growth is buffered by glucose fermentation and the phosphates incorporated in the media (5). Yeast extract, the vitamin source, and a trace of glucose, the minimal carbon source, may be eliminated in formula, but they are necessary to stimulate growth of some organisms (3), especially *Salmonella* (20). Organisms that cannot use ammonium salts or malonate as carbon source **can** grow on these media.

V. QUALITY CONTROL MICROORGANISMS

A. Positive

Enterobacter aerogenes	ATCC 13048
Klebsiella pneumoniae subsp. *pneumoniae*	ATCC 13883

B. Negative

Escherichia coli   ATCC 25922
Uninoculated

VI. RESULTS

> See Figure 25.1 (Appendix 1) for colored photographic results

VII. INTERPRETATION

A. **Malonate**
  1. Positive (+)
     a. Alkaline reaction
     b. Light blue to deep Prussian blue color throughout the medium
  2. Negative (−): no color change (green) or yellow (glucose fermentation **only**)
     In the malonate medium devised by Leifson (12), sodium malonate is the only carbon source available. If an organism uses sodium malonate as its carbon source at the same time that it uses ammonium sulfate as its nitrogen source, alkalinity increases because of formation of sodium hydroxide (NaOH) and sodium bicarbonate ($NaHCO_3$) (14). Since all *Enterobacteriaceae* ferment glucose, those that cannot use malonate acidify the medium (20); bromthymol blue changes to a yellow color.

B. **Phenylalanine**
  1. Positive (+): deep green color
  2. Negative (−): **no** change; medium remains light blue

VIII. PRECAUTIONS

A. According to Oberhofer (14), the malonate test technically tests for alkalinization rather than utilization.
B. Some malonate-positive organisms produce only slight alkalinity, which makes the results difficult to interpret. If in doubt, compare with an uninoculated malonate tube. Any trace of blue denotes a positive test at the end of a 48-h incubation. A final negative interpretation should not be made until the tubes have been incubated for 48 h.
   Take care when interpreting results after prolonged incubation. Slight bluing (blue-green) becomes noticeable and may appear as a weakly positive reaction but should be ignored (14).

C. Some malonate-negative strains produce a yellow color. This is because fermentation of **only** glucose increases acidity, which causes the pH indicator to change to yellow at a pH of 6.0.
D. *E. coli* and the *Klebsiella-Enterobacter* groups do not absolutely require yeast extract and glucose enrichments; however, incorporation of these two enrichments into the malonate medium is recommended for differentiating among the *Salmonella* species.

REFERENCES

1. Burrows W, Moulder JW. Textbook of Microbiology, vol II, ed 19. Philadelphia: WB Saunders, 1968:129–131, 201–202.
2. Cantarow A, Schepartz B. Biochemistry, ed 3. Philadelphia: WB Saunders, 1962:263–264, 674.
3. Cowan ST. Cowan & Steel's Manual for the Identification of Medical Bacteria, ed 2. Cambridge: Cambridge University Press, 1974:152.
4. Difco Manual, ed 10. Detroit: Difco Laboratories, 1984:554.
5. Eiken Manual, ed 3. Tokyo: Eiken Chemical Company, 1969:48.
6. Ewing WH. Edwards and Ewing's Identification of *Enterobacteriaceae,* ed 4. New York: Elsevier, 1986:522.
7. Ewing WH, Davis BR, Reavis RW. Phenylalanine and malonate media and their use in enteric bacteriology. Public Health Lab 1957;15:153–161.
8. Greenberg DM. Metabolic Pathways, vol I, ed 3. New York: Academic Press, 1967:151.
9. Gunsalus IC, Stanier RY. The Bacteria, vol II. New York: Academic Press, 1961:216.
10. Holt JG, Krieg NR, Sneath PHA, et al. Bergey's Manual of Determinative Bacteriology, ed 9. Baltimore: Williams & Wilkins, 1994:203–206, 209–211, 213, 223, 225, 241–242, 247.
11. Koneman EW, Allen SD, Janda WM, et al. Color Atlas and Textbook of Diagnostic Microbiology, ed 4. Philadelphia: JB Lippincott, 1992:150–151.
12. Leifson E. Fermentation of sodium malonate as a means of differentiating *Aerobacter* and *Escherichia.* J Bacteriol 1933;26:329–330.
13. Mahler HR, Cordes EH. Biological Chemistry. New York: Harper & Row, 1966:527.
14. Oberhofer TR. Manual of Nonfermenting Gram-Negative Bacteria. New York: John Wiley & Sons, 1985:82.
15. Pelczar Mr Jr, Reid RD. Microbiology, ed 2. New York: McGraw-Hill, 1965:120–121.
16. Powers DA, McCuen PJ. Manual of BBL Products and Laboratory Procedures, ed 6. Cockeysville, MD: Becton Dickinson Microbiology Systems, 1988:191–192.
17. Quastel JH, Woodridge WR. LXXXIV, Some properties of the dehydrogenating enzymes of bacteria. Biochem J 1928;22:689–702.
18. Shaw C. Distinction between *Salmonella* and *Arizona* by Leifson's sodium malonate medium. Int Bull Bacteriol Nom Tax 1956;6(1):1–4.
19. Shaw C, Clarke PH. Biochemical classification of Proteus and Providence cultures. J Gen Microbiol 1955;13(1):155–161.
20. Washington JA. Laboratory Procedures in Clinical Microbiology, ed 2, New York: Springer-Verlag, 1985:206.

26 Methylene Blue Milk Reduction Test for Enterococci

I. PRINCIPLE

To differentiate organisms by their enzymatic ability to reduce methylene blue in a milk medium

II. PURPOSE

(Also see Chapter 43)

This enzymatic ability is used primarily to differentiate *Enterococcus* spp. from the group D streptococci and other *Streptococcus* spp. The group D *Enterococcus* species formerly in the *Streptococcus* genus and group D *Streptococcus* species are given below.

Group D *Enterococcus* spp. (formerly in the *Streptococcus* genus) (2, 6–8, 10, 12, 13, 17, 19–21, 23, 25, 26)

> *E. asini*   *E. columbae*
> *E. avium*   *E. dispar*
> *E. casseliflavus* *E. durans*
> *E. cecorum*
> *E. faecalis* (former subspecies: *Streptococcus faecalis* subsp. *liquefaciens*, *S. faecalis* subsp. *zymogens*, and *S. faecalis* subsp. *faecalis*, no longer recognized, are lumped into one species, *Enterococcus faecalis* (3, 18).)
> *E. faecium* (former *Streptococcus faecium* subsp. *casseliflavus*, now a separate species of *Enterococcus* (7, 29))
> *E. flavescens*   *E. pseudoavium*
> *E. gallinarum*   *E. raffinosus*
> *E. hirae*   *E. saccharolyticus*
> *E. malodoratus*   *E. solitarius*
> *E. mundtii*   *E. sulfureus*

(*Enterococcus seriolicida*, now *Lactococcus gervieae*)

Group D Streptococcus spp.

> *S. bovis*
> *S. equinus*

III. BIOCHEMISTRY INVOLVED

The cytochrome oxidase system activates the oxidation of reduced cytochrome by molecular oxygen (28), which in turn acts as an electron acceptor in the terminal stage of the electron transfer system (22, 28). When aerobic conditions exist (presence of atmospheric oxygen), oxygen is the final hydrogen ion acceptor, producing either water or hydrogen peroxide (H_2O_2) depending on the bacterial species and its enzyme system. The cytochrome system is usually only present in aerobic organisms (4), which makes them capable of using oxygen as a final hydrogen acceptor to reduce molecular oxygen to hydrogen peroxide, the last link in the chain of aerobic respiration (4, 14).

Artificial substrates such as methylene blue may be substituted for natural electron acceptors anywhere within the electron transport chain where they act as reductants of the cytochrome *c*–cytochrome oxidase system (5, 15, 22, 27). Methylene blue, a basic salt, is an oxidation-reduction indicator which, when incorporated into a medium, denotes changes in the oxidation-reduction potential. Certain organisms can use dissolved oxygen in a medium and thus can reduce the oxidation-reduction potential; reduction is catalyzed by the enzyme reductase (16, 22), a respiratory enzyme concerned with cellular oxidation.

When the synthetic reducible dye methylene blue is added to a medium containing metabolizing organisms, electrons produced from an oxidizable substrate are diverted from their normal pathway (if reductase is produced) and are used to reduce the dye (27). Anaerobically, the blue, oxidized form of methylene blue is reduced by an organism to a colorless, hydrogenated, leucomethylene blue compound (16, 24, 27). This reduction occurs in the presence of either nicotinamide adenine dinucleotide (NADH) (diphosphopyridine nucleotide; DPN or DPNH) or succinate along with the appropriate oxidase system (24). The reductase is classified as a dehydrogenase, since two hydrogens are transferred from their normal substrate to the artificial electron acceptor methylene blue without involvement of molecular oxygen (15). The reduction of methylene blue is shown below (22).

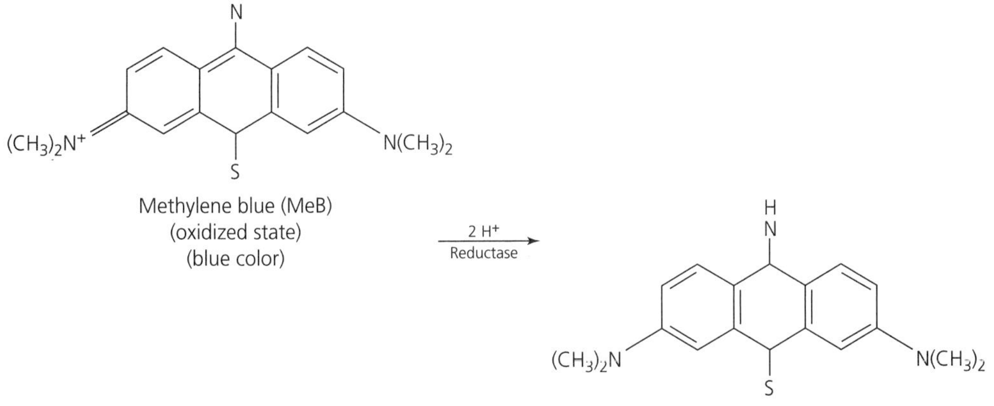

Methylene blue (MeB)
(oxidized state)
(blue color)

Leuco-methylene blue (MeB–H_2)
(reduced state)
(colorless)

$$\text{MeB} + 2\,H^+ \xrightarrow{\text{Reductase}} \text{Meb–}H_2$$

Oxidized state — Reduced state

Aerobically, reduced leucomethylene blue is spontaneously oxidized, and molecular oxygen serves as the terminal hydrogen acceptor (16, 27). Oxidation of reduced methylene blue produces hydrogen peroxide as its final product (15, 27).

$$\text{MeB–}H_2 \xrightarrow[O_2]{\text{Oxidation}} \text{MeB} + H_2O_2$$

Reduced state — Oxidized state — Hydrogen peroxide

Therefore, in the presence of atmospheric oxygen, methylene blue is concerned with electron transport; the cytochrome system is bypassed, and no oxidative phosphorylation takes place (27). In the electron transport system, the transfer of electrons involves a flavoprotein (coenzyme: flavin adenine dinucleotide, FAD) (27).

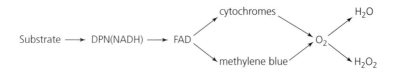

Most organisms contain the enzyme catalase that degrades hydrogen peroxide (4), since its accumulation is toxic. However, *Streptococcus* spp. **do not** produce catalase, and death occurs if hydrogen peroxide is allowed to accumulate. *Enterococcus* spp. are all usually capable of reducing methylene blue to its colorless state; *Streptococcus* spp. fail to decolorize methylene blue milk medium (MBM).

IV. MEDIUM EMPLOYED: MILK MEDIUM, pH 6.4

A. Ingredients, base (1)

Skim milk, dehydrated	100.0 g
Deionized water	1000.0 mL

B. Method of preparation, base
  1. Weigh out amount as directed on the label.
  2. Rehydrate with distilled or deionized water, preferably preheated to 50°C.
  3. Heat **gently** into solution; avoid caramelization of the milk.
C. Preparation of the oxidation-reduction indicator: methylene blue dye
  1. Add a 1% concentration of dye (10 g/L) to the **rehydrated** skim milk medium, or 100 mL of a 1% aqueous solution per 900 mL of base (1).
     a. Oxidized state: blue
     b. Reduced state: colorless
  2. Uninoculated medium, pH 6.4; blue color, oxidized state
D. Dispense the methylene blue milk medium, approximately 10.0 mL per screw-cap tube (16 × 125 mm).
E. Method of sterilization: autoclave; **113–115°C, 8–10 lb, 20 min**
F. Cool before use, screw caps down, and refrigerate for storage (4–10°C); shelf life approximately 6 months.
G. Inoculation
  1. **Heavy** inoculum
  2. Growth from an 18- to 24-h **pure** culture; a single colony on plate medium or a broth culture of a confirmed *Enterococcus/Streptococcus* spp. (catalase-negative Gram-positive cocci, singly, pairs, or in chains; variable hemolytic pattern; bile insoluble; optochin resistant)
  3. Shake the tube **gently** to suspend the bacteria.
H. Incubation: aerobically, 35°C; 18–24 h

V. QUALITY CONTROL MICROORGANISMS

A. Positive (+, R, Reduction): *Enterococcus faecalis,* ATCC 29212
B. Negative (−, NR, No Reduction):
  1. *Streptococcus pyogenes,* ATCC 19615
  2. Uninoculated

VI. RESULTS

> See Figure 26.1 (Appendix 1) for colored photographic results

VII. INTERPRETATION

A. Positive (+)
   1. Reduction (R); colorless medium
   2. Usually an *Enterococcus* sp.
B. Negative (−)
   1. **No** reduction (NR); medium remains blue.
   2. *Streptococcus* spp.

VIII. PRECAUTIONS

A. Other organisms besides the enterococci can reduce methylene blue. Thus, the organism being tested must be confirmed as an *Enterococcus* sp. **prior** to using this test procedure to differentiate within the genus. Also, within the group D organisms, organisms other than enterococci have occasionally been shown to reduce MBM. Facklam (9) showed that all group D enterococci could reduce MBM to its colorless state, while among the nonenterococcal group D streptococci, *S. equinus* was **unable** to reduce MBM. Some 60% of *S. bovis* strains reduced MBM, making its reaction variable, which limits the usefulness of MBM as a means of differentiating between the group D enterococci and group D nonenterococcal organisms (*S. equinus* and *S. bovis*) or between the group D enterococci and other *Streptococcus* spp. not group D. The lactic streptococci, group N, also reduce MBM, as do some strains of groups E and G (11). However, Facklam (9) recommends nonreduction of MBM as a means of identifying *S. avium* (group Q but also weak group D reaction), since physiologically it is similar to *E. faecium*.

To identify the group D enterococci and nonenterococci and to differentiate between them and the nongroup D streptococci, Facklam and Moody (11) recommend the bile esculin test as the test of choice, followed by *S. faecalis* (SF) broth, and then the MBM and salt tolerance tests. Performing a combination of tests or all four test procedures would greatly enhance **presumptive** differentiation between group D and non–group D streptococci and differentiation between enterococcal and nonenterococcal species within group D.

B. Time required for reduction of methylene blue is directly related to the number of bacteria present (4); the heavier the inoculum of a positive organism, the shorter the time to reduction. It is not unusual for reduction to occur within a few hours of incubation.

REFERENCES

1. Baron EJ, Finegold SM. Bailey & Scott's Diagnostic Microbiology, ed 8. Philadelphia: CV Mosby, 1990:A19.
2. Bridge PD, Sneath PHA. *Streptococcus gallinarum* sp. nov. and *Streptococcus oralis* sp. nov. Int J Syst Bacteriol 1982;32:410–415.
3. Bridge PD, Sneath PHA. Numerical taxonomy of *Streptococcus*. J Gen Microbiol 1983;129:565–597.
4. Burrows W, Lewert RM, Rippon JW. Textbook of Microbiology. The Pathogenic Microorganisms, ed 19. Philadelphia: WB Saunders, 1968:110–111, 326.
5. Cantarow A, Schepartz B. Biochemistry, ed 3. Philadelphia: WB Saunders, 1962:385.
6. Collins MD, Farrow JAE, Jones D. *Enterococcus mundtii* sp. nov. Int J Syst Bacteriol 1986;36(1):8–12.

7. Collins MD, Jones D, Farrow JAE, et al. *Enterococcus avium* nom. rev., comb. nov.; *E. casseliflavus* nom. rev., comb. nov.; *E. durans* nom. rev., com. rev., comb. nov.; *E. gallinarum* comb. nov., and *E. malodoratus* sp. nov. Int J Syst Bacteriol 1984;43(2):220–223.
8. Devriese LA, Dutta GN, Farrow JAE, et al. *Streptococcus cecorum*, a new species isolated from chickens. Int J Syst Bacteriol 1983;33:772–776.
9. Facklam RR. Recognition of group D streptococcal species of human origin by biochemical and physiological tests. Appl Microbiol 1972;23(6):1131–1139.
10. Facklam RR, Collins MD. Identification of *Enterococcus* species isolated from human infections by a conventional test scheme. J Clin Microbiol 1989;27(4):731–734.
11. Facklam RR, Moody MD. Presumptive identification of group D streptococci: The bile-esculin test. Appl Microbiol 1970;20(2):245–250.
12. Farrow JAE, Collins MD. *Enterococcus hirae*, a new species that includes amino assay strain NCDO 1258 and strains causing growth depression in young chickens. Int J Syst Bacteriol 1985;35(1):73–75.
13. Farrow JAE, Kruze J, Phillips BA, et al. Taxonomic studies on *Streptococcus bovis* and *Streptococcus saccharolyticus* sp. nov. Int J Syst Bacteriol 1984;5:467–482.
14. Frobisher M. Fundamentals of Microbiology, ed 6. Philadelphia: WB Saunders, 1957:105, 181.
15. Gunsalus IC, Stanier RY. The Bacteria, vol II. New York: Academic Press, 1961:335, 341–342.
16. Harrow B, Mazur A. Textbook of Biochemistry, ed 9. Philadelphia: WB Saunders, 1966:168–169.
17. Holt JG, Krieg NR, Sneath PHA, et al. Bergey's Manual of Determinative Bacteriology, ed 9. Baltimore: Williams & Wilkins, 1994:528, 538–539.
18. Jones D, Sackin MJ, Sneath PHA. A numerical taxonomic study of streptococci of serological group D. J Gen Microbiol 1972;72:439–450.
19. Kalina AP. The taxonomy and nomenclature of enterococci. Int J Syst Bacteriol 1970;20(2):185–189.
20. Knight RG, Shlaes DM. Deoxyribonucleic acid relatedness of *Enterococcus hirae* and *Streptococcus durans* homology group II. Int J Syst Bacteriol 1986;36(1):111–113.
21. Langston CW, Guttierez J, Bouma C. Motile enterococci (*Streptococcus faecium* var *mobilis* N) isolated from grass silage. J Bacteriol 1960;80:714–718.
22. Mahler HR, Cordes EH. Biological Chemistry. New York: Harper & Row, 1966:286, 557–558.
23. Nowlan SS, Deibel RH. Group Q streptococci. I. Ecology, serology, physiology, and relationship to established enterococci. J Bacteriol 1967;94:291–296.
24. Oser BL, ed. Hawk's Physiological Chemistry, ed 14. New York: McGraw-Hill, 1965:423.
25. Schleifer KH, Kilpper-Bälz R. Transfer of *Streptococcus faecalis* and *Streptococcus faecium* to the genus *Enterococcus* nom. rev. as *Enterococcus faecalis* comb. nov. and *Enterococcus faecium* comb. nov. Int J Syst Bacteriol 1984;34(1):31–34.
26. Schleifer KH, Kilpper-Bälz R. Molecular and chemotaxonomic approaches to the classification of streptococci, enterococci, and lactococci: A review. Syst Appl Microbiol 1987;10:1–9.
27. Stanier RY, Doudoroff M, Adelberg EA. The Microbial World, ed 2. Englewood Cliffs, NJ: Prentice-Hall, 1963:266–267.
28. Steel KJ. The oxidase reaction as a taxonomic tool. J Gen Microbiol 1961;25(2):297–306.
29. Vaughan DH, Riggsby WS, Mundt JO. Deoxyribonucleic acid relatedness of strains of yellow-pigmented group D streptococci. Int J Syst Bacteriol 1979;29:204–212.

27 Methyl Red Test

I. PRINCIPLE

A. To test the ability of an organism to produce and maintain stable acid end products from glucose fermentation and to overcome the buffering capacity of the system
B. This is a quantitative test for acid production (pH determination); some organisms produce more acids than others

II. PURPOSE

(Also see Chapters 43 through 45)
Methyl red results are valuable characteristics for the identification of bacterial species that produce strong acids from glucose (13).

A. To aid in differentiation between genera or in species differentiation within a genus among the *Enterobacteriaceae*. The methyl red test is part of the IMViC battery of tests (indole-methyl red-Voges-Proskauer-citrate).
   1. *Escherichia coli* (MR+) from *Enterobacter aerogenes* (MR−) and *Enterobacter cloacae* (MR−)
   2. *Yersinia* species (V, variable, usually +) from other Gram-negative, nonenteric bacilli (MR−)
   3. Differentiate *Edwardsiella ictaluri* (MR−) from *E. hoshinae* (MR+) and *E. tarda* biogroup 1 (MR+) (11)
   4. Differentiate *Leminorella richardii* (MR−) from *L. grimontii* (MR+) (11)
   5. Differentiate *Klebsiella oxytoca* and *K. pneumoniae* subsp. *pneumoniae* (both V, usually MR−) and *K. terrigena* (V) from other *Klebsiella* spp. or subsp. (MR+) (11)
   6. *Budvicia aquatica* (MR+) from other *Enterobacteriaceae* with KIA/TSI results of Acid/Acid, H_2S
B. Other organisms that are methyl red positive.
   1. *Aerococcus urinae* (MR+) from *A. viridans* (MR−)
   2. All *Shigella* spp. (MR+)
   3. *Ewingella americana* (MR+)
   4. *Kluyvera* spp. (MR+)
   5. *Leclercia adecarboxylata* (MR+)
   6. *Citrobacter* spp. (MR+)
   7. *Buttiauxella agrestis* (MR+)
C. Methyl red and Voges-Proskauer tests are used to aid in the identification of
   1. *Aeromonas hydrophila* (MR+/VP+)
   2. *Aeromonas salmonicida* subsp. *masoucida* (MR+/VP+)
   3. *Aeromonas veronii* (MR+/VP+)
   4. *Listeria* spp. (MR+/VP+) (2)
   5. *Vibrio metschnikovii* (MR+/VP+)

III. BIOCHEMISTRY INVOLVED

The methyl red test (MR) is a quantitative test based on the use of a pH indicator, methyl red, to determine the hydrogen ion concentration (pH) when an organism ferments glucose (17). The hydrogen ion concentration depends on the gas ratio (CO_2 and H_2), which in turn is an index to the different pathways of glucose metabolism exhibited by various organisms (5). The different fermentation patterns are due to variations in enzymes concerned with pyruvic acid metabolism in the organism (7).

All *Enterobacteriaceae* are, by definition, glucose fermenters. In MR/Voges-Proskauer (VP) broth, after 18–24 h of incubation, the resulting fermentation produces acidic metabolic byproducts; therefore, **initially** all enterics will give a positive methyl red reaction if tested (3, 4, 6). However, after further incubation required by the test procedure (2–5 days), methyl red–**positive** organisms continue to produce acids, resulting in a low terminal pH that overcomes the phosphate buffering system and maintains an acid environment in the medium (pH 4.2 or less) (3, 6).

Methyl red–**negative** organisms further metabolize the initial fermentation products by decarboxylation to produce neutral acetyl methylcarbinol (acetoin), which results in decreased acidity in the medium and raises the pH toward neutrality (pH 6.0 or above) (3, 6).

E. coli and other MR-positive organisms produce a high yield of acids through the mixed acid fermentation pathway: lactic, succinic, acetic, and formic; formic acid breakdown yields hydrogen and carbon dioxide (15). *E. coli* produces equal amounts (1:1 ratio) of H_2 and CO_2 from glucose metabolism (7). The overall reaction of glucose metabolism by *E. coli* is (10, 16)

$$2\ \text{Glucose} + H_2O \longrightarrow 2\ \text{Lactic acid} + \text{acetic acid} + \text{ethanol}\ 2\ CO_2 + 2\ H_2$$
$$(\text{Formic acid} \longrightarrow H_2 + CO_2)$$

MR-positive organisms produce stable acids (5), maintaining a high concentration of hydrogen ions (17) until a certain concentration is reached, and then all activity ceases (5).

The MR-negative organisms still produce acids (acetic, lactic, and formic), but they have a lower concentration of hydrogen ions because of a **reversion** toward neutrality, caused by further degradation of the organic acids to carbonates and on to carbon dioxide and possibly formation of ammonium compounds from the protein in the medium (15). Also, below pH 6.3, acetic acid is converted to acetoin and 2,3-butanediol (9), neutral end products; H_2 production is suppressed and CO_2 accumulation increases. For example, MR-negative *Klebsiella-Enterobacter* spp. (*E. cloacae* and *E. aerogenes*) produce more ethyl alcohol than *E. coli*, fewer acids, and twice as much CO_2 as H_2 (gas ratio, 2:1). The lack of H_2 production is due to the absence of the enzyme hydrogen lyase (9). The overall reaction of glucose metabolism by the *Klebsiella-Enterobacter* group is (9)

$$\text{Glucose} + \tfrac{1}{2}O \longrightarrow 2,3\text{-Butanediol} + H_2O + 2\ CO_2$$
$$(\text{Acetoin} \rightleftharpoons 2,3\text{-butanediol})$$

The validity of the methyl red test depends upon long enough incubation to let the difference in glucose metabolism occur (14). The organisms to be tested should be incubated **at least** 2 days at 35–37°C (5), which allows all organisms with low gas ratios (MR+) to show their limiting hydrogen ion concentration (low terminal pH), while all those with high gas ratios (MR−) will show a lower hydrogen ion concentration (high terminal pH) (5).

IV. MEDIUM EMPLOYED: CLARK AND LUBS MEDIUM (METHYL RED/VOGES-PROSKAUER BROTH, MR/VP BROTH), pH 6.9 (5)

A. Formulation of Clark and Lubs (5)
B. Ingredients

Polypeptone or buffered meat peptone	7.0 g
or pancreatic digest of casein	3.5 g
and peptic digest animal tissue	3.5 g
Glucose (dextrose)	5.0 g
Dipotassium phosphate buffer, (K_2HPO_4)	5.0 g
Deionized water	1000.0 mL

C. Method of preparation
  1. Weigh out amount accurately as directed on the label. Various company products may vary slightly.
  2. Rehydrate with distilled or demineralized water.
  3. Heat **gently** into solution.
  4. Dispense approximately 5.0 mL per tube (16 × 125 mm).
D. Method of sterilization: autoclave, 121°C, 15 lb, 15 min
E. Cool before use and refrigerate for storage (4–10°C); shelf life 6–8 weeks.
F. Inoculation
  1. Growth from an 18- to 24-h **pure** culture Kligler's iron agar (KIA), triple sugar iron (TSI) agar, MacConkey agar (MAC), or blood agar (BA)
  2. **Light** inoculum below surface of the medium; loose cap
G. Incubation
  1. Absolute minimum: 35°C, 48 h
  2. Recommended (5, 8): 30°C, 3–5 days
H. Add methyl red pH indicator directly to an incubated aliquot **before** attempting to interpret.

Commercial MR/VP medium is a modification of Clark and Lubs' medium (5). Clark and Lubs (5) used 1% peptone and glucose, but a lower concentration, no less than 0.5%, is the minimum that is satisfactory, so that the limiting high hydrogen ion concentration is not reached by MR-negative organisms (5). Using 0.5% peptone gives less color to the medium and makes interpretation of the color reaction easier.

V. REAGENT USED: METHYL RED (MR) pH INDICATOR

A. Method of preparation
  1. Dissolve 0.1 g of methyl red in 300 mL of 95% ethyl alcohol (ethanol).
  2. Add 200.0 mL of deionized water to the alcohol-indicator mixture; total volume, 500 mL.
B. Method of use
  1. Inoculated Clark and Lubs medium is also used for the VP test. The MR result is determined after 48 h or longer incubation, the VP usually after 24 h. If it is necessary to prolong incubation for the MR test, it is recommended that either an aliquot from a single tube be used for the MR test or both tests be inoculated in same medium but in different tubes.
  2. **Aseptically,** by pipette, remove a 2.5 mL-aliquot for methyl red determination.
  3. Add 5 drops of the methyl red indicator.
  4. Interpret color result **immediately.**
C. Storage: store the reagent in a refrigerator (4°C) when not in use; shelf life, 2–3 weeks.
D. Chemistry of reagent action: methyl red is an indicator that is already acidic and will denote changes in acidity by color reactions over a pH range of 4.4–6.0. At pH 4.4 or below in the medium, the reagent remains red, while with decreased acidity at pH 6.0, methyl red

indicator changes to a yellow color. A yellow color still denotes acidity, but the concentration of hydrogen ions is much lower. Various shades of orange occur in the pH range 5.0–5.8 (3).

VI. QUALITY CONTROL MICROORGANISMS

A. MR-**positive** (+)/VP-negative (−): *Escherichia coli* ATCC 25922.
B. MR-**negative** (−)/VP-positive (+): *Enterobacter aerogenes* ATCC 13048.

VII. RESULTS

> See Figure 27.1 (Appendix 1) for colored photographic results

VIII. INTERPRETATION

A. **MR positive** (+): culture is sufficiently acid to allow the methyl red reagent to remain a distinct, stable, bright red color (pH 4.4) at the surface of the medium. MR-positive microorganisms produce more acids with a resultant low terminal pH. They overcome the phosphate buffer system and maintain an acidity in the medium (pH 4.2 or less (40).
B. **MR negative** (−): yellow color (pH 6.0) at the surface of the medium
C. **Delayed reaction** (±): reddish orange color indicates organism produced less acid from test substrate. Continue incubation to 4 days and repeat the test.

IX. RAPID MICROTECHNIQUE

A. Method of Barry, Bernsohn, Adams, and Thrupp (3)
B. Detects MR-positive organisms in 18 h
C. Medium: MR/VP broth (5)
   1. Store in screw-cap tubes (16 × 125 mm)
   2. **Just before** use, **aseptically** pipette 0.5-mL aliquots into small test tubes (13 × 100 mm).
D. Procedure
   1. Inoculum
      a. Pick **center** of a single colony (**pure** culture).
      b. Culture from an 18- to 24-h growth on eosin methylene blue agar (EMB), MacConkey agar (MAC), sheep blood agar (SBA).
   2. Incubation: 35°C, 18–24 h
   3. **After** incubation add **1 drop** of MR reagent to each tube.
   4. Interpretation
      a. Positive MR: bright red color
      b. Negative MR: definite yellow color

The microtechnique of Barry et al. (3) has greatly decreased the incubation period from that required by the standard method (2–5 days). Studies (3) showed that smaller broth volumes gives test organisms better exposure to atmospheric oxygen, and MR-negative organisms revert to the initial acid pH faster.

X. PRECAUTIONS

A. The peptone present in the medium may affect the methyl red results. Before use, each lot should have a quality control check using known MR-positive and MR-negative organisms (12).

B. During sterilization, tubes **must** be placed in a solid-bottomed container to protect them from contact with steam (1); if this is neglected, medium becomes straw-yellow. Medium should be water clear; yellow medium is **un**satisfactory (8).
C. Clark and Lubs medium, either uninoculated or inoculated, looks exactly like indole medium. Be sure that all tubes are labeled correctly **prior** to inoculation, as any media mixup invalidates test results.
D. The methyl red and Voges-Proskauer tests should **not** be relied upon exclusively to differentiate E. coli from most Klebsiella-Enterobacter groups in routine identification or water analysis. Citrate and indole tests (IMViC) **must** be performed in conjunction with the MR/VP tests. There is the possibility that acetoin (in VP test) may be destroyed, invalidating results of the two tests (MR/VP) for identification purposes.
E. The methyl red reaction **cannot** be accelerated by increasing the glucose concentration in the medium (5, 6).
F. **No** attempt should be made to interpret a methyl red result after fewer than 48 h of incubation (8). The validity of the MR test depends upon sufficient incubation to permit the difference in glucose metabolism to occur (14). If the MR test is performed too early, results are often equivocal or falsely positive, since MR-negative organisms may not have had sufficient time to completely metabolize the initial acidic products that accumulated from glucose fermentation (3). After only 18–24 h of incubation **all results are MR positive.**
G. If commercial medium is not available, any medium is satisfactory so long as it contains no less than 0.5% glucose and peptone along with a phosphate buffer and a quality control is performed.
H. Avoid testing an extremely turbid broth-inoculum mixture; bacterial growth is inhibited if the inoculum exceeds a maximum of about 10^9 viable cells per mL (3). Each logarithmic decrease in inoculum size increases the time required for MR-positive organisms to accumulate enough acidic products to overcome the buffering system (3).
I. For optimal and reproducible results a laboratory should standardize the following variables: (a) the inoculum density, (b) the total volume of broth, and (c) the size of test tube used. An orange color reaction often occurs when broth volume is too large, which makes interpretation rather subjective and less reproducible (3).
J. Methyl red pH indicator has a range between 6.0 (yellow) and 4.4 (red). Test organisms **must** produce large quantities of acid from the carbohydrate substrate being used for MR to produce a color change (13).

REFERENCES

1. Abd-el-Malek Y, Gibson T. Studies in the bacteriology of milk. II. The staphylococci and micrococci of milk. J Dairy Res 1948;15(3):249–260.
2. Balows A, Hausler WJ Jr, Herrmann KL, et al. Manual of Clinical Microbiology, ed 5. Washington, DC: American Society for Microbiology, 1991:290.
3. Barry AL, Bernsohn KL, Adams AB, Thrupp LD. Improved 18-hour methyl red test. Appl Microbiol 1970;20(6):866–870.
4. Branson D. Methods in Clinical Bacteriology. Springfield, IL: Charles C Thomas, 1972:32–33.
5. Clark WM, Lubs HA. The differentiation of bacteria of the Colon-Aerogenes family by the use of indicators. J Infect Dis 1915;17(1):160–173.
6. Cowan ST. Cowan & Steel's Manual for the Identification of Medical Bacteria, ed 2. Cambridge: Cambridge University Press, 1974:37, 48.
7. Doelle HW. Bacterial Metabolism. New York: Academic Press, 1969:284–286, 291.
8. Ewing WH. Edwards and Ewing's Identification of Enterobacteriaceae, ed 4. New York: Elsevier, 1986:523.
9. Gunsalus IC, Stanier RY. The Bacteria, vol II. New York: Academic Press, 1961:84–89.
10. Harden A. The chemical action of Bacillus coli communis and similar organisms on carbohydrates and allied compounds. J Chem Soc 1901;79:610.
11. Holt JG, Krieg NR, Sneath PHA, et al. Bergey's Manual of Determinative Bacteriology, ed 9. Baltimore: Williams & Wilkins, 1994:204, 212, 235.
12. Jennens MG. The methyl red test in peptone media. J Gen Microbiol 1954;10(1):121–126.
13. Koneman EW, Allen SD, Janda WM, et al. Color

Atlas and Textbook of Diagnostic Microbiology, ed 4. Philadelphia: JB Lippincott Company, 1992:121, 175.
14. Ruchhoft CC, Kallas JG, Chinn B, Coulter EW. *Coli-Aerogenes* differentiation in water analysis. II. The biochemical differential tests and their interpretation. J Bacteriol 1931;22(1):125–181.
15. Sokatch JR. Bacterial Physiology and Metabolism. New York: Academic Press, 1969:79.
16. Stokes JL. Fermentation of glucose by suspensions of *Escherichia coli*. J Bacteriol 1949;57(2):147–158.
17. Wilson GS, Miles AA. Topley and Wilson's Principles of Bacteriology and Immunity, vol I, ed 5. Baltimore: Williams & Wilkins, 1964:815–816.

28 Motility Test

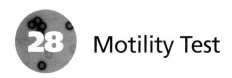

I. PRINCIPLE

A. To determine if an organism is motile or nonmotile
B. Bacteria are motile by means of flagella. Flagella occur primarily among the bacilli (rod-shaped bacteria); however, a few coccal forms are motile (2, 13). Motile bacteria may contain a single flagellum or many flagella, and their location varies with bacterial species and cultural conditions (11). Occasionally, motile bacteria produce nonmotile variants that appear stable and rarely revert to motile forms (2). Nonmotile organisms lack flagella.

II. PURPOSE

(Also see Chapters 43 through 45)

A. **Incubation: 37°C**
   1. To aid in differentiation between genera
      a. *Enterobacter* (V, variable; usually +) from *Klebsiella* (−)
      b. *Vibrio* (V, usually +) from *Actinobacillus* (−)
      c. *Aeromonas media* (−) and *Aeromonas salmonicida* (−) from other *Aeromonas* spp. (+) and *Plesiomonas shigelloides* (+)
   2. To aid in species differentiation
      a. Aerogenic *Escherichia coli* (+) from the anaerogenic (inactive) variety of *E. coli* (−). Old *Alkalescens-Dispar* now classified as anaerogenic (non–gas producing) *E. coli*
      b. *Bacillus anthracis* (−) and *B. mycoides* (−) from other *Bacillus* spp. (V, usually +)
      c. *Bordetella bronchiseptica* (+) and *B. avium* (+) from *B. parapertussis* (−) and *B. pertussis* (−)
      d. *Legionella oakridgenus* (−) from other *Legionella* spp. (+) frequently isolated from human infections
      e. *Edwardsiella ictaluri* (−) from *E. tarda* (+), *E. tarda* biogroup 1 (+), and *E. hoshinae* (l)
      f. *Enterobacter asburiae* (−), *E. dissolvens* (−), and *E. hormaechei* (V) from other *Enterobacter* spp. (+)
B. **Incubation: 22–25°C (room temperature)**
   1. To aid in differentiation between genera: *Listeria monocytogenes* (+) from *Corynebacterium* spp. (V, usually −)
   2. To aid in species differentiation
      a. *Corynebacterium aquaticum* (+) and *C. matruchotii* (+) from other *Corynebacterium* spp. (variable, usually −)
      b. *Yersinia enterocolitica* (+) from other *Yersinia* spp. (−)

III. MEDIA EMPLOYED: MOTILITY TEST MEDIUM (SEMISOLID)

A. Two variants
   1. Ingredients, pH 7.3 (1); formulation of Edwards and Ewing (7)

Beef extract	3.0 g
Peptone	10.0 g
Sodium chloride (NaCl)	5.0 g
Agar	4.0 g
Distilled water	1000.0 mL

2. Ingredients, pH 7.2 (6)

Tryptose	10.0 g
Sodium chloride (NaCl)	5.0 g
Agar	5.0 g
Distilled water	1000.0 mL

B. Commercial products available
C. Method of preparation
   1. Weigh out amounts accurately as directed on the label. Various company products may differ slightly.
   2. Rehydrate with distilled or demineralized water.
   3. Heat **gently** into solution.
   4. Dispense approximately 5.0 mL per tube (13 × 100 mm).
D. Method of sterilization: **autoclave, 121°C, 15 lb, 15 min**
E. **Allow medium to cool in an upright position** and refrigerate for storage (4–10°C).
F. Inoculation
   1. Growth from an 18- to 24-h **pure** culture: Kligler's iron agar (KIA) or other suitable medium
   2. Stab the **center** of the medium with an inoculating needle to a depth of ½ inch.
G. Incubation
   1. 35°C
   2. 24–48 h; if negative, incubate at 21–25°C for 5 days (1, 7)

The incubation temperature is extremely critical, because many motile organisms are motile at 15–25°C but nonmotile at 37°C, which is their optimal growth temperature. If you suspect an organism may exhibit motility at a lower temperature, inoculate two tubes simultaneously; incubate one at 35°C and the other at room temperature (22–25°C).

H. Use tetrazolium salts in motility medium if desired; however, this reagent inhibits certain organisms.
   1. Prepare a 1.0% aqueous solution of 2,3,5-triphenyltetrazolium chloride (TTC).
   2. Two methods of sterilization
      a. Filter
         (1) Seitz filter
         (2) Millipore membrane filter, 0.45-μm pore diameter
         (3) **Aseptically,** add 5.0 mL of **sterile** 1% TTC per liter of **sterile** motility medium.
      b. **Prior** to autoclaving add 0.05 g of TTC per liter of motility medium or 5.0 mL of a 1.0% solution (1, 9). Kelly and Fulton (9) recommend addition of 0.005% tetrazolium salt to help detect motility, particularly when an interpretation is difficult. They state that using TTC minimizes errors and eliminates the need for comparison with an uninoculated motility tube. Tetrazolium salts are colorless, but as the organism grows, the dye is incorporated into the bacterial cells where it is reduced to an insoluble red pigment, formazan (9). The red color forms only in the area of the medium where the bacteria are growing (9).

Tetrazolium salts are monotetrazoles (4) containing two azo group bases (R–N=N–OH). The azo group (–N=N) is a basic chromophore that imparts color to the compound in which it occurs (4). Tetrazolium is a salt of a colored base, usually chloride (4).

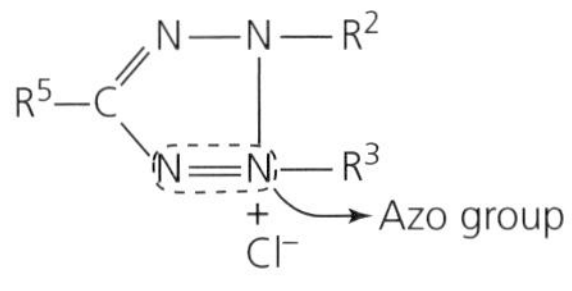

Basic structure

TTC has a benzene ring attached to nitrogen atoms.

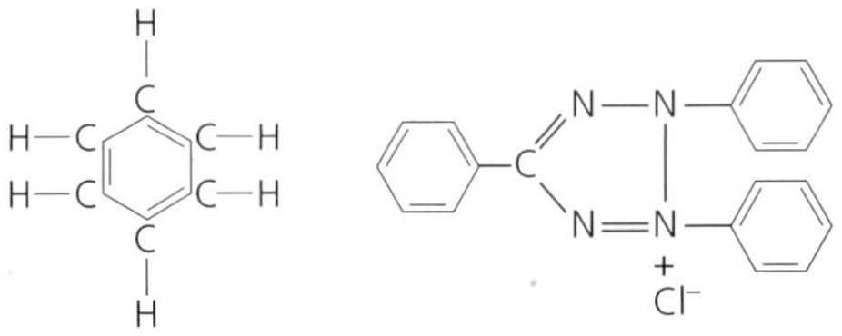

Benzene (C$_6$H$_6$)

2,3,5-Triphenyltetrazolium chloride (TTC)

TTC can act as an artificial electron acceptor for pyridine nucleotide–linked enzymes, i.e., succinic dehydrogenase, cytochrome oxidase, NAD (DPN), and NADP (TPN) (3) in the biological oxidative chain (3, 4). The salt is reduced by either cytochrome *b* or *c*, or it can compete for the electrons of cytochrome oxidase (3). Oxidation is mediated by reduction of specific dehydrogenases via the electron transport system.

Tetrazolium is a colorless, soluble compound that is taken up by bacterial cells and reduced at the site of enzymatic oxidations (4) releasing the acid formazan, a highly pigmented (red), insoluble compound.

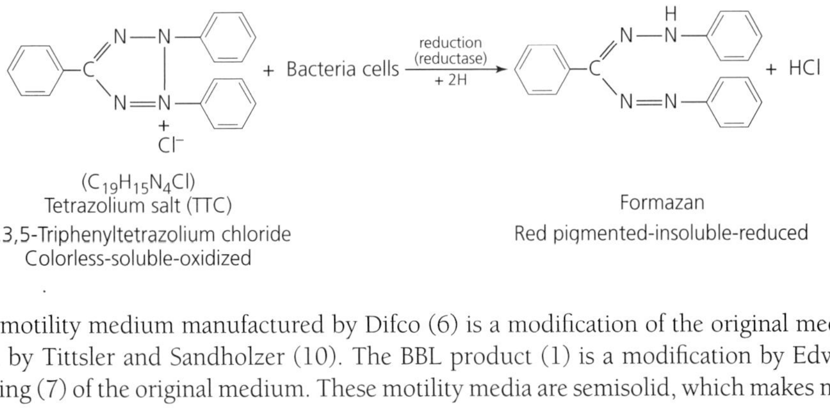

(C$_{19}$H$_{15}$N$_4$Cl)
Tetrazolium salt (TTC)
2,3,5-Triphenyltetrazolium chloride
Colorless-soluble-oxidized

Formazan
Red pigmented-insoluble-reduced

The motility medium manufactured by Difco (6) is a modification of the original medium devised by Tittsler and Sandholzer (10). The BBL product (1) is a modification by Edwards and Ewing (7) of the original medium. These motility media are semisolid, which makes motility interpretations macroscopic (12). Using a semisolid medium, Tittsler and Sandholzer (12) found motile strains of bacteria that were designated nonmotile by the hanging drop procedure. They stated that after 24-h incubation, motility determinations on semisolid media were identical to those determined by hanging drop, but after 48-h incubation, 4% more positive motile cultures were obtained.

An uninoculated control is needed when incorporating TTC into motility medium.

IV. QUALITY CONTROL MICROORGANISMS

A. Positive (+)

Escherichia coli   ATCC 25922
Clostridium sporogenes   ATCC 11437

B. Negative (−)

    Staphylococcus aureus subsp. *aureus*   ATCC 25923
    Uninoculated

V. RESULTS

> See Figure 28.1 (Appendix 1) for colored photographic results

VI. INTERPRETATION—MACROSCOPICALLY

A. **Motility medium**
  1. Positive result (motile): motile organisms migrate from the stab line and diffuse into the medium, causing turbidity. They may exhibit fuzzy streaks of growth (1, 2, 9, 12).
  2. Negative result (nonmotile): bacterial growth accentuated along stab line (1, 2); surrounding medium remains clear.
  3. Control medium (uninoculated): no growth, medium remains colorless and clear.

B. **Motility medium with TTC**
  1. Positive result (motile): motile organisms produce a pink turbid cloud that diffuses throughout the medium (9).
  2. Negative result (nonmotile): bacterial growth produces a bright red line confined to stab line (8); surrounding medium remains clear.
  3. Control medium (uninoculated): no growth, medium remains colorless and clear.

VII. ALTERNATIVE PROCEDURES

A. **Hanging drop**; two methods
  1. Direct drop on a slide
     a. Heavy loopful from an 18- to 24-h **pure** broth culture
     b. View microscopically, low power.
  2. Drop in a hanging drop chamber
     a. May be viewed under higher magnification
     b. Used mainly to detect motility of species that do not grow well in semisolid media

B. **Semisolid selective motility (SSM) medium**
  1. Formulation of Goossens et al. (8)
  2. Purpose: based on swarming of *Campylobacter* spp. from stool specimens
  3. Ingredients

Muller-Hinton broth	1000.0 mL
Agar, 4%	4.0 g
Cefoperazone	30 µg/mL
Trimethoprim	50 µg/mL

Antibiotics cefoperazone and trimethoprim **do not** inhibit swarming.

  4. Inoculation
    a. Direct
    b. Loopful at periphery of agar plate; plate diameter 50 mm (small dish)
  5. Incubation: two choices
    a. Candle jar: 37°C, 18 and 42 h
    b. Special incubator: 42°C, 5% O_2, 6% CO_2, 88% N_2; 18 and 42 h

6. Interpretation
   a. **Read only** for swarming, **not** for organisms.
   b. Typical spiral forms of campylobacters observed exclusively. Commercial kit is available from Institut Virion AG, Zurich, Switzerland.
C. **Combination media** (see Chapter 42, Multitest Systems)
   1. MIL/MILS: motility-indole-lysine-(H_2S)
   2. MIO: motility-indole-ornithine
   3. Motility-nitrate medium (motility medium S)
   4. Motility sulfide medium
   5. Sulfide-indole motility medium (SIM)

VIII. PRECAUTIONS

A. **General**
   1. The organ of locomotion, the flagellum, is protein and subject to denaturation by excessive heat (13). A culture heated prior to testing for motility yields a false-negative result.
   2. Motility results are difficult to determine on anaerobic bacteria. Only a positive result (motile) has any significance (5).
   3. Flagella may be destroyed or broken by violently shaking a bacterial culture tube (11), which may produce weakly positive motility or a false-negative result.
   4. Motile organisms kept as stock cultures on artificial medium over a long period of time tend to lose their motility (2).
   5. Many bacteria are motile at one temperature and nonmotile when cultivated at another (2). An organism that is negative after 48-h incubation at 35°C should be incubated at 22–25°C for 5 days (1, 7) to confirm lack of motility. Most motile bacteria can be tested at 35°C; however, *Y. enterocolitica* develops flagellar proteins at room temperature (22–25°C), but **not at 35°C** (10). *L. monocytogenes* also requires a temperature of 22–25°C (10).
   6. If a motility test is difficult to interpret, compare it with an uninoculated motility tube. Use of a tetrazolium salt in the medium may **aid** interpretation (9). If still in doubt, perform a hanging drop preparation with a heavy loopful of an 18- to 24-h culture.
   7. Occasionally, a motile culture may be temporarily nonmotile, with only a few motile bacteria present. In this case a positive culture may exhibit only a few tufts or rosettes that are often overlooked as motility indicators (9).
   8. Agar concentration in media should be 0.4% or less; a higher concentration makes the gel too firm to permit organisms to spread (10).
   9. *Pseudomonas aeruginosa* grows well only in the presence of oxygen (O_2) and produces a film on surface of motility medium because it does not grow in the deeper, oxygen-deficient portion of the tube (10).
   10. Edwards and Ewing's medium (7) with 4% agar is crystal clear and supports growth of most fastidious bacteria. This medium avoids the possibility of turbidity that may make motility interpretations difficult.
B. **Tetrazolium:** tetrazolium salts aid in visual detection of bacterial growth; however, salts may inhibit certain fastidious bacteria and cannot be used in all cases (10).
C. **Semisolid selective motility (SSM) medium**
   1. Change in agar lot number markedly affected swarming; optimal concentration is 0.28–0.4%, depending on batch and commercial source. Goossens et al. (8) noted significant batch-to-batch variation in Mueller-Hinton broth.
   2. Disadvantage is that nonmotile campylobacters might **not** be identified.

REFERENCES

1. BBL Manual of Products and Laboratory Procedures, ed 6. Cockeysville, MD: Becton Dickinson Microbiology Systems, 1988.
2. Burrows W, Lewert RM, Rippon JW. Textbook of Microbiology. The Pathogenic Microorganisms, ed 19. Philadelphia: WB Saunders, 1968: 44, 223.
3. Cantarow A, Schepartz B. Biochemistry, ed 3. Philadelphia: WB Saunders, 1962:385–386.
4. Conn HJ, Lillie RD, eds. HJ Conn's Biological Stains, ed 9. Baltimore: Williams & Wilkins, 1977:24, 51, 200, 225–227.
5. Cowan ST. Cowan & Steel's Manual for the Identification of Medical Bacteria, ed 2. Cambridge: Cambridge University Press, 1974:21–22.
6. Difco Manual, ed 10. Detroit: Difco Laboratories, 1984:184.
7. Ewing WH. Edwards and Ewing's Identification of Enterobacteriaceae, ed 4. New York: Elsevier, 1986:523.
8. Goossens H, Vlaes L, Galand I, et al. Semisolid blood-free selective-motility medium for the isolation of campylobacters from stool specimens. J Clin microbiol 1989;27(5):1077–1080.
9. Kelly AT, Fulton M. Use of triphenyl tetrazolium in motility test medium. Am J Clin Pathol 1953;23(5):512.
10. Koneman EW, Allen SD, Janda WM, et al. Color Atlas and Textbook of Diagnostic Microbiology, ed 5. Philadelphia: JB Lippincott, 1997:188–189.
11. Oginsky EL, Umbreit WW. An Introduction to Bacterial Physiology, ed 2. San Francisco: WH Freeman, 1959:33.
12. Tittsler RP, Sandholzer LA. The use of semisolid agar for the detection of bacterial motility. J Bacteriol 1936;31:575–580.
13. Wilson G, Miles A, Parker MT, eds. Topley and Wilson's Principles of Bacteriology and Virology, ed 7. Baltimore: Williams & Wilkins, 1983.

29 *Neisseria* Carbohydrate Utilization Tests

I. PRINCIPLE

To determine the ability of *Neisseria* spp. to ferment (degrade) a specific carbohydrate incorporated into a basal medium, producing acid

II. PURPOSE

(Also see Chapter 45)

A. *Neisseria* spp. presently are **presumptively** identified by growth, colony characteristics, Gram stain reaction, cellular morphology, and oxidase activity (62).
B. For epidemiologic, medicolegal, and clinical purposes, it is necessary to **confirm** *Neisseria* pathogenic spp. identification by carbohydrate utilization tests (85).
   1. Carbohydrate use patterns are generally distinctive for differentiation between pathogenic and saprophytic *Neisseria* and **differentiation** and **confirmation** of the two pathogens: *N. meningitidis* (maltose, A) and *N. gonorrhoeae* (maltose, −).
   2. Failure to form acid from one or more carbohydrates is common within the genus (62); e.g., evidence that sulfadiazine-resistant *N. meningitidis* strains do not ferment maltose (59) (see Minitek rapid procedure). Therefore, a number of acceptable carbohydrate utilization tests are included here.
C. The only species of *Neisseria* to demonstrate glycosidase activity is *N. lactamica,* the **only** lactose fermenter (may be delayed), but rapidly *o*-nitrophenyl-β-galactopyranoside (ONPG) positive (see Chapter 11, β-Galactosidase (ONPG and PNPG) Tests).

III. BIOCHEMISTRY INVOLVED

Neisseria spp. are fastidious in their growth requirements but are metabolically active. A number of pathways are involved in the glucose metabolism of various *Neisseria* (3, 65, 78); strains that metabolize glucose do so primarily by an oxidative (oxidation-fermentation (OF) test: O/−) pathway rather than by fermentation (7, 38). Glycolytic formation of lactic acid with subsequent oxidation to pyruvate and then acetate occurs in both *N. gonorrhoeae* and *N. meningitidis* (3, 65); glucose is metabolized by *N. gonorrhoeae* by a combination of the Entner-Doudoroff and pentose phosphate pathways, with carbon dioxide (CO_2) and acetic acid being the major end products during aerobic growth (61). No growth occurs anaerobically, but small amounts of acetic and lactic acid are produced from glucose (65) (see Chapter 5, Carbohydrate Fermentation Tests, for a discussion of carbohydrate degradation pathways).

The use of glucose (dextrose) by *N. gonorrhoeae* occurs in two steps: first, glucose is dissimulated to acetate and CO_2 during active growth; acetic acid (acetate) is oxidized **after** depletion of glucose in the test medium (65). The change in the pH indicator in the test medium (e.g., cysteine Trypticase agar) to acid is due to production of acetic acid and small amounts of lactic acid (65). On prolonged incubation (72 h or longer), the peptone in the medium is deaminated enzymatically to amino acids, and these products **combined** with acetic acid oxidation after depletion of glucose produce **alkaline** byproducts that tend to neutralize the acid produced and may cause glucose test medium to revert from an acid to an alkaline reaction (false negative) (16, 17, 35, 36, 75). In the absence of any carbohydrate usable by a *Neisseria* spp. (e.g., *N. flavescens*), the peptone in the medium is deaminated for a nitrogen source, producing an alkaline reaction and hence a negative carbohydrate test result (35, 36).

The only species of *Neisseria* to demonstrate glycosidase activity is *N. lactamica*, which is limited to galactosidase (18). *N. meningitidis* uses maltose via the phosphorolysis pathway (29); possibly this pathway may be present as means of glycolytic degradation in the absence of glycosidase activity (18). Sulfadiazine-resistant strains of *N. meningitidis* lack permease activity (50), and maltose cannot normally enter the cell for degradation. *N. gonorrhoeae* can use maltose by alternate pathways of 3-carbon fragment metabolism but produces **no** acidic end products (62).

Vanderkerkove et al. (78) also established the production of acetylmethylcarbinol (ACM, VP-positive) from glucose by *N. gonorrhoeae* and other *Neisseria* spp.; similar findings were obtained by Morse et al. (61).

Pathogenic *Neisseria* spp. are extremely fastidious organisms in both their growth and metabolizing abilities, and laboratory identification by carbohydrate oxidation, particularly by *N. gonorrhoeae*, is often complicated by non-acid-producing strains and nonviable or mixed cultures (4). The optimal method of testing carbohydrate use by *Neisseria* spp. incorporates the combined action of **both** preformed enzymes and those formed during growth (85).

IV. MEDIA EMPLOYED

A. **Cystine Trypticase agar (CTA) base medium with carbohydrates** (5, 79)
   1. Enriched semisolid medium for determination of fermentation (really oxidative) reactions of *Neisseria* spp. and other fastidious organisms (79)
   2. Ingredients, pH 7.3

Cystine (an amino acid)	0.5 g
Trypticase (tryptic) peptone (or pancreatic digest of casein)	20.0 g
Sodium chloride, NaCl	5.0 g
Sodium sulfite, Na_2SO_3	0.5 g
Phenol red	0.017 g
Agar	2.5–3.5 g
Distilled water	1000.0 mL

   3. pH indicator; phenol red
      a. Acid: yellow color, pH 6.8
      b. Alkaline: pinkish red color, pH 8.4
      c. Uninoculated medium: pH 7.3, reddish orange color
   4. Commercial products available
      a. BBL: Cystine Trypticase agar (5)
      b. Difco: Cystine Tryptic agar (21)
   5. Method of preparation, CTA base medium
      a. Weigh out amounts accurately as directed on label. Various company products may differ slightly.
      b. Rehydrate with distilled or demineralized water.
      c. Heat **gently** into solution.
   6. Method of sterilization: autoclave, 121°C, **12 lb** (5), 15 min
   7. Cool to 45–50°C in water bath
   8. Carbohydrate solutions
      a. Battery

         Glucose (dextrose) (G, D)
         Maltose (M)
         Sucrose (S)

Lactose (L)
Fructose (F)
Mannitol (Ma)
Levulose (Le)
   b. Final concentration of sugar solution: 1%
   c. Preparation of sugar solutions; two procedures
      (1) **Recommended**
         (a) Prepare 10% solution of desired sugar(s) in distilled water; 10.0 g/100 mL.
         (b) Sterilize by **filtration**; method of choice
            1. Millipore membrane filter method
            2. Membranes: 0.45-µm pore diameter
         (c) **Aseptically,** add 100 mL of a 10% sugar solution to 900 mL of **cooled, sterile** CTA base for each individual sugar and mix thoroughly; final concentration, 1%.
         (d) **Aseptically,** dispense approximately 4.0–5.0 mL per **sterile** screw-capped tube (13 × 100 mm); tighten caps.
      (2) Alternative
         (a) Add individual sugars directly to **unsterile** CTA base; 10.0 g/L of CTA; final concentration, 1%.
         (b) Dispense approximately 4.0–5.0 mL per screw-capped tube (13 × 100 mm); loosen caps.
         (c) Autoclave: 121°C, 15 lb, **3 min**
            1. Used when time is critical
            2. Controls **must** be run **prior** to their use for diagnostic purposes to check for possible breakdown.
9. Cool **before** use.
10. Storage: CTA/carbohydrate medium (5)
    a. Cotton-plugged tubes: room temperature (25°C)
    b. Screw-capped tubes with caps **tightened:** refrigerator (4°C)
11. Inocula
    a. Loopful of a **pure** confluent growth of **presumptively** identified Neisseria spp. subcultured on a chocolate agar plate (CA) from isolation media; incubated 35°C 18–24 h under 6% CO_2
    b. **Heavy** inoculum emulsified in 0.5 of **sterile** saline or **sterile** Trypticase soy broth (TSB)
12. Inoculation
    a. With **sterile** Pasteur pipette, add 2–3 drops of test organism suspension onto surface of CTA medium
    b. With plugged **sterile** capillary pipette, stab **upper** ⅓ of medium several times
    c. Control tubes to run simultaneously with each batch of medium
       (1) **Inoculated** carbohydrate-free tube of CTA basal medium; any saprophytic Neisseria spp.
       (2) **Uninoculated glucose** tube **with** carbohydrate
13. Incubation
    a. 35°C
    b. **Tighten** caps and **no** increased CO_2 **or** candle jar with caps **loosened** and moist paper towel (or filter paper) in bottom of jar (approximately 5–10% increased CO_2).
    c. Examine **daily** for growth (turbidity) and acid production (yellow color upper layer of medium).
       (1) 48–72 h (79); 1–4 days.
       (2) If result is negative and N. gonorrhoeae is suspected, repeat inoculation with

CTA/carbohydrate medium containing either a supplement (improves growth) or increased carbohydrate concentration.
  (a) Carbohydrate: 10%; 100 g/L of CTA base
  (b) Supplements: 10% ascitic fluid (45), 1% rabbit serum (70), heated bovine albumin (66), placenta broth (45, 72), yeast autolysate (27), or hemolyzed erythrocytes (27)

B. **Elrod and Braun (modified) salt solution with carbohydrates** (26)
  1. Nongrowth synthetic medium; nitrogen-free salt solution
  2. Salt solution base
     a. Ingredients, pH 7.0

Magnesium sulfate, $MgSO_4$	0.2 g
Calcium chloride, $CaCl_2$	0.1 g
Sodium chloride, NaCl	0.2 g
Dipotassium phosphate, K_2HPO_4	0.2 g
Bromthymol blue, 0.2% aqueous	20.0 mL
Distilled water	880.0 mL

     b. pH indicator: bromthymol blue (BTB)
        (1) Acid: yellow color, pH 6.0
        (2) Alkaline: deep Prussian blue color, pH 7.6
        (3) Uninoculated: pH 7.0, green color
     c. Sterilize by filtration (see Section IV.A.8.c.(i) for method).
  3. Carbohydrates: standard *Neisseria* battery (see Section IV.A.8.a.)
     a. Concentration 10%; 10.0 g/100 mL of distilled water
     b. Sterilize by filtration.
  4. **Aseptically,** add 1.0 mL of desired 10% sugar concentration to 9.0 mL of salt solution in a **sterile** tube and mix **gently** by swirling.
  5. **Aseptically,** with **sterile** pipette, dispense 0.5 mL aliquots into **sterile** tubes (13 × 100 mm) and cap.
  6. Store at room temperature (25°C).
  7. Inoculation
     a. Growth from a 16- to 20-h **pure** culture on sheep blood agar (SBA)
     b. **Heavy** inoculum well emulsified in salt/carbohydrate solution
     c. Control tube: carbohydrate-**free** solution
  8. Incubation: 35°C water bath; up to 24 h; **preformed enzymes** may produce acid in less than 6 h.

C. **Gonococcus identification medium (GCID)**
  1. Procedure of Graves and Magee (34)
  2. Medium formulation; enriched, bicarbonate-containing carbohydrate medium
     a. Basal gonococcus (GC) medium
        (1) Ingredients

Dehydrated GC medium (Difco)	3.6 g
Phenol red, 0.2%	2.0 mL
Distilled water	50.0 mL

        (2) pH indicator (see Section IV.A.3 for color reactions)
        (3) Autoclave: 121°C, 15 lb, 15 min
        (4) Place in 45–50°C water bath
     b. Hemoglobin (Hb) source: lysed erythrocytes (RBCs)
        (1) **Aseptically** centrifuge defibrinated sheep blood; can substitute cow (bovine) or horse RBCs.
        (2) Remove serum with **sterile** Pasteur pipette and discard.

(3) **Aseptically** with **sterile** pipette, add 2.0 mL of packed RBCs to 80.0 mL of **sterile** distilled water.
(4) Store in refrigerator (4°C) until used; use day prepared.
   c. Nutritional supplement: IsoVitaleX; **sterile**, 2 mL lyophilized vials (BBL)
      (1) IsoVitaleX reconstituting diluent contains glucose; **do not** use accompanying diluent.
      (2) **Aseptically,** substitute diluent with **sterile** distilled water; use manufacturer's volume.
   d. Carbon dioxide source: bicarbonate, $NaHCO_3$
      (1) Concentration: 4%; 4.0 g/100 mL of distilled water
      (2) Autoclave: 121°C, 15 lb, 15 min
      (3) Replacement for gaseous CO_2 (25, 44, 77)
   e. Carbohydrates: 8% concentration
      (1) Battery: glucose, maltose, sucrose, and lactose
      (2) 8.0 g/100 mL of distilled water
      (3) Sterilize by filtration.
3. **Final working GCID medium:** make up in sets of each carbohydrate.
   a. Constituents: use **aseptic** technique

Cooled (50°C) GC basal medium	50.0 mL
Hemoglobin solution	20.0 mL
Single carbohydrate, 8%	25.0 mL
Sodium bicarbonate, 4%	0.5 mL
IsoVitaleX	1.0 mL

   b. Adjust to pH 7.5 with **sterile** 0.2 N NaOH (1.0 mL of 10 N NaOH, brought to **50** mL with distilled water) (see Appendix 4, pH Adjustment, for preparation of 10 N NaOH)
   c. **Aseptically,** dispense 3.0 mL per sterile screw-capped tube (13 × 100 mm).
   d. Cool in **slanted** position.
   e. Storage: refrigerator (4°C)
4. Procedure: each GCID carbohydrate set
   a. With inoculating **loop,** streak slant **lightly** with growth from a 14- to 18-h **pure** culture from chocolate agar (CA).
   b. Control: uninoculated tube to be run simultaneously with **each set** of carbohydrates.
   c. Tighten caps.
5. Incubation: 35°C, 24–48 h

V. QUALITY CONTROL MICROORGANISMS

(Table 29.1)

Table 29.1. Quality Control Organisms for CTA W/Carbohydrates

Organism	ATCC Number	Glucose (Dextrose)	Maltose	Sucrose	Lactose
N. gonorrhoeae	ATCC 19424	+[a]	—	—	—
N. meningitidis	ATCC 13090	+	+[a]	—	—
N. lactamica	ATCC 23970	+	+	—	+[b]
Moraxella catarrhalis	ATCC 25238	—	—	—	—
Enterobacter aerogenes	ATCC 13048	+	+	+	+
Uninoculated					

[a]May be weak or absent.
[b]Slow.

VI. RESULTS

> See Figure 5.2 (Appendix 1) for colored photographic results; CTA color results same as those with any carbohydrate test, except *Neisseria* spp. **do not** produce gas

VII. INTERPRETATION

A. **CTA/carbohydrate medium** (5, 21, 79)
   1. Positive (A, +)
      a. Yellow color first appears at surface and progresses usually only in area of stabs (upper third of medium).
         (1) Small amount of acid because of decreased diffusion
         (2) **No** gas production
      b. Acid production; carbohydrate degraded
      c. If acid (yellow color) throughout medium, a possible contaminant; Gram stain and perform an oxidase test on growth.
   2. Negative (−)
      a. Red (alkaline) to orange (neutral) color; peptones used
      b. Compare with uninoculated tube from same batch
   3. Control tubes; glucose
      a. Uninoculated: **no** change in color (NC); medium remains reddish orange
      b. Inoculated, no carbohydrate: red (alkaline) to orange (neutral) color; peptones used
B. **Elrod and Braun (modified) solution** (26)
   1. Positive (A, +): yellow color; acid production
   2. Negative (−): deep Prussian blue color, alkaline or no change (NC), medium remains green
C. **Gonococcus identification medium (GCID)** (34)
   1. Positive (A, +): yellow or gold color along slant; acid production
   2. Negative: no color change; medium remains deep red (alkaline)

VIII. RAPID COMMERCIAL CARBOHYDRATE TESTS (KITS)

(*Note*: Non–growth-dependent methods. In all tests follow manufacturer's directions.) The influx in new techniques is primarily due to equivocal (+/−) results obtained with the widely used CTA/carbohydrate agar test and the need for more-rapid procedures (85). (See Chapter 42, Multitest Systems)

A. **Minitek disk system** (5, 64)
   1. Manufacturer: BD Biosciences
   2. Confirmatory identification of *N. gonorrhoeae*, *N. meningitidis*, and *N. lactamica*
   3. System apparatus supplied by BBL (5); use only their products for system
   4. Paper disks impregnated with appropriate carbohydrates in individual wells on plastic tray
      a. Dextrose (glucose) without nitrate, maltose, sucrose, and ONPG
      b. Modified CTA broth; added sodium bicarbonate ($NaHCO_3$), 210 μg/mL enhances phenol red color reactions (64).
   5. Inoculum: **heavy** suspension
   6. Results

a. ONPG results within 1 h
   b. Carbohydrate results within 4 h; read hourly.
 7. Interpretation
   a. Positive (A): disk yellow-orange; acid production
   b. Negative (−): disk bright red; alkaline pH

Generally results are equivalent to those with reference methods (27). Studies by Morse and Bartenstein (64) revealed no false-positive results with maltose; maltose could also be detected by sulfadiazine-resistant strains of N. meningitidis. Sulfadiazine-resistant N. meningitidis strains lack maltose permease activity (50); possibly the high concentration of maltose in the Minitek disk allows maltose to enter the bacterial cell by passive diffusion (64).

B. **API Quad-Ferm +**
 1. Manufacturer: bioMerieux
 2. System: plastic strip with seven microcupules with dehydrated buffers and phenol red indicator
   a. Carbohydrates: microcupules 1–4; glucose (dextrose), maltose, sucrose, lactose
   b. Control microcupule 5 **without** carbohydrate
   c. Microcupule 6 contains penicillin and phenol red for acidometric determination of β-lactamase by N. gonorrhoeae and Moraxella catarrhalis.
   d. Microcupule 7 contains acidometric test for DNase production by M. catarrhalis.
 3. Inoculum: **dense** McFarland #3 organism suspension (see Appendix 5)
 4. Results within 2 h. Studies showed excellent agreement with conventional methods for identification of both Neisseria spp. and M. catarrhalis (23, 33, 40).
C. *Neisseria*-**Kwik Test Kit**
 1. Manufacturer: MicroBiologics
 2. Commercial modification of rapid carbohydrate test procedure
 3. System: tray with separate carbohydrate wells
 4. Inoculum: heavy
 5. Results within 3–4 h; results compare well with those by conventional methods (22).
D. **Gonobio Test**
 1. Manufacturer: I.A.F. Productions
 2. Commercial modification of rapid carbohydrate procedures
 3. System: tray of microtubes with carbohydrates in separate wells
 4. Inoculum: **heavy**
 5. Results within 2 h; results compare well with those by conventional methods (22).

IX. CHROMOGENIC ENZYME SUBSTRATE TESTS

A. Principle/systems
 1. Profiles obtained by assaying for presence of a variety of enzymatic activities by use of chromogenic (color producing) substrates (18). These systems are restricted to N. gonorrhoeae, N. meningitidis, and N. lactamica species that can grow on selective media (e.g., MTM, ML, NYC, GC- Lect). M. catarrhalis also grows and uses these systems (53).
 2. Buffered aryl-substituted chromogenic substrates
   a. β-Naphthol
   b. β-Naphthylamine
   c. β-Nitrophenol derivatives (31)
 3. Enzymatic profiles established with **preformed** single enzymes
   a. β-Galactosidase (ONPG): specific for N. lactamica, the only Neisseria spp. with glycosidase activity (18); ONPG disk positive
   b. τ-Glutamylaminopeptidase: specific for N. meningitidis

c. Proyl-hydroxyprolyl aminopeptidase: specific for *N. gonorrhoeae*
4. Enzymatic activities detected (Table 29.2)
   a. **Hydrolysis** of amide or ester linkages detected by liberation of aryl group with resultant color change (67); naphthol or naphthylamine.
   b. Naphthol or naphthylamine chromogen released, detected by coupling with a diazotized indicator (e.g., cinnamalamide); with *p*-nitrophenol, buffering to an alkaline pH
5. Purpose
   a. Differentiation of *N. gonorrhoeae* and *N. meningitidis* from other *Neisseria* spp.
   b. Differentiation of *N. gonorrhoeae* from *N. meningitidis*: N-γ-glutamyl-β-naphthylamide substrate test for separating these two species.
      (1) N-γ-Glutamyl-β-naphthylamide substrate test for separating these two species.
      (2) Examples (16)

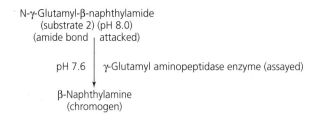

Table 29.2. Enzymatic Profiles for Pathogenic *Neisseria* spp. and *Moraxella catarrhalis*

Organism	β-Galactosidase (ONPG)	γ-Glutamylamino-peptidase	Hydroxyprolylamino-peptidase	Butyrate esterase
N. lactimca	+	−	+	−
N. meningitidis	−	+	V	−
N. gonorrhoeae	−	−	+	−
M. catarrhalis	−	−	−	+

From reference 53; V, variable reaction.

6. Results within 4 h
7. Commercial kits
   a. **Gonochek II**
      (1) Manufacturer: DuPont deNemours
      (2) System: single tube; three dehydrated chromogenic substrates; determines specific hydrolysis
      (3) Inoculum: 5–10 colonies of an oxidase-positive, Gram-negative diplococci from a pure culture grown on selective medium
      (4) Results within 30 min
      (5) Specific colored reactions for confirmation of identification
         (a) τ-Glutamyl-*p*-nitroanilide: hydrolysis end product color yellow; specific for *N. meningitidis*
         (b) 5-Bromo-4-chloro-3-indoxyl-β-D-galactopyranoside: hydrolysis end product color blue; specific for *N. lactamica*
         (c) **If suspension is colorless,** contact with the diazo dye coupler (*o*-aminoazotoluene diazonium salt (Fast Garnet)); detect β-naphthylamine released by hydroxyprolyl amine peptidase activity by a red color; specific for *N. gonorrhoeae*
         (d) At completion, **absence of color presumptively** identifies *M. catarrhalis*. Results comparable to results of conventional methods for *Neisseria* identification (11, 22, 81).

b. **BactiCard Neisseria**
   (1) Manufacturer: REMEL
   (2) System: four chromogenic substrates impregnated on individual test circles in a cardboard holder
      (a) IB circle: indoxyl butyrate esterase substrate (IB-5-bromo-4-chloro-3-indoxyl butyrate): blue to blue-green color **within 2 min**; specific for *M. catarrhalis*. **No further testing required**
      (b) **If IB circle negative:** galactosidase substrate circle BGAL (5-bromo-4-chloro-3-indoxyl-β-D-galactopyranoside) allowed to sit **13 min** more (total 15 min); a blue-green color is specific for *N. lactamica*; no further testing required
      (c) **If BGAL circle negative:** add color developer reagent on PRO (prolyl-aminopeptidase) and GLUT (τ-glutamyl-β-naphthylamide) test circles; a pink-red color **within 30 sec**
         1 PRO positive: *N. gonorrhoeae* and some strains of *N. meningitidis*
         2 GLUT positive: *N. meningitidis*
   (3) Good comparison with conventional methods for *Neisseria* identification (42).
c. **Neisstrip**
   (1) Manufacturer: Lab M Ltd, United Kingdom
   (2) Similar to BactiCard; lacks indoxyl butyrate reagent for identification of *M. catarrhalis*; good comparison with conventional methods (20)

X. ALTERNATIVE TESTS

A. **Identification of *N. gonorrhoeae* by genetic transformation**
   1. Highly specific procedure of Bawdon, Juni, and Britt (4)
   2. Principle: DNA extracted from suspected gonococcal isolate used to genetically transform a nutritionally deficient (uracil and arginine) auxotroph (mutant) to a prototroph
      a. Prototroph: strain with same nutritional requirements as wild-type strain (i.e., a strain found in nature or a standard strain).
      b. Auxotroph: strain derived from prototroph that requires extra growth factors
   3. Advantages: (*a*) no cross-reaction with other *Neisseria* spp., transformation positive **only** with *N. gonorrhoeae*; (*b*) may be used with a mixed and/or nonviable test culture; (*c*) may be identified from a purulent discharge; and (*d*) reaction is **not** influenced by occasional glucose-negative strains (standard testing).
   4. Reaction usually within 36 h
B. **Electron-capture gas-liquid chromatography of metabolites** (see ref. 61)
C. **Direct fluorescent antibody techniques (FA staining)** (47, 53, 68)
   1. Used routinely to identify and confirm *N. gonorrhoeae* (47, 68)
   2. Fast and can identify living or nonviable *Neisseria*
   3. Uses monoclonal antibodies that recognize epitopes on Por, the principle outer membrane protein of *N. gonorrhoeae* (8, 41, 56, 82)
   4. *Neisseria gonorrhoeae* **Culture Confirmation Test**
      a. Manufacturer: Syva Company; monoclonal FA test
      b. Fast; can test colonies directly from primary media
      c. Small amount of growth required
      d. Gonococci appear as apple-green fluorescent diplococci
D. **Coagglutination tests**
   1. Principle
      a. Ability of protein A on *Staphylococcus aureus* subsp. *aureus* cells to bind immunoglobulin G (IgG) molecules by their Fc region
      b. Binding of antigonococcal antibody to killed *S. aureus* subsp. *aureus* cells and subse-

quent mixture with a suspension of gonococci yielding visible agglutination of suspension
   2. Commercial tests available
      a. **Phadebact GC OMNI Test**
         (1) Manufacturer: Karo-Bio, Sweden
         (2) Uses monoclonal antibodies to gonococcal Por (protein I); favorable evaluations (15, 22, 23, 41)
      b. **GonoGen I test**
         (1) Manufacturer: New Horizons Diagnostics
         (2) Uses staphylococcal cells coated with monoclonal antibodies directed against outer membrane protein I of several gonococcal serovars; sensitivities of 86–100% and specificities of 99–100% (41, 49, 57, 60)
      c. **Meritec GC Test**
         (1) Manufacturer: Meridian Diagnostics
         (2) Similar to GonoGen I; sensitivity 92–93% and specificity 99% (41)
E. Probe technology
   1. Purpose: confirmation and direct detection of N. gonorrhoeae
      a. Nucleic acid probes; hybridize specifically with ribosomal RNA (rRNA) from N. gonorrhoeae
      b. Colorimetric, fluorescent, and chemiluminescent hybridization detection methods facilitate introduction of probe techniques in the laboratory (74).
   2. Commercial probes
      a. **AccuProbe *Neisseria gonorrhoeae* Culture Confirmation Test**
         (1) Manufacturer: Gen-Probe
         (2) Identifies organism by detecting rRNA sequence unique to N. gonorrhoeae
            (a) Chemiluminescent hybridization detection method
            (b) Various investigators have found the test 100% accurate (37, 58, 86).
      b. **PACE-2NG (probe assay-chemiluminescence)**
         (1) Manufacturer: Gen-Probe
         (2) Direct detection of gonococci in urogenital specimens
F. **Multi ID Test Kits:** for identification of *Neisseria* spp. and other fastidious Gram-negative microorganisms (see Chapter 42, Multitest Systems)

XI. PRECAUTIONS

A. General
   1. *N. gonorrhoeae* and *N. meningitidis* have been isolated from a variety of clinical sources: *N. gonorrhoeae* from locations other than genitourinary tract and *N. meningitidis* from urinary tract (28, 84). The possibility of isolating pathogenic *Neisseria* from almost any body area or specimen has put an added burden on bacteriology laboratories to isolate, identify, and confirm these pathogens. Medical treatments for these two organisms are entirely different, and they **must** be correctly identified from the clinical source as quickly as possible.
   Since 1948, identifying and confirming the pathogenic *Neisseria* depended completely on growth characteristics on isolation media, fermentation reactions in CTA/carbohydrate media with visual acid detection, and the direct fluorescent antibody (FA) test (79). These tests are still in use in most laboratories today. Much emphasis has been placed on developing reliable systems for biochemical confirmation of *Neisseria* spp. because of frequent equivocal results with strains of *N. gonorrhoeae* that occasionally fail to use glucose (dextrose). The visibility of color reactions in fermentation tests is influenced by the pH indicator used (12, 48), the buffering properties of the medium (12), contamination of com-

mercial maltose with small amounts of glucose (12, 48), and the most uncontrollable problem, inoculum size (27, 48). Faur et al. (27) showed that an effective medium must support the growth of smaller inocula of highly fastidious strains of Neisseria and produce a clear-cut, rapid indicator color change upon metabolism of carbohydrates. Some more fastidious Neisseria require additional growth factors for proper degradation patterns (47, 83).

Methods rely on preformed enzymes and/or are growth dependent. Both methodologies have innate difficulties: (a) the heavy inoculum required necessitates subculture from primary isolation media, with loss of 24 h in identification time; (b) chemically pure carbohydrates must be used to avoid false-positive results; and (c) unreliable results may occur from plates incubated for more than 18 to 24 h or from plates containing antimicrobial agents (47).

2. It is not possible to tailor the size of inoculum to each strain of N. gonorrhoeae; false-negative carbohydrate results occur frequently when tests depend on preformed enzymes **alone** (85). Optimally, carbohydrate utilization testing of Neisseria should incorporate the combined action of performed enzymes and those formed in test medium during growth (84).

3. **All** primary isolates grown on isolation or transport media (e.g., Thayer-Martin (TM), Modified Thayer-Martin (MTM), enriched chocolate agar (ECA), New York City (NYC) agar plates, Modified NYC (MNYC), Transgrow, Neigon plates, Gono-Pak, or JEMBEC plates) **must** be **subcultured** to chocolate agar (CA) plates, since antibiotics in these media can influence bacterial fermentation patterns (46, 64). CA plates should be incubated 18–24 h at 35°C, under 6% CO_2 for use as inocula for carbohydrate test procedures. CO_2 needed for initial isolation of certain strains of N. gonorrhoeae on solid media (39, 69) can be replaced by bicarbonate in isolation media (25, 44, 77).

4. During growth of Neisseria, certain intrinsic enzyme(s) can degrade peptones to alkaline products that may neutralize the acid formed, causing reversion from acidity to alkalinity (19) and a false-negative test result.

5. Morse and Bartenstein (64) reported that the purity of the maltose source is important; commercially prepared maltose is often contaminated with glucose. The maltose used in broth growth and non-growth-dependent test procedures often produces false-positive results due to maltose contamination (12, 18). Maltose-negative organisms can use contaminating glucose, producing a false-positive maltose reaction.

6. Addition of starch neutralizes the toxicity of some types of agar but not others; the toxicity of various commercial agars is the major factor in preventing strains of N. gonorrhoeae from growing on solid agar (43).

7. Sulfadiazine-resistant strains of N. meningitidis lack maltose permease activity (50) and so are usually maltose negative. Morse and Bartenstein (64) found that maltose use by sulfadiazine-resistant strains was detected by the Minitek test system.

8. N. lactamica is the only species of Neisseria to demonstrate glycosidase activity. If a laboratory fails to use lactose in its testing battery, this organism could be misidentified as either N. meningitidis or saprophyte N. subflava.

B. **CTA/carbohydrate medium**
1. CTA deficiencies are (a) **heavy** inoculum required, (b) poor growth of fastidious Neisseria pathogens, (c) delayed results (72 h or longer), and (d) atypical biochemical patterns with N. gonorrhoeae and N. meningitidis (6, 14, 27, 48, 70, 71, 75, 83, 85). Prolonged incubation may lead to changes in pH indicator (27, 68, 75, 83, 85) or abnormal lactose/sucrose reactions with some Neisseria pathogens (1). Inadequate growth in many carbohydrates is due to strains with various nutritional requirements (48, 72). Knapp and Holmes (52) reported that 39% of isolates from nondisseminated gonococcal infections required arginine, hypoxanthine, and uracil. The prevalence of these fastidious auxotrophs may contribute to the large number of isolates that show false reactions on CTA

(67). Various investigators (1, 2, 13, 27, 64, 70, 71, 80, 85) have reported anywhere from 4.0 to 39.1% nonreactivity of *N. gonorrhoeae* and *N. meningitidis* in CTA sugars.
2. Addition of more than 0.5% carbohydrates may necessitate adjusting pH (5) (see Appendix 4).
3. For maximum efficiency, CTA should be **freshly** prepared or boiled (with caps loosened) and cooled just prior to inoculation (5).
4. Test tubes with cotton plugs are **un**satisfactory if the medium is to be held 10 days or longer; appreciable drying may occur (5).
5. Some strains of *N. gonorrhoeae* may exhibit weak or no visible color changes with phenol red pH indicator (12).
6. LaScolea et al. (55) reported that sodium chloride in the medium inhibits *N. gonorrhoeae*.
7. Baron and Saz (2) showed that the cystine:$NaSO_3$ ratio (concentration) may inhibit some enzyme(s) in the glucose metabolic pathway. Inhibition of growth and hence glucose metabolism was also observed by several other investigators (9, 32). Baron and Saz (2) showed that cystine and sulfhydryl compounds are not needed to obtain luxuriant growth and acid production from glucose, since gonococcus cysteine (GCC) medium with no added cystine or sulfhydryl gave equally satisfactory results; even in CTA from which cystine was removed, glucose-negative reactions occurred. By substituting *l*-cysteine and sodium **sulfate** (Na_2SO_4), Baron and Saz (2) eliminated this inhibitory effect. However, Vera (79), who developed CTA, reported that sodium sulfite and cystine enhanced growth of *N. gonorrhoeae* in CTA.
8. *Neisseria* spp. usually produce acid only in the area of stabs (upper third); if there is strong acid (yellow color) throughout the medium, it is a possible contaminant. If in doubt about a tube containing a *Neisseria* sp., perform a Gram stain and oxidase test on the growth (Gram-negative, kidney-shaped diplococci; oxidase positive).
9. Some commercial CTA formulas may be supplemented with ascitic fluid to support growth of more fastidious microorganisms.

C. GCID medium: IsoVitaleX diluent contains glucose; **do not use.** Substitute sterile distilled water for test procedure.

D. **Minitek system**
1. **Do not** use a dextrose-nitrate disk because nitrate markedly inhibits production of acid from glucose by *N. gonorrhoeae* (64), giving a false-negative result.
2. Earlier problems related to medium/inoculum size suspension in the *Neisseria* Minitek method (64, 71) were resolved by special commercial *Neisseria* broth available as part of system (64); **do not substitute.**
3. Occasional false-negative results are due to an inoculum with a low cell density (below McFarland's no. 9 standard) or an inoculum prepared directly from initial isolation on Transgrow or Thayer-Martin plate medium (64).
4. A positive reaction may be delayed or inhibited if the $NaHCO_3$ concentration is too high (>420 µg/mL) (64), leading to a false-negative result. The pH may be increased to alkalinity by production of CO_3^{2-} from HCO_3^- (64) or *Neisseria* may use HCO_3^- as a growth factor (63).
5. The system has noted some weak, glucose-positive reactions with some strains of *N. cinerea,* which may result in misidentification of *N. gonorrhoeae* (10, 24).

E. **FA tests**
1. At present antisera for FA are available commercially only for *N. gonorrhoeae* (76).
2. Some cross-reactions exist between strains of gonococci and meningococci and gonococci and staphylococci; refer to the test procedure for the method of eliminating this cross-reactivity.
3. Syva's MicroTrak is not intended for direct detection and identification of organisms on smears from patient specimens (53).

4. In the Phadebact GC Omni test, an organism suspension heavier than the specified McFarland density may yield false-positive results (53).
5. In the Phadebact GC Omni test, use of saline with a pH above or below 7.4 has been reported to produce false-positive results with some strains of *N. lacyimca, N. cinerea,* and *M. catarrhalis* (15, 22, 41, 51).

REFERENCES

1. Appelbaum PC, Lawrence RB. Comparison of three methods for identification of pathogenic *Neisseria* species. J Clin Microbiol 1979;9(5): 598–600.
2. Baron ES, Saz AK. Effects of types of media on the production of acid from glucose by so-called glucose-negative strains of *Neisseria gonorrhoeae.* J Clin Microbiol 1976;3(3):330–333.
3. Baron ESG, Miller CP. Studies on biological oxidations. I. Oxidations produced by gonococci. J Biol Chem 1932;97(3):691–715.
4. Bawdon RE, Juni E, Britt EM. Identification of *Neisseria gonorrhoeae* by genetic transformation: A clinical laboratory evaluation. J Clin Microbiol 1977;5(1):108–109.
5. BBL Manual of Products and Laboratory Procedures, ed 6. Cockeysville, MD: Becton Dickinson and Company, 1988.
6. Beno DW, Devine LF, Larson GL. Identification of *Neisseria meningitidis* carbohydrate fermentation patterns in Mueller-Hinton broth. J Bacteriol 1968;96(2):563.
7. Berger U. Über den Kohlenhydrat-stoffwechsel von *Neisseria* und *Gemella.* Zentralbl Bakteriol Parasitenk Infektionskr Hyg Abt I Orig 1960; 180(1):147–149.
8. Boehm DM, Bernhardt M, Kurzynski TA, et al. Evaluation of two commercial procedures for rapid identification of *Neisseria gonorrhoeae* using a reference panel of antigenically diverse gonococci. J Clin Microbiol 1990;28(9):2099–2100
9. Boor AK. A difference in metabolic requirements of meningococcus and gonococcus. Proc Soc Exp Biol Med 1942;50(1):22–25.
10. Boyce JM, Mitchell EB. Difficulties in differentiating *Neisseria cinerea* from *Neisseria gonorrhoeae* in rapid systems used for identifying pathogenic *Neisseria* species. J Clin Microbiol 1985;22 (5):731–734.
11. Brown JD, Thomas KR. Rapid enzyme system for the identification of pathogenic *Neisseria* spp. J Clin Microbiol 1985;21(5):857–858.
12. Brown WJ. Modification of the rapid fermentation test for *Neisseria gonorrhoeae.* Appl Microbiol 1974;27(6):1027–1030.
13. Brown WJ. A comparison of three fermentation methods for the confirmation of *Neisseria gonorrhoeae.* Health Lab Sci 1976;13(1):54–58.
14. Carifo K, Catlin BW. *Neisseria gonorrhoeae* auxotyping: Differentiation of clinical isolates based on growth responses on chemically defined media. Appl Microbiol 1973;26(3):223–230.
15. Carlson BL, Calnan MR, Goodman RE, George H. Phadebact monoclonal GC OMNI test for confirmation of *Neisseria gonorrhoeae.* J Clin Microbiol 1987;25(10):1982–1984.
16. Catlin BW. *Neisseria meningitidis* (meningococcus). In: Blair JE, Lennette EH, Truant JP, eds. Manual of Clinical Microbiology. Washington, DC: American Society for Microbiology, 1970: 76–81.
17. Catlin BW. *Neisseria meningitidis* (meningococcus) In: Lennette EH, Spaulding EH, Truant JP, eds. Manual of Clinical Microbiology, ed 2. Washington, DC: American Society for Microbiology, 1974:116–123.
18. D'Amato RF, Eriquez LA, Tomfohrde KM, Singerman E. Rapid identification of *Neisseria gonorrhoeae* and *Neisseria meningitidis* by using enzyme profiles. J Clin Microbiol 1978;7(2):77–81.
19. Davies JA, Mitzel JR, Beam WE Jr. Carbohydrate fermentation patterns of *Neisseria meningitidis* determined by Microtiter method. Appl Microbiol 1971;21(6):1072–1074.
20. Dealler SF, Gough KR, Campbell L, et al. Identification of *Neisseria gonorrhoeae* using the Neisstrip rapid enzyme detection test. J Clin Pathol 1991;44:376–379.
21. Difco Supplementary Literature. Detroit: Difco Laboratories, 1968:81.
22. Dillon JR, Carballo M, Pauz M. Evaluation of eight methods for identification of pathogenic *Neisseria* species: *Neisseria*-Kwik, RIM-N, Gonobio-Test, Minitek, Gonochek I, GonoGen, Phadebact Monoclonal GC OMNI test and Syva MicroTrak test. J Clin Microbiol 1988;26(3): 493–497.
23. Dolter J, Bryant L, Janda JM. Evaluation of five rapid systems for the identification of *Neisseria gonorrhoeae.* Diagn Microbiol Infect Dis 1990; 13:265–267.
24. Dossett JH, Applebaum PC, Knapp JS, Totten PA. Proctitis associated with *Neisseria cinerea* misidentified as *Neisseria gonorrhoeae* in a child. J Clin Microbiol 1985;21(4):575–577.
25. Earl RG, Dennison D, Whadford V, et al. Preliminary studies in the clinical use of bicarbonate containing growth medium for *Neisseria gonorrhoeae.* J Am Vener Dis Assoc 1976;3(1):40–42.
26. Elrod RP, Braun AC. *Pseudomonas aeruginosa:* Its role as a plant pathogen. J Bacteriol 1942;44(6): 633–645.
27. Faur YC, Weisburd MH, Wilson ME. Carbohydrate fermentation plate medium for confirma-

28. Faur YC, Weisburd MH, Wilson ME. Isolation of *Neisseria meningitidis* from the genito-urinary tract and anal canal. J Clin Microbiol 1975;2(3):178–182.
29. Fitting C, Doudoroff M. Phosphorolysis of maltose by enzyme preparations from *Neisseria meningitidis*. J Biol Chem 1952;199(1):153–163.
30. Germer JJ, Washington JA II. Evaluation of a rapid identification method for *Neisseria* spp. J Clin Microbiol 1985;21(6):987–988.
31. Goldstein TP, Plapinger RE, Nachlas MM, Seligman AM. Synthesis of chromogenic substrates for the assay of aminopeptidase activity. J Med Pharm Chem 1962;5(4):852–857.
32. Gould RG. Glutathione as an essential growth factor for certain strains of *Neisseria gonorrhoeae*. J Biol Chem 1944;153(1):143–162.
33. Gradus MD, Ng CM, Silver KJ. Comparison of the QuadFERM + 2-hr identification system with conventional carbohydrate degradation test for confirmatory identification of *Neisseria gonorrhoeae*. Sex Transm Dis 1989;16:57–59.
34. Graves JO, Magee LA. *Neisseria* confirmation by an enriched, bicarbonate-containing carbohydrate medium. J Clin Microbiol 1978;8(5):525–528.
35. Holten E. Glutamate dehydrogenase in genus *Neisseria*. Acta Pathol Microbiol Scand 1973;81:49–58.
36. Holten E, Jyssum K. Glutamate dehydrogenases in *Neisseria meningitidis*. Acta Pathol Microbiol Scand 1973;81:43–48.
37. Hornyik G, Platt JH Jr. Cerebrospinal fluid shunt infection by *Neisseria sicca*. Pediatr Neurosurg 1994;21:189–191.
38. Hugh R, Leifson E. The taxonomic significance of fermentative versus oxidative metabolism of carbohydrates by various Gram negative bacteria. J Bacteriol 1953;66(1):24–26.
39. James-Holmquest AN, Wende RD, Mudd RL, Williams RP. Comparison of atmospheric conditions for culture of clinical specimens of *Neisseria gonorrhoeae*. Appl Microbiol 1973;26:466.
40. Janda WM, Montero M. Premarket evaluation of the BactiCard Neisseria. Proc 95th general meeting, American Society for Microbiology, Washington, DC, abstr C-303, 1995:53.
41. Janda WM, Wilcoski LM, Mandel KL, et al. Comparison of monoclonal antibody-based methods and a ribosomal ribonucleic acid probe test for *Neisseria gonorrhoeae* culture confirmation. Eur J Clin Microbiol Infect Dis 1993;12:177–184.
42. Janda WM, Zigler KL, Bradna JJ. API QuadFerm + with rapid DNase identification of *Neisseria* spp. and *Branhamella catarrhalis*. J Clin Microbiol 1987;25(2):203–206.
43. Jones RT, Talley RS. Simplified complete medium for the growth of *Neisseria gonorrhoeae*. J Clin Microbiol 1977;5(1):9–14.
44. Jones RT, Talley RS. Effects of gaseous CO_2 and bicarbonate on the growth of *Neisseria gonorrhoeae*. J Clin Microbiol 1978;5(4):427–432.
45. Juhlin I. A new fermentation medium for *N. gonorrhoeae*. HAP medium. Influence of different constituents on growth and indicator colour. Acta Pathol Microbiol Scand 1963;58(1):51–71.
46. Kellogg DS Jr. *Neisseria gonorrhoeae* (gonococcus). In: Lennette EH, Spaulding EH, Truant JP, eds. Manual of Clinical Microbiology, ed 2. Washington, DC: American Society for Microbiology, 1974:124–129.
47. Kellogg DS Jr, Holmes KK, Hill GA. Cumitech 4: Laboratory Diagnosis of Gonorrheae. Washington, DC: American Society for Microbiology, 1976.
48. Kellogg DS Jr, Turner EM. Rapid fermentation confirmation of *Neisseria gonorrhoeae*. Appl Microbiol 1973;25(4):550–552.
49. Kellogg JA, Orwig LK. Comparison of GonoGen, GonoGen II, and MicroTrak direct fluorescent antibody test with carbohydrate fermentation for confirmation of culture isolated of *Neisseria gonorrhoeae*. J Clin Microbiol 1995;33(2):474–476.
50. Kingsbury DT. Relationship between sulfadiazine resistance and the failure to ferment maltose in *Neisseria meningitidis*. J Bacteriol 1967;94(3):557–561.
51. Knapp JS. Historical perspectives and identification of *Neisseria* and related species. Clin Microbiol Rev 1988;1:415–431.
52. Knapp JS, Holmes KK. Disseminated gonococcal infections caused by *Neisseria gonorrhoeae* with unique nutritional requirements. J Infect Dis 1975;132:204.
53. Koneman EW, Allen SD, Janda WM, et al. Color Atlas and Textbook of Diagnostic Microbiology, ed 5. Philadelphia: JB Lippincott, 1997:510–513.
54. Lairscey RC, Kelly MT. Evaluations of a one-hour test for identification of *Neisseria* species. J Clin Microbiol 1985;22(2):238–240.
55. LaScolea LJ Jr, Dul MJ, Young FE. Stability of pathogenic colony types of *Neisseria gonorrhoeae* in liquid culture by using the parameters of colony morphology and deoxyribonucleic acid transformation. J Clin Microbiol 1975;1(2):165–170.
56. Laughon BE, Ehret JM, Tanino TT, et al. Fluorescent monoclonal antibody for confirmation of *Neisseria gonorrhoeae* cultures. J Clin Microbiol 1987;25(12):2388–2390.
57. Lawton WD, Battiaglioli GJ. GonoGen coagglutination test for *Neisseria gonorrhoeae*. J Clin Microbiol 1983;18(5):1264–1265.
58. Lewis JS, Kranig-Brown D, Trainor DA. DNA probe confirmatory test for *Neisseria gonorrhoeae*. J Clin Microbiol 1990;28(10):2349–2350.
59. Martin JE Jr, Lester A. Transgrow, a medium for transport and growth of *Neisseria gonorrhoeae* and *Neisseria meningitidis*. HSMHA Health Service Rep 1971;86(1):30–33.
60. Minshew BH, Beardsley JL, Knapp JS. Evalua-

tion of GonoGen coagglutination test for serodiagnosis of *Neisseria gonorrhoeae:* Identification of problem isolates by auxotyping, serotyping, and with fluorescent antibody reagent. Diagn Microbiol Infect Dis 1985;3:41–46.
61. Morse CD, Brooks JB, Kellogg DS. Electron capture gas chromatographic detection of acetylmethylcarbinol produced by *Neisseria gonorrhoeae.* J Clin Microbiol 1976;3(1):34–41.
62. Morse CD, Brooks JB, Kellogg DS Jr. Identification of *Neisseria* by electron capture gas-liquid chromatography of metabolites in a chemically defined growth medium. J Clin Microbiol 1977; 6(5):474–481.
63. Morse SA, Bartenstein L. Growth and survival of *Neisseria gonorrhoeae* in liquid medium. Proc annual meeting, American Society for Microbiology, abstr. G86, 1972:44.
64. Morse SA, Bartenstein L. Adaptation of the Minitek System for the rapid identification of *Neisseria gonorrhoeae.* J Clin Microbiol 1976;3 (1):8–13.
65. Morse SA, Stein S, Hines J. Glucose metabolism in *Neisseria gonorrhoeae.* J Bacteriol 1974;120 (2):702–714.
66. Mullaney PJ. A simple fermentation medium for *Neisseria gonorrhoeae.* J Pathol Bacteriol 1956;71 (2):516–517.
67. Nardon P, Monget D, Didier-Fichet ML, de-The G. Comparison of zymogram of three lymphoblastoid cell lines with a new microtechnique. Biomedicine 1976;24:183–190.
68. Peacock WL Jr, Welch BG, Martin JE Jr, Thayer JD. Fluorescent antibody technique for identification of presumptively positive gonococcal cultures. Public Health Rep 1968;83(4):337–339.
69. Platt DJ. Carbon dioxide requirement of *Neisseria gonorrhoeae* growing on a solid medium. J Clin Microbiol 1976;4(2):129–132.
70. Pollock HM. Evaluation of methods for the rapid identification of *Neisseria gonorrhoeae* in a routine clinical laboratory. J Clin Microbiol 1976;4 (1):19–21.
71. Reddick A. A simple carbohydrate fermentation test for identification of the pathogenic *Neisseria.* J Clin Microbiol 1975;2(1):72–73.
72. Reyn A, Bentzon MW. Possible effects of antibiotic treatment on the sensitivity and growth requirements of *Neisseria gonorrhoeae.* Bull WHO 1961;24(2):333–342.
73. Robinson A, Griffith SB, Moore DG, Carlson JR. Evaluations of the RIM system and GonoGen test for identification of *Neisseria gonorrhoeae* from clinical specimens. Diagn Microbiol Infect Dis 1985;3:125–130.
74. Rossau R, Vanmechelen E, De Ley J, Van Heuverswijn H. Specific *Neisseria gonorrhoeae* DNA probes derived from ribosomal RNA. J Gen Microbiol 1989;135:1735–1745.
75. Shtibel R, Toma S. *Neisseria gonorrhoeae:* Evaluation of some methods used for carbohydrate utilization. Can J Microbiol 1978;24(1):177–181.
76. Strauss RR, Holderbach J, Friedman H. Comparison of a radiometric procedure with conventional methods for identification of *Neisseria.* J Clin Microbiol 1978;7(5):419–422.
77. Talley RS, Baugh CL. Effects of bicarbonate on growth of *Neisseria gonorrhoeae:* Replacement of gaseous CO_2 atmosphere. Appl Microbiol 1975; 29(4):469–471.
78. Vanderkerkove M, Faucon R, Andiffren P, Oddon A. Metabolism of carbohydrates by *Neisseria intracellularis.* V. Evidence of acetylmethylcarbinol produced from glucose. Med Trop 1965;25:457.
79. Vera HD. A simple medium for identification and maintenance of the gonococcus and other bacteria. J Bacteriol 1948;55(4):531–536.
80. Wallace R, Ashton F, Charron F, Diena BB. An improved sugar fermentation technique for the confirmation of *Neisseria gonorrhoeae.* Can J Public Health 1975;66:251–252.
81. Welborn PP, Uyeda CT, Ellison-Birang N. Evaluation of Gonochek-II as a rapid identification system for pathogenic *Neisseria* species. J Clin Microbiol 1984;20(4):680–683.
82. Welch WD, Cartwright G. Fluorescent monoclonal antibody compared with carbohydrate utilization for rapid identification of *Neisseria gonorrhoeae.* J Clin Microbiol 1988;26(2):293–296.
83. White LA, Kellogg DS Jr. An improved fermentation medium for *Neisseria gonorrhoeae* and other *Neisseria.* Health Lab Sci 1970;2(4):238–241.
84. Willmott FE. Meningococcal salpingitis. Br J Vener Dis 1976;52(3):182–183.
85. Yong DCT, Prytula A. Rapid micro-carbohydrate test for confirmation of *Neisseria gonorrhoeae.* J Clin Microbiol 1978;8(6):643–647.
86. Young LS, Moyes A. Comparative evaluation of AccuProbe culture identification test for *Neisseria gonorrhoeae* and other rapid methods. J Clin Microbiol 1993;31(8):1996–1999.

30 Nitrate/Nitrite Reduction Tests

I. PRINCIPLE

To determine the ability of an organism to reduce nitrate to nitrites or free nitrogen gas

II. PURPOSE

(Also see Chapters 43–45)

A. **Nitrate reduction**
   1. **To aid in species differentiation**
      a. *Afipia felis* (+) from *A. broomeae* (−) and *A. clevelandensis* (−)
      b. *Alcaligenes faecalis* (−) from *A. latus* (+)
      c. *Bartonella felis* (+) from other *Bartonella* spp. (−) most frequently isolated
      d. *Bordetella bronchiseptica* (+) from *B. avium* (−), *B. parapertussis* (−), and *B. pertussis* (−)
      e. *Capnocytophaga sputigena* (+) and *C. cynodegmi* (V, variable) from *C. canimorsus* (−), *C. gingivalis* (−), and *C. ochracea* (−)
      f. *Helicobacter cinaedi* (+) and *H. mustelae* (+) from *H. fennelliae* (−), and *H. pylori* (V)
      g. *Kingella denitrificans* (+) from *K. kingae* (−)
      h. *Microbacterium lacticum* (+) from *M. arborescens* (−), *M. imperiale* (−), and *M. laevaniformens* (−)
      i. *Mobiluncus curtisii* subsp. *holmesii* (+) from *M. curtisii* subsp. *curtisii* (−) and *M. milieris* (−)
      j. *Moraxella atlantae* (−), *M. lincolnii* (−), and *M. osloensis* (V) from *M. catarrhalis* (V, usually +) and *M. bovis* (V)
      k. *Neisseria canis* (+), *N. mucosa* (+), *M. polysaccharea* (+) from other *Neisseria* spp. (−) most frequently isolated
      l. *Pasteurella lymphangitis* (−) from other *Pasteurella* spp. (+)
      m. *Peptostreptococcus indolicus* (+) and *P. prevotii* (V) from other *Peptostreptococcus* spp. (−) that may cause human infections
      n. *Sphingobacterium thalpophilum* (+) from *S. multivorum* (−) and *S. spiritivorum* (−)
      o. *Vibrio harveyi* (−) and *V. metschnikovii* (−) from other *Vibrio* spp. (+) most frequently isolated
   2. **To aid in differentiation between genera**
      a. *Haemophilus* spp. (+), *Neisseria gonorrhoeae* (−), *Kingella denitrificans* (+) and *Moraxella catarrhalis* (V, usually +) (20)
      b. All *Enterobacteriaceae* (+) except certain biotypes of *Pantoea agglomerans* and certain species of *Serratia* and *Yersinia* (20)
   3. To differentiate *Mycobacterium* spp.: *M. tuberculosis* (+), *M. kansasii* (+), *M. szulgai* (+), and *M. fortuitum* (+) from other *Mycobacterium* spp. (−)

B. **Nitrate and nitrite reduction**
   1. *Gemella haemolysans* (NO_3+/NO_2+) from *G. morbillorum* (NO_3-/NO_2-)
   2. Differentiation between *Neisseria* spp. and *Moraxella* spp. of animal origin; not useful for differentiation between human spp. (3, 19, 23) (Table 30.1)

Table 30.1. Differentiation between *Neisseria* and *Moraxella* spp. of Animal Origin

Organism	NO_3	NO_2
Neisseria canis	+	V−
Neisseria weaveri	V−	+
Neisseria iguanae	+	V
Moraxella caviae[a]	+	+
Moraxella ovis[a]	+	V−
Moraxella cuniculi[a]	V−	V−

Data from refs 3, 19, 23, 24.
[a]Formerly in the genus *Neisseria*; species of animal origin.

III. BIOCHEMISTRY INVOLVED

Reduction of nitrate (NO_3^-) to nitrite (NO_2^-) and to nitrogen gas (N_2) usually takes place under anaerobic conditions, in which an organism derives its oxygen from nitrate (12, 30). The oxygen serves as a hydrogen acceptor (30); i.e., the final proton and electron acceptor (35). Most aerobic bacteria are facultative anaerobes and can only reduce nitrate in the absence of oxygen (35). This anaerobic respiration is an oxidation process in which inorganic substances (mainly nitrate and sulfate, rarely carbonate) furnish oxygen to serve as an electron acceptor to provide energy (35). In nitrate reduction, bacterial cytochromes transport electrons to specific acceptor molecules (17, 35). Gunsalus and Stanier (17) state that nitrate acts as the ultimate oxidant in the cytochrome systems. Nitrate reduction characteristic of a particular species is more or less constant (41).

Nitrate to Nitrite Reduction (35)

Nitrate to Nitrite Reduction (24)

$$NO_3^- + 2\bar{e} + 2H^+ \rightarrow NO_2^- + H_2O$$
Nitrate → Nitrite

The end product possibilities of nitrate reduction are many: nitrite (NO_2), ammonia (NH_3), molecular nitrogen (N_2), nitric oxide (NO), nitrous oxide (N_2O), or hydroxylamine (R·NH·OH) (6, 10, 11, 17, 25, 34). Which product is formed depends upon the bacterial species (25). The more common end product is molecular nitrogen (a gas) via nitrite reduction (35). Depending upon environmental conditions, these products are usually not further oxidized or assimilated into cellular metabolism, but are excreted into the surrounding medium (25, 34). Reduction of nitrate to nitrogen gas (N_2) or nitrous oxide (N_2O) is called **denitrification** (32, 35). Nitrate serves as an electron acceptor; for each molecule of nitrate reduced, five electrons are accepted (35).

Nitrate to Molecular Nitrogen (35)

$$2NO_3^- + 10\bar{e} + 12H^+ \rightarrow N_2 + 6H_2O$$

In the dentrification process, nitrous oxide (an intermediate) may accumulate if the concentration of nitrate is high; when the concentration of nitrate is low, nitrous oxide is further reduced to molecular nitrogen (35). In nitrate reduction several processes may occur for the use of the end products formed. Ammonia or hydroxylamine may be assimilated into nitrogen-containing cell components (proteins and nucleic acids) for synthesis of new compounds (25,

34). Reduction, therefore, in the nitrate reduction test, is evidenced by either presence of a catabolic end product or absence of nitrate in the medium.

IV. MEDIA EMPLOYED: POTASSIUM NITRATE MEDIUM, TWO VARIANTS

A. **Nitrate broth**: pH 7.0 (12)
B. **Nitrate agar**: pH 6.8 (12)
C. Ingredients: either medium

Beef (meat) extract	3.0 g
Gelatin peptone	5.0 g
Potassium nitrate, KNO_3, 0.1%	1.0 g
Agar (**agar medium only**), nitrite-free	12.0 g
Deionized water	1000.0 mL

D. Commercial products available: BBL, Difco, nitrate broth
E. Method of preparation
   1. Weigh out amount accurately as directed on the label.
   2. Rehydrate with distilled or demineralized water.
   3. Heat **gently** into solution.
   4. Dispense approximately
      a. Nitrate agar: 5.0 mL per tube (13 × 100 mm)
      b. Nitrate broth: 1.0 mL per tube (13 × 100 mm) (2); add **inverted** Durham tubes to detect gas production
F. Method of sterilization: autoclave, 121°C, 15 lb, 15 min
G. Allow **nitrate agar** medium to solidify in a **slanted position**.
H. Cool either medium before use and refrigerate for storage (4–10°C). Shelf life approximately 6 months
I. Inoculation
   1. Growth from an 18- to 24-h **pure** culture Kligler's iron agar (KIA) or other suitable culture
   2. Broth medium: **heavy** inoculum (42)
   3. Agar slant medium: **fishtail slant** and **stab butt** (12)
   4. Two controls should be tested simultaneously
      a. Control tube 1: inoculated with a known nitrate-positive **organism** (39)
      b. Control tube 2: **uninoculated**, but run under the same conditions as those inoculated. Check to determine if nitrite is present in the medium (39).
J. Incubation: 35°C, 12–24 h (12); rarely, incubation prolonged up to 5 days may be required (10)
K. Add nitrate reagents before attempting an interpretation. Most organisms capable of reducing nitrate do so within 24 h. Nitrate medium may be used as either broth or an agar slant. However, ZoBell (41) and Hitchens (18) recommend using a semisolid medium containing 0.2–0.4% agar. ZoBell (41) states that a semisolid medium enhances reproduction, permits movement of motile organisms, readily diffuses nutrients and waste byproducts, and enhances an organism's reducing activities. ZoBell also states that (*a*) many organisms fail to reduce nitrate in liquid or solid medium but do so in a semisolid and (*b*) some microaerophilic pathogens only reproduce in a semisolid medium (41). ZoBell (41) found nitrate reduction to be **highest** in both degree and percentage positive reactions when organisms were cultivated on semisolid medium and **lowest** on liquid medium. Hitchens (18) made two observations about the use of semisolid medium for cultivation: (*a*) many fastidious organisms reproduce that fail to do so in a liquid or solid medium, and (*b*) a semisolid medium retards oxygen diffusion, providing all degrees of aerobiosis in some area of the tube. Any basal medium is satisfactory that contains 0.1% potassium nitrate

(KNO_3) (41), supports growth (41), and provides conditions sufficiently anaerobic for the oxygen-sensitive enzyme nitratase (39).

An uninoculated control tube should be incubated and tested for nitrate reduction in conjunction with inoculated tubes, and a comparison should be made before interpreting results (12).

V. REAGENTS EMPLOYED

A. **Acetic acid, 5 N, 30%**

Glacial acetic acid, CH_3COOH	30.0 mL
Deionized water to bring to	1000.0 mL

(*Note:* Nitrate reagents were developed by a German chemist, Griese, in the 19th century (16).)

B. **Reagent A**: two choices (2, 10)
 1. α-Naphthylamine, 0.5%: α-Naphthylamine was determined to be carcinogenic; as a precaution, *N,N*-dimethyl-α-naphthylamine is preferred (1).
 2. **N,N-dimethyl-α-naphthylamine, 0.6%**; Eastman Chemical Company (see Appendix 11)
    a. Ingredients

N,N-Dimethyl-α-naphthylamine, $C_{10}H_7N(CH_3)_2$ (or α-naphthylamine, $C_{10}H_7NH_2$ 5.0 g)	6.0 g
Glacial acetic acid, 5 N, 30%	1000.0 mL

    b. Method of preparation
       (1) Dissolve either chemical in less than 1000 mL of 5 N acetic acid by **gently** heating.
       (2) Transfer solution to a 1-L volumetric flask and bring to 1000 mL with 5 N acetic acid.
       (3) Filter solution through washed absorbent cotton.
       (4) Store in glass-stoppered brown bottle (1).
       (5) Label correctly.

C. **Reagent B: sulfanilic acid, 0.8%** (2, 10); dry crystalline chemical, Sigma-Aldrich (see Appendix 11)
 1. Ingredients

Sulfanilic acid (*p*-aminobenzene sulfonic acid), $H_2NC_6H_4SO_3H \cdot H_2O$	8.0 g
Glacial acetic acid, 5 N, 30%	1000.0 mL

 2. Method of preparation
    a. Dissolve sulfanilic acid in less than 1000 mL of 5 N acetic acid.
    b. Transfer solution to a 1-L volumetric flask and bring to 1000 mL with 5 N acetic acid.
    c. Store in glass-stoppered bottle (2).
    d. Label correctly.

D. **Nessler's reagent** (10)
 1. Dissolve 5.0 g of potassium iodide (KI) in 5.0 mL deionized water; water **must** be ammonia (NH_3) free.
 2. Add cold **saturated** mercuric chloride ($HgCl_2$) solution until a slight precipitate remains after shaking.
 3. Add 40 mL of 9 N sodium hydroxide (NaOH) (see Appendix 6 for preparation).
 4. Dilute with deionized water to 100 mL.
 5. Allow solution to stand 24 h **before** use. A slight precipitate will settle to the bottom; **do not** disturb sediment when using reagent.
 6. Store in a paraffin-lined glass bottle or a dark brown bottle; avoid exposure to light.
 7. Label correctly.

E. Method of use

1. First, check for gas production in Durham tube or agar butt.
   a. If **gas is present** and the organism is a **nonfermenter**, result is positive for **denitrification**.
   b. If **gas is present** and the organism is a **fermenter, proceed to phase 1**.
   c. If there is no gas, **proceed to phase 1**.
2. **Phase 1**
   a. To an incubated nitrate culture, directly add reagents; two procedures
      (1) Preferred
         (a) **Immediately before testing,** mix equal parts of reagents A and B (26).
         (b) Add approximately 10 drops of mixture to culture.
      (2) Alternative
         (a) Reagent A: 5 drops
         (b) Reagent B: 5 drops
         (c) Shake culture **gently** to mix reagents.
   b. A positive result (red color) within 1–2 min denotes a **completed test**; discard tube(s).
   c. If result is **negative** (no color development), **proceed to phase 2**.
3. **Phase 2: zinc reduction method**
   a. To the tube containing reagents A and B, directly add a pinch (approximately 20 mg on tip of an applicator stick) of zinc dust (Zn) (9, 10).
   b. Zinc dust **must** be nitrate-nitrite free (9).
   c. Observe for final interpretation. Color occurs within 5–10 min.
E. Quality control: reagents A and B **must** both be tested with known positive and negative cultures before being put into general use.
F. Store reagent A in refrigerator (4°C) when not in use; store reagent B at room temperature. These reagents are usually stable for at least 3 months (2). Periodically, however, they should be given a quality control check and discarded when demonstrating a negative or weak reaction with a known positive organism.
G. Chemistry of reagents actions: reduction of nitrate (NO_3^-) to nitrite (NO_2^-) is denoted by color development when nitrite reacts with the two reagents: sulfanilic acid and dimethyl-α-naphthylamine (or α-naphthylamine). The resulting color reaction is due to formation of a diazonium compound (28), p-sulfobenzene-azo-α-naphthylamine (37).

Phase 1 reaction (13, 37)

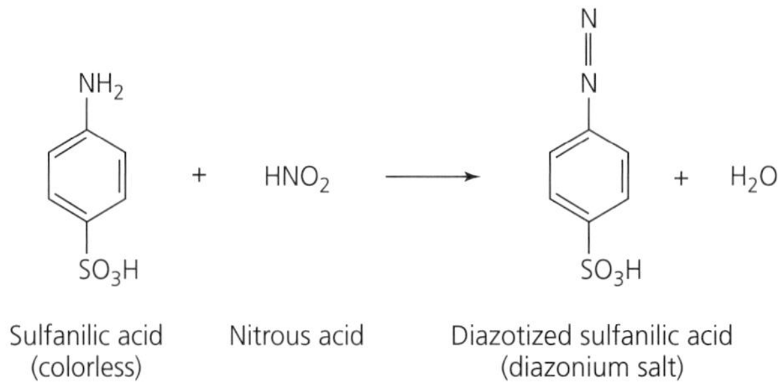

Sulfanilic acid (colorless) + Nitrous acid (HNO_2) → Diazotized sulfanilic acid (diazonium salt) + H_2O

(continued)

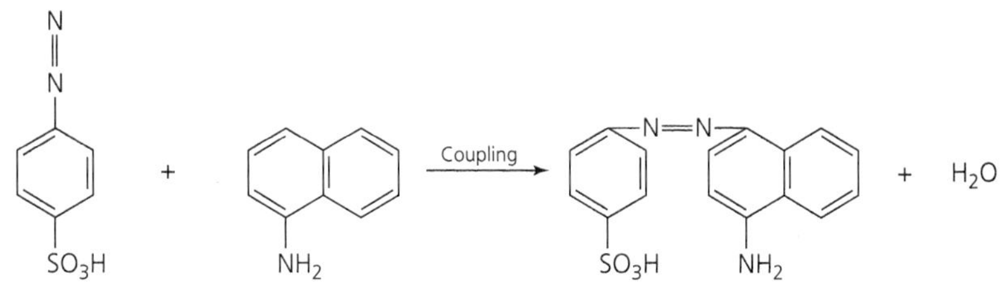

Diazotized sulfanilic acid (colorless) + **α-Naphthylamine** (colorless) →[Coupling] **p-Sulfobenzene-azo-α-naphthylamine** (red azo dye) (water soluble) + H_2O

The –N=N–azo group linkage yields a colored compound (28) via a nitroso reaction (7). Diazonium dye compounds are formed by coupling through an azo link of an aromatic amine with a phenolic type compound usually at the *para* position to a hydroxyl (OH) or amino group (NH_2) (2, 28). In this case coupling occurs *para* to an amino group.

Phase 2 reaction (27)

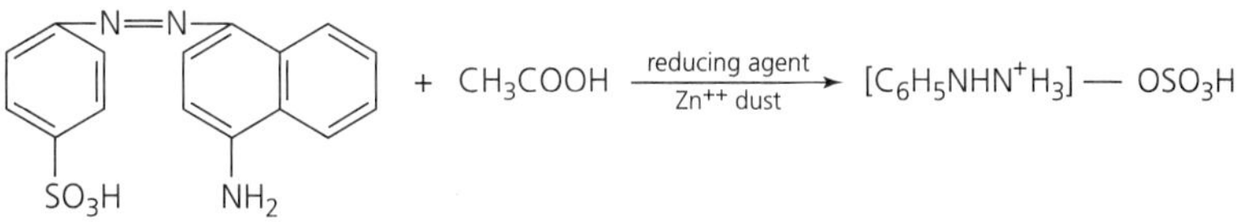

p-Sulfobenzene-azo-α-naphthylamine (Diazonium colored compound) + CH_3COOH (Acetic acid) →[reducing agent / Zn^{++} dust] $[C_6H_5NHN^+H_3]$ — OSO_3H **Arylhydrazine** (colored compound)

Reduction of the diazonium salt by the reducing agent zinc dust in the presence of acetic acid produces a colored compound, arylhydrazine (27). The sulfanilic acid-α-naphthylamine nitrate procedure developed by Conn (8) often exhibits fading or disappearance of color in a positive result (37). Fading is denoted by a brownish yellow color (39). Wallace and Neave (37) found this color instability to be correlated with production of hydrogen sulfide (H_2S), determined by the lead acetate strip procedure, which is quite sensitive. They stated that maximum color development stops in organisms able to reduce nitrate and at the same time produce H_2S, probably because part of the nitrous acid (HNO_2) molecule is destroyed. However, H_2S production does not cause the fading color directly (37). H_2S production is eliminated by using cysteine-free peptone to prepare the medium (36). Cysteine contains –SH (sulfide) bonds and removing them from the medium eliminates H_2S formation.

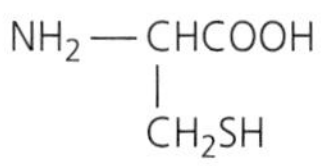

$$NH_2-CHCOOH$$
$$|$$
$$CH_2SH$$

Cysteine

Wallace and Neave (37) also noted that fading occurs more readily with a strong nitrate-positive organism when a single drop of each reagent gave a positive reaction. Increasing the amounts of each reagent kept the color stable. Nitrite (NO_2^-) concentration increases when H_2S is formed, which completely destroys the color reaction. This excess nitrous acid directly destroys the color by acting on the *p*-amino group of the diazonium salt and causing a breakdown to a hydroxyazo derivative (37).

354 Biochemical Tests for Identification of Medical Bacteria

Due to problems that may occur, Wallace and Neave (37) recommend substituting dimethyl-α-naphthylamine for the standard α-naphthylamine in the coupling reaction for color development. Dimethyl-α-naphthylamine **does not fade,** nor is it destroyed in the presence of an increased concentration of nitrite (NO_2) since the amino group is protected (37). However, with an increased NO_2^- concentration, this colored compound may precipitate out, but a positive test will still give a red color (37). A low concentration of NO_2 causes the color development to form at a slower rate (37).

Both α-naphthylamine and dimethyl-α-naphthylamine are sensitive to 1 part nitrite nitrogen in 100 million parts of solution (37).

VI. QUALITY CONTROL ORGANISMS

A. Positive (+)

    Escherichia coli   ATCC 11775
    Pseudomonas aeruginosa   ATCC 10145
    NO_3+/Gas+

B. Negative (−)

    Acinetobacter lwoffii   ATCC 15309
    NO_3-/Gas−
    Uninoculated

VII. RESULTS

> See Figure 30.1 (Appendix 1) for colored photographic results

VIII. INTERPRETATION (10, 41)

(*Note:* Add nitrate reagent **before** attempting an interpretation.)

A. **First check for gas production**
  1. Positive (G)
     a. Gas bubbles in Durham tube, at surface, or throughout semisolid medium
     b. A **single** bubble is significant; record as gas production.
     c. If test organism is a **nonfermenter**
        (1) **Test completed;** discard tubes
        (2) Report **denitrification.**
        (3) Production of N_2, N_2O, or nongaseous breakdown products other than NO_2
     d. If test organism is a **fermenter** (e.g., *Enterobacteriaceae*)
        (1) Gas is hydrogen so **must** test with nitrate reagents.
        (2) **Proceed to phase 1.**
  2. **Negative (NG):** no gas; **proceed to phase 1.**
B. **Phase 1**
  1. Positive result (+)
     a. Pink to a deep red color within 1–2 min
     b. Nitrate (NO_3^-) **reduced** to nitrite (NO_2^-) by organism
     c. Test completed
  2. Negative result (−)
     a. No color development

b. Nitrite (NO_2^-) **not present**
c. **Proceed to phase 2** to test for presence of unreduced nitrate (NO_3-).
C. **Phase 2: Zinc reduction test**
  1. Positive result
     a. No color development
     b. Absence of nitrite (NO_2^-) in the medium
     c. Organism **reduced** nitrate (NO_3^-) to nitrite (NO_2^-) and then further reduced nitrite to nongaseous products; denitrification (N_2). Test for ammonia (NH_3) by adding a few drops of Nessler's reagent; positive result, a deep orange color (14)
  2. Negative result
     a. Pink to deep red within 5–10 min
     b. Confirms negative result of phase 1
     c. Nitrate present; **not reduced** by organism
     d. Zinc reduced nitrate (NO_3^-) to nitrite (NO_2^-).

IX. NITRATE REDUCTION TESTS FOR *MYCOBACTERIUM* SPP.

(*Note:* Certain mycobacteria can reduce nitrate via the enzyme nitroreductase. Nitrate reaction is key test in the identification of M. tuberculosis, M. kansasii, M. fortuitum, and M. szulgai (Table 30.2).)

Table 30.2. Some *Mycobacterium* spp.: Nitrate Reduction Results

Organism	Runyon Group	Nitrate Reduction
M. flavescens	I. Photochromogen	+
M. fortuitum	IV. Rapid growers	+
M. kansasii	I. Photochromogen	+
M. szulgai	I. Photochromogen, 25°C	+
	II. Scotochromogen, 37°C	+
M. thermoresistible	II. Scotochromogen	+
M. triviale	III. Nonphotochromogen	+
M. tuberculosis	Slow grower	+
M. africanum	Slow grower	V
M. terrae complex	III. Nonphotochromogen	V
M. asiaticum	I. Photochromogen	−
M. avium complex	III. Nonphotochromogen	−
M. celatum	II. Scotochromogen	−
M. chelonae	IV. Rapid growers	−
M. gastri	III. Nonphotochromogen	−
M. genavense	III. Nonphotochromogen	−
M. gordonae	II. Scotochromogen	−
M. haemophilum	III. Nonphotochromogen	−
M. malmoense	III. Nonphotochromogen	−
M. mariunum	I. Photochromogen	−
M. shimoidei	III. Scotochromogen	−
M. simiae	I. Photochromogen	−
M. ulcerans	III. Scotochromogens	−
M. xenopi	III. Nonphotochromogen	−

Data from reference 20.

A. **Commercial nitrite test strips** (15)
  1. Manufacturers: Difco, Bacto-nitrite strips
  2. Procedure; modified Kilburn nitrite procedure (32); used primarily for *Mycobacterium* identification, but may be used with other organisms

a. To a **sterile** screw-cap tube (13 × 100 mm), add 0.5 mL **sterile** distilled water.
b. Specimens
   (1) *Mycobacterium* spp.
      (a) 3- to 4-week-old specimen cultured on Lowenstein-Jensen medium or a co-agulated egg medium
      (b) Rapid growers can be tested within 2 weeks.
      (c) Slow growers can be tested after 3–4 weeks of luxuriant growth (15).
   (2) Other genera
      (a) Enteric organisms: growth from triple sugar iron agar (TSI)
      (b) Other organisms: tryptic soy agar (TSA)
      (c) With **sterile** forceps, insert a nitrite test strip according to manufacturer's directions. The strip should touch only the fluid at the bottom, **not the sides**, and remain in an upright position.
         1. In distal end (marked by arrow) buffered sodium nitrate ($NaNO_3$)
         2. A and B reagents in upper portion of strip
         3. Strip stable 1 year refrigerated (2–8°C)
d. Inoculum: enough growth to form a heavy suspension around distal end of strip; **avoid wetting upper portion.**
e. Incubation: set up uninoculated control (distilled water and strip **only**) along with strong-positive, weakly positive, and negative *Mycobacterium* spp. (20) (see TB Nitrate Reduction Broth for Mycobacteria).
f. Incubation
   (1) Specimen/controls: screw cap down tightly, incubate in water bath, 35°C, 2 h, with periodic **gentle** shaking in a tilting motion.
   (2) At the end of the 2 h, **gently** rotate tube several times to wet the entire strip.
   (3) At the end of 2 h, place tube in a slanted position 10 min to allow liquid to cover the entire strip; this permits reagents in upper portion of strip to react.
g. Results
   (1) Positive (+): **any** blue color at top portion of strip; organism produced nitroreductase. Color appears on paper strip, **not in liquid.**
   (2) Negative (−): no color change; lack of nitroreductase.

Commercial strips yield acceptable results only with strong nitrate-positive mycobacteria such as *M. tuberculosis*. *M. tuberculosis* control tube **must be strongly positive** or results are **unreliable** (15). If either paper strip is negative or positive control tube is **not** strongly positive, chemical procedure (broth) **must** be performed with strong and weakly positive controls (15).

B. **TB nitrate reduction broth for mycobacteria** (35)
   1. Specimen: emulsify two large clumps of a 4 week-old *Mycobacterium* culture in saline to milky turbidity.
   2. Substrate: 0.01 M in M/45 phosphate buffer (0.02 M, pH 7.0)
      a. Ingredients; pH 7.0

Sodium nitrate, $NaNO_3$	0.8 g
Potassium phosphate, monobasic, KH_2PO_4	1.17 g
Sodium phosphate, dibasic, Na_2HPO_4	1.93 g
Deionized water to bring to	999.0 mL

      b. Sterilization: autoclave, 121°C, 15 lb, 15 min
      c. Dispense: aliquots of 2.0 mL in **sterile** screw-cap tubes (13 × 100 mm)
      d. Storage: refrigerator (2–8°C); shelf life, 1–2 months
   3. Reagents
      a. 0.2% Sulfanilimide: 0.1 g in 50 mL deionized water

(1) May be necessary to warm to 50°C to put into solution
(2) Store in brown glass bottle (2–8°C) away from direct light; shelf life, 1 month
b. 0.1% N-(1-naphthyl)ethylenediamine dihydrochloride ($C_{10}H_7NHCH_2CH_2NH_2 \cdot 2HCl$)
(1) 0.05 g in 50 mL deionized water
(2) Store in brown glass bottle (2–8°C) away from direct light; shelf life, 1 month
c. Hydrochloric acid, HCl, concentrated; 1:2 dilution with deionized water. **Always** add concentrated acid to water; **never** water to acid, as splattering may occur resulting in burns to the skin or eyes. **Use Pro pipette** to measure HCl.
4. Method of use
a. **Sterile** screw-cap tube (13 × 100 mm)
(1) Emulsify 1 loopful of *Mycobacterium* culture to be tested (first brought to room temperature, 22–25°C).
(2) Add 2.0 ml of TB buffered broth solution to test suspension and shake **gently.**
5. Incubation: 35°C, 2 h
6. Add reagents in the following order
a. 1 drop concentrated HCl to acidify culture; shake **gently**
b. 2 drops 0.2% sulfanilamide
c. 2 drops 0.1% N-(1-naphthyl)ethylenediamine dihydrochloride
7. Quality control organisms
a. Positive (+)

Mycobacterium tuberculosis	ATCC 25618 (H37R), strongly positive
Mycobacterium kansasii	ATCC 12478, weakly positive

b. Negative(−)

Mycobacterium avium	ATCC 25291
Uninoculated	

8. Results
a. Positive (+): red or pink color
b. If no color change; confirm negative results by adding a small amount of zinc dust. Pink to red color: nitrate reduced. Ability of mycobacteria to reduce nitrate is influenced by age of colonies, temperature, pH, and enzyme inhibitors (15).

X. NITRATE MEDIUM FOR *NEISSERIA* SPP.

A. Purpose: identification of nonpathogenic *Neisseria* spp.; if inability to grow on selective media, if clinically significant, or if isolated in pure culture (20)
B. Media: tryptic soy broth (TSB) or heart infusion broth (HIB) with 0.1% (w/v) potassium nitrate (KNO_3) and 0.01% (w/v) potassium nitrite (KNO_2) (21, 22)
C. Results: see Table 30.3

Table 30.3. Key Reactions in Identifying Most Frequently Isolated Nonpathogenic *Neisseria* spp.

Organism	NO$_3$	NO$_2$	Polysaccharide from sucrose	Fructose	Sucrose
N. subflava					
biovar *subflava*	−	+	−	−	−
biovar *flava*	−	+	−	+	−
biovar *perflava*	−	+	+	+	+
N. sicca	−	+	+	+	+
N. mucosa	+	+	+	+	+

Data from reference 20.

XI. DISK METHOD FOR ANAEROBES

A. Procedure of Wideman, Citronbaum, and Sutter (38)
B. Disks impregnated with 6-mg solution of potassium nitrate (KNO$_3$) in aqueous 0.1% sodium molybdate (Na$_2$MoO$_4$)
C. Determines nitrate reductase production in anaerobes
D. Incubation: 48 h
E. Agreement with conventional indole-nitrate medium, 89%

XII. RAPID TESTS

A. **Rapid procedure of Blazevic, Koepcke, and Matsen (5), and Schreckenberger and Blazevic (33)**
   1. Inoculate 0.5 mL of nitrate broth **heavily**.
   2. Incubation: water bath 35°C, 2 h
   3. Add 1 drop each of reagents A and B **directly** to tube and shake.
   4. Interpretation same as standard test (see Section VIII)
B. **Spot test on standard procedure broths**
   1. Transfer 0.5 mL of incubated broth(s) (see Sections IV–VIII) to spot plate (containing wells/depressions) or small test tubes.
   2. Add 1 drop each of reagents A and B.
      a. Performed during early growth stage
      b. Observe for **tentative** results.
      c. Aliquot of broth culture leaves enough growth medium for later testing by standard procedure if spot test is negative.
C. **Nitrate disks/tablets**
   1. Tablets
      a. Manufacturer: Key Scientific (see Appendix 11)
      b. Reagent tablets; rehydrate to make nitrate A and B reagents.
         (1) 1 drop nitrate reagent A (sulfanilic acid)
         (2) 1 drop reagent B (1,6-Cleve's acid, 1-naphthalamine-6-sulfonic acid)
      c. Media; two choices
         (1) Standard nitrate agar/broth. If this medium used, add a few drops of 5 N acetic acid to broth **before** adding nitrate reagents to compensate for any alkaline products.
         (2) FMN medium
   2. **Disks** (see Appendix 11)
      a. Key Scientific Company: performed on plate or tubed media
      b. BBL: Nitrate Reductase Minitek Discs
      c. Positive (+): pink to red color; nitrate reduced to nitrite. If no color, add zinc dust on disk to confirm a negative result.

XIII. FLUORESCENCE-DENITRIFICATION (FN) MEDIUM

A. Purpose: identification of pseudomonads and other nonfermenting bacilli
B. Principle
   1. Ability to produce fluorescein pigment
   2. Reduce nitrate to nitrite or nitrite completely to nitrogen gas
C. Media; two choices
   1. **Fluorescence denitrification (FN) medium** (20)
      a. Ingredients, pH 7.2

Peptone peptone no. 3, Difco	1.0 g
Magnesium sulfate, $MgSO_4 \cdot 7H_2O$	0.15 g
Dipotassium hydrogen phosphate, K_2HPO_4	0.15 g
Potassium nitrate, KNO_3	0.2 g
Sodium nitrite, $NaNO_2$	0.05 g
Agar	1.5 g
Deionized water	100.0 mL

      b. Method of preparation
         (1) Suspend all ingredients **except** magnesium sulfate in deionized water.
         (2) Dissolve magnesium sulfate in a small amount of deionized water **before** adding to agar medium; this avoids formation of insoluble precipitate.
   2. **Fluorescent lactose nitrate (FLN) medium**
      a. To FN medium add
         (1) Lactose, 2.0 g to aid in identification of lactose fermenters
         (2) Phenol red, 0.002 g; pH indicator
   3. **Nitrate/nitrite reduction medium**

Heart infusion broth	25.0 g
Potassium nitrate, KNO_3	2.0 g
Deionized water	1000.0 mL

   4. Dispense (any of the 3 media): 4.0 mL FN medium in screw-cap tubes (13 × 100 mm); permit to solidify to give a "deep" and a slant of equal length
   5. Inoculum: **heavy** suspension; stab deeply and streak slant
   6. Incubation: 35°C, 24–48 h
   7. Quality control organisms
      a. Fluorescence positive/denitrification positive: *Pseudomonas aeruginosa* ATCC 10145
      b. Fluorescence negative
         (1) Denitrification positive: *Pseudomonas stutzeri* ATCC 17588
         (2) Denitrification negative: *Escherichia coli* ATCC 11775
   8. Results
      a. **Fluorescence positive**
         (1) Ultraviolet light source (Wood's lamp)
         (2) Bright yellow-green glow
      b. Gas: gas bubbles in deep of medium
      c. FLN medium: lactose fermentation, acid production: yellow slant
      d. Broth medium: gas bubble in upper portion of inverted Durham insert: nitrogen gas formation

Fluorescent colonies are **not** detected on ordinary isolation media such as blood agar (BA) and MacConkey's (MAC); require media with cationic salts that act as activators or coactivators to intensify luminescence. Sellers medium may be substituted for FN or FLN for determination of fluorescence and denitrification.

XIV. PRECAUTIONS

A. **Standard nitrate reduction tests**
1. When performing the nitrate reduction test using α-naphthylamine, the color produced in a positive reaction may fade quickly (37). Interpret results immediately, particularly when performing a number of determinations. Wallace and Neave (37) also noted that fading occurred more readily with strongly nitrate-positive organisms when a single drop of each reagent gave a positive reaction. Increasing the amounts of each reagent kept the color stable. Nitrite (NO_2^-) concentration is increased when H_2S is formed, which completely destroys the color reaction. These authors recommended substituting dimethyl-α-naphthylamine in the coupling reaction for color development; this compound neither fades nor is destroyed in the presence of increased nitrite concentration, since the amino group is protected. With increased NO_2 concentration, this colored compound may precipitate, but a positive result is still red. A low concentration of NO_2 causes color to develop more slowly. Both α-naphthalamine and dimethyl-α-naphthylamine are sensitive to 1 part nitrogen in 100 million parts of solution (37).
2. Eliminate fading or destruction of color development by H_2S-producing organisms by using a sulfur-free peptone medium (37).
3. A strongly nitrate-positive reducing organism may exhibit a brown precipitate immediately after addition of the reagents. This is due to the effect of excess nitrite upon the *p*-amino group of the azo dye and may be reduced by using dimethyl-α-naphthylamine instead of α-naphthylamine (4).
4. The nitrate test is very sensitive, and an **uninoculated** nitrate tube **should be** tested with reagents to ensure that the medium is nitrite free (31, 37).
5. Some organisms reduce nitrate to nitrite but destroy the nitrite as fast as it is formed, yielding a false-negative result (41). This nitrite destruction is evident in quite a few bacteria, particularly some *Salmonella* and *Pseudomonas* spp. and *Brucella suis* (41). ZoBell and Meyer (42) tested 400 *Brucella* cultures and found that all reduced nitrates.
6. A positive zinc reduction result (41) indicates that nitrate was reduced to nitrite and then further reduced. There is no evidence of nitrite accumulation. However, the nitrate, on reduction, may have been assimilated into the bacterial cell or have been converted directly to cell nitrogen but not reduced (8, 38, 41).
7. ZoBell (41) stated that some organisms can destroy the 0.01% KNO_3 in the medium after a 2-day incubation period.
8. Conn (8) stated that in some instances nitrate may only be partially reduced or an organism may temporarily lose its ability to reduce nitrate.
9. In **all cultures** where nitrite is absent, when using α-naphthylamine (or dimethyl-α-naphthylamine) and sulfanilic acid reagents, **add zinc dust** directly to tube **before** making a final interpretation.
10. α-Naphthylamine was determined to be carcinogenic (29); therefore, substitution of *N*,*N*-dimethyl-α-naphthylamine is recommended along with such safety precautions as avoiding aerosols, mouth pipetting, and contact with skin (27).
11. When adding zinc, **do not** use an excess; if too much Zn is added, the large amount of hydrogen gas produced may reduce the nitrite (formed from unreduced nitrate) to ammonia (NH_3), which could give a false-negative result (no color) or just a fleeting color reaction (31).
12. Test organism(s) must grow enough to reduce nitrate **before** reagents are added; 48 h should suffice (4).
13. Glassware or reagent contaminated with nitrous oxide may give a false-positive result; avoid this possibility by testing an uninoculated control tube for a negative reaction (4).
14. Both α-naphthalamine and sulfanilic acid are relatively unstable; perform quality con-

trol tests frequently. The diazonium compound that forms from the reduced nitrate is also relatively unstable, and color tends to fade; interpretations should be made soon after addition of reagents.
15. Any basal medium is satisfactory that contains 0.1% potassium nitrate (KNO_3) (42).
16. To prevent delay in initiating growth and the medium reaction, the inoculum should **not** be taken from a liquid or broth suspension of the organism.
17. If a precipitate forms in sulfanilamide reagent, discard it. Discard naphthylenediamine reagent if color changes; it should be yellow.
18. Occasionally colors may be pale and difficult to interpret; alleviate this problem by preparing color standards for comparisons.

B. *Mycobacterium* testing
1. Care **must** be taken **not to shake** tubes too vigorously after nitrite strips have been added; reaction in various degrees may take place in middle portion of the strip if it becomes wet, and the reaction may **not** occur later at the top of the strip (32).
2. No single test suffices for identification of mycobacteria; a group of standard tests are necessary.
3. Commercial strips yield acceptable results only with strongly nitrate-positive mycobacteria such as *M. tuberculosis*. The *M. tuberculosis* control tube **must be strongly positive** or results are **unreliable** (15). If either the paper strip is negative or the positive control tube is **not** strongly positive, chemical procedure (broth) **must** be performed using strong and weakly positive controls (15).
4. If there is brown discoloration at the distal end of the nitrate test strip, discard it; this indicates deterioration of the reagent (12).

C. **Fluorescence-denitrification**: fluorescent colonies are not detected on ordinary isolation media such as blood agar (BA) and MacConkey's (MAC); they require media with cationic salts that act as activators or coactivators to intensify luminescence.

REFERENCES

1. American Public Health Association, Committee on Laboratory Standards and Practices. Bacterial nitrate reduction test: Suggestions for use of alternate (noncarcinogenic) reagents. Am Soc Microbiol News 1975;41:225–227.
2. Bachmann B, Weaver RH. Rapid microtechnics for identification of cultures. V. Reduction of nitrates to nitrites. Am J Clin Pathol 1951;21(2): 195–196.
3. Barrett SJ, Schlater LK, Montall RJ, Sneath PHA. A new species of *Neisseria* from iguanid lizards, *Neisseria iguanae* sp. nov. Lett Appl Microbiol 1994;18:200–202.
4. Blazevic DJ, Ederer GM. Principles of Biochemical Tests in Diagnostic Microbiology. New York: John Wiley & Sons, 1975:79–82.
5. Blazevic DJ, Koepcke MH, Matsen JM. Incidence and identification of *Pseudomonas fluorescens* and *Pseudomonas putida* in the clinical laboratory. Appl Microbiol 1973;25(1):107–110.
6. Breed RS, Murray EGD, Smith NR. Bergey's Manual of Determinative Bacteriology, ed 7. Baltimore: Williams & Wilkins, 1957:336, 466–467.
7. Burrows W, Lewert RM, Rippon JW. Textbook of Microbiology. The Pathogenic Microorganisms, ed 19. Philadelphia: WB Saunders, 1968:15, 141.
8. Conn HJ. On the detection of nitrate reduction. J Bacteriol 1936;31:225–233.
9. Conn HJ, Harding HA, Kligler IJ, et al. Methods of pure culture study. Preliminary report of the committee on the chart for identification of bacterial species. J Bacteriol 1918;3(2):115–128.
10. Cowan ST. Cowan & Steel's Manual for the Identification of Medical Bacteria, ed 2. Cambridge: Cambridge University Press, 1974:38–39, 167.
11. Daubner I. Die Reduktion der Nitrate durch Bakterien der Familie *Enterobacteriaceae*. Arch Hyg Bakt (Berlin) 1962;146:147–150.
12. Difco Manual, ed 10. Detroit, Difco Laboratories, 1984:616–618.
13. Feigl F. Spot Tests in Organic Analysis, ed 7. New York: Elsevier, 1966:90–91.
14. Finegold SM, Baron EJ. Bailey and Scott's Diagnostic Microbiology, ed 7. St. Louis: CV Mosby, 1986:490.
15. Forbes BA, Sahn DF, Weissfeld AS. Bailey & Scott's Diagnostic Microbiology, ed 10. St. Louis: CV Mosby, 1998:738–739, 748.
16. Griess P: Uebereinige Azoverbindungen. Ber Deutsch Chem Gesellsch 1879;12:426.
17. Gunsalus IC, Stanier RY. The Bacteria, vol II. New York: Academic Press, 1961:375, 416–417, 452–453.

18. Hitchens AP. Advantages of culture mediums containing small percentages of agar. J Infect Dis 1921;29:390–407.
19. Holmes B, Costas M, On SLW, et al. *Neisseria weaverii* sp. nov. (formerly CDC group M-5) from dog bite wounds of humans. Int J Syst Bacteriol 1993;43:687–693.
20. Koneman EW, Allen SD, Janda WM, Color Atlas & Textbook of Diagnostic Microbiology, ed 5. Philadelphia: JB Lippincott, 1997:335, 519, 913, 916–917, 1335, 1366.
21. Knapp JS. Reduction of nitrite by *Neisseria gonorrhoeae*. Int J Syst Bacteriol 1984;34:376–377.
22. Knapp JS. Historical perspectives and identification of *Neisseria* and related species. Clin Microbiol Rev 1988;1:415–431.
23. Knapp JS. Laboratory methods for the detection and phenotypic characterization of *Neisseria gonorrhoeae* strains resistant to antimicrobial agents. Sex Transm Dis 1988;15:225–233.
24. Knapp JS, Hook EW III. Prevalence and persistence of *Neisseria cinerea* and other *Neisseria* spp. in adults. J Clin Microbiol 1988;26(5):896–900.
25. Mahler HR, Cordes EH. Biological Chemistry, New York: Harper & Row, 1966:655–656.
26. Murray PR, Baron EJ, Pfaller MA, Manual of Clinical Microbiology, ed 6. Washington, DC: American Society for Microbiology, 1995:335, 422.
27. Noller CR. Chemistry of Organic Compounds, ed 3. Philadelphia: WB Saunders, 1965:544–545, 743.
28. Nussenbaum S. Organic Chemistry. Boston, Allyn & Bacon, 1963:441–445.
29. Occupational Safety and Health Administration (OSHA), Department of Labor. Federal Register 1974;39(20).
30. Pelczar MJ Jr, Reid RD. Microbiology, ed 2. New York: McGraw-Hill, 1965:567.
31. Porres JM, Porter V. Rapid nitrate reduction test. Am J Med Technol 1974;40(6):257–259.
32. Quigley HJ Jr, Elston HR. Nitrite test strips for detection of nitrate reduction by mycobacteria. Am J Clin Pathol 1970;53(4):663–665.
33. Schreckenberger PC, Blazevic DJ. Rapid methods for biochemical testing of anaerobic bacteria. Appl Microbiol 1974;28(5):759–762.
34. Smith DT, Conant NF, Willett HP. Zinsser's Microbiology, ed 14. New York: Appleton-Century-Crofts, 1968:116–117.
35. Stanier RY, Doudoroff M, Adelberg EA. The Microbial World, ed 2. Englewood Cliffs, NJ: Prentice-Hall, 1963:271–272.
36. Virtanen S. A study of nitrate reduction by mycobacteria. The use of the nitrate reduction test in the identification of mycobacteria. Acta Tuberc Scand (Suppl) 1960;48:1–119.
37. Wallace GI, Neave SL. The nitrite test as applied to bacterial cultures. J Bacteriol 1927;14(6):377–384.
38. Wideman PA, Citronbaum DM, Sutter VL. Simple disk technique for detection of nitrate reduction by anaerobic bacteria. J Clin Microbiol 1977;5(3):315–319.
39. Wilson G, Miles A, Parker MT, eds. Topley and Wilson's Principles of Bacteriology, Virology, and Immunology, ed 7. Baltimore: Williams & Wilkins, 1983:8.
40. Yu P, Birk RJ, Washington JA II. Evaluation of a reagent-impregnated strip for detection of nitrate reduction by bacterial isolates. Am J Clin Pathol 1969;52(6):791–793.
41. ZoBell CE. Factors influencing the reduction of nitrates and nitrites by bacteria in semisolid media. J Bacteriol 1932;24:273–281.
42. ZoBell CE, Meyer KF. Reduction of nitrates and nitrites by representatives of the *Brucella* group. Proc Soc Exp Biol Med 1932;29(2):116–118.

31 Optochin Disk Test

I. PRINCIPLE

To test an organism's susceptibility to the chemical optochin. Optochin susceptibility tests the fragility of the bacterial cell membrane.

II. PURPOSE

(Also see Chapter 44)

The optochin disk is used specifically to differentiate between *Streptococcus pneumoniae* (sensitive, S, Sens) and other α-*Streptococcus* (viridans) species (resistant, R); a phenotypic method.

III. BIOCHEMISTRY INVOLVED

Optochin is a chemical, ethylhydrocupreine hydrochloride (3). Ethylhydrocupreine, the base for the optochin disk (13), is insoluble in water (4, 17). However, ethylhydrocupreine hydrochloride is completely soluble in water (4). Optochin is a derivative of the alkaloid hydroquinine (13), which is prepared by hydrogenation, demethylation, and ethylation of quinine (17).

Ethylhydrocupreine hydrochloride (optochin)

Each filter paper disk is impregnated with approximately 0.02 mL of a 1:4000 aqueous dilution of the chemical (4, 7) and dried at 37°C (4). This is the optimal concentration of optochin for *S. pneumoniae* differentiation (3). Optochin has approximately 95% specific sensitivity for *S. pneumoniae* (3, 11, 18) and is bacteriostatic at a 1:500,000 to 1:100,000 concentration (13). The other α-*Streptococcus* spp. require a 1:5000 (or greater) concentration to inhibit growth (11, 16). *S. pneumoniae* cells lyse because of changes in surface tension, and a zone of inhibition is produced by contact with optochin (11).

IV. PROCEDURE

A. Inoculation of organism to be tested
  1. **Pure** colony
  2. Medium: 5% blood agar plate
     a. Recommended: sheep blood
     b. Alternative: outdated human blood (blood bank). Blood agar plate medium **must** be

used for optochin testing since all *Streptococcus* spp. are fastidious and require additional enrichments for growth.
3. Method of inoculating for maximum growth; two choices
   a. Subculture to Trypticase soy broth (TSB); **single** colony
      (1) Incubation: 35°C, 18–24 h
      (2) Application of organism
         (a) **Sterile** swab
         (b) Swab **entire** blood agar plate; four directions.
   b. Direct inoculation
      (1) **Single** colony
      (2) Streak entire blood agar plate with an inoculating loop; four directions.
      (3) Four-direction streaking procedure. If several organisms are to be tested for optochin sensitivity, a single blood agar plate may be divided into four quadrants (pie plate) for four separate determinations.

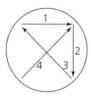

Mark a blood agar plate into four quadrants on the bottom half of the plate, which contains the medium. **Before inoculation,** label each pie area appropriately to avoid any mixup in interpreting results.

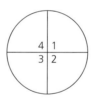

Do not attempt to use more than four disks per plate. The use of a pie plate still requires streaking for maximum growth.

B. Optochin disk (5 μg)
   1. Commercial products available; approximately 5 μg/disk
      a. Difco: Bacto-Differentiation discs, optochin (8)
      b. BBL: Taxo P discs (2)
   2. Storage: refrigerator (4–10°C); screw-cap bottles.

Bowers and Jeffries (4) state that optochin disks are stable for 9 months, either refrigerated (4°C) or stored at room temperature (25°C). However, it is recommended that they be kept refrigerated at all times when not in use. Periodically, optochin disks should be given a quality control check and removed from use when they demonstrate a negative or weak reaction with a known sensitive *S. pneumoniae* strain. If commercially prepared disks are not reacting properly, as evidenced by quality control, the entire lot may be returned to the company for replacement.

   3. Application of disks
      a. **Aseptically,** with alcohol-flamed forceps, remove an optochin disk and apply to the center of a streaked blood agar plate or pie area.
         (1) **Do not** place near edge of plate.

(2) **Gently** apply pressure to disk so that it adheres to the surface of the plate but does not press down into the medium.
b. A drop of **sterile** distilled water may be placed on the disk after application. Bowen et al. (3) showed that the zone of inhibition of a sensitive organism is 2–3 mm larger in diameter with wet disks than with dehydrated disks. The moisture causes optochin to diffuse into the medium faster.
c. Keep the top on the bottle of disks at all times when not in use.
C. Incubation
1. **Inverted plate** (lid down)
2. Candle jar; 3–5% increased CO_2 (10)
3. 35°C
4. 18–24 h

V. QUALITY CONTROL MICROORGANISMS

A. Sensitive (S, sen): *Streptococcus pneumoniae* ATCC 33400
B. Resistant (R): *Enterococcus faecalis* ATCC 19433

VI. RESULTS

> See Figures 31.1–31.3 (Appendix 1) for colored photographic results

VII. INTERPRETATION

(*Note:* Disk diameter and zones of inhibition **must** be measured **before** making an interpretation (11). **Measure from edge of disk.**)

A. Sensitive (S): presumptive identification of *S. pneumoniae*
  1. Growth inhibited around disk
     a. 6-mm disk (BBL): zone 14 mm or greater
     b. 10-mm disk (Difco): zone 16 mm or greater
     c. If zone is smaller, perform alternative procedures (e.g., bile solubility, serologic testing)
  2. Clear zone around disk
  3. Alpha (α) hemolysis
B. Resistant (R): other α-*Streptococcus* spp.
  1. Growth **not** inhibited around disk
  2. Growth up to and around disk

The size of the zone of inhibition exhibited by *S. pneumoniae* varies from 15 to 30 mm with a clear-cut margin (3, 10).

VIII. PRECAUTIONS

A. The terms *sensitive* or *resistant* **must** be used for interpretations of the optochin disk test. Abbreviations *S* and *R* are acceptable to denote results as long as your laboratory has given previous explanations to requesting physicians. Never use *positive* (+) or *negative* (−) to denote optochin results. A positive result does not explain sufficiently; it could mean inhibited growth or simply that the organism grew on blood agar but did not act with optochin.
B. The optochin test is used only to differentiate α-hemolytic *S. pneumoniae* from other α-

Streptococcus (viridans) spp. However, if in doubt as to the hemolytic pattern exhibited by a possible *Streptococcus* sp., set up an optochin test. α-*Streptococcus* spp. and *S. pneumoniae* are often difficult to differentiate by Gram morphology and colony morphology and thus **require** additional tests for differentiation (optochin and/or bile solubility tests). However, *S. pneumoniae* and all other *Streptococcus* spp., regardless of their hemolytic pattern, are catalase negative, and this determination should be made **before** performing an optochin test.

C. Bowen et al. (3) state there is no correlation between the size of the zones of inhibition exhibited by *S. pneumoniae* and their serologic types.

D. Cruickshank (7) notes that occasionally a few scattered optochin-resistant colonies of *S. pneumoniae* may be observed in a wide zone of inhibition. To ensure that you have a pure culture, subculture the resistant colonies onto a blood agar plate and determine the following: catalase reaction, Gram-stain morphology, and colony morphology. Then repeat the optochin test before making a final interpretation.

E. Cowan and Steel (6) state that occasionally an α-*Streptococcus* spp. may exhibit a very small zone (1–2 mm diameter) of inhibition. If zone of inhibition is smaller than 14 mm, alternative tests should be performed since some non-pneumo-viridans streptococci and aerococci may show small zones of inhibition (11).

Bowers and Jeffries (4) state that if the ethylhydrocupreine hydrochloride used for disks is less than a 1:8000 concentration, inexperienced microbiologists may overlook small zones of inhibition. For routine diagnostic use, a concentration of 1:4000 is used, which gives a wide zone of inhibition with *S. pneumoniae* to distinguish it from strains of bile-insoluble α-*Streptococcus* that may exhibit a slight zone of inhibition (5).

Ragsdale and Sanford (15) showed that *S. pneumoniae* may exhibit a **decrease** in the size of zone of optochin inhibition when plates are incubated under 5% CO_2. The mean diameter of zone inhibition was 21.9 mm on plates incubated in room air; under CO_2 (5%), the mean diameter was 16.3 mm. However, streptococci are fastidious organisms, and initial growth (metabolism) is greatly enhanced by incubation under at least 2–3% CO_2. A CO_2 incubator or candle jar may be used that replaces part of the nitrogen with CO_2.

Austrian and Collins (1) showed that 8% of *S. pneumoniae* strains require higher CO_2 tension than that supplied by the atmosphere for **initial** isolation on plate media. Martin and Niven (12) and Wright (19) showed that CO_2 enters the metabolic pathway to facilitate growth of *S. pneumoniae* via condensation of a one-carbon compound with a three-carbon compound, forming oxaloacetic acid, which in turn is aminated to aspartic acid. When oxaloacetic acid is absent, pneumococci require increased CO_2 for synthesis of aspartic acid (12). Pneumococci require either oleic acid or increased CO_2 tension for growth in casein hydrolyzate medium (12). Martin and Niven (12) showed that streptococci grown in a casein hydrolyzate medium lacking oleate but containing aspartic acid required CO_2 for growth. The increased CO_2 was necessary for aspartate synthesis (12). However, the same studies showed that when oleate and aspartic acid were both present, no aspartate synthesis occurred, since the aspartate in the medium was sufficient for growth. The mechanism is undefined; however, either oleic acid (oleate) or increased CO_2 is necessary for streptococcal growth (11).

F. Scant growth of an isolate makes accurate interpretation difficult. The minimal criterion for *S. pneumoniae* to be considered optochin sensitive is usually a 14- to 16-mm or greater zone of inhibition (measured from edge of disk). If the zone of inhibition is less than 14 mm, it is wise to do a bile solubility test for confirmation.

Ragsdale and Sanford (15) recommend **initial isolation** of *Streptococcus* spp. under 5% O_2, but incubation for optochin susceptibility in a room air incubator with **no** increased CO_2 tension. Then, if there is no growth on agar at room temperature, a bile solubility test should be performed (12). If incubation is performed under increased CO_2, Ragsdale and Sanford (15) recommend determining standard zone sizes.

Branson (5) recommends setting up optochin susceptibility tests on azide blood agar, since the zones of inhibition are more clearly defined.

G. Optochin-resistant *S. pneumoniae* isolates have been reported but rarely encountered (9, 14).

REFERENCES

1. Austrian R, Collins P. Importance of carbon dioxide in the isolation of pneumococci. J Bacteriol 1966;92(5):1281–1284.
2. BBL Manual of Products and Laboratory Procedures, ed 5. Cockeysville, MD: BBL Microbiology Systems, Division of Becton Dickinson and Company, 1988.
3. Bowen MK, Thiele LC, Stearman BD, Schaub IG. The optochin sensitivity test: A reliable method for identification of pneumococci. J Lab Clin Med 1957;49(4):641–642.
4. Bowers EF, Jeffries LR. Optochin in the identification of *Str. pneumoniae*. J Clin Pathol 1955;8(1):58–60.
5. Branson D. Methods in Clinical Bacteriology. Springfield IL: Charles C Thomas, 1972:39.
6. Cowan ST. Cowan & Steel's Manual for the Identification of Medical Bacteria, ed 2. Cambridge: Cambridge University Press, 1974:26–27.
7. Cruickshank R. Medical Microbiology, ed 11. London: Livingstone, 1968:166.
8. Difco Supplementary Literature. Detroit: Difco Laboratories, 1968:81.
9. Fenoll A, Martinez-Suarez JV, Munoz R, et al. Identification of atypical strains of *Streptococcus pneumoniae* by a specific DNA probe. Eur J Clin Microbiol Infect Dis 1990;9:396–401.
10. Forbes BA, Sahn DF, Weissfeld AS. Bailey & Scott's Diagnostic Microbiology, ed 10. St. Louis: CV Mosby, 1998:442.
11. Koneman EW, Allen SD, Janda WM, et al. Color Atlas & Textbook of Diagnostic Microbiology, ed 5. Philadelphia: JB Lippincott, 1997:609, 1359.
12. Martin WR, Niven CF Jr. Mode of CO_2 fixation by the minute streptococci. J Bacteriol 1960;79(2):295–298.
13. Moore HF. The action of ethylhydrocupreine (optochin) on type strains of pneumococci in vitro and in vivo, and on some other microorganisms in vitro. J Exp Med 1915;22(3):269–285.
14. Munoz R, Fenoll A, Vicioso D, Casal J. Optochin-resistant variants of *Streptococcus pneumoniae*. Diagn Microbiol Infect Dis 1989;13:63–66.
15. Ragsdale AR, Sanford JP. Interfering effect of incubation in carbon dioxide on the identification of pneumococci by optochin discs. Appl Microbiol 1971;22(5):854–855.
16. Smith DT, Conant NF, Willett HP. Zinsser's Microbiology, ed 14. New York: Appleton-Century-Crofts, 1968:728.
17. The Merck Index, ed 7. Rahway, NJ: Merck and Company, 1960:756.
18. Whitmore FC. Organic Chemistry. New York: Van Nostrand, 1937:943.
19. Wright DE. The metabolism of carbon dioxide by *Streptococcus bovis*. J Gen Microbiol 1960;22(3):713–725.

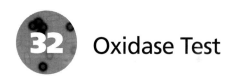

32 Oxidase Test

I. PRINCIPLE

To determine the presence of the oxidase enzymes

II. PURPOSE

(Also see Chapters 43–45)

A. The oxidase test, originally devised to identify all *Neisseria* spp., was later used to distinguish the *Pseudomonadaceae* from the oxidase-negative members of the *Enterobacteriaceae* (12, 30, 43).
B. Most Gram-positive bacteria are oxidase negative (42).
C. Among the *Enterobacteriaceae* **only** *Plesiomonas shigelloides* is oxidase positive.
D. To aid in differentiation between genera
   1. *Moraxella* (+) and *Neisseria* (+) from *Acinetobacter* (−)
   2. *Aeromonas* (+), *Plesiomonas shigelloides* (+), and *Vibrio* (V, variable, usually +) from other *Enterobacteriaceae* (−)
E. To aid in species differentiation among the Gram-negative nonenteric bacteria
   1. *Bacteroides distasonis* (+), *B. eggerthii* (+), and *B. ureolyticus* from other *Bacteroides* spp. (−) most frequently isolated
   2. *Bartonella felis* (+), *B. quintana* (+w), and *B. vinsonii* (+w) from *B. bacilliformis* (−), *B. elizabethae* (−), and *B. henselae* (−); most frequently isolated species (*B. quintana* and *B. vinsonii* are weakly positive with Kovacs' modification, negative by the routine method (47)).
   3. *Bordetella parapertussis* (+) from other *Bordetella* spp. (−)
   4. Most frequently isolated species: *Burkholderia gladioli* (−) and *B. mallei* (variable) from *B. cepacia* (+) and *B. pseudomallei* (+)
   5. Most frequently isolated species: *Capnocytophaga canimorsus* (+w) and *C. cynodegmi* (+) from *C. gingivalis* (−), *C. ochracea* (−), and *C. sputigena* (−)
   6. *Haemophilus aphrophilus* (−), *H. paragallinarum* (−), *H. parasuis* (−), and *H. segnis* (−) from other *Haemophilus* spp. (+)
   7. *Pseudomonas syringae* (−), *P. viridiflava* (−) from other *Pseudomonas* spp. (+) most frequently isolated
   8. *Vibrio gazogenes* (−) and *V. metschnikovii* (−) from other *Vibrio* spp. (+) most frequently isolated
F. To aid in identification of Gram-negative **nonenteric** bacteria:

Acidovorax spp. (+)
Actinobacillus spp. (V, usually +)
Aeromonas spp. (+)
Afipia spp. (+)
Agrobacterium spp. (V, usually +)
Alcaligenes spp. (+)
Brevundimonas spp. (+)
Brucella spp. (+)

Campylobacter spp. (+)
Cardiobacterium hominis (+)
Chromobacterium violaceum (V, usually + with Kovacs' reagent; violet pigment may interfere with reading. Oxidase-negative strains may be mistaken for enteric species, and oxidase-positive strains may be mistaken for *Aeromonas* and *Vibrio* species (41).)
Comamonas spp. (+)
Eikenella corrodens (+)
Flavobacterium spp. (+)
Helicobacter spp. (+)
Janthinobacterium lividum (+) (V, usually + by Kovacs'; violet pigment may interfere with interpretation.)
Kingella spp. (+) (*K. denitrificans* and *K. kingae* weakly positive with dimethyl reagent; positive with tetramethyl-*p*-phenylalanine reagent)
Methylobacterium spp. (+)
Moraxella spp. (+)
Morococcus cerebrosus (+)
Neisseria spp. (+) (oxidase test key for identification of *Neisseria* spp.)
Ochrobactrum spp. (+)
Oligella spp. (+)
Pasteurella spp. (+)
Psychrobacter spp. (+)
Ralstonia spp.
Roseomonas spp. (+)
Shewanella spp. (+)
Sphingomonas (V)
Suttonella indologenes (+)
Taylorella equigenitalis (+)
Weeksiella spp. (+)
Wolinella succinogenes (+)
Xanthobacter spp. (+)

III. BIOCHEMISTRY INVOLVED

The oxidase test is based on bacterial production of an intracellular oxidase enzyme. This oxidase reaction is due to a cytochrome oxidase system that activates oxidation of reduced cytochrome by molecular oxygen (43, 49), which in turn acts as an electron acceptor in the terminal stage of the electron transfer system (34, 43).

All aerobic bacteria obtain their energy by respiration, a process responsible for oxidation of various substrates. The respiratory chain is a sequence of enzymes and carriers responsible for transport of reducing equivalents from substrates to molecular oxygen (26). Molecular oxygen oxidizes a substrate via intervention by the electron transport system (16). Oxygen is the final hydrogen acceptor, producing either water or hydrogen peroxide from the hydrogen, depending upon the bacterial species and its enzyme system (22). Oxidases catalyze removal of hydrogen from a substrate but use only oxygen as a hydrogen acceptor (26).

$$AH_2 \text{ (Reduced)} \to A \text{ (Oxidized)}$$
$$\tfrac{1}{2}O_2 \xrightarrow{\text{Oxidase}} H_2O$$

(24)

The cytochrome system, usually present only in aerobic organisms (6), allows them to use oxygen as a final hydrogen acceptor to reduce molecular oxygen to hydrogen peroxide, the last link in the chain of aerobic respiration (8, 22). Steel (43) found that all oxidase-positive organisms he studied were either aerobic or facultatively anaerobic, except *Vibrio fetus* (now in genus *Campylobacter*), which has a microaerophilic oxygen requirement. Gordon and McLeod (24) state that a positive oxidase reaction is limited to organisms that can grow in the presence of oxygen and produce the enzyme catalase. Catalase degrades hydrogen peroxide (8) whose accumulation is toxic.

$$2 H_2O_2 \xrightarrow{catalase} 2 H_2O + O_2$$
Hydrogen peroxide

Obligate anaerobes lack oxidase activity; they cannot live in the presence of atmospheric oxygen and do not possess a cytochrome oxidase system (8, 13, 22, 43). Deibel and Evans (13) showed that *Lactobacillus* spp. lacked this enzyme activity.

The cytochrome oxidase system varies among bacterial species (38); some organisms possess only one oxidase while others may produce two or three (40, 43). Cytochromes other than terminal cytochrome oxidase are b → c_1 → c enzymes responsible for a positive oxidase test result; production of these two enzymes differs in various genera. *Neisseria* spp. were thought to produce indophenol oxidase, while cytochrome oxidase was produced by *Pseudomonas* spp. Spectrophotometric studies proved that Warburg's cytochrome oxidase and indophenol oxidase are the same (39). Gaby and Hadley (23) state that cytochrome oxidase has been referred to by many other names: Atmungsferment, cytochrome c oxidase, cytochrome a_3 oxidase, and cytochrome a oxidase. Castor and Chance (11) showed photochemically that four bacterial pigments act as terminal cytochrome oxidase respiratory enzymes: cytochrome a_1, cytochrome a_2, cytochrome a_3, and a carbon monoxide–binding pigment (CO-binding) designated cytochrome o. Two cytochromes (a and a_3) are combined in the same protein, and the complex is called cytochrome aa_3 (24). A mixture of cytochrome a and cytochrome a_3 is termed *cytochrome c oxidase* (25, 26). The cytochromes are respiratory pigments containing iron-porphyrin compounds (43). Cytochrome aa_3 contains two molecules of heme A, each having one Fe (iron) atom that swings back and forth between Fe^{3+} (ferric) and Fe^{2+} (ferrous) during oxidation and reduction, and two atoms of Cu^{2+} (copper) associated with cytochrome oxidase activity and reaction of electrons with molecular oxygen (26).

$$\text{Cytochrome-Fe}^{+++} + \bar{e} \rightleftharpoons \text{Cytochrome-Fe}^{++}$$

(oxidized-removal of electrons)   (reduced-gain of electrons)

(ferric)   (ferrous)

All *Pseudomonas* and *Neisseria* spp. produce an oxidase enzyme which, in the presence of atmospheric oxygen, cytochrome c, and an oxidase reagent, oxidize the reagent to a colored compound, indophenol (4, 23). Electrons from cytochrome c are taken up by oxidized cytochrome oxidase; which passes them to an oxygen molecule (45). Free oxygen is necessary for indirect regeneration of oxidized cytochrome c (45). The test really determines the presence of cytochrome c and results are positive only for bacteria containing cytochrome c as a respiratory enzyme (6).

$$2 \text{ Reduced cytochrome c} + 2H^+ + \tfrac{1}{2} O_2 \xrightarrow{\text{cytochrome oxidase}} 2 \text{ Oxidized cytochrome c} + H_2O$$

A positive oxidase result consists of a series of reactions, with an autooxidizable component of the cytochrome system as the final catalyst (25). Artificial substrates may be substituted for natural electron acceptors anywhere within the electron transport chain where they reduce the cytochrome c–cytochrome oxidase system (9, 25). The various oxidase test reagent dyes are artificial electron acceptors; p-phenylenediamine reagent and indophenol are both acceptors and donors of electrons (9). These artificial substrates are either colorless or colored, depending on their state (9); the final oxidase reaction yields a colored product.

IV. REAGENTS EMPLOYED

A. Oxidase reagents, several choices (Eastman Chemical Co.; see Appendix 11)
  1. **Kovacs' reagent**: 1% (30), 0.5% (5) tetramethyl-p-phenylenediamine dihydrochloride (TPD) (N,N,N,N-tetramethyl-p-phenylenediamine dihydrochloride); solution colorless
  2. **Gordon and McLeod's reagent** (24, 43): 1–1.5% dimethyl-p-phenylenediamine hydrochloride (also called N,N-dimethyl-p-phenylenediamine monohydrochloride (HCl) or p-aminodimethylaniline monohydrochloride); solution light purple
  3. **Gaby and Hadley reagents** (23), modified by Ewing and Johnson (18)
     a. Reagent A, 1% α-naphthol in 95% ethyl alcohol (ethanol) and reagent B, 1% p-aminodimethylaniline HCl (or oxalate) (also called dimethyl-p- phenylenediamine oxalate)
     b. Also referred to as indophenol oxidase reagent
     c. Original "nadi" reaction; *na* from naphthol and *di* from diamine.
  4. **Carpenter, Suhrland, and Morrison reagent** (10): 1% p-aminodimethylaniline oxalate
  5. **Oxidase impregnated disks/strips**
     a. Difco (15)
        (1) Bacto-differentiation disks, oxidase; reagent: p-aminodimethylaniline oxalate
        (2) Dryslide oxidase test; reagent N,N,N', N'-tetramethyl-p-phenylenediamine dihydrochloride
     b. BBL (4): Taxo N Discs; reagent: p-aminodimethylaniline
     c. Key Scientific Products (see Appendix 11)
        (1) Disks and strips
        (2) Reagent: N,N,N', N'-tetramethyl-p-phenylenediamine dihydrochloride
     d. REMEL: Microdase test disks
        (1) Modified oxidase; separates *Staphylococcus* (−) from *Micrococcus* (+)
        (2) Filter paper disks with tetra (oxidase reagent) in dimethyl sulfoxide (DMSO); DMSO renders cell permeable to reagent.
        (3) Inoculum: colony removed from growth medium with applicator stick and rubbed onto disk
        (4) Results
           (a) All *Staphylococcus* are negative **except** strains of *S. caseolyticus, S. sciuri, S. lentus,* and *S. vitulus* (2, 19).
           (b) *Nesterenkonia halobia, Dermacoccus nishinomiyaenis,* and *Arthrobacter agilis* modified oxidase positive (28, 42); all species formerly in genus *Micrococcus*
B. Method of preparation, reagents
  1. Dissolve 1.0 g of desired reagent in less than 100 mL of distilled water (exception α-naphthol)
     α-Naphthol (1-naphthol)   1.0 g
     Ethyl alcohol (ethanol), 95%   100.0 mL
  2. Warm **gently** to put into solution.
  3. Transfer to a volumetric flask and bring to 100 mL with appropriate diluent (water or ethanol).
  4. Allow to stand 15 min before use (1).

5. Store in a dark glass-stoppered bottle. Avoid undue exposure to light (12).
6. Label correctly.

Kovac's reagent, a 1% aqueous solution of tetramethyl-*p*- phenylenediamine, is less toxic and more sensitive than the dimethyl compound, but more expensive (1, 14, 17, 30, 43). This reagent gives oxidase-positive colonies a lavender color which gradually turns dark purple-black, but it may also impart color to the surrounding medium (1). Gordon and McLeod's reagent (24), a 1–1.5% aqueous solution of dimethyl-*p*-phenylenediamine, is more stable than the tetramethyl compound (32). All of the *p*-phenylenediamine compounds are relatively **unstable** (3, 43).

The *p*-aminodimethylaniline oxalate reagent has an advantage over either Kovacs' or Gordon and McLeod's reagents in being extremely stable both in powder form and in solution; an aqueous solution is stable at least 6 months (14). *p*-Aminodimethylaniline is a little less soluble than the hydrochloride salt reagents, but gentle warming puts it into solution. Another advantage is that the oxalate salt does not form a black precipitate when it is flooded on colonies growing on chocolate agar, as sometimes occurs with hydrochloride reagents (14).

The use of commercially impregnated oxidase disks or strips eliminates the necessity of making up fresh reagents.

None of these reagents interfere with the Gram staining reaction (1).

C. Method of use
  1. **Reagent solutions**
     a. Direct **slant** procedure; indophenol reagents (nadi reaction) (18, 21, 23)
        (1) Growth medium: **nutrient** agar slant: 18–24 h; **do not** incubate longer.
        (2) Add 2–3 drops of each reagent (A and B) to slant; **tilt** tube(s) to permit reagents to mix and flow over growth.
        (3) Observe for color change; blue color on growth **within 2 min.**
     b. Direct **plate** procedure
        (1) Add 2–3 drops of reagent directly to a **few suspected colonies** growing on plate medium, e.g., blood agar (BA) or chocolate agar.
        (2) **Do not** flood the entire plate with reagent.
        (3) **Do not** invert plate.
        (4) Observe for color changes.
            (a) Kovacs' reagent: color reaction within 10–15 **sec** (1, 30)
            (b) Gordon and McLeod's reagent: color reaction within 10–30 **min** (24, 43)
            (c) Kovacs' indirect filter paper procedure (30)
                1. Place a 6-cm^2 piece of Whatman no. 1 filter paper in a Petri dish.
                2. Add 2–3 drops of Kovacs' reagent to the center of the paper.
                3. With a **platinum** wire inoculating **needle**, smear a loopful of a suspected colony onto the reagent-impregnated paper in a line 3–6 cm long.
                4. A positive color reaction occurs within 5–10 **sec.**
  2. **Oxidase disks**
     a. Direct plate procedure (4, 15)
        (1) Moisten impregnated disks with **sterile** distilled water.
        (2) Place disk on a few **suspected colonies** growing on plate medium, e.g., blood agar (BA) or chocolate agar.
        (3) **Do not** invert plate.
        (4) Return plate to a 35°C incubator for 20–30 **min.** The test may be incubated at room temperature (25°C) or in a refrigerator (4–10°C), but the reaction is slower.
        (5) Observe for color changes: immediately, rose to purple; after 20–30 min incubation, red to black.
     b. Indirect procedure (4, 15)
        (1) Two variations

(a) Moisten disk with **sterile** distilled water, place in a Petri dish, and add a loopful of a suspected colony growing on solid medium.
(b) Moisten disk with a broth culture of the suspected organism.
(2) Observe for color changes; a positive reaction should occur within **seconds**: pink to black.
3. Swab test (29)
   a. For testing fastidious bacteria
   b. Reagent: tetramethyl-*p*-phenylenediamine hydrochloride
   c. Use a white cotton swab instead of bacteriological loop, needle, or applicator stick.
   d. Colony picked up with swab and rubbed onto piece of filter paper containing reagent.
   e. Interpret **on swab, not** filter paper.
      (1) Positive reaction within 10–15 sec; delayed or weak reaction when color develops over 30 sec but within 1 min.
      (2) Swab test result may be positive when result on filter paper is negative.
D. Quality control: any reagents or disks must be tested with known positive and negative cultures before being put into general use.
E. Storage: store all reagents and disks in a refrigerator (4°C) when not in use; warm reagents before use (13). Barry and Bernsohn (3) recommend freezing reagents (−20°C) in 1- to 2-mL amounts and thawing 3–4 h **before** use to reduce autooxidation and prolong their activity. **Do not** use more than 1 day after thawing (5, 35). All reagents **should be freshly prepared just before use**; in solution they become deactivated rapidly. If they are refrigerated they **may** remain stable anywhere from 5 days to 2 weeks (29, 43). Difco Laboratories (14) state that the *p*-aminodimethylaniline **oxalate** reagent is stable for at least 6 months. However, since the stability of these reagents varies, it is advisable that reagents and disks be given a weekly quality control check and discarded when they give a negative or weak reaction with a known positive organism. Oxidase activity decreases if disks become darkened upon extended storage (3). If commercially prepared disks are not reacting properly, as evidenced by quality control, the entire lot may be returned to the company for replacement.
F. Chemistry of reagent action: the *p*-phenylenediamine dyes are primary aromatic amines (36), diamino derivatives of benzene (20). Cytochrome oxidase does not react directly with *p*-phenylenediamine reagent but oxidizes cytochrome *c*, which in turn oxidizes the reagent (4, 23, 27, 43).

(1) 2 Reduced cytochrome *c* + 2H$^+$ + ½ O$_2$ $\xrightarrow{\text{cytochrome oxidase}}$ 2 Oxidized cytochrome *c* + H$_2$O

(2) 2 Oxidized cytochrome *c* + Reagent $\xrightarrow{\text{oxidized}}$ Colored compound

The basic compound of reagents, phenylenediamine, is methylated. The more methyl groups introduced into the amino (NH$_2$) radical, the bluer the color; and if three phenyl groups (C$_6$H$_5$) are introduced instead of methyl, the color is even deeper (33). Oxidation of aromatic amines produces quinones (37). If oxidase reagent is prepared with α-naphthol, indophenol blue is formed (48); however, α-naphthol is not necessary for the reaction to take place. Naphthol is an azoic coupling component: –N=N-azo group (37).

Aniline (phenylamine) ← Aromatic amines → *p*-Phenylenediamine

There are two main types of oxidase tests using different reagents but the mechanism and results are comparable (5).

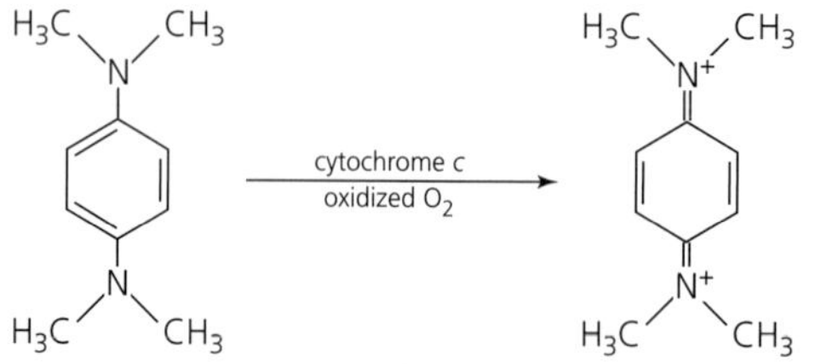

Tetramethyl-*p*-phenylenediamine (Wurster's reagent) → (cytochrome c, oxidized O₂) → Wurster's blue (formed in presence of ozone (O) or hydrogen peroxide (H₂O₂))   (26)

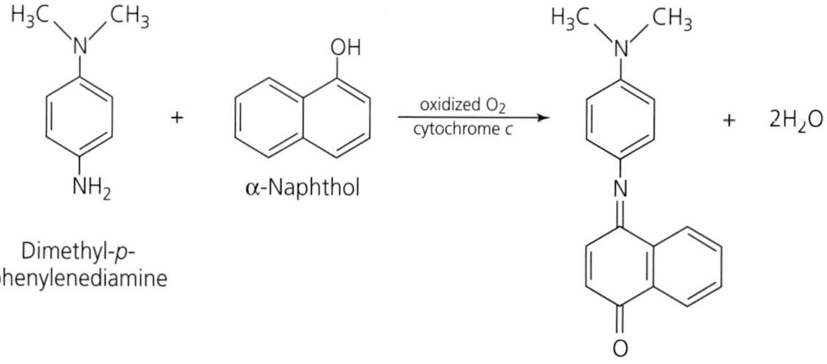

Dimethyl-*p*-phenylenediamine + α-Naphthol → (oxidized O₂, cytochrome c) → Indophenol blue (37) (insoluble in water) + 2H₂O

Indophenol is a dye, an N-analog of quinone in which the =N replaces one or both of the =O groups (48).

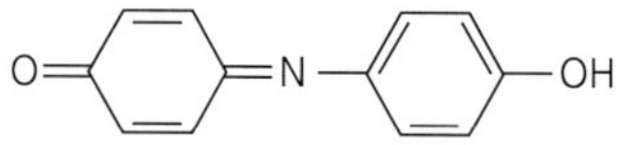

Indophenol (34)
(benzenone indophenol (31))

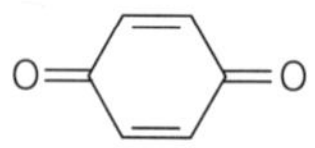

Quinone

The reagent phenylenediamine hydrochloride forms a dichlorimide group (ClN=C_6H_4 =NCl); the =NCl is either reduced to –NH$_2$ or hydrolyzed to =O (48).

V. QUALITY CONTROL ORGANISMS

A. Positive (+)

    Neisseria mucosa   ATCC 19696
    Pseudomonas aeruginosa   ATCC 10145

B. Negative (−)

Escherichia coli   ATCC 11775
Uninoculated

VI. RESULTS

> See Figures 32.1–32.3 (Appendix 1) for colored photographic results

VII. INTERPRETATION

A. **Oxidase-positive colonies:** colony becomes pink, then maroon (dark red), and finally black (purplish black)
   1. Pink colonies
      a. Viable bacteria
      b. Stage for subculturing
   2. Black colonies
      a. Within **10–15 sec**
      b. Bacteria **non**viable

When using a dimethyl-*p*-phenylenediamine-α-naphthol reagent mixture, a positive result is denoted by a blue color (23, 42) **within 1–2 min.**

B. **Oxidase-negative colonies**
   1. No color change in colonies or a light pink color due to the reagent
   2. Black discoloration of the surrounding medium may occur

With Kovacs' reagent, a positive result is denoted by a purplish black color that develops within 10 sec; a positive reaction within 10–60 sec is considered a delayed result (43). Steel (43) states that development of color after 60 sec denotes a negative result.

VIII. BARRY AND BERNSOHN REAGENT IMPREGNATED OXIDASE TEST STRIPS (3)

A. Strip preparation
   1. Whatman no. 1 filter paper
      a. Cut into strips 6–8 cm in diameter.
      b. Saturate with a 1.0% aqueous solution of dimethyl-*p*-phenylenediamine oxalate.
   2. Dry **rapidly**.
      a. Hang on strings or glass rods.
      b. Avoid contact with metal clips, tacks, etc.
   3. Store in screw-cap jars containing a generous amount of desiccant.
   4. Store in refrigerator; stable up to 6 months.
B. Procedure
   1. Smear a **pure** colony onto a **dry** strip.
   2. A number of colonies may be tested simultaneously on the same strip.
C. Interpretation
   1. Results within 10 sec
   2. Positive: red color

IX. PRECAUTIONS

A. The oxidase test is used routinely to identify members of the genus *Neisseria*. However, other genera also yield a positive oxidase result (see II. Purpose). Ellingworth et al. (17)

found that *Haemophilus influenzae* was oxidase negative with dimethyl-*p*-phenylenediamine but positive with the more sensitive Kovacs' reagent, tetramethyl-*p*-phenylenediamine. Castor and Chance (11) state that *Pseudomonas maltophilia* is often delayed oxidase positive and that not all *Pseudomonas* spp. are positive. They recommend **not** using the oxidase reaction to describe the genus *Pseudomonas*.

Using the oxidase test to aid in identifying the genus *Neisseria* **requires** doing a Gram stain on all oxidase-positive colonies. All *Neisseria* spp. are Gram-negative, coffee bean–shaped diplococci, while other organisms that may exhibit a positive oxidase result are Gram-negative bacilli or Gram-negative coccobacilli. However, *Oligella urethralis* (formerly *Moraxella urethralis*) may exhibit a Gram morphology similar to *Neisseria*. Thus, carbohydrate fermentation tests **must** be used for final identification of *Neisseria* spp.

B. **Do not** attempt to perform an oxidase test on any colonies growing on medium containing glucose; its fermentation inhibits oxidase activity, which may result in false negatives. An oxidase test on Gram-negative bacilli should use **only** colonies from **nonselective** and/or **nondifferential** media to ensure valid results: blood agar (BA), Trypticase soy agar (TSA), heart infusion agar (HIA), nutrient agar (NA), etc.; **not** EMB, MAC, XLD, and BGA agar plates.

C. Lautrop (31) states that false positives may occur with *B. pertussis* cultivated on media containing a high concentration of blood.

D. Use of a platinum inoculating loop or needle or applicator sticks to remove colonies for oxidase testing is recommended by Steel (43), who states that any trace of iron (Nichrome) can **alone** oxidize the phenylenediamine reagent, yielding a false-positive result.

E. False-negative results occur if a mixed culture contains the two genera *Pseudomonas* and *Neisseria*. An inhibitory substance is produced by *Pseudomonas* spp. that interferes with production of oxidase by *Neisseria* spp. (46).

F. A negative oxidase result may exhibit black discoloration in the medium surrounding the colonies but **not on** the colonies. This discoloration has **no significance.** A black precipitate may occur in the surrounding chocolate agar when an old hydrochloride reagent is used (14). Observe the reaction **on the colony** (colonies) being tested, **not** in the medium beneath the colony. The oxalate salt does not form this precipitate (14). The oxalate salt is preferred over mono- or dihydrochloride reagents; oxalate is more stable and is usually prepared weekly, while hydrochloride **must** be prepared daily.

G. **Do not** label the tetramethyl-*p*-phenylenediamine dihydrochloride reagent simply *Kovacs' reagent,* but *Kovacs' oxidase reagent.* There is also a Kovacs' indole reagent.

H. The oxidase reagents quickly autooxidize (with free oxygen in air) and lose sensitivity. Autooxidation is reduced by adding a 0.1% solution of ascorbic acid directly to the reagent (44) during its preparation. Reagents should be discarded if any precipitate forms (14). Avoid any undue exposure of the reagents to light. Kovacs' tetramethyl reagent should be discarded if it turns deep blue; it should be colorless (12).

Time periods for color development **must** be adhered to, since a purple-black color may develop **later** because of autooxidation of reagents **and/or** a weakly positive organism containing a small quantity of cytochrome *c*; it is impossible to interpret accurately, which may cause a false-positive result.

I. Kovacs' tetramethyl reagent is reliable only as long as the time-limiting period for a positive result to occur is adhered to (up to 60 **sec**) (43). Kovacs' reagent is very sensitive with a final reading within 10 sec; any results **after** 10–60 sec are **not typical** of *Neisseria* spp. (35). However, the dimethyl reagent may require anywhere from 10 to 30 min for a positive result (24, 43); with a delayed reaction, the test should be repeated using an 18- to 24-h culture from blood agar (BA, SBA) (35).

J. Spectrophotometric studies showed that cytochrome oxidase and indophenol oxidase are the same (39).

K. Using indophenol (nadi) test reagents A and B, **disregard** any weak or doubtful reactions **after 2 min** (35).

L. Dimethyl-*p*-phenylenediamine hydrochloride (DPM) is less sensitive, and viscid (sticky) colonies may appear oxidase negative because of poor penetration by reagent (35).
M. Use of the disk or indirect filter paper procedure (30) provides sufficient viable growth for subculturing and inoculation for additional biochemical procedures.
N. The oxidase test is an oxidizing reaction, and oxygen **must** reach colonies; after flooding growth or a portion of colony growth, tilt slants or plates to permit the reagent to run, exposing colonies to air.
O. The oxidase test should be performed on **all** Gram-negative bacilli (7). If the test is not performed on *Enterobacteriaceae* (all oxidase negative except *P. shigelloides*), it is possible to misidentify *Aeromonas hydrophilia* (+) as *E. coli* or *Serratia* sp. and *P. shigelloides* (oxidase +) (formerly *Aeromonas shigelloides*) as *Shigella sonnei*.

REFERENCES

1. Bailey RW, Scott EG. Diagnostic Microbiology, ed 2. St. Louis: CV Mosby, 1966:329–330.
2. Baker JS. Comparison of various methods for differentiation of staphylococci and micrococci. J Clin Microbiol 1984;19(6):875–879.
3. Barry AL, Bernsohn KL. Methods for storing oxidase test reagents. Appl Microbiol 1969;17(6):933–934.
4. BBL Manual of Products and Laboratory Procedures, ed 6. Cockeysville, MD: BBL Microbiology Systems, Division of Becton Dickinson and Company, 1988.
5. Blazevic DJ, Ederer GM. Principles of Biochemical Tests in Diagnostic Microbiology. New York: John Wiley & Sons, 1975:91–93, 127.
6. Blazevic DJ, Schreckenberger PC, Matsen JM. Evaluation of the PathoTec "Rapid I-D System." Appl Microbiol 1973;26(6):886–889.
7. Branson D. Methods in Clinical Bacteriology. Springfield, IL: Charles C Thomas, 1972:41.
8. Burrows W, Lewert RM, Rippon JW. Textbook of Microbiology. The Pathogenic Microorganisms, ed 19. Philadelphia: WB Saunders, 1968:110–111.
9. Cantarow A, Schepartz B. Biochemistry, ed 3. Philadelphia: WB Saunders, 1962:385.
10. Carpenter CM, Suhrland LG, Morrison M. The oxalate salt of *p*-aminodimethylaniline, an improved reagent for the oxidase test. Science 1947;105:649–650.
11. Castor LN, Chance B. Photochemical determinations of the oxidases of bacteria. J Biol Chem 1959;234(6):1587–1592.
12. Cowan ST. Cowan & Steel's Manual for the Identification of Medical Bacteria, ed 2. Cambridge: Cambridge University Press, 1974:22, 148–149.
13. Deibel RH, Evans JB. Modified benzidine test for the detection of cytochrome containing respiratory systems in microorganisms. J Bacteriol 1960;79(3):356–360.
14. Difco Manual, ed 10. Detroit: Difco Laboratories, 1984:71, 298, 603.
15. Difco Supplementary Literature. Detroit: Difco Laboratories, 1968:83.
16. Dubos RJ, Hirsch JG, eds. Bacterial and Mycotic Infections of Man, ed 4. Philadelphia: JB Lippincott, 1965:93–94.
17. Ellingworth S, McLeod JW, Gordon J. Further observations on the oxidation by bacteria of compounds of the *para*-phenylene diamine series. J Pathol Bacteriol 1929;32(2):173–184.
18. Ewing WH, Johnson JG. The differentiation of *Aeromonas* and C27 cultures from *Enterobacteriaceae*. Int Bull Bacteriol Nomencl Taxon 1960;10(3):223–230.
19. Faller A, Schleifer KH. Modified oxidase and benzidine tests for separation of staphylococci and micrococci. J Clin Microbiol 1981;13(6):1031–1035.
20. Fieser LF, Fieser M. Organic Chemistry, ed 3. New York: Reinhold, 1956:601–602.
21. Finegold SM, Baron EJ. Bailey and Scott's Diagnostic Microbiology, ed 7. St. Louis: CV Mosby, 1986:491.
22. Frobisher M. Fundamentals of Bacteriology, ed 3. Philadelphia: WB Saunders, 1944:181.
23. Gaby WL, Hadley C. Practical laboratory test for the identification of *Pseudomonas aeruginosa*. J Bacteriol 1957;74(3):356–358.
24. Gordon J, McLeod JW. The practical application of the direct oxidase reaction in bacteriology. J Pathol Bacteriol 1928;31(2):185–190.
25. Gunsalus IC, Stanier RY. The Bacteria, vol II. New York: Academic Press, 1961:335, 371.
26. Harper HA, Rodwell VW, Mayes PA. Review of Physiological Chemistry, ed 16. Los Altos, CA: Lange Medical Publications, 1977:225–228.
27. Keilin D, Hartree EF. Cytochrome oxidase. Proc Roy Soc 1938;B125:171–186.
28. Koch C, Schumann P, Stackebrandt E. Reclassification of *Micrococcus agilis* (Ali-Cohen 1889) to the genus *Arthrobacter* as *Arthrobacter agilis* comb. nov. and emendation of the genus *Arthrobacter*. Int J Syst Bacteriol 1995;45:837–839.
29. Koneman EW, Allen SD, Janda WM, Schreckenberger PC, Winn WC Jr. Color Atlas & Textbook of Diagnostic Microbiology, ed 5. Philadelphia: JB Lippincott, 1997:449.
30. Kovacs N. Identification of *Pseudomonas py-*

ocyanea by the oxidase reaction. Nature 1956;178:703.
31. Lautrop H. Laboratory diagnosis of whooping-cough or *Bordetella* infections. Bull WHO 1960;23(1):15–35.
32. LeClerc H, Beerens H. Une technique simple de mise en évidence de l'oxydase chez les bactéries. Ann Inst Pasteur (Lille) 1962;13:187.
33. Lillie RD. HJ Conn's Biological Stains, ed 9. Baltimore: Williams & Wilkins, 1977:29, 374.
34. Mahler HR, Cordes EH. Biological Chemistry. New York: Harper & Row, 1966:286.
35. Murray PR, Baron EJ, Pfaller MA, et al. Manual of Clinical Microbiology, ed 6. Washington, DC: American Society for Microbiology, 1995.
36. Noller CR. Chemistry of Organic Compounds, ed 3. Philadelphia: WB Saunders, 1965:533, 554–555.
37. Nussenbaum S. Organic Chemistry. Boston: Allyn & Bacon, 1963:441.
38. Oginsky EL, Umbreit WW. An Introduction to Bacterial Physiology, ed 2. San Francisco: WH Freeman, 1959:215.
39. Oser BL, ed. Hawk's Physiological Chemistry, ed 14. New York: McGraw-Hill, 1965:424–425.
40. Smith DT, Conant NF, Willett HP. Zinsser's Microbiology, ed 14. New York: Appleton-Century-Crofts, 1968:106.
41. Sneath PHA, Mair NS, Sharpe ME, Holt JG, eds. Bergey's Manual of Systematic Bacteriology, vol 2. Baltimore: Williams & Wilkins, 1986.
42. Stackebrandt E, Koch C, Gvozdiak O, Schumann P. Taxonomic dissection of the genus *Micrococcus: Kocuria* gen. nov., *Nesterenkonia* gen. nov., *Kytococcus* gen. nov., *Dermacoccus* gen. nov., and *Micrococcus* Cohen 1872 gen. amend. IJSB 1995;45:682–692.
43. Steel KJ. The oxidase reaction as a taxonomic tool. J Gen Microbiol 1961;25(2):297–306.
44. Steel KJ. The oxidase activity of staphylococci. J Appl Bacteriol 1962;25(3):445–447.
45. Summer JB, Somers BF. Chemistry and Methods of Enzymes, ed 2. New York: Academic Press, 1947:225.
46. TM-227–5, Laboratory Procedures in Clinical Bacteriology. Washington, DC: Department of the Army, 1963:6–11.
47. Weyant RS, Moss CW, Weaver RE, et al. Identification of Unusual Pathogenic Gram-Negative Aerobic and Facultatively Anaerobic Bacteria. Baltimore: Williams & Wilkins, 1996.
48. Whitmore FC. Organic Chemistry. New York: Van Nostrand, 1937:805–806.
49. Wilson G, Miles A, Parker MT, eds. Topley and Wilson's Principles of Bacteriology, Virology, and Immunology, ed 7. Baltimore: Williams & Wilkins, 1983:493.

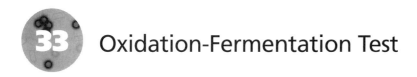

33 Oxidation-Fermentation Test

I. PRINCIPLE

To determine the oxidative or fermentative metabolism of a carbohydrate or its nonuse

II. PURPOSE

(Also see Chapters 44–45)

A. Determination of the oxidation-fermentation (O/F, Oxi/Ferm) reaction early in the laboratory diagnosis greatly aids identification of aerobic/facultative anaerobic bacteria.
   1. Primarily to differentiate enteric and nonenteric, Gram- negative, aerobic to facultative anaerobic, **bacilli** from the *Enterobacteriaceae*, which are all fermenters (F). Not all bacteria listed below are normal or abnormal inhabitants of the intestinal tract as are the *Enterobacteriaceae*; however, any bacteria can be found in any area of the body under certain conditions.
      a. Fermentation (F, Ferm) or fermentation and oxidation (F & O):

Actinobacillus spp.	*Gardnerella vaginalis*	*Succinivibrio dextrinosolvens*
Aeromonas spp.	*Haemophilus* spp.	*Suttonella indologenes*
Capnocytophaga spp.	*Helicobacter* spp.	*Vibrio* spp.
Cardiobacterium hominis	*Kingella* spp.	*Xanthomonas* spp.
Chromobacterium violaceum	*Megamonas hypermegas*	

      b. Oxidation (O, Oxi) and/or inert (−, NR, nonreactive):

Acidovorax spp.	*Comamonas* spp.	*Pseudomonas* spp.
Acinetobacter spp.	*Eikenella corrodens*	*Ralstonia* spp.
Afipia spp.	*Flavimonas oryzihabitans*	*Roseomonas* spp.
Agrobacterium spp.	*Flavobacterium* spp.	*Shewanella* spp.
Alcaligenes spp.	*Legionella* spp.	*Sphingomonas* spp.
Bartonella spp.	*Methylobacterium* spp.	*Stenotrophomonas* spp.
Brevundimonas spp.	*Moraxella* spp.	*Taylorella equigenitalis*
Brucella melitensis	*Ochrobactrum anthropi*	*Weeksella* spp.
Campylobacter spp.	*Oligella* spp.	*Wolinella succinogenes*
Chryseomonas luteola	*Pasteurella* spp.	*Xanthobacter* spp.

   2. To aid in differentiation between genera *Staphylococcus* and *Micrococcus*
      a. *Staphylococcus* spp.: glucose fermenters; **exception:** *S. saprophyticus*, weak fermenter or nonreactive (neither fermentation nor oxidation)
      b. *Micrococcus* spp.: usually glucose oxidizers
   3. To aid in identification of other organisms
B. Determination of motility and gas production (CO_2 and H_2) because of the semisolid medium

III. BIOCHEMISTRY INVOLVED

Bacteria use carbohydrates metabolically by one of two processes, fermentative or oxidative. Some bacteria can metabolize a carbohydrate (as exhibited by acid production) only under aerobic conditions, while others produce acid both aerobically and anaerobically (10). Bacteria that can grow, metabolize, and reproduce under either aerobic (presence of atmospheric oxygen) or anaerobic (absence of atmospheric oxygen) conditions are termed *facultative anaerobes*. Most medical bacteria are facultative anaerobes.

Fermentation (F, Ferm)

Fermentation is an **anaerobic process** and bacteria that ferment a carbohydrate are usually facultative anaerobes (10). In fermentation, a carbohydrate is split into two triose molecules (10) that are further converted to a number of 1-, 2-, 3-, or 4-carbon compounds (3); the key intermediate is pyruvic acid. The final products of fermentation vary with each bacterial species, depending upon its enzyme system and environmental conditions (5). The important criterion is that **prior** to its breakdown, the sugar glucose is phosphorylated to glucose 6-phosphate (3). Fermentation requires an organic compound as the terminal electron acceptor (5).

The main fermentative pathway of glucose is the Embden-Meyerhof-Parnas (EMP) pathway, although degradation may occur via or in combination with the pentose shunt or the Entner-Doudoroff (ED) pathway (3). However, all three pathways require phosphorylation of glucose as the **initial** step before degradation can occur (11). The Embden-Meyerhof-Parnas (EMP) pathway is also called the glycolytic, or anaerobic, pathway or fermentation pathway. The Entner-Doudoroff pathway is also called the aerobic pathway.

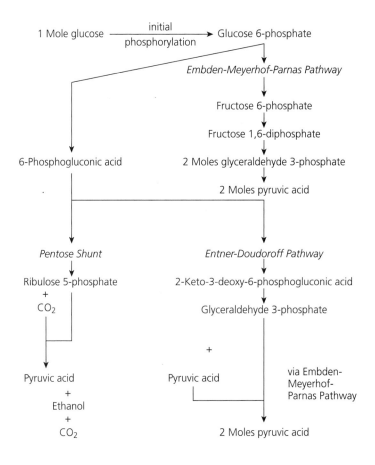

Three Phosphorylated Fermentation Pathways (4)

Oxidation (O/Oxi)

Oxidation of glucose via one of the shunt pathways is an **aerobic** process, and bacteria that oxidize carbohydrates are usually obligate (strict) aerobes (10). In the oxidation process, glucose or other carbohydrates are not degraded and split into two trioses (10); instead, the aldehyde group is directly oxidized to a carboxyl group, forming gluconic acid, which is further oxidized to a 2-ketogluconic acid (10, 14, 16). 2-Ketogluconic acid may accumulate or be further degraded (15) into two molecules of pyruvic acid. In contrast to fermentation, Sebek and Randles (15) and Norris and Campbell (14) found that oxidation requires **no initial** phosphorylation of a carbohydrate prior to degradation. Sebek and Randles (15) attribute the lack of phosphorylation in the initial stage of oxidation to the inability of adenosine triphosphate (ATP) to penetrate the bacterial cell. Oxidation requires oxygen or an inorganic compound as the terminal electron acceptor (6).

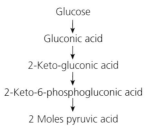

Oxidative Pathway: No Initial Phosphorylation (4)

The main difference between fermentative and oxidative metabolism of a carbohydrate is the requirement for atmospheric oxygen and initial phosphorylation. Fermentation is an **anaerobic process** requiring initial phosphorylation of glucose prior to degradation to relatively strong mixed acids, whereas oxidation, in the absence of inorganic compounds such as nitrate and sulfate, is a **strict aerobic process** involving direct oxidation of a nonphosphorylated glucose molecule (initially) (10). Fermentation produces higher acidity than oxidation (10).

IV. MEDIA EMPLOYED

A. Media; two choices depending on morphology of test organisms
  1. **Hugh and Leifson's OF basal medium (OFBM)**; Gram-negative bacilli (enteric OF) (1, 5, 7, 10)
     a. Semisolid basal medium ingredients, pH 7.1

Casein peptone (Tryptone), 0.2%	2.0 g
Sodium chloride, NaCl	5.0 g
Dipotassium phosphate, (K_2HPO_4)	0.3 g
Agar	2.0–3.0 g
Bromthymol blue (BTB)	0.03–0.08 g
Deionized water	1000 mL

     b. pH indicator: bromthymol blue (BTB)
        (1) Acid: yellow color, pH 6.0
        (2) Alkaline: deep Prussian blue color, pH 7.6
        (3) Uninoculated medium: pH 7.1; green color
     c. Commercial products available
        (1) Difco: Bacto-OF basal medium (5)
        (2) BBL: OF basal medium (1)

2. **Staph OF**: fermentation medium for differentiating Gram-positive *Staphylococcus* and *Micrococcus* (8)
   a. Semisolid basal medium ingredients, pH 7.0

Pancreatic digest of casein (Tryptone), 1%	10.0 g
Yeast extract	1.0 g
Agar	2.0 g
Bromcresol purple (BCP)	0.001 g
Deionized water	1000.0 mL

   b. pH indicator: bromcresol purple (BCP)
      (1) Acid: yellow, pH 5.2
      (2) Alkaline: purple, pH 6.8
      (3) Uninoculated medium: pH 7.0; **purple**

Alternate pH indicators such as Andrades acid fuchsin and phenol red may substitute (see Appendix 3 for their color reactions).

B. Method of preparation, basal medium; either medium
   1. Weigh out amount accurately as directed on the label. Various company products may differ slightly.
   2. Rehydrate with distilled or demineralized water.
   3. Heat **gently** into solution.
C. Method of sterilization, basal medium; either medium
   1. Autoclave
   2. 121°C, 15 lb, 15 min
D. Cool sterile basal medium to 40–45°C in a water bath.
E. Addition of carbohydrates, 2 choices
   1. Aqueous solutions, 10% (10 g/100 mL)
      a. Carbohydrates
         (1) Enteric OF: glucose, maltose, lactose, mannitol, sucrose, xylose
         (2) Staph OF: **only** glucose and mannitol
      b. Method of sterilization
         (1) Filtration, recommended (11)
            (a) Millipore membrane filter method
            (b) Membranes: 0.45-μm pore diameter
         (2) Alternative procedure (1)
            (a) 1% concentration of desired carbohydrate added to the basal medium **prior** to sterilization (10 g/L)
            (b) Autoclave: 118°C, 10 min

If the carbohydrate is added to the basal medium prior to autoclaving, the temperature may cause the carbohydrate to break down (10). However, Hugh and Leifson (10) state that carbohydrates may be autoclaved if a 10% aqueous solution is used. Still, it is recommended that all carbohydrates be sterilized by filtration.

   c. To a 100-mL aliquot of **sterile** melted basal medium add 10 mL of the **sterile** (filtered) 10% concentration of carbohydrate desired (1, 5, 10); **final concentration of carbohydrate, 1%.**
   d. **Aseptically** dispense approximately 5.0 mL per **sterile screw-cap tube** (1, 5).
   2. **Sterile**, commercial carbohydrate disks
      a. Manufacturer: BBL, Difco, Key Scientific (C.O.T. tablets)
      b. Basal medium
         (1) Same as used for aqueous solutions of carbohydrates

(2) Add carbohydrate disks to **sterile, tubed** medium.
  (a) **Aseptically**
  (b) Follow manufacturer's directions.
F. Cool before use and refrigerate for storage (4–10°C).
G. Inoculation, standard two-tube test
  1. Inoculum: growth from 18- to 24-h **pure** culture
    a. **Enteric OF**: Kligler's iron agar (KIA) or other suitable agar slant (2)
    b. **Staph OF**: blood agar plate (BA, SBA) or other suitable isolation plate medium; **do not** inoculate from mannitol salt agar medium.
  2. For each carbohydrate, inoculate a **pair** of OF tubes for each organism being tested. Label one "open" and the other "covered" (or "sealed"). Also set up control sets: one **inoculated** set with **no** carbohydrate added and one **uninoculated** set **with** carbohydrate.
  3. **Light** inoculum (2, 7)
    a. Inoculating **needle**
    b. **Stab** both tubes to approximately ¼ inch from the bottom.
  4. Overlay **all** tubes labeled "covered" (or "sealed") with approximately 1.0–2.0 mL of **sterile** melted petrolatum or **sterile** Vaspar to exclude all oxygen.
    a. Sealants (2)
      (1) Mineral oil or paraffin oil
        (a) In a 200-mL bottle, add 1 mL of water to 100 mL mineral oil or paraffin.
        (b) Sterilization; two choices
          1 Autoclave: 121°C, 15 lb, 15 min
          2 Hot air oven: 160–170°C, 1 h
      (2) Vaspar: more effective; it **does not** retract from glass as does paraffin and is a solid so less possibility of air diffusion
        (a) Mixture 1:1 of petroleum jelly and paraffin
        (b) To a 100-mL bottle, add 50 mL of mixture.
        (c) Sterilization: for **each 50-mL aliquot**, autoclave, 121°C, 15 lb, 1 h
        (d) **After** sterilization, place in dry oven at 110°C to drive off entrapped water.
    b. Recommend **not** using mineral oil; a heavy liquid petroleum, it increases air diffusion.
H. Incubation: 35°C, 48 h or longer (1, 5). Slow growers may require 3–4 days (2, 7) or even up to 14 days of prolonged incubation (4). **Loosen caps.** A low carbohydrate:protein ratio reduces formation of alkaline amines that may neutralize small quantities of weak acids that may form from oxidative metabolism (11). Large amounts of carbohydrates increase the amount of acid found (11).

Enteric OF medium of Hugh and Leifson (10) contains a high concentration of carbohydrate with a low concentration of peptone to overcome the possibility of an aerobic organism using peptone and thus producing an alkaline condition that neutralizes any slight acidity produced by an oxidative organism. These authors state that certain peptones may not be satisfactory; they recommend a pancreatic digest of casein. Dipotassium phosphate in the medium promotes fermentation and acts as buffer to control the pH (10). Sodium chloride enhances growth of *Brucella* spp. (10).

The semisolid agar concentration used also allows determination of motility in addition to the oxidative or fermentative ability of an organism. The agar also helps distribute the acid produced at the surface throughout the tube, which makes pH interpretation easier (10, 11). Glucose is used routinely in the OF basal medium; however, some organisms being tested are unable to metabolize glucose but can attack other carbohydrates (11). A battery of glucose, lactose, and sucrose should be used, and at times, maltose (6), mannitol, and xylose (10).

On storage, a small amount of oxygen may be absorbed by the medium, but Hugh and Leifson (10) state that this small amount does not affect OF reactions appreciably. Cowan and Steel (4) advise that the oxygen absorbed by stored OF medium may be removed by first steaming, and then quickly cooling, the medium just prior to use.

V. QUALITY CONTROL MICROORGANISMS

A. **Enteric OF**
   1. Growth with fermentation (F, Ferm):

Proteus vulgaris	ATCC 13315
Escherichia coli	ATCC 8677

   2. Growth with oxidation (O, Oxi):

Pseudomonas aeruginosa	ATCC 10145

   3. Growth with neither F nor O (NC):

Alcaligenes faecalis	ATCC 8750

B. **Staph OF**
   a. Growth with fermentation (F/Ferm):

Staphylococcus aureus subsp. *aureus*	ATCC 12600

   b. Growth with oxidation (O/Oxi):

Micrococcus luteus	ATCC 4698

   c. Control tube: OF basal medium without carbohydrate

VI. RESULTS

> See Figures 33.1 and 33.2 (Appendix 1) for colored photographic results

VII. INTERPRETATION: TWO-TUBE TEST

A. Besides carbohydrate use, gas production and motility may be detected with OF medium (5). Record gas and/or acid production and motility reaction for each tube, using the following abbreviations.
   1. **Carbohydrate reactions**

      Acid: A
      Acid and gas: AG, Ⓐ
      No change or alkaline reaction: NC

   2. **OF determinations**

      Fermentative: F, Ferm
      Oxidative: O, Oxi
      Neither oxidative nor fermentative: NR (nonreactive), − (inert), F (nonfermentative)

   3. **Motility**

      Motile: + (growth diffused away from stab line)
      Nonmotile: − (growth confined along stab line)

   If organisms exhibit **no growth** in either OF medium, report **no growth** (NG) (9).

B. **Enteric OF**: carbohydrate utilization patterns (2, 10) (Tables 33.1 and 33.2)

Table 33.1. Enteric OF Carbohydrate Patterns

Reaction	Tube with Reaction	Open Tube	Covered (Sealed Tube)
Oxidation (O, OX)	Open	Yellow (A)[a]	Green (−)
Fermentation (F)			
Anaerogenic	Covered	Yellow (A)	Yellow (A)
Aerogenic	Covered	Yellow (AG)	Yellow (AG)
Neither fermentation nor oxidation (NR, −)	Neither[b]	Blue or green (−)	Purple (−)
Both fermentation and oxidation (O + F, O/F)	Both	Yellow (A or AG)	Yellow (A or AG)

[a]A; acid production.
[b]**Uninoculated** carbohydrate control reading; no change in color.

Table 33.2. Staph OF Carbohydrate Utilization Patterns

Staph OF	Tube with Reaction	Open Tube	Covered (Sealed Tube)
1. Oxidation (O, Ox)	Open	Yellow (A)[a]	Purple (−)
2. Fermentation (F) (anaerogenic)	Covered	Yellow (A)	Yellow (A)
3. Neither fermentation nor oxidation (NR, −)	Neither[b]	Purple (−)	Purple (−)

Micrococcus: oxidative (O) or neither fermentative nor oxidative (nonreactive, NR, or −).
Staphylococcus aureus and *S. epidermidis:* fermentative (F).
Staphylococcus saprophyticus: weakly fermentative (WF) or nonreactive (NR, −).
[a]A; acid production.
[b]**Uninoculated** carbohydrate control reading; no change in color.

VIII. PRECAUTIONS

A. Correct abbreviations **must** be used in recording OF reactions. Do not use positive (+) or negative (−) to denote oxidation (O, Oxi) or fermentation (F, Ferm). This could be misleading, possibly indicating the motility result or making it impossible to deduce whether the carbohydrate result was negative for oxidation, fermentation, or both.

B. In most textbooks, OF reactions of many organisms are stated as +/−, which indicates that these organisms vary in their OF reaction and are either oxidative or neither oxidative nor fermentative (no **glucose** utilization, inert).

C. At times an aqueous (water) solution of the pH indicator is added to the medium, 3.0 mL of a 1% concentration per liter. Alcoholic solutions must **not** be used, because an organism may produce acid from the alcohol (11), yielding a false-positive fermentation or oxidation result.

D. Cowan and Steel (4) state that some organisms cannot grow in Hugh and Leifson's medium. If this occurs, repeat the OF test with Hugh and Leifson's (10) basal medium with added enrichment, either 2.0% serum or 0.1% yeast extract (4).

E. Hugh and Leifson (10) state that nitrate is reduced by most fermentative organisms; however, nonreduction of nitrate is common among nonfermenters.

F. Hugh and Leifson (10) found that an organism that **only** oxidizes glucose will not ferment any other carbohydrate (only oxidize it); therefore, when testing with other carbohydrates, the covered (sealed) tube may be omitted.

G. An organism that is neither oxidative nor fermentative (−) will produce a slight alkalinity in the open tube (blue-green color), but the covered tube will not exhibit a color change (green) (10).

H. Some organisms may grow in both OF tubes without any acid production. If this occurs, Cowan and Steel (4) recommend confirming the negative reaction by using another basal medium containing glucose.

I. Some organisms require prolonged incubation before acid production is visible (4, 7). Lederberg (13) attributed the delayed reaction to inability of a carbohydrate to penetrate the bacterial cell. He recommended performing the galactosidase test (ONPG test) to determine potential fermentative ability.

J. Hugh and Leifson (10) showed that the OF reaction of most Gram-negative bacteria is either oxidative or fermentative; however, their reactions may cause some confusion because they are often slow or weak.

K. Hugh and Leifson (10) stated that the paracolon bacteria may both oxidize and ferment carbohydrates, and in this case oxidation is not evident unless fermentation is weak or slow. The paracolon bacteria *Salmonella choleraesuis* subsp. *arizonae* (formerly *Arizona*) and *Citrobacter* spp. can either oxidize lactose, ferment it, or both (10).

L. Fermentative organisms exhibit an acid reaction throughout the medium in both tubes. However, acid production by an oxidative organism is first evident **only** at the surface of the open tubed medium and gradually spreads throughout the tube (10). If the oxidative reaction is delayed or weak, alkalinity may be observed on the surface of the open tube, often resulting in misinterpretation of the OF reaction as negative (neither oxidative nor fermentative). However, on prolonged incubation of several days, the alkaline reaction reverts to acid (10). Therefore, all negative OF reactions should undergo prolonged incubation of 3–4 days.

M. **Heavy inoculum** is essential to detect biochemical products from many nonfermenters that are strict aerobes; the environment within the confined OF tube **may not** support optimal growth (12).

N. Medium is stabbed in the center of the tube, so surface growth is lacking. This may make it difficult to determine whether a negative result reflects biochemical inactivity or inability of organism to grow in the medium (12).

O. Highest percentage of discrepancies with the O/F test occurs with fastidious or rarely encountered bacterial strains; this often leads to false-negative results (12).

P. The use of packaged commercial identification kits by microbiologists and bypassing inoculation of **unknown** to either KIA or TSI may make it impossible to determine whether to select an F or O system. Koneman et al. (12) recommend first assessing O/F characteristics of all **unknown isolates** of **Gram-negative bacilli** on KIA/TSI.

Q. Loosen caps to permit air exchange; if caps are tightened, control tubes with unoxidized carbohydrate might not become alkaline (9).

R. Utilization patterns of several other carbohydrates (e.g., lactose, maltose, sucrose, and xylose) are often required to aid in identifying an organism's genus or species (9).

S. If one suspects an unknown, nonfermentative, Gram-negative bacillus; look for three main identifying characteristics: (*a*) no evidence of glucose fermentation, (*b*) cytochrome oxidase positivity, and (*c*) failure to grow on MacConkey (MAC) medium (13).

REFERENCES

1. BBL Manual of Products and Laboratory Procedures, ed 6. Cockeysville, MD: BBL Microbiology Systems, Division of Becton Dickinson and Company, 1988:216–217.
2. Branson D. Methods in Clinical Bacteriology. Springfield, IL: Charles C Thomas, 1972:12, 135.
3. Burrows W, Lewert RM, Rippon JW. Textbook of Microbiology. The Pathogenic Microorganisms, ed 19. Philadelphia: WB Saunders, 1968: 118–121, 135.
4. Cowan ST. Cowan & Steel's Manual for the Identification of Medical Bacteria, ed 2. Cambridge: Cambridge University Press, 1974:28, 170.
5. Difco Supplementary Literature. Detroit: Difco Laboratories, 1968:255.
6. Doelle HW. Bacterial Metabolism. New York: Academic Press, 1969:130, 257.
7. Ewing WH. Edwards and Ewing's Identification of Enterobacteriaceae, ed 4. New York: Elsevier, 1986.
8. Facklam RR, Smith PB. The Gram positive cocci. Hum Pathol 1976;7(2):187–194.

9. Forbes BA, Sahn DF, Weissfeld AS. Bailey & Scott's Diagnostic Microbiology, ed 10. St. Louis: CV Mosby, 1958:174, 443.
10. Hugh R, Leifson E. The taxonomic significance of fermentative versus oxidative metabolism of carbohydrates by various gram negative bacteria. J Bacteriol 1953;66(1):24–26.
11. Hugh R, Ryschenkow E. *Pseudomonas maltophilia*, an *Alcaligenes*-like species. J Gen Microbiol 1961;26(1):123–132.
12. Koneman EW, Allen SD, Janda WM, et al. Color Atlas & Textbook of Diagnostic Microbiology, ed 5. Philadelphia: JB Lippincott, 1997:254–261, 304.
13. Lederberg J. The beta-D-galactosidase of *Escherichia coli*, strain K-12. J Bacteriol 1950;60(4):381–392.
14. Norris FC, Campbell JJR. The intermediate metabolism of *Pseudomonas aeruginosa*. III. The application of paper chromatography to the identification of gluconic and 2-ketogluconic acids, intermediates in glucose oxidation. Can J Res 1949;27C:253–261.
15. Sebek OK, Randles CI. The oxidative dissimilation of mannitol and sorbitol by *Pseudomonas fluorescens*. J Bacteriol 1952;63(6):693–700.
16. Stokes FC, Campbell JJR. The oxidation of glucose and gluconic acid by dried cells of *Pseudomonas aeruginosa*. Arch Biochem Biophysics 1951;30(1):121–125.

34 Phenylalanine Deaminase Test

I. PRINCIPLE

To determine the ability of an organism to deaminate phenylalanine to phenylpyruvic acid enzymatically, with resulting acidity

II. PURPOSE

(Also see Chapters 43–45)

A. Phenylalanine deaminase activity is characteristic of *Morganella morganii* biogroups 1 and 2 and all *Proteus* and *Providencia* spp. It is used to separate these genera from **most** other members of the *Enterobacteriaceae* most frequently isolated. Other *Enterobacteriaceae* spp. that exhibit deaminase activity are

Rare isolates of *Enterobacter* (15)
Pantoea agglomerans (V, variable, usually +)
Rahnella aquatilis (+)
Tatumella ptyseos (+)

B. To aid in species differentiation: *Afipia felis* (+) from *A. broomeae* (−) and *A. clevelandensis* (−)

III. BIOCHEMISTRY INVOLVED

The aromatic amino acid phenylalanine is oxidatively deaminated by an amino acid oxidase, a flavoprotein (20), to yield the keto acid, phenylpyruvic acid. Oxidative deamination removes the amino group (NH_2) of the amino acid to form a double-bond α-keto acid and free ammonia (NH_3). This is a two-step process: initially, hydrogen is removed, yielding an imino acid, and the hydrogen combines with oxygen to form water; then the imino acid is hydrolyzed to a keto acid (17).

$$RCHNH_2COOH + \tfrac{1}{2}O \xrightarrow[\text{enzyme}]{-2H} RCNHCOOH \xrightarrow{+H_2O} RCOCOOH + NH_3$$

Amino acid → Imino acid → Keto acid

Net Reaction

Phenylalanine + $\tfrac{1}{2}O$ $\xrightarrow[\text{flavoprotein}]{-2H}$ Phenylpyruvic acid + NH_3 (Ammonia)

Phenylalanine is deaminated to phenylpyruvic acid and may be further reduced to phenyllactic acid upon additional incubation. Phenyllactic acid can be reconverted to phenylalanine, and the deamination cycle occurs again. A small amount of phenylpyruvic acid can be decarboxylated to phenylacetic acid, which can also be reconverted to phenylalanine (4, 12).

(Redrawn from Harrow, B., and Mazur, A. *Textbook of Biochemistry,* 9th ed., p. 405, with permission of W. B. Saunders Co., Philadelphia.)

IV. MEDIUM EMPLOYED: PHENYLALANINE (PA) MEDIUM (2, 3, 6, 9)

A. **Ingredients, pH 7.3**

DL-Phenylalanine	2.0 g
Yeast extract	3.0 g
Sodium chloride, NaCl	5.0 g
Disodium phosphate, Na_2HPO_4	1.0 g
Agar	12.0 g
Deionized water	1000.0 mL

Yeast extract provides both carbon and nitrogen sources.

B. Commercial products available
C. Method of preparation
   1. Weigh out amount accurately as directed on the label.
   2. Rehydrate with distilled or demineralized water.
   3. Heat **gently** into solution.
   4. Dispense approximately 4.0 mL per tube, **long slant,** (16 × 120 mm).
D. Method of sterilization: autoclave, 121°C, 15 lb, 15 min
E. Allow medium to solidify in **slanted** position.

F. Cool before use and refrigerate for storage (4–10°C).
G. Inoculation
   1. **Heavy** inoculum (8)
   2. Growth from an 18- to 24-h **pure** culture (Kligler's iron agar, KIA)
H. Incubation: 35°C; 4 h or 18–24 h
I. Add reagent **directly** to the incubated tube **before** attempting to interpret, and roll reagent **gently** over the slant to dislodge surface colonies.

If commercial phenylalanine medium is not available and if L- phenylalanine is used instead of the DL isomer mixture, only 1.0 g (1%) is required (5). The L (+) form of phenylalanine is more rapidly degraded by *Proteus* and *Providencia* than the DL mixture (14).

V. REAGENTS EMPLOYED: TWO CHOICES

A. **Aqueous ferric chloride (FeCl$_3$), 10%**
   1. Ingredients, two types
      a. Acidic, **recommended**

Ferric chloride, FeCl$_3$	12.0 g
Concentrated hydrochloric acid, HCl	2.5 mL
Deionized water to bring to	100.0 mL

      b. Nonacidic

Ferric chloride, FeCl$_3$	10.0 g
Deionized water	100.0 mL

B. **Iron (III) ammonium sulfate (ferric ammonium sulfate)**, FeSO$_4$(NH$_4$)$_2$SO$_4$ · 6H$_2$O, half saturated (5)
C. **Methods of use**
   1. **Ferric chloride, either type**
      a. Add 4–5 drops of FeCl$_3$ **directly** to an 18- to 24-h incubated tube. If the tube is inoculated heavily, a 4-h incubation should suffice (2).
      b. **Gently** rotate the tube to loosen the growth.
      c. A positive green color reaction occurs within 1–5 min on the slant and in the syneresis fluid (8).
   2. **Ferric ammonium sulfate** (5)
      a. Acidify with 10% sulfuric acid (H$_2$SO$_4$), using phenol red as an indicator.

         Alkaline: red

         Acid: yellow

      b. Add 4–5 drops of half-saturated ferric ammonium sulfate.
      c. Shake tube **gently**.
      d. A positive green color reaction occurs within 1 min.
   3. Either reagent: interpret reaction **immediately**, because the color is unstable and fades quickly (5, 19).
D. Quality control: reagents **must** be tested with known positive and negative cultures before being put into general use.
E. Storage: store reagents in a refrigerator (4°C) when not in use. These reagents should be placed in **dark bottles** to avoid exposure to light. Their stability varies; therefore, each week they should be given a quality control check and discarded when yielding a negative or weak reaction with a known positive organism.
F. Chemistry of reagent action: since phenylalanine is deaminated, the color produced by addition of 10% FeCl$_3$ is due to formation of a keto acid, phenylpyruvic acid (19). Henecka (13) showed that α- and β-keto acids give a positive color reaction with either an alcoholic or aqueous solution of FeCl$_3$. Phenylpyruvic acid is an α-keto acid.

Singer and Volcani (19) attribute a positive $FeCl_3$ reaction to formation of a hydrazone. A hydrazine ($RNHNH_2$) is an ammonia derivative added to a carbonyl group; one of the hydrogens is bound to oxygen, while a nitrogen is bound to a carbon atom (17). When an aldehyde or a ketone is condensed with a hydrazine, a hydrazone or hydrazone-type compound (an unsaturated nitrogen-containing derivative) is produced, and water is eliminated (10, 11, 17).

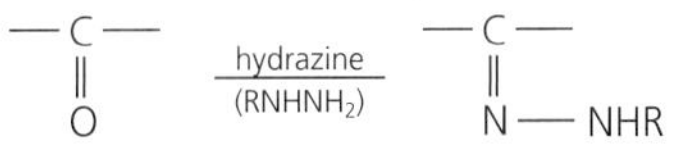

Ketone Hydrazone

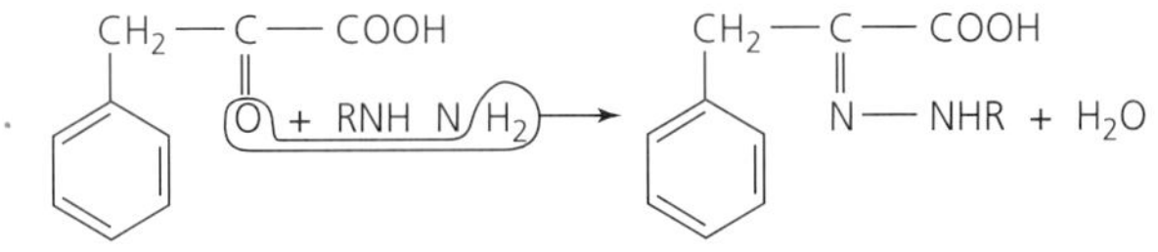

Phenylpyruvic acid Hydrazine Phenylhydrazone

The guanidine nucleus in peptone $[C(NH)(NH_2)_2]$ is an ammonia and hydrazine derivative of carbonic acid (1). Ketone-type compounds are colorless, but if a keto group (C=O) is conjugated with another keto group or with –C–C– or other double bonds, color may result (17).

$FeCl_3$ is an oxidizing agent, and in an acid solution with hydrazine, the ferric ion (Fe^{3+}) will form (via a hydrazone) nitrogen and ammonia as its end products (1), reducing the ferric ion.

$$N_2H_5^+ + Fe^{+++} \longrightarrow NH_4^+ + \tfrac{1}{2} N_2 + H^+ + Fe^{++}$$

$FeCl_3$ is a chelating agent; it chelates with phenylpyruvic acid to form a green color (11). Exposing a phenylalanine culture tube to atmospheric oxygen after addition of $FeCl_3$, increases the rate of production and the strength of a positive reaction (14).

VI. QUALITY CONTROL ORGANISMS

A. Positive (+): *Proteus vulgaris* ATCC 13315

B. Negative (−):

Escherichia coli ATCC 11775

Uninoculated

VII. RESULTS

See Figure 34.1 (Appendix 1) for colored photographic results

VIII. INTERPRETATION

A. Positive result (+): light to deep green color on the slant and in the syneresis fluid (6)

B. Negative result (−): no color change; remains yellow because of the color of the $FeCl_3$ reagent

IX. ALTERNATIVE TESTS

A. **Phenylalanine-Malonate Broth Medium**
   1. Formulation of Shaw and Clark (18); combined phenylalanine medium of Buttiaux, Osteux, Fresnoy, and Moriamex (3), later modified by Ewing (7), and malonate medium of Leifson (16), later modified by Ewing, Davis and Reaves (9)
   2. Differentiates by ability to use sodium malonate and carbon source and/or deaminate phenylalanine to phenylpyruvic acid
   3. Ingredients; pH 6.3

Yeast extract	1.0 g
DL-phenylalanine	2.0 g
Sodium malonate	3.0 g
Sodium chloride, NaCl	2.0 g
Ammonium sulfate, $(NH_4)_2SO_4$	2.0 g
Dipotassium phosphate, K_2HPO_4	0.6 g
Monopotassium phosphate, KH_2PO_4	0.4 g
Bromthymol blue (BTB)	
Deionized water	1000 mL

   4. pH indicator: bromthymol blue
      a. Acid: pH 6.0, yellow
      b. Alkaline: pH 7.6, deep Prussian blue
   5. Dispense: screw-cap tubes; 6–8 mL/tube (16 × 125 mL)
   6. Sterilization: autoclave, 121°C, 15 lb, **10 min**
   7. Inoculation: growth from an 18- to 24-h **pure** culture; **heavy** inoculum
   8. Incubation: aerobically, 35°C, 18–24 h
   9. Interpretation (*Note:* first test for malonate utilization)
      a. **Malonate**
         (1) Positive (+): dark blue color; alkaline reaction
         (2) Negative (−): no change; medium remains light green
      b. **Phenylalanine**
         (1) Add ferric chloride reagent **prior to** interpretation; $FeCl_3$, 0.8 g/10 mL sterile distilled water; to slant add
            (a) $FeCl_3$ solution, 8%: 3–5 drops
            (b) HCl_3, 0.1 N: 3–5 drops
         (2) Positive (+)
            (a) Immediate intense dark green color
            (b) Phenylalanine deaminated to phenylpyruvic acid
         (3) Negative (−): Yellow color

B. **Commercial disks or tablets** (*Note:* follow manufacturer's directions)
   1. Key IPA tablets
      a. Manufacturer: Key Scientific Products
      b. Determines two biochemical reactions: indole and phenylalanine
   2. Urea-PDA Disk
      a. Manufacturer: REMEL
      b. Determines two biochemical reactions: phenylalanine deaminase and urease
   3. Minitek disks
      a. Manufacturer: BD Biosciences
      b. Phenylalanine deaminase

X. PRECAUTIONS

A. A positive phenylalanine result **must** be interpreted immediately after addition of the $FeCl_3$ reagent, because the green color fades quickly (20). An interpretation of either positive or negative must be made within the first 5 min. Rolling the $FeCl_3$ over the slant helps to obtain a faster reaction with a more pronounced color.
B. The letters *PA* are often used by laboratories to denote phenylalanine medium. However, *PA* can also stand for peptone agar, and peptone and phenylalanine agars appear identical. If in doubt about which medium *PA* represents, run a quality control with a known positive phenylalanine organism before putting the medium into general use.
C. Meat extracts or protein hydrolysates **cannot** be used for medium preparation because they vary naturally in phenylalanine content (15).

REFERENCES

1. Audrieth LF, Ackerson B. The Chemistry of Hydrazine. New York: John Wiley & Sons, 1951: 214–215.
2. BBL Manual of Products and Laboratory Procedures ed 6. Cockeysville, MD: BBL Microbiology Systems, Division of Becton Dickinson and Company, 1988.
3. Buttiaux R, Osteux R, Fresnoy R, Moriamez J. Les propriétés biochimiques caracteristiques du genre *Proteus*. Inclusion sorihaitable des Providencia dans celui-ci. Ann Inst Pasteur Lille 1954;87(4):375–386.
4. Cantarow A, Schepartz B. Biochemistry, ed 3. Philadelphia: WB Saunders, 1962:584–585.
5. Cowan ST. Cowan & Steel's Manual for the Identification of Medical Bacteria, ed 2. Cambridge: Cambridge University Press, 1974:39–40, 152.
6. Difco Supplementary Literature. Detroit: Difco Laboratories, 1968:280.
7. Ewing WH. *Enterobacteriaceae:* Biochemical method for group differentiation. Public Health Service publ. no. 743. Washington, DC: US Government Printing Office, 1962:19.
8. Ewing WH. Edwards and Ewing's Identification of *Enterobacteriaceae*, ed 4. New York: Elsevier, 1986:253.
9. Ewing WH, Davis BR, Reavis RW. Phenylalanine and malonate media and their use in enteric bacteriology. Public Health Lab 1957;15: 153–161.
10. Fieser LF, Fieser M. Organic Chemistry, ed 3. New York: Reinhold, 1956:211.
11. Handbook of Clinical Laboratory Data, ed 2. Cleveland: Chemical Rubber Company, 1958: 321.
12. Harrow B, Mazur A. Textbook of Biochemistry, ed 9. Philadelphia: WB Saunders, 1966:405.
13. Henecka H. Chemie der-Beta-Decarbonyl-Verbindungen. Berlin: Springer, 1950:110–129.
14. Henriksen SD, Closs K. The production of phenylpyruvic acid by bacteria. Acta Pathol Microbiol Scand 1938;15:101–113.
15. Koneman EW, Allen SD, Janda WM, et al. Color Atlas & Textbook of Diagnostic Microbiology, ed 5. Philadelphia: JB Lippincott, 1997:187, 1375.
16. Leifson E. Fermentation of sodium malonate as a means of differentiating *Aerobacter* and *Escherichia*. J Bacteriol 1933;26:329–330.
17. Nussenbaum S. Organic Chemistry. Boston: Allyn & Bacon, 1963:351, 358, 597.
18. Shaw C, Clarke PH. Biochemical classification of *Proteus* and *Providencia* cultures. J Gen Microbiol 1955;13(1):155–161.
19. Singer J, Volcani BE. An improved ferric chloride test for differentiating *Proteus-Providencia* group from other *Enterobacteriaceae*. J Bacteriol 1955;69(3):303–306.
20. Smith DT, Conant NF, Willett HP. Zinsser's Microbiology, ed 14. New York: Appleton-Century-Crofts, 1968:117.

35 Phosphatase Test

I. PRINCIPLE

To determine the ability of an organism to produce sufficient phosphatase enzyme to split phenolphthalein diphosphate (PDP)

II. PURPOSE

(Also see Chapters 43 and 44)

A. **PDP media**
   1. Initially, primarily to determine pathogenic strains of *Staphylococcus* spp. (coagulase-positive *Staphylococcus aureus* subsp. *aureus*)
   2. To differentiate species
      a. *Actinobacillus muris* (−) and *A. seminis* (−) from other *Actinobacillus* spp. (+) most frequently isolated
      b. *Haemophilus haemoglobinophilus* (−) from other *Haemophilus* spp. (+)
      c. *Pasteurella testudinis* (−) from other *Pasteurella* spp. (+)
      d. *Kurthia zopfii* (−) from *K. gibsonii* (+) and *K. sibirica* (+)
      e. *Corynebacterium diphtheriae* subsp. *gravis* (+) from other *Corynebacterium* spp. (−)
   3. To differentiate predominate constituents of oral mycoplasma flora, *Mycoplasma salivarium* (+) from *M. orale* (−) (19)
B. **Methyl green phosphatase test (MGP)**: to differentiate members of the *Enterobacteriaceae* (+) from other Gram-negative intestinal bacteria (−) (15–18)

III. BIOCHEMISTRY INVOLVED

Phosphatase production is determined by liberation of phenolphthalein, indicated by a color change in the medium (11). The liberated phenolphthalein reacts with an alkali to give a bright pink-red color.

$$\text{Phenolphthalein diphosphate (sodium salt)} \xrightarrow{\text{phosphatase}} \text{Free phenolphthalein} \quad (1)$$

$$\text{Phenolphthalein} + \text{alkali (NaOH or NH}_3\text{)} \longrightarrow \text{Bright pink-red color} \quad (2)$$

Phthalein is a compound of phthalic anhydride with a phenol or phenolic derivative (5) containing a five-sided lactone ring. Phthalic anhydride combined with two molecules of phenol makes the compound phenolphthalein.

[Reaction scheme: Phthalic anhydride + 2 Phenol → Phenolphthalein]

When phenolphthalein is neutralized, the alkali attaches to the C=O group, breaking the lactone ring and forming a quinoid in one of the benzene rings (5).

[Structures: Benzine ring C_6H_6; Quinoid structure (quinone) $C_6H_4O_2$; Lactone ring (five sided)]

[Reaction: Phenolphthalein (colorless in acid) $C_{20}H_{14}O_4$ + NaOH → Phenolphthalein (red in alkaline) $C_{20}H_{13}O_4$]

Certain fundamental radicals known as **chromophores** are responsible for the color produced by certain compounds: C=C, C=O, C=S, C=N, N=N, N=O, and NO_2 (5). The more of these groups in the same compound, the more intense is the color produced (5).

In benzene compounds, the chromophore radicals are termed **chromogens**, colored compounds but not dyes, since they have no affinity for tissue or fibers (5). In phenolphthalein the chromogen has the quinoid (or quinone) structure containing two C=O groups. The quinoid structure gives the compound a pink-red color; however, this color disappears if the solution is again acidified, because of loss of the quinoid structure and reestablishment of the phenolic form (5).

Phenolphthalein is capable of salt formation, usually the sodium salt, which is more stable (2). **Auxochromes** are the salt-forming group of dyes and chromogens, either acidic or basic (5). The acidic carboxyl group (–COOH) of phenolphthalein is present but in a sodium salt as –COONa, the characteristic auxochrome. Phenolphthalein is primarily used as an acid-base indicator; it is colorless in an acid or neutral environment and pink to red when alkaline (5). However, be aware that this indicator has a variety of colors, depending upon the pH (4, 12).

Phenolphthalein Color Range (10)

(Redrawn from Nussenbaum, S. *Organic Chemistry: Principles and Applications,* p. 458, 1963, with permission of Allyn and Bacon, Inc., Boston.)

IV. MEDIA EMPLOYED: PHENOLPHTHALEIN DIPHOSPHATE MEDIUM (PDP)

A. **Phenolphthalein substrate**
   1. Manufacturer: Sigma-Aldrich (see Appendix 11)
   2. Ingredients; 0.5% concentration

Phenolphthalein diphosphate sodium salt, PDP	0.5 g
Distilled or deionized water	100.0 mL

   3. Method of sterilization (4): filtration (Millipore or Seitz), membrane filter, 0.22 μm
   4. Storage: −20°C

B. **Media**; two choices
   1. **PDP nutrient broth** (3, 7)
      a. Ingredients, pH 7.5

Beef extract	3.0 g
Peptone	5.0 g
Deionized water	1000.0 mL

  b. Commercial products available: BBL, Difco
  c. Method of preparation
     (1) Weigh out amount accurately as directed on the label.
     (2) Rehydrate with distilled or demineralized water.
     (3) Heat **gently** into solution.
     (4) Dispense approximately 3.0 mL per tube (13 × 100 mm).
  d. Method of sterilization: autoclave, 115°C, 15 lb, 15 min
  e. Cool before use and refrigerate for storage (4–10°C).
  f. Just prior to use add 0.5% PDP solution.
     (1) **Aseptically**
     (2) One drop (0.05 mL) to each tube (4, 11)
     (3) Mix **gently**; agitate the bottom of the tube back and forth with your fingers.
  g. Inoculation
     (1) Simultaneously, two tubes for each organism being tested.
     (2) Label tubes A and B.
     (3) Growth from an 18- to 24-h **pure** culture
     (4) **Heavy** inoculum
  h. Incubation, **both** tubes: 35°C, 6 h
  i. **After** incubation, add sodium hydroxide (NaOH) **before** attempting to make an interpretation.
2. **PDP nutrient agar** (3, 7, 11)
  a. Ingredients, pH 7.3; 1.5%

Beef extract	3.0 g
Peptone	5.0 g
Sodium chloride, NaCl	8.0 g
Agar	15.0 g
Deionized water	1000.0 mL

  b. Commercial products available: BBL, Difco
  c. Method of preparation
     (1) Weigh out amount accurately as directed on the label.
     (2) Rehydrate with distilled or demineralized water.
     (3) Heat **gently** into solution.
  d. Method of sterilization: autoclave, 115°C, 15 lb, 15 min
  e. Cool to 45–50°C.
     (1) Water bath, 37°C
     (2) Watch temperature drop closely to avoid resolidification.
  f. Add substrate
     (1) **Aseptically**
     (2) Final dilution: 1/10,000
        (a) PDP sodium salt, 5%, 2.0–20.0 mL
        (b) Melted nutrient agar, 45–50°C, 98.0–980.0 mL
     (3) Mix **gently**.
        (a) Swirl flask slowly.
        (b) Avoid formation of bubbles.
  g. **Aseptically** pour into Petri dishes, approximately 12–15 mL per plate
  h. Cool before use and refrigerate for storage (4–10°C).
     (1) Cool: upright position (**lid up**)

(2) Store: inverted position (**lid down**)
  i. Inoculation
     (1) Growth from an 18- to 24-h **pure** culture
     (2) **Light** inoculum (6)
     (3) Streak for isolation (discrete colonies) (6).
  j. Incubation: 35°C, 18–24 h (2); inverted position, **lid on bottom**

According to studies by Baird-Parker (1), more positive cultures are obtained when incubation is extended to 3–5 days at 30°C.

  k. **After** incubation, expose colonies to ammonia vapor **before** attempting to interpret.

V. REAGENTS

A. **10 N Sodium hydroxide (NaOH) (40%)**
  1. Ingredients

     NaOH, carbonate free, R.G.   40.0 g
     Deionized water   100.0 mL
  2. Method of preparation
     a. **Rapidly** weigh the NaOH and dissolve in less than 100 mL of distilled water in a beaker. This reagent is highly hygroscopic.
     b. Place beaker in a circulating cold water bath to control the temperature.
     c. Cool and transfer the NaOH solution to a 100-mL volumetric flask and bring to 100 mL with distilled water.
     d. Store in a polyethylene or paraffin-lined glass reagent bottle.
  3. Method of utilization
     a. **Broth** tubed medium
     b. After incubation, add 1 drop of 40% NaOH to tube A.
        (1) If positive, record results.
        (2) If negative, continue incubation of tube B; 35°C, 18–24 h
           (a) Add reagent to tube B.
           (b) Record results.

B. **Ammonia vapor (NH_3)**
  1. Concentrated ammonium hydroxide (NH_4OH), specific gravity 0.880
  2. Method of utilization
     a. **Plate** medium
     b. Two methods; exposure of colonies to ammonia vapors
        (1) Hold growth **over** an open bottle of ammonia vapor.
        (2) Add 1.0 mL of ammonia to lid of Petri dish and **invert medium above it. Sodium hydroxide and ammonium hydroxide are both extremely caustic, so avoid exposure to skin, as painful burns may occur.**

VI. QUALITY CONTROL ORGANISMS

A. Positive (+)

Staphylococcus aureus subsp. *aureus*   ATCC 25923
Staphylococcus epidermidis   ATCC 12228

B. Negative (−)

Staphylococcus saprophyticus   ATCC 15305
Staphylococcus hominis   ATCC 27844

VII. INTERPRETATION (2): EITHER REAGENT

A. Positive (+): bright pink-red colored broth or colonies
B. Negative (−): no color change; broth or colonies remain clear or white.

According to Lewis (11), the tube and plate methods are equally sensitive for coagulase-positive staphylococci. However, his studies showed that the plate method gives **no** indication of pathogenic strains, but is better than the broth method for coagulase-negative staphylococci, while the broth method showed fewer phosphatase-positive coagulase-negative strains. The broth procedure can be used for phosphatase and coagulase testing (8).

VIII. ALTERNATE MEDIA/PROCEDURES

A. **Phosphate blood agar (PDPBA)**
   1. Useful as a differentiation medium for screening staphylococcal isolates
   2. Base: Columbia agar: BBL, Difco
      a. From scratch, base ingredients:

Casein/meat (50/50) peptone	10.0 g
Casein/yeast (50/50) peptone	10.0 g
Heart peptone	3.0 g
Sodium chloride, NaCl	5.0 g
Corn starch	1.0 g
Agar	13.5 g
Deionized water	1000.0 mL

      b. Substrate: phenolphthalein diphosphate tetrasodium salt (Sigma-Aldrich)
         (1) Sterilized by membrane filtration and added at 1:10 dilution to sterile (autoclaved) and cooled (50°C) agar base.
      c. Final medium

Columbia agar base	4%
Defibrinated **sterile** sheep blood	5%
Phenolphthalein diphosphate tetrasodium salt	0.05%

      d. Dispense 15–20 mL/Petri dish.
B. **Methyl green phosphate (MGP) procedure** (15–18)
   1. Procedure of Satta et al. (16); originally developed for identification of Gram-positive bacteria; modified to work well with Gram-negative *Enterobacteriaceae* (16).
   2. **Dye**: methyl green (MG)
      a. Manufacturer: Carlo Erba, Milan, Italy
      b. Sterilized by Seitz filter, 0.22-μm pore size
      c. 50 μg/mL
   3. **Phosphate substrates**: three choices; 500 μg/mL
      a. Phenolphthalein diphosphate (PDP), 0.5 M
      b. Phenolphthalein monophosphate (PMP)
      c. 6-Benzylnaphthyl phosphate (6-BNP)
   4. **Medium**: Tryptose phosphate agar (TPA)
      a. Difco: Tryptose phosphate broth (TPB)
      b. Add 15.0 g agar/L medium.
      a. Cool prepared TPA to 44°C and add methyl green and desired phosphate substrate.
   5. Dispense: 20 mL/Petri dish
   6. Inoculum: isolated colonies picked and deposited on agar surface
   7. Incubation: 35°C, 24 h
   8. Interpretation

a. Positive (+)
   (1) **Any** colonies exhibiting **any blue-green color; due to bacterial phosphatase activity** (17).
   (2) **Any** blue-green staining of agar surrounding colonies or beneath colony itself is recorded as a halo (17). Enzyme released in medium by growing bacteria accounts for stained halos (15).

Double strength agar is used to prevent swarming of *Proteus* spp. (15). Sensitivities of procedure for Gram-negative bacteria vary with different phosphate substrates (15). Higher sensitivity with PMP and even better with 6-BNP when either are substituted for conventional PDP (15). According to Satta et al. (16), all strains of *Enterobacteriaceae* except some *Leminorella richardii* formed green-stained colonies. Strains of intestinal Gram-negative bacteria *Acinetobacter calcoaceticus*, *Alcaligenes faecalis*, *Pseudomonas aeruginosa*, and other pseudomonads that grow on MacConkey (MAC) agar and ferment glucose were all phosphatase negative and all failed to produce stained colonies on MGP (17).

Extracellular activity is readily detected by methyl green phosphatase procedure but **not** by conventional tests (15). *Proteeae* strains produce both an exocellular and an intracellular phosphatase (17). *Morganella morganii* and *Providencia stuartii* have much higher intracellular activity than all other members of the *Enterobacteriaceae*; these are readily detected by MGP but **not** by conventional tests (17).

C. **Hydrolysis of *p*-nitrophenylphosphate (PNP)**
   1. Colorless PNP acted upon by alkaline phosphatase to yield inorganic phosphate (P_i) and yellow *p*-nitrophenol.
   2. Several procedures for phosphatase reaction of coagulase-negative staphylococci
      a. Procedure of Penny and Huddy (13)
         (1) 0.5 mL 0.1% PNP per tube
         (2) **Heavy** inoculum from blood agar
         (3) Positive: yellow color within 4 h; liberation of *p*-nitrophenol. *S. aureus* subsp. *aureus*, *S. hyicus*, *S. intermedius*, *S. schleiferi*, and most strains of *S. epidermidis* are positive for alkaline phosphatase.
      b. Procedure of Geary and Stevens, PNP agar (8)
         (1) Muller-Hinton agar buffered to pH 5.6–5.8 with addition of 0.495 mg/mL PNP
         (2) Spot inoculated and incubated 18–24 h
         (3) Positive: bright yellow color under and around inoculum
D. **Spot test** (14)
   1. Primary purpose: identification of coagulase-negative *S. saprophyticus* (+) from *S. epidermidis* (−) in urine cultures. Procedure recommended by Pickett (14) for urine cultures to identify *S. saprophyticus*; organism is second to coliforms as the most common cause of acute urethral syndrome in women (10, 21).
   2. Inoculum: colony from PDP blood agar
      a. Colony that appears to be a staphylococcal isolate
      b. **First** perform catalase and coagulase tests.
      c. Filter paper saturated with 1 N NaOH
      d. Colony removed and touched to filter paper
   3. Results
      a. Positive (+)
         (1) Bright pink within seconds; free phenolphthalein
         (2) *S. epidermidis*
      b. Negative (−)
         (1) No color

(2) *S. saprophyticus.* Identification based on a negative phosphatase result along with resistance to a 5-μg novobiocin disc (<17 mm) (14).

Major advantage is the elimination of *S. epidermidis,* which usually has no clinical significance in urine cultures (14).

E. **Commercial tablets/disks**
   1. Alkaline phosphatase tablets (PO_4) or PNP: Key Scientific Company
   2. Phosphate disks: BBL

IX. PRECAUTIONS

A. The color produced by the indicator phenolphthalein varies with the pH (4). Add reagents in their correct quantities because too little or an excess of alkali may give false-positive or false-negative results.
B. Colonies tested for phosphatase production with ammonia vapor are viable for a very short period and any required subculturing should be done **immediately** after recording results (4).
C. Try to avoid labeling the two broth tubes *tube 1* and *tube 2* when they are set up simultaneously on a single organism; when most laboratories log in their specimens they give them a working laboratory number. Use of *A* and *B* or other comparable letters avoids the possibility of confusing the laboratory specimen number with the tube number.
D. The broth method can only be used after the organism has been isolated in **pure** culture (11).
E. The phosphatase test for the determination of *Staphylococcus* pathogenicity **must not** be confused with the phosphatase test used to determine the effect of pasteurization on milk; the two tests are not the same (6).
F. PDP is relatively **unstable.** Degradation may occur in media or original substance if not stored at −20°C, dissociating phenolphthalein phosphate and giving false-positive results
G. Soro et al. (20) showed phosphatase activity to be a property of **all** *Staphylococcus* spp. whose strains are most frequently isolated from human origin. Production of phosphatase is affected by pH and presence of P_i in growth medium (9). Soro et al. (20) found that **all** strains of *Staphylococcus* were phosphatase positive at pH 8.0 when grown without P_i; however, when grown on medium supplemented with 0.3% P_i at low or high pH, **only** *S. aureus* subsp. *aureus,* most *S. epidermidis,* and *S. xylosus* were phosphatase positive, and none of the other *Staphylococcus* spp. tested were phosphatase positive (20). The phosphatases of various staphylococci have different properties. (20). The activity is constitutive in some species and repressed by phosphatase in others (20).

REFERENCES

1. Baird-Parker AC. A classification of micrococci and staphylococci based on physiological and biochemical tests. J Gen Microbiol 1963;30(3):409–427.
2. Barber M, Kuper SWA. Identification of *Staphylococcus pyogenes* by the phosphatase reaction. J Pathol Bacteriol 1951;63(1):65–68.
3. BBL Manual of Products and Laboratory Procedures, ed 6. Cockeysville, MD: BBL Microbiology Systems, Division of Becton Dickinson and Company, 1988.
4. Branson D. Methods in Clinical Bacteriology. Springfield, IL: Charles C Thomas, 1972:43–44.
5. Conn HJ, Lillie RD, eds. HJ Conn's Biological Stains, ed 9. Baltimore: Williams & Wilkins, 1977:21, 307.
6. Difco Manual, ed 10. Detroit: Difco Laboratories, 1984:29, 127.
7. Edwards PR, Ewing WH. Identification of Enterobacteriaceae, ed 3. Minneapolis: Burgess, 1972.
8. Geary C, Stevens M. Detection of phosphatase production by *Staphylococcus* species. Med Lab Sci 1991;48:99–105.
9. Koneman EW, Allen SD, Janda WM, et al. Color Atlas & Textbook of Diagnostic Microbiology, ed 5. Philadelphia: JB Lippincott, 1997:555.
10. Latham RH, Running HK, Stamm WE. Urinary tract infections in young adult women caused by

Staphylococcus saprophyticus. JAMA 1983;250: 3063–3066.
11. Lewis B. Phosphatase production by staphylococci—a comparison of two methods. J Med Lab Technol 1961;18:112–113.
12. Nussenbaum S. Organic Chemistry. Boston, Allyn & Bacon, 1963:458.
13. Penny CA, Huddy RB. Phosphatase reaction of coagulase-negative staphylococci and micrococci. J Pathol Bacteriol 1967;93:685–688.
14. Pickett DA, Welch DF. Recognition of *Staphylococcus saprophyticus* in urine cultures by screening colonies for production of phosphatase. J Clin Microbiol 1985;21(3):310–313.
15. Pompei R, Cornaglia G, Ingianni A, Satta G. Use of a novel phosphatase test for simplified identification of species of the tribe *Proteeae*. J Clin Microbiol 1990;28(6):1214–1218.
16. Satta G, Grazi G, Varaldo PE, Fontana R. Detection of bacterial phosphatase activity by means of an original and simple test. J Clin Pathol 1979;32:391–395.
17. Satta G, Pompei R, Grazi G, Cornaglia G. Phosphatase activity is a constant of all isolates of all major species of the family *Enterobacteriaceae*. J Clin Microbiol 1988;26(12):2637–2641.
18. Satta G, Pompei R, Ingianni A. The selective staining mechanism of phosphatase producing colonies in the diphosphate-phenolphthalein-methyl green method for the detection of bacterial phosphatase activity. Microbiologica 1984; 7:159–170.
19. Shibata K-I, Totsuka M, Watanabe T. Phosphatase activity as a criterion for differentiation of oral mycoplasmas. J Clin Microbiol 1986; 23(5):970–972.
20. Soro O, Grazi G, Varaldo PE, Satta G. Phosphatase activity of staphylococci is constitutive in some species and repressed by phosphatase in others. J Clin Microbiol 1990;28(12):2707–2710.
21. Stamm WE, Wagner KF, Amsel R, et al. Causes of the acute urethral syndrome in women. N Engl J Med 1980;303:409–415.

36 Porphyrin-δ-Aminolevulinic Acid (ALA) Test

I. PRINCIPLE

To test whether non-hemin-requiring *Haemophilus* species have the enzyme necessary to synthesize heme precursors from δ-(delta)-aminolevulinic acid (ALA); detection of porphyrin synthesis (3)

II. PURPOSE

Speciation of *Haemophilus* species

III. BIOCHEMISTRY INVOLVED

Most *Haemophilus* spp. require X factor, V factor, or both for growth.

X Factor

The X factor is hemin (also called *protoporphyrin*), a heat-stable compound that is necessary for synthesizing respiratory enzymes. Some species of *Haemophilus* lack the enzyme necessary to convert ALA to protoporphyrin and are X dependent (7).

ALA

The ALA test originally described by Kilian (3) detects the ability of *Haemophilus* strains to synthesize protoporphyrin intermediates in the biosynthetic pathway to hemin from the precursor ALA (4). ALA is the precursor for porphobilinogen, porphyrins, and heme; enzyme porphobilinogen synthase converts ALA into porphobilinogen with no requirement for heme factor X for growth. Two molecules of ALA are condensed to form the pyrrole-ringed compound porphobilinogen (PGB).

Two molecules of δ-aminolevulinate → (ALA Dehydratase, −2H$_2$O) → Porphobilinogen (first precursor pyrrole) (6)

Next, four molecules of PGB combine to form uroporphyrinogen, which subsequently undergoes side-chain substitution to form coproporphyrinogen and protoporphyrin IV. Protoporphyrin IV is the immediate precursor of the heme moiety (5). Through oxidation, uroporphyrin and coproporphyrin are formed as byproducts of the reaction (5).

IV. TEST PROCEDURES; TWO CHOICES

A. **ALA enzyme substrate solution** (1)
 1. Ingredients

δ-Aminolevulinic acid hydrochloride (Sigma Co), (2 mol/L)	0.34 g
Magnesium sulfate, $MgSO_4$ (0.08 mol/L)	0.0096 g
Phosphate buffer, (0.1 mol/L), pH 6.9	1000.0 mL

 2. Dispense
    a. Small, plastic snap-top tubes (12 × 75 mm)
    b. 0.5 mL/tube

The magnesium sulfate **must** be prepared in a more concentrated solution and diluted to the desired final concentration.

B. **ALA Disk**
 1. Manufacturer: REMEL.
 2. Rapid detection of porphobilinogens and porphyrins
 3. Method of use; follow manufacturer's directions.
    a. Rehydrate disk.
       (1) Remove from manufacturer's vial only the number of disks being used at one time and bring to room temperature **before** use.
       (2) Place "A" side of disk down directly on agar surface or in **sterile** Petri dish.
       (3) Rehydrate with 40 µL of **sterile** water. **Do not** oversaturate disk.
 4. Inoculum
    a. **Heavy** inoculum of an isolated 18- to 24-h colony of **suspected** *Haemophilus* sp.
    b. Place filter paper, moistened with **sterile** water, in lid of specimen container to keep disk moist.
 5. Incubation: 35°C
 6. Results: examine disk for red fluorescence at 1 h and up to 6 h in a darkened room with long-wave ultraviolet light (Wood's lamp); approximately 360 nm.
 7. Chemistry of reaction: various porphyrinogens are colorless; whereas, various porphyrins when dissolved in strong mineral acids or organic solvents and illuminated by ultraviolet light emit a strong red fluorescence (6). The double bonds in the porphyrins are responsible for characteristic absorption and fluorescence (6).

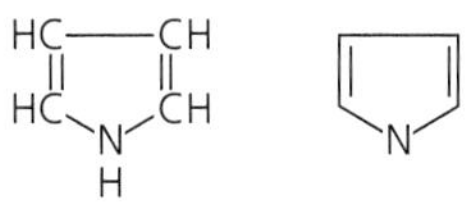

Pyrrole

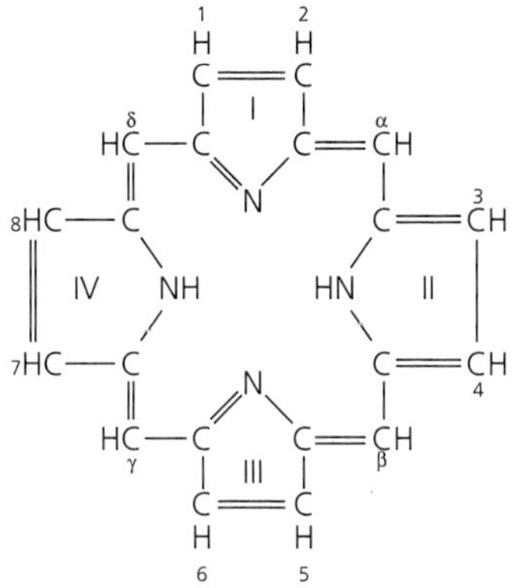

Porphin
($C_{20}H_{14}N_4$)

The porphin molecule. Rings are labeled I, II, III, IV.
Substituent positions on rings are labeled 1, 2, 3, 4, 5, 6, 7, 8.
Methenyl bridges are labeled α, β, γ, δ. (6)

Reduction (by addition of hydrogen) of the methenyl (–HC=) bridges to methylene (–CH$_2$–) leads to formation of colorless compounds termed *porphyrinogens* (6).

8. Storage
    a. ALA solution: −20°C until use
    b. ALA disk: in original container, 2–8°C; protected from light

V. QUALITY CONTROL ORGANISMS

A. Positive (+): *Haemophilus parahaemolyticus*   ATCC 10014
B. Negative (−): *Haemophilus influenzae*   ATCC 10211

VI. RESULTS

See Figure 36.1 (Appendix 1) for photographic results

VII. INTERPRETATIONS

A. Positive (+)
   1. **ALA solution**: development of a brick red to orange fluorescence in lower aqueous phase under ultraviolet light (Wood's lamp)
   2. **ALA disk**: development of an red-orange fluorescence under ultraviolet light

3. Presence of porphyrins
4. *Haemophilus* strains that **do not** require exogenous X factor for growth possess enzymes that synthesize protoporphyrin compounds from ALA (4).

B. Negative (−)
1. No color change either in reagent layer or on disk when examined under ultraviolet light
2. Cannot synthesize heme
3. *Haemophilus* strains that **require** exogenous X factor for growth cannot synthesize protoporphyrins from ALA (4).

VIII. PRECAUTIONS

A. **General**
1. Fluorescence observations **must** be made in a darkened room or black box.
2. Oxidase-positive and catalase-positive bacteria commonly found in the oropharynx can make heme and heme precursors from ALA and thus yield false-positive results. The morphology of the organism being tested must be consistent with *Haemophilus* spp. (2). Also, organisms that give a strong oxidase or catalase-positive reaction may give a false-positive result because such organisms make heme and its precursors from ALA in the process of synthesizing oxidase and catalase. Test **only** *Haemophilus* spp. with ALA.
3. **Always test** fresh subcultures of quality control microorganisms each time test is performed (1).
4. Cultures being tested **must not** be older than 24 h.
5. Inoculum **must** be heavy; the heavier the better.

B. **ALA disk**
1. Store in original container at 2–8°C and protect from light; substrate is highly light sensitive.
2. *Haemophilus* spp. being tested should be 18–24 h old, no older.
3. Protect disks from moisture; remove only the number of disks needed. Let disks come to room temperature (22–25°C) **before** use.
4. **Do not** use disks if (*a*) color changes from white (*b*) expiration date has expired, or (*c*) desiccant in vial has changed from blue to pink.

REFERENCES

1. Baron EJ, Peterson LR, Finegold SM. Bailey & Scott's Diagnostic Microbiology, ed 9. St. Louis: CV Mosby, 1994:415–417.
2. Gadbury JL, Amos MA. Comparison of a new commercially prepared porphyrin test and the conventional satellite test for the identification of *Haemophilus* species that require the X factor. J Clin Microbiol 1986;23(3):637–639.
3. Kilian M. A rapid method for the differentiation of *Haemophilus* strains. Acta Pathol Microbiol Scand Sect B 1974;82:835–842.
4. Koneman EW, Allen SD, Janda WM, et al. Color Atlas & Textbook of Diagnostic Microbiology, ed 5. Philadelphia: JB Lippincott, 1997:379.
5. Lund ME, Blazevic DJ. Rapid speciation of *Haemophilus* with the porphyrin production test versus the satellite test for X. J Clin Microbiol 1977;5(2):142–144.
6. Murray RK, Granner DK, Mayes PA, Rodwell VW. Harper's Biochemistry, ed. 21. San Mateo, CA: 1988:319–325.
7. White DC, Granick S. Hemin biosynthesis in *Haemophilus*. J Bacteriol 1963;85:842–850.

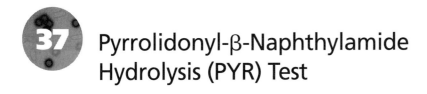

37 Pyrrolidonyl-β-Naphthylamide Hydrolysis (PYR) Test

I. PRINCIPLE

To detect the presence of enzyme L-pyrrolidonyl arylamidase (PYR)

II. PURPOSE

PYR test is a modification of test described by Godsey, Schulman, and Enriquez (4).

A. Specific presumptive test for both group A β-hemolytic streptococci (*S. pyogenes*) and most group D *Enterococcus* spp.; differentiates group A streptococci from other *Streptococcus* spp. Highly sensitive test; replaces bacitracin and salt tolerance (growth in 6.5% NaCl) (3)
B. Preliminary characterization of *Streptococcus, Enterococcus,* and streptococcus-like organisms. PYR is often used in conjunction with leucine aminopeptidase (LAP) and other biochemical tests (6) (Table 37.1).

Table 37.1. Characteristics of *Streptococcus, Enterococcus,* and Streptococcus-like Organisms (3)

Organism	Catalase	LAP	PYR	Esculin Hydrolysis	Growth in 6.5% NaCl	Vancomycin
β-*Streptococcus*						
S. pneumoniae	−	+	V	V	−	S
S. pyogenes, Group A	−	+	+	+	−	S
Other β-*Streptococcus* spp.	−	−	−	−	−	S
Enterococcus spp., group D.	−	+	+	+	V+	S
Aerococcus						
A. viridans	−	−	+	V	+	S
A. urinae	−	+	−	V	+	S
Alloiococcus otitis	+	+	+	−	+[a]	S
Gemella						
G. hemolysans	−	V	+	−	−	S
G. morbillorum	−	+	+[wb]	−	−	S
Globicatella sanguis	−	−	+	V	+	S
Helcococcus kunzii	−	−	+	+	V	S
Lactococcus spp.	−	+	+	+	−	S
Leuconostoc spp.	−	−	−	−	V	R
Nutrionally variant streptococci						
Abiotrophia adiacens	−	+	V	−	−	S
Abiotrophia defectiva	−	+	V	−	−	S
Pediococcus spp.	−	+	−	+	V	R
Tetragenacoccus spp.	−	+	−	NR	NR	S
Vagacoccus spp.	−	+	+	+	+	S

NR, no results; +[w] weakly positive; S, susceptible (sensitive); R, resistant.
[a]May take 2–7 days.
[b]Large inoculum **must** be used.

C. Characterization of *Staphylococcus* spp. (5, 9, 12); *S. haemolyticus, S. intermedius, S. lugdunensis,* and *S. schleiferi* are all usually PYR positive (9).

III. ENZYME/SUBSTRATE

Enzyme

Bacterial aminopeptidase (EC 3.4.11.8) L-pyrrolidonyl arylamidase, also called pyrrolidonase, L-pyroglutamylaminopeptidase, and L-pyroglutamylpeptidase hydrolase (9)

Substrate

A. L-pyrrolindonyl-β-naphthylamine; also called pyrroglutamyl-β-naphthylamide or L-pyroglutamic acid-β-naphthylamide
B. Manufacturer: Sigma
C. Dissolve in methyl alcohol (CH_3OH) and dilute with **sterile** distilled water. Adjust pH to 5.7–6.0; final concentration, 0.02%

IV. REAGENT *p*–DIMETHYLAMINOCINNAMALDEHYDE (DMACA)

(*Note:* Same reagent as used for LAP test (Chapter 21).)

A. **Properties**
   1. Commercially available
   2. DMACA is a diazo dye coupler; a vinyl analogue of *p*-dimethylaminobenzaldehyde (DMABA).
   3. Reagent couples with naphthylamide to form a red Shiff base (2, 6).
   4. **Not** a dye or stain, but upon hydrolysis yields a substance that is converted into an insoluble azo dye (7)
   5. Acid solution; concentration 1% in 10% concentrated hydrochloric acid (HCl); final concentration, 0.01%
   6. Prepare fresh every 2 months.
B. **Chemistry of reagent action**: PYR/LAP reagent is an acid solution containing detergent that forms a red Shiff base with free β-naphthylamide. β-Naphthylamines are not reactive, since the amino group is involved in amide bond (3).
   1. **Step 1**: substrate L-pyrrolindonyl-β-naphthylamide is hydrolyzed by enzyme L-pyroglutamylaminopeptidase to L-pyrrolidone and free β-naphthylamine; a colorless substance.
   2. **Step 2**: β-naphthylamine reacts with DMACA, which acts as a diazo dye coupler, and a red color forms.

Step 1

L-Pyrrolindonyl-β-naphthylamide $\xrightarrow{\text{L-pyrrolidonyl arylamidase, enzyme hydrolysis}}$ L-Pyrrolidone + free β-naphthylamine

Substrate C_4H_9N $C_{10}H_7NH_2$
                                                      (colorless)   (colorless)

Step 2

β-naphthylamine + *p*-Dimethylaminocinnamaldehyde $\xrightarrow{\text{Diazo dye coupler}}$ Red color

Substrate   PYR reagent   Shiff base

When a chromophore azo group –N=N– is formed by coupling with enzymatically released naphthols or naphthylamine, color results (7). Diazo compounds combine with aromatic amines or phenols (e.g., β-naphthylamine). Azo group –N=N– (or diazo group if an N is connected to an element other than carbon) results in a colored compound (7) that contains **unsaturated** structures; e.g., –N=N– (azo).

V. RAPID TESTS

(*Note:* Adaptations are commercially available from REMEL; both media and reagent.)

A. **PYR broth** (1, 6, 9, 10)
   1. Basal medium: Todd-Hewitt broth
      a. Substrate L-pyrrolidonyl-β-naphthylamide, 0.01%
      b. Dispense 0.02 mL/screw cap tube (13 × 100 mm).
   2. Inoculum: with **sterile** inoculating loop, pick 2–3 morphologically similar colonies and emulsify in PYR broth/substrate; turbidity of McFarland no. 2 standard (see Appendix 5).
   3. Incubation: 35°C, 2 h
   4. **After** incubation, add 1 drop PYR/LAP reagent to each tube **without mixing.** Observe for color change after 2 min.
B. **PYR agar** (3, 11)
   1. Medium: Tryptic soy agar (TSA) with 0.01% substrate
   2. Inoculum/incubation: same as listed above under PYR broth; streak for isolation
   3. **After** incubation add 1 drop of PYR/LAP reagent directly to surface growth on plate. Observe for color change after 2 min.
C. **PYR strips** (2, 8)
   1. Preparation of strips
      a. Whatman no. 3 filter paper cut into strips approximately 1.0 × 0.5 cm
      b. Saturate strips with PYR/LAP reagent, 0.02%.
      c. Dry at room temperature (22–25°C) and store desiccated at 2–6°C; shelf life more than 1 year
   2. Test organisms: isolate on sheep blood agar (SBA) 18–24 h, 35°C, **prior** to testing
   3. Inoculum
      a. Place strip in Petri dish and moisten with **sterile** distilled water, pH 5.7–6.0.
      b. With **sterile** inoculating loop, pick several morphologically similar colonies and rub onto strip.
   4. Incubation: 35°C, **10 min**
   5. Add 1 drop PYR/LAP reagent directly to strip and observe for color change.

VI. COMMERCIAL DISK SPOT TESTS

A. Manufacturers; follow manufacturer's directions.
   1. PYR/esculin disks: REMEL (11)
   2. PYR disks: Key Scientific Products
B. Procedures
   1. Rehydrate disk; two methods
      a. Moisten with **sterile** distilled water.
      b. Place disk on agar surface; e.g., sheep blood agar (SBA).
   2. With wooden applicator stick or inoculating loop, heavily rub several **pure** colonies from an 18- to 24-h agar plate onto disk. If slow-growing isolate, incubate 2–3 days for sufficient inoculum.
   3. Incubate room temperature (22–25°C), 5 min

4. **After** incubation, add **1 drop** of detection reagent to disk; allow **1 min** for color development.

VII. QUALITY CONTROL ORGANISMS

A. Positive (+)

Streptococcus pyogenes	ATCC 19615
Enterococcus faecalis	ATCC 29212

B. Negative (−)

Streptococcus agalactiae	ATCC 12386
Streptococcus bovis	ATCC 9809

VIII. RESULTS

> See Figures 37.1 and 37.2 (Appendix 1) for colored photographic results

IX. INTERPRETATIONS

A. Positive (+)
   1. Cherry red to dark-purple red color
   2. PYR hydrolyzed
   3. Group A β-streptococci and group D enterococci
B. Negative (−)
   1. Pink, orange, or yellow (no change) color
   2. Group B streptococci, β-streptococci not A, B, or D, viridans streptococci

X. PRECAUTIONS

A. **General**
   1. DHEW publication no. (NIH) 76–900 lists amino acid β- naphthylamines as known carcinogens. Prepare and store PYR/LAP substrates carefully.
   2. **Before** performing the PYR test, confirm that organism is a β-hemolytic, Gram-positive coccus and is catalase negative. Other catalase-negative, Gram-positive cocci are PYR positive (Table 37.1.).
   3. Clinical isolates of possible streptococci are preferably tested before 48-h incubation or subcultured prior to testing. Isolates PYR negative after more than 48 h should be resolved by using fresh isolates or by conventional methods (8).
   4. Test each new batch of PYR reagent each day test is performed.
   5. Further biochemical and serologic testing may be necessary for definitive identification.
B. **Disks** (11)
   1. Store disks in original container at 2–8°C; **do not** freeze or overheat. Allow to come to room temperature before use; **do not** incubate.
   2. Color development after 1 min **should be disregarded.**
   3. False-negative results may occur if inadequate inoculum is used.
C. **PYR strips**: discard if desiccant has changed from blue to pink.

REFERENCES

1. Bosley GS, Facklam RR, Grossman D. Rapid identification of enterococci. J Clin Microbiol 1983;18(5):1275–1277.
2. Ellner PD, Williams DA, Hosmer ME, Cohenford A. Preliminary evaluation of a rapid colorimetric method for the presumptive identification of group A streptococci and enterococci. J Clin Microbiol 1985;22(5):880–881.
3. Facklam RR, Thacker LG, Fox B, Eriquez L. Presumptive identification of streptococci with a new test system. J Clin Microbiol 1982;15(6):987–990.
4. Godsey J, Schulman R, Enriquez l. The hydrolysis of L-pyrrolidonyl-β-naphthylamide as an aid in the rapid identification of *Streptococcus pyogenes, S. avium,* and group D enterococci. Abstr Annu Meet Am Soc Microbiol, C84, 1981:276.
5. Hébert GA, Crowder CG, Hancock GA, et al. Characterization of coagulase-negative staphylococci that help differentiate these species and other members of the family *Micrococcaceae.* J Clin Microbiol 1988;26(10):1939–1949.
6. Koneman EW, Allen SD, Janda WM, et al. Color Atlas & Textbook of Diagnostic Microbiology, ed 5. Philadelphia: JB Lippincott, 1997:609, 614–615, 1375.
7. Lillie RD. H J Conn's Biological Stains, ed. 9. Baltimore: Williams & Wilkins, 1977:200.
8. Morgan JW. Evaluation of a rapid method for the determination of L-pyrrolidonyl-β-naphthylamide hydrolysis. Lab Med 1987;18(10):682–683.
9. Murray PR, Baron EJ, Pfaller MA, et al. Manual of Clinical Microbiology, ed 6. Washington, DC: American Society for Microbiology, 1995:289–290.
10. Oberhofer TR. Value of the L-pyrrolidonyl-β-naphthylamide hydrolysis test for identification of select gram-positive cocci. Diagn Microbiol Infect Dis 1986;4:43–47.
11. REMEL. PYR/Esculin Disk, TI no. 21138, 1998.
12. Tierno PM, Stotzky G. Differentiation of strains of *Staphylococcus epidermidis* by aminopeptidase profiles. Ann Clin Lab Sci 1978;8:111.

38 Starch Hydrolysis Test

I. PRINCIPLE

A. To determine the ability of an organism to hydrolyze starch enzymatically
B. Test for disappearance of starch by use of iodine reagent

II. PURPOSE

(Also see Chapters 43 and 44)

A. To aid in species differentiation among various aerobic genera: *Bacillus* spp. and *Streptococcus* spp.
   1. *Bacillus pumilis* (−), *B. sphaericus* (−) from other *Bacillus* spp. (+) most frequently isolated
   2. *Streptococcus bovis* (+), nonenterococci, group D (+) from other group D *Streptococcus* spp. (usually −) (29)
B. To aid in species differentiation among various anaerobic genera
   1. *Clostridium butyrium* (+), *C. baratii* (+), *C. fallax* (+), *C. perfringens* (+), and *C. sphenoides* (variable) from other most frequently isolated *Clostridium* spp. (−) with subterminally located spores
   2. *Prevotella oulora* (−), and *P. intermedia* (variable, usually +) from other *Prevotella* spp. (+) most frequently isolated
C. To aid in species differentiation
   1. *Corynebacterium diphtheriae* type gravis (+) from other *Corynebacterium* spp. (usually −).
   2. *Pseudomonas saccharophila* (+) and *P. stutzeri* (+) from other *Pseudomonas* spp. (−) most frequently isolated
   3. *Brevundimonas vesicularis* (+() from *B. diminuta* (−) (20)
   4. *Chryseobacterium meningosepticum* (−) from *C. indologenes* (+) (20)
D. To aid in identification of genera where **all species are**
   1. *Methylobacterium* spp. (+)
   2. *Mobiluncus* spp. (+)
   3. *Roseomonas* spp. (+)

III. BIOCHEMISTRY INVOLVED

Starch is a homopolysaccharide, a condensation product (23) of many monomers (molecular units) of a single type of monosaccharide, α-D-glucose, forming a polymer of many units united by α-glucosidic (acetal) linkages (14). Polysaccharides $(C_6H_{10}O_5)_n$ such as starch and dextrins, by definition yield more than six molecules of monosaccharides on hydrolysis (14). The basic structure of starch is a mixture of two polyglucose polysaccharide molecules: linear amylose (10–20%) and branched amylopectin (80–90%) (17), usually in a ratio of 1:4 to 1:5 (22). Starch that yields only glucose on hydrolysis is called a *glucosan* (14).

Starch is a class of carbohydrates of high molecular weight with low solubility in their native state, only slightly soluble in water (5, 7) and insoluble in aqueous ethanol and usually in organic solvents (5). The glucose (dextrose) residues of starch, α-amylose and amylopectin, are all α-D-glucose (glucopyranose) molecules. Glucose ($C_6H_{12}O_6$), is a 6-carbon monosaccharide; a hexose.

Since the ring resembles the six-member heterocyclic compound pyran it may also be called a *pyranose* (23); α-glucopyranose. The structural difference between α- and β-glucose is the position (projection) of the OH groups on carbon number 1: α, downward (below the plane) in the Haworth formula or to right in straight chain; β, upward (above the plane) or to the left (18, 23). The ordinary form found in starch is α. The difference in this case with cellulose is digestibility. Cellulose is composed of indigestible β-glucose units; starch of digestible α-units (18).

Naturally occurring glucose is the D isomer; however, two optical isomers exist, D and L. The two forms are mirror images of each other but are not identical; they are asymmetric and **cannot** be superimposed. The D form occurs naturally; the L form is manmade (18).

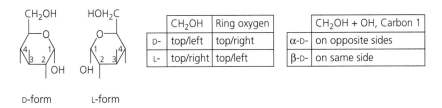

	CH₂OH	Ring oxygen
D-	top/left	top/right
L-	top/right	top/left

	CH₂OH + OH, Carbon 1
α-D-	on opposite sides
β-D-	on same side

Glucose contains an aldehyde group (CHO or O=C–H) and hence is also an *aldose* or *aldohexose* (23). It is a polyhydroxyaldehyde possessing properties of aldehydes (23). Glucose exists in three readily interconvertible forms; in aqueous solution all exist, and an equilibrium is established between open and cyclic forms (18).

α-Glucose
(cyclic hemiacetal)
(36%)

Open form
(polyhydroxyaldehyde)
(0.02%)

β-Glucose
(cyclic hemiacetal)
(64%)

The aldehyde form is unstable and exists only as a transient intermediate in carbohydrate reactions (18). Aldehydes react with one alcohol group to form an unstable hemiacetal compound that does not involve a loss of water or with two alcohol groups (e.g., glucose residues) with water split out by acetal formation (18, 23). Glucose possesses a hemiacetal linkage to which an ether (–C–O–C–) linkage and an –OH group are attached; OH in hemiacetal is activated by the ether linkage attached at the same site (18).

Aldehyde + Alcohol ⇌ Hemiacetal +HOR'/Second alcohol ⇌ Acetal + H_2O

R' and R" in starch are identical; α, D-glucose residues.

Hemiacetal (glucose residue) + Alcohol (glucose residue) ⇌ Acetal (α-maltose) + H_2O

Acetalization blocks any possible opening of the ring to form aldehydro sugar (5). In starch, acetal oxygen bridges (–C–O–R–) linking glucose units together are easily hydrolyzed, especially in the presence of acids or certain enzymes, e.g., amylases (3, 18, 23). Hydrolase, the digestive enzyme specific for starch hydrolysis was formerly called *diastase* (1); it is now termed *amylase*. Two types of amylases exist: α-amylase, or endoamylase (5, 13), excreted by many bacteria (16, 27) and β-amylase, or exoamylase, present in higher plants (5).

The optimal pH for α-amylase activity is 6.9–7.2 (3, 24), but it varies from 5.5 to 6.5 with different substrates and is unstable below pH 4.5 (5). Its optimal temperature is 50–55°C, but the reaction appears satisfactory at 37°C (16). Animal α-amylases require chloride (Cl^-) or related anions (Br^-, I^-, NO_3^-) in at least 0.01 M concentration (3) for their activity (5).

Enzymatic hydrolysis occurs at the α-1,4- and α-1,6-acetal linkages that hold the starch polymer together (27). α-Amylase catalyzes hydrolysis of the α-1,4-glucosidic (acetal) linkages of polysaccharides such as starch (3). It attacks the interior of polysaccharide chains, either amylose or amylopectin, at random points, forming a mixture of fragments (15, 23) of 5 to 9 units (15) of the α configuration (5). Amylose is split completely by amylase (5). Complete hydrolysis of starch requires another enzyme, which acts on 1,6-branch-points in amylopectin molecule such as oligo-1,6-glucosidase (5). Dextrins and maltose are absorbed by the cells from the medium and further hydrolyzed by specific intracellular enzymes (27): e.g., branching dextrin enzyme, 1,4-α-d-glucan; 6-α(1,4-α-glucano)-transferase (30); maltase (glycosidase), a glycoside-splitting enzyme with group specificity hydrolyzing compounds and with α-glycosidic linkage (23).

Takeshita and Hehre (28) first showed that digestion of starch or glycogen by α-amylases can lead, under certain circumstances, to products differing structurally from those obtained by hydrolysis. α-Amylase converts starch to products other than hemiacetal-bearing entities (dextrins, maltose, glucose). These authors also showed that although sugars and maltodextrins formed by α- amylase digestion of α-glucans are formed predominantly by hydrolysis, they do not arise exclusively in that way or necessarily represent segments as they preexisted in substrate molecules. To some extent their formation also involves redistribution of glycosyl units from one saccharide molecule to another.

Starch may also be hydrolyzed by acid hydrolysis, with the same intermediate products formed and glucose as the end product; this is an example of the catalytic action of the hydrogen ion (24). Overall hydrolysis of soluble starch forms single glucose residues in a step-by-step process (5, 14, 17, 22–25):

$$(C_6H_{10}O_5)_n^* \xrightarrow[\text{H}_2\text{O}]{\alpha\text{-amylase}} \alpha\text{-Amylose} + \text{Amylopectin} \quad (1)$$

Starch
(nonreducing
carbohydrate)

(blue soluble color
with iodine)

(bluish-red to red-brown insoluble color
with iodine)

$$(C_6H_{10}O_5)_x \xrightarrow[\text{H}_2\text{O}]{\alpha\text{-amylase}} \text{Dextrins: } (C_6H_{10}O_5)_y \longrightarrow (C_6H_{10}O_5)_z \quad (2)$$

Amylopectin

Erythrodextrins
(blue → violet → red-brown
color with iodine)

Achroodextrins
(colorless with
iodine)

* Molecule gets smaller and smaller as hydrolysis progresses; n larger number than x, x larger than y, and y larger than z.

$$(C_6H_{10}O_5)_z \xrightarrow[\text{H}_2\text{O}]{\alpha\text{-amylase} \atop \text{oligo-1,6-glucosidase}} \alpha\text{-Maltose} \quad (3)$$

Achroodextrins

α-Maltose

(4-α-D-glucopyranose-α-D-glucopyranoside)
(α-D-glucopyranosyl-4-α-D-glucopyranose)
(glucose-4-α-glucoside)
(colorless with iodine)

$$\alpha\text{-Maltose} \xrightarrow[\text{H}_2\text{O}]{\text{maltase}} \alpha\text{-Glucose} \quad (\text{two molecules glucose per molecule maltose hydrolyzed}) \quad (4)$$

α-Maltose
($C_{12}H_{22}O_{11}$)
Disaccharide
(reducing sugar)
(colorless with iodine)

α-Glucose (dextrose)
($C_6H_{12}O_6$)
Monosaccharide
(reducing sugar)
(colorless with iodine)

The two constituents of starch, amylose and amylopectin, are composed of a number of α-glucose residues united by 1,4-linkages in chains of amylose and amylopectin and 1,6-branch-point linkages in amylopectin (14). α-Glucosidic linkages are analogous to α-hydroxyl groups (OH); glucosidic links connect the anomeric (potential carbonyl) carbon of one monosaccharide with any carbon of a second monosaccharide (23).

α-Amylose is a polysaccharide, with a molecular weight of 69,000 to 1 million, composed of long, linear polymers of α-D-glucose linked by 1,4-α-glucosidic (acetal) bonds (3, 5, 17). α-Linkage gives the amylose chain a spiral conformation; molecules are wound in a nonbranching helix with 6 glucose residues per turn (23). With the spiral conformation, hydrogen bonds cannot be formed as easily between different chains; thus, starch has no strength and is more soluble in water than cellulose, since its OH groups can interact with water molecules (23). The helical structure is responsible for a blue soluble color with iodine reagent (5, 24).

The amylopectin molecule is larger than amylose, with a molecular weight of 200,000 to many million, composed of a highly branched network of α-D-glucose units (3); it is estimated that there is one branch for every 24–30 glucose units linked in a chain by 1,4-bonds. Each of the 1,6-α-glucosidic (acetal) linked residues is the origin of a side chain (3, 5, 23); highly branched chains give a red insoluble color with iodine (24) because they do not coil effectively (14).

Further hydrolysis of amylopectin occurs through a series of partially digested starch molecules called *dextrins* of decreasing molecular weight (5); these are partial random breakdown products of about 4% of amylopectin acetal oxygen bridges (17, 18). Dextrins are still large molecules (17), consisting of fewer glucose polymers (27), with a marked reduction in viscosity (5, 14). Dextrins are soluble, nonfermentable (5), linear, or branched molecules that undergo slower hydrolysis (5). The first dextrin formed is erythrodextrin, which gives a color progressing from blue to violet to red-brown with iodine (5, 18). As hydrolysis proceeds, the iodine color is no longer produced because of formation of achroodextrins that are colorless (5, 14). Terminal molecules of maltose are successively split off with gradual, more or less complete, degradation of intermediate dextrins to maltose and a smaller amount of glucose (5). Monosaccharides such as glucose cannot be converted into simpler carbohydrates by hydrolysis (23).

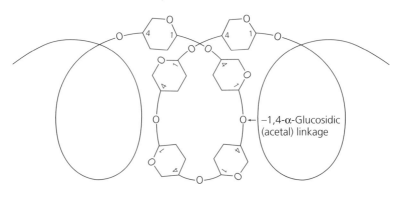

Amylose
(Helical coil structure)

(continued)

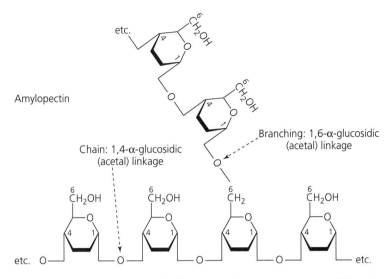

(Redrawn and modified from Harper, H. A. Rodwell, V. W., and Mayes, R. A. *Review of Physiological Chemistry,* 16th ed., 1977, p. 103, with permission of Lange Medical Publications, Los Altos, Calif.)

Some reducing sugars and fermentable substances are produced throughout the reaction; however, the main course of reaction is the breakdown of polysaccharides first to dextrins followed by the slower phase of maltose formation (5).

IV. MEDIUM EMPLOYED: STARCH MEDIUM

A. Medium appropriate to type of organism being tested (1)
   1. Broth
   2. Agar plates or slants
B. Ingredients; pH 7.2 (12)
   1. **Basal medium**

Peptone	5.0 g
Beef extract	3.0 g
Sodium chloride, NaCl	5.0 g
Agar (omit for broths)	20.0 g
Deionized water	1000.0 mL

   2. **Soluble (potato) starch**
      a. Preferred: 0.2% (1, 10, 11)
         (1) 20.0 g per liter of basal medium
         (2) Recommended for anaerobes (10)
      b. Other concentrations: 1% (20) or 5% (26)
C. **Commercial products available**
   1. Basal medium
      a. BBL (2)
         (1) Infusion agar/broth
         (2) Mueller-Hinton agar broth
      b. Difco (9)
         (1) Heart Infusion agar (HIA)
         (2) Mueller-Hinton agar/broth
         (3) Protease no. 3 agar: 2% proteose to 1% starch
         (4) Tryptose blood agar base

2. Soluble starch: Difco and Merck; BBL, starch Minitek disks
D. Method of preparation (21)
  1. Weigh out amounts accurately as directed on the label; various company products may vary slightly.
  2. Rehydrate basal medium in 500 mL of distilled or demineralized water.
  3. Heat **gently** into solution.
  4. Dissolve 20.0 g of starch (0.2%) in 250 mL of distilled or demineralized water.
     a. Native starch slightly soluble in water (5, 17)
     b. A heat labile supplement (10)
     c. **Carefully** bring to just boiling; do not boil **excessively,** as overheating may hydrolyze starch (7).
  5. Combine (steps 2 and 4) and mix well by **gently** swirling flask.
  6. Make up to 1 L volume.
  7. Adjust pH, if necessary.
E. Method of sterilization: autoclave, 121°C, 15 lb, 15 min
F. **Aseptically,** dispense into screw-cap tubes (16 × 125 mm) (12).
  1. 15 to 20 mL per tube
  2. Agar slants: allow medium to solidify in **slanted** position.
  3. Plate agar medium
     a. Dispense into tubes for storage; they need not be slanted.
        (1) **Before** use, melt tubes as required in boiling water bath.
        (2) Pour into individual Petri dishes.
        (3) Allow to **cool before** inoculation.
     b. If poured plates of starch agar are refrigerated, medium becomes opaque.
G. Cool before use, **tighten caps,** and refrigerate for storage (4–10°C).
H. Inoculation
  1. Growth from an 18- to 24-h **pure** culture
  2. Slanted tubed medium: fishtail slant
  3. Plate agar medium: several cultures can be tested on one agar plate (6).
     a. A single starch agar plate may be divided into four quadrants (pie plate) for four separate determinations.
     b. See procedure in Chapter 31, Optochin Disk Test, Section IV, Procedure.
I. Incubation
  1. 35°C, 18–24 h (1, 6), 48 h (11), or until sufficient growth has occurred (1)
  2. 20°C: 5 days (1)
J. Add reagent **directly** to the incubated tube(s)/plate(s) **before** attempting to interpret; record results **immediately.**

V. REAGENTS EMPLOYED

A. Two choices
  1. **Aqueous Gram's iodine** (4)
     a. Ingredients

Iodine crystals, I_2	1.0 g
Potassium iodide, KI	2.0 g
Distilled water	300.0 mL

     b. Method of preparation
        (1) Grind solids in about 20 mL of distilled water in mortar.
        (2) Add remainder of water, rinsing out mortar with smaller portions of water until required volume is reached, and shake flask until dissolved.
        (3) Filter into brown, pharmacy, medicine-dispensing bottles, 5 ounce capacity.

2. **Aqueous Lugol's iodine** (21)
   a. Ingredients

Iodine, powdered crystals, I_2	5.0 g
Potassium iodide, KI	10.0 g
Distilled or deionized water	100.0 mL

   b. Method of preparation
      (1) Stock solution
         (a) Dissolve KI in distilled water.
         (b) Add I_2 crystals **slowly** and shake until dissolved.
         (c) Filter into **tightly** stoppered brown bottle.
      (2) Working solution (7)
         (a) Dilute 1:5 with distilled water.
         (b) Dispense into brown, pharmacy, medicine-dispensing bottles, 5 ounce capacity.
         (c) Prepare fresh every 3 weeks.
3. Either reagent is a deep yellow solution.

B. Method of use; either reagent (1, 3, 6)
   1. Media
      a. Broth
         (1) Add a few drops of reagent
         (2) Shake tube **gently** to distribute reagent throughout medium
      b. Plates/slanted tube medium: **flood** with reagent
   2. Interpret reaction **immediately**; blue color formed with starch may fade (1).

Iodine (I_2) dissolved in an aqueous solution of potassium iodide (KI), like iodine alone, is only slightly soluble in water, but when iodide ion is present, it combines with iodine molecules to form a triiodide ion, I_3, which liberates iodine easily on demand (17). The iodine test can detect minute traces of starch in solution (17).

C. Quality control: the reagents **must** be tested with known positive and negative cultures **before** being put into general use.

D. Storage: store reagents in a refrigerator (4°C) when not in use. These reagents should be placed in dark bottles to avoid exposure to light. Their stability varies, as the solution fades on standing; therefore, each week they should be given a quality control check and discarded when they give a negative or weak reaction with a known positive organism.

E. **Chemistry of reagent action:** amylose and amylopectin behave differently toward iodine (23); the amylose starch fraction combines with much more iodine (23) and produces an intense, deep blue complex (5, 14, 22, 23, 24). The amylose-iodine complex is an adsorption complex of starch and iodine rather than a definite compound (24). Iodine molecules are trapped within the nonbranching helix of glucose units of the amylose chain to form a blue inclusion compound (17, 22, 23). If this network disintegrates, as it does during starch hydrolysis, the blue color is lost (17). The course of starch hydrolysis in a test tube (plate) can be followed by use of iodine reagent, for as the reaction proceeds the color produced by iodine gradually changes from an intense blue to purple to no color if starch is being hydrolyzed (17, 24).

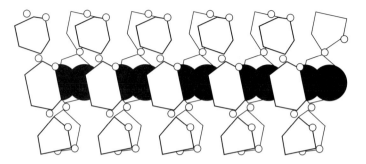

Helix of amylose enclosing iodine molecules (Iodine—dark shading spaces)

(Redrawn from Nussenbaum, S. *Organic Chemistry: Principles and Applications,* 1963, p. 522, with permission of Allyn and Bacon, Inc., Boston.)

The highly branched chains of amylopectin give only a red color with iodine because they do not coil effectively (14, 22). The color is reddish brown to colorless with dextrin, depending on the type of dextrin and whether or not the preparation contains some starch (partial hydrolysis), as many preparations do (24). In performing this test, the solution must always be neutral or acid in reaction (24).

VI. QUALITY CONTROL ORGANISMS

A. **Anaerobes**
   1. Positive (+)

      Bacteroides fragilis   ATCC 25285
      Clostridium perfringens   ATCC 13124

   2. Negative (−)

      Clostridium bifermentans   ATCC 638
      Eikenella corrodens   ATCC 23834

B. **Aerobes**
   1. Positive (+)

      Bacillus subtilis   ATCC 6633

   2. Negative (−)

      Escherichia coli   ATCC 25922

VII. RESULTS

> See Figure 38.1 (Appendix 1) for colored photographic results

VIII. INTERPRETATION

A. **Positive (+)**
   1. Media (1, 3, 6, 10, 11)
      a. **Broth: no** color throughout medium; medium remains colorless or has a slight yellow tinge due to color of iodine reagent.
      b. **Plates/slanted tubes:** medium purple-blue with **colorless** area (hydrolysis zone) around growth

2. Relative **absence** of starch; 6 or fewer glucose units still present (16)
3. Starch completely **hydrolyzed** to glucose with acids (24).
4. See Section XII, Precautions, when testing *Bacillus* spp. for hydrolysis.

B. **Partial hydrolysis**
   1. Color observed may give a rough estimation of the extent of hydrolysis (16); violet to red to red-brown.
   2. Temporary red color
      a. Presence of 18–12 glucose units (16)
      b. Erythrodextrins (14)
   3. Continue incubation and retest; flooding plates with iodine reagent **does not** contaminate plate, and it may be reincubated and subsequently retested if necessary (21).

C. **Negative (−)** (1, 3, 6, 10, 11)
   1. Media
      a. Broth: **blue** color throughout medium
      b. Plates/slanted tubes: medium **purple-blue** color right up to (around) growth
   2. **Presence** of starch; more than 30 glucose units present (16)
   3. Starch **not hydrolyzed**; most still present.
   4. Blue color may fade after a while; interpret test results **immediately** after adding iodine reagent (1).

IX. RAPID MICROMETHOD

A. Procedure of Clark and Cowan (6)
B. Testing for preformed enzyme of bacterial cells in 4 h
C. Growth medium
   1. Favorable solid medium, preferably without blood or fermentable substance
   2. 35°C; 18–24 h
D. Test suspension
   1. Wash growth from plate/slant in tap water.
   2. Glassware need not be sterile but **must** be chemically clean.
   3. Centrifuge, and if using growth from blood agar medium, wash once more to remove hemoglobin.
   4. Resuspend sedimented cells in small volume of water.
E. Procedure
   1. Pipette 0.04 mL of test suspension into each of **two** Durham tubes containing 0.4 mL of starch-agar base (0.2% agar, 0.05% potato starch).
   2. Run blank control simultaneously containing uninoculated starch agar.
   3. Incubation: 37°C, 4 **and** 24 h; if 4-h result is negative, continue incubation of second tube and test again at end of 24-h period.
   4. Add 1 drop Lugol's iodine; read after **30 min** at room temperature (22–25°C) against blank tube.
   5. Interpretation
      a. Hydrolysis: **no** color on column
      b. No hydrolysis: **blue** color on column

The micromethod of Clark and Cowan (6) is not complicated by side effects or multiple reactions that may occur in cultures growing in a nutrient medium containing test substrate; it gives reasonably rapid results, and sterile technique is not required. Clark and Cowan (6) showed that a positive result is obtained in 2 h with more-active starch-hydrolyzing organisms, but the test uses 4- and 24-h incubations to detect weaker reactors.

X. ALTERNATIVE TESTS

A. **Ethanol Procedure of Kellerman and McBeth** (19)
   1. Medium: starch agar plates (BBL)
   2. Reagent
      a. 95% ethanol (ethyl alcohol)
      b. Flood incubated plate with reagent
   3. Interpretation
      a. Hydrolysis: **clear** zones around growth
      b. No hydrolysis: **white** areas around growth
      c. Reaction **not** instantaneous; observe reaction **30 min** after addition of reagent
B. **Detection of end product, glucose; reducing sugar**
   1. Benedict's reagent or Clinitest tablets
   2. Preparation, method of use, and interpretation, see Chapter 13, Gluconate Test, Section V.

XI. PRECAUTIONS

A. **Enzyme**: α-Amylase is not stable below pH 4.5 (5).
B. **Media/starch**
   1. Avoid overheating starch when dissolving into basal medium; it may hydrolyze by itself and give false-positive results (7). Heating disrupts granules and yields amylose and amylopectin (15).
   2. Starch is **not** a reducing carbohydrate (17), and the soluble starch substrate preparation should be free of reducing sugars (8).
   3. The starch medium **must** be neutral or acid in reaction (24); the optimal pH for the medium is 7.2.
   4. Avoid using dextrose starch agar medium; some streptococci produce enough acid from starch to make test results unsatisfactory (9).
   5. Starch agar gives the best results if used before it is 2 weeks old; after that period, starch changes, and reddish purple spots may develop on addition of iodine solution (1).
   6. Nutrient agar is often recommended for the basal medium; however, chloride ion is necessary for α-amylase activity (3, 14), and many commercial nutrient broths/agars do not contain chloride (NaCl) or other anions. Any medium used to detect starch hydrolysis **must** contain at least 0.01 M chloride (as sodium chloride) (3). Use caution in selecting basal medium for starch hydrolysis testing.
   7. It is advisable not to store and refrigerate **poured** starch agar plates; the medium becomes opaque, which may cause difficulty in interpreting results. Store the medium in screw-cap tubes and, just prior to use, melt in a water bath, **pour,** and **cool before** inoculation.
C. **Reagents**
   1. Record results **immediately** after adding iodine reagent because any blue color formed may fade, giving a false-positive result of absence of starch (1).
   2. Lugol's **stock** iodine reagent **must** be diluted 1:5 to a working solution; failure to do so makes the reagent too strong, so that too much iodine is trapped by the amylose helix and excess (free) iodine is present throughout medium, and hence, true starch hydrolysis is not detected yielding a false-negative test result.
D. **Interpretation/results**
   1. Test organisms giving a red-violet color with iodine reagent (partial hydrolysis) should be retested after additional incubation; flooding of plates;/slants with iodine **does not** contaminate growth (21).
   2. Some strains of *Bacillus* spp. produce only restricted zones of hydrolysis that may not be obvious until bacterial growth has been scraped away from agar before interpreting results (8).

E. **Micromethod**: Clark and Cowan's (6) procedure does not require sterile equipment, but glassware **must** be chemically clean to avoid introducing any substance that might interfere with, or change, results.

REFERENCES

1. Allen PW. A simple method for the classification of bacteria as to diastase production. J Bacteriol 1918;3(1):15–17.
2. BBL Manual of Products and Laboratory Procedures, ed 6. Cockeysville, MD: BBL Microbiology Systems, Division of Becton Dickinson and Company, 1988.
3. Blazevic DJ, Ederer GM. Principles of Biochemical Tests in Diagnostic Microbiology. New York: John Wiley & Sons, 1975:99–101.
4. Branson D. Methods in Clinical Bacteriology. Springfield, IL: Charles C Thomas, 1972:176–177.
5. Cantarow A, Schepartz B. Biochemistry, ed 3. Philadelphia: WB Saunders, 1962:1, 7, 10, 16, 29, 242, 271–274.
6. Clarke PH, Cowan ST. Biochemical methods for bacteriology. J Gen Microbiol 1952;6(2):187–197.
7. Cowan ST. Cowan & Steel's Manual for the Identification of Medical Bacteria, ed 2. Cambridge: Cambridge University Press, 1974:12, 148, 162.
8. Cowan ST, Steel KJ. Manual for the Identification of Medical Bacteria. Cambridge: Cambridge University Press, 1966:104, 129, 163.
9. Difco Manual, ed 10. Detroit: Difco Laboratories, 1984:879.
10. Dowell VR. Anaerobic infections. In: Bodily HL, Updyke EL, Manson JO, eds. Diagnostic Procedures for Bacterial, Mycotic, and Parasitic Infections, ed 5. New York: American Public Health Association, 1970:510, 520–522.
11. Facklam RR. Recognition of group D streptococcal species of human origin by biochemical and physiological tests. Appl Microbiol 1972;23(6):1131–1139.
12. Finegold SM, Baron EJ. Bailey and Scott's Diagnostic Microbiology, ed 7. St. Louis: CV Mosby, 1986:466.
13. Fisher EH, Stein E. Alpha-Amylase. In: Boyer PD, Lordy H, Myrbach K, eds. The Enzymes, vol 4. New York: Academic Press, 1960:313–344.
14. Harper HA, Rodwell VW, Mayes PA. Review of Physiological Chemistry, ed 16. Los Altos, CA: Lange Medical Publications, 1977:93, 95, 101–103, 106, 204.
15. Harrow B, Mazur A. Textbook of Biochemistry, ed 9. Philadelphia: WB Saunders, 1966:214, 217.
16. Henry RJ. Clinical Chemistry: Principles and Technics. New York: Hoeber Medical Division, Harper & Row, 1968:469.
17. Holum JR. Principles of Physical, Organic, and Biological Chemistry. New York: John Wiley & Sons, 1969:451–453.
18. Holum JR. Elements of General and Biological Chemistry, ed 4. New York: John Wiley & Sons, 1975:285–286, 324–326, 331–334.
19. Kellerman KF, McBeth IG. The fermentation of cellulose. Zentralbl Bakteriol II Abt 1912;34:485–494.
20. Koneman EW, Allen SD, Janda WM, et al. Color Atlas & Textbook of Diagnostic Microbiology, ed 5. Philadelphia: JB Lippincott, 1997:270, 283.
21. Lennette EH, Balows A, Hausler WJ Jr, Shadomy HJ. Manual of Clinical Microbiology, ed 4. Washington, DC: American Society for Microbiology, 1985:918–919, 945.
22. Noller CR. Chemistry of Organic Compounds, ed 3. Philadelphia: WB Saunders, 1965:396.
23. Nussenbaum S. Organic Chemistry. Boston: Allyn & Bacon, 1963:504–506, 508, 510–511, 521–523, 527, 541.
24. Oser BL, ed. Hawk's Physiological Chemistry, ed 14. New York: McGraw-Hill, 1965:94–95, 105–106.
25. Porter JR. Bacterial Chemistry and Physiology. New York: John Wiley & Sons, 1946:497.
26. Skerman VB. A Guide to the Identification of the Genera of Bacteria, ed 2. Baltimore: Williams & Wilkins, 1967.
27. Stanier RY, Doudoroff M, Adelberg EA. The Microbial World, ed 2. Englewood Cliffs, NJ: Prentice-Hall, 1963:301–302.
28. Takeshita M, Hehre EJ. The capacity of alpha-amylases to catalyze the nonhydrolytic degradation of starch and glycogen with formation of novel glycosylation products. Arch Biochem Biophys 1975;169(2):627–637.
29. Trepeta RW, Edberg SC. Measurement of microbial alpha-amylases with p-nitrophenyl glycosides as the substrate complex. J Clin Microbiol 1984;19(1):60–62.
30. Umeki K, Yamamoto T. Structures of multi-branched dextrins produced by saccharifying α-amylase from starch. J Biochem 1975;78(5):897–903.

39 Urease Test

I. PRINCIPLE

To determine the ability of an organism to split urea into two molecules of ammonia by the action of the enzyme urease, with resulting alkalinity

II. PURPOSE

(Also see Chapters 44 through 45.)

A. Originally this enzymatic activity was characteristic of all *Proteus* spp. and was used primarily to differentiate the rapidly urease-positive *Proteus* organisms from other members of the *Enterobacteriaceae;* other genera may have been delayed positive.
   1. *Proteus* (usually + and rapid)

      P. inconstans: urease −
      P. mirabilis: urease +
      P. myxofaciens: urease +
      P. penneri: urease +
      P. rettgeri: urease +
      P. vulgaris: urease +

   2. *Providencia* (V, variable; usually −)

      P. heimbachae: urease −
      P. stuartii: urease V
      P. rustigianii: urease −

   3. *Morganella morganii* biogroups 1 and 2: urease weakly +
B. To aid in species differentiation
   1. *Actinobacillus seminis* (−) from other *Actinobacillus* spp. (+) most frequently isolated
   2. *Bartonella felis* (+) from other *Bartonella* spp. (−) frequently isolated
   3. *Bordetella avium* (−) from *B. bronchiseptica* (+), *B. parapertussis* (+), and *B. pertussis* (+)
   4. *Pasteurella aerogenes* (+), *P. dagmatis* (+), *P. lymphangitidis* (+), *P. mairii* (+), and *P. pneumotropica* (+) from other *Pasteurella* spp. (−)
   5. Christensen's urease
      a. *Enterobacter dissolvens* (+), *E. gergoviae* (+), *E. hormaechae* (V, usually +), *E. cloacae* (V), and *E. absuriae* (V, usually +) from other *Enterobacter* spp. (−)
      b. *Klebsiella ornithinolytica* (+), *K. oxytoca* (+), *K. planticola* (+), and *K. pneumoniae* subsp. *pneumoniae* (+) from other *Klebsiella* spp. (−)
   6. *Oligella ureolytica* (+) from *O. urethralis* (−)
   7. *Weeksella zoohelcum* (+) from *W. virosa* (−)
   8. T-strain *Mycoplasma urealyticum* (+); T-mycoplasmas are the only mycoplasmas known to contain urease (see Section VIII.A)
   9. *Peptostreptococcus tetradius* (+), *P. lactolyticus* (+), and *P. prevotii* (V, usually −) from other *Peptostreptococcus* spp. − frequently isolated

10. Viridans *Streptococcus vestibularis* (+) and *S. salivarius* (V, usually +) from other viridans *Streptococcus* −
11. Human *Haemophilus* spp., *H. influenzae* biotypes I, II, II, IV (+), *H. influenzae* biogroup *aegyptius* (+), *H. parainfluenzae* biotypes II, III, IV, VII (+), *H. haemolyticus* (+), *H. paracuniculus* (+), *H. parahaemolyticus* (+), and *H. paraphrophaemolyticus* (+) from other *Haemophilus* spp. −

C. To aid in the identification of
1. *Vibrio parahaemolyticus* urease variable, usually + (25)
2. *Helicobacter cinaedi* rapidly urease + (20, 24, 32)
3. *Mycobacterium* spp. (V); (see Section VIII.B)
4. *Cryptococcus* spp. (yeast) (+, 1–2 days) (35)

III. BIOCHEMISTRY INVOLVED

The substrate urea, a diamide of carbonic acid, is often referred to as a carbamide (8, 29). All amides
$$\begin{pmatrix} O \\ \parallel \\ RC-NH_2 \end{pmatrix}$$
are readily hydrolyzed (30). Urea is hydrolyzed by a specific enzyme, urease (or urea amidohydrolase), to yield two molecules of ammonia. In solution, urea hydrolyzes to ammonium carbonate as the end product (8, 29).

$$\begin{array}{c} H_2N \\ \diagdown \\ C=O \\ \diagup \\ H_2N \end{array} + 2\,HOH \xrightarrow{\text{urease}} CO_2 + H_2O + 2\,NH_3 \rightleftharpoons (NH_4)_2CO_3$$

Urea   Carbon dioxide   Ammonia   Ammonium carbonate

Urease is an important microbial enzyme concerned with decomposition of organic compounds (21). Bacterial enzymes are classified as either constitutive or adaptive. An adaptive, or induced, enzyme is produced only when its specific substrate is present (7). Urease is considered constitutive because it is synthesized by certain bacteria regardless of the presence or absence of its substrate urea (7, 46).

There are two broad divisions of enzymes: (a) hydrolases, which are concerned with the hydrolysis (addition of water) of esters, carbohydrates, proteins, and amides, and (b) those that are concerned with various oxidation-reduction reactions (17). Urease is classified as an amidase, catalyzing the hydrolysis of amides (8). Oppenheimer (31) included among the amidases all enzymes that can break the bond between nitrogen and carbon by hydrolysis.

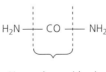

Urease (an amidase)

In the case of urease, nitrogen is dissociated as ammonia (NH_3) (31). Urease (27, 44) acts on the C-N bonds in compounds, except those that contain peptide bonds (27).

The optimal pH for urease activity is 7.0 (22).

426 Biochemical Tests for Identification of Medical Bacteria

IV. MEDIA EMPLOYED

A. **Rustigian and Stuart's urea broth,** pH 6.8 (1, 13, 15, 40)
   1. Ingredients

Monopotassium phosphate, KH_2PO_4	9.1 g
Disodium phosphate, Na_2HPO_4, (Sorensen buffer)	9.5 g
Yeast extract	0.1 g
Urea, highest purity, 20%	20.0 g
Phenol red	0.01 g
Deionized water	1000.0 mL

   2. pH indicator: phenol red
      a. Acid: yellow color, pH 6.8
      b. Alkaline: pinkish red color, pH 8.4
      c. Uninoculated medium: pH 6.8, yellow-orange color
   3. Commercial products available: BBL, urease test broth (1); Difco, urea broth (13)
   4. Method of preparation
      a. Weigh out amount accurately as directed on the label.
      b. Rehydrate with distilled or demineralized water.
      c. **Do not** heat into solution; on heating, urea decomposes.
   5. Recommended method of sterilization
      a. Filtration
         (1) Millipore membrane filter
         (2) Membranes: 0.45-μm pore diameter
      b. **Aseptically,** dispense approximately 3.0 mL (8) per **sterile** tube (13 × 100 mm)
      c. If the medium is prepared and inoculated **immediately,** reliable results can be obtained without filtration (1).
      d. The basal medium may be rehydrated in 900 mL of distilled or demineralized water and sterilized by autoclave at 121°C, 15 lb, for 15 min. On cooling, 100 mL of a 20% solution of **sterile** urea (filtered) is added, and the broth is dispensed in tubes (3 mL per **sterile** 13 × 100 mm tube) (15).
   6. Cool before use and refrigerate for storage (4–10°C).
   7. Inoculation
      a. Growth from an 18- to 24-h **pure** culture, Kligler's iron agar (KIA) or other suitable culture
      b. **Heavy** inoculum: 3 loopfuls (2-mm loop) (1, 15, 40)
      c. Shake the tube **gently** to suspend the bacteria (40).
   8. Incubation
      a. 35°C incubator or water bath (15, 40)
      b. Observe reactions after 8, 12, 24, and 48 h of incubation.
      c. Changes in temperature change the rate of urease production (40).

Rustigian and Stuart's urea broth is a highly buffered medium in which detection of urea use after 48 h or less of incubation was originally restricted to urease production by **only** *Proteus* spp. (40). Now the medium gives positive results for most *Proteus, Morganella,* and a few *Providencia stuartii* strains (5). Other organisms, particularly *Enterobacter* spp. can attack urea slowly and weakly, but with Rustigian and Stuart's urea broth urease activity is **not** detected within 48 h of incubation (40).

The yeast extract incorporated in the medium provides the growth factors required by the strongly urease-positive genera (formerly all included in a single genus, *Proteus*); these organisms can use urea nitrogen, but other urease-producing organisms require an additional nitrogen source (12).

The hydrogen ion indicator, phenol red, shows production of urease by the *Proteeae* by demonstrating decreased hydrogen ion concentration because of formation of two molecules of ammonia (NH_3).

B. **Christensen's urea agar**, pH 6.8 (1, 10, 13, 15)
   1. Ingredients

Peptone	1.0 g
Sodium chloride, NaCl	5.0 g
Monopotassium phosphate, KH_2PO_4	2.0 g
Glucose (dextrose), 0.1%	1.0 g
Urea, 20%, highest purity	20.0 g
Phenol red	0.012 g
Agar	15.0 20.0 g
Deionized water	1000.0 mL

   2. pH indicator: phenol red
      a. Acid: yellow color, pH 6.8
      b. Alkaline: pinkish red color, pH 8.4
      c. Uninoculated medium: pH 6.8, yellow to buff color
   3. Commercial products available
      a. BBL and Difco, Urea agar base (1, 13)
      b. BBL: Urea agar base (1)
   4. Method of preparation and sterilization (1, 13)
      a. Dehydrated urea base (29%)
         (1) Weigh out accurately 29.0 g of the dehydrated base and dissolve in 100 mL of distilled or demineralized water.
         (2) **Do not** heat into solution. Urea decomposes when exposed to heat.
         (3) Sterilize by Millipore membrane filter, 0.45-μm pore diameter
      b. Agar
         (1) Dissolve 15.0 g of agar in 900 mL of distilled or demineralized water.
         (2) Autoclave: 121°C, 15 lb, 15 min
         (3) Cool to 50°C.
      c. Add 100 mL of **sterile** urea base aseptically to the 900 mL agar and water mixture; final concentration of urea is 10%.
      d. Dispense the medium **aseptically** into **sterile** tubes, approximately 4.0–5.0 mL per 13 × 100 mm tube (long slant, short butt) (1, 13, 15).
      e. This medium may be used in liquid form if desired (15).
   5. Allow medium to cool in a **slanted** position.
   6. Cool before use and refrigerate for storage (4–10°C).
   7. Inoculation
      a. Growth from an 18- to 24-h **pure** culture, Kligler's iron agar (KIA) or other suitable culture
      b. **Heavy** inoculum (5, 10, 15); **fishtail** the entire surface of the slant
      c. **Do not** stab the butt; it serves as a color control (1).
      d. For *Brucella* spp. hold at **room temperature** (22–25°C) 2 h, then incubate with 2–10% CO_2 (4).
   8. Incubation: 35°C, 6 and 24 h and every day thereafter for 6 days (11). Longer periods may be necessary.

Christensen's urea agar is used to detect urease activity by all rapidly urease-positive *Proteus* organisms. This medium also detects definite urease activity in *Enterobacter* spp. and other members of the *Enterobacteriaceae* (10) that exhibit a delayed urease reaction. *Enter-*

obacter spp. can use urea as a sole source of nitrogen (43); they can lose this ability, but can either retain or regain their ability to hydrolyze urea (10). Christensen's medium eliminates the organism's need to use the byproduct of urea (ammonia) as its sole nitrogen source and also exhibits urease activity in organisms with more complex nitrogen requirements (10). The urea medium of Rustigian and Stuart (34) has so few nutrients that if an organism cannot use ammonia, it must rely on the yeast extract in the medium for its nitrogen and carbon sources.

Christensen's medium eliminates the need for an organism to use ammonia as its sole source of nitrogen (10) and permits detection of urea hydrolysis by other *Enterobacteriaceae* whose urease activity is slight and delayed (10). This is accomplished by (a) adding glucose to the medium, (b) decreasing the peptone concentration, and (c) decreasing the buffering system; the less-buffered medium detects a smaller amount of alkali (16). All *Enterobacteriaceae* ferment glucose by definition, and the resulting acidity will counteract the alkalinity generated by peptone decomposition; therefore, the glucose furnishes a source of energy, leaving the peptone intact (10). Addition of glucose eliminates possible false-negative results and stimulates urease activity in organisms that hydrolyze urea slowly (10). The energy provided by glucose fermentation stimulates urease by increasing the rate of metabolism and cell reproduction (10). Addition of glucose does not appreciably increase urease activity in *Proteus* spp., suggesting that their urease is constitutive (10).

On Christensen's medium the rate of urea hydrolysis differentiates rapid-urease *Proteeae* organisms (*Proteus* spp., *M. morganii*, and some *P. stuartii*) and other urease-positive organisms. Positive *Proteeae* organisms exhibit a positive reaction on the slant within 1–6 h of incubation (10), with the characteristic red-violet (pinkish red) color extending throughout the medium at the end of 6 h of incubation. It is not unusual for these *Proteeae* organisms to exhibit a positive result after only 30 min of incubation—their urease activity is so rapid on Christensen's medium. The extent and rate of color penetration throughout the medium is a measure of an organism's urease activity (10). All urease-positive *Proteeae* give a 4+ reaction after 24 h of incubation. The speed of urea hydrolysis does not differ among the positive *Proteeae* organisms on Christensen's medium (10).

Delayed urease-positive organisms such as *Klebsiella* or *Enterobacter* spp. vary in their rate of urea hydrolysis. Some go from a 1+ positive reaction after 6 h of incubation to a 4+ reaction after 3–5 days of incubation, while others may exhibit only a 1+ reaction after 6 days (10).

C. **Urea R (rapid) broth** (14)
1. Ingredients; pH 6.9

Yeast extract	0.1 g
Urea	20.0 g
Monopotassium phosphate, KH_2PO_4	0.091 g
Disodium phosphate, Na_2HPO_4	0.095 g
Phenol red	0.01 g
Deionized water	1000.0 mL

Monopotassium phosphate and disodium phosphate have low buffering capacity.

2. Sterilization: filtration (Millipore); 0.45-μm pore diameter
3. Dispense: 3.0 mL per **sterile** borosilicate screw-cap tube (13 × 100 mm)
4. Storage: refrigerator, 2–8°C; shelf life maximum, 48 h; recommend use on day prepared (14)
5. Inoculum: 3 loopfuls (2-mm loop) (1, 15, 40)
6. Incubation: aerobically, 35°C, water bath; observe at 10 min, 1 h, and 2 h.

V. QUALITY CONTROL ORGANISMS

A. Positive (+); **rapid and strong**

    Proteus mirabilis   ATCC 29906
    Proteus vulgaris   ATCC 13315

B. Positive (+); **weak**

    Klebsiella pneumoniae subsp. *pneumoniae*   ATCC 13883

C. Negative −

    Escherichia coli   ATCC 11775
    Uninoculated

VI. RESULTS

> See Figures 39.1–39.4 (Appendix 1) for colored photographic results

VII. INTERPRETATION

A. **Stuart's urea broth**
 1. Positive (+)
    a. Intense pink-red color throughout the broth
    b. Certain *Proteeae* spp.:

    P. mirabilis
    P. myxofaciens
    P. penneri
    P. rettgeri (now *Providencia rettgeri*)
    P. vulgaris
    M. morganii biogroups 1 & 2
    Few *P. stuartii* strains

 2. Negative −: no color change (yellow-orange)

B. **Christensen's urea agar**
 1. Positive (+): intense pink-red (red-violet) color on the slant. Color may penetrate into the agar; the extent of color indicates rate of urea hydrolysis (2).
    a. Degree of hydrolysis
       (1) 4+; entire tube pink-red
       (2) 2+; slant pink, butt no change
       (3) Weakly +; top of slant pink, remainder no change
    b. Rapid positive: 1–6 h for **all positive** *Proteeae* organisms
    c. Delayed positive: 24 h to 6 days of incubation or longer

    Some *Klebsiella* strains
    Some *Enterobacter* strains
    Some *Citrobacter* strains
    Bacteria other than the *Enterobacteriaceae*

 2. Negative −: no color change (buff to pale yellow)

C. **Urea R broth**: positive (+), cerise (reddish purple) color

VIII. ALTERNATIVE TEST MEDIA

A. **U-9 broth (urease color test medium)**
   1. Formulation of Shepard and Lunceford (36)
   2. Purpose: selective isolation of T-strain mycoplasmas from clinical specimens; aid in identification of *Ureaplasma urealyticum* (37) in culture; the **only** mycoplasma to contain urease
   3. Ingredients
      a. **Stock solutions**
         (1) Urea solution, 10%
            (a) Highest purity grade; 3.0 g/30 mL distilled water
            (b) Dispense 0.7 mL per screw-cap tube (13 × 100 mm).
         (2) Phenol red solution: 1.0%, 100 mg sodium phenolsulfonphthalein/10 mL distilled water
         (3) Penicillin G potassium
            (a) 0.63 g/10 mL **sterile** distilled water
            (b) Final concentration: 100,000 units/mL
      b. **Base**

Trypticase soy broth (TSB) or tryptic digest broth	0.75 g
Sodium chloride, NaCl	0.5 g
Monopotassium phosphate, KH_2PO_4	0.02 g
Deionized water	100.0 mL

      c. **Completed medium**; pH 5.0

U-9 base, **sterile**, cooled 45–50°C	95.0 mL
Horse serum, **unheated** (normal), 4%, **sterile**	5.0 mL
Urea solution, 10% **sterile**	0.5 mL
Phenol red solution, 1%, **sterile**	0.1 mL
Penicillin G, **sterile**	1.0 mL.

   4. Modifications with additives
      a. **U-9 broth with amphotericin** (38)
         (1) Purpose: isolation of ureaplasmas from female genitourinary tract specimens; suppresses growth of *Candida* spp. and filamentous fungi
         (2) To **sterile** U-9 broth, **aseptically** add 2.5 μg/mL **sterile** amphotericin (Fungizone).
      b. **U-9B broth** (38)
         (1) Added growth supplement
         (2) To completed U-9 medium, add 0.5 mL of a 2% L-cysteine·HCl stock solution **prior to** sterilization.
      c. **U-9C broth**; ingredients

Trypticase soy broth (TSB)	1.5 g
Yeast extract	0.1 g
Magnesium chloride, $MgCl_2·6H_2O$	0.2 g
Deionized water	90.0 mL

         Adjust pH to 5.5 with 2 N HCl.

         After sterilization, add

Horse serum, **unheated** (normal), **sterile**	10.0 mL
Urea, 10%, **sterile**	0.3 mL
L-Cysteine·HCl·H_2O, **sterile**	0.5 mL
GHL tripeptide, 20 μg/mL, **sterile**	0.1 mL
Phenol red solution, 1%, **sterile**	0.1 mL
Penicillin G solution, 100,000 units/mL, **sterile**	1.0 mL

(*Note:* GHL tripeptide is glycyl-L-histidyl-L-lysine acetate; Calbiochem-Novabiochem; see Appendix 11)

5. Sterilization
   a. Filtration (Millipore), 0.22-μm pore diameter: urea solution, L-cysteine, GHL peptide, horse serum, and antimicrobial agents
   b. Autoclave, 121°C, 15 lb, 15 min: base and phenol red solution
6. Dispense
   a. Screw-cap tubes: 1.8 mL/tube (13 × 100 mm)
   b. Vials: 1.8 mL/vial (Wheaton)
7. Storage
   a. Base: refrigerator, 2–8°C
   b. Frozen
      (1) Stock solutions, horse serum, L-cysteine, and GHL tripeptide: -20°C
      (2) Original specimen extract: -70°C
      (3) Shelf life, completed media: approximately 1 month
8. Inoculation
   a. Specimens extracted in 1.8 mL U-9 broth (original extract). Save (frozen, -70°C) for possible subculturing.
   b. A 10^{-1} dilution of original extract is made by transferring 0.2 mL to vial containing 1.8 mL U-9 broth (or U9-B or C) (37).
9. Incubation
   a. Both original and dilution vials
   b. Aerobically, 35°C, 18–24 h
   c. Observe throughout incubation period for first change in pH indicator. Continue incubation for 7 days with daily observations before reporting as urease negative.
10. Quality control organisms
    a. Positive (+)

       Ureaplasma urealyticum ATCC 27618

    b. Negative −

       Mycoplasma pneumoniae ATCC 15531
       Staphylococcus aureus subsp. *aureus* ATCC 12600
       Uninoculated
11. Interpretation (also see Table 39.1)
    a. Positive (+)
       (1) Pink–deep red color starts at bottom of tube and spreads throughout medium during continued incubation.
       (2) Hydrolysis of urea and accumulation of ammonia (NH_3)
       (3) Alkaline pH
       (4) **No turbidity** (cloudiness) **evident in broth medium**
    b. Negative −
       (1) No color change; medium remains straw colored.
       (2) **No** hydrolysis of urea

Table 39.1. Urease Activity: pH/Time

pH Reaction	Incubation Period (h)
6.9–7.2	4
7.2–8.0	8
9.2–9.4[a]	24

[a]All urease-positive *Proteeae* organisms.

B. **Urea broth for mycobacteria** (39)
   1. Ingredients

Peptone	1.0 g
Glucose (dextrose)	1.0 g
Sodium chloride, NaCl	5.0 g
Potassium phosphate, monobasic, K_2HPO_4	0.4 g
Urea	20.0 g
Phenol red, sodium, 1.0%	1.0 mL
Tween 80	1.1 mL
Deionized water	1000.0 mL

   2. Inoculum
      a. Young, actively growing culture on Lowenstein-Jensen medium
      b. Moderate turbidity
   3. Incubation: 35°C, **without CO_2**; interpret after 1–7 days.
   4. Quality control organisms
      a. Positive (+): *Mycobacterium fortuitum* ATCC 35931
      b. Negative −: Uninoculated
   5. Interpretation; change from bright yellow to

      1+: light pink; negative
      2+: dark pink; positive
      3+: light red; positive
      4+: dark red; positive

C. **Aid in differentiation of *Mycobacterium* spp.**: *M. scrofulaceum* (+) from pigmented strains *M. intracellulare-avium* complex (−); Runyon group I (*M. tuberculosis, M. bovis, M. kansasii,* and *M. marinum*) usually +; other groups variable to negative (23)
   1. Test media; three choices
      a. **Urease disk test** (28)
         (1) Urea disks (Difco) impregnated with Ewing's urea R broth (15) added to 0.5 mL of **sterile** distilled water in screw-cap tubes (13 × 100 mm)
         (2) Nonspecific color changes are observed in uninoculated medium in some brands of disposable tubes; problem eliminated with multiple-use tubes (28).
      b. Either tubed media; dispense 3.0-mL aliquots into **sterile** borosilicate screw-cap tubes (13 × 100 mm).
         (1) Medium of Toda, Hagihara, and Takeya (42)
            (a) Phosphate buffer system, 0.01 M, pH 6.7
            (b) Autoclave and while **still hot** add 3.0 g of urea and 1.0 mL of 0.1% phenol red pH indicator per 100 mL of buffer.
         (2) Medium of Wayne and Doubek (45): Christensen's urea agar base (Difco) **without** agar, diluted 1:10 in **sterile** distilled water
   2. All three procedures (28)
      a. **Heavy** inoculum (emulsion) from 21-day-old egg base culture
      b. Incubation: 35°C; observe results in 1 h and then at 24-h intervals up to 72 h
      c. Positive: cerise (reddish purple) color

D. **Buffered urea medium, azide free**
   1. Rapid urease detection of *Helicobacter (Campylobacter) pylori* (19)
   2. Ingredients; pH 6.3–6.5

Urea	2.0 g
Aqueous phenol red, 0.4%, (wt/vol)	2.5 mL
Sodium phosphate, NaH_2PO_4, 10 mmol, pH 6.3	0.14 g
Oxoid agar no. 4	0.4 g
Deionized water	**100.0 mL**

3. Dispense: 200 μL/well in Linborough flat-bottomed, 96-well microtiter trays; shelf life, 10 days refrigerated (2–8°C).
4. Inoculation: 5 μL (**heavy**) stabbed into wells with multipipette
5. Incubation
   a. Room temperature (22–25°C)
   b. Avoid exposure to light; place in cupboard. Exposed to light, culture may develop peroxide, which may interfere with urease reaction.
6. Interpretation
   a. Observe for color change after 5 and 30 min and 1, 2, 3, 12, and 18 h.
   b. *H. pylori* shows an immediate, persistent, deep red reaction.

E. **Nonselective medium (NSM)**
  1. Purpose: rapid screening test for isolation and detection of urease by *H. pylori* (9); may be used for antral biopsies
  2. Ingredients; pH 6.8

Columbia agar base	39.0 g
IsoVitaleX, 2%	20.0 mL
Hemin	10.0 mg
Urea	20.0 g
Phenol red	1.2 mg
Granulated agar	4.0 g
Deionized water	**980.0 mL**

  3. Selective medium (SM): optional antimicrobial additives; eliminates contaminating flora

Trimethoprim	5.0 mg
Vancomycin	10.0 mg
Amphotericin B	5.0 mg
Cefsulodin	5.0 mg

  4. Sterilization
     a. Urea and phenol red: filtration (Millipore); 0.22-μm pore diameter
     b. Columbia agar: autoclave, 121°C, 15 lb, 15 min; cool and add urea, phenol red, and antibiotics.
  5. Dispense: 15–20 mL/plate (15 × 100 mm)
  6. Inoculation: biopsy specimens maintained in 0.4 mL brucella broth; homogenized and plated **within 2 h**.
  7. Incubation: 35°C, in microaerophilic atmosphere (Campy Pak jar)
  8. Quality control microorganisms
     a. Positive (+): *Helicobacter pylori*, ATCC 11637, NCTC 11637; color change within 1 h
     b. Negative −

        Proteus vulgaris ATCC 13315; color change in 24 h
        Pseudomonas aeruginosa ATCC 27853; color change in 48 h
        Campylobacter jejuni ATCC 32292; **no** color change

  9. Interpretation
     a. Check for color change in 5 and 30 min and 1, 2, 3, 6, 24, 36, and 48 h.
     b. Positive (+)
        (1) Yellow to red color
        (2) Bacterial growth visible after 3 days
     c. Negative: **no** color change

H. pylori gives an immediate reaction within 1 h, and medium is completely red at 3 h. *H. pylori* has a highly active urease, of high molecular weight, and produces copious amounts of urease when cultured on solid medium (20, 24, 32).

434 Biochemical Tests for Identification of Medical Bacteria

F. **Balanced salt solution** (27)
   1. Purpose: biotyping of human *Haemophilus* spp. (26)
   2. Ingredients; pH 7.0

Monopotassium phosphate KH_2PO_4	0.1%
Potassium phosphate, dibasic KH_2PO_4	0.1%
Sodium chloride, NaCl	0.5%
Phenol red, 2%	0.5 mL
Total volume,	**100 mL**

   Sterilize: autoclave, 121°C, 15 lb, 15 min and add **sterile** (Millipore filter) aqueous urea 10.0 mL

   3. Dispense: small amounts in **sterile** tubes (13 × 100 mm)
   4. Inoculum: **heavy** suspension
   5. Incubation: 35°C, 4 h
   6. Results
      a. Positive (+): red color

      Haemophilus influenzae biotypes I, II, III, IV, and biotype *aegyptius*
      Haemophilus parainfluenzae biotypes II, III, IV, VII
      Haemophilus haemolyticus
      Haemophilus parahaemolyticus
      Haemophilus paraphrophaemolyticus

IX. RAPID TESTS

A. **Key Urease Test Tablets**
   1. Manufacturer: Key Scientific Products
   2. Formula of Christensen
   3. Results within 6–12 h of incubation
   4. Procedure: follow manufacturer's directions.
B. **Urea disks**
   1. Manufacturers
      a. BBL, urease (UR) Minitek disks; in conjunction with Gram stain and oxidase, can be used for rapid confirmation of *H. pylori* (41)
      b. Difco, urea disks
   2. Results within 1–4 h of incubation
C. **Urea-phenylalanine disks (PDA disks)**
   1. Manufacturer: REMEL
   2. Procedure: follow manufacturer's directions.
   3. See Figures 39.3 and 39.4 (Appendix 1).
   4. **Heavy** inoculum from 18- to 24-h agar slant
   5. Incubation: 37°C water bath; observe at 10 min, 1 and 2 h.
   6. Positive: cerise (reddish purple) color
D. **CLO Striptest**
   1. Manufacturer: Delta West Ltd, Western Australia, Australia
   2. Rapid urease for *H. pylori* (3, 11)
   3. Follow manufacturer's directions.
   4. Read after 15 min, and 1, 3, and 20 h.

X. ALTERNATIVE PROCEDURES

A. **Liquid scintillation counting**; cumulative radiometric technique of Buddemeyer (6)
B. **Noninvasive [^{13}C] and [^{14}C] urea breath tests** (23)

1. ^{14}C
   a. Manufacturer: Pytest, Ballard Medical Products, Draper, Utah
   b. Uses ^{14}C to measure bicarbonate given off by urea-producing *H. pylori*
2. ^{13}C
   a. Manufacturer: Meretek UBT, Nashville, TN
   b. Urea breath test; [^{13}C]urea contained in prinactin, a clear colorless solution

C. **Detection of *H. pylori* using [^{15}N]urea as a tracer**; measures NH_4 excretion

XI. PRECAUTIONS

A. General
   1. **All** urea test media, both broth and slant agar, rely on demonstration of alkalinity; hence, they are **not specific for urease**. The use of peptones, especially in slant agar (e.g., *P. aeruginosa*), or other proteins in the medium **may** raise the pH to alkalinity because of protein hydrolysis and release of excessive amino acid residues and yield false-positive results. To eliminate possible protein hydrolysis, run a control using the same test medium **without urea** (2).
   2. The sensitivity of urease testing may be adjusted with buffers. Stuart's broth is strongly buffered, 10 times that of Christensen's slant agar, and usually **only** urease-positive *Proteeae* organisms break down urea in Stuart's broth to produce alkalinity because the excessive amount of NH_3 produced cannot be neutralized by buffer (2).
   3. **Do not** heat or reheat urea base into solution; urea decomposes on heating.
   4. Urea media exposed to light may develop peroxide, which could interfere with the urease reaction (12).
   5. Urea is known to undergo autohydrolysis; therefore, it is advisable to store media in the refrigerator 4–8°C. Color change may take slightly longer when media is refrigerated (12).
   6. **Un**buffered media are less specific (13, 15, 16).

B. **Stuart's urea broth**
   1. The strong buffering system masks urease activity in organisms that are delayed positive; this medium is designed only for detection of urease activity in all *Proteus* spp., *M. morganii*, *P. rettgeri*, and urease-positive *P. stuartii* organisms (10).
   2. *M. morganii* hydrolyzes urea slowly (10), and after 24 h of incubation the reaction may only show a faint pink color. If in doubt as to the result, compare with an uninoculated tube of medium or reincubate for an additional 24 h. *M. morganii* usually requires approximately 36-h incubation to develop a strong positive urease reaction (40). A strong positive urease result for *Proteeae* occurs when the pH reaches 8.1 or above (40). There are variations in the pH reaction depending upon the incubation period and the urease-positive *Proteeae* being tested (Table 39.1). *P. vulgaris* and *P. mirabilis* give a positive urease reaction (pH 8.1) after approximately 8 h of incubation. *P. rettgeri* attacks urea rapidly, giving a positive result in about 12 h. *M. morganii* requires approximately 36 h of incubation to develop a strong positive urease reaction (40).
   3. The pH of positive reactions can vary because of differences in the size of the inoculum used or differences in rates of urease activity of various *Proteeae* positive strains (34). Increasing a bacteria-saline suspension inoculum of *Proteeae* from 0.01 to 0.1 mL, **decreases** the time required to reach pH 8.1; however, a heavier inoculum produces no further acceleration (40). The accepted standard inoculum of 0.1 gives a positive result approximately 3 h faster than a 0.01-mL inoculum (40).
   4. The amount of substrate used and/or the incubation temperature can alter the rate of urease production by urease-positive *Proteeae* (40). Stuart et al. used a constant inoculum and varied the amount of medium per tube from 1.5 to 3.0 to 4.5 and 6.0 mL and

found that the time required to develop a positive result **increased** with the volume. The minimum acceptable amount of medium per tube for an accurate reading is 1.5 mL (40).
5. False-negative results may occur if the amount of NH_3 formed is too low to change the hydrogen ion concentration of the high buffering system to an alkaline pH that would cause the phenol red indicator to change color (46).
6. Both prepared and dehydrated **broth base** should be refrigerated; if the seal is broken, the bottle is preferable stored with a desiccant in a sealed container.
7. If nutrients furnished by yeast extract are depleted before the organism shows noticeable growth, its ability to hydrolyze urea **cannot** be accurately determined (10).
8. If an organism can hydrolyze urea but **cannot** use the ammonia (NH_3) as a source of nitrogen, growth **does not** occur and a false-negative result could occur (10).

C. Christensen's urea agar
1. Urease-positive *Proteeae* cause Christensen's medium to turn alkaline (pinkish red) soon after inoculation. For the results to be valid for detection of *Proteeae*, they **must** be read within the first 2–6 h of incubation. *Citrobacter freundii* and *K. pneumoniae* subsp. *pneumoniae* may convert Christensen's urea agar within 24–48 h. This medium detects rapid urease activity of only the urease-positive *Proteeae*.
2. Christensen's urea medium is **not** used to determine the absolute rate of urease activity (10). Many urease-positive organisms other than *Proteeae* may hydrolyze urea within 24 h and then slowly further break down urea. This is evident by the alkaline color penetrating throughout the medium slant and butt. The further degrading of urea may be due to a lack of tolerance of some organisms to the increased alkalinity, which subsequently decreases urease activity (10).

D. **Urea R broth must** be prepared on the day of use since the buffer will not maintain desired pH longer than 48 h.

E. **U-9 media**
1. Basal broth preparation, conversion to complete U-9 medium, and dispensing should always be accomplished on the same day (37).
2. **Remember: growth and urease** activity by ureaplasmas in U-9 broth medium occur **without** detectable turbidity (cloudiness) **at any time** (37).
3. On rare occasions, ureaplasmas exhibit delayed positive urease reactions after 3–5 days of incubation (37).
4. *Ureaplasma* spp. are the **only** members of *Mycoplasmatales* known to contain urease; therefore, the urease reaction is specific for ureaplasmas (37).
5. L forms of *Proteus* can be induced to hydrolyze urea in U-9 medium (37). A heavy inoculum is required and an incubation period of 48–72 h (37). However, if *Proteus* L forms are in a clinical specimen and succeed in breaking through the penicillin barrier in the medium, they multiply in the bacillary form and produce obvious bacterial-type turbidity and yield a false-positive urease result for ureaplasmas (37).
6. False-positive urease results may also occur if fungi are present in the clinical specimen (primarily *Candida* spp. and certain filamentous fungi); however, **except** for *Candida humicola* (35), these organisms are urease negative. They can multiply in the presence of penicillin and release alkaline byproducts from basal medium alone that produce strong alkaline reactions and red color changes in the medium (37). False-positive results due to *Candida* are recognized by obvious turbidity and/or heavy sediment and a yeastlike odor (35). False-positive results due to filamentous fungi are evidenced by development of characteristic fluffy, cottonlike balls of growth (36). Usually these fungi can be suppressed by incorporating 2.5 μg/mL of the antifungal agent amphotericin B; however, a few strains of *Candida* may fail to be inhibited (35).
7. Robertson (33) showed that phenol red in U-9 turns from straw color to pale pink at pH 7.0, and by pH 8.2 the medium is deep pink. Color change is **not** evident until station-

ary growth is reached (33). Subcultures **must** be made when the pink-red color change is **first detected**; subcultures made **after** development of **full red color** (usually 9–12 h (33)) generally yield negative agar cultures due to the high alkalinity (pH 8.0–9.0) reached in the medium, which is lethal to *Ureaplasma* spp. (18). If inactivation occurs, a frozen aliquot of the original extract may be thawed and used to inoculate agar.

8. Both *M. hominis* and *U. urealyticum* grow in U-9 broth; however, **only** *U. urealyticum* changes the color of the medium (33).

REFERENCES

1. BBL Manual of Products and Laboratory Procedures, ed 6. Cockeysville, MD: BBL Microbiology Systems, Division of Becton Dickinson and Company, 1988:154.
2. Blazevic DJ, Ederer GM. Principles of Biochemical Tests in Diagnostic Microbiology. New York: John Wiley & Sons, 1975:103–104, 132–133.
3. Borromeo M, Lambert JR, Pinkard KJ. Evaluation of "CLO-test" to detect *Campylobacter pyloridis* in gastric mucosa. J Clin Pathol 1987;40:462–463.
4. Branson D. Methods in Clinical Bacteriology. Springfield, IL: Charles C Thomas, 1972:46–49.
5. Brenner DJ, Farmer JJ III, Hickman FW, et al. Taxonomic and Nomenclature Changes in *Enterobacteriaceae*. Atlanta, GA: CDC, Public Health Service, HEW publ no. 78-8356, Jun 1978.
6. Buddemeyer EU. Liquid scintillation vial for cumulative and continuous radiometric measurement of in vitro metabolism. Appl Microbiol 1974;28(2):177–180.
7. Burrows W, Moulder JW. Textbook of Microbiology, vol II, ed 19. Philadelphia: WB Saunders, 1968:115.
8. Cantarow A, Schepartz B. Biochemistry, ed 3. Philadelphia: WB Saunders, 1962:247–248.
9. Cellini L, Allocati N, Piccolomini R, et al. New plate medium for growth and detection of urease activity of *Helicobacter pylori*. J Clin Microbiol 1992;30(5):1351–1353.
10. Christensen WB. Urea decomposition as a means of differentiating *Proteus* and paracolon cultures from each other and from *Salmonella* and *Shigella* types. J Bacteriol 1946;52(4):461–466.
11. Coudron PE, Kirby DF. Comparison of rapid urease tests, staining techniques, and growth on different solid media for detection of *Campylobacter pylori*. J Clin Microbiol 1989;27(7):1527–1530.
12. Cowan ST. Cowan & Steel's Manual for the Identification of Medical Bacteria, ed 2. Cambridge: Cambridge University Press, 1974:180.
13. Difco Supplementary Literature, ed 10. Detroit: Difco Laboratories, 1968:1040–1045.
14. Ewing WH. *Enterobacteriaceae*. Biochemical Methods for Group Differentiation. US Public Health Service publ no. 174, 1962.
15. Ewing WH. Edwards and Ewing's Identification of Enterobacteriaceae, ed 4. New York: Elsevier, 1986:527.
16. Farmer JJ III, McWhorter AC, Huntley GA, Catignani J. Unusual *Enterobacteriaceae*: A *Salmonella cubana* that is urease positive. J Clin Microbiol 1975;1(1):106–107.
17. Fieser LF, Fieser M. Organic Chemistry, ed 3. New York: Reinhold, 1956:460.
18. Ford DK, MacDonald J. Influence of urea on growth of T-strain mycoplasmas. J Bacteriol 1967;93(5):1509–1512.
19. Goldie J, van Zanten SJOV, Jalali S, et al. Optimization of a medium for the rapid urease test for detection of *Campylobacter pylori* in gastric antral biopsies. J Clin Microbiol 1989;27(9):2080–2082.
20. Goodwin CS, Armstrong JA, Marshall BJ. *Campylobacter pyloridis*, gastritis and peptic ulceration. J Clin Pathol 1986;39:353–365.
21. Gunsalus IC, Stanier RY. The Bacteria, vol II. New York: Academic Press, 1961:151.
22. Harrow B, Mazur A. Textbook of Biochemistry, ed 9. Philadelphia: WB Saunders, 1966:104.
23. Jicong W, Guolong L, Zhenhua Z, et al. $^{15}NH_4^+$ excretion test: A new method for detection of *Helicobacter pylori* infection. J Clin Microbiol 1992;30(1):181–184.
24. Jones DM, Lessells AM, Eldridge J. Campylobacter-like organisms on the gastric mucosa: Culture, histological and serological studies. J Clin Pathol 1984;37:1002–1006.
25. Kelly MT, Stroh EMD. Urease-positive, Kanagawa-negative *Vibrio parahaemolyticus* from patients and the environment in the Pacific northwest. J Clin Microbiol 1989;27(12):2820–2822.
26. Koneman EW, Allen SD, Janda WM, et al. Color Atlas & Textbook of Diagnostic Microbiology, ed 5. Philadelphia: JB Lippincott, 1997:380–381.
27. Mahler HR, Cordes EH. Biological Chemistry. New York: Harper & Row, 1966:284.
28. Murphy DB, Hawkins JE. Use of urease test disks in the identification of mycobacteria. J Clin Microbiol 1975;1(5):465–468.
29. Noller CR. Chemistry of Organic Compounds, ed 3. Philadelphia: WB Saunders, 1965:333–335.
30. Nussenbaum S. Organic Chemistry. Boston: Allyn & Bacon, 1963:415, 597.
31. Oppenheimer C. Die Fermente und ihre Wirkungen, ed 5. Leipzig: FCW Vogel, 1926.
32. Owen RJ, Martin SR, Borman P. Rapid urea hy-

drolysis by gastric campylobacter. Lancet 1985; ii:111.
33. Robertson JA. Bromthymol blue broth: Improved medium for detection of *Ureaplasma urealyticum* (T-strain mycoplasma). J Clin Microbiol 1978;7(2):127–132.
34. Rustigian R, Stuart CA. Decomposition of urea by *Proteus*. Proc Soc Exp Biol Med 1941;47(1):108–112.
35. Seeliger HRP. Use of a urease test for screening and identification of cryptococci. J Bacteriol 1956;72(2):127–131.
36. Shepard MC, Lunceford CD. Occurrence of urease in T strains of *Mycoplasma*. J Bacteriol 1967;93(5):1513–1520.
37. Shepard MC, Lunceford CD. Urease color test medium U-9 for the detection and identification of "T" mycoplasmas in clinical material. Appl Microbiol 1970;20(4):539–543.
38. Shepard MC, Lunceford CD. Differential agar medium (A7) for identification of *Ureaplasma urealyticum* (human T mycoplasmas) in primary cultures of clinical material. J Clin Microbiol 1976;3(6):613–625.
39. Steadham JE. Reliable urease test for identification of mycobacteria. J Clin Microbiol 1979;10(2):134–137.
40. Stuart CA, Van Stratum E, Rustigian R. Further studies on urease production by *Proteus* and related organisms. J Bacteriol 1945;49(5):437–444.
41. Sweeney L, Garcia LP, Talbert M, et al. Minitek urea disk test, a sensitive and cost-effective method to screen for *Campylobacter pylori* in gastric biopsies. J Clin Microbiol 1989;27(12):2684–2686.
42. Toda T, Hagihara Y, Takeya K. A simple urease test for the classification of mycobacteria. Am Rev Respir Dis 1961;83(5):757–761.
43. Vaughn RH, Levine M. Differentiation of the "intermediate" coli-like bacteria. J Bacteriol 1942;44(4):487–505.
44. Vuye A, Pijck J. Urease activity of *Enterobacteriaceae*: Which medium to choose. Appl Microbiol 1973;26(6):850–854.
45. Wayne LG, Doubek JR. Diagnostic key to mycobacteria encountered in clinical laboratories. Appl Microbiol 1968;16(6):925–931.
46. White EC, Hill JH. Bacterial urease. I. A critique of methods heretofore used for demonstrating bacterial urease and presentation of a valid and more sensitive test. II. A study of the ureolytic action of bacteria or significance in genito-urinary infection. J Urol 1941;45(5):744–759.

40 Voges-Proskauer Test

I. PRINCIPLE

To determine the ability of some organisms to produce a neutral end product, acetylmethylcarbinol (AMC, acetoin), from glucose fermentation. Voges-Proskauer (VP) is a double eponym; Voges and Proskauer (41) were the first bacteriologists to observe a red color reaction on culture media after treatment with potassium hydroxide.

II. PURPOSE

(Also see Chapters 43 through 45.)

A. To aid in differentiation between genera
   1. *Klebsiella pneumoniae* subsp. *pneumoniae* (+) and *Enterobacter* (usually +) from *Escherichia coli* (−)
   2. *Staphylococcus* (usually +) from *Micrococcus* (−)
B. To aid in species differentiation
   1. *Klebsiella pneumoniae* subsp. *pneumoniae* (+), *K. oxytoca* (+), *K. planticola* (+), and *K. terrigena* (+) from *K. pneumoniae* subsp. *ozaenae* (−) and *K. pneumoniae* subsp. *rhinoscleromatis* (−)
   2. *Aeromonas hydrophila* (+), *A. salmonicida* subsp. *masoucida* (+), *A. veronii* (+), and *A. sobria* (V, variable; usually +) from other *Aeromonas* spp. (−) most frequently isolated
   3. Commonly isolated viridans streptococci: *S. mutans* (+), *S. milleri* group (V), *S. bovis* (+), and *S. salivarius* (variable, usually positive) from *S. sanguis* (−) and *S. mitis* (−) (29)
C. To aid in the identification of
   1. *Hafnia alvei*: 22–25°C (+); 37°C (V)
   2. *Yersinia enterocolitica*: 22–25°C (V, usually +), 37°C (−)
   3. *Listeria monocytogenes* (20)
      a. Coblentz reagents (+)
      b. O'Meara reagent (−)
D. **Both** methyl red (MR+) and Voges-Proskauer (VP+)
   1. All *Listeria* spp. (MR+/VP+)
   2. *Brochothrix campestris* and *B. thermosphacta* (both MR+/VP+)

III. BIOCHEMISTRY INVOLVED

The Voges-Proskauer (VP) test is based on detection of acetoin, a neutral end product derived from glucose metabolism. Glucose is metabolized to pyruvic acid, the key intermediate in glycolysis. From pyruvic acid there are many pathways a bacterium may follow; production of acetoin is one pathway for glucose degradation in bacteria (1).

The Voges-Proskauer test for acetoin is used primarily to separate *Escherichia coli* from the *Klebsiella-Enterobacter* groups, although other *Enterobacteriaceae* may produce a positive VP result. The *Enterobacteriaceae* are characteristically classified as mixed acid or formic acid fermenters, indicating that their end products of glucose fermentation are acidic: formic acid, acetic acid, succinic acid, ethanol, hydrogen, and carbon dioxide (15, 34).

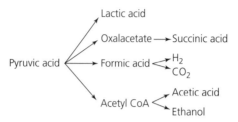

Mixed acid fermenters can be further divided into two groups: (a) those that produce acids but no 2,3-butanediol (or 2,3-butylene glycol), such as E. coli (VP−), and (b) those that produce 2,3-butanediol as their major end products, such as the *Klebsiella-Enterobacter* groups (VP+).

The major end product of pyruvate utilization by the *Klebsiella-Enterobacter* groups, *Serratia* spp., *Bacillus* spp., and many other microorganisms is 2,3-butanediol. However, the Voges-Proskauer test is based on the detection of acetoin, a precursor in 2,3-butanediol production (15, 23, 34). One molecule of acetoin is formed by decarboxylation of two molecules of pyruvic acid. Harden and Walpole (23) state that acetoin is an intermediate stage in the conversion to 2,3-butanediol. Both acetoin and 2,3-butanediol are neutral products of glucose fermentation (25).

$$2 \text{ Pyruvate} \longrightarrow \text{Acetoin} + 2 \text{ CO}_2$$

Harden and Walpole (23) found that when glucose is fermented, only a small amount of the precursor, acetoin, is formed; a larger portion of the glucose carbon is further used to form 2,3-butanediol. Paretsky and Werkman (32) found that acetoin accumulates when an organism is cultured under aerobic conditions. Walpole (42) also found that *Enterobacter aerogenes* accumulates more acetoin produced from 2,3-butanediol when the culture is exposed to atmospheric oxygen.

Acetoin can be metabolized by one of two means: (a) reduction to 2,3-butanediol, which accumulates unless reoxidation occurs, or (b) rarely by oxidation to diacetyl, which can be further catabolized (17). Stahly and Werkman (37) found that acetoin and 2,3-butanediol formation is a reversible reduction or oxidation system, acetoin to 2,3-butanediol by reduction of 2,3-butanediol oxidized to acetoin; exposure to atmospheric oxygen and alkali, slowly reverses the reaction (34). Studying two organisms, *E. aerogenes* and *Staphylococcus aureus* subsp. *aureus*, Strecker and Harary (38) isolated two enzymes responsible for the oxidation-reduction of acetoin and 2,3-butanediol.

$$\underset{\text{Pyruvate}}{\begin{array}{c}CH_3\\|\\C=O\\|\\COO^-\end{array}} + \text{lipoate} \xrightarrow[\text{dehydrogenase}]{\text{lipoate}} \underset{\text{Acetyllipoate}}{\begin{array}{c}CH_3\\|\\C=O\\|\\\text{Lipoate}\end{array}} + CO_2$$

$$\underset{\text{Acetyl CoA}}{\begin{array}{c}CH_3\\|\\C=O\\|\\sCoA\end{array}} \xrightarrow{\substack{\text{Oxidation}\\\text{Acetoin dehydrogenase}}} \qquad \xleftarrow{\substack{\text{Pyruvate}\\\text{enzyme}}} \underset{\text{Pyruvate}}{\begin{array}{c}CH_3\\|\\C=O\\|\\COO^-\end{array}}$$

$$\underset{\text{Diacetyl}}{\begin{array}{c}CH_3\\|\\C=O\\|\\C=O\\|\\CH_3\end{array}} + \text{Lipoate} + \text{HSCoA} \qquad\qquad \underset{\alpha\text{-Acetolactate}}{\begin{array}{c}CH_3\\|\\HO-C-COO^-\\|\\C=O\\|\\CH_3\end{array}} + \text{Lipoate} \quad \substack{\text{pH 6.0}\\\text{Acetolactate enzyme}}$$

$$\text{NADH} + H^+ \searrow \underset{\substack{\text{Acetoin}\\\text{dehydrogenase}}}{\updownarrow} \qquad \underset{\substack{\text{Acetoin}\\\text{dehydrogenase}}}{\nearrow} \qquad \xrightarrow{\substack{\text{Decarboxylation}\\\text{Acetolactate decarboxylase}}}$$

$$\underset{\substack{\text{Acetoin}\\\text{(acetylmethylcarbinol)}}}{\begin{array}{c}CH_3\\|\\H-C-OH\\|\\C=O\\|\\CH_3\end{array}} \qquad\qquad \underset{\substack{\text{Acetoin}\\\text{(acetylmethylcarbinol)}}}{\begin{array}{c}CH_3\\|\\H-C-OH\\|\\C=O\\|\\CH_3\end{array}} + CO_2$$

$$\text{NADH} + H^+ \searrow \substack{\text{Butanediol dehydrogenase}}$$

$$\underset{\text{2,3-Butanediol (2,3-butylene glycol) (9,15,21)}}{\begin{array}{c}CH_3\\|\\H-C-OH\\|\\H-C-OH\\|\\CH_3\end{array}} + NAD^+$$

$$\text{2,3-Butanediol} \xrightarrow[\text{2,3-butanediol dehydrogenase}]{\text{oxidation}} \text{Acetoin} \qquad (1)$$

$$\text{Acetoin} \xrightarrow[\text{diacetyl (acetoin) reductase}]{\text{reduction}} \text{2,3-Butanediol} \qquad (2)$$

Formation of 2,3-butanediol from glucose fermentation is usually of the "diol hydrogen" type (25).

$$\text{Glucose} \longrightarrow \text{2,3-Butanediol} + 2\,CO_2 + H_2$$

Production of 2,3-butanediol increases production of carbon dioxide, resulting in formation of fewer acids and accumulation of acetoin (25). The balance between acetoin and 2,3-butanediol is determined by the amount of available hydrogen (25), or differences in the oxidation-reduction potentials (43). In the presence of atmospheric oxygen and alkali, the neutral end products acetoin and 2,3-butanediol are oxidized to diacetyl, the reactant for the color produced in the Voges-Proskauer test (36, 39). Therefore, diacetyl is an oxidation product of acetoin.

A cyclic pathway was postulated by Juni and Heym (24–26) for the breakdown of 2,3-butanediol, acetoin, and diacetyl by organisms capable of using acetoin and 2,3-butanediol as the sole sources of carbon.

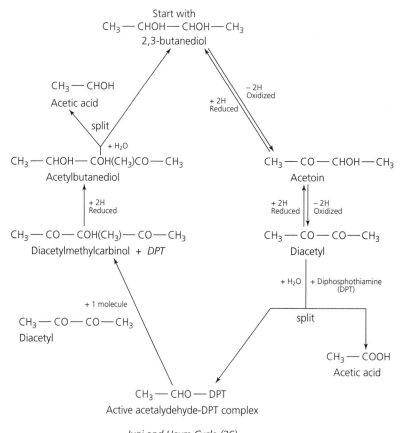

Juni and Heym Cycle (26)

(Reproduced from Juni, E., and Heym, G. (1956) J. Bacteriol. *71*, p. 427, with permission of The American Society for Microbiology.)

Starting with 2 molecules of 2,3-butanediol, 1 molecule of 2,3-butanediol is regenerated and 2 molecules of acetic acid are formed (24–26), which accounts for the rise in acidity.

The pH of the Voges-Proskauer medium is extremely important; an acid pH should be avoided. Above pH 6.3, acetic and formic acids accumulate with suppressed production of

CO_2, H_2, acetoin, and 2,3-butanediol. Below pH 6.3, acetic acid is converted to acetoin and 2,3-butanediol, and H_2 production is suppressed while CO_2 production is increased (15, 21). The *Klebsiella-Enterobacter* groups produce more ethanol than *E. coli*, fewer acids, and twice as much CO_2 as H_2 (a gas ratio of 2:1). *E. coli* cannot form acetoin from pyruvate in the normal incubation period and has a $CO_2:H_2$ ratio of 1:1 (21).

The overall reaction of glucose metabolism by the *Klebsiella-Enterobacter* groups follows (21).

$$\text{Glucose} \longrightarrow \text{2,3-Butanediol} + 2\,CO_2 + H_2$$

IV. MEDIUM EMPLOYED: MODIFIED CLARK AND LUBS MEDIUM (MR/VP BROTH) (10)

A. Ingredients; pH 6.9

Polypeptone or a buffered peptone	7.0 g
Dextrose (glucose)	5.0 g
Dipotassium phosphate buffer, K_2HPO_4	5.0 g
Deionized water	1000.0 mL

Commercial MR/VP medium is a modification of Clark and Lubs medium. Clark and Lubs used a 1% concentration of peptone and glucose, but a concentration of no less than 0.5% is the **minimum** that is satisfactory, so that the limiting hydrogen ion concentration is not reached by methyl red–negative organisms (4). A concentration of 0.5% peptone gives less color to the medium, which makes it easier to interpret the reaction.

B. Commercial products available: BBL, Difco, Merck, Oxoid
C. Method of preparation
   1. Weigh out amount accurately as directed on the label. Various company products may vary slightly.
   2. Rehydrate with deionized water.
   3. Heat **gently** into solution.
   4. Dispense approximately 5.0 mL per screw-cap tube (16 × 125 mm).
D. Method of sterilization: autoclave, 121°C, 15 lb, 15 min
E. Cool before use and refrigerate for storage (4–10°C). Shelf life, 6–8 weeks
F. Inoculation
   1. Growth from an 18- to 24-h **pure** culture (Kligler's iron agar (KIA)/triple sugar iron agar (TSI))
   2. **Light** inoculum (8); except **heavy** for Coblentz test procedure (14)
G. Incubation
   1. Absolute minimum: 35°C, 18–24 h
   2. Recommended (5, 9): 30°C, 3–5 days; may require longer incubation, up to 10 days (1)

Some bacteria, particularly *H. alvei*, are VP variable at 35°C, but positive at 25–30°C. If *H. alvei* is suspected, repeat the VP culture and incubate at 22–25°C (13, 18). Cowan (13) found that incubation at 30°C for 5 days is the minimum time to detect all VP-positive organisms among the *Enterobacteriaceae* with Barritt's (2) VP reagents (α-naphthol in ethanol and 40% KOH). However, for most VP-positive *Enterobacteriaceae*, 18–24 h of incubation at 35°C suffices.

H. Add the Voges-Proskauer reagents **directly** to an incubated **aliquot before** attempting an interpretation.

V. REAGENTS EMPLOYED: THREE CHOICES

A. **Barritt's VP reagents** (2)
   1. Reagent A: 5% α-naphthol in **absolute** ethyl alcohol (ethanol)
   2. Reagent B: 40% potassium hydroxide (KOH)
B. **Coblentz VP reagents** (12)
   1. Reagent A: 5% α-naphthol in **95%** ethanol
   2. Reagent B: 0.3% creatine in 40% KOH. Creatine: N-methyl-N-guanylglycine; NH:C (NH$_2$)N(CH$_3$)CH$_2$COOH
C. **O'Meara's (modified) single VP reagent**: 0.3% creatine in 40% KOH (33)
D. Method of preparation; all reagents above
   1. **α-Naphthol 5%, color intensifier**
      a. Ingredients

α-Naphthol (1-naphthol)	5.0 g
Ethanol (absolute or 95% depending on test procedure used)	100.0 mL

      b. Dissolve the α-naphthol in less than 100 mL of absolute (or 95%) ethanol.
      c. Transfer solution to a 100-mL volumetric flask and bring to 100 mL with absolute (or 95%) ethanol.
   2. **Potassium hydroxide (KOH), 40%, oxidizing agent**
      a. Ingredients

KOH	40.0 g
Creatine (Coblentz and O'Meara's reagents **only**)	0.3 g
Deionized water	100.0 mL

      b. **Rapidly** weigh out the KOH and dissolve in less than 100 mL of distilled water in a beaker. This reagent is highly hygroscopic. Add creatine **except** with Barritt reagent.
      c. Place beaker in a circulating cold water bath to control the temperature.
      d. Cool and transfer the KOH solution to a 100-mL volumetric flask and bring to 100 mL with distilled water.
      e. Store in a polyethylene or paraffin-lined glass reagent bottle. Shelf life, 2–3 weeks (6)
      f. Label correctly.

Sodium hydroxide (NaOH), 40%, may be substituted for 40% KOH. The ingredients and preparation are the same as those for potassium hydroxide. **Sodium and potassium hydroxide are extremely caustic solutions; avoid exposure to the skin as painful burns may occur.**

E. Method of Utilization

(*Note:* One medium is used for both MR and VP tests; MR test result (see Chapter 27) is determined after 48 h or longer incubation, the VP result usually after 24 h; therefore, one must test aliquots for the VP reaction in case it is necessary to prolong incubation for the MR test. However, use of an aliquot for the MR test is also recommended.

   1. **Aseptically** (by pipette) **remove an aliquot** for the Voges-Proskauer determination.
      a. Barritt's test: 2.5 mL (2)
      b. Coblentz test: 2.0 mL (12)
      c. O'Meara test: 1.0 mL (30)
   2. Add the VP reagents **directly to the aliquots** in the following order
      a. Barritt's or Coblentz reagents; **reagents appropriate to the test procedure being used** (2, 12)
         (1) **First:** 0.6 mL (6 drops) of reagent A
         (2) **Second:** 0.2 mL (2 drops) of reagent B
      b. O'Meara's procedure: Add 1 mL of reagent (30).

c. Shake tube(s) **gently** 30 sec to 1 min so the medium is exposed to atmospheric oxygen to oxidize the acetoin and obtain a color reaction.
3. Allow tube(s) to stand for an appropriate time **before** attempting to interpret the color.
   a. Barritt tubes: at least 10–15 min; reaction is often immediate (2).
   b. Coblentz tubes: 10–20 min (12)
   c. O'Meara tubes: 35°C or room temperature (22–25°C), final reading 4 h; if equivocal results (±), repeat tests with broth cultures incubated at 25°C, 48 h (20).

O'Meara's test depends on formation of acetoin, which is oxidized in alkaline medium in presence of air to form diacetyl; diacetyl reacts with creatine to produce a pinkish red compound (30).

F. **Storage:** Store reagent in a refrigerator (4°C) when not in use; O'Meara's reagent deteriorates rapidly, and should be stored no longer than 2–3 weeks (20).
G. **Chemistry of reagent action:** The Barritt reagents for detection of acetoin in the Voges-Proskauer test act in a three-step procedure (6, 11).

$$C_6H_{12}O_6 \xrightarrow{\text{Fermentation}} \underset{\substack{\text{Acetoin} \\ \text{(acetylmethylcarbinol, AMC)}}}{CH_3-CO-CHOH-CH_3} \quad (1)$$

$$\underset{\substack{\alpha\text{-Naphthol} \\ \text{(Catalyst)}}}{\text{C}_{10}H_7OH} + \underset{\text{Acetoin}}{CH_3-CO-CHOH-CH_3} \xrightarrow[O_2 \text{ (oxidized)}]{40\% \text{ KOH}} \underset{\text{Diacetyl}}{CH_3-CO-CO-CH_3} + 2 H_2O \quad (2)$$

$$\underset{\substack{\text{Diacetyl} \\ \text{(Substrate)}}}{CH_3-CO-CO-CH_3} + \underset{\substack{\text{Guanidine nucleus} \\ \text{present in peptone} \\ \text{(arginine: } NH{:}C(NH_2){\cdot}NH{\cdot}(CH_2)_3 - CH(NH_2)COOH)}}{C(NH_2)({=}NH)(NH{\cdot}R)} \xrightarrow{\text{condensation}} \text{Pinkish-red color} \quad (3)$$

The three main ingredients in the VP test are α-naphthol, a nitrogenous substance present in peptone, and diacetyl.

The **first reagent** added to an incubated aliquot is the catalyst α-naphthol. An alcoholic solution of α-naphthol is essential because it acts as a color intensifier, which increases the sensitivity of the reaction with no loss of specificity (2). α-Naphthol combines with the product of the reaction of diacetyl and the guanidine-type compound, arginine, present in peptone early in the reaction; thus it must be added first (2).

The **second reagent** is 40% KOH (or 40% NaOH), which in the VP medium aids in absorption of CO_2 (17). The exact amount of 0.2 mL should not be exceeded. **These two reagents,** α-naphthol and 40% KOH, must be added in the right order. KOH reacts with peptone to yield a salmon-pink color, and subsequent addition of α-naphthol will not alter the color (2).

After addition of α-naphthol and KOH, the tube **must be shaken gently** to expose the medium to atmospheric oxygen to oxidize any acetoin present to diacetyl. Branen and Keenan (5) showed that aeration by agitation greatly enhances diacetyl accumulation. KOH acts as an oxidizing agent and hastens oxidation of acetoin to diacetyl (2). Diacetyl is the essential reactant that gives a color reaction with KOH and peptone. With the use of an oxidizing agent, the color disappears rapidly, primarily because the reacting diacetyl-peptone complex may be rapidly oxidized further to a colorless compound (2).

Diacetyl is the active reacting substance, **not** p-xyloquinone ($C_6H_6O_2(CH_3)_2$), which can be formed from diacetyl by the action of KOH (19). The VP test is based on the reaction between diacetyl and the guanidine nucleus ($NH{:}C(NH_2){\cdot}NH{\cdot}R$) present in peptone under alkaline conditions (15). Harden and Norris (22) showed that diacetyl can react with compounds that contain the guanidine nucleus, such as arginine, agmatine, creatine, dicyanamide, and guanidineacetic acid. The guanidine nucleus–containing compound here is arginine ($NH{:}C(NH_2){\cdot}(NH){\cdot}(CH_2)_3^-\ CH(NH_2)COOH$) (2, 6). A free NH_2 group on the guanidine moiety available from arginine in peptone is necessary for color development (4). O'Meara (30) and Coblentz (12) reagents incorporate an additional source of guanidine nucleus, creatine ($H_2N{\cdot}C(NH){\cdot}N(CH_3){\cdot}(CH_2){\cdot}COOH$); an additional free NH_2 group intensifies color development, usually within 15 min.

Therefore, when diacetyl, peptone, and α-naphthol are mixed in correct proportions, a red color develops almost instantly (2) at the surface of the medium; the rate of color development depends on the amount of acetoin in the test culture (11). Harden and Walpole (23) postulated that this coloration only on the surface suggested an oxidation process. A positive reaction usually occurs within 2–5 min, exhibiting a faint pink color; however, marked coloration (deep red) occurs upon standing for 30 min. **Maximum color** is reached after 1 h (2). A 1-h or longer exposure of a negative VP culture to the reagents may show a copperlike color caused by the action of KOH on α-naphthol (2).

When acetoin and 2,3-butanediol are oxidized in the presence of alkali and peptone, to diacetyl and acetoin and then diacetyl, respectively, they yield a positive VP result (2, 15). Harden and Walpole (23) showed that neither 2,3-butanediol nor acetoin exhibits any coloration with KOH alone. However, acetoin and peptone without an alkali exhibits a positive VP result. The Barritt reagents are quite sensitive and specific, and this test has revealed that acetoin is produced by many bacteria previously considered VP negative (2). Eddy (17) used sensitive methods of detecting acetoin to show that the differences between bacteria (e.g., the *Enterobacteriaceae*) that were previously regarded as qualitative, may actually be quantitative.

VI. QUALITY CONTROL ORGANISMS

A. VP positive (+)

    Enterobacter cloacae   ATCC 13047

B. VP negative (−)

    Escherichia coli   ATCC 11775

    Uninoculated

VII. RESULTS

> See Figure 40.1 (Appendix 1) for colored photographic results

VIII. INTERPRETATION

A. VP positive (+): pinkish red color at the surface of the medium (acetoin present)
B. VP negative (−): yellow color at the surface of the medium (same color as the reagent). A copperlike color may form, but it is still a negative result (due to action of the reagents when mixed).

IX. ALTERNATIVE TESTS (REFER TO REFERENCES)

A. Gas-liquid chromatography (GLC); measures diacetyl (8, 14, 16, 27, 33).
B. Electron capture gas-liquid chromatography (EC-GLC) (28)
C. Gas chromatography–chemical ionization mass spectrometry (GC-CMS) (28)
D. Colorimetric method for diacetyl measurement (7)

X. RAPID VP TEST OF BARRY AND FEENEY (3)

A. MR/VP broth: **aseptically** pipette 0.2 mL into a 10 × 75 mm test tube.
B. Inoculum: loopful of growth from an 18- to 24-h **pure** culture from KIA, TSI, MacConkey agar (MAC), blood agar (BA), chocolate agar (CA); **not** from eosin methylene blue agar (EMB) (4)
C. Incubation: 35°C water bath, 4 h
D. Add reagents; shake well between each addition.
   1. Creatine solution: 0.3%; 2 drops
   2. Barritt's reagents: A **then** B, 2–3 drops of each
E. Positive (+): cherry red color within 15 min

XI. PRECAUTIONS

A. **General**
   1. Clark and Lubs (MR/VP) medium, either uninoculated or inoculated, looks exactly like indole medium. Be sure the tubes are labeled correctly before inoculation, as any mixup of media invalidates all test results.
   2. If commercial medium is not available, any medium is satisfactory that contains no less than 0.5% glucose and peptone and a phosphate buffer. Quality control tests **must** be performed.
   3. The methyl red and Voges-Proskauer tests should **not** be considered sufficient to differentiate *E. coli* from the *Klebsiella-Enterobacter* groups in routine identification or water analysis. Citrate and indole tests **must** be performed in conjunction with the MR/VP tests. There is the possibility that acetoin may be destroyed, making the two tests (MR and VP) invalid for identification purposes.
B. **Voges-Proskauer (VP) test medium**
   1. All members of the *Enterobacteriaceae* can produce acetoin from glucose, but not all strains can ferment acetoin, e.g., all strains of *E. aerogenes* (39). Some bacteria can me-

tabolize acetoin by either reduction or oxidation, thus reducing the amount of substrate for detection by the VP procedure (17). Acetoin may be reduced to 2,3-butanediol, which gives a negative VP reaction (17). The intermediate metabolism of strains varies (39).

2. Acetoin present in Clark and Lubs medium gives a positive reaction within 1–3 days of incubation. Some VP-positive organisms can produce an acid condition in the medium after prolonged incubation and yield weakly positive or false-negative VP results (31, 39). Some members of the *Escherichia-Enterobacter* groups can destroy acetoin (19, 38, 43); acid is produced when acetoin is used as the sole source of carbon (39, 44). Tittsler (39), working with strains of *E. aerogenes,* showed that this organism can produce acid and gas when cultivated in a synthetic medium containing acetoin as the sole source of carbon. Negative reactions are **not** due to depletion of peptone in the medium (39). As a carbon source, acetoin is fermented or converted into VP-negative compounds such as 2,3-butanediol by reduction or by oxidation to diacetyl, which is further metabolized (17, 39). However, the VP test can still be useful to distinguish *E. coli* from the *Klebsiella-Enterobacter* groups as long as the incubation period does not exceed 3 days (39).

3. Many laboratory personnel have the erroneous impression that an organism that is VP positive is automatically MR negative, or vice versa. It is true that most members of the *Enterobacteriaceae* give opposite reactions (increased alkalinity results in a negative MR and a positive VP due to the formation of acetoin (6)), but certain organisms such as *H. alvei* (when incubated at 37°C) and *Proteus mirabilis* may give both a positive MR and VP reaction, although the VP reaction is often delayed.

4. When performing the VP test to identify other organisms such as *Bacillus* and *Staphylococcus* spp., the phosphate present in Clark and Lubs medium may interfere with acetoin production (39). Smith et al. (35) recommend substituting sodium chloride (NaCl) for the phosphate, while Abd-el-Malek and Gibson (1) recommend a plain glucose-peptone broth without sodium chloride or phosphate.

5. The order of adding Barritt's VP reagents is extremely important. First add α-naphthol, then KOH. Reversing the order of reagent addition may give a weak positive or false-negative result. α-Naphthol combines **early** in the reaction with the product of the reaction of diacetyl and the guanidine-type compound present in peptone (2).

6. An exact amount, **0.2 mL**, of 40% KOH should not be exceeded, since excess KOH may mask a weakly positive VP reaction by exhibiting a copperlike color due to its reaction with α-naphthol alone (2).

7. The maximum color for detection of minimal quantities of acetoin is produced in a positive VP tube after 1 h of standing (2, 39). After exposure to the reagents for **over** 1 h, a negative VP culture may show a copperlike color because of the action of KOH on α-naphthol (2), causing a microbiologist to interpret the result as positive. Vaughn et al. (40) also found that completed tests may give a false-positive result after exposure to the reagents for more than 1 h and that these results occur more frequently with incubation at 30°C than at 37°C.

8. Meat infusion broth should **not** be used to grow the test organism because the acetoin, diacetyl, and related substances in muscle extract produce a false-positive test result (2).

9. Upon addition of α-naphthol and KOH, the tube(s) **must** be shaken **gently** to expose the medium to atmospheric oxygen to oxidize any acetoin present to diacetyl. Branen and Keenan (5) showed that aeration by agitation greatly enhanced oxidation of acetoin to diacetyl (2). Diacetyl is the essential reactant needed to produce the red color with KOH and peptone. With use of an oxidizing agent, the color disappears rapidly, primarily because the reacting diacetyl-peptone complex can be rapidly oxidized further to a colorless compound (2).

REFERENCES

1. Abd-el-Malek Y, Gibson T. Studies in the bacteriology of milk. II. The staphylococci and micrococci of milk. J Dairy Res 1948;15(3):249–260.
2. Barritt MM. The intensification of the Voges-Proskauer reaction by the addition of α-naphthol. J Pathol Bacteriol 1936;42(2):441–454.
3. Barry AL, Feeney KL. Two quick methods for Voges-Proskauer test. Appl Microbiol 1967;15(5):1138–1141.
4. Blazevic DJ, Ederer GM. Principles of Biochemical Tests in Diagnostic Microbiology. New York: John Wiley & Sons, 1975:105–107.
5. Branen AL, Keenan TW. Diacetyl and acetoin production by Lactobacillus casei. Appl Microbiol 1971;22(4):517–521.
6. Branson D. Methods in Clinical Bacteriology. Springfield IL: Charles C Thomas, 1972:49–51.
7. Brenner MW, Blick SR, Frenkel G, Siebenberg J. New light on diacetyl. Proc Eur Brew Conv 1964;9:233–235.
8. Brooks JB, Kellogg DS, Thacker L, Turner EM. Analysis by gas chromatography of hydroxy acids produced by several species of Neisseria. Can J Microbiol 1972;18(2):157–168.
9. Bryn K, Ulstrup JC, Størmer FC. Effect of acetate upon the formation of acetoin in Klebsiella and Enterobacter and its possible practical application in a rapid Voges-Proskauer test. Appl Microbiol 1973;25(3):511–512.
10. Clark WM, Lubs HA. The differentiation of bacteria of the colon-aerogenes family by the use of indicators. J Infect Dis 1915;17(1):160–173.
11. Clarke PH, Cowan ST. Biochemical methods for bacteriology. J Gen Microbiol 1952;6(2):187–197.
12. Coblentz LM. Rapid detection of the production of acetyl-methyl-carbinol. Am J Public Health 1943;33(7):815–817.
13. Cowan ST. Cowan & Steel's Manual for the Identification of Medical Bacteria, ed 2. Cambridge: Cambridge University Press, 1974:29, 37–38, 148.
14. Doelle HW. Gas chromatographic separation of micro quantities of acetone, C_1-C_7 alcohols, and diacetyl. J Gas Chromatogr 1967;5:582–584.
15. Doelle HW. Bacterial Metabolism. New York: Academic Press, 1969:284–291, 293–298, 368–369.
16. Drucker DB. Analysis of lactic acid and volatile fatty acids extracted from bacterial fermentations. J Chromatogr Sci 1970;8:489–490.
17. Eddy BP. The Voges-Proskauer reaction and its significance: A review. J Appl Bacteriol 1961;24(1):27–41.
18. Ewing WH. Edwards and Ewing's Identification of Enterobacteriaceae, ed 4. New York: Elsevier, 1986.
19. Feigl F. Spot Tests in Organic Analysis, ed 7. New York: Elsevier, 1966:446.
20. Finegold SM, Baron EJ. Bailey and Scott's Diagnostic Microbiology, ed 7. St. Louis: CV Mosby, 1986:159, 216, 495.
21. Gunsalus IC, Stanier RY. The Bacteria, vol II. New York: Academic Press, 1961:84–89, 92–93.
22. Harden A, Norris D. The bacterial production of acetylmethylcarbinol and 2,3-butyleneglycol from various substances. Proc R Soc 1911–1912;84:492–499.
23. Harden A, Walpole GS. Chemical action of Bacillus lactis aerogenes (Escherichia) on glucose and mannitol production of 2,3-butyleneglycol and acetylmethylcarbinol. Proc R Soc B 1906;77:399–405.
24. Juni E, Heym GA. A cyclic pathway for the bacterial dissimulation of 2,3-butanediol, acetylmethylcarbinol, and diacetyl. I. General aspects of the 2,3-butanediol cycle. J Bacteriol 1956;71(4):425–432.
25. Juni E, Heym GA. A cyclic pathway for the bacterial dissimulation of 2,3-butanediol, acetylmethylcarbinol, and diacetyl. II. The synthesis of diacetylmethylcarbinol from diacetyl, a new diphosphothiamin catalyzed reaction. J Bacteriol 1956;72(6):746–753.
26. Juni E, Heym GA. A cyclic pathway for the bacterial dissimulation of 2,3-butanediol, acetylmethylcarbinol, and diacetyl. III. A comparative study of 2,3-butanediol dehydrogenase from various microorganisms. J Bacteriol 1957;74(6):757–767.
27. Lee SM, Drucker DB. Analysis of acetoin and diacetyl in bacterial culture supernatants by gas-liquid chromatography. J Clin Microbiol 1975;2(3):162–164.
28. Morse CD, Brooks JB, Kellogg DS. Electron capture gas chromatographic detection of acetylmethylcarbinol produced by Neisseria gonorrhoeae. J Clin Microbiol 1976;3(1):34–41.
29. Murray PR, Baron EJ, Pfaller MA, et al. Manual of Clinical Microbiology, ed 6. Washington, DC: American Society for Microbiology, 1995:302–304.
30. O'Meara RAQ. A simple delicate and rapid method of detecting the formation of acetylmethylcarbinol by bacteria fermenting carbohydrate. J Pathol Bacteriol 1931;34(4):401–406.
31. Paine FS. The destruction of acetylmethylcarbinol by members of the colon-aerogenes group. J Bacteriol 1927;13(4):269–274.
32. Paretsky D, Werkman CH. The conversion of 2,3-butyleneglycol to acetylmethylcarbinol in bacterial fermentation. Arch Biochem Biophys 1947;14(1):11–25.
33. Rigby R. Reagent for the oxidation of acylions to diketones. J Chem Soc 1951:793–795.
34. Smith DT, Conant NF, Willett HP. Zinsser's Microbiology, ed 14. New York: Appleton-Century-Crofts, 1968:113.

35. Smith NR, Gordon RE, Clark FE. Aerobic mesophilic sporeforming bacteria. U.S. Department of Agriculture, misc. publ no. 559, 1946.
36. Sokatch JR. Bacterial Physiology and Metabolism. New York: Academic Press, 1969:78.
37. Stahly GL, Werkman CH. Origin and relationship of acetylmethylcarbinol to 2,3-butyleneglycol in bacterial fermentations. Biochem J 1942;36:575–581.
38. Strecker HJ, Harary I. Bacterial butylene glycol dehydrogenase and diacetyl reductase. J Biol Chem 1954;211(1):263–270.
39. Tittsler RP. The fermentation of acetylmethylcarbinol by the *Escherichia-Aerobacter* group and its significance in the Voges-Proskauer reaction. J Bacteriol 1938;35:157–162.
40. Vaughn R, Mitchell NB, Levine M. The Voges-Proskauer and methyl red reactions in the coli-aerogenes group. J Am Water Works Assoc 1939;31:993–1001.
41. Voges O, Proskauer B. Beitrag zur Ernärungsphysiologie und zur Differential-diagnose der Bakterien der hämorrhagischen Septicemia. Z Hyg Infektkr 1898;28:20–37.
42. Walpole GS. The action of *Bacillus lactis* aerogenes on glucose and mannitol. II. The investigation of the 2:3 butanediol and the acetylmethylcarbinol formed; the effect of free oxygen on their production; The action of *B. lactis* aerogenes on fructose. Proc R Soc B 1910–1911;83:272–286.
43. Werkman CH. An improved technic for the Voges-Proskauer test. J Bacteriol 1930;20(2):121–125.
44. Williams OB, Morrow MB. The bacterial destruction of acetyl-methylcarbinol. J Bacteriol 1928;16(1):43–48.

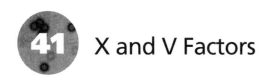

41 X and V Factors

I. PRINCIPLE

Determine the requirement for X and V growth factors to support growth of *Haemophilus* spp. in vitro

II. PURPOSE

Qualitative procedure for isolation and differentiation of *Haemophilus* spp.; growth depends partially on the presence of the X or V factors or both (5).

III. BIOCHEMISTRY INVOLVED

X Factor

The heme portion of hemoglobin (protoporphyrin) necessary for synthesis of respiratory enzymes; also called hemin and hematin; **heat stable**

V Factor

Coenzyme nicotinamide adenine dinucleotide (NAD); **heat labile**

X and V Factors

Both X and V factors remain within **intact** red blood cells (RBCs). They are **not** readily available to *Haemophilus* spp. on **un**heated sheep blood agar (SBA) media (6).

IV. MEDIA/REAGENTS EMPLOYED

A. Media
   1. Inoculum medium: brain-heart infusion broth (BHIB)
   2. Test media; agar media **without** growth factors
      a. Trypticase soy agar (TSA)
      b. Brain-heart infusion agar (BHIA).
B. Reagents
   1. Paper strips or disks impregnated with X and V factors
   2. Commercially available; BBL: Taxo X, V, and XV strips (6)

V. PROCEDURE

A. From a **pure** agar culture of **suspected** *Haemophilus* sp., prepare a **light** suspension of growth in BHIB.
   1. With a **sterile** swab, inoculate the surface of either TSA or BHIA (factor-deficient agars).
   2. Swab surface for maximum growth.
   3. Allow a few minutes for agar surface to dry.
B. Place X and V strips (or disks) on agar in area of inoculum.

1. Place strips approximately 1 cm apart.
2. **Gently** press down on strips so that they adhere to agar surface.

C. Incubation: 3–5%, CO_2, 35°, 18–24 h.

VI. QUALITY CONTROL ORGANISMS

    X factor only: *Haemophilus haemoglobinophilus*   ATCC 19416
    V factor only: *Haemophilus parainfluenzae*   ATCC 33392
    X and V factors: *Haemophilus influenzae*   ATCC 33391

VII. INTERPRETATION

Visually inspect agar surface for visible growth **between** or **around** one or more of the strips (or disks) (Fig. 41.1; Table 41.1). X factor requirement may occasionally be observed on primary isolation but is best on subculture (2).

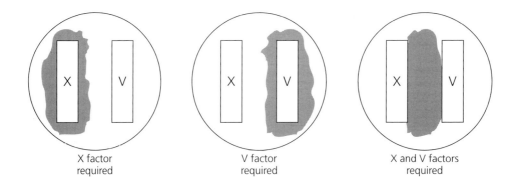

X factor required   V factor required   X and V factors required

Table 41.1. Growth of *Haemophilus* spp. with X and/or V factors

	Factor	
Organism	X	V
H. actinomycetem-comitans	−	−
H. aphrophilus	−	−
H. ducreyi	+	−
H. haemoglobinophilus	+	−
H. haemolyticus	+	+
H. influenzae	+	+
H. paracuniculus	−	+
H. paragallinarum	−	+
H. parahaemolyticus	−	+
H. parainfluenzae	−	+
H. paraprohaemophilus	−	+
H. parasuis	−	+
H. segnis	−	+

VIII. PRECAUTIONS

A. Perform tests on all isolates **suspected** of being *Haemophilus* on the basis of growth characteristics and colony morphology on chocolate agar (CA).
B. Strips or disks should be separated on the plates so that synergy of growth because of diffusion of growth factors is prevented (4).

C. Mueller-Hinton agar should **not** be used for the test since it supports a small amount of growth of some *Haemophilus* strains (4).
D. The X and V growth test should **not** be performed on blood agar because the RBCs bind V factor, making it unavailable to the test organism and markedly inhibiting growth of *H. influenzae* (4).
E. A **light suspension** of the test organism in saline or broth is **essential** to reduce the carryover of nutrients from chocolate agar; a heavy inoculum increases the chance of some visible growth around the V strip (disk) before the organism can be considered to be *H. parainfluenzae* (4).
F. *Eikenella corrodens* may exhibit growth around the X strip; a useful diagnostic test (40).
G. When transferring growth from isolation medium to inoculum broth avoid any pickup of hemin-containing medium from primary isolation plate (3). Many X factor–requiring organisms can carry over enough factor from primary isolation medium to give a false-negative result (e.g., growth occurs so far from the X strip that it falsely indicates that the organism **does not** require X factor (1). Testing for these factors has largely been replaced by the porphyrin test (ALA) (Chapter 36), which establishes an organisms's X factor requirement without the problem of carryover from primary isolation media.
H. Allow inoculum on test medium to dry thoroughly before placing strips/disks on agar surface.
I. **Do not** place strips too close to one another; results may be confusing.

REFERENCES

1. Forbes BA, Sahm DF, Weissfeld AS. Bailey & Scott's Diagnostic Microbiology, ed. 10. St. Louis: CV Mosby, 1998:559.
2. Kilian M. A taxonomic study of the genus *Haemophilus* with the proposal of a new species. J Gen Microbiol 1976;93:9–62.
3. Koneman EW, Allen SD, Janda WM, et al. Color Atlas & Textbook of Diagnostic Microbiology, ed. 5. Philadelphia: JB Lippincott, 1997:1383–1384.
4. Oberhof TR. Manual of Practical Medical Microbiology and Parasitology. New York: John Wiley & Sons, 1985:282–284.
5. Parker RH, Doeprich PD. Disc method for rapid identification of *Haemophilus* sp. Am J Clin Pathol 1962;37:319–327.
6. Power DA, McCuen PJ. Manual of BBL Products and Laboratory procedures, ed 6. Cockeysville, MD: Becton Dickinson Microbiology Systems, 1988:328.

SECTION II

Multitest Systems

# 42 Multitest Systems

A number of commercial multitest systems (kits) and molecular microbiology techniques, as well as numerous other media with combined tests, are on the market. Most have undergone extensive testing by various laboratories, resulting in modifications of some to enhance their usefulness.

Most commercial multitest kits use a microtechnique, with a number of tests incorporated into a single unit. This may create problems not usually encountered with standard macrotechniques currently still in use: carryover of substrate during inoculation causes problems, both age and concentration of the inoculum can be critical (some tests require a light inoculum while others a heavy inoculum), and primarily, problems arise from the use of these kits and combined media by laboratory personnel **not** experienced enough in bacteriology to be aware of their limitations and/or potential problems. This is especially seen in small laboratories in doctors' offices where the tests are performed by nursing or administrative staff who are not trained in bacteriology.

Many commercial kits are primarily used to differentiate and identify members of the *Enterobacteriaceae*, a family of bacteria that requires the utmost in knowledge and experience for accurate identification, since it includes many organisms that can vary far from the norm in biochemical activity.

The past saw increased interest in the Gram-negative, nonfermenting bacilli (rods) (NF, NFB). These organisms have been found with increased frequency in clinical specimens and hospital environments, and because of their multiple drug resistance, accurate identification has put a burden on many laboratories. Identification of nonfermenters requires extensive biochemical testing with interpretation by experienced bacteriology personnel; however, the main problem is the lengthy incubation required and the dire need for rapid identification. Many laboratories are not equipped with either the means or the experienced personnel to identify nonfermenters. Many multitest systems kits are on the market. As with any of the multitest systems there are precautions. The multitest systems for nonfermenters are an **aid** but do **not** usually suffice for definitive identification; supplemental tests are often required, and their selection and interpretation require experienced judgment.

When these kits are used, the results obtained **must** be correlated with other identifying characteristics such as specimen source and colony morphology on both differential and selective media before a **presumptive** identification is made. Also, many of the results may **not** suffice for confirmation, and further biochemical and serologic testing may be required.

The manufacturer's direction must be followed explicitly. Read directions carefully to become familiar with the kit's primary purpose and its limitations.

The more frequently used multitest systems kits and automated instruments are listed here. Listing all systems and techniques in any detail here is not feasible (see the American Society for Microbiology (ASM) Manual (169) and Koneman's book (132)). Information about these systems can usually be acquired from the manufacturer upon request (for addresses see Appendix 11).

Molecular microbiology is the newest field for bacteria identification: nucleic acid amplification techniques (probe, signal, and target amplifications), DNA sequencing and typing, direct molecular probe techniques, nucleic acid quantitation, and gene chip technology (166, 167, 188, 211).

I. MISCELLANEOUS COMBINED TEST MEDIA

(*Note:* Refer to test reference(s) for procedures; most media are commercially available.)
A. **Coagulase mannitol agar/broth**
   1. Combined plate media of Esber and Faulconer (70)
   2. Purpose: isolation of pathogenic *Staphylococcus* spp. (Fig. 42.1, Appendix 1)
   3. Reactions are not sufficient to speciate staphylococci; additional tests required (e.g., coagulase, DNase)
B. **FN medium (fluorescence-denitrification medium)/fluorescence-lactose-nitrate medium (FLN)**
   1. Tubed medium of Pickett and Pedersen (191–193)
   2. Differentiates pseudomonads from other nonfermentative bacilli by ability to reduce nitrate to nitrite (denitrification) and possession of fluorescein pigment
C. **Indole-nitrate medium (Trypticase nitrate broth)**
   1. Differential by ability to reduce nitrate and/or produce indole; supports growth of aerobes and facultative and obligate anaerobes
   2. One tube combined test medium for indole and/or nitrate determination for bacteria other than the *Enterobacteriaceae* (57)
   3. Not recommended for coliforms and other enterics (57)
      a. False-negative indole results
      b. Rapid reduction of nitrates and formation of sodium nitrate may inhibit indole production (222)
D. **Lecithin-lactose anaerobic agar (anaerobic lecithin-lactose agar)**
   1. Formulation of Ellner and O'Donnell (68, 69)
   2. Purpose
      a. Differential by the ability to ferment lactose and/or produce lecithinase
      b. Selective for isolation and differentiation of histotoxic *Clostridium* spp.
E. **Lecithin-lipase anaerobic agar, modified McClung-Toabe agar)**
   1. Modification of McClung and Toabe agar (156)
   2. Differential by ability to produce lecithinase and/or demonstrate lipase activity
F. **Lombard-Dowell (LD) media**: Presumpto plate media of Dowell and Lombard (56–58); single plate with four quadrants of different media; aids in identification of **anaerobic** bacteria
   1. LD agar
      a. Evaluates degree of growth and indole and catalase production
      b. Differentiates *Bacteroides* and *Fusobacterium* spp.
   2. LD bile agar: differentiates *Bacteroides* spp. by ability to grow in the presence of bile with/without formation of a precipitate
   3. LD egg yolk agar: detects lipase, lecithinase, and proteolytic activity of both sporeforming and nonsporeforming obligate anaerobes, e.g., *Bacteroides, Fusobacterium, Clostridium* spp. and nonsporeforming Gram-positive anaerobes
   4. LD esculin agar: determines esculin hydrolysis, hydrogen sulfide (H_2S), and catalase production of *Bacteroides* and *Fusobacterium* spp.
   5. LD gelatin agar: determines gelatinase activity of *Clostridium* spp.
G. **Lysine-ornithine-mannitol (LOM) agar**
   1. Formulation of Bucher and von Graevenitz (26); modification of Rimler-Shotts medium (220)
   2. Differentiates by ability to ferment mannitol and decarboxylate lysine and/or ornithine
   3. Detects and aids in identifying *Pantoea agglomerans* (formerly in *Enterobacter* genus)

H. **Methyl red–Voges-Proskauer broth medium (MR/VP broth, Clark and Lubs medium)**
   1. Formulation of Clark and Lubs (35)
   2. Aids in differentiation between genera or between species within a genus
I. **Motility-indole-lysine (MIL)/motility-indole-lysine-sulfate (MILS) media**
   1. MIL formulation of Reller and Mirrett (198); MILS formulation of Ederer, Lund, Blazevic, Reller, and Mirrett (64)
   2. Five biochemical determinations: indole, H_2S, lysine decarboxylase, lysine deaminase, and motility
   3. Together with KIA or TSI and urea permits early presumptive identification of *Enterobacteriaceae* pathogens from fecal specimens
J. **Motility-indole-ornithine (MIO) medium**
   1. Formulation of Ederer and Clark (63), and Oberhofer and Hajkowski (176)
   2. Single-tube test medium
   3. Aids in identification of *Enterobacteriaceae*
K. **Motility-nitrate medium (motility S, motility medium S)**
   1. Formulation of Ball and Sellers (8)
   2. Determination of motility, gelatin liquefaction, and nitrate (NO_3) reduction
L. **Motility-sulfide medium**
   1. Formulation of Hajna (88); modification of Edwards and Bruner (65)
   2. Determination of motility and H_2S
M. **Sulfide indole motility medium (SIM)**
   1. Differentiates by ability to produce indole and H_2S and exhibit motility
   2. Aids in identification of Gram-negative *Enterobacteriaceae* especially *Salmonella* and *Shigella* following presumptive identification evidence on differential tubed medium (KIA/TSI)
   3. Reactions **not** sufficient to speciate; additional biochemical and serologic tests are required for confirmation.
   4. H_2S reactions are intensified with motile cultures.
N. **Trehalose-mannitol broth**
   1. Formulation of Knapp and Washington (130)
   2. Differentiates *Staphylococcus epidermidis* from other coagulase-negative staphylococci in 2 h
O. **Trehalose-mannitol-phosphate agar (TMPA)**
   1. Formulation of Stevens and Jones (229)
   2. Identifies and differentiates *S. epidermidis* and *Staphylococcus saprophyticus* when used in conjunction with novobiocin disk
   3. Other human species of coagulase-negative staphylococci produce variable reactions.

II. MICROTECHNIQUES: MULTITEST SYSTEMS, KITS WITH/WITHOUT AUTOMATION

(*Note:* Most kits are miniaturized, and interpretation of reactions generates a biotype number that is used along with a computer-assisted database to identify organism(s).)
(*Note:* Becton Dickinson Microbiology Systems has been renamed BD Biosciences.)
A. ***Actinobacillus* identification:** polymerase chain reaction (PCR) (54)
B. ***Actinobacillus actinomycetemcomitans* identification**
   1. PAGE; polyacrylamide gel electrophoresis
   2. PCR (85)
C. **Anaerobe identification** (56)
(*Note:* Except for API-ZYM, all systems provide numeric codes, computer databases, and identification tables.)

1. API-ZYM: manufacturer, bioMerieux
2. API-An-Indent: manufacturer, bioMerieux
3. ATB 32A: manufacturer, bioMerieux
4. API 20A: manufacturer, bioMerieux
5. IDS RapID-ANA II: manufacturer, REMEL (Fig. 42.2, Appendix 1)
6. Minitek Anaerobe II: manufacturer, BD Biosciences
7. Rapid ID ANA: manufacturer, bioMerieux
8. MicroScan Rapid Anaerobic Identification System: manufacturer, Dade/MicroScan
9. Vitek Anaerobe Identification (ANI) card: manufacturer, bioMerieux
10. BBL Crystal Anaerobe (ANR) ID panel (31)

D. ***Bordetella pertussis* identification**
   1. Direct fluorescent antibody (DFA): tests nasopharyngeal smears directly
   2. ELISA (enzyme-linked immunosorbent assay): tests isolated colonies (87, 212)
   3. PCR (27, 86, 95, 141, 241): identification of *B. pertussis* and *B. parapertussis*
   4. Pulsed-field gel electrophoresis (13, 50)

E. ***Brucella* spp. identification**: Biolog (255)
   1. Manufacturer, Biolog
   2. Carbon substrate utilization test

F. ***Burkholderia* identification**
   1. Latex agglutination (228)
   2. Pulsed-field gel electrophoresis (34)
   3. RapID NF Plus

G. ***Campylobacter* spp. identification**
   1. Latex agglutination tests
      a. Meritec-Campy (jcl) (171)
         (1) Manufacturer, Meridian Diagnostics
         (2) Culture isolate identifies *C. jejuni, C. coli,* and *C. lari*
      b. Campslide (100)
         (1) Manufacturer, BD Biosciences
         (2) Used for genus-level culture confirmation of four major pathogens: *C. jejuni, C. coli, C. lari,* and *C. fetus* subsp. *fetus*
   2. AccuProbe *Campylobacter* culture identification test
      a. Manufacturer, Gen-Probe
      b. DNA probe-based test for rapid identification of *C. jejuni, C. coli,* and *C. lari* directly from bacterial colonies
   3. API Campy (108); manufacturer, bioMerieux
   4. PCR (80, 145, 160, 164)
   5. Pulsed-field gel electrophoresis (91)

H. ***Corynebacterium* spp. identification**
   1. API Coryne system (76, 123)
      a. Manufacturer, bioMerieux
      b. Identify to genus or species level
   2. API 20 NEC: manufacturer, bioMerieux (76)
   3. IDS RapID CB Plus (107): manufacturer, REMEL (Fig. 42.3, Appendix 1)
   4. Carbon substrate assimilation (199)

I. ***Clostridium difficile* identification** (4, 149, 179)
   1. EIAs (enzyme immunoassays) to detect enterotoxin (toxin A), cytotoxin (toxin B), or both
   2. Six commercial systems available; detection from feces (159, 253).
      a. Cytoclone A and B: manufacturer, Cambridge Biotech
      b. Premier Toxin A test: manufacturer, Meridian Diagnostics

c. Primatoxin A: manufacturer, Bartels
   d. Toxin CD EIA: manufacturer, BD Biosciences
   e. TechLab Toxin A test: manufacturer, Tech Lab
   f. VIDAS *C. difficile* Toxin A test: manufacturer, bioMerieux
  3. PCR (36)
  4. ImmunoCard: manufacturer, Meridian Diagnostics (225)
J. ***Enterococcus* spp. identification** (72)
  1. API Rapid Strep; manufacturer, bioMerieux
  2. MicroScan Pos ID panel (133, 236, 257): manufacturer, Dade/MicroScan
  3. Genetic and molecular methods (67)
     a. DNA hybridization methods (55)
     b. Contour-clamped homogeneous electric field electrophoresis
     c. Ribotyping
     d. Pulsed-field gel electrophoresis (40, 81, 84, 150)
     e. PCR (33, 60)
K. ***Enterobacteriaceae* identification**
  1. *Escherichia coli* identification
     a. Screening procedures to detect isolates of toxic serotype 0157:147 strains responsible for hemorrhagic colitis
     b. Tests: indole, ONPG, and 4-methylumbeliferyl-(β-D-glucuronide (MUG)
     c. Systems
        (1) Lyfo-Kwik OMI: manufacturer, MicroBioLogics
        (2) MUG Plus: Difco (235)
        (3) BactiCard *E. coli:* REMEL (62, 127)
  2. Detection of urinary tract pathogens
     a. Purpose: detection of bacteria most commonly encountered in urinary tract infections: *E. coli, Proteus, Klebsiella, Serratia, Enterobacter, Pseudomonas* spp. and coagulase-negative staphylococci, enterococci, and others (176)
     b. Systems
        (1) IDS RapID SS/u System
            (a) Manufacturer, REMEL
            (b) 12 single chromogenic substrates
        (2) OMP and NGP-Wee Tabs (106)
            (a) Manufacturer, Key Scientific Products
            (b) Two substrate tablets provide 8 enzymatic tests that combined with urease identify 95% of the *Enterobacteriaceae*
        (3) Commercial screening agars: combination of chromogenic agars and rapid spot tests
            (a) CPS ID 2: manufacturer, bioMerieux (155)
            (b) Rainbow Agar UTI System: manufacturer, Biolog (18, 214)
  3. Specific ID systems
     a. API 20 E (30, 174, 180)
        (1) Manufacturer, bioMerieux
        (2) **Reference method against which the accuracy of other systems is compared; most frequently used in clinical laboratories; has large database including common and atypical strains**
        (3) 21 characteristics determined
        (4) Read with API Profile with computer assistance or can be read manually
     b. API Rapid 20 E (RE) (174, 180)
        (1) Manufacturer, bioMerieux

(2) Differs from API 20 E in that substrates are not buffered; therefore yields faster reactions (4 h) and smaller cupules (wells)
  c. BBL Crystal Enteric/Nonfermenter (E/NF) D System (206, 245)
    (1) Manufacturer, BD Biosciences
    (2) Purpose: identification of clinically significant aerobic, Gram-negative *Enterobacteriaceae* plus more-frequently isolated Gram-negative, glucose fermenting and nonfermenting bacilli of human origin
    (3) Miniaturized; modified and conventional chromogenic substrates (Fig. 42.4, Appendix 1)
    (4) Tests for fermentation, oxidation, degradation, and hydrolysis.
  d. BBL Crystal Rapid Stool/Enteric ID Panel
    (1) Manufacturer, BD Biosciences
    (2) 4-h identification from stool specimens
  e. IDS RapID ONE System (128)
    (1) Manufacturer, REMEL
    (2) Purpose: identification of selected oxidase-negative, Gram-negative *Enterobacteriaceae* isolated from human clinical specimens and other selected oxidase-negative, Gram-negative bacteria (Fig. 42.5, Appendix 1)
  f. Enterotube II (110, 121, 175, 181, 234)
    (1) Manufacturer, BD Biosciences
    (2) Easiest to inoculate (132); risk of contamination minimal
    (3) 15 biochemical determinations; computer coding and ID system (CCIS) (Fig. 42.6, Appendix 1)
  g. Micro-ID (11, 79, 121)
    (1) Manufacturer, REMEL
    (2) 15 reaction chambers; results in 4–6 h
  h. Minitek (92, 126, 252)
    (1) Manufacturer, BD Biosciences
    (2) Highly recommended; choice in selection of characteristics for identification (132)
    (3) 40 different reagent-impregnated disks
    (4) Identification of organisms other than the enterics, e.g. nonfermenters and anaerobes
  i. r/b Enteric Differential System: manufacturer, REMEL
  j. Rapid Gram-Neg ID Type 2: manufacturer, Dade International/Dade MicroScan
4. Replicator system (75)
  a. Identification of enterics, Gram-positive cocci, and other organisms
  b. Backbone Steers replicator; seed plate with 32–36 wells; standard agar
5. Biolog GN MicroPlate
  a. Manufacturer, Biolog
  b. Tests 95 different carbon sources in presence of a redox indicator
  c. Problems with some strains of *Klebsiella, Enterobacter,* and *Serratia* spp.; least biochemically active are *Moraxella* and *Neisseria* strains (102)
6. Automated systems
  a. MicroScan System (48, 202, 215)
    (1) Manufacturer, Dade/MicroScan
    (2) Identification of *Enterobacteriaceae* and other Gram-positive, Gram-negative bacilli
    (3) 32 reagent substrates; urinary tract panel and antimicrobic panel for susceptibility tests available
    (4) AutoScan-4-automated reader

b. Septor System (258)
      (1) Manufacturer, BD Biosciences
      (2) Substrate panels
   c. Sensititre Gram-Negative Autoidentification System (224)
      (1) Manufacturer, AccuMed International
      (2) Fluorescent technology to detect bacterial growth and enzyme activity; 32 biochemical tests
      (3) Manual enteric system or Automated-Sensititre AutoReader
   d. Vitek System (AMS) (22, 142)
      (1) Manufacturer, bioMerieux
      (2) Reliable approach to rapid identification of commonly encountered Gram-negative bacilli (132)
      (3) *Enterobacteriaceae*-plus Biochemical Card (EBC+)
      (4) GNI+ Card (Gram-negative identification): identification of glucose-fermenting organisms within 2–8 h; glucose-nonfermenting organisms within 4–12 h (168)
   e. MicroScan Walkaway/Auto SCAN-W/A (122, 177, 178, 189, 200, 260)
      (1) Manufacturer, Dade/MicroScan
      (2) Rapid fluorescein panels in additional to 96 conventional tests available for use with the Walkaway automated instrument
      (3) Rapid Gram Negative Identification Panel 3: 36 newly formulated tests and new database (1)
   7. PCR (74, 232)
   8. Premier EHEC (119, 182)
      a. Manufacturer, Meridian Diagnostics
      b. Detects Shiga toxin–producing *Shigella* and *E. coli;* enzyme-linked immunosorbent assay
   9. Pulsed-field gel electrophoresis (161, 219)
L. **Gram-negative bacteria identification**: identifies glucose nonfermenting, Gram-negative bacteria and selected glucose-fermenting Gram-negative bacteria other than the *Enterobacteriaceae*
   1. API 20 E (185): manufacturer, bioMerieux
   2. BBL Crystal F/NF (186): manufacturer, BD Biosciences (103) (Fig. 42.7, Appendix 1)
   3. MicroScan Walkaway System: manufacturer, Dade/MicroScan (200)
   4. Rapid Gram-Neg ID type 3: manufacturer, Dade/MicroScan (12)
   5. IDS RapID NF Plus panel; manufacturer, REMEL; used to identify Gram-negative bacteria other than the *Enterobacteriaceae;* glucose-nonfermenting Gram-negative bacteria and selective glucose-fermenting Gram-negative bacteria
   6. Radiometer Sensititre AO 80 (226)
   7. Rapid NFT; manufacturer, Analytab Products (226)
M. **Gram-positive rods**
   1. Minitek Gram-Pos kit
      a. Manufacturer, BD Biosciences
      b. Filter paper disks impregnated with various substrates
   2. BBL Crystal Gram-Positive ID panel
      a. Manufacturer, BD Biosciences
      b. Identifies clinical specimens in 4 h (Fig. 42.8, Appendix 1)
   3. MicroScan Gram-Positive Breakpoint Combo panel
      a. Manufacturer, Dade/MicroScan
      b. Simultaneous identification and antimicrobial susceptibility results; microtiter format
   4. Vitek Gram-Positive Identification (GPI) card
      a. Manufacturer, bioMerieux

b. Same system used to identify coagulase-negative staphylococci and certain non-sporeforming, facultatively Gram-positive bacilli
   5. Gas liquid chromatography (GLC)
   6. High-pressure liquid chromatography (HPLC) of
      a. Mycolic acids (28, 47)
      b. Menaquinones (16, 38, 39, 259)
N. *Francisella tularensis* identification: Microbial Identification (MIDI) System
   1. Manufacturer, MIDI
   2. Cellular fatty acid analysis
O. **Fastidious Gram-negative rods**
   1. IDS RapID NH system; manufacturer, REMEL
   2. Vitek *Neisseria-Haemophilus* Identification (NHI) card; manufacturer, bioMerieux
   3. MicroScan *Haemophilus-Neisseria* Identification (HNID) panel; manufacturer, Dade/MicroScan
P. *Fusobacterium nucleatum* identification: PCR (21)
Q. *Haemophilus* spp. identification
   1. RIM-H (Rapid Identification Method) (183)
      a. Manufacturer, Ortho Diagnostics Systems
      b. Two systems
         (1) *Haemophilus* 1/RIM
            (a) Carbohydrates, ALA (δ-aminolevulinic acid) porphyrin test
            (b) Species identification
         (2) 2/RIM: indole, ornithine, and urease for biotypes of *H. influenzae* and *H. parainfluenzae*
   2. Systems used for identification within 4 h with pure cultures (53, 112)
      a. IDS RapID NH: manufacturer, REMEL
      b. *Neisseria-Haemophilus* Identification (NHI) Card; manufacturer, bioMerieux
      c. HNID: manufacturer, Dade/MicroScan
      d. BBL Crystal *Neisseria/Haemophilus* ID panel
         (1) Manufacturer, BD Biosciences
         (2) Identification of *Neisseria*, *Haemophilus* spp., and fastidious *Gardnerella vaginalis*
   3. Systems also used to identify enterics (7, 61, 106): to biotype *Haemophilus* strains
      a. API 20E; bioMerieux
      b. Micro ID (61); Dade/MicroScan
      c. Minitek system; BD Biosciences
   4. *Haemophilus influenzae* type b immunologic identification techniques (151, 204, 208, 218, 249)
      a. Polyribosyl-ribitol-phosphate (PRP) capsular antigen in urine and serum
      b. Directigen Meningitis Test
         (1) Manufacturer, BD Biosciences
         (2) Latex particle agglutination
      c. Wellcogen bacterial antigen kit: manufacturer, Murex Diagnostics (109)
      d. Phadebact *H. influenzae* type b: manufacturer, Karo Bio AB (37)
      e. Coagglutination tests
      f. Counterimmunoelectrophorsis tests
      g. PCR (54, 203)
R. *Helicobacter pylori* identification
   1. Biopsy urease test (CLO test) (157)
      a. Medium containing urea and a pH-sensitive dye inoculated with a mucosal biopsy specimen
      b. Test may give false-negative results if small number of organisms present (157)

c. False-positive results if other urea-splitting organisms are present (159)
 2. Urease breath test (UBT) (43, 153)
   a. Noninvasive test
   b. Patient ingests ^{13}C-labeled urea dissolved in water followed by collection of breath samples after 60 min to be analyzed for the presence of $^{13}CO_2$
 3. Radio-labeled urea test (43)
   a. Oral ingestion of urea containing ^{15}N
   b. Urea is broken down by *H. pylori* in the stomach and excreted in the urine; amount and rate of excretion are determined.
 4. PCR (134, 147, 247)
 5. EIA kits
   a. HM-CAPEIA; manufacturer, Enteric Products
   b. PYLORI STAT EIA kit; manufacturer, Bio Whittaker
   c. G.A.P. kit; manufacturer, Bio-Rad Laboratories/Biomerica
 6. Immunologic dot blot assay (20)
 7. Pulsed-field gel electrophoresis (213)
 8. ELISA (158)
 9. Pyloriset Dry rapid latex agglutination test (146)
S. **Lactococcus and Leuconostoc identification** (66–67): sodium dodecyl sulfate–polyacryamide gel electrophoresis. SDS-PAGE: analysis of soluble whole-cell proteins
T. **Neisseria and Moraxella catarrhalis identification**
 (*Note: M. catarrhalis* formerly in genera *Neisseria* and *Branhamella*)
 1. Commercial carbohydrate utilization tests
   a. Minitek *Neisseria* Test
     (1) Manufacturer, BD Biosciences
     (2) Paper disks impregnated with carbohydrates
     (3) Precaution: weak glucose-positive results for some strains of *N. cinerea* may result in misidentification of *N. gonorrhoeae* (23)
   b. API QUAD-FERM + (82, 117)
     (1) Manufacturer, bioMerieux
     (2) Series of microcupules (wells) containing glucose, sucrose, lactose, and maltose, plus control without a carbohydrate
     (3) One cupule with penicillin for acidometric determination of β-lactamase in *N. gonorrhoeae* and *M. catarrhalis*
     (4) One cupule for acidometric determination of DNase production by *M. catarrhalis*
   c. *Neisseria*-Kwik test kit (51)
     (1) Manufacturer, MicroBioLogics
     (2) Commercial modification of carbohydrate procedures
   d. Gonobio test
     (1) Manufacturer, I.A.F. Production
     (2) Commercial modification of carbohydrate procedures
 2. Chromogenic enzyme substrate tests
   a. Gonochek II (24, 51, 115, 248)
     (1) Manufacturer, E-Y Laboratories
     (2) Identification of *Neisseria* pathogens: *N. gonorrhoeae, N. meningitidis,* and *N. lactamica* plus *M. catarrhalis*
     (3) Single tube with three chromogenic substrates: γ-glutamyl-*p*-itroanilide, 5-bromo-4-chloro-3-indoxyl-β-D-galactopyranoside, and (β-naphthylamine; detection of glycosidase and aminopeptidase enzymes
   b. BactiCard *Neisseria* (113)

(1) Manufacturer, REMEL
(2) Identification of pathogenic *Neisseria* spp.: *N. gonorrhoeae, N. meningitidis,* and *N. lactamica* plus *M. catarrhalis*
(3) Four chromogenic substrates: indoxyl butyrate esterase, β-galactoside (BGAL), prolylaminopeptidase (PRO), and γ-glutamyl-β-naphthylamide (GLUT)
  c. Neisstrip (46)
    (1) Manufacturer, Lab. M Ltd., Bury, United Kingdom
    (2) Similar to BactiCard but lacks indoxyl esterase substrate; rapid enzyme detection kit
3. Immunologic methods
  a. Fluorescent Monoclonal Antibody Test (FA); *N. gonorrhoeae* culture confirmation test (15, 19, 116, 136, 243, 250)
    (1) Manufacturer, Syva
    (2) Rapid; can identify viable and dead organisms
4. Coagglutination tests
  a. Principle: binding antigonococcal antibody to killed *Staphylococcus aureus* cells; mixed with a suspension of gonococci gives a viable agglutination of suspension
  b. Gono Gen I test: manufacturer, New Horizons Diagnostics (5, 118, 122, 139, 164, 206)
  c. Meritec GC test: manufacturer, Meridian Diagnostics
  d. Gono Gen II: manufacturer, New Horizons Diagnostics (116, 120)
  e. Phadebact GC OMNI test: manufacturer, Karo-Bio (5, 19, 29, 51, 116, 131)
5. Kit systems: identification of *Neisseria* and other fastidious Gram-negative organisms encountered in clinical specimens; all kits are modified conventional tests: carbohydrates, urease, indole, ornithine, and chromogenic substrates. Results within 2–4 h
  a. IDS RapID NH (Neiss-Haem) system
    (1) Manufacturer, REMEL
    (2) Microtray system identifies both *Neisseria* and *Haemophilus* spp.; provides biotype designation for *H. influenzae* and *H. parainfluenzae*
    (3) 7 substrates; results in 4 h
  b. Vitek HHI (Neiss-Haem Identification) card: manufacturer, bioMerieux
  c. Haem-Neiss Identification (HNID) panel: manufacturer, Dade/MicroScan (111)
  d. API NH system: manufacturer, bioMerieux, La Balme-les-Grottes, France (10, 112)
6. Miscellaneous
  a. Probe technology: nucleic acid probes for cultural confirmation of *N. gonorrhoeae*; identifies specific rRNA sequences unique to *N. gonorrhoeae*
    (1) AccuProbe: manufacturer, Gen-Probe (116, 139, 262)
    (2) PACE (probe assay–chemiluminescence enhanced); DNA probe assay, manufacturer, Gen-Probe
      (a) PACE 2 NG system: direct detection of *N. gonorrhoeae* (32, 89, 90, 138, 140, 238)
      (b) PACE 2 CT: direct detection of *Chlamydia trachomatis* (89)
      (c) PACE 2C: direct detection of *N. gonorrhoeae* and *C. trachomatis*
  b. PCR: molecular techniques; direct detection of *N. gonorrhoeae* from clinical specimens (42, 99, 124, 194)
  c. Liquid chain reaction (LCR); amplification technique for detection of *N. gonorrhoeae* (17, 221)
  d. Cx *Neisseria gonorrhoeae* assay (105, 118)
    (1) Manufacturer, Abbott Laboratories
    (2) Ligase chain reaction
  e. Ligase chain reaction (221)

U. *Staphylococcus* identification
  1. Commercial identification kits
     a. Staph ASE test
        (1) Manufacturer, bioMerieux
        (2) Modified slide/tube coagulase test in microcupule
        (3) Dehydrated rabbit plasma; clumping (positive) within 2 min
     b. API Staph
        (1) Formerly API Staph-Trac; manufacturer, bioMerieux
        (2) Identification of *Staphylococcus* spp. and *Micrococcus* spp.
        (3) 19 biochemical tests
        (4) According to Perl et al. (187), system performed poorly with less common isolates such as *S. haemolyticus, S. hominis, S. simulans,* and *S. warneri*.
     c. API STAPH-INDENT
        (1) Manufacturer, bioMerieux
        (2) Identification of *Staphylococcus, Micrococcus,* and *Stomatococcus mucilaginosus*
        (3) Battery of 10 miniaturized biochemical tests
        (4) Species identification by a four-digit octal code
        (5) Inadequate for identification of commonly encountered and uncommon species in family *Micrococcaceae* (201)
     d. ID 32 Staph
        (1) Manufacturer, bioMerieux
        (2) Identification of staphylococci and micrococci; 26 biochemical tests (25)
     e. Staph-ZYM (244)
        (1) Manufacturer, ROSCO
        (2) 10 dehydrated chromogenic and modified conventional substrates
        (3) Evaluated for ability to identify bovine isolates, but not investigated for identification of human staphylococcal isolates
     f. Staf-Sistem 18-R
        (1) Manufacturer, Liofilchem s.r.l.
        (2) 18 modified conventional substrates (190)
     g. BBL Crystal MRSA ID panel (129, 197)
        (1) Manufacturer, BD Biosciences
        (2) Screening for detection of methicillin-resistant *S. aureus* from isolated colonies
        (3) Results in 4 h
  2. Fluorogenic chromogenic methods
     a. RapiDEC Staph (242)
        (1) Manufacturer, bioMerieux, Marcy l'Etoile, France
        (2) Identification of *S. aureus, S. epidermidis,* and *S. saprophyticus* within 2 h
        (3) Determination of coagulase, alkaline phosphatase, and β-galactosidase (BGAL)
        (4) Fluorogenic coagulase test; proteolytic enzyme of coagulation reacts with prothrombin to form a complex called staphylothrombin, which enzymatically cleaves a fluorogenic peptide present in test cupule (77, 114, 154, 165)
     b. MicroScan Rapid Pos Combo Panel (246)
        (1) Manufacturer, Dade/MicroScan
        (2) 22 fluorogenic substrates; contains metabolites conjugated to fluorophores (83, 231)
        (3) Tests read manually or with AutoScan Walk/Away automated system
  3. Sceptor Gram-Positive MIC/ID Panel
     a. Manufacturer, BD Biosciences
     b. Combination substrate identification and antimicrobial susceptibilities
  4. Vitek Gram-Positive Identification (GPI) Card

a. Manufacturer, bioMerieux
b. Identification of *Staphylococcus, Streptococcus, Corynebacterium* spp., *Erysipelothrix rhusiopathiae,* and *Listeria monocytogenes* (9)
c. 28 biochemical tests; identification with Vitek automated bacterial identification susceptibility testing system
5. Minitek Gram-Pos Panel (Modified)
    a. Manufacturer, BD Biosciences
    b. Filter paper disks impregnated with various test substrates and carbohydrates (41)
    c. Identification of *Staphylococcus, Streptococcus,* and *Micrococcus* spp.
6. Disk susceptibility procedures
    a. Furazolidone and bacitracin
        (1) Manufacturer, BD Biosciences
        (2) Differentiation of micrococci from staphylococci
        (3) Disks
            (a) Furazolidone (FX): 100 μg
            (b) Bacitracin (A): Taxo A disk (BBL): 0.04 U
            (c) Novobiocin, 5 μg: **presumptive** identification of *S. saphrophyticus;* important agent of urinary tract infections
            (d) *Staphylococcus* spp.: FX susceptible (S) and bacitracin resistant (R)
            (e) **Presumptive** *S. saphrophyticus:* FX susceptible (S), bacitracin (A), resistant (R), novobiocin, resistant (R)
    b. Desferrioxamine susceptibility (143, 144)
        (1) Identification of *S. epidermidis* and *S. hominis*
        (2) Susceptibility to desferrioxamine, a siderophore produced by *Streptomyces pilosus*
        (3) Desferrioxamine, 1 mg (Desferal), manufacturer, Ciba-Geigy, Switzerland
7. Latex agglutination tests
    a. Principle: latex spheres (beads) are coated with plasma; fibrinogen bound to latex detects clumping factors. Immunoglobulin also present on latex detects protein A on surface of *S. aureus* cells.
    b. Commercial systems (148, 254)
        (1) StaphAurex Plus: manufacturer, Murex Diagnostics
        (2) Slidex Staph: manufacturer, bioMerieux
        (3) Staphlatex: manufacturer, Dade/MicroScan
        (4) Staph RapID: manufacturer, Roche
        (5) Pastorex Staph-Plus: manufacturer, Sanofi
        (6) Avistaph: manufacturer, Omega Diagnostics
        (7) Staphlase: manufacturer, Oxoid, Unipath, England
        (8) Ser-STAT: manufacturer, Adams Scientific
    c. Precaution: some strains of *Staphylococcus lugdunensis* and *Staphylococcus schleiferi* subsp. *schleiferi* produce clumping factor and may give positive results with these rapid procedures.
8. Miscellaneous procedures
    a. Passive hemagglutination
        (1) Principle: sheep erythrocytes (RBCs) coated (sensitized) with fibrinogen and bacterial cells react to give visible clumping.
        (2) Commercial systems (2, 170, 186, 196, 208)
            (a) Staphyloside: manufacturer, BD Biosciences
            (b) Staphyslide: manufacturer, bioMerieux
        (3) Precaution: nonsensitized RBC cell suspension must be included as negative control

b. Microbial Identification System MIS or MIDI
   (1) Manufacturer, MIDI Labs
   (2) High resolution gas-liquid chromatography (GLC) of cellular fatty acid derivatives for identification of bacteria (230)
c. GP Biolog MicroPlate Identification System
   (1) Manufacturer, Biolog
   (2) Gram-positive identification based on oxidation of various substrates; 95 substrates (163)
d. Pulsed-field gel electrophoresis (217)
e. PCR (14, 152, 239, 240)

V. *Streptococcus* spp. **Identification**
1. Direct detection of group A streptococci from throat swabs (71)
   a. EIA tests (44, 52, 78, 93, 97, 101, 135, 184, 207, 217, 233)
      (1) TestPack Strep A-Plus: manufacturer, Abbott Laboratories (6)
      (2) CARD O.S.: manufacturer, Pacific Biotech
   b. Q Test Strep kit: manufacturer; Becton Dickinson, Franklin Lakes, NJ
   c. Strep A OIA: manufacturer, Biostar, optical immunoassay (44, 45, 49, 93, 94, 97)
   d. Group A Streptococcus Direct Test (GASD) (96, 195, 227)
      (1) Manufacturer, Gen-Probe
      (2) Nonisotopic method; uses DNA probe to detect complementary rRNA sequence
   e. Latex agglutination tests (237) procedures have essentially replaced Lancefield extraction–capillary precipitin technique as reference method for serogrouping of β-hemolytic streptococci (132).
      (1) Streptex: manufacturer, Murex
      (2) Patho-Dx Strep Grouping kit: manufacturer, Diagnostic Products
      (3) Slidex Strep: manufacturer, bioMerieux
2. *Streptococcus pneumoniae* identification: rapid serologic identification (coagglutination) (223, 251)
   a. Phadebact Pneumococcus: manufacturer, Karo Bio
   b. Pneumoslide: manufacturer, BD Biosciences
   c. PCR (264)
3. Viridans streptococci identification: Fluo-Card Milleri; manufacturer, Key Scientific (73)
   a. Impregnated filter paper strips
   b. 3 reagents: β-D-fucoside, β-glucosidase, and α-glucosidase
4. IDS RapidID STR (261)
   a. Manufacturer, REMEL
   b. 14 biochemical tests; identifies streptococci and streptococcus-like organisms
5. API Rapid Step system (98, 210)
   a. Manufacturer, bioMerieux
   b. Identification of viridans and veterinary pathogens
   c. 20 physiologic and chromogenic tests
   d. Caution: some misidentification; must consider other preliminary tests along with biochemical reactions
6. Rapid ID 32 Strep system (3)
   a. Manufacturer, bioMerieux, La Balme les Grottes, France
   b. Identification of streptococci and streptococcus-like organisms
   c. 32 test strips
7. PCR (59, 209)

W. *Ureaplasma urealyticum* **identification**: PCR (125, 173)

X. *Vibrio* spp. identification
   1. DNA probes (172)
   2. Pulsed-field gel electrophoresis (256)

III. MOLECULAR MICROBIOLOGY

A. **Nucleic acid amplification techniques**
   1. Probe amplification: probe molecule itself is replicated enzymatically
      a. QB-replicase
      b. Ligase chain reaction
   2. Signal amplification: signal generated from each probe molecule is increased by use of compound probes or branched-probe technology
   3. Target amplification
      a. Nucleic acid sequence–based amplification; recommended as a standard for laboratory diagnosis of some infections (166)
      b. Transcription-mediated amplification
      c. PCR based on ability of DNA polymerase to copy and amplify a strand of DNA (211)
B. **Gene chip technology**: analyze specific nucleic acid sequences and identify nucleotide base changes such as point mutation and polymorphism (167)

REFERENCES

1. Achondo K, Bascomb S, Bobolis J, et al. New improved MicroScan Rapid Negative identification panel. Abstr Annu Meet Am Soc Microbiol C307 (95), 1995:53.
2. Adams J, Vanenk R. Use of commercial particle agglutination systems for rapid identification of methicillin-susceptible and methicillin-resistant *Staphylococcus aureus*. Eur J Clin Microbiol Infect Dis. 1994;13:86–89.
3. Ahmet Z, Warren M, Houang ET. Species identification of members of the *Streptococcus milleri* group isolated from the vagina by ID 32 Strep system and differential phenotypic characteristics. J Clin Microbiol 1995;33(6):1592–1595.
4. Allen SD, Siders JA, Marler LM. Current issues and problems in dealing with anaerobes in the clinical laboratory. Clin Lab Med 1995;15:333–364.
5. Anand CM, Gubash SM, Shaw H. Serological confirmation of *Neisseria gonorrhoeae* by monoclonal antibody-based coagglutination procedures. J Clin Microbiol 1988;26(11):2283–2286.
6. Anhalt JP, Heiter BJ, Naumovitz DW, Bourbeau PP. Comparison of three methods for detection of group A streptococci in throat swabs. J Clin Microbiol 1992;30(8):2135–2138.
7. Back AE, Oberhofer TR. Use of the Minitek system for biotyping *Haemophilus* species. J Clin Microbiol 1978;7(3):312–313.
8. Ball RJ, Sellers W. Improved motility medium. Appl Microbiol 1966;14(4):670–673.
9. Bannerman TL, Kleeman KT, Koos WE. Evaluation of the Vitek systems gram-positive identification card for species identification of coagulase-negative staphylococci. J Clin Microbiol 1993;31(5):1322–1325.
10. Barbe G, Babolat M, Boeufgras JM, et al. Evaluation of API NH, a new 2 hour system for identification of *Neisseria* and *Haemophilus* species and *Moraxella catarrhalis* in a routine clinical laboratory. J Clin Microbiol 1994;32(1):187–189.
11. Barry AL, Badal RE. Rapid identification of *Enterobacteriaceae* with the Micro-ID System versus API 20E and conventional media. J Clin Microbiol 1979;10(3):293–298.
12. Bascomb S, Abbott SL, Bobolis JD, et al. Multicenter evaluation of the MicroScan Rapid Gram-negative identification type 3 panel. J Clin Microbiol 1997;35(10):2531–2536.
13. Beall B, Cassiday PK, Sanden GN. Analysis of *Bordetella pertussis* isolates from an epidemic by pulsed-field gel electrophoresis. J Clin Microbiol 1995;33(12):3083–3086.
14. Becker K, Roth R, Peters G. Rapid and specific detection of toxigenic *Staphylococcus aureus:* Use of two multiplex PCR enzyme immunoassays for amplification and hybridization of staphylococcal enterotoxin genes, exfoliative toxin genes, and toxic shock syndrome toxin 1 gene. J Clin Microbiol 1998;36(9):2548–2553.
15. Beebe JL, Rau MP, Flageolle S, et al. Incidence of *Neisseria gonorrhoeae* isolates negative by Syva direct fluorescent-antibody test but positive by Gen-Probe Accuprobe test in a sexually transmitted disease clinic population. J Clin Microbiol 1993;31(9):2535–2537.
16. Bendinger B, Kroppenstedt RM, Klatte S, Altendorf K. Chemotaxonomic differentiation of coryneform bacteria isolated from biofilters. Int J Syst Bacteriol 1992;42:474–486.
17. Birkenmeyer L, Armstrong AS. Preliminary evaluation of the ligase chain reaction for specific de-

tection of *Neisseria gonorrhoeae*. J Clin Microbiol 1992;30(12):3089–3094.
18. Bochner B. Rainbow UTI System: A rapid and simple multicolor diagnostic system for common urinary tract pathogens. Abstr Annu Meet Am Soc Microbiol C374, 1995:65.
19. Boehm DM, Bernhardt M, Kurzynski TA, Pennell DR, Schell RF. Evaluation of two commercial procedures for rapid identification of *Neisseria gonorrhoeae* using a reference panel of antigenically diverse gonococci. J Clin Microbiol 1990;28(9):2099–2100.
20. Bolin I, Lonroth F, Svennerholm AM. Identification of *Helicobacter pylori* by immunological dot blot method based on reaction of a species-specific monoclonal antibody with a surface-exposed protein. J Clin Microbiol 1995;33(2):381–384.
21. Bolstad AI, Jensen HB. Polymerase chain reaction-amplified nonradioactive probes for identification of *Fusobacterium nucleatum*. J Clin Microbiol 1993;31(3):528–532.
22. Bourbeau PP, Heiter BJ. Comparison of Vitek GNI and GNI+ cards for identification of gram-negative bacteria. J Clin Microbiol 1998;36(9):2775–2777.
23. Boyce JM, Mitchell EB Jr. Difficulties in differentiating *Neisseria cinerea* from *Neisseria gonorrhoeae* in rapid systems used for identifying pathogenic *Neisseria* species. J Clin Microbiol 1985;22(5):731–734.
24. Brown JD, Thomas KR. Rapid enzyme system for the identification of pathogenic *Neisseria* spp. J Clin Microbiol 1985;21(5):857–858.
25. Brun Y, Bes M, Boeufgras JM, et al. Internal collaborative evaluation of the ATB 32 Staph gallery for identification of the *Staphylococcus* species. Int V Med Microbiol Virol Parasitol Infect Dis 1990;273:(3)
26. Bucher C, von Graevenitz A. Evaluation of three different media for detection of *Enterobacter agglomerans (Erwinia herbicola)*. J Clin Microbiol 1982;15(6):1164–1166.
27. Buck GE. Detection of *Bordetella pertussis* by rapid-cycle PCR and colorimetric microwell hybridization. J Clin Microbiol 1996;34(6):1355–1358.
28. Buter WR, Kilburn JO, Kubica GP. Gram positive bacilli high-performance liquid chromatography analysis of mycolic acids as an aid in laboratory identification of *Rhodococcus* and *Nocardia* species. J Clin Microbiol 1987;25:2126–2131.
29. Carlson BL, Calnan MR, Goodman RE, George H. Phadebact monoclonal GC OMNI test for confirmation of *Neisseria gonorrhoeae*. J Clin Microbiol 1987;25(10):1982–1984.
30. Castillo CB, Bruckner DA. Comparative evaluation of the Eiken and API 20E Systems and conventional methods for identification of members of the family *Enterobacteriaceae*. J Clin Microbiol 1984;20(4):754–757.
31. Cavallaro JJ, Wiggs LS, Miller JM. Evaluation of the BBL Crystal anaerobe identification system. J Clin Microbiol 1997;35(12):3186–3191.
32. Chapin-Roberston K, Reece EA, Edberg SC. Evaluation of the Gen-Probe PACE II assay for the direct detection of *Neisseria gonorrhoeae* in endocervical specimens. Diagn Microbiol Infect Dis 1992;15:645–649.
33. Cheng S, McCleskey FK, Gress MJ, et al. A PCR for identification of *Enterococcus faecium*. J Clin Microbiol 1997;35(5):1248–1250.
34. Chetoui H, Melin P, Struelens MJ, et al. Comparison of biotyping, ribotyping, and pulsed-field gel electrophoresis for investigation of a common-source outbreak of *Burkholderia pickettii* bacteremia. J Clin Microbiol 1997;35(6):1398–1403.
35. Clark WM, Lubs HA. The differentiation of bacteria of the Colon-Aerogenes family by the use of indicators. J Infect Dis 1915;17(1):160–173.
36. Collier MC, Stock F, DeGirolami PC, et al. Comparison of PCR-based approaches to molecular epidemiologic analysis of *Clostridium difficile*. J Clin Microbiol 1996;34(5):1153–1157.
37. Collins JK, Kelly MT. Comparison of Phadebact coagglutination, Bactogen latex agglutination, and counterimmunoelectrophoressis for detection of *Haemophilus influenzae* type b antigens in cerebrospinal fluid. J Clin Microbiol 1983;17(6):1005–1008.
38. Collins MD, Goodfellow M, Minnikin DE, Anderson G. Menaquinone composition of mycolic acid-containing actinomyces and some sporo-actinomycetes. J Appl Bacteriol 1985;58:77–86.
39. Collins MD, Pirouz T, Goodfellow M, Minnikin DE. Distribution of menaquinones in actinomyces and corynebacteria. J Gen Microbiol 1977;100(2):221–230.
40. Coque TM, Murray BE. Identification of *Enterococcus faecalis* strains by DNA hybridization and pulsed-field gel electrophoresis. J Clin Microbiol 1995;33(12):3368–3369.
41. Couch SF, Pearson TA, Parham DM. Comparison of Modified Minitek system with Staph-Ident system for species identification of coagulase-negative staphylococci. J Clin Microbiol 1987;25(9):1626–1628.
42. Crotchfelt KA, Welsh LE, DeBonville D, et al. Detection of *Neisseria gonorrhoeae* and *Chlamydia trachomatis* in genitourinary specimens from men and women by a coamplification PCR assay. J Clin Microbiol 1997;35(6):1536–1540.
43. Cutler AF, Havstad S, Maa CK, Blasee MJ, Perez-Perez GI, Schubert TT. Accuracy of invasive and noninvasive tests to diagnose *Helicobacter pylori* infection. Gastroenterology 1995;109:136–141.
44. Dale JC, Vetter EA, Contezac JM, et al. Evaluation of two rapid antigen assays, BioStar Strep A OIA and Pacific Biotech CARDS O.S. and culture for detection of group A streptococci in throat swabs. J Clin Microbiol 1994;32(11):2698–2701.
45. Daly JA, Korgenski EK, Munson AC, Llausas-Magana E. Optical immunoassay for streptococcal pharyngitis: Evaluation of accuracy with rou-

46. Dealer SF, Gough KR, Campbell L, et al. Identification of *Neisseria gonorrhoeae* using the Neisstrip rapid enzyme detection test. J Clin Pathol 1991;44:376–379.
47. De Briel D, Couderc F, Riegel P, Minck R. High-performance liquid chromatography of corynomycolic acids as a tool in identification of *Corynebacterium* species and related organisms. J Clin Microbiol 1992;30(6):1407–1417.
48. DeGirolami PC, Eichelberger KA, Salfity LC, Rizzo MF. Evaluation of the AutoSCAN-3, a device for reading microdilution trays. J Clin Microbiol 1983;18(6):1292–1295.
49. Della-Latta P, Whittier S, Hosmer M, Agre F. Rapid detection of group A streptococcal pharyngitis in a pediatric population with optical immunoassay. Pediatr Infect Dis J 1994;13:742–743.
50. de Moissac YR, Ronald SL, Peppler MS. Use of pulse-field gel electrophoresis for epidemiological study of *Bordetella pertussis* in a whooping cough outbreak. J Clin Microbiol 1991;32(2):398–402.
51. Dillon JR, Carballo M, Pauze M. Evaluation of eight methods for identification of pathogenic *Neisseria* species: *Neisseria*-Kwik, RIM-N, Gonobio-Test, Minitek, Gonochek II, GonoGen, Phadebact Monoclonal GC OMNI Test, and Syva MicroTrak test. J Clin Microbiol 1988;26(3):493–497.
52. Dobkin D, Schulman ST. Evaluation of an ELISA for group A streptococcal antigen for diagnosis of pharyngitis. J Pediatr 110(1987;4):566–569.
53. Doern GV, Chapin KC. Laboratory identification of *Haemophilus influenzae*: Effects of basal media on the results of the satellitism test and evaluation of the RapID NH system. J Clin Microbiol 1984;20(3):599–601.
54. Dogan B, Asikainen S, Jousimies-Somer H. Evaluation of two commercial kits and arbitrarily primed PCR for identification and differentiation of *Actinobacillus actinomycetemcomitans*, *Haemophilus aphrophilus*, and *Haemophilus paraphrophilus*. J Clin Microbiol 1999;37(3):742–747.
55. Donabedian S, Chow JW, Shales DM, et al. DNA hybridization and contour-clamped homogeneous electric field electrophoresis for identification of enterococci to the species level. J Clin Microbiol 1995;33(1):141–145.
56. Dowell V, Lombard G. Presumptive Identification of Anaerobic Non-sporeforming Gram-negative Bacilli. Atlanta, GA: U.S. DHEW, Centers for Disease Control (CDC), June 1977.
57. Dowell VR Jr, Hawkins TM. Laboratory Methods in Anaerobic Bacteriology. CDC Laboratory Manual, U.S. DHEW Publ no. (CDC) 74–8272, Washington, DC: U.S. Government Printing Office, 1974:3–4.
58. Dowell VR Jr, Lombard GL, Thompson FS, Armfield AY. Media for Isolation, Characterization, and Identification of Obligately Anaerobic Bacteria. Atlanta, GA: U.S. DHEW, Centers for Disease Control (CDC), Nov 1977.
59. du Plessis M, Smith AM, Klugman KP. Rapid detection of penicillin-resistant *Streptococcus pneumoniae* in cerebrospinal fluid by a seminested-PCR strategy. J Clin Microbiol 1998;36(2):453–457.
60. Dutka-Malen S, Evers S, Courvalin P. Detection of glycopeptide resistance genotypes and identification to the species level of clinically relevant enterococci by PCR. J Clin Microbiol 1995;33(1):24–27.
61. Edberg SC, Melton E, Singer JM. Rapid biochemical characterization of *Haemophilus* species by using the Micro-ID. J Clin Microbiol 1980;11(1):22–26.
62. Edberg SC, Trepeta RW. Rapid and economical identification and antimicrobial susceptibility test methodology for urinary tract infections. J Clin Microbiol 1983;18(6):1287–1291.
63. Ederer GM, Clark M. Motility-indole-ornithine medium. Appl Microbiol 1970;20(5):849–850.
64. Ederer GM, Lund ME, Balazevic DJ, et al. Motility-indole-lysine-sulfide medium. J Clin Microbiol 1975;2(3):266–2267.
65. Edwards PR, Bruner DW. Serological identification of *Salmonella*. Circulation of the Kentucky Agricultural Experimental Station, no. 54, 1942.
66. Elliott JA, Facklam RR. Identification of *Leuconostoc* spp. by analysis of soluble whole cell protein patterns. J Clin Microbiol 1993;31(5):1030–1033.
67. Elliott JA, Gllins MD, Pigott NE, Facklam RR. Differentiation of *Lactococcus lactis* and *Lactococcus garvieae* from humans by comparison of whole-cell protein patterns. J Clin Microbiol 1991;29(1):2731–2734.
68. Ellner PD, O'Donnell ED. A selective differential medium for histotoxic clostridia. Am J Clin Pathol 1971;56(2):197–200.
69. Ellner PD, Granato PA, May CB. Recovery and identification of anaerobes: A system suitable for the routine clinical laboratory. Appl Microbiol 1973;26(6):904–913.
70. Esber RJ, Faulconer RJ. A medium for initial visual demonstration of production of coagulase and fermentation of mannitol by pathogenic staphylococci. Am J Clin Pathol 1959;32(2):192–194.
71. Facklam RR. Specificity study kits for detection of group A streptococci directly from throat swabs. J Clin Microbiol 1987;25(3):508.
72. Facklam RR, Collins MD. Identification of *Enterococcus* species isolated from human infections by a conventional test scheme. J Clin Microbiol 1989;27(4):731–734.

73. Flynn CE, Ruoff KL. Identification of "Streptococcus milleri" group isolates to the species level with a commercially available rapid test system. J Clin Microbiol 1995;33(10):2704–2706.

74. Fratamico PM, Sackitey SK, Wiedman M, Deng MY. Detection of *Escherichia coli* 0157:H7 by multiplex PCR. J Clin Microbiol 1995;33(8):2188–2191.

75. Fuchs PC. The replicator method for identification and biotyping of common bacterial isolates. Lab Med 1975;6(5):6–11.

76. Funke G, Renaud FN, Freney J, Riegel P. Multicenter evaluation of the updated and extended API (RAPID) Coryne database 2.0. J Clin Microbiol 1997;35(12):3122–3126.

77. Geary C, Stevens M. Detection of phosphatase production by *Staphylococcus* species: A new method. Med Lab Sci 1989;46(4):291–294.

78. Gerber MA, Randolph MF, DeMeo KK. Liposome immunoassay for rapid identification of group A streptococci directly from throat swabs. J Clin Microbiol 1990;28(6):1463–1464.

79. Gooch WM III, Hill GA. Comparison of Micro-ID and API 20E in rapid identification of *Enterobacteriaceae*. J Clin Microbiol 1982;15(5):885–890.

80. Gonzalez I, Grant KA, Richardson PT, et al. Specific identification of the enteropathogens *Campylobacter jejuni* and *Campylobacter coli* by using a PCR test based on the *ceuE* gene encoding a putative virulence determinant. J Clin Microbiol 1997;35(3):759–763.

81. Gordillo ME, Singh KV, Murray BE. Comparison of ribotyping and pulsed-field gel electrophoresis for subspecies differentiation of strains of *Enterococcus faecalis*. J Clin Microbiol 1993;31(6):1570–1574.

82. Gradus MD, Ng CM, Silver KJ. Comparison of the QuadFERM 1 2-hr identification system with conventional carbohydrate degradation test for confirmatory identification of *Neisseria gonorrhoeae*. Sex Transm Dis 1989;16:57–59.

83. Grant CE, Sewell DL, Pfaller M, et al. Evaluation of two commercial systems for identification of coagulase negative staphylococci to species level. Diagn Microbiol Infect Dis 1994;18(1):1–5.

84. Green M, Barbadora K, Donabedian S, Zervos MJ. Comparison of field inversion gel electrophoresis with contour-clamped homogeneous electric field electrophoresis as a typing method for *Enterococcus faecium*. J Clin Microbiol 1995;33(6):1554–1557.

85. Griffen AL, Leys EJ, Fuerst PA. Stain identification of *Actinobacillus actinomycetemcomitans* using the polymerase chain reaction. Oral Microbiol Immunol 1992;7:240–243.

86. Grimprel E, Begue P, Anjak I, et al. Comparison of polymerase chain reaction, culture, and western immunoblot serology for diagnosis of *Bordetella pertussis*. J Clin Microbiol 1993;31(10):2745–2750.

87. Gustafsson BA, Askelof P. Monoclonal antibody-based sandwich enzyme-linked immunosorbent assay for detection of *Bordetella pertussis* filamentous hemagglutinin. J Clin Microbiol 1988;26(10):2077–2082.

88. Hajna AA. A semi-solid medium suitable for both motility and hydrogen sulfide tests. Public Health Lab 1950;8:36.

89. Hale YM, Melton ME, Lewis JS, Willis DE. Evaluation of the PACE 2 *Neisseria gonorrhoeae* assay by the public health laboratories. J Clin Microbiol 1993;31(2):451–453.

90. Hanks JW, Scott CT, Butler CE, Wells DW. Evaluation of a DNA probe assay (Gen-Probe PACE 2) as the test of cure for *Neisseria gonorrhoeae* genital infections. J Pediatr 1994;125(1):161–162.

91. Hanninen ML, Pajarre S, Klossner ML, Rautelin H. Typing of human *Campylobacter jejuni* isolates in Finland by pulsed-field gel electrophoresis. J Clin Microbiol 1998;36(6):1787–1789.

92. Hanson CW, Cassorla R, Martin WJ. API and Minitek systems in identification of clinical isolates of anaerobic gram-negative bacilli and *Clostridium* species. J Clin Microbiol 1979;10(1):14–18.

93. Harbeck RJ. Evaluation of two rapid antigen assays, BioStar Strep A OIA and Pacific Biotech CARDS O.S., and culture for detection of group A streptococci in throat swabs. J Clin Microbiol 1995;33(12):3365–3367.

94. Harbeck RJ, Teague J, Crossen GR, et al. Novel, rapid optical immunoassay technique for detection of group A *streptococci* from pharyngeal specimens: Comparison with standard culture methods. J Clin Microbiol 1993;31(4):839–844.

95. He Q, Mertsola J, Soini H, et al. Comparison of polymerase chain reaction with culture and enzyme immunoassay for diagnosis of pertussis. J Clin Microbiol 1993;31(3):642–645.

96. Heiter BJ, Bourbeau PP. Comparison of the Gen-Probe group A *Streptococcus* direct test with culture and a rapid streptococcal antigen assay for diagnosis of streptococcal pharyngitis. J Clin Microbiol 1993;31(8):2070–2073.

97. Heiter BJ, Bourbeau PP. Comparison of two rapid streptococcal antigen 176 detection assays with culture for diagnosis of streptococcal pharyngitis. J Clin Microbiol 1995;33(5):1408–1410.

98. Hinnebusch CJ, Nikilai DM, Bruckner DA. Comparison of API Rapid STREP, Baxter-MicroScan Rapid POS ID Panel, BBL Minitek Differential Identification system, IDS RapID STR system, and Vitek GBI to conventional biochemical tests for identification of viridans streptococci. Am J Clin Pathol 1991;96(4):455–463.

99. Ho BS, Feng WG, Wong BKC, Egglestone SI. Polymerase chain reaction for the detection of *Neisseria gonorrhoeae* in clinical samples. J Clin Pathol 1992;45:439–442.

100. Hodinka RL, Gilligan PH. Evaluation of the

100. Campyslide agglutination test for confirmatory identification of selected *Campylobacter* species. J Clin Microbiol 1988;26(1):47–49.
101. Hoffmann S. Detection of group A streptococcal antigen from throat swabs with five diagnostic kits in general practice. Diagn Microbial Infect Dis 1990;13(2):209–215.
102. Holmes B, Costas M, Ganner M, On SLW, Stevens M. Evaluation of Biolog system for identification of some gram-negative bacteria of clinical importance. J Clin Microbiol 1994; 32(8):1970–1975.
103. Holmes B, Costas M, Thaker T, Stevens M. Evaluation of two BBL Crystal systems for identification of some clinically important gram-negative bacteria. J Clin Microbiol 1994; 32(9):2221–2224.
104. Holmes RL, DeFranco LM, Otto M. Novel method of using biotyping *Haemophilus influenzae* that use API 20E. J Clin Microbiol 1982;15(6):1150–1152.
105. Hook EW III, Ching SF, Stephens J, et al. Diagnosis of *Neisseria gonorrhoeae* infections in women by using the ligase chain reaction on patient-obtained vaginal swabs. J Clin Microbiol 1997;35(8):2129–2132.
106. Hudspeth MK, Gerardo SH, Citron DM, Goldstein EJ. Growth characteristics and a novel method for identification (the WEE-AB system) of *Porphyromonas* species isolated from infected dog and cat bite wounds in humans. J Clin Microbiol 1997;35(10):2450–2453.
107. Hudspeth MK, Gerardo SH, Citron DM, Goldstein EJ. Evaluation of the RapID CB Plus system for identification of *Corynebacterium* species and other gram-positive rods. J Clin Microbiol 1998; 36(2):543–547.
108. Huysmans MB, Turnidge JD, Williams JH. Evaluation of API Campy in comparison with conventional methods for identification of thermophilic campylobacters. J Clin Microbiol 1995;33(12):3345–3346.
109. Ingram DL, Pearson AW, Occhitui AR. Detection of bacterial antigens in body fluids with the Wellcogen *Haemophilus influenzae* b, *Streptococcus pneumoniae,* and *Neisseria meningitidis* (ACYW135) latex agglutination tests. J Clin Microbiol 1983;18:1119–1121.
110. Isenberg HD, Scherber JS, Cosgrove JO. Clinical laboratory evaluation of the further improved Enterotube and Encise II. J Clin Microbiol 1975;2(2):139–141.
111. Janda WM, Bradna JJ, Ruther P. Identification of *Neisseria* spp., *Haemophilus* spp., and other fastidious gram-negative bacteria with the MicroScan *Haemophilus-Neisseria* identification panel. J Clin Microbiol 1989;27(5):869–873.
112. Janda WM, Malloy PJ, Schreckenberger PC. Clinical evaluation of the Vitek *Neisseria-Haemophilus* Identification Card. J Clin Microbiol 1987;25(1):37–41.
113. Janda WM, Montero M. Premarket evaluation of the BactiCard Neisseria. Abstr Annu Meet Am Soc Microbiol C303, 1995:53.
114. Janda WM, Ristow K, Novak D. Evaluation of RapiDEC Staph for identification of *Staphylococcus aureus, Staphylococcus epidermidis,* and *Staphylococcus saprophyticus.* J Clin Microbiol 1994;32(9):2056–2059.
115. Janda WM, Ulanday MG, Bohnhoff M, LeBeau LJ. Evaluation of the RIM-N, Gonochek II, and Phadebact systems for the identification of pathogenic *Neisseria* spp. and *Branhamella catarrhalis.* J Clin Microbiol 1985;21(5):734–737.
116. Janda WM, Wilcoski LM, Mandel KL, et al. Comparison of monoclonal antibody-based methods and a ribosome ribonucleic acid probe test for *Neisseria gonorrhoeae* culture confirmation. Eur J Clin Microbiol Infect Dis 1993; 12(3):177–184.
117. Janda WM, Zigler KL, Brandna JJ. API Quad-FERM + with Rapid DNase for identification of *Neisseria* spp. and *Branhamella catarrhalis.* J Clin Microbiol 1987;25(2):203–206.
118. Kehl SC, Georgakas K, Swain GR, et al. Evaluation of the Abbott LCx assay for detection of *Neisseria gonorrhoeae* in endocervical swab specimens from females. J Clin Microbiol 1998;36(12):3549–3551.
119. Kehl KS, Havens P, Behnke CE, Acheson DW. Evaluation of the premier EHEC assay for detection of Shiga toxin-producing *Escherichia coli.* J Clin Microbiol 1997;35(8):2051–2054.
120. Kellogg JA, Orwig LK. Comparison of Gono-Gen, GonoGen II, and MicroTrak direct fluorescent antibody test with carbohydrate fermentation for confirmation of culture isolated of *Neisseria gonorrhoeae.* J Clin Microbiol 1995;33(2):474–476.
121. Kelly MT, Latimer JM. Comparison of the AutoMicrobic system with API, Enterotube Micro-ID, Micro-Media systems and conventional methods for identification of *Enterobacteriaceae.* J Clin Microbiol 1980;12(5):659–662.
122. Kelly MT, Leicester C. Evaluation of the Autoscan Walkaway system for rapid identification and susceptibility testing of gram-negative bacilli. J Clin Microbiol 1992;30(6):1568–1571.
123. Kerr KG, Hawkey PM, Lacey RW. Evaluation of the API Coryne system for identification of *Listeria* spp. J Clin Microbiol 1993;31(3):749–750.
124. Kertesz DA, Byrne SK, Chow AW. Characterization of *Neisseria meningitidis* by polymerase chain reaction and restriction endonuclease digestion of the porA gene. J Clin Microbiol 1993;31(10):2594–2598.
125. Kessler HH, Dodge DE, Pierer K, et al. Rapid detection of *Mycoplasma pneumoniae* by an assay based on PCR and probe hybridization in a nonradioactive microwell plate format. J Clin Microbiol 1997;35(6):1592–1594.

126. Kiehn TE, Brennan K, Ellner PD. Evaluation of the Minitek System for identification of *Enterobacteriaceae*. Appl Microbial 1974;28(4):668–671.
127. Kilian M, Bulow P. Rapid diagnosis of *Enterobacteriaceae*. I. Detection of bacterial glycosidases. Acta Pathol Microbiol Scand Sect B 1976;84:245–251.
128. Kitch TT, Jacobs MR, Appelbaum PC. Evaluation of RapID ONE system for identification of 379 strains in the family *Enterobacteriaceae* and oxidase-negative, gram-negative nonfermenters. J Clin Microbiol 1994;32(4):931–934.
129. Knapp CC, Ludwig MD, Washington JA. Evaluation of BBL Crystal MRSA ID system. J Clin Microbiol 1994;32(10):2588–2589.
130. Knapp CC, Washington JA. Evaluation of trehalose-mannitol broth for differentiation of *Staphylococcus epidermidis* from other coagulase-negative staphylococcal species. J Clin Microbiol 1989;27(11):2624–2625.
131. Knapp JS. Historical perspectives and identification of *Neisseria* and related species. Clin Microbiol Rev 1988;1(1):415–431.
132. Koneman EW, Allen SD, Janda WM, Schreckenberger PC, Washington CW Jr. Color Atlas & Textbook of Diagnostic Microbiology, ed 5. Philadelphia: JB Lippincott, 1997.
133. Knudtson LM, Hartman PA. Routine procedures for isolation and identification of enterococci and fecal streptococci. Appl Environ Microbiol 1992;58:3027–3031.
134. Lage AP, Godfroid E, Fauconnier A, et al. Diagnosis of *Helicobacter pylori* infection by PCR: Comparison with other invasive techniques and detection of *cagA* gene in gastric biopsy specimens. J Clin Microbiol 1995;33(10):2752–2756.
135. Laubscher B, van Melle G, Dreyfuss N, deCrousaz H. Evaluation of a new immunologic test kit for rapid detection of group A streptococci, the Abbott Testpack Strep A Plus. J Clin Microbiol 1995;33(1):260–261.
136. Laughton BE, Ehret JM, Tanino TT, et al. Fluorescent monoclonal antibody for confirmation of *Neisseria gonorrhoeae* cultures. J Clin Microbiol 1987;25(12):2388–2390.
137. Lawton WD, Battiaglioli GJ. GonoGen coagglutination test for *Neisseria gonorrhoeae*. J Clin Microbiol 1983;18(5):1264–1265.
138. Lewis JS, Fakile O, Foss E, et al. Direct DNA probe assay for *Neisseria gonorrhoeae* in pharyngeal and rectal specimens. J Clin Microbiol 1993;31(10):2783–2785.
139. Lewis JS, Kranig-Brown D, Trainor DA. DNA probe confirmatory test for *Neisseria gonorrhoeae*. J Clin Microbiol 1990;28(10):2349–2350.
140. Limberger RJ, Biega R, Evancoe A, et al. Evaluation of culture and the Gen-Probe ACE 2 assay for detection of *Neisseria gonorrhoeae* and *Chlamydia trachomatis* in endocervical specimens transported to a state health laboratory. J Clin Microbiol 1992;30(5):1162–1166.
141. Lind-Brandberg L, Welinder-Olsson C, Lagergard T, et al. Evaluation of PCR for diagnosis of *Bordetella pertussis* and *Bordetella parapertussis* infectious. J Clin Microbiol 1998;36(3):679–683.
142. Linde HJ, Neubauer H, Meyer H, et al. Identification of *Yersinia* species by the Vitek GNI card. J Clin Microbiol 1999;37(1):211–214.
143. Lindsay JA, Aravena-Roman MA, Riley TV. Identification of *Staphylococcus epidermidis* and *Staphylococcus hominis* from blood cultures by testing susceptibility to desferrioxamine. Eur J Microbiol Infect Dis 1993;12:127–131.
144. Lindsay JA, Riley TV. Susceptibility to desferrioxamine: A new test for the identification of *Staphylococcus epidermidis*. J Med Microbiol 1991;35(1):45–48.
145. Linton D, Lawson AJ, Owen RJ, Stanley J. PCR detection identification to species level, and fingerprinting of *Campylobacter jejuni* and *Campylobacter coli* direct from diarrheic samples. J Clin Microbiol 1997;35(10):2568–2572.
146. Lozniewski A, Korwin JD, Conroy MC, et al. Evaluation of Pyloriset Dry, a new rapid agglutination test for *Helicobacter pylori* antibody detection. J Clin Microbiol 1996;34(7):1773–1775.
147. Lu JJ, Perng CL, Shyu RY, et al. Comparison of five PCR methods for detection of *Helicobacter pylori* DNA in gastric tissue. J Clin Microbiol 1999;37(3):772–774.
148. Luijendijka A, van Belkum A, Verbrugh H, Kluytmans J. Comparison of five tests for identification of *Staphylococcus aureus* from clinical samples. J Clin Microbiol 1996;34(9):2267–2269.
149. Lyerly DM. *Clostridium difficile* testing. Clin Microbiol Newslett 1995;17:17.
150. Malathum K, Singh KV, Weinstock GM, Murray BE. Repetitive sequence-based PCR versus pulsed-field gel electrophoresis for typing of *Enterococcus faecalis* at the subspecies level. J Clin Microbiol 1998;36(1):211–215.
151. Marcon MJ, Hamoudi AC, Cannon HJ. Comparative laboratory evaluation of three antigen detection methods for diagnosis of *Haemophilus influenza* type b disease. J Clin Microbiol 1984;19(3):333–337.
152. Marcos JY, Soriano AC, Salazar MS, et al. Rapid identification and typing of *Staphylococcus aureus* by PCR-restriction fragment length polymorphism analysis of the *aroA* gene. J Clin Microbiol 1999;37(3):570–574.
153. Marchildon PA, Ciota LM, Zamaniyan FZ, et al. Evaluation of three commercial enzyme immunoassays compared with the ^{13}C urea breath test for detection of *Helicobacter pylori*

infection. J Clin Microbiol 1996;34(5):1147–1152.
154. Mathew D, Picard V. Comparative evaluation of five agglutination techniques and a new miniaturized system for rapid identification of methicillin-resistant strains of *Staphylococcus aureus*. Zentralbl Bakteriol 1991;276:46–53.
155. Mazoyer MA, Orenga S, Doleans F, Freney J. Evaluation of CPS ID2 medium for detection of urinary tract bacterial isolates in specimens from a rehabilitation center. J Clin Microbiol 1995;33(4):1025–1027.
156. McClung LS, Toabe R. The egg yolk plate reaction for the presumptive diagnosis of *Clostridium sporogenes* and certain species of the gangrene and botulinum groups. J Bacteriol 1947;53(2):139–147.
157. McNulty CAM, Dent JC, Uff JS, et al. Detection of *Campylobacter pylori* by the biopsy urease test. An assessment in 1445 patients. Gut 1989;30:1058–1062.
158. Meijer BC, Thijs JC, Kleibeuker JH, et al. Evaluation of eight enzyme immunoassays for detection of immunoglobulin G against *Helicobacter pylori*. J Clin Microbiol 1997;35(1):292–294.
159. Merz CS, Kramer C, Forman M, et al. Comparison of four commercially available rapid enzyme immunoassays with cytotoxin assay for detection of *Clostridium difficile* toxin(s) from stool specimens. J Clin Microbiol 1994;32(5):1142–1147.
160. Metherell LA, Logtan JM, Stanley J. PCR-enzyme-linked immunosorbent assay for detection and identification of *Campylobacter* species: Application to isolates and stool samples. J Clin Microbiol 1999;37(2):433–435.
161. Miller JM, Biddle JW, Quenzer VK, McLaughlin JC. Evaluation of Biolog for identification of members of the family *Micrococcaceae*. J Clin Microbiol 1993;31(12):3170–3173.
162. Minshew BH, Beardsley JL, Knapp JS. Evaluation of GonoGen coagglutination test for serodiagnosis of *Neisseria gonorrhoeae*: Identification of problem isolates by auxotyping, serotyping, and with fluorescent antibody reagent. Diagn Microbiol Infect Dis 1985;3(1):41–46.
163. Miranda G, Kelly C, Solorzano F, et al. Use of pulsed-field gel electrophoresis typing to study an outbreak of infection due to *Serratia marcescens* in a neonatal intensive care unit. J Clin Microbiol 1996;34(12):3138–3141.
164. Misawa N, Allos BM, Blaser MJ. Differentiation of *Campylobacter jejuni* serotype 019 strains from non-019 strains by PCR. J Clin Microbiol 1998;36(12):3567–3573.
165. Mitchell CJ, Geary C, Stevens M. Detection of *Staphylococcus aureus* in blood cultures: Evaluation of a two-hour method. Med Lab Sci 1991;48(2):106–109.
166. Mitchell PS, Espy MJ, Smith TF, et al. Laboratory diagnosis of central nervous system infections with herpes simplex virus by PCR performed with cerebrospinal fluid specimens. J Clin Microbiol 1997;35:2873–2877.
167. Mitchell PS, Persing DH. Current trends in molecular microbiology. Lab Med 1999;30(4):263–270.
168. Moss NS, Wilder D, Combs D, Monroe D, Mayer J, Morris R. Evaluation of the Vitek GNI + Card. Abstr Annu Meet Am Soc Microbiol 1996;C389(96):70.
169. Murray PR, Tenover FC, Baron EJ, Yolken RH. Manual of Clinical Microbiology, ed. 7. Washington, DC: American Society for Microbiology, 1999.
170. Myrick BA, Ellner PD. Evaluation of the latex agglutination test for identification of *Staphylococcus aureus*. J Clin Microbiol 1982;15(2):275–277.
171. Nachmkin I, Barbagallo S. Culture confirmation of *Campylobacter* spp. by latex agglutination. J Clin Microbiol 1990;28(5):817–818.
172. Nair GB, Bag PK, Shimada T, et al. Evaluation of DNA probes for specific detection of *Vibrio cholerae* 0139 Bengal. J Clin Microbiol 1995;33(8):2186–2187.
173. Nelson S, Matlow A, Johnson G, et al. Detection of *Ureaplasma urealyticum* in endotracheal tube aspirates from neonates by PCR. J Clin Microbiol 1998;36(5):1236–1239.
174. Neubauer H, Sauer T, Becker Hl, Aleksic S, Meyer H. Comparison of systems for identification and differentiation of species within the genus *Yersinia*. J Clin Microbiol 1998;36(11):3366–3368.
175. Nord C-E, Lindberg AA, Dahlback A. Evaluation of five test kits—API, AuxoTab, Enterotube, PathoTec and R-B—for identification of *Enterobacteriaceae*. Med Microbiol Immunol 1974;159(3):211–220.
176. Oberhofer TR, Hajkowski R. Evaluation of non-lactose-fermenting members of the *Klebsiella-Enterobacter-Serratia* division. I. Biochemical characteristics. Am J Clin Pathol 1970;54(11):720–725.
177. O'Hara CM, Miller JM. Evaluation of the autoSCAN-W/A system for rapid (2-hour) identification of members of the family *Enterobacteriaceae*. J Clin Microbiol 1992;30(6):1541–1543.
178. O'Hara CM, Tenover FC, Miller JM. Parallel comparison of accuracy of API 20E, Vitek GNI, MicroScan Walk/Away Rapid ID, and Becton Dickinson Cobas Micro ID-E/NF for identification of members of the family *Enterobacteriaceae* and common gram-negative, non-glucose-fermenting bacilli. J Clin Microbiol 1993;31(12):3165–3169.
179. Onderdonk AB, Allen SD. *Clostridium*. In: Murray PR, Baron EJ, Pfaller MA, et al., eds. Manual of Clinical Microbiology, ed 6. Washington, DC: American Society for Microbiology, 1995:574–586.

180. Overman TL, Plumley D, Overman SB, Goodman NL. Comparison of the API Rapid E four-hour system with the API 20E overnight system for the identification of routine clinical isolates of family *Enterobacteriaceae*. J Clin Microbiol 1985;21(4):542–545.
181. Painter G, Isenberg HD. Clinical laboratory experience with the improved Enterotube. Appl Microbiol 1973;25(6):896–899.
182. Pal T, Al-Sweih NA, Herpay M, Chug TD. Identification of enteroinvasive *Escherichia coli* and *Shigella* strains in pediatric patients by an IpaC-specific enzyme-linked immunosorbent assay. J Clin Microbiol 1997;35(7):1757–1760.
183. Palladino S, Leahy BJ, Newall TL. Comparison of the RIM-H Rapid Identification kit with conventional tests for the identification of *Haemophilus* spp. J Clin Microbiol 1990;28(8):1862–1863.
184. Patrick MR, Lewis D. Short of a length: *Streptococcus sanguis* knee infection from dental source. Br J Rheumatol 1992;31(8):569.
185. Peele D, Bradfield J, Pryor W, Vore S. Comparison of identifications of human and animal source gram-negative bacteria by API 20E and Crystal E/NF systems. J Clin Microbiol 1997;35(1):213–216.
186. Pennell DR, Rott-Petri JA, Kurzynski TA. Evaluation of three commercial agglutination tests for the identification of *Staphylococcus aureus*. J Clin Microbiol 1984;20(4):614–617.
187. Perl TM, Rhomberg PR, Bale MJ, et al. Comparison of identification systems for *Staphylococcus epidermidis* and other coagulase-negative *Staphylococcus* species. Diagn Microbiol Infect Dis 1994;18(3):151–155.
188. Persing DH. In vitro nucleic amplification techniques. In: Persing DH, Smith TF, Tenover FC, et al., eds. Diagnostic Molecular Biology: Principles and Applications. Washington, DC: American Society for Microbiology, 1993:51–87.
189. Pfaller MA, Sahm D, O'Hara C, et al. Comparison of the AutoSCAN-W/A Rapid Bacterial Identification system and the Vitek AutoMicrobic system for identification of gram-negative bacilli. J Clin Microbiol 1991;29(7):1422–1428.
190. Piccolomini R, Catamo G, Picciani C, D'Antonio D. Evaluation of Staf-Sistem 18-R for identification of staphylococcal clinical isolates to the species level. J Clin Microbiol 1994;32(3):649–653.
191. Pickett MJ, Pedersen MM. Screening procedure for partial identification of nonfermentive bacilli associated with man. Appl Microbiol 1968;16(10):1631–1632.
192. Pickett MJ, Pedersen MM. Characterization of saccharolytic nonfermentative bacteria associated with man. Can J Microbiol 1970;16(5):351–362.
193. Pickett MJ, Pedersen MM. Nonfermentative bacilli associated with man. II. Detection and identification. Am J Clin Pathol 1970;54(8):164–177.
194. Poh CL, Ramachandran V, Tapsall JW. Genetic diversity of *Neisseria gonorrhoeae* IB-2 and IB-6 isolates revealed by whole-cell repetitive element sequence-based PCR. J Clin Microbiol 1996;34(2):292–295.
195. Pokorski SJ, Vetter EA, Wollan PC, Cockerill FR III. Comparison of Gen-Probe Group A *Streptococcus* Direct test with culture for diagnosing streptococcal pharyngitis. J Clin Microbiol 1994;32(6):1440–1443.
196. Qadri SMH, Akhter J, Qadri SGM. Latex agglutination and hemagglutination tests for the rapid identification of methicillin-sensitive and methicillin-resistant *Staphylococcus aureus*. J Hyg Epidemol Microbiol Immunol 1991;35:65–71.
197. Qadri SM, Ueno Y, Imambaccus H, Almodovar E. Rapid detection of methicillin-resistant *Staphylococcus aureus* by Crystal MRSA ID system. J Clin Microbiol 1994;32(7):1830–1832.
198. Reller LB, Mirrett S. Motility-indole-lysine medium for presumptive identification of enteric pathogens of *Enterobacteriaceae*. J Clin Microbiol 1975;2(3):247–252.
199. Renaud FN, Dutaur M, Daoud S, et al. Differentiation of *Corynebacterium amycolatum, C. minutissimum,* and *C. striatum* by carbon substrate assimilation tests. J Clin Microbiol 1998;36(12):3698–3702.
200. Rhoads S, Marinelli L, Imperatrice CA, Nachamkin I. Comparison of MicroScan WalkAway system and Vitek system for identification of gram-negative bacteria. J Clin Microbiol 1995;33(11):3044–3046.
201. Rhoden DL, Miller JM. Four-year prospective study of STAPH-IDENT system and conventional methods for reference identification of *Staphylococcus, Stomatococcus,* and *Micrococcus*. J Clin Microbiol 1995;33(1):96–98.
202. Rhoden DL, Smith PB, Baker CN, Schable B. AutoScan-4 system for identification of gram-negative bacilli. J Clin Microbiol 1985;22(6):915–918.
203. Riggio MP, Lennon A. Rapid identification of *Actinobacillus actinomycetemcomitans, Haemophilus aphrophilus,* and *Haemophilus paraphrophilus* by restriction enzyme analysis of PCR-amplified 13 S rRNA genes. J Clin Microbiol 1997;35(6):1630–1632.
204. Rivera L. Detection of *Haemophilus influenzae* type b antigenuria by Bactigen and Phadebact kits. J Clin Microbiol 1985;21(4):638–640.
205. Robinson A, Griffith SB, Moore DG, Carlson JR. Evaluations of the RIM system and Gono-Gen test for identification of *Neisseria gonorrhoeae* from clinical specimens. Diagn Microbiol Infect Dis 1985;3(2):125–130.
206. Robinson A, McCarter YS, Tetreault J. Comparison of Crystal Enteric/Nonfermenter system, API 20E system, and Vitek automicrobic

system for identification of gram-negative bacilli. J Clin Microbiol 1995;33(2):364–370.
207. Roe M, Kishiyama C, Davidson K, et al. Comparison of BioStar Strep A OIA optical immunoassay, Abbott Test-Pack Plus Strep A, and culture with selective media for diagnosis of group A streptococcal pharyngitis. J Clin Microbiol 1995;33(6):1551–1553.
208. Rossney AS, English LF, Keane CT. Coagulase testing compared with commercial kits for routinely identifying *Staphylococcus aureus.* J Clin Pathol 1990;43(3):246–252.
209. Rudolph KM, Parkinson AJ, Black CM, Mayer LW. Evaluation of polymerase chain reaction for diagnosis of pneumococcal pneumonia. J Clin Microbiol 1993;31(10):2661–2666.
210. Ruoff KL, Kunz LJ. Use of rapid STREP system for identification of viridans streptococcal species. J Clin Microbiol 1983;18(5):1138–1140.
211. Saiki RK, Gelfand DH, Stoffel S, et al. Primer-directed enzyme amplification of DNA with a thermostable DNA polymerase. Science 1988; 239:487–491.
212. Sanden GN, Cassiday PK, Barbaree JM. Rapid immunoblot technique for identifying *Bordetella pertussis.* J Clin Microbiol 1993;31(1): 170–172.
213. Saunders KE, McGovern KJ, Fox JG. Use of pulsed-field gel electrophoresis to determine genomic diversity in strains of *Helicobacter hepaticus* from geographically distant locations. J Clin Microbiol 1997;35(11):2859–2863.
214. Schieven BC. Evaluation of Rainbow UTI system for rapid isolation and identification of urinary pathogens. Abstr Annu Meet Am Soc Microbiol C375, 1995;65.
215. Schieven BC, Hussain Z, Lannigan R. Comparison of American MicroScan dry and frozen microdilution trays. J Clin Microbiol 1985;22 (4):495–496.
216. Schlichting C, Branger C, Fournier JM, et al. Typing of *Staphylococcus aureus* by pulsefield gel electrophoresis, zymotyping, capsular typing, and phage typing: Resolution of clonal relationships. J Clin Microbiol 1993;31(2):227–232.
217. Schwabe LD, Small MT, Randall SL. Comparison of TestPack Strep A test kit with culture technique for detection of group A streptococci. J Clin Microbiol 1987;25(2):309–311.
218. Shaw ED, Darker RJ, Feldman WE, et al. Clinical studies of a new latex particle agglutination test for detection of *Haemophilus influenzae* type b polyribose phosphate antigen in serum, cerebrospinal fluid and urine. J Clin Microbiol 1982;15(6):1153–1156.
219. Shi ZY, Liu PY, Lau YJ, et al. Use of pulsed-field gel electrophoresis to investigate an outbreak of *Serratia marcescens.* J Clin Microbiol 1997; 35(1):325–327.
220. Shotts EB, Rimler R. Medium for the isolation of *Aeromonas hydrophila.* Appl Microbiol 1973; 26(4):550.
221. Smith KR, Ching S, Lee H, et al. Evaluation of ligase chain reaction for use with urine for identification of *Neisseria gonorrhoeae* in females attending sexually transmitted disease clinic. J Clin Microbiol 1995;33(2):455–457.
222. Smith RF, Rogers RR, Bettge CL. Inhibition of the indole test reaction by sodium nitrite. Appl Microbiol 1972;23(2):423–424.
223. Smith SK, Washington JA II. Evaluation of the Pneumoslide latex agglutination kit test for identification of *Streptococcus pneumoniae.* J Clin Microbiol 1984;20(3):592–593.
224. Staneck JL, Vincelette J, Lamothe F, Polk EA. Evaluation of the Sensititre system for identification of *Enterobacteriaceae.* J Clin Microbiol 1983;17(4):647–654.
225. Staneck JL, Weckbach LS, Allen SD, et al. Multicenter evaluation of four methods for *Clostridium difficile* detection: ImmunoCard *C. difficile,* cytotoxin assay, culture, and latex agglutination. J Clin Microbiol 1996;34(11): 2718–2721.
226. Staneck JL, Weckbach LS, Tilton RC, et al. Collaborative evaluation of the Radiometer Sensititre AP80 for identification of gram-negative bacilli. J Clin Microbiol 1993;31(5):1179–1184.
227. Steed LL, Korgenski EK, Daly JA. Rapid detection of *Streptococcus pyogenes* in pediatric patient specimens by DNA probe. J Clin Microbiol 1993;31(11):2996–3000.
228. Steinmetz I, Reganzerowski A, Brenneke B, et al. Rapid identification of *Burkholderia pseudomallei* by latex agglutination based on an exopolysaccharide-specific monoclonal antibody. J Clin Microbiol 1999;37(1):225–228.
229. Stevens DL, Jones C. Use of trehalose-mannitol-phosphatase agar to differentiate *Staphylococcus epidermidis* and *Staphylococcus saprophyticus* from other coagulase-negative staphylococci. J Clin Microbiol 1984;20(5):977–980.
230. Stoakes L, John MA, Lannigan R, et al. Gas-liquid chromatography of cellular fatty acids for identification of staphylococci. J Clin Microbiol 1994;32(8):1908–1910.
231. Stoakes L, Schieven BC, Ofori E, et al. Evaluation of MicroScan Rapid Pos Combo panels for identification of staphylococci. J Clin Microbiol 1992;30(1):93–95.
232. Stone GG, Oberst RD, Hays MP, et al. Combined PCR-oligonucleotide ligation assay for rapid detection of *Salmonella* serovars. J Clin Microbiol 1995;33(11):2888–2893.
233. Tenjarla G, Jumar A, Dyke JW. TestPack Strep A kit for throat swabs in a clinical pathology laboratory. Am J Clin Pathol 1991;96(6):759–761.
234. Tomfohrde KM, Rhoden DL, Smith PB, Balows A. Evaluation of the redesigned Enterotube—a

system for the identification of *Enterobacteriaceae*. Appl Microbiol 1973;25(2):301–304.
235. Trepeta RW, Edberg SC. Methylumbelliferyl-β-D-glucuronidase-based medium for rapid isolation and identification of *Escherichia coli*. J Clin Microbiol 1984;19(2):172–174.
236. Tritz DM, Iwen PC, Woods GL. Evaluation of MicroScan for identification of *Enterococcus* species. J Clin Microbiol 1990;28(6):1477–1478.
237. Truant AL, Satishchandran V. Comparison of Streptex versus PathoD for group D typing of vancomycin resistant *Enterococcus*. Diagn Microbiol Infect Dis 1993;16(1):89–91.
238. Vlaspolder F, Mutsaers JAEM, Blog F, Notowicz A. Value of a DNA probe assay (Gen-Probe) compared with that of culture for diagnosis of gonococci infection. J Clin Microbiol 1993;31:107–110.
239. van Belkum A, Kluytmans J, van Leeuwen W, et al. Multicenter evaluation of arbitrarily primed PCR typing of *Staphylococcus aureus* strains. J Clin Microbiol 1995;33(6):1537–1547.
240. Vandenbroucke-Gruls CM, Kusters JG. Specific detection of methicillin-resistant *Staphylococcus* species by multiplex PCR. J Clin Microbiol 1996;34(6):1599.
241. van der Zee A, Agterberg C, Peeters M, et al. Polymerase chain reaction assay for pertussis: Simultaneous detection and discrimination of *Bordetella pertussis* and *Bordetella parapertussis*. J Clin Microbiol 1993;31(8):2134–2140.
242. van Griethuysen A, Buiting A, Goessens W, et al. Multicenter evaluation of a modified protocol for the RAPIDEC staph system for direct identification of *Staphylococcus aureus* in blood cultures. J Clin Microbiol 1998;36(12):3707–3709.
243. Walton DT. Fluorescent-antibody-negative penicillinase-producing *Neisseria gonorrhoeae*. J Clin Microbiol 1989;27(8):1885–1886.
244. Watts JL, Washbrun PJ. Evaluation of the Staph-Zym system with staphylococci isolated from bovine intramammary infections. J Clin Microbiol 1991;29(1):59–61.
245. Wauters G, Boel A, Voorn GP, et al. Evaluation of a new identification system, Crystal Enteric/Nonfermenter, for gram-negative bacilli. J Clin Microbiol 1995;33(4):845–849.
246. Weinstein MP, Mirrett S, Van Pelt L, et al. Clinical importance of identifying coagulase-negative staphylococci isolated from blood cultures: Evaluation of MicroScan Rapid and Dried Overnight Gram-Positive panels versus conventional reference method. J Clin Microbiol 1998;36(7):2089–2092.
247. Weiss J, Mecca D, da Silva E, Gassner D. Comparison of PCR and other diagnostic techniques for detection of *Helicobacter pylori* infection in dyspeptic patients. J Clin Microbiol 1994;32(7):1663–1668.
248. Welborn PP, Uyeda CT, Ellison-Birang N. Evaluation of Gonochek-II as a rapid identification system for pathogenic *Neisseria* species. J Clin Microbiol 1984;20(4):680–683.
249. Welch DF, Hensel D. Evaluation of Bactogen and Phadebact for detection of *Haemophilus influenzae* type b antigen in cerebrospinal fluid. J Clin Microbiol 1982;16(5):905–908.
250. Welch WD, Cartwright G. Fluorescent monoclonal antibody compared with carbohydrate utilization for rapid identification of *Neisseria gonorrhoeae*. J Clin Microbiol 1988;26(2):293–296.
251. Wellstood S. Evaluation of a latex test for rapid detection of pneumococcal antigens in sputum. Eur J Microbiol Infect Dis 1992;11(5):448–451.
252. Wellstood-Nuesse S. Comparison of the Minitek system with conventional methods for identification of nonfermenative and oxidase-positive fermentative gram-negative bacilli. J Clin Microbiol 1979;9(4):511–516.
253. Whittier S, Shapiro DS, Kelly WF, et al. Evaluation of four commercially available enzyme immunoassays for laboratory diagnosis of *Clostridium difficile*-associated diseases. J Clin Microbiol 1993;31(11):2861–2865.
254. Wilkerson M, McAllister S, Miller JM, et al. Comparison of five agglutination tests for identification of *Staphylococcus aureus*. J Clin Microbiol 1997;35(1):148–151.
255. Wong HC, Lu KT, Pan TM, et al. Subspecies typing of *Vibrio parahaemolyticus* by pulsed-field gel electrophoresis. J Clin Microbiol 1996;34(6):1535–1539.
256. Wong JD, Janda JM, Duffey PS. Preliminary studies on the use of carbon substrate utilization patterns for identification of *Brucella* species. Diagn Microbiol Infect Dis 1992;15(2):109–113.
257. Woods GL, DiGiovanni B, Levison M, et al. Evaluation of MicroScan rapid panels for detection of high-level aminoglycoside resistance in enterococci. J Clin Microbiol 1993;31(10):2786–2787.
258. Woolfrey BF, Lally RT, Quall CO. Evaluation of the AutoScan-3 and Septor systems for *Enterobacteriaceae* identification. J Clin Microbiol 1983;17(5):807–813.
259. Yassin AF, Brzezinka H, Schaal KP, et al. Menaquinone composition in the classification and identification of aerobic actinomycetes. Zentralbl Bakteriol Mikrobiol Hyg 1988;[A]267:339–356.
260. York MK, Brooks GF, Fiss EH. Evaluation of the AutoSCAN-W/A rapid system for identification and susceptibility testing of gram-negative fermentative bacilli. J Clin Microbiol 1992;30(11):2903–2910.
261. You MS, Facklam RR. New test system for

identification of *Aerococcus, Enterococcus,* and *Streptococcus* species. J Clin Microbiol 1986; 24(4):607–611.
262. Young LS, Moyes A. Comparative evaluation of AccuProbe culture identification test for *Neisseria gonorrhoeae*. J Clin Microbiol 1993;31(8): 1996–1999.
263. Zhang Y, Isaacman DJ, Wadowsky RM. Detection of *Streptococcus* in whole blood by PCR. J Clin Microbiol 1995;33(3):596–601.

SECTION III

Identification Schemas

43 Gram-Positive Bacteria

Classification 483
Changes in Nomenclature/References 487
Genera Descriptions/Tables 502
Warning 573
Diagrams
  Bacilli
Gram-Positive Aerobes/Facultative Anaerobes 576
    Gram-Positive Anaerobes 589
  Cocci
    Gram-Positive Aerobes/Facultative Anaerobes 604
    Gram-Positive Anaerobes 620
    References 622

(*Note:* All genera covered are listed alphabetically.)

CLASSIFICATION: PROPOSED OUTLINE OF *BERGEY'S MANUAL OF SYSTEMATIC BACTERIOLOGY*, 2ND EDITION

Volume 1 The Archae, Cyanobacteria, Phototrophs and Deeply Branching Genera

The Bacteria (Eubacteria)
Section VIII: The Deinos
Kingdom: Deincocci
  Division: Deinococci
    Order I: *Deinococcales*
      Family: *Deinococcaceae*
        Deinococcus: 7 species

Volume 2 The Proteobacteria

Bacteria
Kingdom: *Proteobacteria*
Section XV: α-*Proteobacteria*
  Class I: *Rhodospirillales*
    Family II: *Acetobacteraceae*
      Frateuria: 1 species
    Order VI: *Rhizobiales*
      Family X: *Hyphomicrobiaceae*
        Xanthobacter: 4 species

Volume 3 Bacteria: The Low G + C Gram Positives: Low guanine-plus-cytosine content of DNA; bacteria more regular in shape

Section XX: Clostridia and Relatives
    Class: Clostridia
        Order I: *Clostridiales*
            Family I: *Clostridiaceae*
                Clostridium: 131 species
                Sarcina: 2 species
                Oxobacter: 1 species
                Caloramator: 2 species
            Family II: *Peptostreptococcaceae*
                Peptostreptococcus: 16 species
                Filifactor: 1 species
            Family III: *Eubacteriaceae*
                Eubacterium: 51 species
                Pseudoramibacter: 1 species
            Family IV: *Lachnospiraceae*
                Butyrivibrio: 2 species
                Ruminococcus: 12 species
                Coprococcus: 3 species
            Family V: *Peptococcaceae*
                Peptococcus: 1 species
            Family VI: *Syntrophomonadaceae*
                Syntrophospora: 1 species
                Moorella: 2 species
                Thermoanaerobacter: 10 species
        Order II: *Haloanaerobiales*
            Family II: *Halobacteroidaceae*
                Sporohalobacter: 1 species
Section XXI-The Mollicutes
    Class: *Mollicutes*
        Order: *Mycoplasmatales*, walled relatives of mycoplasmas
            Erysipelothrix: 2 species
Section XXII: The Bacilli and Lactobacilli
    Class: *Bacilli*
        Order I: *Bacillales*
            Family I: *Bacillaceae*
                Bacillus: 73 species
                Exiguobacterium: 2 species
                Aneurinibacillus: 2 species
                Brevibacillus: 10 species
            Family II: *Planococcaceae*
                Kurthia: 3 species
            Family V: *Paenibacillaceae*
                Paenibacillus: 15 species
            Family VI: *Alicyclobacillaceae*
                Alicyclobacillus: 3 species
        Order II: *Lactobacillales*
            Family I: *Lactobacillaceae*
                Lactobacillus: 80 species

Family II: *Leuconostocaceae*
    Leuconostoc: 11 species
    Oenococcus: 1 species
    Weissella: 7 species
Family III: *Streptococcaceae*
    Pediococcus: 7 species
    Streptococcus: 45 species
    Lactococcus: 8 species
Family IV: *Enterococcaceae*
    Enterococcus: 18 species
    Vagococcus: 2 species
    Melissococcus: 1 species
Family V: *Carnobacteriaceae*
    Carnobacterium: 6 species
    Alloiococcus: 1 species
    Lactosphaera: 1 species
Family VI: *Aerococcaceae*
    Aerococcus: 2 species
    Globicatella: 1 species
    Tetragenococcus: 1 species
    Abiotrophia: 2 species
Family VII: *Listeriaceae*
    Listeria: 8 species
    Brochothrix: 2 species
Family VIII: *Staphylococcaceae*
    Staphylococcus: 47 species
    Gemella: 2 species
    Genera of low G + C Gram positives
    Acetobacterium: 7 species
    Oxalophagus: 1 species
    Pasteuria: 3 species

Volume 4 Bacteria: The High G + C Gram Positives: High guanine-plus-cytosine content of DNA; bacteria irregular cell shape

Section XXIII: Class *Actinobacteria*
  Subclass II: *Rubrobacteridae*
    Order: *Rubrobacterales*
      Family: *Rubrobacteraceae*
        Rubrobacter: 2 species
  Subclass III: *Coriobacteridae*
    Order: *Coriobacterales*
      Family: *Coriobacteriaceae*
        Atopobium: 3 species
  Subclass V: *Actinobacteridae*
    Order I: *Actinomycetales*
      Suborder I: *Actinomycineae*
        Family: *Actinomycetaceae*
          Actinomyces: 20 species
          Arcanobacterium: 4 species
          Mobiluncus: 4 species

Suborder II: *Micrococcineae*
  Family I: *Micrococcaceae*
    Micrococcus: 2 species
    Arthrobacter: 24 species
    Kocuria: 3 species
    Leucobacter: 1 species
    Nesterenkonia: 1 species
    Rothia: 1 species
    Stomatococcus: 1 species
  Family II: *Brevibacteraceae*
    Brevibacterium: 12 species
  Family III: *Cellulomonadaceae*
    Cellulomonas: 10 species
  Family IV: *Dermabacteraceae*
    Dermabacter: 1 species
  Family V: *Dermatophilaceae*
    Dermacoccus: 1 species
    Kytococcus: 1 species
  Family VII: *Jonesiaceae*
    Jonesia: 1 species
  Family VIII: *Microbacteriaceae*
    Microbacterium: 6 species
    Agromyces: 8 species
    Aureobacterium: 13 species
    Clavibacter: 10 species
    Curtobacterium: 6 species
    Rathayibacter: 3 species
  Family IX: *Promicromonosporaceae*
    Terrabacter: 1 species
Suborder III: *Corynebacterineae*
  Family I: *Corynebacteriaceae*
    Corynebacterium: 42 species
  Family II: *Dietziaceae*
    Dietzia: 1 species
  Family III: *Gordoniaceae*
    Gordonia: 8 species
    Skermania: 1 species
  Family IV: *Mycobacteriaceae*
    Mycobacterium: 83 species
  Family V: *Norcardiaceae*
    Nocardia: 14 species
    Rhodococcus: 12 species
  Family VI: *Tsukamurellaceae*
    Tsukamurella: 5 species
Suborder V: *Propionibacterineae*
  Family I: *Propionibacteriaceae*
    Propionibacterium: 12 species
    Propioniferax: 1 species
  Family II: *Nocardioidaceae*
    Nocardioides: 5 species
Suborder VI: *Pseudonocardineae*

Family: *Pseudonocardiaceae*
    ***Pseudonocardia*:** 9 species
    ***Amycolatopsis*:** 11 species
    ***Saccharothrix*:** 16 species
Suborder VII: *Streptomycineae*
  Family: *Streptomycetaceae*
    ***Streptomyces*:** 509 species
Suborder VIII: *Streptosporangineae*
  Family II: *Nocardiopsaceae*
    ***Nocardiopsis*:** 9 species
Order II: *Bifidobacteriales*
  Family: *Bifidobacteriaceae*
    ***Bifidobacterium*:** 33 species
    ***Gardnerella*:** 1 species
    ***Falcivibrio*:** 2 species
  Unknown affiliation
    ***Turicella*:** 1 species

(*Note:* Bergey's outline of classification is listed only for organisms covered in this chapter or new genera and species listed in New Nomenclature. Outline courtesy of Dr. George Garrity, Editor-in-Chief, Bergey's Manual Trust.)

CHANGES IN NOMENCLATURE: GRAM-POSITIVE RODS (BACILLI) AND GRAM-POSITIVE COCCI (SPHERES)

(*Note:* Bergey's Manual of Determinative Bacteriology, 9th edition, was printed in 1994; therefore, references to new genera or new species are listed from 1995 to 1997.)

Definitions

Basonym: original name of a new combination
Synonym:
    Objective: more than 1 name
    Subjective: different name to different types; first published, senior; later, junior
comb. nov.: new combination; species transferred to another genus or subsp. transferred to another species
gen. nov.: new genus
sp. non.: new species
nomen dubium: doubtful name

Current Name	Old Name (Basonym(s)/Synonym(s))
Abiotrophia, gen. nov.[1]	
Abiotrophia adiacens[1]	*Streptococcus adiacens*
Abiotrophia defectiva[1]	*Streptococcus defectivus*
Acetobacterium bakii, sp. nov.[2]	
Acetobacterium fimetarium, sp. nov.[2]	
Acetobacterium paludosum, sp. nov.[2]	
Actinobaculum, gen. nov.[3]	
Actinobaculum schaalii, sp. nov.[3]	
Actinobaculum suis, comb. nov.[3]	*Actinomyces suis; Eubacterium suis; Corynebacterium suis*
Actinomyces europaeus, sp. nov.[4]	CDC coryneform sp 2 bacteria
Actinomyces georgiae[5]	*Actinomyces D08*

Actinomyces gerencseriae	*Actinomyces israelii* serotype II
Actinomyces graevenitzii, sp. nov.[6]	
Actinomyces meyeri	*Actinobacterium meyeri*
Actinomyces radingae, sp. nov.[7]	
Actinomyces turicensis, sp. nov.[7]	
Aerococcus urinae, sp. nov.[8]	*Aerococcus*-like organisms (ALOs)
Agromyces mediolanus	*Corynebacterium mediolanum*
Alicyclobacillus acidocaldarius	*Bacillus acidocaldarius*
Alicyclobacillus acidoterrestris	*Bacillus acidoterrestris*
Alicyclobacillus cycloheptanicus	*Bacillus cycloheptanicus*
Alloiococcus otitidis	*Alloiococcus otitis*
Amycolatopsis azurea	*Pseudonocardia azurea*
Amycolatopsis fastidiosa	*Pseudocardia fastidiosa*
Amycolatopsis coloradensis, sp. nov.[9]	
Amycolatopsis japonica, sp. nov.[10]	Incorrect name, *Amycolatopsis japonicum*
Amycolatopsis mediterranei	*Nocardia mediterranei*; *Actinomyces mediterranei*; *Streptomyces mediterranei*
Amycolatopsis methanolica	*Nocardia* sp. strain 239
Amycolatopsis orientalis	*Actinomyces orientalis*; *Streptomyces orientalis*; *Proactinomyces orientalis*
Amycolatopsis orientalis subsp. *lurida*	*Nocardia lurida*
Amycolatopsis orientalis subsp. *orientalis*	*Nocardia orientalis*
Amycolatopsis rugosa	*Nocardia rugosa*; *Proactinomyces rugosa*
Amycolatopsis sulphurea	*Nocardia sulphurea*
Aneurinibacillus, gen. nov.[11]	
Aneurinibacillus aneurinilyticus, comb. nov.[11]	*Bacillus aneurinolyticus*
Aneurinibacillus migulanus, comb. nov.[11]	*Bacillus migulanus*
Aneurinibacillus thermoaerophilus, comb. nov.[12]	*Bacillus thermoaerophilus*
Arcanobacterium bernardiae, comb. nov.[13]	*Actinomyces bernardiae*; CDC coryneform group 2 bacteria
Arcanobacterium haemolyticum	*Corynebacterium haemolyticum*
Arcanobacterium phocae, sp. nov.[13]	
Arcanobacterium pyogenes	*Actinomyces pyogenes*; *Corynebacterium pyogenes*
Arthrobacter agilis, comb. nov.[14]	*Micrococcus agilis*
Arthrobacter cumminsii, sp. nov.[15]	
Arthrobacter ilicis	*Corynebacterium ilicis*
Arthrobacter protophormiae	*Brevibacterium protophormiae*
Arthrobacter woluwensis, sp. nov.[15]	
Atopobium minutum	*Lactobacillus minutus*
Atopobium parvulum	*Peptostreptococcus parvulus*; *Streptococcus parvulus*
Atopobium rimae	*Lactobacillus rimae*
Aureobacterium barkeri	*Corynebacterium barkeri*
Aureobacterium esteraromaticum	*Flavobacterium esteraromaticum*
Aureobacterium flavescens	*Arthrobacter flavescens*
Aureobacterium liquefaciens	*Microbacterium liquefaciens*
Aureobacterium saperdae	*Brevibacterium saperdae*; *Curtobacterium saperdae*
Aureobacterium terregens	*Arthrobacter terregens*

Aureobacterium testaceum	*Brevibacterium testaceum;* *Curtobacterium testaceum*
Bacillus agaradhaerens, sp. nov.[16]	
Bacillus amyloliquefaciens	*Bacillus amylolyticus*
Bacillus carbonifilus, sp. nov.[17]	
Bacillus chitinolyticus, sp. nov.[18]	
Bacillus clarkii, sp. nov.[16]	
Bacillus clausii, sp. nov.[16]	
Bacillus dipsosauri, sp. nov.[19]	
Bacillus ehimensis, sp. nov.[18]	
Bacillus fusiformis	*Bacillus sphaericus* subsp. *fusiformis*
Bacillus gibsonii, sp. nov.[16]	
Bacillus halmapalus, sp. nov.[16]	
Bacillus haloalkaliphilus, sp. nov.[20]	
Bacillus halodurans, comb. nov.[16]	*Bacillus alcalophilus* subsp. *halodurans*
Bacillus horikoshii, sp. nov.[16]	
Bacillus infernus, sp. nov.[21]	
Bacillus marinus	*Bacillus globisporus* subsp. *marinus*
Bacillus oleronius, sp. nov.[22]	
Bacillus pseudalcaliphilus, sp. nov.[16]	
Bacillus pseudofirmus, sp. nov.[16]	
Bacillus salexigens, sp. nov.[23]	
Bacillus sporothermodurans, sp. nov.[24]	
Bacillus thermoamylovorans, sp. nov.[25]	
Bacillus thermocloacae	Misspelled *"thermocloaceae"*
Bacillus thermosphaericus, sp. nov.[26]	
Bacillus vallismortis, sp. nov.[27]	
Bacillus vedderi, sp. nov.[28]	
Bifidobacterium denticolens, sp. nov.[29]	
Bifidobacterium dentium	*Bifidobacterium appendicitis;* *Bifidobacterium eriksonii*
Bifidobacterium inopinatum, sp. nov.[29]	
Bifidobacterium lactis, sp. nov.[30]	
Bifidobacterium pseudolongum subsp. *globosum*	*Bifidobacterium globosum*
Bifidobacterium thermophilum	*Bifidobacterium thermophilium;* incorrect name
Brevibacillus, gen. nov.[11]	CDC groups B1 and B3
Brevibacillus agri, sp. nov.[11]	*Bacillus agri; Bacillus galactophilus*
Brevibacillus borstelensis, comb. nov.[11]	*Bacillus borstelensis*
Brevibacillus brevis, comb. nov.[11]	*Bacillus brevis*
Brevibacillus centrosporus, comb. nov.[11]	*Bacillus centrosporus*
Brevibacillus choshinensis, comb. nov.[11]	*Bacillus choshinensis*
Brevibacillus formosus, comb. nov.[11]	*Bacillus formosus*
Brevibacillus laterosporus, comb. nov.[11]	*Bacillus laterosporus*
Brevibacillus parabrevis, comb. nov.[11]	*Bacillus parabrevis*
Brevibacillus reuszeri, comb. nov.[11]	*Bacillus reuszeri*
Brevibacillus thermoruber, comb. nov.[11]	*Bacillus thermoruber*
Brevibacterium liquefaciens	Erroneously classified as *Corynebacterium liquefaciens*
Brochothrix thermosphacta	*Mycobacterium thermosphactum*
Caloramator fervidus	*Clostridium fervidus*
Carnobacterium divergens	*Lactobacillus divergens*

Carnobacterium piscicola	*Lactobacillus piscicola; Lactobacillus carnis*
Cellulomonas cellulans	*Oerskovia xanthineolytica; Brevibacterium fermentans; Brevibacterium lyticum; Cellulomonas cartae; Nocardia cellulans*
Cellulomonas hominis, sp. nov.[31]	
Cellulomonas turbata	*Oerskovia turbata; Nocardia turbata;* CDC groups A3 and A4 (in part)
Clavibacter michiganense subsp. *insidiosum*	*Corynebacterium insidiosum*
Clavibacter michiganense subsp. *michiganense*	*Corynebacterium michiganense*
Clavibacter michiganense subsp. *nebraskense*	*Corynebacterium nebraskense*
Clavibacter michiganense subsp. *sepedonicum*	*Corynebacterium sepedonicum*
Clavibacter michiganense subsp. *tessellarius*	*Corynebacterium michiganense* subsp. *tessellarius*
Clostridium acetireducens, sp. nov.[32]	
Clostridium algidicarnis, sp. nov.[33]	
Clostridium argentinense	*Clostridium botulinum* toxin type G; *Clostridium hastiforme* (some strains); *Clostridium subterminale* (some strains)
Clostridium baratii	*Clostridium paraperfringens; Clostridium perennet; Clostridium perenne*
Clostridium butyricum	*Clostridium pseudotetanicum*
Clostridium cadaveris	*Clostridium capitovale*
Clostridium chartatabidum, sp. nov.[34]	
Clostridium chauvoei	*Clostridium feseri*
Clostridium clostridioforme	*Clostridium clostridiiforme*
Clostridium cochlearium	*Clostridium lentoputrescens*
Clostridium difficile	*Clostridium difficilis*
Clostridium fallax	*Clostridium pseudofallax*
Clostridium fimetarium, sp.nov.[2]	
Clostridium gohnii	*Clostridium gohni*
Clostridium grantii, sp.nov.[35]	
Clostridium haemolyticum	*Clostridium novyi* type D
Clostridium herbivorans, sp. nov.[36]	
Clostridium laramiense	Incorrect name, *Clostridium laramie*
Clostridium neopropionicum, sp. nov.[37]	
Clostridium oroticum	*Zymobacterium oroticum*
Clostridium pascui, sp. nov.[38]	
Clostridium perfringens	*Clostridium welchii*
Clostridium piliforme	*Bacillus piliformis*
Clostridium polysaccharolyticum	*Fusobacterium polysaccharolyticum*
Clostridium proteoclasticum, sp. nov.[39]	
Clostridium quinii, sp. nov.[40]	
Clostridium ramosum	*Eubacterium ramosum; Actinomyces ramosus*
Clostridium symbiosum	*Fusobacterium biacutus; Bacteroides biacutus; Fusobacterium symbiosum; Bacteroides symbiosum*
Clostridium ultunense, sp. nov.[41]	

Clostridium vincentii, sp. nov.[42]
Clostridium viride, sp. nov.[43]
Corynebacterium accolens   CDC group 6
Corynebacterium afermentans   CDC group ANF-1
Corynebacterium ammoniagenes   *Brevibacterium ammoniagenes*
Corynebacterium argentoratense, sp. nov.[44]
Corynebacterium auris, sp. nov.[45]   CDC ANF-1-like bacteria
Corynebacterium coyleae, sp. nov.[46]
Corynebacterium cystitis   *Corynebacterium renale* type III
Corynebacterium durum, sp. nov.[47]
Corynebacterium glucuronolyticum, sp. nov.[48]
Corynebacterium glutamicum   *Brevibacterium flavumu*; *Brevibacterium divaricatum*; *Brevibacterium lactofermentumu*; *Corynebacterium lilium*

Corynebacterium imitans, sp. nov.[49]
Corynebacterium jeikeium   CDC JK group
Corynebacterium lipophiloflavum, sp. nov.[50]
Corynebacterium macginleyi, sp. nov.[51]
Corynebacterium mastitidis, sp.nov.[52]
Corynebacterium matruchotii   *Bacterionema matruchotii*
Corynebacterium mucifaciens, sp. nov.[53]
Corynebacterium pilosum   *Corynebacterium renale* (in part)
Corynebacterium propinquum   CDC group ANF-3
Corynebacterium pseudodiphtheriticum   *Corynebacterium hofmanni*
Corynebacterium seminale, sp. nov.[54]
Corynebacterium singulare, sp. nov.[55]
Corynebacterium striatum   nomen dubium, wrong & lost strain, *Corynebacterium flavidum*

Corynebacterium ulcerans, sp. nov.[56]
Corynebacterium urealyticum   CDC group D2
Corynebacterium variabilis   *Caseobacter polymorphus*; *Arthrobacter variabilis*

Corynebacterium vitaeruminis   *Brevibacterium vitarumen*; incorrect name, *Corynebacterium vitarumen*

Curtobacterium albidum   *Brevibacterium albidum*
Curtobacterium citreum   *Brevibacterium citreum*
Curtobacterium flaccumfaciens   *Corynebacterium betae*; *Corynebacterium flaccumfaciens*

Curtobacterium luteum   *Brevibacterium luteum*
Curtobacterium flaccumfaciens   *Corynebacterium oortii*; *Corynebacterium poinsettiae*

Curtobacterium pusillum   *Brevibacterium pusillum*
Deinococcus, gen. nov.[57]
Deinococcus geothermalis, sp. nov.[58]
Deinococcus grandis, comb. nov.[57]   *Deinobacter grandis*
Deinococcus murrayi, sp. nov.[58]
Deinococcus proteolyticus   *Micrococcus radioproteolyticus*
Deinococcus radiodurans   *Micrococcus radiodurans*
Deinococcus radiophilus   *Micrococcus radiophilus*
Dermabacter hominis   CDC groups 3 & 5
Dermacoccus gen. nov.[59]

Dermacoccus nishinomiyaenis, comb. nov.[59]	*Micrococcus nishinomiyaensis*
Dietzia, gen. nov.[60]	
Dietzia maris, comb. nov.	*Rhodococcus maris*; *Flavebacterium maris*
Enterococcus avium	*Streptococcus avium*
Enterococcus casseliflavus	*Streptococcus casseliflavus*; *Streptococcus faecium* subsp. *casseliflavus*
Enterococcus cecorum	*Streptococcus cecorum*
Enterococcus durans	*Streptococcus durans*
Enterococcus faecalis	*Streptococcus faecalis*
Enterococcus gallinarum	*Streptococcus gallinarum*
Enterococcus malodoratus	*Streptococcus faecalis* subsp. *malodoratus*
Enterococcus saccharolyticus	*Streptococcus saccharolyticus*
Erysipelothrix rhusiopathiae	*Erysipelothrix insidiosa*
Eubacterium barkeri	*Clostridium barkeri*
Eubacterium exiguum, sp. nov.[61]	*Eubacterium* group S strains
Eubacterium infirmum, sp. nov.[62]	
Eubacterium minutum, sp. nov.[63]	
Eubacterium oxidoreducens	Incorrect name, *Eubacterium oxidoreducans*
Eubacterium plautii	*Fusobacterium plautii*
Eubacterium tarantellae	Incorrect name, *Eubacterium tarantellus*
Eubacterium tardum, sp. nov.	
Exiguobacterium acetylicum [62]	*Brevibacterium acetylicum*
Filifactor villosus	*Clostridium villosum*
Frateuria aurantia	*Acetobacter aurantinum*
Fusobacterium plauti	*Eubacterium plautii*
Gardnerella vaginalis	*Haemophilus vaginalis*; *Corynebacterium vaginalis*
Gamella haemolysans	*Neisseria haemolysans*
Gemella morbillorum	*Streptococcus morbillorum*; *Diplococcus morbillorum*; *Diplococcus rubeolae*; *Peptostreptococcus morbillorum*
Globicatella, gen. nov.[64]	
Globicatella sanguinis, sp. nov.[64]	Incorrect name, *Globicatella sanguis*; salt-tolerant viridans streptococci
Gordona	Incorrect genus name
Gordonia, gen. nov.	
Gordonia aichiensis	Incorrect name, *Gordona aichiensis*; *Rhodococcus aichiensis*
Gordonia amarae	Incorrect name, *Gordon amarae*; *Nocardia amarae*
Gordonia aichiensis	*Rhodococcus aichiensis*
Gordonia bronchialis	Incorrect name, *Gordona bronchialis*; *Rhodococcus bronchialis*
Gordonia hirsuta, sp. nov.[65]	Incorrect name, *Gordona hirsuta*
Gordonia hydrophobica	Incorrect name, *Gordona hydrophobica*
Gordonia rubropertinctus	Incorrect name, *Gordona rubropertinctus*; *Rhodococcus corallinus*; *Rhodococcus rubropertinctus*
Gordonia sputi	Incorrect name, *Gordona sputi*; *Rhodococcus chubuensis*; *Rhodococcus sputi*; *Rhodococcus obuensis*

Gordonia terrae	Incorrect name, *Gordona terrae*; *Rhodococcus terrae*
Holdemania, gen. non.[66]	
Holdemania filiformis, sp. nov.[66]	*Eubacterium*-like strains sp. S 14
Jonesia denitrificans	*Listeria denitrificans*
Kocuria, gen. nov.[59]	
Kocuria erythromyxa, comb. nov.[59]	*Deinococcus erythromyxa*; *Sarcina erythromyxa*
Kocuria kristinae, comb. nov.[59]	*Micrococcus kristinae*
Kocuria rosea, comb. nov.[59]	*Micrococcus roseus*
Kocuria varians, comb. nov.[59]	*Micrococcus varians*
Kytococcus, gen. nov.[59]	
Kytococcus sedentarius, comb. nov.[59]	*Micrococcus sedentarius*
Lactobacillus acidophilus	CDC group A3
Lactobacillus curvatus subsp. *melibiosus*, subsp. nov.[67]	
Lactobacillus delbrueckii subsp. *bulgaricus*	*Lactobacillus bulgaricus*
Lactobacillus delbrueckii subsp. *lactis*	*Lactobacillus lactis*; *Lactobacillus leichmannii*
Lactobacillus fructivorans	*Lactobacillus heterohiochii*; *Lactobacillus trichodes*
Lactobacillus kefiri	Incorrect name, *Lactobacillus kefir*
Lactobacillus lactis subsp. *hordniae*	*Lactobacillus hordniae*
Lactobacillus lactis subsp. *lactis*	*Lactobacillus xylosus*
Lactobacillus lindneri, sp. nov [68]	
Lactobacillus mali	*Lactobacillus yamanashiensis*
Lactobacillus panis, sp. nov.[69]	
Lactobacillus paracasei subsp. *paracasei*	*Lactobacillus paracasei* subsp. *alactosus*; *Lactobacillus casei* subsp. *pseudoplantarum*; *Lactobacillus casei* subsp. *alactosus*
Lactobacillus paracasei subsp. *tolerans*	*Lactobacillus casei* subsp. *tolerans*
Lactobacillus paraplantarum, sp. nov.[70]	
Lactobacillus rhamnosus	*Lactobacillus casei* subsp. *rhamnosus*
Lactobacillus sakei	*Lactobacillus bavaricus*; incorrect name, *Lactobacillus sake*
Lactobacillus sakei subsp. *carnosus*	Incorrect name, *Lactobacillus sake* subsp. *carnosus*
Lactobacillus sakaei subsp. *sakei*	Incorrect name, *Lactococcus sake* subsp. *sake*
Lactobacillus sanfranciscensis	Incorrect name, *Lactobacillus sanfrancisco*
Lactobacillus zeae, sp. nov.[71]	
Lactococcus garvieae	*Enterococcus seriolicida*; *Streptococcus garvieae*
Lactococcus lactis subsp. *cremoris*	*Streptococcus cremoris*; *Streptococcus lactis* subsp. *cremoris*
Lactococcus lactis subsp. *hordniae*	*Lactobacillus hordniae*
Lactococcus lactis subsp. *lactis*	*Lactobacillus xylosus*; *Streptococcus lactis* subsp. *diacitilactis*; *Streptococcus diacetilactis*; *Streptococcus lactis*
Lactococcus plantarum	*Streptococcus plantarum*

Lactococcus raffinolactis	*Streptococcus raffinolactis*
Lactosphaera, gen. nov.[72]	
Lactosphaera pasteurii, comb. nov.[72]	*Ruminococcus pasteurii*
Leucobacter, gen. nov.[73]	
Leucobacter komagatae, sp. nov.[73]	
Leuconostoc citreum	*Leuconostoc amelibiosum*
Leuconostoc mesenteroides subsp. *cremoris*	*Leuconostoc cremoris*
Leusonostoc mesenteroides subsp. *dextranicum*	*Leuconostoc dextranicum*
Listeria grayi	*Listeria murrayi*
Melissococcus pluton	Misspelled, *Melisococcus*; *Streptococcus pluton*
Microbacterium arborescens	*Flavobacterium arborescens*
Microbacterium imperiale	*Brevibacterium imperiale*
Microbacterium laevaniformans	*Corynebacterium laevaniformans*
Moorella thermoacetica	*Clostridium thermoaceticum*
Moorella thermoautotrophica	*Clostridium thermoautotrophicum*
Mycobacterium abscessus	*Mycobacterium chelonae* subsp. *abscessus*
Mycobacterium avium subsp. *paratuberculosis*	*Mycobacterium paratuberculosis*
Mycobacterium branderi, sp. nov.[74]	
Mycobacterium chelonae subsp. *chelonae*	Incorrect name, *Mycobacterium chelonei*
Mycobacterium chlorophenolicum	*Rhodococcus chlorophenolicus*
Mycobacterium conspicuum, sp. nov.[75]	
Mycobacterium gordonae	Rejected name, *Mycobacterium aquae*
Mycobacterium hassiacum, sp. nov.[76]	
Mycobacterium hodleri, sp. nov.[77]	
Mycobacterium interjectum, sp. nov.[78]	
Mycobacterium lentiflavum, sp. nov.[79]	
Mycobacterium mageritense, sp. nov.[80]	
Mycobacterium mucogenicum, sp. nov.[81]	
Mycobacterium novocastrense, sp. nov.[82]	
Mycobacterium triplex, sp. nov.[83]	
Nesterenkonia, gen. nov.[59]	
Nesterenkonia halobia, comb. nov.[59]	*Micrococcus halobius*
Nocardia alborubida	*Actinomyces alborubidus*
Nocardia brevicatena	*Micropolyspora brevicatena*
Nocardia otitidiscaviarum	Incorrect name, *Nocardia otitidis-caviarum*
Nocardia pseudobrasiliensis, sp. nov.[84]	
Nocardioides simplex	*Arthrobacter simplex*; *Pimelobacter simplex*
Nocardiopsis alborubidus	*Actinomyces alborubidus*
Oenococcus, gen. nov.[85]	
Oenococcus oeni, comb. nov.[85]	*Leuconostoc oenos*
Oxalophagus oxalicus	*Clostridium oxalicum*
Oxobacter pfennigii	*Clostridium pfennigii*
Paenibacillus, gen. nov.[86]	
Paenibacillus alginoluticus, comb. nov.[86]	*Bacillus alginolyticus*
Paenibacillus alvei, comb. nov.[86]	*Bacillus alvei*

Paenibacillus amycololyticus, comb. nov.[87]	*Bacillus amylolyticus*
Paenibacillus apiarius, sp. nov.[88]	
Paenibacillus azotofixans	*Bacillus azotofixans*; *Clostridium azotofixans*; *Paenibacillus durum*; *Clostridium durum*
Paenibacillus chibensis, sp. nov.[89]	
Paenibacillus chondroitinus, comb. nov.[88]	*Bacillus chondroitinus*
Paenibacillus curdlanolyticus, comb. nov.[86]	*Bacillus curdlanolyticus*
Paenibacillus glucanolyticus, comb. nov.[86]	*Bacillus glucanolyticus*
Paenibacillus illinoisensis, sp. nov.[89]	
Paenibacillus kobensis, comb. nov.[86]	*Bacillus kobensis*
Paenibacillus larvae, comb. nov.[90]	*Bacillus larvae*
Paenibacillus larvae subsp. larvae, comb. nov.[90]	
Paenibacillus larvae subsp. pulvifaciens, comb. nov.[90]	*Bacillus pulvifaciens*; *Paenibacillus pulvifaciens*
Paenibacillus lautus, comb. nov.[91]	*Bacillus lautus*
Paenibacillus marcerans, comb. nov.[87]	*Bacillus marcerans*
Paenibacillus macquariensis, comb. nov.[87]	*Bacillus macquariensis*
Paenibacillus pabuli, comb. nov.[87]	*Bacillus pabuli*
Paenibacillus peoriae, comb. nov.[91]	*Bacillus peoriae*
Paenibacillus polymyxa, comb. nov.[92]	*Bacillus polymyxa*
Paenibacillus thiaminolyticus, comb. nov.[86]	*Bacillus thiaminolyticus*
Paenibacillus validus, comb. nov.[93]	*Bacillus validus*; *Bacillus gordonae*; *Paenibacillus gordonae*
Pasteuria penetrans	*Bacillus penetrans*
Pediococcus urinaeequi	*Pediococcus urinae equi*
Peptococcus niger	*Peptostreptococcus saccharolyticus*; *Ataphylococcus saccharolyticus*; *Micrococcus niger*
Peptostreptococcus asaccharolyticus	*Peptococcus asaccharolyticus*
Peptostreptococcus harei, sp. nov.[94]	
Peptostreptococcus heliotrinreducens	*Peptococcus heliotrinreducens*
Peptostreptococcus indolicus	*Peptococcus indolicus*
Peptostreptococcus ivorii, sp. nov.[94]	
Peptostreptococcus magnus	*Peptococcus magnus*
Peptostreptococcus micros	*Peptococcus glycinophilus*
Peptostreptococcus octavius, sp. nov.[94]	
Peptostreptococcus prevotii	*Peptococcus prevotii*
Peptostreptococcus tetradius	*Gaffkya anaerobius*; *Micrococcus tetragenus anaerobius*
Propionibacterium acidipropionici	Incorrect name, *Propionibacterium acid-propionici*
Propionibacterium cyclohexanicum, sp. nov.[95]	
Propionibacterium propionicus	*Arachnia propionica*
Propioniferax innocua	*Propionibacterium innocuum*
Pseudonocardia autotrophica	*Nocardia autotrophica*
Pseudonocardia hydrocarbonoxydans	*Nocardia hydrocarbonoxydans*
Pseudonocardia petroleophila	*Nocardia petroleophila*
Pseudonocardia saturnea	*Nocardia saturnea*

Pseudoramibacter, gen. nov.[96]	
Pseudoramibacter alactolyticus, comb. nov.[96]	*Eubacterium alactolyticum*
Rathayibacter iranicus	*Corynebacterium iranicum*
Rathayibacter rathayi	*Corynebacterium rathayi*
Rathayibacter tritici	*Corynebacterium tritici*
Rhodococcus equi	*Corynebacterium equi*; *Nocardia restricta*
Rhodococcus erythropolis	*Arthrobacter picolinophilus*; *Nocardia calcarea*
Rhodococcus fascians	*Corynebacterium fascians*; *Rhodococcus luteus*; *Mycobacterium luteum*
Rhodococcus opacus, sp. nov.[97]	
Rhodococcus percolatus, sp. nov.[98]	
Rhodococcus rhodochrous	*Rhodococcus roseus*; *Bacterium rosea*
Rothia dentocariosa	CDC group 4, Rothia-like organism
Rubrobacter radiotolerans	*Arthrobacter radiotolerans*
Rubrobacter xylananophilus, sp. nov.[99]	
Ruminococcus productus	*Peptostreptococcus productus*
Ruminococcus hansenii	*Streptococcus hansenii*
Saccharothrix aerocolonigenes	*Nocardia aerocolonigenes*
Saccharothrix mutabilis subsp. *capreolus*	*Nocardia capreola*
Skermania piniformis	*Nocardia pinensis*
Sporohalobacter lortetii	*Clostridium lortetii*
Staphylococcus aureus subsp. *aureus*	*Staphylococcus aureus*
Staphylococcus capitis subsp. *capitis*	*Staphylococcus capitis*
Staphylococcus epidermidis	*Staphylococcus albus*
Staphylococcus chonii subsp. *cohnii*	*Staphylococcus chonii*
Staphylococcus chromogens	*Staphylococcus hyicus* subsp. *chromogenes*
Staphylococcus lentus	*Staphylococcus sciuri* subsp. *lentus*
Staphylococcus lutrae, sp. nov.[100]	
Staphylococcus pulvereri, sp. nov.[101]	
Staphylococcus saccharolyticus	*Peptococcus saccharolyticus*
Staphylococcus saprophyticus subsp. *bovis*, subsp. nov.[102]	
Staphylococcus saprophyticus subsp. *saprophyticus*	*Staphylococcus saprophyticus*
Staphylococcus schleiferi subsp. *schleiferi*	*Staphylococcus schleiferi*
Staphylococcus sciuri subsp. *carnaticus*, subsp. nov.[103]	
Staphylococcus sciuri subsp. *rodentium*, subsp. nov.[103]	
Staphylococcus sciuri subsp. *sciuri*, subsp. nov.[103]	
Stomatococcus mucilaginosus	*Micrococcus mucilaginous*; *Staphylococcus mucilaginous*
Streptococcus anginosus	"*Streptococcus milleri*"; *Streptococcus constellatus*; *Streptococcus intermedius*
Streptococcus cristatus	Incorrect name, *Streptococcus crista*
Streptococcus difficile, sp. nov.[104]	
Streptococcus downei	*Streptococcus mutans* serotype h

Streptococcus dysgalactiae subsp. *dysgalactiae*	*Streptococcus dysgalactiae*; Lancefield groups C G L
Streptococcus dysgalactiae subsp. *equisimilis*, subsp. nov.[105]	
Streptococcus equi subsp. *zooepidemicus*	*Streptococcus zooepidemicus*
Streptococcus ferus	*Streptococcus mutans* subsp. *ferus*
Streptococcus gallolyticus, sp. nov.[106]	*Streptococcus caprinus*
Streptococcus hyovaginalis, sp. nov.[107]	
Streptococcus iniae	*Streptococcus shiloi*
Streptococcus intermedius	*Streptococcus anginosus*
Streptococcus parasanguinis	Incorrect name, *Streptococcus parasanguis*
Streptococcus pneumoniae	*Diplococcus pneumoniae*
Streptococcus ratti	Incorect name, *Streptococcus rattus*
Streptococcus sanguinis	Incorrect name, *Streptococcus sanguis*
Streptococcus sobrinus	*Streptococcus mutans*subsp. *sobrinus*
Streptococcus thermophilus	*Streptococcus salivarius* subsp. *thermophilus*, revived name
Streptococcus thoraltensis, sp. nov.	
Streptomyces asterosporus	*Actinomyces asterosporus*
Streptomyces atrovirens	*Actinomyces atrovirens*
Streptomyces aureorectus	*Actinomyces aureorectus*
Streptomyces candidus	*Actinomyces candidus*
Streptomyces caniferus	*Actinomyces caniferus*
Streptococcus cristatus	Incorrect name, *Streptococcus crista*
Streptomyces enissocaesilis	*Actinomyces enissocaesilis*
Streptomyces flavofungini	*Actinomyces flavofungini*
Streptomyces flavovariabilis	*Actinomyces flavovariabilis*
Streptomyces flavoviridis	*Actinomyces flavoviridis*
Streptococcus gallolyticus	*Streptococcus caprinus*
Streptomyces glaucosporus	*Actinomyces glaucosporus*
Streptomyces glaucus	*Actinomyces glaucus*
Streptomyces heliomycini	*Actinomyces flavochromogenes* subsp. *heliomycini*
Streptomyces malachitospinus	*Actinomyces malachitospinus*
Streptomyces megasporus	*Actinomyces megasporus*
Streptomyces rectiviolaceus	*Actinomyces rectiviolaceus*
Streptomyces rubrogriseus	*Actinomyces rubrogriseus*
Streptomyces sporocinereus	*Actinomyces sporocinereus*
Streptomyces sporoclivatus	*Actinomyces sporoclivatus*
Streptomyces spororaveus	*Actinomyces spororaveus*
Streptomyces sporoverrucosus	*Actinomyces sporoverrucosus*
Streptomyces tauricus	*Actinomyces tauricus*
Streptomyces viridobrunneus	*Actinomyces viridobrunneus*
Streptomyces wedmorensis	*Actinomyces wedmorensis*
Syntrophospora bryantii	*Clostridium bryantii*
Terrabacter tumescens	*Arthrobacter tumescens*; *Pimelobacter tumescens*
Tetragenococcus halophilus	*Enterococcus solitaris*; *Pediococcus halophilus*
Thermoanaerobacter thermocopriae	*Clostridium thermocopriae*
Thermoanaerobacter thermohydrosulfuricus	*Clostridium thermohydrosulfuricum*

Thermoanaerobacterium thermosaccharolyticum	Clostridium thermosaccharolyticum
Thermoanaerobacterium thermosulfurigenes	Clostridium thermosulfurogenes
Tsukamurella inchonensis, sp. nov.[108]	
Tsukamurella paurometabolum	Corynebacterium paurometabolum; Rhodococcus aurantiacus
Tsukamurella pulmonis, sp. nov.[109]	
Tsukamurella tyrosinosolvens, sp. nov.[110]	
Tsukamurella wratislaviensis, sp. nov.[111]	
Vagococcus salmoninarum	Carnobacterium divergens; Carnobacterium piscicola; Carnobacterium gallinorum; Carnobacterium mobile
Weissella confusa	Lactobacillus confusus
Weissella halotolerans	Lactobacillus halotolerans; Lactobacillus viridescens subsp. halotolerans
Weissella kandleri	Lactobacillus kandleri
Weissella minor	Lactobacillus minor; Lactobacillus viridescens subsp. minor
Weissella paramesenteroides	Leuconostoc paramesenteroides
Weissella viridescens	Lactobacillus viridescens
Xanthobacter tagetidis, sp. nov.[112]	

(*Note:* In 2000, the *International Journal of Systematic Bacteriology* (IJSB) will become the *International Journal of Systematic and Evolutionary Microbiology* (IJSEM).)

REFERENCES

[1] Kawamura Y, Hou XG, Sultana F, et al. Transfer of *Streptococcus adjacens* and *Streptococcus defectivus* to *Abiotrophia* gen. nov. as *Abiotrophia afiacens* comb. nov. and *Abiotrophia defectiva* comb. nov., respectively. Int J Syst Bacteriol 1995;45(4):798–803.

[2] Kotsyurbenko OR, Simankova MV, Nozhevnikova AN, et al. Validation list no. 60. Int J Syst Bacteriol 1997;47(2):242.

[3] Lawson PA, Falsen E, Akervall E, et al. Characterization of some *Actinomyces*-like isolates from human clinical specimens: Reclassification of *Actinomyces suis* (Soltys and Spratling) as *Actinobaculum suis* comb. nov. and description of *Actinobaculum schaalii* sp. nov. Int J Syst Bacteriol 1997;47(3):899–903.

[4] Funke G, Alvarez N, Pascual C, et al. *Actinomyces europaeus* sp. nov., isolated from human clinical specimens. Int J Syst Bacteriol 1997;47(3):687–692.

[5] Johnson JL, Moore LVH, Kaneko B, Moore WEC. *Actinomyces georgiae* sp. nov., *Actinomyces gerencseriae* sp. nov., designation of two genospecies of *Actinomyces naeslundii*, and inclusion of *A. naeslundii* serotypes II and III and *Actinomyces viscosus* serotype II in *A. naeslundii* genospecies 2. Int J Syst Bacteriol 1990;40(3):273–286.

[6] Ramos CP, Falsen E, Alvarez N, et al. *Actinomyces graevenitzii* sp. nov., isolated from human clinical specimens. Int J Syst Bacteriol 1997;47(3):885–888.

[7] Wüst J, Stubbs S, Weiss N, et al. Validation list no. 54. Int J Syst Bacteriol 1995;45(3):619–620.

[8] Christensen JJ, Whitney AM, Teixeira LM, et al. *Aerococcus urinae*: Intraspecies genetic and phenotypic relatedness. Int J Syst Bacteriol 1997;47(1):28–32.

[9] Labeda DP. *Amycolatopsis coloradensis* sp. nov., the avoparcin (LL-AV290)-producing strain. Int J Syst Bacteriol 1995;45(1):124–127.

[10] Goodfellow M, Brown AB, Cai J, et al. Validation list no. 62. Int J Syst Bacteriol 1997;47(4):915–916.

[11] Shida O, Takagi H, Kadowaki K, Komagata K. Proposal for two new genera, *Brevibacillus* gen. nov. and *Aneurinibacillus* gen. nov. Int J Syst Bacteriol 1996;46(4):939–946.

[12] Heyndrickx M, Lebbe L, Vancanneyt M, et al. A polyphasic reassessment of the genus *Aneurinibacillus*, reclassification of *Bacillus thermoaerophilus* (Meier-Srauffer et al. 1996) as *Aneurinibacillus thermoaerophiluis* comb. nov., and emended descriptions of *A. aneurinilyticus* corrig., and *A. migulanus*, and *A. thermoaerophilus*. Int J Syst Bacteriol 1997;47(3):808–817.

[13] Ramos CP, Foster G, Collins MD. Phylogenetic analysis of the genus *Actinomyces* based on 16S rRNA gene sequences: Description of *Arcanobacterium phocae* sp. nov., *Arcanobacterium bernardiae* comb. nov., and *Arcanobacterium pyogenes* comb. nov. Int J Syst Bacteriol 1997;47(1):46–53.

[14] Koch C, Schumann P, Stackebrandt E. Reclassification of *Micrococcus agilis* (Ali-Cohen 1889) to the genus *Arthrobacter* as *Arthrobacter agilis* comb.

nov. and emendation of the genus *Arthrobacter*. Int J Syst Bacteriol 1995;45(4):837–839.

[15] Funke G, Hutson RA, Bernard KA, et al. Validation list no. 60. Int J Syst Bacteriol 1997;47(2):242.

[16] Nielsen P, Fritze D, Priest FG. Validation list no. 55. Int J Syst Bacteriol 1995;45(4):879–880.

[17] Fujita T, Shida O, Takagi H, et al. Description of *Bacillus carboniphilus* sp. nov. Int J Syst Bacteriol 1996;46(1):116–118.

[18] Kuroshima KI, Sakane T, Takata R, Yokota A. *Bacillus ehimensis* sp. nov. and *Bacillus chitinolyticus* sp. nov., new chitmolytic members of the genus *Bacillus*. Int J Syst Bacteriol 1996;46(1):76–80.

[19] Lawson PA, Deutsch CE, Collins MD. Validation list no. 59. Int J Syst Bacteriol 1996;46(4):1189–1190.

[20] Fritze D. *Bacillus haloalkaliphilus* sp. nov. Int J Syst Bacteriol 1996;46(1):98–101.

[21] Boone DR, Liu Y, Zhao ZJ, et al. *Bacillus infernus* sp. nov., an Fe (III)- and Mn (IV)-reducing anaerobe from the deep terrestrial subsurface. Int J Syst Bacteriol 1995;45(3):441–448.

[22] Kuhnigk T, Borst EM, Breunig A, et al. Validation list no. 57. Int J Syst Bacteriol 1996;46(2):625–626.

[23] Garabito MJ, Arahal DR, Mellado E, et al. *Bacillus salexigens* sp. nov., as new moderately halophilic *Bacillus* species. Int J Syst Bacteriol 1997;47(3):735–741.

[24] Pettersson B, Lembe F, Hammer P, et al. *Bacillus sporothermodurans*, a new species producing highly heat-resistant endospores. Int J Syst Bacteriol 1996;46(3):759–764.

[25] Combet-Blanc Y, Ollivier B, Streicher C, et al. *Bacillus thermoamylovorans* sp. nov., a moderately thermophilic and amylolytic bacterium. Int J Syst Bacteriol 1995;45(1):9–16.

[26] Andersson M, Laukkanen M, Nurmiaho-Lassila EL, et al. Validation list no. 56. Int J Syst Bacteriol 1996;46(2):362–363.

[27] Roberts MS, Nakamura LK, Cohan FM. *Bacillus vallismortis* sp. nov., a close relative of *Bacillus subtilis*, isolated from soil in Death Valley, California. Int J Syst Bacteriol 1996;46(2):470–475.

[28] Agnew MD, Koval SF, Jarrell KF. Validation list no. 56. Int J Syst Bacteriol 1996;46(2):362–363.

[29] Crociani F, Biavati B, Alessandrini A, et al. *Bifidobacterium inopinatum* sp. nov. and *Bifidobacterium denticolens* sp. nov., two new species isolated from human dental caries. Int J Syst Bacteriol 1996;46(2):564–571.

[30] Meile L, Ludwig N, Rueger J, et al. Validation list no. 62. Int J Syst Bacteriol 1997;47(4):915–916.

[31] Funke G, Ramis CP, Collins MD. Validation list no. 56. Int J Syst Bacteriol 1996;46(2):362–363.

[32] Örlygsson J, Krooneman J, Collins MD, et al. *Clostridium acetireducens* sp. nov., a novel amino acid-oxidizing, acetate-reducing anaerobic bacterium. Int J Syst Bacteriol 1996;46(2):454–459.

[33] Lawson PA, Dainty RH, Kristiansen N, et al. Validation list no. 52. Int J Syst Bacteriol 1995;45(1):197–198.

[34] Kelly WJ, Asmundson RV, Hopcroft DH. Validation list no. 57. Int J Syst Bacteriol 1996;46(2):625–626.

[35] Montfort DO, Rainey FA, Burghardt J, Stackebrandt E. Validation list no. 57. Int J Syst Bacteriol 1996;46(2):625–626.

[36] Varel VH, Tanner RS, Woese CR. *Clostridium herbivorns* sp. nov., a cellulolytic anaerobe from the pig intestine. Int J Syst Bacteriol 1995;45(3):490–494.

[37] Tholozan JL, Touzel JP, Samain E, et al. Validation list no. 55. Int J Syst Bacteriol 1995;45(4):879–880.

[38] Wilde E, Collins MD, Hippe H. *Clostridium pascui* sp. nov., a new glutamate-fermenting sporeformer from a pasture in Pakistan. Int J Syst Bacteriol 1997;47(1):164–170.

[39] Attwood GT, Reilly K, Patel BK. *Clostridium propteoclasticum* sp. nov., a novel proteolytic bacterium from the bovine rumen. Int J Syst Bacteriol 1996;46(3):753–758.

[40] Svensson BH, Dubourguier HC, Prensier G, Zehnder AJB. Validation list no. 55. Int J Syst Bacteriol 1995;45(4):879–880.

[41] Schnürer A, Schink B, Svensson BH. *Clostridium ultunense* sp. nov., a mesophilic bacterium oxidizing acetate in syntrophic association with a hydrogenotrophic methanogenic bacterium. Int J Syst Bacteriol 1996;46(4):1145–1152.

[42] Mountford DO, Rainey FA, Burghardt J, et al. Validation list no. 62. Int J Syst Bacteriol 1997;47(4):915–916.

[43] Buckel W, Janssen PH, Schuhmann A, et al. Validation list no. 54. Int J Syst Bacteriol 1995;45(3):619–620.

[44] Riegel P, Ruimy R, De Briel D, et al. *Corynebacterium argentoratense* sp. nov., from the human throat. Int J Syst Bacteriol 1995;45(3):533–537.

[45] Funke G, Lawson PA, Collins MD. Heterogeneity within human-derived Centers for Disease Control and Prevention (CDC) coryneform group ANF-1-like bacteria and description of *Corynebacterium auris* sp. nov. Int J Syst Bacteriol 1995;45(4):735–739.

[46] Funke G, Ramos CP, Collins MD. *Corynebacterium coyleae* sp. nov., isolated from human clinical specimens. Int J Syst Bacteriol 1997;47(1):92–96.

[47] Riegel P, Heller R, Prevost G, et al. *Corynebacterium durum* sp. nov., from human clinical specimens. Int J Syst Bacteriol 1997;47(4):1107–1111.

[48] Funke G, Brnard KA, Bucher C, et al. Validation list no. 55. Int J Syst Bacteriol 1995;45(4):879–880.

[49] Funke G, Efstratiou A, Kuklinska D, et al. Validation list no. 63. Int J Syst Bacteriol 1997;47(4):1274.

[50] Funke G, Hutson RA, Hilleringmann M, et al. Validation list no. 63. Int J Syst Bacteriol 1997;47(4):274.

[51] Riegel P, Ruimy R, de Briel D, et al. Genomic diversity and phylogenetic relationships among lipid-requiring diphtheroids from humans and characterization of *Corynebacterium macginleyi* sp. nov. Int J Syst Bacteriol 1995;45(1):128–133.

[52] Fernandez-Garayzabal JF, Collins MD, Hutson RA, et al. *Corynebacterium mastitidis* sp. nov., isolated from milk of sheep with subclinical mastitis. Int J Syst Bacteriol 1997;47(4):1082–1085.

[53] Funke G, Lawson PA, Collins MD. *Corynebacterium mucifaciens* sp. nov., an unusual species from human clinical material. Int J Syst Bacteriol 1997;47(4):952–957.

[54] Riegel P, Ruimy R, De Briel D, et al. Validation list no. 56. Int J Syst Bacteriol 1996;46(2):362–363.

[55] Riegel P, Ruimy R, Renaud FN, et al. *Corynebacterium singulare* sp. nov., a new species for urease-positive strains related to *Corynebacterium minutissimum*. Int J Syst Bacteriol 1997;47(4):1092–1096.

[56] Riegel P, Ruimy R, De Briel D, et al. Validation list no. 54. Int J Syst Bacteriol 1997;45(3):619–620.

[57] Rainey FA, Nobre MF, Schumann P, et al. Phylogenetic diversity of the deinococci as determined by 16S ribosomal DNA sequence comparison. Int J Syst Bacteriol 1997;47(2):510–514.

[58] Ferreira AC, Nobre MF, Rainey FA, et al. *Deinococcus geothermalis* sp. nov. and *Deinococcus murrayi* sp. nov., two extremely radiation-resistant and slightly thermophilic species from hot springs. Int J Syst Bacteriol 1997;47(4):939–947.

[59] Stackebrandt E, Koch C, Gvozdiak O, Schumann P. Taxonomic dissection of the genus *Micrococcus*: *Kocuria* gen. nov., *Nesterenkonia* gen. nov., *Kytococcus* gen. nov., *Dermacoccus* gen. nov., and *Micrococcus* Cohn 1872 gen. emend. Int J Syst Bacteriol 1995;45(4):682–692.

[60] Rainey FA, Klatte S, Kroppenstedt RM, Stackebrandt E. *Dietzia*, a new genus including *Dietzia maris* comb. nov., formerly *Rhodococcus maris*. Int J Syst Bacteriol 1995;45(1):32–36.

[61] Poco SE Jr, Nakazawa F, Ikeda T, et al. *Eubacterium exiguum* sp. nov., isolated from human oral lesions. Int J Syst Bacteriol 1996;46(4):1120–1124.

[62] Cheeseman SL, Hiom SJ, Weightman AJ, Wade WG. Phylogeny of oral asaccharolytic *Eubacterium* species determined by 16S ribosomal DNA sequence comparison and proposal of *Eubacterium infirmum* sp. nov. and *Eubacterium tardum* sp. nov. Int J Syst Bacteriol 1996;46(4):957–959.

[63] Poco SE Jr, Nakazawa F, Sato M, Hoshino E. *Eubacterium minutum* sp. nov., isolated from human periodontal pockets. Int J Syst Bacteriol 1996;46(1):31–34.

[64] Collins MD, Aguirre M, Facklam RR, et al. Validation list no. 53. Int J Syst Bacteriol 1995;45(2):418–419.

[65] Klatte S, Kroppenstedt Rm, Schumann P, et al. *Gordona hirsuta* sp. nov. Int J Syst Bacteriol 1996;46(4):876–880.

[66] Willems A, Moore WE, Weiss N, Collins MD. Phenotypic and phylogenetic characterization of some *Eubacterium*-like isolates containing a novel type B wall murein from human feces: Description of *Holdemania filiformis* gen. nov., sp. nov. Int J Syst Bacteriol 1997;47(4):1201–1204.

[67] Torriani S, Van Reenen GA, Klein G, et al. *Lactobacillus curvatus* subsp. *curvatus* subsp. nov. and *Lactobacillus curvatus* subsp. *melibiosus* subsp. nov. and *Lactobacillus sake* subsp. *sake* subsp. nov. and *Lactobacillus sake* subsp. *carnosus* subsp. nov., new subspecies of *Lactobacillus curvatus* Abo-Elnaga and Kandler 1965 and *Lactobacillus sake* Katagiri, Kitahara, and Fukami 1934 (Klein et al. 1996, emended descriptions), respectively. Int J Syst Bacteriol 1996;46(4):1158–1163.

[68] Back W, Bohak I, Ehrmann M, et al. Validation list no. 61. Int J Syst Bacteriol 1997;47(2):601–602.

[69] Wiese BG, Strohmar W, Rainey FA, Diekmann H. *Lactobacillus panis* sp. nov., from sourdough with a long fermentation period. Int J Syst Bacteriol 1996;46(2):449–463.

[70] Curk MC, Hubert JC, Bringel F. *Lactobacillus paraplantarum* sp. nov., a new species related to *Lactobacillus plantarum*. Int J Syst Bacteriol 1996;46(2):595–598.

[71] Dicks LMT, Du Plessis EM, Dellaglio F, Lauer E. Reclassification of *Lactobacillus casei* subsp. *casei* ATCC 393 and *Lactobacillus rhamnosus* ATCC 15820 as *Lactobacillus zeae* nom. rev., designation of ATCC 334 as the neotype of *L. casei* subsp. *casei*, and rejection of the name *Lactobacillus paracasei*. Int J Syst Bacteriol 1996;46(1):337–340.

[72] Janssen PH, Evers S, Rainey FA, et al. *Lactosphaera* gen. nov., a new genus of lactic acid bacteria, and transfer of *Ruminococcus pasteurii* Schink 1984 to *Lactosphaera pasteurii* comb. nov. Int J Syst Bacteriol 1995;45(3):565–571.

[73] Takeuchi M, Weiss N, Schumann P, Yokota A. *Leucobacter komagatae* gen. nov., sp. nov., a new aerobic Gram-positive, nonsporulating rod with 2,4-diaminobutyric acid in the cell wall. Int J Syst Bacteriol 1996;46(4):967–971.

[74] Koukila-Kähkölä P, Springer B, Böttger EC, et al. *Mycobacterium branderi* sp. nov., a new potential human pathogen. Int J Syst Bacteriol 1995;45(3):549–553.

[75] Springer B, Tortoli E, Richtek I, et al. Validation list no. 56. Int J Syst Bacteriol 1996;46(2):362–363.

[76] Schröder KH, Naumann L, Kroppenstedt RM, Reisch U. *Mycobacterium hassiacum* sp. nov., a rapidly growing thermophilic mycobacterium. Int J Syst Bacteriol 1997;47(1):86–91.

[77] Kleespies M, Kroppenstedt RM, Rainey FA, et al. *Mycobacterium hodleri* sp. nov., a new member of the fast-growing mycobacteria capable of degrading polycyclic aromatic hydrocarbons. Int J Syst Bacteriol 1996;46(3):683–687.

[78] Springer B, Kirschner P, Rost-Meyer G, et al. Validation list no. 52. Int J Syst Bacteriol 1995;45(1):197–198.

[79] Springer B, Wu WK, Bodmer T, et al. Validation list no. 58. Int J Syst Bacteriol 1996;46(3):836–837.

[80] Domenech P, Jimenez MS, Menendez MC, et al. *Mycobacterium mageritense* sp. nov. Int J Syst Bacteriol 1997;47(2):535–540.

[81] Springer B, Bottger EC, Kirschner P, Wallace RJ Jr. Phylogeny of the *Mycobacterium chelonae*-like organism based on partial sequencing of the 16S rRNA gene and proposal of *Mycobacterium mucogenicum* sp. nov. Int J Syst Bacteriol 1995;45(2):262–267.

[82] Shojaei H, Goodfellow M, Magee JG, et al. *Mycobacterium novocastrense* sp. nov., a rapidly growing photochromogenic mycobacterium. Int J Syst Bacteriol 1997;47(4):1205–1207.

[83] Floyd MM, Guthertz LS, Silcox VA, et al. Validation list no. 61. Int J Syst Bacteriol 1997;47(2):601–602.

[84] Ruimy R, Riegel P, Carlotti A, et al. *Nocardia pseudobrasiliensis* sp. nov., a new species of *Nocardia* which groups bacterial strains previously identified as *Nocardia brasiliensis* and associated with invasive diseases. Int J Syst Bacteriol 1996;46(1):259–264.

[85] Dicks LMT, Dellaglio F, Collins MD. Proposal to reclassify *Leuconostoc oenos* as *Oenococcus oeni* [corrig] gen. nov., comb. nov. Int J Syst Bacteriol 1995;45(2):395–397.

[86] Shida O, Takagi H, Kadowaki K, et al. Transfer of *Bacillus alginolyticus, Bacillus chondroitinus, Bacillus curdlanolyticus, Bacillus glucanolyticus, Bacillus kobensis,* and *Bacillus thiaminolyticus* to the genus *Paenibacillus* and emended description of the genus *Paenibacillus.* Int J Syst Bacteriol 1997;47(2):289–298.

[87] Ash C, Priest FG, Collins MD. Validation list no. 52. Int J Syst Bacteriol 1995;45(1):197–198.

[88] Nakamura LK. *Paenibacillus apiarius* sp. nov. Int J Syst Bacteriol 1996;46(3):688–693.

[89] Shida O, Takagi H, Kadowaki K, et al. Emended description of *Paenibacillus amylolyticus* and description of *Paenibacillus illinoisensis* sp. nov. and *Paenibacillus chibensis* sp. nov. Int J Syst Bacteriol 1997;47(2):299–306.

[90] Heyndrickx M, Vandemeulebroecke K, Hoste B, et al. Reclassification of *Paenibacillus* (formerly *Bacillus*) *pulvifaciens* (Nakamura 1984) Ash et al. 1994, a later subjective synonym of *Paenibacillus* (formerly *Bacillus*) *larvae* (White 1906) Ash et al. 1994, as a subspecies of *P. larvae*, with emended descriptions of *P. larvae* as *P. larvae* subsp. *larvae* and *P. larvae* subsp. *pulvifaciens.* Int J Syst Bacteriol 1996;46(1):270–279.

[91] Heyndrickx M, Vandemeulebroecke K, Scheldeman P, et al. A polyphasic reassessment of the genus *Paenibacillus*, reclassification of *Bacillus lautus* (Nakamura 1984) as *Paenibacillus lautus* comb. nov. and of *Bacillus peoriae* (Montefusco et al. 1993) as *Paenibacillus peoriae* comb. nov., and emended description of *P. lautus* and of *P. peoriae.* Int J Syst Bacteriol 1996;46(4):988–1003.

[92] Ash C, Priest FG, Collins MD. Validation list no. 51. Int J Syst Bacteriol 1994;44(4):852.

[93] Heyndrickx M, Vandemeulebroecke K, Scheldeman P, et al. *Paenibacillus* (formerly *Bacillus*) *gordonae* (Pichinoty et al. 1986) Ash et al. 1994 is a later subjective synonym of *Paenibacillus* (formerly *Bacillus*) *validus* (Nakamura 1984) Ash et al. 1994: Emended description of *P. validus.* Int J Syst Bacteriol 1995;45(4):661–669.

[94] Murdoch DA, Collins MD, Willems A, et al. Description of three new species of the genus *Peptostreptococcus* from human clinical specimens: *Peptostreptococcus harei* sp. nov., *Peptostreptococcus ivorii* sp. nov., and *Peptostreptococcus octavius* sp. nov. Int J Syst Bacteriol 1997;47(3):781–787.

[95] Kusano K, Yamada H, Niwa M, Yamasato K. *Propionibacterium cyclohexanicum* sp. nov., a new acid-tolerant omega-cyclohexyl fatty acid-containing propionibacterium isolated from spoiled orange juice. Int J Syst Bacteriol 1997;47(3):825–831.

[96] Willems A, Collins MD. Phylogenetic relationship of the genera *Acetobacterium* and *Eubacterium* sensi stricto and reclassification of *Eubacterium alactolyticum* as *Pseudoramibacter alactolyticus* gen. nov., comb. nov. Int J Syst Bacteriol 1996;46(4):1083–1087.

[97] Klatte S, Kroppenstedt RM, Rainey FA. Validation list no. 52. Int J Syst Bacteriol 1995;45(1):197–198.

[98] Briglia M, Rainey FA, Stackebrandt E, et al. *Rhodococcus percolatus* sp. nov., a bacterium degrading 2,4,6-trichlorophenol. Int J Syst Bacteriol 1996;46(1):23–30.

[99] Carreto L, Moore E, Nobre MF, et al. *Rubrobacter xylanophilus* sp. nov., a new thermophilic species isolated from a thermally polluted effluent. Int J Syst Bacteriol 1996;46(2):460–465.

[100] Foster G, Ross HM, Hutson RA, Collins MD. *Staphylococcus lutrae* sp. nov., a new coagulase-positive species isolated from otters. Int J Syst Bacteriol 1997;47(3):724–726.

[101] Zakrzewska-Czerwinska-Mastalarz A, Lis B, Gamian A, Mordarski M. *Staphylococcus pulvereri* sp. nov., isolated from human and animal specimens. Int J Syst Bacteriol 1995;45(1):169–172.

[102] Hájek V, Meugnier H, Bes M, et al. *Staphylococcus saprophyticus* subsp. *bovis* subsp. nov., isolated from bovine nostrils. Int J Syst Bacteriol 1996;46(3):792–796.

[103] Kloos WE, Ballard DN, Webster JA, et al. Ribotype delineation and description of *Staphylococcus sciuri* subspecies and their potential as reservoirs of methicillin resistance and staphylolytic enzyme genes. Int J Syst Bacteriol 1997;47(2):313–323.

[104] Eldar A, Bejerano Y, Bercovier H. Validation list no. 52. Int J Syst Bacteriol 1995;45(1):197–198.

[105] Vandamme P, Pot B, Falsen E, et al. Taxonomic study of Lancefield streptococcal groups C, G, and L *(Streptococcus dysgalactiae)* and proposal of *S. dysgalactiae* subsp. *equisimilis* subsp. nov. Int J Syst Bacteriol 1997;46(3):774–781.

[106] Osawa R, Fujisawa T, Sly LL. Validation list no. 56. Int J Syst Bacteriol 1996;46(2):362–363.

[107] Devriese LA, Pot B, Vandamme P, et al. *Streptococcus hyovaginalis* sp. nov. and *Streptococcus thoraltensis* sp. nov., from the genital tract of sows. Int J Syst Bacteriol 1997;47(4):1073–1077.

[108] Yassin AF, Rainey FA, Brzezinka H, et al. *Tsukamurella inchonensis* sp. nov. Int J Syst Bacteriol 1995;45(3):522–527.

[109] Yassin AF, Rainey FA, Brzezinka H, et al. *Tsukamurella pulmonis* sp. nov. Int J Syst Bacteriol 1996;46(2):429–436.

[110] Yassin AF, Rainey FA, Burghardt J, et al. *Tsukamurella tyrosinosolvens* sp. nov. Int J Syst Bacteriol 1997;47(3):607–614.

[111] Goodfellow M, Zakrzewska-Czerwinska J, Thomas EG, et al. Validation list no. 53. Int J Syst Bacteriol 1995;45(2):418–419.

[112] Padden AN, Rainey FA, Kelly DP, Wood AP. *Xanthobacter tagetidis* sp. nov., an organism associated with *Tagetes* species and able to grow on substituted thiophenes. Int J Syst Bacteriol 1997;47(2):394–401.

GENUS: *ABIOTROPHIA* (19)
Gram-positive cocci/coccobacilli; long chains in broth media
Nonsporeforming
Facultatively anaerobic
Catalase negative
Nonencapsulated
6.6% NaCl: no growth
10°C: no growth
45°C: no growth
LAP (leucine aminopeptidase) positive
PYR (pyrrolidonylarylamidase) variable
Bile esculin negative
Vancomycin: S (sensitive)
2 species: *S. adjacens, S. defectivus*

Does not grow on blood or chocolate agars unless supplemented with vitamin B_6 (0.001% pyridoxal hydrochloride/thiol) either by an impregnated disk, cross-streaking with staphylococcus, or supplemented culture media (19).

Formerly "nutritionally variant" or "satelliting" streptococci; may satellite around staphylococci colonies on 5% sheep blood agar (BA) or chocolate agar

GENUS: *ACETOBACTERIUM* (26, 30)
Gram-positive ovoid or short rods arranged singly, in pairs, and occasionally **short chains.** Cells are tapered to blunt ends.
Nonsporeforming
Obligate (strict) anaerobes
Catalase negative
Nonencapsulated
Motile by 1 or 2 subterminal flagella
O/F glucose: F (fermentative)
Optimal growth temperature 30°C
7 species: *A. bakii, A. carbinolicum, A. fimetarium, A. malicum, A. paludosum, A. wieringae, A. woodii*
Type species: *A. woodii* ATCC 29683
Resemble streptococci; β-hemolytic

GENUS: *ACTINOMYCES* (26, 40)
Gram-positive rods that often stain irregularly and rise to a beaded appearance. Slender, straight or slightly curved rods and filaments with **true branching**, but no conidia. Rods often have clubbed ends. Arranged singly and in pairs; V and Y arrangements and palisades.
Nonsporeforming
Facultative anaerobes; require CO_2 for maximum growth aerobically or anaerobically. Some species grow poorly in air even with CO_2.
Catalase variable
Nonencapsulated
Nonmotile
O/F glucose: F (fermentative)
Nitrate reduction variable
Indole negative
CAMP positive: *A. neuii* subsp. *anitratus* and *A. neuii* subsp. *neuii*
Optimal growth temperature 35–37°C
Not acid-fast
20 species: *A. bovis, A. denticolens, A. europaeus, A. georgia, A. gerencseriae, A. gravenitzii,*

A. hordeovulneris, A. howellii, A. humiferus, A. hyovaginalis, A. israelii, A. meyeri, A. naeslundii, A. neuii subsp. anitratus, A. neuii subsp. neuii, A. odontolyticus, A. radingae, A. slackii, A. turicensis, A. viscosus

Type species: A. bovis ATCC 13683
Species best differentiated by protein gel electrophoresis

Table 43.1. Differential Characteristics of the Most Frequently Isolated *Actinomyces* spp. (33)

Test	A. israelii	A. meyeri	A. naeslundii	A. neuii subsp. anitratus	A. neuii subsp. neuii	A. odontolyticus	A. viscosus
Catalase	−	−	V	+	+	−	+
NO$_3$→NO$_2$	V	−	+	−	+	+	V$^+$
Pink-red pigmentation (BA)	−	−	−	NR	NR	V^{+a}	−
H$_2$S (TSI)	+	−	+	NR	NR	+	+
CAMP	−	NR	−	+	+	−	−
Esculin hydrolysis	+	−	+	NR	NR	V	V
Urease	−	V	+	NR	NR	−	V
Glucose	A	NR	A	A	A	A	A
Maltose	A	NR	A	A	A	V	A
Mannitol	V	−	V	A	A	−	−
Sucrose	A	NR	A	A	A	A	A
Xylose	A	A	V	A	A	V	V

V, variable reaction; V$^+$, variable, usually positive, NR, no results; A, acid production (+) BA, blood agar.
^{a} If positive, may take 7–10 days; exposure to oxygen enhances pigment production.

GENUS: *AEROCOCCUS* (26, 33, 40)

Gram-positive cocci arranged singly or in pairs; large clusters or characteristic **tetrads in liquid media** (thioglycolate)

Microaerophilic to facultatively anaerobic; best growth at reduced oxygen tension. Poor growth anaerobically (may be slow)

Nonsporeforming

Catalase negative or weak (pseudocatalase reaction) due to nonheme catalase (32)

Nonencapsulated

Nonmotile

Oxidase negative

Nitrate reduction negative

O/F glucose: F (fermentative)

Optimal growth temperature 30°C

Resemble enterococci

Alpha (α) hemolysis on 5% sheep blood agar (SBA)

2 species

Type species: A. viridans ATCC 11563, NCTC 8251

Table 43.2. Differentiation of *Aerococcus* spp.

Test	A. urinae	A. viridans
Catalase	+	−
Growth at 10°C	NG	NG
Growth at 45°C	NG	NG
6.5% NaCl	G	G
40% bile	NR	G
Mannitol	NR	A
Arginine	NR	−
Bile esculin hydrolysis	V	V
Gelatin liquefaction, 22°C	NR	−
Hippurate hydrolysis	NR	+
Voges-Proskauer (VP)	NR	−
LAP	+	−
PYR	−	+
Vancomycin (30 μg)	S	S

G, growth; NG, no growth, A, acid production (+); V, variable reactions; S, sensitive (susceptible); LAP, leucine aminopeptidase; PYR, pyrrolidonylarylamidase.

GENUS: *ALLOIOCOCCUS* (19)
Gram-positive large cocci arranged in pairs and tetrads
Nonsporeforming
Obligate (strict) aerobe; no growth anaerobically
Catalase positive but weak; catalase negative only when cultivated on media devoid of whole blood (e.g., chocolate agar)
Nonencapsulated
Oxidase negative
6.5% NaCl: growth; may take 2–7 days
10°C: no growth
45°C: no growth
LAP (leucine aminopeptidase) positive
PYR (pyrrolidonylarylamidase) positive
Bile esculin negative
Hippurate positive
Vancomycin: S (sensitive)
1 species: *A. otitidis* (formerly *A. otitis*)
Type species: DSM 7252, NCFB 2890
Resemble viridans streptococci

GENUS: *AMYCOLATOPSIS* (26, 40)
Gram-positive rods; aerial hyphae; branching hyphae; long chains
Nonsporeforming
Facultative anaerobes
Catalase positive
12 species: *A. alba, A. azurea, A. coloradensis, A. fastidiosa, A. japonica, A. mediterranei, A. methanolica, A. orientalis, A. orientalis* subsp. *lurida, A. orientalis* subsp. *orientalis, A. rugosa, A. sulphurea*
Type species: *A. orientalis* ATCC 19795

GENUS: *ARACHNIA* (26, 33, 40)
One species: *A. propionica*; transferred to genus *Propionibacterium* as *Propionibacterium propionicus* (5) and genus *Arachnia* now eliminated.
See *Propionibacterium* species for biochemical results

GENUS: *ARCANOBACTERIUM* (26, 33, 40)

Gram-positive slender, irregular rods; may show clubbed ends. Stain unevenly after 48 hrs. Occasionally arranged in **V formation**; no filaments. Occasional rudimentary branching that is more pronounced when cultured anaerobically (19). Older cultures exhibit short, irregular rods and cocci. Difficult to distinguish from *Corynebacterium* spp.

Nonsporeforming
Facultative anaerobe; anaerobic growth better than aerobic
Catalase Variable, usually negative; some strains exhibit weak activity
Nonencapsulated
Nonmotile
Nitrate reduction: most strains usually positive
O/F glucose: F (fermentative)
Optimal growth temperature 37°C
Not acid-fast
Delayed β-hemolysis on sheep and rabbit blood agars; resemble streptococci
4 species: *A. bernardiae, A. haemolyticum, A. phocae, A. pyogenes*
Type species: *A. haemolyticum* ATCC 9345, NCTC 8452

Table 43.3. Biochemical Characteristics of Three *Arcanobacterium* Species

Test	*A. haemolyticum*	*A. pyogenes*	*A. bernardiae*
Hemolysis, 5% SBA[a]	β	β[b]	γ
Reverse CAMP	+	−	−
Pigmentation	−	−	−
H_2S (KIA/TSI)	−	−	−
Glucose	A	A	A
Maltose	A	V	A
Mannitol	−	V	−
Sucrose	V	V	−
Xylose	−	A	−
Gelatin liquefaction	−[c]	+[c]	NR
Indole	−	−	−
Urease	−	−	−
Phospholipase D		NR	NR
Pyrazinamidase	+	NR	NR

V, variable reaction; v+, variable, usually positive; A, acid production (+); β, beta hemolysis; γ, gamma (no) hemolysis.
Data from references 19, 33.
[a]β-Hemolysis stronger on agar that contains human or rabbit blood (19).
[b]May exhibit β-hemolysis on brain-heart infusion agar with human blood (19).
[c]After 48 h.

GENUS: *ARTHROBACTER* (26, 33, 40)

Gram-positive easily decolorized rods; young culture has irregular rods, often **V shaped with clubbed ends;** no filaments. As growth proceeds (after 72 h), cells appear as small cocci arranged singly or in pairs or irregular clumps. In the stationary phase almost all cells are coccoid; typical coryneform.

Nonsporeforming
Aerobic
Catalase positive
Nonencapsulated
Motility variable, usually negative; some rod species are motile (19)
Nitrate reduction variable
O/F glucose: O (oxidative)
Optimal growth temperature 25–30°C

DNase positive
Esculin variable
CAMP negative
Gelatin liquefaction, 22°C positive
Not acid-fast
Lacks mycolic acid in cells
24 species: A. agilis, A. atrocyaneus, A. aurescens, A. citreus, A. crystallopoietes, A. cumminsii, A. duodecadis, A. globiformis, A. histidinolovorans, A. ilicis, A. mysorens, A. nicotianae, A. nicotinovorans, A. oxydans, A. pascens, A. polychromogenes, A. protophormiae, A. ramosus, A. siderocapsulatus, A. sulfureus, A. uratoxydans, A. ureafaciens, A. viscosus, A. woluwensis
Type species: A. globiformis ATCC 8010

GENUS: *AUREOBACTERIUM* (19, 26, 40)
Gram-positive, irregular, short rods arranged singly and in pairs. Many cells arranged in V formation
Nonsporeforming
Aerobic
Catalase positive
Nonencapsulated
Motility variable
O/F glucose: O (oxidative); slow and weak
Optimal growth temperature 25–30°C
Nitrate reduction variable
CAMP negative
Esculin variable
Gelatin liquefaction, 22°C variable
Urease negative
Not acid-fast
Mycolic acid absent in cells
13 species: A. arabinogalactanolyticum, A. barkeri, A. esteraromaticum, A. flavescens, A. keratanolyticum, A. liquefaciens, A. luteolum, A. saperdae, A. schleiferi, A. terrae, A. terregens, A. testaceum, A. trichothecenolyticum
Type species: A. liquefaciens ATCC 43647

Table 43.4. Differentiation of Some *Aureobacterium* Species

Test	A. barberi	A. flavescens	A. liquefaciens	A. saperdae	A. terregens	A. testaceum
Motility	+	−	−	+	−	+
Gelatin liquefaction	NR	+	+	−	−	+
Tellurite (0.05% w/v reduced)	+	NR	−	−	NR	+

NR, no test results.

GENUS: *BACILLUS* (19, 26, 32, 40)
Gram-positive or Gram-variable rods with rounded or square ends, arranged in pairs or chains. Some species are Gram positive **only** in young cultures.

Endospores; oval or occasionally round or cylindrical. **only one** spore per cell and sporulation is **not** repressed by exposure to air. Heat resistant. Aerobic to facultatively anaerobic; some species are strict (obligate) aerobes (e.g., B. brevis, B. firmus, B. megaterium, B. sphaericus, and B. subtilis (33).

Catalase variable, usually positive; a few species are negative, but are seldom seen in a clinical laboratory

Encapsulated; *B. anthracis* **only**

Motility usually positive **except** *B. anthracis* and *B. mycoides*; flagella peritrichous. Motility depends on growth medium (40).

Nitrate reduction variable

Oxidase variable

O/F glucose: F (fermentative) or O (oxidative) or both (F/O)

Optimal growth temperature 35°C; exception: *B. stearothermophilus* no growth at 35°C, growth at 65°C. Capsule of *B. anthracis* destroyed at 42–43°C making organism avirulent.

75 species: *B. agaradhaerens, B. alcalophilus, B. amyloliquefaciens, B. anthracis, B. atrophaeus, B. azotoformans, B. badius, B. benzoevorans, B. carboniphilus, B. cereus, B. chitinolyticus, B. circulans, B. clarkii, B. clausii, B. coagulans, B. cohnii, B. edaphicus, B. ehimensis, B. fastidiosus, B. firmus, B. flexus, B. fusiformis, B. gibsonii, B. globisporus, B. halmapalus, B. haloalkaliphilus, B. halodenitrificans, B. halodurans, B. halophilus, B. horikoshii, B. horti, B. infernus, B. insolitus, B. kaustophilus, B. laevolacticus, B. lentus, B. licheniformis, B. marinus, B. marismortui, B. megaterium, B. methanolicus, B. mojavensis, B. mucilaginosus, B. mycoides, B. naganoensis, B. niacini, B. oleronius, B. pallidus, B. pasteuri, B. pseudalcaliphilus, B. pseudofirmus, B. pseudomycoides, B. psychrophilus, B. psychrosaccharolyticus, B. pumilus, B. schlegelii, B. silvestris, B. simplex, B. smithii, B. sphaericus, B. sporothermodurans, B. stearothermophilus, B. subtilis* subsp. *spizizenii, B. subtilis* subsp. *subtilis, B. thermoamylovorans, B. thermocatenulatus, B. thermocloacae, B. thermoglucosidasius, B. thermoleovorans, B. thermosphaericus, B. thuringiensis, B. tusciae, B. vallismortis, B. vedderi, B. weihenstephanensis*

Type species: *B. subtilis* subsp. *subtilis* ATTC 6051, CCM 2216, NCIB 3610

Catalase production and aerobic endospore formation distinguishes *Bacillus* spp. from *Clostridium* spp. (33).

At the present time, no commercial identification systems are available for routine use in the clinical laboratory (19).

Table 43.5. Differential Characteristics of the Most frequently Isolated *Bacillus* spp.[a]

Test	B. anthracis[b]	B. cereus[c]	B. circulans	B. coagulans	B. firmus[d]	B. licheniformis	B. megaterium	B. pumilis	B. sphaericus[d]	B. stearothermophilus[e]	B. subtilis subsp. subtilis
Gram, stain reaction	+	+	V	+	+	+	+	+	V	V	+
Catalase[f]	+	+	+	+	+	+	+	+	+	+	V
Nitrate reduction	+	+	V+	V	V	+	V	–	–	–	V+
Spores[g]											
Ellipsoidal	+	+	+	+	+	+	+	+	–	+	+
Spherical	–	–	–	–	–	–	–	–	+	–	–
Central	–	+	V	V	V	+	+	+	–	–	+
Terminal or subterminal	+	–	V	V	V	–	–	–	+	+	–
Swelling of sporangia	–	–	+	V	–	–	–	–	+	+	–
β-hemolysis, 5% SBA	–	V+h	–	V	–	+	–	V	–	–	V
Capsule	+[i]	–	+	–	–	–	NR	–	NR	NR	–
Motility	–	V+	V+	+	V+	+	+[k]	+	+	+	+
OF glucose	F	F	F/O	F	O	F	O	O	O	F/O	F
Growth											
Anaerobic	G	G	V	G	NG	G	NG	NG	NG	NG	NG
7.5% NaCl	G	G	V	NG	G	G	G	G	V	NG	G
Carbohydrates											
Glucose	A	A	A	A	A	A	A	A	–	A	A
Arabinose	–	–	–	V	V	A	V+	A	–	V	A
Mannitol	–	–	–	V	A	A	V+	A	–	V	A
Xylose	–	–	V	V	V	A	V+	A	–	V	A

Misc. tests									
Gelatin liquefaction, 22°C	+[l]	+	+	−	+	+[l]	+[m]	V	+[l]
Indole	−	−	−	−	−	−	−	−	−
Lecithinase	+[n]	+	−[n]	−	−	−[n]	−[n]	−	−
Phenylalanine deaminase	−	−	−	−	+	−	V	+	−
Simmons citrate	V	+	−	−	−	+	+	−	+
Starch hydrolysis	+	+	+	+	+	+	+	−	+
Urease	V	V	−	−	−	V	V	V	V
Voges-Proskauer[o]	+	+	−	−	−	+	−	−	+

V, Variable; V[+], variable, usually positive; G, growth; NG, no growth; +[w], weakly positive; SBA, sheep blood agar.

Data from references 26, 36, 40.

[a]Generally it is **not** necessary to identify species, except for *B. anthracis*, causative agent of anthrax, and *B. cereus* and *B. licheniformis*, causative agents of food poisoning. A few other species listed here may be implicated in food poisoning and in human infections.

[b]Virulent and **a**virulent strains.

[c]*B. cereus* and *B. cereus* var. *mycoides*. *B. cereus* is frequently β-lactamase positive (19).

[d]Strict aerobe. *Bacillus* spp. that are strict aerobes **may** appear as nonfermentative Gram-negative bacilli on Kligler's iron agar (KIA) or triple sugar iron agar (TSI).

[e]*B. stearothermophilus* **no growth** at 35°C; growth at 65°C.

[f]Catalase usually positive; exceptions exist but are **not** likely to be seen in clinical specimen isolates.

[g]One endospore per mother cell (sporangium) in the presence of oxygen.

[h]On 5% sheep blood agar (SBA), *B. cereus* positive β-hemolysis; *B. cereus* var. *mycoides* is variable, usually positive.

[i]Virulent *B. anthracis* has a capsule; **a**virulent *B. anthracis*, no capsule. Capsule is formed under appropriate conditions (with HCO$_3$ and anaerobic or CO$_2$). Capsule is visible when stained with a polychrome methylene blue (MI Fadyean) stain.

[j]*B. cereus* is motile; *B. cereus* var. *mycoides* is usually nonmotile; motility depends on growth medium used.

[k]*B. megaterium* requires free aeration for a **slow** positive motility.

[l]Slow.

[m]Rapid.

[n]A weak positive lecithinase reaction, visible only beneath colony when growth is scraped away.

[o]Incubate an additional 24 h at 37°C.

GENUS: *BIFIDOBACTERIUM* (26)

Gram-positive rods that often stain irregularly; varied shapes; somewhat curved and clubbed; often branched. Arranged singly, in pairs, and V arrangement. At times appear as **chains in palisades of parallel cells or rosettes.** Often swollen coccoid forms

Nonsporeforming

Anaerobic; few species can grow in air with 10% CO_2 (26)

Catalase negative; rare positive reaction when grown in air with CO_2 (19, 26)

Nonencapsulated

Nonmotile

O/F glucose: F (fermentative)

Optimal growth temperature 37–41°C

Not acid-fast

Nitrate reduction negative; however, cells grown in the presence of lysed red cells may be capable of nitrate reduction (33)

Urease: usually positive

Usually nonpathogenic

Closely related to *Lactobacillaceae*

32 species: *B. adolescentis, B. angulatum, B. animalis, B. asteroides, B. bifidum, B. boum, B. breve, B. catenulatum, B. choerinum, B. coryneforme, B. cuniculi, B. denticolens, B. dentium, B. gallicum, B. gallinarum, B. indicum, B. infantis, B. inopinatum, B. lactis, B. longum, B. magnum, B. merycicum, B. minimum, B. pseudocatenulatum, B. pseudolongum* subsp. *globosum, B. pseudolongum* subsp. *pseudolongum, B. pullorum, B. ruminantium, B. saeculare, B. subitile, B. suis, B. thermophilum*

Type species: *B. bifidum* ATCC 29521, DSM 20456

Require specialized techniques for strict anaerobiosis and metabolic studies.

Identification unreliable unless special procedures are used; most direct and reliable characteristic is demonstration of F6PPK in cellular extracts.

GENUS: *BREVIBACILLUS* (19)

Gram-positive rods

Sporeforming; spores swell sporangia

Aerobic

Glucose negative

Mannitol: acid (+)

Xylose negative

Citrate variable

Indole negative

Lecithinase negative

Voges-Proskauer (VP) negative

10 species: *B. agri, B. borstelenis, B. brevis, B. centrosporus, B. choshinensis, B. formosus, B. laterosporus, B. parabrevis, B. reuszeri, B. thermoruber*

Type species: *B. brevis* ATCC 8246, NCIB 9372, NCTC 2611

GENUS: *BREVIBACTERIUM* (26, 33, 40)

Gram-positive irregular rods that are easily decolorized. Arranged singly, in pairs, and often **V formations.** Mycelium **not** formed. Older cultures appear coccoid.

Nonsporeforming

Obligate (strict) aerobes

Catalase positive

Nonencapsulated

Nonmotile

Oxidase variable

O/F glucose: O (oxidative) or inert (−)

Optimal growth temperature: B. casei and B. epidermidis 20–37°C; B. linens and B. iodinum 20–30°C (21)

Not acid-fast

No mycolic acid in cells

CAMP negative

All strains proteolytic

10 species: B. casei, B. epidermidis, B. frigoritolerans, B. halotolerans, B. iodinum, B. linens, B. liquefaciens, B. mcbrellneri, B. otitidis, B. stationis

Type species: B. linens ATCC 9172, ATCC 14929

Table 43.6. Differentiation of the Most Frequently Isolated *Brevibacterium* species

Test	B. casei[a,b]	B. epidermidis[b,c]	B. iodinum[d,e,f]	B. linens[a]
Colony pigmentation[g,h]	White-yellow	Grey-white	Grey-white	Yellow-orange
Oxidase	−	−	+[i]	+[w]
$NO_3 \rightarrow NO_2$	−	+	+	−
TSI (ALK/NC)	+	+	NR	+
Color reaction w/KOH	+	−	−	−
Crystals of iodinin formed	−	+	−	−
Growth 37°C	G	G	NG[j]	NG[k]
Growth 42°C	G	G	NR	NG
Growth 6.5% NaCl	G	G	G	G
Casein hydrolysis	+	+	+[w]	+
DNase	+	+	+	+
Esculin hydrolysis	−	−	NR	−
Gelatin liquefaction	+	+	+	+
Hippurate hydrolysis	+	+	−	+
Starch hydrolysis	−	−	−	−
Urease	−	−	−	−
Voges-Proskauer (VP)	−	−	NR	−

ALK/NC, alkaline/no change; G, growth; NG, no growth; NR, no results; +[w], weakly positive.

Data from references 21, 26.

[a]Found in cheese; *B. casei* has a cheese odor.

[b]Differentiation between *B. casei* and *B. epidermidis* only by menaquinone composition mol %, G:C ratio, and DNA-DNA base-pairing values.

[c]Normal skin flora; not usually pathogenic.

[d]Found only in milk.

[e]Formerly *Chromobacterium iodinum*.

[f]May show intracellular crystals of iodinin; shimmering metallic, purple color (phenazine derivative).

[g]On nutrient agar.

[h]When incubated in light; pigment production is light dependent. Pigment does not develop if plates are exposed to light after colonies are fully developed and growth has ceased (40).

[i]Strong.

[j]Some growth may occur.

[k]Rare strains may exhibit growth.

GENUS: *BROCHOTHRIX* (26, 40)

(*Note*: Genus may be confused with genus *Kurthia*; *Brochothrix* spp. produce acid from a wide variety of sugars; *Kurthia* is **not** saccharolytic (40).)

Gram-positive unbranched rods arranged singly, in chains, or **long filamentous chains that fold into knotted masses.** In older culture appear coccoid. Some cells lose their ability to retain Gram stain.

Nonsporeforming

Facultative anaerobe

Catalase positive (depending on medium and with incubation at 20°C)

Nonencapsulated
Nonmotile at 22°C
Oxidase negative
O/F glucose: F (fermentative)
Optimal growth temperature 20–25°C; usually **cannot** grow at 35–37°C
Nonpigmented
Nonhemolytic on blood agar (BA)
Absence of mycolic acid in cells
Not acid-fast
2 species
Type species: *B. thermosphacta*; ATCC 11509

Table 43.7. Differentiation of *Brochothrix* spp.

Test	*B. campestris*	*B. thermosphacta*[a]
$NO_3 \rightarrow NO_2$	−	−
6.5% NaCl	G	G
H_2S	+	+
Rhamnose	A	−
Hippurate hydrolysis	+	−
Indole	+	+
Methyl red (MR)	+	+
Voges-Proskauer (VP)	+	+

A, acid production (+); G, growth.

[a]Formerly *Microbacterium thermosphactum*. Strains of *B. thermosphacta* most likely to be confused with genera *Lactobacillus* and *Listeria* (40).

GENUS: *BUTYRIVIBRIO* (26, 33, 40)

Gram-positive and Gram-negative curved rods arranged singly, chains, and filaments that may be helical. Stain Gram negative but cell wall is Gram- positive type.
Nonsporeforming
Obligate (strict) anaerobes
Catalase negative
Nonencapsulated
Motile; few polar or subpolar flagella; rapid and vibratory
O/F glucose: F (fermentative)
Optimal growth temperature 37°C; slow < 30°C
Nonpathogenic
2 species
Type species: *B. fibrisolvens* ATCC 19171

Table 43.8. Differentiation of *Butyrivibrio* spp.

Test	*B. crossotus*	*B. fibrisolvens*
Single polar flagellum	−	+
$NO_3 \rightarrow NO_2$	−	−
Butyrate produced	+	+
H_2 produced	−	+
Indole	−	−
Esculin hydrolysis	−	V
Glucose	A[w]	A
Sucrose	−	A

A, acid production (+); w, weak reaction; V, variable reaction.

GENUS: *CASEOBACTER* (26, 40)
C. polymorphus moved to genus *Corynebacterium* as *Corynebacterium polymorphus* (11)

GENUS: *CELLULOMONAS* (19, 26)
Gram-positive but easily decolorized, irregular, straight or slightly curved rods in young cultures. Arranged in pairs and rods and often exhibit V formation. Occasional branching but **no** mycelium. Cells in older cultures may be short rods or cocci.

Nonsporeforming

Facultative anaerobes; some strains grow poorly anaerobically.

Catalase positive

Nonencapsulated

Motility variable; usually positive with 1 to a few flagella

Oxidase negative

O/F glucose: F (fermentative) and O (oxidative)

Optimal growth temperature 30°C

Not acid-fast

No mycolic acid in cells

Nitrate reduction positive

CAMP negative

Casein negative

Esculin hydrolysis positive

Gelatin liquefaction, 22°C, positive

10 species: *C. biazotea, C. cellasea, C. cellulans, C. fermentans, C. fimi, C. flavigena, C. gelida, C. hominis, C. turbata, C. uda*

Type species: *C. flavigena* ATCC 482, CCM 1926, NCIB 8073

GENUS: *CLOSTRIDIUM* (26, 33, 40)
Gram-positive rods in young cultures arranged in short chains with round or pointed ends.

Commonly pleomorphic

Oval or spherical endospores

Obligate (strict) anaerobes; a few species can grow in air (e.g., *C. carnis, C. histolyticum,* and *C. tertium;* aerotolerant)

Catalase variable, usually negative; trace amounts may be detected in some strains (40)

Nonencapsulated

Motility variable; peritrichous flagella

O/F glucose: F (fermentative)

Optimal growth temperature 10–65°C

131 species: *C. absonum, C. aceticum, C. acetireducens, C. acetobutylicum, C. acidiurici, C. aerotolerans, C. aldrichii, C. algidicarnis, C. aminophilum, C. aminovalericum, C. arcticum, C. argentinense, C. aurantibutyricum, C. baratii, C. beijerinckii, C. bifermentans, C. botulinum, C. butyricum, C. cadaveris, C. carnis, C. celatum, C. celerecrescens, C. cellobioparum, C. cellulofermentans, C. cellulolyticum, C. cellulosi, C. cellulovorans, C. chartatabidum, C. chauvoei, C. clostridioforme, C. coccoides, C. cochlearium, C. cocleatum, C. colinum, C. collagenovorans, C. cylindrosporum, C. difficile, C. disporicum, C. estertheticum, C. fallax, C. felsineum, C. fimetarium, C. formicoaceticum, C. ghoni, C. glycolicum, C. grantii, C. haemolyticum, C. halophilum, C. hastiforme, C. herbivorans, C. histolyticum, C. homopropionicum, C. hydroxybenzoicum, C. indolis, C. innocuum, C. intestinalis, C. irregularis, C. josui, C. kluyveri, C. laramiense, C. lentocellum, C. leptum, C. limosum, C. litorale, C. lituseburense, C. ljungdahlii, C. magnum, C. malenominatum, C. mangenotii, C. mayombei, C. methylpentosum, C. neopropionicum, C. nexile, C. novyi, C. oceanicum, C. orbiscindens, C. oroticum, C. oxalicum, C. papyrosolvens, C. paradoxum, C. paraputrificum, C. pascui, C. pasteurianum, C. perfringens, C. piliforme, C. polysaccharolyticum, C. populeti, C. propionicum, C. proteoclasticum, C. proteolyticum, C. puniceum, C. purinolyticum, C. putrefaciens, C. putrificum, C. quercicolum, C.*

quinii, C. ramosum, C. rectum, C. roseum, C. saccharolyticum, C. sardiniensis, C. sartagoformum, C. scatologenes, C. scindens, C. septicum, C. sordellii, C. sphenoides, C. spiroforme, C. sporogenes, C. sporosphaeroides, C. stercorarium, C. sticklandii, C. subterminale, C. symbiosum, C. termitidis, C. tertium, C. tetani, C. tetanomorphum, C. thermoaceticum, C. thermoalcaliphilum, C. thermobutyricum, C. thermocellum, C. thermolacticum, C. thermopalmarium, C. thermopapyrolyticum, C. thermosuccinogenes, C. tyrobutyricum, C. ultunense, C. vincentii, C. viride, C. xylanolyticum

Type species: C. butyricum ATCC 19398, NCIB 7423, NCTC 7423

Table 43.9. Differential Characteristics of the Most Frequently Isolated *Clostridium* spp. with Subterminally Located Spores

Test	C. argentinense[a]	C. baratii	C. bifermentans	C. botulinum	C. butyricum	C. celatum	C. chauvoeri[b]	C. clostridioforme	C. difficile[c]
Aerotolerant	−	−	−	−	−	−	−	−	−
Toxigenic	Yes	Yes	Yes	Yes	Yes	No	Yes	No	Yes
Hemolysis, 5% SBA	γ	α, β, γ	V⁺ β	β	γ	α,β	β	γ	γ
Spore location/shape	So[i,j]	So[i,k]	So[l]	So[i]	So[l]	SO[m]	So[i,m]	So[i,m,n]	So[i,o]
NO₃→NO₂	−	V	V	−	V	V	+	V	−
Growth									
6.5% NaCl	NG	NG	NG	NG	NG	NG	NG	NG	NR
20% Bile	NG	NG	NG	NG	NR	NG	NG	V	NR
Cooked meat digestion	V	NR	+	V	−	NR	−	NR	−
Milk	V D	C	D	V D	ACG[w]	AC	−	C	−
H₂S	+	NR	V	V	−	+	−	V	V
Motility	+	−	+[x]	+	+	+	+	V	+
Indole	−	−	+	−	−	NR	−	V	−
Gelatin liquefaction, 22°C	+	−	+	+	−	NR	+	−	+[y]
Lecithinase	−	+	+	V⁻	−	−	−	−	−
Lipase	−	−	−	+	−	−	−	−	−
Esculin hydrolysis	−	+	−	−	V	+	−	+	−
Starch hydrolysis	−	+	−	−	+	−	−	−	−
Christensen's urease	+	NR	−[z]	−	−	+	−	NR	−
Voges-Proskauer (VP)	−	NR	−	−	−	NR	−	NR	−

So, subterminal oval spores; Sr, subterminal round spores; SBA, sheep blood agar; NG, no growth; NR, no results; V, variable results; V⁺, variable, usually positive; V⁻, variable, usually negative; D, digestion; C, curd; A, acid production; (+) G, gas.

Data from references 2, 26, 30, 33, 40.

[a]Formerly *Clostridium botulinum* G and some nontoxigenic strains of *Clostridium hastiforme* and *Clostridium subterminale* (43).
[b]*Clostridium chauvoei* classification or *Clostridium feseri*. Pathogenic for herbivores (plants).
[c]Most common toxigenic clostridia species. *C. difficile* easily distinguished from *C. sporogenes*, which it closely resembles phenotypically, by its ability to ferment mannitol, and **in**ability to digest meat or milk or to produce lipase (40).
[d]*C. haemolyticum* and *C. novyi* are among the most fastidious and oxygen-sensitive bacterial pathogens known (43).
[e]Most common gas gangrene clostridia isolated: *C. novyi*, *C. perfringens*, and *C. septicum*; *C. perfringens* is most widely occurring pathogenic bacterium (39).
[f]Synergistic hemolysis (CAMP phenomenon) between *C. perfringens* and *Streptococcus agalactiae* (39).
[g]Most clostridia are obligate anaerobes; however, *C. histolyticum*, *C. carnis*, and *C. tertium* grow in air on enriched media; often confused with aerobic bacilli (e.g., lactobacilli) because they are catalase-negative and do not form spores under aerobic conditions (2).
[h]Double zone of hemolysis; α and β.
[i]Spores may swell cells.
[j]Spores rarely observed.

(continued)

Most common toxigenic species is *C. difficile*.
Most common invasive pathogen is *C. perfringens*.
Nagler positive: *C. perfringens, C. baratii, C. sordelli, and C. bifermentans*
Nagler negative: presumptive *C. difficile*
If no spores are present, ethanol spore or heat spore test will distinguish *Clostridium* spp. from nonsporeforming anaerobic bacilli. *C. clostridioforme, C. ramosum,* and *C. perfingens* may not produce spores or survive spore test.

C. fallax	*C. glycolicum*	*C. haemolyticum*[d]	*C. histolyticum*	*C. malenominatum*	*C. novyi*[d,e]	*C. perfringens*[e,f]	*C. putrifiaim*	*C. septicum*[e]	*C. sordellii*	*C. sphenoides*	*C. sporogenes*[e]	*C. subterminale*	*C. symbiosum*
−	−	−	+[g]	−	−	−	−	−	−	−	−	−	−
No	No	Yes	Yes	No	Yes	Yes	No	Yes	Yes	No	No	No	No
β	γ	γ	β	V	β[i,m]	γ,β[h]	V+ β	β	Vβ	γ	V+β	V+β	β
So[i,m]	So[p]	So[j]	So[m,r]	So/Sr[j,l]	So[i,m]	So[m,r,s,t]	So/Sr[j,k]	So[r]	So[l,q,u]	So[i,k]	So[r]	So[r,v]	So/Sr
−	−	−	−	V−	V	V	−	V	V	V−	−	−	−
NG	NG	NG	NG	NG	NG	NG	NG	NR	NG	NR	V	NG	NG
NG	NG	NG	NG	NG	NG	G	NG	NR	NG	NG	V	NG	NG
−	NR	−	+	−	V	−	−	−	+	NR	+	+	V−C
AC	−	AC	D	−	V	ACD[w]	CD	AC	D	C	D	DC	C
+	NR	−	V	NR	−	−	+	−	V+	+	+	V+	NR
+	V	+	+[x]	V	V+	−	+	+	+	+	+	V+	V+
−	NR	+	−	+	V−	−	−	+	+	+	−	−	−
−	NR	+	+	−	+	+	NR	+	+	−	+	+	NR
−	−	+	−	−	V+	+	−	−	+	−	−	V−	−
−	−	−	−	−	V	−	−	−	−	−	+	−	−
−	V	−	−	−	−	V	V	−	−	+	+	−	−
+	−	−	−	−	−	+	−	−	−	V	−	−	−
−	NR	−	−	NR	−	V	NR	−	+	NR	NR	−	NR
−	NR	−	−	NR	−	V	NR	−	−	V	NR	−	NR

[k]Spores may also be terminal.
[l]Central to subterminal spores.
[m]Spores terminal to subterminal to centrally located.
[n]Spores often difficult to demonstrate.
[o]Rarely seen terminally.
[p]Spores often terminal; often occurring as free spores.
[q]Slight swelling.
[r]Distended cells.
[s]Spores rarely seen in vivo or usual in vitro conditions; cells usually Gram negative (33).
[t]*C. perfringens* has nonsporeforming strains.
[u]Often occurring as free spores.
[v]Spores occasionally centrally located.
[w]Stormy fermentation.
[x]Sluggish.
[y]Slow.
[z]*C. bifermentans* differentiated from *C. sordelli,* which it resembles closely phenotypically, by urease-negative reaction (40).

Table 43.10. Differentiation of *C. botulinum*

Test	Toxin Types	
	ABCDF	BCDEF
H₂S	+	−
Cooked meat	D	−
Milk	D	−
Lecithinase	−	V[a]

V, variable reaction; D, digestion.
[a]If positive, very small amounts.

Table 43.11. Carbohydrate Differentiation of *C. novyi* Types

Test	A	B[a]	C
NO₃→NO₂	V	V	−
Meat	−	V	NR
Milk	AC	D	NR
Motility	+	+	−
Indole	−	−	V
Lecithinase	+	+	−
Lipase	+	−	−

AC, acid, clot; D, digestion; NR, no results; V, variable results.
[a]*C. novyi* B results are variable and long delayed.

Table 43.12. Carbohydrate Characteristics of *Clostridium* spp. with Subterminally Located Spores

Testing Media	*C. argentinene*	*C. baratii*	*C. bifermentans*	*C. botulinum*	*C. butyricum*	*C. celatum*	*C. chauvdei*	*C. clostridioforme*	*C. difficile*	*C. fallax*
Arabinose	−	−	−	V⁻	V	−	−	V	V	−
Cellobiose	−	A	−	−	A	A	−	V	Aʷ	−
Dulcitol	−	NR	−	−	−	NR	V	NR	−	−
Galactose	−	Aʷ	−	V⁻	A	A	A	Aʷ	−	A
Glucose	−	A	A	A	A	NR	A	NR	A	A
Inositol	−	NR	−	V⁻	V	NR	−	NR	V	−
Lactose	−	Aʷ	−	−	A	A	A	V	−	−
Melibiose	−	−	−	−	A	−	−	−	−	−
Maltose	−	Aʷ	A	V	A	A	A	Aʷ	−	A
Mannitol	−	−	−	−	V	−	−	−	−	−
Mannose	−	A	V⁻	V⁻	A	A	A	A	A	A
Raffinose	−	−	−	−	A	−	−	V	−	−
Rhamnose	−	−	−	−	−	−	−	NR	−	−
Ribose	−	−	V	V⁻	A	V	A	V	V	V
Salicin	−	Aʷ	−	V⁻	A	A	−	V	V	−
Sorbitol	−	−	V	V⁻	−	−	−	−	V	V
Sucrose	−	A	−	V	A	A	A	Aʷ	−	−
Trehalose	−	−	−	V⁻	A	A	−	A	V	−
Xylose	−	−	V	−	A	−	−	Aʷ	A	A

A, acid production (+); Aʷ, weakly acidic; V, variable results; V⁺, variable, usually positive; V⁻, variable, usually negative; NR, no results.
Data from references 2, 26, 33, 40.

(continued)

Table 43.13. Differentiation of *C. botulinum* Toxin Types

	C. botulinum Proteolytic ABCDF	*C. botulinum* Saccharolytic BCDEF
Arabinose	−	V
Galactose	−	V
Inositol	−	V
Mannose	−	A
Ribose	−	V
Sorbitol	−	V
Trehalose	−	V

A, acid production (+); V, variable results.

Table 43.14. Carbohydrate Differentiation of *C. novyi* Types

Test	*C. novyi* A	*C. novyi* B	*C. novyi* C
Arabinose	V	−	−
Glucose	A	A	A^w
Inositol	V	A	A^w
Maltose	V	A	−
Mannose	−	V	−
Raffinose	V	−	−
Ribose	V	V	A^w
Sucrose	V	−	−

A, acid production (+); W, weak reaction; V, variable reaction.

C. glycolicum	*C. haemolyticum*	*C. histolyticum*	*C. malenominatum*	*C. novyi*	*C. perfringens*	*C. putrificum*	*C. septicum*	*C. sordellii*	*C. sphenoides*	*C. sporogenes*	*C. subterminale*	*C. symbiosum*
−	−	−	NR	V$^−$	−	−	−	V	V	−	−	V
−	−	NR	−	−	V	−	A^w	−	A	−	−	−
NR	−	−	NR	−	V	A	A	−	−	−	−	NR
−	−	−	NR	−	A	V	V	−	V	−	−	A^w
NR	A	−	NR	A	A	A	A	A	A	A	−	NR
NR	V	−	NR	V$^+$	A	−	−	−	V	−	−	NR
−	−	−	−	−	A	A	−	−	V	−	−	V$^−$
−	−	−	NR	−	V	−	−	−	−	−	−	−
V	−	−	V	V	A	A	A	A	A	V	−	−
−	−	−	NR	−	−	−	−	−	A	−	−	V
−	V	−	NR	V$^−$	A	A	A	V	A	−	−	V
−	−	−	NR	V$^−$	V	−	−	V	A	−	−	−
−	NR	−	−	NR	−	NR	−	−	A	−	−	−
−	−	−	−	V	V	V	V	V	V	−	−	−
−	−	V	NR	−	V	V	V	−	A	V	−	−
V	−	−	NR	−	−	−	−	−	−	V	−	−
−	−	−	−	V	A	−	−	−	A	V	−	−
−	−	−	−	−	V	V	V	−	V	V	−	−
V	−	−	−	−	−	−	−	V	A	−	−	−

Table 43.15. Differential Characteristics of the Most Frequently Isolated *Clostridium* spp. with Terminally Located Spores

Test	*C. baratii*	*C. cadaveris*	*C. carnis*	*C. celatum*	*C. cochlearium*	*C. hastiforme*	*C. indolis*
Aerotolerant	−	−	+[a]	−	−	−	−
Toxigenic	Yes	No	No	No	No	No	No
Hemolysis, 5% SBA	α,β,γ[b]	V	β[c]	α,γ	V	Vβ	γ
Spore shape location	To/Tr[e]	To[f,g]	To[e,f]	To[h]	To/Tr[f,g]	To[f]	To/Tr[f,g]
NO$_3$→NO$_2$	V	−	−	V	−	NR	V
Growth							
6.5% NaCl	NG	NG	NG	NG	NG	NG	NG
20% Bile	NG	V−	NG	NG	NG	NG	NG
Cooked meat digestion	NR	+	−	NR	−	+[i]	NR
Milk	C	C,D	−	A,C	−	VD	C
H$_2$S	NR	+	−	+	+	+	+
Motility	−	V+	+	+	V+	NR	+
Indole	−	+	−	NR	V−	NR	+
Gelatin liquefaction, 22°C	−	+	−	NR	Vw	+[n]	NR
Lecithinase	+	−	−	−	−	NR	−
Lipase	−	−	−	−	−	NR	−
Esculin hydrolysis	+	−	−	+	−	NR	+
Starch hydrolysis	V	−	−	−	−	NR	V
Christensen's urease	NR	NR	−	+	−	NR	NR
Voges-Proskauer (VP)	V	NR	−	NR	−	NR	V

To, terminal, oval spores; Tr, terminal, round spores; SBA, sheep blood agar; NG, no growth; G, growth; NR, no results; V, variable results; V+, variable, usually positive; V−, variable, usually negative; Vw, variable, weak reaction if positive; C, clot; D, digestion; A, acid production (+).

Data from references 2, 26, 30, 33, 40.

[a]Grown in air on enriched media; aerotolerant clostridia are often confused with aerobic bacilli (e.g., lactobacilli) since they are catalase negative and **do not** form spores under aerobic conditions (2).
[b]Most are β-hemolytic.
[c]Slightly.
[d]Narrow zone.
[e]Spores may also be subterminal.
[f]Spores swell cell.
[g]Occasionally subterminal spores.
[h]Spores terminal, subterminal, and central.
[i]Spores terminal, subterminal, or free.

(continued)

	C. innocuum	C. leptum	C. malenominatum	C. paraputrificum	C. putrefaciens	C. putrificum	C. ramosum	C. tertium	C. tetani
	—	—	—	—	—	—	—	+[a]	—
	No	No	No	No	No	No	No	No	Yes
	V	γ	V	γ	β	Vβ	γ	β,γ	β[d]
	To[j]	To[j]	To/Tr[e,f]	To[f,h]	To/Tr[e,f]	To/Tr[e,f]	To/Tr[f,j]	To[g]	Tr[k]
	—	—	NR	V	—	—	—	V	—
	NR	NG	NG	V−	NG	NG	NG	NG	NG
	NR	NG	NG	G	NG	NG	NG	V	NG
	—	—	—	NR	—	V	—	—	V
	−[m]	—	—	C	—	NR	C	AC	V
	—	+	+	NR	—	+	—	—	V
	—	—	NR	V	—	+	—	+	+
	—	—	V	—	—	—	—	—	V
	—	V−[o]	V−[w]	—	+	NR	—	—	+
	—	V	—	—	—	—	—	—	—
	—	V−	—	—	—	—	—	—	—
	—	V	—	+	NR	V	+	V	NR
	—	—	—	+	NR	—	NR	+	NR
	—	V−	NR	NR	—	NR	—	—	—
	—	NR	NR	V	—	NR	V	—	—

[j]Rarely seen.
[k]Occasionally oval or subterminal, or both.
[l]Slow.
[m]May be weakly acidified.
[n]Rapid.
[o]If positive, after 3 weeks.

Table 43.16. Carbohydrate Characteristics of *Clostridium* spp. with Terminally Located Spores

Testing Media	C. baratii	C. cadaveris	C. carnis	C. celatum	C. cochlearium	C. hastiforme	C. indolis	C. innocuum	C. leptum	C. malenominatum	C. paraputrificum	C. putrefaciens	C. ramosum	C. tertium	C. tetani
Arabinose	–	–	–	–	–	–	–	V–	NR	NR	–	–	V	V	NR
Cellobiose	A	–	Aw	A	–	–	Aw	A	–	–	A	–	A	A	NR
Dulcitol	NR	NR	–	NR	–	–	NR	–	NR	NR	–	NR	V	V	NR
Galactose	Aw	–	A	A	–	–	Aw	A	NR	NR	A	V	A	A	NR
Glucose	A	A	A	NR	–	–	NR	–	NR	NR	–	A	A	A	–
Inositol	NR	–	–	NR	–	–	NR	–	NR	NR	A	–	–	–	–
Lactose	Aw	–	V	A	–	–	Aw	A	V	–	–	–	A	Aw	–
Melibiose	–	–	–	–	–	–	–	–	NR	–	A	–	A	A	–
Maltose	Aw	–	Aw	A	–	–	Aw	A	A	V	–	–	A	Aw	–
Mannitol	–	–	–	–	–	–	–	A	NR	NR	A	–	V	A	–
Mannose	A	–	Aw	A	–	–	V	A	NR	NR	A	Vw	A	V	–
Raffinose	–	–	V–	–	NR	–	Aw	–	NR	NR	–	NR	A	–	NR
Rhamnose	–	–	–	–	NR	–	V	A	NR	–	–	NR	V	–	–
Ribose	–	–	V–	V	–	–	–	V	Vw	–	V–	NR	V	A	NR
Salicin	Aw	–	A	A	–	–	–	A	NR	NR	A	–	A	A	–
Sorbitol	–	–	–	–	–	–	–	–	NR	NR	V–	NR	–	V	NR
Sucrose	A	–	Aw	A	–	–	V	A	V	–	A	–	A	A	–
Trehalose	–	–	A	A	–	–	–	A	V–w	–	V	NR	A	A	NR
Xylose	–	–	–	–	–	–	V	V	V–w	–	V–	Vw	V	A	–

A, acid production (+); w, weak reaction; NR, no results; V, variable results; V–, variable, usually negative.

Data from references 2, 30, 33, 40.

GENUS: *COPROCOCCUS* (25, 33, 40)

Gram-positive cocci; occasionally ovoid, arranged in pairs or short chains
Nonsporeforming
Strict (obligate) anaerobes
Catalase negative
Nonencapsulated
Nonmotile
O/F glucose: F (fermentative)
Optimal growth temperature: 37°C
Carbohydrates required for growth
3 species
Type species: *C. eutactus* ATCC 27759; rarely isolated from clinical specimens (25)

Table 43.17. Differentiation of *Coprococcus* species

Tests	C. catus	C. comes	C. eutactus
Sucrose	−	A	A
Melezitose	−	−	A
Xylose	−	A	A
Esculin	−	V	+

V, variable results; A, acid production (+).

GENUS: *CORYNEBACTERIUM* (26, 33, 40)

Gram-positive rods that may stain unevenly, giving a beaded appearance; metachromatic granules of polymetaphosphate commonly found in cells. Rods are straight or slightly curved, at times ellipsoidal, ovoid slender rods with tapered or clubbed ends. Middle or ends are slightly wider giving appearance of club cells barred or segmented. *C. matruchotii* has a whip-handle morphology. Arranged singly, pairs, or often V formation or palisades of several parallel cells appearing as "Chinese letters"
Nonsporeforming
Facultative anaerobic
Catalase positive
Nonencapsulated
Nonmotile except *C. aquaticum* and *C. matruchotii*
O/F glucose: F (fermentative) or O (oxidative) or inert (−)
Optimal growth temperature 35–37°C
Not acid-fast
Lipase positive: **only** *C. pseudotuberculosis* and *C. ulcerans*
Possess mycolic acid in cells; smallest and simplest *C. amycolatum* (19) (C_{22}–C_{38}); exceptions: *C. amycolatum*, *C. asperum*, and CDC groups F2 and F12 lack mycolic acid. Plant *Corynebacterium* spp. **do not** possess mycolic acids in cells.
42 species: *C. accolens, C. afermentans, C. afermentans* subsp. *afermentans, C. afermentans* subsp. *lipophilum, C. ammoniagenes, C. amycolatum, C. argentoratense, C. auris, C. beticola, C. bovis, C. callunae, C. coyleae, C. cystitidis, C. diphtheriae, C. durum, C. flavescens, C. glucuronolyticum, C. glutamicum, C. hoagii, C. imitans, C. jeikeium, C. kutscheri, C. lipophiloflavum, C. macginleyi, C. mastitidis, C. matruchotii, C. minutissimum, C. mucifaciens, C. mycetoides, C. pilosum, C. propinquum, C. pseudodiphtheriticum, C. pseudotuberculosis, C. renale, C. seminale, C. singulare, C. striatum, C. ulcerans, C. urealyticum, C. variabilis, C. vitaeruminis, C. xerosis*
Type species: *C. diphtheriae* ATTC 27010
    Lipophilic species (19): *C. accolens, C. afermentans* subsp. *lipophilum, C. jeikeium, C. mcgin-*

leyi, *C. urealyticum*, and CDC F-1 and G. Lipophilic species are slow growers; 3 or more days for growth on routine isolation media (19).

Modified Tinsdale medium: positive species (halo): *C. diphtheriae* biotypes *gravis, mitis, intermedius, belfanti,* and *C. pseudotuberculosis* and *C. ulcerans*

CAMP positive: *C. auris, C. bovis, C. coylae* (strong), *C. glucuronolyticum*.
CAMP variable: *C. afermentans* subsp. *afermentans* and *C. striatum*

Barreau et al. (3) and De Briel et al. (13) have shown that any bacterium lacking mycolic acid cannot be classified in the genus *Corynebacterium*. If no mycolic acid with corynebacterium-type morphology, called **coryneform bacteria**; replaces diphtheroid term

C. pseudotuberculosis and *C. ulcerans* possess phospholipase D activity; a distinct marker within the genus *Corynebacterium* (1).

Table 43.18. Differentiation of *Corynebacterium* species That May Cause Human Infections, *Erysipelothrix rhusiopathiae*, and *Listeria monocytogenes*

Test	*C. amycolatum*[a]	*C. afermentans*[b]	*C. accolens*[c]	*C. bovis*[d]	*C. callionae*	*C. cystitidis*[e]	*C. diphtheriae* biotype gravis[f]	*C. diphtheriae* biotype mitis	*C. diphtheriae* biotype intermedius	*C. diphtheriae* biotype belfantii	*C. flavescens*	*C. glutamicum*
Catalase	+	+	+	+	+	+	+	+	+	+	+	+
Hemolysis, 5% SBA[o]	NR	β	NR	NR	NR	NR	γ[p]	β	γ	γ		
NO$_3$→NO$_2$	−	−	+	−	−	−	+	+	+	−	−	+
H$_2$S (TSI)	−	−	−	−	−	−	−	−	−	−	−	−
O F glucose	F	NF	F	NF	NR	F	F	F	F	F	NR	NR
Motility, 22°C	−	−	−	−	−	−	−	−	−	−	−	−
Carbohydrates												
Arabinose	−	−	−	−	−	−	−	−	NR	NR	−	−
Dextran	NR	NR	V	V−	A	A	NR	NR	NR	NR	−	−
Fructose	A	NR	NR	A	A	A	A	NR	NR	NR	A	A
Galactose	−	NR	NR	A	−	−	A	NR	NR	NR	A	−
Glucose	A	−	A	A	A	A	A	A	A	A	A	A
Lactose	−	NR	NR	V	−	−	−	−	NR	NR	−	−
Maltose	V+	−	−	A	A	A	A	A	A	A	−	A
Mannose	A	NR	NR	−	A	−	A	NR	NR	NR	A	A
Raffinose	−	NR	NR	−	−	−	V	NR	NR	NR	−	−
Ribose	A	−	−	−	NR	NR	A	V+	A	A	NR	NR
Salicin	−	NR	NR	−	A	−	A	−	NR	NR	−	−
Sucrose	V−	−	−	−	A	−	−[aa]	−[z]	−[z]	−[z]	−	A
Trehalose	V	NR	NR	V	A	A	−	NR	NR	NR	−	A
Xylose	−	−	NR	−	−	A	−	−	NR	NR	−	−
Misc. tests												
Alkaline phosphatase	+	V	NR	+	NR	−	−	−	−	−	−	NR
Esculin hydrolysis	−	NR	NR	−	−	−	−	−	−	−	NR	−
Gelatin liquefaction, 22°C	−	NR	−	−	−	−	−	NR	NR	NR	−	−
Glycogn	−	−	+	−	+	+	+	−	−	+		
Hippurate hydrolysis	V	NR	NR	+	+	+	−	NR	NR	NR	−	+
Methyl red (MR)	+	NR	NR	−	+	−	+	NR	NR	NR	+	+
Pyrazinamidase	−	V	NR	V+	NR	+	−	−	−	−	−	NR
Urease	V+	−	−	V−	+	+	−	−	−	−	−	+

(continued)

	C. jeikeium[g]	C. kutscheri[h]	C. matruchotii	C. minutissimum	C. mycetoides	C. pilosum	C. pseudodiphtheriae[i]	C. pseudotuberculosis[j]	C. renale[k]	C. striatum[l]	C. vitarumen	C. xerosis[m]	C. aquaticum[n]	Erysipelothrix rhusiopathiae	Listeria monocytogenes
	+	+	+	+	+	+	+	+	+	+	+	+	+	−	+
		Vβ					V	Vβ[q]	Vβ	+[r]	NR	γ	γ	α	β
	−	+[s]	+	−	−	+	+	V[t]	−	−	+	+	V	−	−
	−	−	−	−	−	−	−	−	−	−	−	−	−	+	−
	NF	F	NF	F	NR	F	F	F	F	F	F	F	O/−[u]	O	F
	−	−	+	−	−	−	−	−	−	−	−	−	+	−	−
	−	−	−	NR	−	−	−	V	−	−	NR	−	−		
	−	A	A	NR	−	A	−	V	A	A	NR	−	NR		
	−	A	A	A	NR	A	−	A	A	A	A	A	A		
	A	−	−	NR	−	−	−	A	−	V	A	A	A		
	A	A	A	A	A	A	−	A	A	A	A	A	A[v]	V	A
	−	−	−	−	−	−	−	−	−	V	V	−	V	A	V
	V	A	A	A	−	A	−	A	V	A	A	−[w]	A[v]	−	A
	−	A	A	V	−	A	−	A	A	A	A	A[x]	A[v]		
	−	−	V[y]	−	−	−	−	−	−	−	−	NR	−		
	A	NR	NR	V	NR	NR	NR	−	A	NR	V	NR	NR		
	−	A	A	NR	NR	−	−	−	−	−	A	A	NR		
	−	A	A	A[bb]	NR	−	V+	−	A[v]	A	A	A[v]	−	V	
	−	V	−	−	V	A	−	−	V	V	A	−[w]	NR	−	A
	−	−	−	−	−	−	−	−	−	−	NR	−	V	A	−
	−	−	−	+	+	−	−	V−	−	+	−	−	NR		
	−	−	+	−	−	−	−	−	−	−	+	−	+	−	+
	−	−	−	−	−	−	−	V[cc]	−	V	−	−	V	−	−
	NR	+	+	+	NR	+	+	−	+	+	−	+	NR		
	−	−	−	−	−	−	−	+	−	+	+	−	NR		
	+	+	+	+	NR	+	+	−	+	NR	+	+	NR		
	−	+	V	−	−	+	+	+	+	−	+	−	−	−	−

(continued)

Table 43.18. Differentiation of *Corynebacterium* species That May Cause Human Infections, *Erysipelothrix rhusiopathiae*, and *Listeria monocytogenes* (continued)

Test	C. amycolatum[a]	C. afermentans[b]	C. accolens[c]	C. bovis[d]	C. callionae	C. cystitidis[e]	C. diphtheriae biotype gravis[f]	C. diphtheriae biotype mitis	C. diphtheriae biotype intermedius	C. diphtheriae biotype belfantii	C. flavescens	C. glutamicum
ONPG						+						
CAMP												
Requires serum	−	V	+	V	NR	−	−	−	+	−	NR	NR

β, beta; γ, gamma (no hemolysis); NR, no results; A, acid production (+); V, variable reaction; V+, variable, usually positive; V−, variable usually negative; SBA, sheep blood agar.

Data from references 19, 26, 33, 40.

[a]*C. amycolatum* is possibly synonymous with CDC groups F2 and F12, I1, I2, G1, and G2.
[b]*C. afermentans* CDC group ANF1; *C. afermentans* subsp. *fermentans* and *C. afermentans* subsp. *lipophilum*.
[c]*C. accolans* CDC group 6.
[d]*C. bovis* is a veterinary pathogen in cows.
[e]*C. cystitis* formerly *C. renale* type III (40).
[f]*C. ulcerans* now in *C. diphtheriae* group (31). *C. ulcerans* no longer a valid species; however, clinical literature often retains the name.
[g]*C. jeikeium* (formerly CDC JK gp.) most common corynebacterial pathogen isolated from clinical specimens (33).
[h]Formerly *Corynebacterium murium*; found in rats.
[i]*C. pseudodiphtheriae* formerly *Corynebacterium hofmannii*; rare human pathogen. Can be lysogenized by bacteriophages of *C. diphtheriae* and thus can produce diphtheria toxin (12).
[j]Found in sheep, goats, horses, and other warm-blooded animals but rarely humans. Formerly *Corynebacterium ovis*. Toxin inhibits action of staphylococcal β-lysin (1).
[k]Found in cattle, pigs, and sheep.
[l]Formerly *Corynebacterium flavidum*; rarely pathogenic.
[m]Halo **not** produced on Tinsdale medium.

(*continued*)

C. jeikeium[g]	C. kutscheri[h]	C. matruchotii	C. minutissimum	C. mycetoides	C. pilosum	C. pseudodiphtheriae[i]	C. pseudotuberculosis[j]	C. renale[k]	C. striatum[l]	C. vitarumen	C. xerosis[m]	C. aquaticum[n]	Erysipelothrix rhusiopathiae	Listeria monocytogenes
													+	
+	−	−	V	NR	NR	−	−	−	−	NR	V[dd]	NR		

[n]Proposed move to a different genus.
[o]When β, slight hemolysis with a narrow zone.
[p]C. diphtheriae biotype gravis occasionally exhibits weak β-hemolysis.
[q]Narrow zone of slight β-hemolysis after 18–24 hr.
[r]Slight hemolysis around deep colonies (40).
[s]Nitrate reduction negative in strains from sheep and goats and positive in strains from horses and cattle (12).
[t]Studies by Knight (29) and Biberstein and Knight (4) showed equine strains reduced nitrate while ovine strains were negative.
[u]In ordinary carbohydrate media, inert (−).
[v]Aerobically only.
[w]Occasional strains are positive.
[x]Occasional strains are negative.
[y]Occasional strains are positive (40).
[z]C. diphteriae's inability to ferment sucrose cannot be taken as proof of nontoxinogenicity; some toxigenic strains ferment sucrose (40). C. diphtheriae produces halos on Tinsdale medium.
[aa]Rarely sucrose positive.
[bb]Occasional strains are negative; approximately 50% of strains are positive (40).
[cc]Gelatin negative at 35°C and 25°C, but positive at 30°C after 14 days.
[dd]DNA groups D and E are positive; DNA groups C and F are negative (33).

GENUS: *DEINOCOCCUS* (2, 40)

Gram-positive cocci in **pairs, or tetrads**; larger spherical cells than most cocci; may be elongated
Nonsporeforming
Aerobic
Catalase positive
Nonencapsulated
Nonmotile
O/F glucose: F (fermentative)
Red to orange pigmented colonies (red pigmented cells often confused with red pigmented *Micrococcus roseus* and *M. agilis*)
Optimal growth temperature 30–37°C
Most strains highly resistant to radiation
7 species: *D. geothermalis, D. grandis, D. murrayi, D. proteolyticus, D. radiodurans, D. radiophilus, D. radiopugnans*
Type species: *D. radiodurans* ATCC 13939, NCIB 9279, CCM 1700

Table 43.19. Differentiation of Most Frequently Encountered *Deinococcus* Species

Test	*D. proteolyticus*	*D. radiodurans*	*D. radiophilus*	*D. radiopugnans*
Colony color	Orange-red	Red	Orange-red	Orange-red
Nitrate reduction	−	V	−	+
Growth 6.5% NaCl	NG	V	G	NG
Esculin in hydrolysis	+	−	−	−
ONPG	−	−	−	+

V, variable reactions; G, growth; NG, no growth.

GENUS: *DERMABACTER* (26, 33, 40)

Gram-positive short, irregular rods; may be rounded coccoid shape; difficult to distinguish from *Corynebacterium* spp.
Nonsporeforming
Facultative anaerobes
Catalase positive
Nonencapsulated
Nonmotile
Oxidase negative
O/F glucose: F (fermentative)
Optimal growth temperature 37°C
No mycolic acid in cells
Not acid-fast
1 species: *D. hominus* ATCC 49369; not included in *Bergey's Manual*; established by Jones and Collins (28). CDC groups 3 and 5

Table 43.20. Characteristics of *Dermabacter hominus*

NO$_3$→NO$_2$	−	CAMP	−
Hemolysis, 5% SBA	γ	Esculin	+
Glucose	A	Gelatin	+
Lactose	A	Hippurate	−
Maltose	A	Lysine	+
Mannose	−	Ornithine	−
Sucrose	A	Voges-Proskauer (VP)	−
Xylose	−		

γ, gamma (no hemolysis); A, acid production (+).

GENUS: *ENTEROCOCCUS* (26, 33, 36, 40)

Gram-positive cocci in pairs, short chains, or singly in liquid media Occasionally coccobacilli when cultivated and Gram-stained from agar growth

Nonsporeforming

Facultative anaerobes

Catalase negative

Nonencapsulated

Motility variable; scanty flagella

O/F glucose: F (fermentative)

Optimal growth temperature 37°C; however, growth at both 10°C and 45°C at pH 9.6.

All PYR positive

All bile insoluble

Usually Lancefield group D

18 species: *E. avium, E. casseliflavus, E. cecorum, E. columbae, E. dispar, E. durans, E. faecalis, E. faecium, E. flavescens, E. gallinarum, E. hirae, E. malodoratus, E. mundtii, E. pseudoavium, E. raffinosus, E. saccharolyticus, E. solitarius, E. sulfureus*

Type species: *E. faecalis* ATCC 19433, NCTC 775, NCIB 775

(*Note: E. faecalis* and *E. faecium* account for over 95% of clinically important strains.)

Table 43.21. Differentiation of Enterococcus[a]

Test	Group I[b]				Group II				
	E. avium	E. malodoratus	E. pseudoavium	E. raffinose	E. faecalis	E. faecium	E. casseliflavus[c]	E. flavescins	E. gallinakium
Lancefield group	Q(D)[f]	D	D	VD	D	D	D	D	D
Catalase[g]	−	−	−	−	−	−	−	−	−
Hemolysis, 5% SBA	α	−	α	−	α, Vβ[h]	Vα	−	NR	α,β
Yellow pigmented colonies	−	−	−	−	−	−	+	+	−
H$_2$S (KIA/TSI)	+	+	−	−	−	−	−	−	−
Growth at									
10°C	V$^{−i}$	G	G	G	G	G	G	G	G
45°C	G	NG	G	G	G	G	G	G	G
50°C	NG	NG	NR	NR	V	V$^+$	NG	NR	NG
Growth in									
Methylene blue milk, 0.1%	V	NR	NR	NR	G	NR	NR	NR	V
NaCl, 6.5% at 45°C	G	G	NG	G	G	G	G	G	G
Tellurite, 0.04%	NG	NG	NG	NG	G	NG	G	NG	V$^+$
Tetrazolium, 0.01%	NG	NG	NR	NG	G	NG	NR	NR	G
Key identification tests									
Mannitol	A	A	A	A	A	V$^+$	A	A	A
Sorbitol	A	A	A	A	V	−	−	−	−
Sorbose	A	A	A	A	−	−	−	−	−
Arginine	−	−	−	−	+	+	V$^+$	+	+
LAP	+	+	+	+	+	+	+	+	+
PYR	+	+	+	+	+	+	+	+	+
Carbohydrates									
Lactose	A	A	A	A	A	A	A	NR	A
Adonitol	A	A	NR	NR	−	−	−	NR	−
Arabinose	A	−	−	A	A	A	A	−	A
Glycerol	A	V	−	A	A	A	−	NR	A
Melezitose	A	−	−	NR	V$^+$	−	−	NR	−
Melibiose	−	A	−	A	−	V	A	NR	A
Raffinose	−	A	−	A	−	−	A	A	A
Ribose	A	A	A	A	A	A	A	−	A
Rhamnose	A	A	NR	NR	V	−	V$^+$	NR	−
Sucrose	A	A	−	A	A	V	A	A	A

(continued)

Group II	Group III				Group IV	Misc.	Atypical		
E. mundtii[c]	*E. dispar*	*E. durans*	*E. faecialis* variant	*E. hirae*	*E. sulfureus*	*E. solitarius*[d]	*E. cecorum*[e]	*E. saccharolyticus*	*E. columbae*[e]
D	ND	D	D	D	NR	D	ND	ND	NR
—	—	—	—	—	—	—	—	—	NR
—	NR	α,β	—	—	NR	NR	α	—	NR
+	—	—	—	—	+	—	—	—	NR
—	—	—	—	NR	NR	NR	NR	NR	NR
G	G	G	G	G	G	G	G[j]	G	G
G	NG	NG	NR	G	NR	G	G	G	G
NG	NG	NG	NR	NG	NR	NR	NR	NG	NR
NR	NR	G	NR	NR	NR	NR	V	NR	NR
G	G	G	G	G	G	G	NG	G	G
NG	NG	NG	G	NG	NG	NR	NR	NR	NR
NR	NR	NG	NR	NR	NR	NR	NR	NR	NR
A	—	V⁻	—	—	—	A	—	A	—
V	—	—	—	—	—	A	—	A	—
—	—	—	—	—	—	—	—	A	—
+	+	+	+	+	—	+	—	—	—
+	+	+	+	+	+	+	+	+	+
+	+	+	+	+	+	+	—	—	—
A	A	A	—	A	NR	—	A	A	NR
A	NR	—	—	—	NR	—	—	—	NR
A	—	—	—	—	—	NR	NR	NR	NR
V	A	—	—	V	NR	NR	—	—	NR
—	NR	—	—	V	NR	A	A	A	NR
A	A	—	—	A	NR	NR	A	A	NR
V⁺	A	—	—	V	A	NR	A	NR	NR
A	NR	NR	NR	NR	A	NR	A	A	A
V⁺	NR	—	—	—	NR	—	—	—	NR
A	A	—	—	A	A	A	A	A	NR

(*continued*)

Table 43.21. Differentiation of *Enterococcus*[a] (continued)

Test	Group I				Group II				
	E. avium	*E. malodoratus*	*E. pseudoavium*	*E. raffinose*	*E. faecalis*	*E. faecium*	*E. cassel, flavus*[c]	*E. flavescins*	*E. gallinakium*
Misc. tests									
Bile esculin (40%)[k]	+	+	+	+	+	+	+	+	+
Bile solubility	Insol	Insol	Insol	Insol	Insol	Insol	Insol	Insol	Insol
Hippurate hydrolysis	V	V	+	−	V	+	−	NR	+
Motility	−	−	−	−	V	V	+	+	−
PYU[l]	+	+	+	+	+	−	−	−	−
Voges-Proskauer (VP)	−	−	+	+	NR	NR	+	NR	NR
Vancomycin susceptibility[m] (30μg)	S	S	S	S	S	S	S	S	S
Isolated from human sources	Rare	No	No	Yes	Yes[n]	Yes[o]	Rare	Rare	Rare

α, alpha; β, beta; V, variable; V[+], variable, usually positive; V[−], variable, usually negative; NaCl, sodium chloride; NR, no results; G, growth; A, acid production (+); S, sensitive (susceptible); LAP, leucine aminopeptidase; PYR, pyrrolidonyl-β-naphthylamide; PYU, pyruvate; SBA, sheep blood; ND, not group D.

Data from references 26, 33, 40.

[a]Not included as separate genus in *Bergey's Manual of Systematic Bacteriology*. Transferred to genus *Enterococcus* by various investigators (33).

[b]*Enterococcus* spp. are separated into 4 main groups plus a misc. group on the basis of 4 tests: mannitol, sorbitol, sorbase, and arginine (33).

[c]*E. casseliflavus* and *E. mundtii* are the only two species that exhibit yellow pigmentation in their colonies; separated by motility: *E. casseliflavus* positive motility; *E. mundtii* nonmotile (30). All other *Enterococcus* species are nonmotile and lack pigmentation (7, 9, 37).

[d]According to Williams, Rodrigues, and Collins (45), *E. solitarius* is more closely related to *Tetragenococcus halophilus* than to any species of *Enterococcus*; DNA homology studies indicate that *E. solitarius* is equally related to the reference strains of *Enterococcus* and *Tetragenococcus*. According to Domenech et al. (14), the rRNA sequence of *E. seriolicida* is identical to that of *Lactococcus garvieae*, protein profiles of *E. seriolicida* and *L. graviae* are identical.

[e]Recent new species: *E. cecorum* and *E. columbae* are more similar to *Streptococcus bovis* strains than to typical *Enterococcus* strains (33).
fGroup Q but may cross-react with group D. Care should be taken in the interpretation of Lancefield typing. Most strains of Pediococcus and half of Leuconostoc isolates from humans also have group D antigens (15).

(continued)

Group II	Group III				Group IV	Misc.	Atypical		
E. mundtii[c]	*E. disper*	*E. durans*	*E. faecialis* variant	*E. hirae*	*E. sulfureus*	*E. solitarius*[d]	*E. cecorum*[e]	*E. saccharolyticus*	*E. columbae*[e]
+	+	+	+	+	+	+	+	+	+
Insol	Insol	Insol	Insol	Insol	Insol	Insol	Insol	Insol	Insol
−	V	V	NR	−	NR	NR	−	−	NR
−	−	−	−	−	−	−	−	−	NR
−	+	−	+	−	−	NR	NR	NR	NR
+	NR	NR	NR	+	NR	V	+	−	NR
S	S	S	S	S	S	S	S	S	S
Rare	Rare	Rare	Rare	Rare	No	No	No	No	No

[g]Enterococci **do not** contain cytochromes. At times, a pseudocatalase is produced (33, 37) that gives a weak catalase reaction.

[h]Some strains of *E. faecalis* are β-hemolytic on rabbit or horse blood but α on sheep blood.

[i]*E. avium* grows poorly if at all at 10°C (37, 38).

[j]Grows very slowly; may require 7–10 days of incubation (33).

[k]According to Murray et al. (33), **presumptive** identification of *Enterococcus* by the bile esculin reaction and growth in 6.5% NaCl is erroneous since strains of *Lactococcus, Leuconostoc,* and *Pediococcus* isolated from human infections may also be positive for bile esculin and growth in NaCl.

[l]PYR is a **presumptive** test for group D enterococci (16) and group A streptococci; it replaces the bacitracin test and salt tolerance for group A streptococci and *Enterococcus* species, respectively. However, some *Lactococcus, Aerococcus, Gamella,* and staphylococci are also PYR positive.

[m]Genetic elements that confer inducible resistance to vancomycin are present in both *E. faecalis* and *E. faecium* (6, 15, 18, 27, 30–32, 46).

[n]Most commonly isolated enterococcal species from human infections; 80–90% (32).

[o]Second most common isolate from human infections; 10–15% (32).

GENUS: *ERYSIPELOTHRIX* (19, 26, 30)

Gram-positive short rods; easily decolorized; slender nonbranching rods, straight or slightly curved; tendency to form long filaments. Old cultures may be Gram negative.
Nonsporeforming
Aerobic to facultative anaerobic; microaerophilic especially on initial isolation
Catalase negative
Nonencapsulated
Nonmotile (22°C)
Oxidase negative
Coagulase positive
O/F glucose: weakly F (fermentative)
Optimal growth temperature 30–37°C
Not acid-fast
Narrow-zone alpha (α) hemolysis on blood agar (BA); **no β-hemolysis**
No mycolic acid in cells
Veterinary pathogen
2 species: *E. rhusiopathiae, E. tonsillarum*
Type species: *E. rhusiopathiae* ATCC 19414
 Alpha (α) hemolysis on sheep blood agar (SBA) after prolonged incubation

H_2S (TSI) positive; most significant biochemical test; may vary with medium used; best TSI; lead acetate (PbAc) **not** reliable. Only catalase-negative, Gram-positive, nonsporeforming rods that produce H_2S. *E. rhusiopathiae* is related to other Gram-positive organisms in *Bacillus-Clostridium* group (33). *E. rhusiopathiae* is distinguished from other Gram-positive rods such as *Listeria, Lactobacillus,* and *Corynebacterium* spp. by type of hemolysis, presence or absence of motility and catalase. *E. rhusiopathiae* is the only catalase-negative, Gram-positive, aerobic bacillus to produce H_2S (TSI/KIA).

A second species, *E. tonsillarum,* from swine, described by Takahashi et al. (43), differentiated primarily by DNA-DNA homology, differs by ability to ferment sucrose.

Table 43.22. Characteristics of *Erysipelothrix rhusiopathiae*

β-hemolysis	—		
$NO_3 \rightarrow NO_2$	—	Esculin	—
Glucose	V	Gelatin liquefaction, 22°C	—
Lactose	A	Urease	—
Maltose	—		
Mannose	—		
Sucrose	—		
Xylose	—		

V, variable reactions; V⁺, variable, usually positive; A, acid production.

GENUS: *EUBACTERIUM* (19, 26, 30, 40)

Gram-positive pleomorphic rods in young cultures. Rods irregular in size appearing as cocci to long rods with swollen or tapered ends; occasionally curved. Arranged singly, in pairs, and chains. *E. nodatum* exhibits beading filaments and branching.
Nonsporeforming
Obligate (strict) anaerobes
Catalase negative; occasional strain of *E. lentum* is catalase positive
Nonencapsulated
Motility variable; peritrichous flagella
O/F glucose: F (fermentative)
Optimal growth temperature 37°C

51 species: *E. acidaminophilum, E. aerofaciens, E. angustum, E. barkeri, E. biforme, E. brachy, E. budayi, E. callanderi, E. cellulosolvens, E. combesii, E. contortum, E. coprostanoligenes, E. cylindroides, E. desmotans, E. dolichum, E. eligens, E. exiguum, E. fissicatena, E. formicigenerans, E. fossor, E. hadrum, E. hallii, E. infirmum, E. lentum, E. limosum, E. minutum, E. moniliforme, E. multiforme, E. nitritogenes, E. nodatum, E. oxidoreducens, E. plautii, E. plexicaudatum, E. ramulus, E. rectale, E. ruminantium, E. saburreum, E. saphenum, E. siraeum, E. tarantellae, E. tardum, E. tenue, E. timidum, E. tortuosum, E. uniforme, E. ventriosum, E. xylanophilum, E. yurii, E. yurii* subsp. *margaretiae, E. yurii* subsp. *schtitka, E. yurii* subsp. *yurii*

Type species: *E. limosum* ATCC 8486, NCIB 9763

Poorly sporing strains of *Clostridium* are readily confused with *Eubacterium* spp. (26).

Easily confused with other anaerobic Gram-positive rods; gas liquid chromatography of metabolic end products useful in differentiation.

Table 43.23. Differentiation of *Eubacterium* Species That May Cause Human Infections[a]

Test	*E. aerofaciens*[b]	*E. biforme*	*E. brachy*[c,d]	*E. combesii*[d]	*E. contortum*	*E. cylindroides*[e]	*E. dolichum*[d,f]	*E. eligens*	*E. formicigenerans*	*E. hadrum*
Butyrate produced	−	+	+	+	−	+	+	−	−	+
NO$_3$→NO$_2$	−	−	+	−	−	−	−	−	−	−
H$_2$S (SIM)	−	NR	NR	V	NR	NR	NR	−	NR	NR
Motility	−	−	−	NR	−	−	NR	+	−	−
Indole	−	−	−	−	−	−	−	−	−	−
Esculin hydrolysis	V	V	+	V	+	+	−	V⁻	−	V⁺
Starch hydrolysis	−	−	V⁻	NR	−	V	NR	−	−	−
Gelatin digestion	−	−	−	+	−	−	V⁻ʷ	V⁻ʷ	−	−

V, variable result; V⁺, variable, usually positive; V⁻, variable, usually negative; w, weak reaction; SIM, sulfide-indole-motility medium. Data from reference 30.

[a]Genus divided into 3 groups: (a) butyric acid producers, (b) nonproducers of butyric acid, and (c) little or no fatty acids produced. *Eubacterium* spp. are easily confused with other anaerobic Gram-positive rods; gas liquid chromotographic analysis of metabolic end products useful in differentiation (23, 24).

[b]*E. aerofaciens* on isolation often appear as pleomorphic cocci to short rods and may be confused with anaerobic streptococci or lactobacilli (40). Three phenotypic groups of *E. aerofaciens* are isolated from feces: *E. aerofaciens* II strains that do not ferment sucrose and *E. aerofaciens* III that do not ferment cellobiose and produce little or no acid in salicin (31).

[c]*E. brachy* resembles *Peptostreptococcus anaerobius* because of short cells in chains; does not grow well on usual isolation media (30). Lecithinase produced.

(continued)

	E. hallii	E. lentum[d]	E. limosum	E. moniliforme[g]	E. nitritogenes[g]	E. nodatum[d,h]	E. ramulus	E. rectale	E. saburreum	E. siraeum	E. tenue	E. timidum	E. tortuosum	E. ventriosum
	+	−	+	+	+	+	+	+	+	−	−	−	+	+
	−	+	−	V	+	−	−	−	−	−	−	−	V	−
	−	−[i]	V	+	NR	−	NR	−	−	NR	+	NR	−	−
	−	NR	−	+	−	−	−	V	−	V−	V+	NR	−	−
	−	−	−	−	−	−	−	−	+	−	+	NR	−	−
	−	−	+	−	+	−	+	+	+	V+	−	−	+	+
	−	NR	V−	−	−	NR	−	+	−	V+	−	NR	−	−
	−	−	V	V−w	V−w	−	−	−	−	−	+	−	−	−

[d]Nonsaccharoclastic.

[e]Easily decolorized and may be confused with *Fusobacterium prausnitzii*; differentiated in that *E. cylindroides* produces acid (<pH 5.5) in mannose, usually from glucose and fructose, and at times from salicin and sucrose; *F. prausnitizii* does not lower pH in these sugar media below pH 5.5.

[f]Fails to grow on blood agar plates.

[g]Lecithinase may be produced.

[h]Morphologically, *E. nodatum* resembles members of genus *Actinomyces* (40).

[i]H_2S (SIM)-negative; TSI, positive H_2S in butt.

GENUS: *EXIGUOBACTERIUM* (19)

Gram-positive cocci; coryneform bacteria
Nonsporeforming
Facultative anaerobic
Catalase positive
Nonencapsulated
Motile
Oxidase variable, usually positive
O/F glucose: F (fermentative)
Nitrate reduction variable
Esculin positive
Gelatin liquefaction variable, usually positive
Urease negative
Lactose negative
Mannose acid (+)
Maltose acid (+)
Sucrose acid (+)
Xylose negative
No mycolic acid in cell wall
2 species: *E. acetylicum* and *E. aurantiacum*
Type species: *E. aurantiacum* ATCC 35652, NCIB 11798

GENUS: *FALCIVIBRIO* (26, 40)

Gram-positive slender, curved rods of variable size and shape; may show clubbed or tapered ends. Arranged singly or in pairs; pairs show sickle configuration. Older cultures are Gram negative with Gram-positive granules.
Nonsporeforming
Anaerobic
Catalase negative
Nonencapsulated
Motile; polar, subpolar, or lateral flagella
Oxidase negative
O/F glucose: F (fermentative)
Optimal growth temperature 37°C
Weak greening (α) or weak β-hemolysis on blood agar (BA)
2 species
Type species: *F. grandis* ATCC 43064
Not included in *Bergey's Manual of Systematic Bacteriology*; proposed by Hammann et al. (22). Genus may be a later synonym of *Mobiluncus*.

Table 43.24. Biochemical Characteristics of *Falcivibrio* spp.

Test	E. grandis	E. vaginalis
$NO_3 \rightarrow NO_2$	—	V
Esculin hydrolysis	—	—
Carbohydrates[a]		
Galactose	A	—
Glucose	A	—
Fructose	A	—
Maltose	A	—
Ribose	A	—
Starch	A	—
D-Xylose	A	—

A, acid production (+); V, variable reaction, usually positive.
[a]Acid production in carbohydrates often weak.

GENUS: *GARDNERELLA* (26, 40)

Gram-positive, Gram-negative **pleomorphic** rods
Nonsporeforming
Facultative anaerobes
Catalase negative
Nonencapsulated
Nonmotile
Oxidase negative
O/F glucose: F (fermentative)
Optimal growth temperature 35–37°C
Human blood but **not** sheep blood hemolyzed
Not acid-fast
Single species: *G. vaginalis* ATCC 14018; NCTC 10287

Table 43.25. Biochemical Characteristics of *Gardnerella vaginalis*

Nitrate reduction	—	H_2S	—
Hippurate hydrolysis	+	Indole	—
Starch hydrolysis	+	Lysine	—
ONPG	V	Phenylalanine	—
Methyl red (MR)	+	Ornithine	—
Arginine dihydrolase	—	Tween 80	—
Esculin hydrolysis	—	Urease	—
Gelatin liquefaction	—	Voges-Proskauer (VP)	—
Carbohydrates			
L-Arabinose	A	Mannitol	—
Cellobiose	—	Mannose	A
Dextrin	A	Melibiose	—
Fructose	A	Raffinose	—
Galactose	A	Ribose	A
Inositol	—	Rhamnose	—
Inulin	A	Salicin	—
Lactose	A	Sucrose	A
Maltose	A	Xylose	A

A, acid production (+); V, variable reaction.

GENUS: *GEMELLA* (26, 33, 40)

Gram-positive or **Gram-variable** (easily decolorized) spherical or elongated cells; often in pairs (diplococci) with flattened adjacent sides or in pairs of unequal size. Resemble *Neisseria* spp. in morphology when Gram negative.
Nonsporeforming
Facultative anaerobes
Catalase negative
Nonencapsulated
Nonmotile
Oxidase negative
O/F glucose: F (fermentative)
Optimum growth temperature 37°C; *no growth* at 10° and 45°C.
2 species
Type species: *G. haemolysans* ATCC 10379, NCTC 5414
Often confused with species within *Neisseria*, *Veillonella*, and *Streptococcus* genera.

Table 43.26. Differentiation of *Gemella* species

Tests	*G. haemolysans*	*G. morbillorum*
10°C	NG	NG
45°C	NG	NG
6.5% NaCl	G	G
Esculin	−	−
PYR	+	+wa
LAP	−	V
Vancomycin (30 μg)	S	S

NG, no growth; G, growth; V, variable results; +w, weakly positive; S, sensitive (susceptible); LAP, leucine aminopeptidase; PYR, pyrrolidonylarylamidase.
aAccording to Facklam and Washington (17), to avoid a false-negative PYR result, a large inoculum **must be used.**

GENUS: *GLOBICATELLA* (19)

Gram-positive cocci arranged in pairs and chains
Nonsporeforming
Facultative anaerobe
Catalase negative
Nonencapsulated
6.5% NaCl: variable growth
10°C: no growth
45°C: variable growth
LAP negative
PYR positive
Bile esculin: variable growth
Vancomycin: S (sensitive)
Single species: *G. sanguis* ATCC 51173, NCFB 2835
Resembles viridans streptococci

GENUS: *GORDONIA* (26, 40)

Gram-positive or Gram-variable short rods or cocci; may appear as coccobacilli
Filamentous bacteria that can fragment into rods and cocci (19)
Nonsporeforming
Aerobic
Catalase positive
Nonmotile

Nitrate reduction positive
Urease positive
Usually partially acid-fast
Possess mycolic acid in cells
8 species: G. aichiensis, G. amarae, G. bronchialis, G. hirsuta, G. hydrophobica, G. rubropertinctus, G. sputi, G. terrae
Type species: G. bronchialis ATCC 25592, NCTC 10667
Genus not included in Bergey's Manual of Systematic Bacteriology; genus reintroduced by Stackebrandt et al. (42).

GENUS: *HELCOCOCCUS* (19)
Gram-positive cocci; may appear as coccobacilli; arranged in chains and clusters
Nonsporeforming
Facultative anaerobic
Catalase negative
Nonencapsulated
6.5% NaCl: growth
10°C: no growth
45°C: no growth
LAP negative
PYR positive
Bile esculin: growth
Single species: H. kunzii NCFB 2900, DSM 1054
Resembles viridans streptococci

GENUS: *JONESIA* (26, 40)
Gram-positive irregular, slender rods arranged singly or **branched Y and clublike forms.** Older cultures readily decolorize and appear filamentous or coccoid; coccoid forms always stain Gram positive
Nonsporeforming
Facultative anaerobic
Catalase positive
Nonencapsulated
Motile by peritrichous flagella
Oxidase negative
O/F glucose: F (fermentative)
Optimal growth temperature 30°C
Not acid-fast
Single species: J. denitrificans ATCC 14870; formerly Listeria denitrificans; not in Bergey's Manual of Systematic Bacteriology; created by Rocourt et al. (34)

Table 43.27. Biochemical Characteristics of *Jonesia denitrificans*

Nitrate reduction	+	Hippurate hydrolysis	Weakly + or −
5% NaCL	Growth	Methyl red (MR)	+
10% NaCL	Growth	Voges-Proskauer (VP)	−
Gelatin liquefaction	−	Starch hydrolysis	+

GENUS: *KURTHIA* (26, 33, 40)
Gram-positive nonbranched rods with rounded ends. Arranged in **long chains,** often parallel in young cultures. May exhibit long parallel chains of rods in loops and whorls giving characteristic "Medusa-head" appearance. Older cultures (>3 days), coccoid cells

Nonsporeforming
Strict (obligate) aerobes
Catalase positive
Nonencapsulated
Motility usually positive at 20–25°C; occasional nonmotile strains; peritrichous flagella
Oxidase negative
O/F glucose: NF (nonfermentative)
Optimal growth temperature 25–30°C
Not acid-fast
No mycolic acid in cells
May exhibit H_2S in TSI butt (19)
Characteristic "bird-feather" growth on nutrient gelatin slants
Rarely implicated in human infections; however, resemble *Bacillus* spp.
3 species
Type species: *K. zopfii* ATCC 33403, NCTC 10597, NCIB 9878

Table 43.28. Differentiation of *Kurthia* spp.

Test	*K. gibsonii*	*K. sibirica*	*K. zopfii*
Colonies cream-colored or yellow	G	NG	NG
Growth at 45°C	G	NG	G
Growth in 7.5% NaCl	G	G	NG
$NO_3 \rightarrow NO_2$	−	−	−
Esculin	−	−	−
Gelatin liquefaction, 22°C[a]	−	−	−
Phosphatase	+	+	−

G, growth; NG, no growth.

[a]Concentration and brand of gelatin used for nutrient gelatin slants are important; not all brands permit typical outgrowth (40).

Meat extract (Lab Lemco powder, Oxoid)	4.0 g
Peptone (Difco)	5.0 g
Yeast extract (Difco)	2.5 g
NaCl	5.0 g
Gelatin (BDH)	100 g
Distilled water	1 L
pH	7.0
Sterilize	115°C, 30 min for quantities up to 100 mL

Inoculate with reference strain *K. zopfii*, NCIB 9878

GENUS; *LACTOBACILLUS* (26, 33, 40)

Gram-positive **long slender rods** (bacilli); some short coccobacilli or spiral forms (coryneform coccobacilli) commonly in short chains or singly. Some strains exhibit bipolar bodies, internal granulations, or a bearded appearance.
Nonsporeforming
Facultative or strict (obligate) anaerobes; 20% are obligate anaerobes; occasionally microaerophilic. Grow poorly in air; enhanced growth with reduced oxygen tension. Isolation of some anaerobes enhanced by carbon dioxide (CO_2).
Catalase and cytochrome negative; some positive strains (26)
Nonencapsulated
Nitrate reduction negative; occasionally positive, but only when terminal pH is >6.0 (40).
Motility rare; peritrichous flagella
O/F glucose: F (fermentative)
Optimal growth temperature 30–40°C

Rarely pathogenic; identification to species level difficult and given low pathogenicity, rarely indicated; however, resemble catalase-negative Gram- positive coccoid organisms

80 species: *L. acetotolerans, L. acidophilus, L. agilis, L. alimentarius, L. amylophilus, L. amylovorus, L. animalis, L. aviarius, L. aviarius* subsp. *araffinosus, L. aviarius* subsp. *aviarius, L. bifermentans, L. brevis, L. buchneri, L. casei, L. casei* subsp. *casei, L. catenaformis, L. cellobiosus, L. collinoides, L. coryniformis, L. coryniformis* subsp. *coryniformis, L. coryniformis* subsp. *torquens, L. crispatus, L. curvatus, L. curvatus* subsp. *curvatus, L. curvatus* subsp. *melibiosus, L. delbrueckii, L. delbrueckii* subsp. *bulgaricus, L. delbrueki* subsp. *dulbrueckii, L. delbrueckii* subsp. *lactis, L. farciminis, L. fermentum, L. fructivorans, L. fructosus, L. gallinarum, L. gasseri, L. graminis, L. hamsteri, L. helveticus, L. hilgardii, L. homohiochii, L. intestinalis, L. jensenii, L. johnsonii, L. kefiranofaciens, L. kefirgranum, L. kefiri, L. lindneri, L. malefermentans, L. mali, L. maltaromicus, L. murinus, L. oris, L. panis, L. parabuchneri, L. paracasei, L. paracaseii* subsp. *paracaseii, L. paracaseii* subsp. *tolerans, L. parakefir, L. paraplantarum, L. pentosus, L. plantarum, L. pontis, L. reuteri, L. rhamnosus, L. rogosae, L. ruminis, L. sakei, L. sakei* subsp. *carnosus, L. sakei* subsp. *sakei, L. salivarius, L. salivarius* subsp. *salicinius, L. salivarius* subsp. *salivarius, L. sanfranciscensis, L. sharpeae, L. suebicus, L. uli, L. vaccinostercus, L. vaginalis, L. vitulinus, L. zeae.*

Type species: *L. delbrueckii* subsp. *delbrueckii* ATCC 9649, NCIB 8130.

(See *Bergey's Manual of Systematic Bacteriology*, volume 2, for complete biochemical reactions.)

Table 43.29. Frequently Isolated *Lactobacillus* Species from Clinical Specimens

Test	*L. acidophilus*	*L. casei*	*L. plantarum*
β-Hemolysis	−	−	−
NO$_3$→NO$_2$	−	−	−
H$_2$S (TSI/KIA)	−	−	−
Growth 10°C	G	G	G
Growth 45°C	NG	G	V
Mannitol	−	A	V
Raffinose	V	−	A
Arginine	−	−	−
Esculin	−	−	−
Gelatin liquefaction, 22°C	−	−	−
Indole	−	−	−
PYR	−	−	−

NG, no growth; G, growth; V, variable reaction; A, acid production (+); PYR, pyrrolidonylarylamidase.

GENUS: *LACTOCOCCUS* (26)

Gram-positive spherical to ovoid cocci in pairs; arranged in short chains in liquid media
Nonsporeforming
Facultative anaerobes
Catalase negative
Nonencapsulated
Nonmotile
Oxidase negative
O/F glucose: F (fermentative)
Optimal growth temperature 30°C
Usually Lancefield group N
8 species: *L. garvieae, L. lactis, L. lactis* subsp. *cremoris, L. lactis* subsp. *hordniae, L. lactis* subsp. *lactis, L. piscium, L. plantarum, L. raffinolactis*
Type species: *L. lactis* subsp. *lactis* ATCC 19435, NCTC 6681, NCIB 668

Table 43.30. Differentiation of *Lactococcus* spp.

Test	*L. garviae*	*L. lactis* subsp. *cremoris*	*L. lactis* subsp. *holdniae*	*L. lactis* subsp. *lactis*[a]	*L. piscium*	*L. plantarum*	*L. raffinolactis*
Hemolysis, 5% SBA	α	α	α	α	α	α	α
Growth[b] at							
10°C	G	G	G	G	G	G	G
40°C	G	NG	NG	V+	NG	NG	NG
45°C[c]	NG	NG	NG	NG	NG	NG	NG
Growth in							
0.5% NaCl	NG	NG	NG	NG	NG	NG	NG
4.0% NaCl	G	NG	NG	G	NR	G	NG
Lactose	A	A	—	A	A	—	A
Mannitol	V+	—	—	V−	A	A	V
Raffinose	—	—	—	—	A	—	A
Arginine	+	—	+	+	—	—	V−
Bile esculin	+	+	+	+	+	+	+
LAP	+	+	+	+	+	+	+
PYR	+	+	+	+	+	+	+
Vancomycin (30 μg)	S	S	S	S	S	S	S

α, Alpha; G, growth; NG, no growth; NR, no results; SBA, sheep blood agar; V, variable results; V+, variable, usually positive; V−, variable, usually negative; A, acid production (+); S, sensitive (susceptible); LAP, leucine aminopeptidase; PYR, pyrrolidonylarylamidase.
Data from reference 26.
[a]*Streptococcus lactis* subsp. *diacetilactis* and *Lactobacillus xylosus* are synonymous with *Lactobacillus lactis* subsp. *lactis* (20).
[b]Recommend growth temperature tests to differentiate lactococci from streptococci and enterococci.
[c]Most strains will **not** growth at 45°C in ≤ 48 h (19).

GENUS: *LEUCONOSTOC* (26, 33, 40)

Gram-positive cocci that are **longer than broad when in characteristic pairs and chains**; occasionally short rods with rounded ends in long chains
Nonsporeforming
Facultative anaerobes
Catalase negative
Nonencapsulated
Nonmotile
O/F glucose: F (fermentative)
Optimal growth temperature 20–30°C
Slow growth; small colonies; slimy growth on sucrose-containing media
Resemble viridans streptococci morphologically
11 species: *L. argentinum, L. carnosum, L. citreum, L. fallax, L. gelidum, L. lactis, L. mesenteroides, L. mesenteroides* subsp. *cremoris, L. mesenteroides* subsp. *dextranicum, L. mesenteroides* subsp. *mesenteroides, L. pseudomesenteroides*
Type species: *L. pseudomesenteroides* subsp. *mesenteroides* ATCC 8293, NCIB 8023

Table 43.31. Differentiation of the Most Frequently Isolated *Leuconostoc* spp.

Test	*L. carnosum*	*L. citreum*	*L. gelidum*	*L. lactis*	*L. mesenteroides* subsp. *cremoris*	*L. mesenteroides* subsp. *dextranicum*	*L. mesenteroides* subsp. *mesenteroides*	*L. pseudomesenteroides*
Growth at 37°C	V	V	V−	G	NG	G	V	G
Pigmentation (lemon-yellow)	−	+	−	−	V−	−	+	−
NO₃→NO₂	−	−	−	−	−	−	−	−
Hemolysis 5% SBA	γ	γ	γ	γ	γ	γ	γ	γ
Arabinose	−	A	A	−	−	−	A	V
Fructose	A	A	A	A	−	A	A	A
Maltose	−	A	V	A	V	A	A	A
Melibiose	V−	−	A	V	V	A	A	V+
Salicin	−	A	A	V	−	V	V−	V
Sucrose	A	A	A	A	−	A	A	V
Trehalose	A	A	A	−	−	A	A	A
Arginine	−	−	−	−	−	−	−	−
Indole	−	−	−	−	−	−	−	−
Esculin	V	+	+	−	−	V	V	V
LAP	−	−	−	−	−	−	−	−
PYR	−	−	−	−	−	−	−	−
Vancomycin (30 μg)	R	R	R	R	R	R	R	R

V, variable reactions; V+, variable, usually positive; V−, variable, usually negative; G, growth, A, acid production (+); R, resistant; LAP, leucine aminopeptidase; PYR, pyrrolidonylamidase; NR, no result; γ, gamma (no) hemolysis.
Data from references 26 and 33.

GENUS: *LISTERIA* (26, 33, 40)

Gram-positive, short, nonbranching rods with rounded ends; somewhat smaller than most Gram-positive bacilli. Older cells are Gram variable. May appear coccoid. Arranged singly and in short chains; rarely long filaments except in older cultures. May be arranged in pairs that cause confusion with *Streptococcus pneumoniae*.
Nonsporeforming
Aerobic to facultative anaerobic
Catalase positive; cytochromes produced; rare strains negative (26)
Nonencapsulated
Motile when grown at 20–25°C (room temperature) in nutrient broth; characteristic end-over-end tumbling motility in wet mount; 5 peritrichous flagella
Oxidase negative
O/F glucose: F (fermentative) or O (oxidative)
Optimal growth temperature 30–37°C
Not acid-fast
Absence of mycolic acid in cells
8 species: *L. grayi, L. innocua, L. ivanovii, L. ivanovii* subsp. *ivanovii, L. ivanovii* subsp. *londoniensis, L. monocytogenes, L. seeligeri, L. welshimeri*
Type species: *L. monocytogenes* ATCC 15313, NCTC 10357 (not hemolytic)
  Colonies bluish gray by normal illumination and on nutrient agar, characteristic blue-green sheen under oblique transmitted light
  L. monocytogenes: **narrow-zone β-hemolysis and positive CAMP test.** *L. monocytogenes* differentiated from group B streptococci (*S. agalactiae*) by positive catalase and positive esculin

hydrolysis. Only *L. monocytogenes* causes infection in humans (33); *L. ivanovii* causes occasional abortion in animals; questionable in humans. Other species are nonpathogenic. Proposed that *L. monocytogenes* and *L. ivanovii* be considered CAMP positive with *R. equi* (exhibiting circular or racket and semicircular or shovel shapes respectively).

Table 43.32. Differentiation of *Listeria* spp.[a]

Test	*L. grayi*[b]	*L. innocua*	*L. ivanovii*[c]	*L. monocytogenes*[d]	*L. seeligeri*	*L. welshimeri*
Catalase	+	+	+	+	+	+
β-Hemolysis, 5% SBA	−	−	+[e]	+[f,g]	+[wf]	−
CAMP w/*S. aureus*[h]	−	−	−	+	+	−
CAMP w/*R. equi*[h]	−	−	+	−	−	−
H$_2$S/TSI	−	−	−	−	−	−
H$_2$S PbAc[i]	+[j]	−	−	−	−	−
Nitrate reduction	−	−	−	−	NR	NR
Carbohydrates						
Glucose	A	A	A	A	A	A
Lactose	A	A	A	V	NR	NR
Mannitol	A	−	−	−	−	−
α-Methyl-D-mannoside	A	A	−[c]	A	−	A
Ribose	V	−	A[c]	−	−	−
Rhamnose	−	V	−	A	−	V
Soluble starch	+	−	−	−	NR	NR
Xylose	−	−	A	−	A	A
Misc. tests						
Esculin hydrolysis[k]	+	+	+	+	+	+
Gelatin liquefaction, 22°C	−	−	−	−	−	−
Hippurate hydrolysis	−	+	+	+	NR	NR
Indole	−	−	−	−	−	−
Methyl red (MR)	+	+	+	+	+	+
Urease	−	−	−	−	−	−
Voges-Proskauer (VP)	+	+	+	+	+	+
Pathogenicity for mice	−	−	+	+	−	−

+[w], weakly positive; A, acid production (+); V, variable results; NR, no results.
Data from references 26, 33, 40.

[a]*Listeria* spp. are often confused with *Bronchothrix*, *Erysipelothrix*, *Lactobacillus* and *Kurthia* (49); *Listeria denitrificans* was transferred to genus *Jonesia*, *Jonesia denitrificans*.
[b]*L. grayi* and *L. murrayi* are combined into a single species, *L. grayi*.
[c]*L. ivanovii* separated into *L. ivanovii* and *L. ivanovii* subsp. *londoniensis*; separated by two carbohydrates; *L. ivanovii* is ribose positive (A) and mannosamine negative (−); *L. ivanovii* subsp. *londoniensis* is ribose negative (−) and mannosamine positive (A).
[d]Only species pathogenic for humans; however, must identify to species because all species can contaminate foods, but only *L. monocytogenes* is a public health concern.
[e]Wide or multiple zones.
[f]Narrow zones.
[g]Occasional strains are negative for beta-hemolysis.
[h]CAMP test with *Staphylococcus aureus* and *Rhodococcus equi*.
[i]Lead acetate test is more sensitive than TSI medium for H$_2$S detection.
[j]Small amount.
[k]Positive result within a few hours.

GENUS: *MICROBACTERIUM* (26, 33)

Gram-positive slender, irregular rods in young cultures; arranged singly or pairs with some arranged at angle to give a V formation.
Nonsporeforming
Aerobic; weak anaerobic growth possible
Catalase positive
Nonencapsulated
Motility variable, usually negative; if positive, 1–3 flagella. **Only** orange-pigmented species *M. imperiale* and *M. arborescens* are motile at 28°C (19).
O/F glucose: O (oxidative) or F (weakly fermentative)
Optimal growth temperature 30°C
Not acid-fast
Absence of mycolic acid in cells
CAMP variable; **occasionally** *M. arborescens* is CAMP positive (19)
Esculin positive, but may be delayed
6 species: *M. arborescens, M. aurum, M. dextranolyticum, M. imperiale, M. lacticum, M. laevaniformans*
Type species: *M. lacticum* ATCC 8180, NCIB 8540

Table 43.33. Differentiation of Some *Microbacterium* spp.

Tests	*M. arborescens*	*M. imperiale*	*M. lacticum*	*M. laevaniformans*
NO$_3$→NO$_2$	−	−	+	−
H$_2$S	+	−	−	+
DNase	+	+	+	+
Arabinose	A^w	A	−	−
Sucrose	A^w	A	−	A
Xylose	A^w	V	−	−

A, acid production (+); A^w, weakly acidic.

GENUS: *MICROCOCCUS* (26, 33, 40)

Gram-positive cocci arranged in **pairs, tetrads, or irregular clusters; not in chains**
Nonsporeforming
Strict (obligate) aerobes
Catalase positive
Nonencapsulated
Nonmotile
Oxidase variable; usually positive but weak
O/F glucose: O (oxidative)
Optimal growth temperature 25–37°C
Red-yellow pigmented colonies variable
Resistant to lysostaphin
2 species
Type species: *Micrococcus luteus* ATCC 4698, NCIB 9278, NCTC 2665

Table 43.34. Differentiation of *Micrococcus* spp.

Test	M. luteus	M. lylae		M. luteus	M. lylae
Catalase	+	+	Acid aerobically from		
Hemolysis, 5% SBA	γ	γ	Glucose	−	−
Pigmentation, 5% SBA	Yellow	Cream-White	Glycerol	−	−
Oxidase	+	+	Lactose	−	−
			Galactose	−	−
$NO_3 \rightarrow NO_2$	−	−	Mannose	−	−
Growth 37°C	G	G	Arginine dehydrolase	−	−
Growth on			Citrate (Simmons)	−	−
6.5% NaCl	G	G	ONPG	−	−
7.5% NaCl	G	G	Esculine hydrolysis	−	−
10% NaCl	V	V	Gelatin liquefaction	+	+
			Motility	−	−
			Lysozyme	S	RS
			Bacitracin (0.04 U)[a]	S	S

γ, Gamma (no hemolysis); SBA, sheep blood agar; V, variable results; G, growth; S, sensitive; RS, slightly resistant; U, units.
Data from references 26, 33, 40.
[a]Susceptibility to bacitran ≥ 10 mm.

GENUS: *MOBILUNCUS* (26, 41)

Gram variable, slender, curved rods with tapered ends. Gram variable or Gram negative, but cell wall is Gram-positive type. Variable in shape and size and arranged singly, but at times in **pairs with gullwing appearance.**
Nonsporeforming
Anaerobic
Nonencapsulated
Catalase negative
Motile by multilateral or subpolar flagella
Oxidase negative
O/F glucose: F (fermentative); weak
Optimal growth temperature 37°C
Presence of mycolic acid in cells; largest and most complex (C_{60}–C_{90})
4 species: *M. curtisii*, *M. curtisii* subsp. *curtisii*, *M. curtisii* subsp. *holmesii*, *M. mulieris*
Type species: *M. curtisii* subsp. *curtisii* ATCC 35241
Not in *Bergey's Manual of Systematic Bacteriology*; established by Spiegel and Roberts (41); **genus** may be a synonym of *Falcivibrio* (41).

Table 43.35. Differentiation of *Mobiluncus* spp.

Test	M. curtisii subsp. *curtisii*	M. curtisii subsp. *holmesii*	*M. mulieris*
$NO_3 \rightarrow NO_2$	−	+	−
H_2S	−	−	−
Glucose	A^w	V^{-vw}	V
Fructose	V^{vw}	V^{vw}	V
Lactose	V^{vw}	−	V^{-vw}
Maltose	A^w	V^{-vw}	A
Mannitol	−	−	−
Ribose	−	−	V^w
Starch	−	V^{vw}	V
Arginine-NH	+	+	−
Esculin hydrolysis	−	−	−
Hippurate hydrolysis	+	+	−
Indole	−	−	−
Starch hydrolysis	+	+	+

A, acid production (+); w, if positive, weak reaction; vw, if positive, very weak reaction; V, variable results; V$^−$, variable, usually negative.

GENUS: *MYCOBACTERIUM* (26, 33, 40)

Gram-positive slender rods, straight or slightly curved. **Not readily stained by Gram stain; weakly positive, but not usually performed.** Sometimes exhibits **branching filaments or mycelium-like growth only visible by magnification.**
Nonsporeforming
Aerobic; slow growing, 2–60 days
Catalase positive
Nonencapsulated
Nonmotile
O/F glucose: O (oxidative)
Optimal growth temperature 30–45°C
Acid-fast
83 species
Some species are fastidious and require special supplements for growth (e.g., *M. paratuberculosis*) or noncultivable on routine mycobacteria media (e.g., *M. leprae*)
Type species: *M. tuberculosis* ATCC 27294
(*Note:* The cultivation and identification of mycobacteria are not routine in most laboratories; they are usually done in larger laboratories (e.g., public health laboratories). Identification to species requires extensive biochemical testing. See *Bergey's Manual of Systematic Bacteriology*, volume 2, for species and identification tests.)

GENUS: *NOCARDIA* (26, 40)

Gram-positive to Gram-variable rods; may be coccoid
Mycelium production and **aerial hyphae**; some branching filaments. Bacteria can fragment into rods and cocci (19).
Nonsporeforming
Obligate (strict) aerobes; mesophilic
Catalase positive
O/F glucose: O (oxidative)
Nonmotile
Acid-fastness variable, usually positive
Nitrate variable
Presence of mycolic acid in cells

14 species: N. asteroides, N. brasiliensis, N. brevicatena, N. carnea, N. coeliaca, N. corynebacterioides, N. farcinica, N. globerula, N. nova, N. otitidiscaviarum, N. pseudobrasiliensis, N. seriolae, N. transvalensis, N. vaccinii

Type species: N. asteroides ATCC 19247

Table 43.36. Biochemical Characteristics of the Most Frequently Isolated Nocardia spp.

Test	N. asteroides	N. brasiliensis	N. farcinia	N. nova	N. otitidiscaviarum	N. transvalensis
42°C[a]	V+	NG	G	NG	V+	G
Casein hydrolysis	−	+	−	−	−	V−
Tyrosine hydrolysis	−	+	−	−	+	V−
Xanthine hydrolysis	−	−	−	−	−	V+
Rhamnose	V−	−	V+	−	−	−
Arylsulfatase[b]	−	−	−	+	−	+
Gelatin hydrolysis	−	+	−	−	−	−

G, growth; NG, no growth; V, variable reaction, usually positive; V, variable reaction, usually negative.
Data from reference 19.
[a]After 3-day incubation.
[b]After 14-day incubation.

GENUS: *OERSKOVIA* (26, 40)

Oerskovia species have been moved to the genus Cellulomonas and genus Oerskovia eliminated.

GENUS: *PAENIBACILLUS* (19)

Gram-positive rods
Sporeforming; spores swell sporangia
Aerobic

26 species: P. aliginolyticus, P. alvei, P. amylolyticus, P. apiarius, P. azotofixans, P. campinasensis, P. chibensis, P. chondroitinus, P. curdlamolyticus, P. denitritiformis, P. glucanolyticus, P. illinoisensis, P. kobensis, P. larvae, P. larvae subsp. larvae, P. larvae subsp. pulvifaciens, P. lautus, P. lentimorbus, P. macerans, P. macquariensis, P. pabuli, P. peoriae, P. polymyxa, P. popilliae, P. thiaminolyticus, P. validus

Type species: P. polymyxa ATCC 842, CCM 1459, NCTC 10343

Table 43.37. Biochemical Characteristics of the Most Frequently Encountered Paenibacillus spp.

Tests	P. alvei	P. macerans	P. polymyxa
Anaerobic	G	G	G
Glucose	−	A	A
Mannitol	−	A	V
Xylose	−	A	A
Citrate	−	−	−
Indole	+	−	−
Lecithinase	−	−	−/w[a]

A, acid production (+); G, growth; V, variable reaction.
[a]Weak; only visible under colonies.

GENUS: *PEDIOCOCCUS* (26, 33, 40)

Gram-positive cocci; arranged in pairs or tetrads; **never elongated**

Nonsporeforming

Facultative anaerobes

Usually catalase negative; cytochromes absent

Nonencapsulated

Nonmotile

O/F glucose: F (fermentative)

Optimal growth temperature 25–40°C

6.5% NaCl: variable growth

No growth at 10° and 45°C

LAP positive

PYR negative

Bile esculin positive

Nonpathogenic for humans; often confused with micrococci; morphologically similar. **Most commonly isolated species are arginine positive.**

7 species: *P. acidilactici, P. damnosus, P. dextrinicus, P. inopinatus, P. parvulus, P. pentosaceus, P. urinaeequi*

Type species: *P. damnosus* ATCC 29358, NCDO 1832

Table 43.38. Differentiation of *Pediococcus* spp.

Test	P. acidilactici	P. damnosus	P. dextrinicus	P. inopinatus	P. parvulus	P. pento saceus	P. urinaeequi
Catalase	+	−	−	−	−	+	−
NO$_3$→NO$_2$	−	−	−	−	−	−	−
Growth at							
10°C	NG	NG	NG	NG	NG	NG	NG
35°C	G	NG	G	G	G	G	G
40°C	G	NG	G	NG	NG	G	G
50°C	G	NG	NG	NG	NG	NG	NG
Growth at							
pH 4.2	G	G	NG	NG	G	G	NG
pH 7.5	G	NG	G	V	G	G	G
pH 8.5	V	NG	NG	NG	NG	V	G
Growth with							
4% NaCl	G	NG	G	G	G	G	G
6.5% NaCl	G	NG	NG	V	G	G	G
18% NaCl	NG	NG	NG	NG	NG	NG	NG
L-Arabinose	V	−	−	−	−	A	V
Dextran	−	−	A	V	−	−	A
Glycerol	−	−	−	−	−	−	−
Starch	A	−	A	−	−	−	−
Indole	−	−	−	−	−	−	−
Arginine	+	−	−	−	−	+	−
Esculin hydrolysis	+	+	+	+	+	+	+
Hippurate hydrolysis	−	−	−	−	−	−	−
LAP	+	+	+	+	+	+	+
PYR	−	−	−	−	−	−	−
Vancomycin (30 µg)	R	R	R	R	R	R	R

G, growth; NG, no growth; V, variable results; A, acid production (+), LAP, leucine aminopeptidase; PYR, pyrrolidonylarylamidase; R, resistant.
Data from references 26, 40.

GENUS: *PEPTOCOCCUS* (26, 33, 40)

Gram-positive spherical cocci arranged in pairs, tetrads, clumps, irregular masses, or short chains

Nonsporeforming

Strict (obligate) anaerobes

Catalase usually negative; may be weakly positive

Nonencapsulated

Nonmotile

O/F glucose: F (weakly fermentative) or − (inert)

Optimal growth temperature 37°C

Indole negative

Nitrate not reduced

Coagulase negative

Esculin negative

Starch negative

Urease negative

Carbohydrates not attacked

H_2S produced from peptones (sulfide-indole-motility medium)

Requires nutritionally enriched media

Black pigmentation on blood agar; may vary from black to olive green to a mustard color. Pigmentation may not be visible by the naked eye; use dissecting microscope. Pigmentation fades quickly when exposed to air. Weak or older colonies exhibit a mustard color.

1 species: *P. niger* ATCC 27731. Rarely recovered from human sources (86)

P. niger differentiated from *Peptostreptococcus* spp. by black pigmentation and catalase reaction

GENUS: *PEPTOSTREPTOCOCCUS* (26, 33, 40)

Gram-positive or Gram-variable cocci that are occasionally ovoid in shape with variable arrangement: **pairs, tetrads, clumps, or chains**

Young cells of *P. anaerobius* are elongated in chains (33). *P. productus* cells may be elongated; resemble coccobacilli (33). *P. vaginalis, P. lacrimalis, P. lactolyticus,* and *P. hydrogenalis,* short chains or masses

Nonsporeforming

Anaerobes

Catalase negative; few strains weak or produce *pseudocatalase* reactions (e.g., *P. asaccharolyticus*)

Nonencapsulated

Nonmotile

O/F glucose: F (fermentative)

Optimal growth temperature 37°C

Require nutritionally enriched media

16 species: *P. anaerobius, P. asaccharolyticus, P. barbesae, P. harei, P. heliotrinreducens, P. hydrogenalis, P. indolicus, P. ivorii, P. lacrimalis, P. lactolyticus, P. magnus, P. micros, P. octavius, P. prevotii, P. tetradius, P. vaginalis*

Type species: *P. anaerobius* ATCC 27337

Table 43.39. Differentiation of *Peptostreptococcus* spp. That May Cause Human Infections

Test	P. anaerobius[a,b]	P. asaccharolyticus[b,c]	P. hydrogenalis	P. indolicus	P. lacrimalis	P. lactolyticus	P. magnus[b]	P. micios	P. prevotii	P. tetradius	P. vaginalis
Catalase	−	V	NR	−	NR	NR	V	−	V	V	NR
Coagulase	−	−	−	+[d]	−	−	−	−	−	−	−
$NO_3 \rightarrow NO_2$	−	−	−	+[d]	−	−	−	−	V	−	−
Glucose	− or A[w]	−	A	−	−	A	− or A[w]	−	A[w]	A	A[w]
Lactose	−	−	−	−	−	A	−	−	−	−	−
Cellobiose	−	−	−	−	−	−	−	−	−	−	−
Maltose	− or A[w]	−	A	−	−	A	−	−	A[w] or −	A	A[w]
D-Mannose	−	−	NR	−	NR	NR	−	−	V	A	NR
Sucrose	− or A[w]	−	A	−	−	A	−	−	− or A[w]	A	NR
Indole	−	+[d]	−	+	−	−	−	−	−	−	−
Esculin	−	−	NR	−	NR	NR	−	−	− or +[w]	− or +[w]	NR
Urease	−	−	−	−	−	+	−	−	V	+	NR
Alkaline phosphatase	−	−	NR	+	NR	NR	V	+	+	−	NR
α-Glucosidase	+	−	NR	−	NR	NR	−	−	−	+[w]	NR
β-Glucuronidase	−	−	NR	−	NR	NR	−	−	−	+	NR
Ammonia from:											
Glutamate	−	+	NR	+	NR	NR	−	−	−	−	NR
Glycine	−	−	NR	−	NR	NR	+	+[w]	−	−	NR

V, variable results; NR, no results; A, acid production (+); A[w], weakly acid.
Data from references 26, 33, 40.
[a]*P. anaerobius* has pungently sweet odor (33).
[b]Most common (33): *P. mangus, P. anaerobius,* and *P. asaccharolyticus.*
[c]*P. asaccharolyticus* slight yellow pigmentation of blood agar (BA) (33).
[d]Occasional strains are negative.

GENUS: *PROPIONIBACTERIUM* (2, 26, 33, 40)

Gram-positive, short, straight, uniform or pleomorphic rods with rounded ends; "anaerobic diphtheroids." Slender branching in young cultures; in older cultures, short rods with one end rounded, other tapered or coccobacillary, may resemble streptococci. Stains less intensely; may have a beaded appearance. Arranged in pairs, in **Y and V configuration, parallel rows forming palisades, swollen spherical cells,** or **clumps with "Chinese character" arrangement**

Nonsporeforming
Obligate (strict) anaerobes; some strains aerotolerant but grow best anaerobically
Catalase variable; usually positive
Nonencapsulated
Nonmotile
Nitrate reduction variable
O/F glucose: F (fermentative)
Optimal growth temperature 30–37°C
CAMP positive: *P. acnes;* **CAMP variable:** *P. granulosum*
Not acid-fast
12 species: *P. acidipropionici, P. acnes, P. avidum, P. cyclohexanicum, P. freudenreichii, P. freudenreichii* subsp. *freudenreichii, P. freudenreichii* subsp. *shermanii, P. granulosum, P. jensenii, P. lymphophilum, P. propionicus, P. thoenii*
Type species: *P. freudenreichii* subsp. *freudenreichii* ATCC 6207, CCM 1857, NCTC 10470.

Table 43.40. Differential Characteristics of the Most Frequently Isolated *Propionibacterium* spp.

Test	P. propionicus[a]	P. acidipropionici	P. acnes	P. avidum	P. feundenreichii	P. granulosum	P. jensenii	P. lymphophilum	P. thoenii
Colony pigmentation	White-gray white	Cream-white-yellow	White-gray	White-cream	Cream-tan or pink	White-gray	Cream-white-pink	White	Orange-red-brown
Catalase	–	V+	V+	+	+	+	V+	V+	+
β-hemolysis 5% SBA	–	–	V	+	–	V–	–	–	+
NO$_3$ → NO$_2$	+	+	+	–	V	–	–	V–	–
Carbohydrates									
Amygdalin	V	–	–	–	–	V	V+	–	V+
L-Arabinose	–	A	–	V+	A	–	–	–	–
Cellobiose	–	A	–	–	–	–	V–	–	–
Glucose	A	A	A	A	A	A	A	A	A
Glycerol	V[b]	A	V+	A	A	A	A	–	A
Maltose	A	A	–	A	–	A	A	A	A
Mannitol	A	A	V–	V–	–	V+	A	V	–
Sucrose	A	A	–	A	–	A	A	–	A
Misc. tests									
Indole	–	–	+	–	–	–	–	–	–
Esculin hydrolysis	–	+	–	+	+	–	+	–	+
Gelatin liquefaction	V	–	+[c]	+[c]	–	–	–	–	–
CAMP w/*S. aureus*	–	–	+	–	–	+	–	–	–

V, variable results; V+, variable, usually positive; V–, variable, usually negative; SBA, sheep blood agar; A, acid production (+).

Data from references 26, 33, 40.

[a]Formerly *Actinomyces propionica* and later a single species in the genus *Arachnia*. Charfreitag, Collins, and Strackebrandt (5) recommend that the genus *Arachnia* be eliminated and the single species be transferred to genus *Propionibacterium* as *P. propionicus*

[b]Serovar 1 variable; serovar 2 usually negative.

[c]Strong.

GENUS: *RODOCOCCUS* (26, 40)

Gram-positive rods or cocci; rods to extensively branched vegetative **mycelium;** fragments of rods
Nonsporeforming
Aerobic
Catalase positive
Nonmotile
O/F glucose: NF (nonfermentative)
Nitrate reduction variable
Urease: variable
Presence of mycolic acid in cells
Usually partially acid-fast
12 species: *R. coprophilus, R. equi, R. erythropolis, R. fascians, R. globerulus, R. marinonascens, R. opacus, R. percolatus, R. rhodnii, R. rhodochrous, R. ruber, R. zopfii*
Type species: *R. rhodochrous* ATCC 13808, NCTC 10210
Closely related to *Corynebacterium, Mycobacterium,* and *Nocardia* spp.

GENUS: *ROTHIA* (26, 33, 40)

Gram-positive, evenly stained, irregular rods; irregular swelling and clubbed ends give a coccobacillar appearance; coryneform bacteria. May be filamentous rods with branching after several days of incubation in broth media
Nonsporeforming
Facultative anaerobes
Catalase positive
Nonmotile
O/F glucose: F (fermentative)
Optimal growth temperature 35–37°C
Presence of mycolic acids
Not acid-fast
1 species: *R. dentocariosa* ATCC 17931
Differentiate from *Nocardia* spp. by ability to ferment carbohydrates
CDC Group 4: *Rothia*-like microorganism: H_2S positive and gelatin liquefaction positive

Table 43.41. Biochemical Characteristics of *Rothia dentocariosa*

$NO_3 \rightarrow NO_2$	+	Esculin	+
Lactose	−	Gelatin liquefaction, 22°C	V
Maltose	A	Indole	−
Mannose	−	Urease	−
Sucrose	A	Voges-Proskauer (VP)	+
Xylose	−		

V, variable results; A, acid production (+).

GENUS: *SARCINA* (26)

Gram-positive cocci arranged **in cuboidal packets of eight or more;** some cells singly, pairs, and tetrads; usually flattened in areas that contact adjacent cells
Nonsporeforming
Strict (obligate) anaerobes
Catalase negative
Nonencapsulated
Nonmotile
O/F glucose: F (fermentative)
Optimal growth temperature 30–37°C
2 species
Type species: *S. ventriculii* ATCC 19633

Table 43.42. Differentiation of *Sarcina* spp.

Test	*S. ventriculii*	*S. maxima*
Cellulose formation	+	−
Ethanol production	+	−
Butyrate production	−	+
Melibiose	A	−
Xylose	−	A

A, acid production (+).

GENUS: *STAPHYLOCOCCUS* (26, 33, 40)

Gram-positive cocci arranged **singly, in pairs, or in irregular grapelike clusters**
Coagulase variable
Nonsporeforming
Facultative anaerobes (except *S. saccharolyticus* exhibits more rapid and abundant growth under aerobic conditions (40))
Catalase variable; usually positive (*S. aureus* subsp. *anaerobius* and *S. saccharolyticus* are catalase negative and usually only grow anaerobically)
Capsule variable; usually negative, but if present, limited capsule formation
Nonmotile
Oxidase variable; usually negative (*S. caseolyticus, S. lentus, S. sciuri,* and *S. vitulus* are modified oxidase positive)
O/F glucose: F (fermentative)
Optimal growth temperature 30–37°C
Susceptible to lysis by lysostaphin, but resistant to lysozyme
44 species: *S. arlettae, S. aureus* subsp. *anaerobius, S. aureus* subsp. *aureus, S. auricularis, S. capitis* subsp. *capitis, S. capitis* subsp. *ureolyticus, S. caprae, S. carnosus, S. caseolyticus, S. chromogenes, S. cohnii* subsp. *cohnii, S. cohnii* subsp. *urealyticum, S. delphini, S. epidermidis, S. equorum, S. felis, S. gallinarum, S. haemolyticus, S. hominis, S. hyicus, S. hyicus* subsp. *hyicus, S. intermedius, S. kloosii, S. lentus, S. lugdunensis, S. lutrae, S. muscae, S. pasteuri, S. piscifermentans, S. pulvereri, S. saccharolyticus, S. saprophyticus* subsp. *bovis, S. saprophyticus* subsp. *saprophyticus, S. schleiferi, S. schleiferi* subsp. *coagulans, S. schleiferi* subsp. *schleiferi, S. sciuri, S. sciuri* subsp. *carnaticus, S. sciuri* subsp. *rodentium, S. sciuri* subsp. *sciuri, S. simulans, S. vitulus, S. warneri, S. xylosus*
Type species: *S. aureus* subsp. *aureus* ATCC 12600, NCTC 8532
(Notes: *S. aureus* subsp. *aureus, S. epidermidis, S. haemolyticus, S. lugdunensis, S. saprophyticus* subsp. *saprophyticus* are the most commonly isolated *Staphylococcus* spp. associated with human infections. *S. lutrae* is a new species that is coagulase positive.)

Table 43.43. Differentiation of the Most Commonly Isolated Species of *Staphylococcus* That May Cause Human Infections

Test	*S. aureus* subsp. *anaerobius*	*S. aureus* subsp. *aureus*	*S. epidermidis*	*S. haemolyticus*	*S. lugdunensis*	*S. saprophyticus* subsp. *saprophyticus*	*S. schleiferi* subsp. *coagulans*	*S. schleiferi* subsp. *schleiferi*
Catalase[a]	−	V+	+	+	+	+	+	+
Oxidase[b]	−	−	−	−	−	−	−	−
NO$_3$→NO$_2$	−	+	+^{w}	V+	+	−	+	+
Colony pigment[c]	−	+	−	V	V	V	−	−
Capsule	−	+[d]	−	−	−	−	−	−
Growth								
Aerobic	V^{we}	G	G	G	G	G	G	G
Anaerobic[f]	G^g	G	G	V	G	V+	G	G
Growth in NaCl agar:								
10% (wt/vol)	G	G	G^w	G	G	G	NR	G
15% (wt/vol)	V	G^w	NG	V	G	V	NR	G
Growth at								
15°C	NR	G	V^{-w}	V^{-w}	NR	+	NR	NR
45°C	NG	G	V	G	G	V	NR	G
Staphylocoagulase[h]	+	+	−	−	−	−	+	−
Clumping factor[i]	−	+	−	−	+^{g}	−	−	+
Fibrinolysin	NR	DE[j]	V	NR	−	NR	NR	−
Heat-stable nuclease	+	+	V	−	−	−	+	+
Hemolysins (hemolysis)	+	+	V	V	+	−	+[k]	+[k]
DNase	+	+	V^{-w}	DS	NR	−	NR	NR
Acid (aerobically) from								
L-Arabinose	−	−	−	−	−	−	−	−
D-Cellobiose	−	−	−	−	−	−	−	−
β-D-Fructose	A	A	A	V	A	A	NR	NR
D-Fructose	NR	−	−	−	NR	−	NR	NR
D-Galactose	−	A	V	V	NR	−	A	NR
α-Lactose	−	A	V	V	A	V	V	−
Maltose	A	A	A	A	A	A	−	−
D-Mannitol	−	A	−	V	−	V	V	−
D-Mannose	−	A	V	−	A	−	A	A
D-Melezitose	−	−	V	−	NR	−	−	NR
Raffinose	−	−	−	−	−	−	−	−
D-Ribose	−	A	V	V	−	−	A	−
Salicin	−	−	−	−	NR	−	NR	NR
Sucrose	A	A	A	A	A	A	V	−
Trehalose	−	A	−	A	A	A	−	V
D-Turanose	NR	A	V	V	V	A	−	−
Xylitol	−	−	−	−	−	V	−	−
D-Xylose	−	−	−	−	−	−	−	−

(continued)

Table 43.43. Differentiation of the Most Commonly Isolated Species of *Staphylococcus* That May Cause Human Infections (*continued*)

Test	*S. aureus* subsp. *anaerobius*	*S. aureus* subsp. *aureus*	*S. epidermidis*	*S. haemolyticus*	*S. lugdunensis*	*S. saptophyticus* subsp. *saprophyticus*	*S. schleiferi* subsp. *coagulans*	*S. schleiferi* subsp. *schleiferi*
Misc. tests[m]								
Alkaline phosphatase	+	+	V[+n]	−	−	−	+	+
Argininedihydrolase	NR	+	+	+	−	V[−w]	+	+
Hyaluronidase	+	+	V	NR	NR	NR	NR	NR
Ornithine decarboxylase	NR	−	V	−	+	−	−	−
Pyrrolidonyl arylamidase	NR	−	−	+	+	−	NR	+
Esculin hydrolysis	−	−	−	−	−	−	−	−
Urease	NR	+	+	−	V	+	NR	−
Voges-Proskauer (VP)[o]	−	+	+	V[+]	+	+	+	+
β-Glucosidase	−	+	V	V	+	V	NR	+[k]
β-Glucuronidase	−	−	−	V	−	−	NR	−
β-Galactosidase	−	−	−	−	−	V[+]	NR	V[+]
Sensitivity tests								
Novobiocin resistance[p]	−	−	−	−	−	+	−	−
Polymyxin B resistance[q]	NR	+	+	−	V	−	NR	NR

V, variable reactions; V[+], variable, usually positive; V[−], variable, usually negative, w, weak reaction; NR, no test result; A, positive result with acid production (+); wt/vol, weight per volume; DE, differentiates ecotypes; DS, differentiated subspecies not separated out in above table. Data from references 26, 33, 40.

[a]Produced by cells growing aerobically; occasional strains are catalase negative; absent in respiratory deficient mutants. *S. aureus* subsp. *anaerobius* is catalase negative and usually only grows anaerobically.

[b]Modified oxidase test for detection of cytochrome c.

[c]Positive indicates visual detection of carotenoid pigments (e.g., yellow, yellow-orange, orange) during colony development at normal or room temperature. Pigmentation is not always a reliable characteristic for identification.

[d]Encapsulated strains produce colonies that are smaller and more convex than those of nonencapsulated strains and that have a glistening wet appearance (4).

[e]On P agar, or bovine, sheep, or human blood agar at 34 to 37°C, *S. aureus* subsp. *anaerobius* grows very slowly in the presence of air; requires addition of blood, serum, or egg yolk for growth on primary isolation agar.

[f]Semisolid thioglycolate medium symbols: G, growth moderate or heavy down tube within 18–24 h; V, heavier growth in upper portion of tube and less growth in lower anaerobic portion; −, no visible growth upper portion of tube in 48 h, but weak diffuse growth or a few scattered cells in lower portion in 72–96 h.

[g]If growth, may be delayed.

[h]Free coagulase; tube test; rabbit plasma.

[i]Bound coagulase; slide test; rabbit or human plasma.

[j]DE: differentiates ecotypes.

[k]Delayed.

[l]DS: test-differentiated subspecies not separated in table.

[m]Detected primarily by commercial, rapid, differential tests.

[n]Alkaline phosphatase activity negative for approximately 6–15% of strains of *S. epidermidis* depending on population samples.

[o]Acetoin.

[p]Positive: MIC ≥ 1.6 μg/mL or a growth inhibition zone diameter ≤ 16 mm with 5-μg novobiocin disk.

[q]Positive: growth inhibition zone diameter < 10 mm with 300-U polymyxin disk.

Table 43.44. Differentiation of Other Less Common Species of *Staphylococcus* That May Cause Human and Other Primate Infections

Test	*S. arlettae*	*S. auricularis*	*S. capitis* subsp. *capitis*[a]	*S. capitis* subsp. *ureolyticus*	*S. caprae*	*S. cohnii* subsp. *cohnii*	*S. cohnii* subsp. *urealyticum*
Catalase[c]	+	+	+	+	+	+	+
Oxidase[d]	−	−	−	−	−	−	−
NO$_3$ → NO$_2$	−	V[e]	V	V	+	−	−
Colony pigment[f]	+	−	−	V[e]	−	−	V
Capsule	−	−	−	−	−	−	−
Growth							
Aerobic	G	G[e]	G	G	G	G	G
Anaerobic[g]	NG	V^{-w}	G[e]	G[e]	G[e]	V	G[e]
Growth in NaCl agar							
10% (wt/vol)	NR	G	G	NR	NR	G	G
15% (wt/vol)	NR	G	V^{-w}	NR	NR	V	V
Growth at							
15°C	NR	NG	NG	NR	NR	G	G
45°C	NR	G	G	NR	G	V	V
Staphylocoagulase[h]	−	−	−	−	−	−	−
Clumping factor[i]	−	−	−	−	−	−	−
Fibrinolysin	−	NR	NR	NR	−	NR	NR
Heat-stable nuclease	−	−	−	−	−	−	−
Hemolysins (hemolysis)	−	NR	V^{-w}	V[e]	+[e]	V[e]	V[e]
DNase	−	V^{-w}	+	NR	+	V$^-$	V$^-$
Acid (aerobically) from							
L-Arabinose	A	−	−	−	−	−	−
D-Cellobiose	−	−	−	−	−	−	−
β-D-Fructose	A^w	A	A	NR	−	A	A
β-D-Fucose	A	−	−	NR	−	−	−
D-Galactose	V	−	−	NR	A	−	V
α-Lactose	A	−	−	V[e]	A	−	A
Maltose	A	A[e]	−	A	V[e]	V[e]	V[e]
D-Mannitol	A	−	A	A	V	V	V
D-Mannose	A^w	−	A	A	A	V[e]	A
D-Melezitose	A	−	−	NR	−	−	−
Raffinose	A	−	−	−	−	−	−
D-Ribose	A	−	−	NR	−	−	−
Salicin	NR	−	−	NR	−	−	−
Sucrose	A	V	A[e]	A	−	−	−
Trehalose	A	A[e]	−	−	A[e]	A	A
D-Turanose	A	V[e]	−	V	−	−	−
Xylitol	−	−	−	NR	−	V[e]	V[e]
D-Xylose	A	−	−	−	−	−	−
Misc. tests[j]							
Alkaline phosphatase	+[e]	−	−	−	+[e]	−	+
Arginine dihydrolase	−	V	V	+	+	−	V^{-w}
Hyaluronidase	−	NR	NR	NR	−	NR	NR
Ornithine decarboxylase	−	−	−	−	−	−	−
Pyrrolidonylarylamidase	−	V	−	V[e]	V	−	V
Esculin hydrolysis	−	−	−	−	−	−	−
Urease	−	−	−	+	+	−	+

(continued)

	S. hominis	S. pasteuri	S. saccharolyticus	S. schleiferi subsp. coagulans[b]	S. schleiferi subsp. schleiferi[b]	S. simulans	S. warneri	S. xylose
	+	+	−	+	+	+	+	+
	−	−	−	−	−	−	−	−
	V	V	+	+	+	+	V	V
	V	V	−	−	−	−	V	V
	−	−	−	−	−	−	−	−
	G	G	V−w	G	G	G	G	G
	V−w	G	G	G	G	G	G	V
	G	NR	NR	NR	G	G	G	G
	NG	NR	NR	NR	G	Gw	Gw	V
	V−w	NR	V−w	NR	NR	G	V	G
	G	NR	G	NR	G	G	G	V−w
	−	−	−	+	−	−	−	−
	−	−	−	−	+	−	−	−
	NR	NR	NR	NR	−	NR	NR	NR
	−	−	NR	+	+	V	−	−
	V−w	V[e]	−	+[e]	+[we]	V−w	V[e]	V−w
	V−	NR	NR	NR	NR	V	+	V
	−	−	−	−	−	−	−	A
	−	−	−	−	−	−	−	−
	A	NR	A[e]	A	Aw	A	A	A
	−	NR	NR	NR	NR	−	−	−
	V	NR	NR	A	NR	V−w	V	V
	V	V	−	V	−	A	V	V
	A	V[e]	−	−	−	V−w	A[e]	A
	−	V	−	V	V	A	V	V
	−	−	A[e]	A	A	V	−	A
	V	NR	NR	−	NR	−	V	−
	−	−	−	−	−	−	−	−
	−	NR	NR	A	−	V	V	V
	−	NR	NR	NR	NR	−	−	V
	A[e]	A	−	V	−	A	A	A
	V	A	−	−	V	V	A	A
	V	V[e]	NR	−	−	−	V[e]	V
	−	NR	−	−	−	−	−	V−w
	−	−	−	−	−	−	−	A
	−	−	V	+	+	+[e]	−	V
	V	V	+	+	+	+	V	−
	NR	NR	NR	−	NR	NR	NR	NR
	−	NR	−	−	−	−	−	−
	−	NR	−	NR	+	+	−	V
	−	−	NR	−	−	−	−	V
	+	+	NR	+	−	+	+	+

(continued)

Table 43.44. Differentiation of Other Less Common Species of *Staphylococcus* That May Cause Human and Other Primate Infections (*continued*)

Test	*S. arlettae*	*S. auricularis*	*S. capitis* subsp. *capitis*[a]	*S. capitis* subsp. *ureolyticus*	*S. caprae*	*S. cohnii* subsp. *cohnii*	*S. cohnii* subsp. *urealyticum*
Voges-Proskauer (VP)[k]	−	V	V	V	+	V	V
β-Glucosidase	NR	−	−	−	−	−	−
β-Glucuronidase	+	−	−	−	−	−	+
β-Galactosidase	V[e]	V[e]	−	−	−	−	+
Sensitivity tests							
Novobiocin resistance[l]	+	−	−	−	−	+	+
Polymyxin B resistance[m]	NR	−	−	−	−	−	−

V, variable reactions; V+, variable, usually positive; V−, variable, usually negative, w, weak reaction; NR, no test result; A, positive result with acid production (+); wt/vol, weight per volume.

Data from references 26, 33, 40.

[a]Rarely encountered in clinical specimens.

[b]Pathogen in European countries but seldom in the United States (33).

[c]Produced by cells growing aerobically; occasional strains are catalase-negative; absent in respiratory deficient mutants. *S. saccharolyticus* is catalase negative and usually only grows anaerobically.

[d]Modified oxidase test for detection of cytochrome c.

[e]If positive, usually delayed.

[f]Positive means visual detection of carotenoid pigments (e.g., yellow, yellow-orange, orange) during colony development at normal or room temperature. Pigmentation is not always a reliable characteristic.

(*continued*)

S. hominis	S. pasteuri	S. saccharolyticus	S. schleifer subsp. coagulens[b]	S. schleifer subsp. schleifer[b]	S. similans	S. warneri	S. xylose
V	V	NR	+	+	V−w	+	V
−	+	NR	NR	−	−	+	+
−	+	NR	N R	−	V	V	V
−	−	NR	NR	V	+	−	+
−	−	−	−	−	−	−	+
−	NR	NR	NR	−	−	−	−

[g]Semisolid thioglycolate medium symbols: G, growth moderate or heavy down tube within 18–24 h; V, heavier growth upper portion of tube and less growth in lower anaerobic portion; −, no visible growth upper portion of tube in 48 h, but weak diffuse growth or a few scattered cells in lower portion in 72–96 h.
[h]Free coagulase; tube test; rabbit plasma.
[i]Bound coagulase; slide test; rabbit or human plasma.
[j]Detected primarily by commercial, rapid, differential tests.
[k]Acetoin.
[l]Positive: MIC ≥ 1.6 μg/mL or a growth inhibition zone diameter ≤ 16 mm with 5-μg novobiocin disk.
[m]Positive: growth inhibition zone diameter < 10 mm with 300-U polymyxin disk.

Table 43.45. Differentiation of *Staphylococcus* spp. That May Be Found in Foods or Cause Animal Infections

Test	*S. caseolyticus*[a,b]	*S. carnosus*[c]	*S. chromogenes*[a,d]	*S. delphini*[e]	*S. equorum*[f]	*S. felis*[g]	*S. gallmarium*[h]
Catalase[q]	+	+	+	+	+	+	+
Oxidase[r]	+	−	−	−	−	−	−
NO$_3$ → NO$_2$	+	+	+	+	+	+	+
Colony pigment[s]	V	−	+	−	−	−	V
Capsule	−	−	−	−	−	−	−
Growth							
Aerobic	G	G	G	G	G[t]	G	G
Anaerobic[u]	V−w	G	G	G[t]	NG	G	G[t]
Growth in NaCl agar							
10% (wt/vol)	NR	G	G	G	NR	G	NR
15% (wt/vol)	NR	G	V−w	G	NR	G	NR
Growth at							
15°C	NR	G	G	V−w	NR	G[w]	NR
45°C	NR	G	V−w	G	NG	G	G[w]
Staphylocoagulase[v]	−	−	−	+	−	−	−
Clumping factor[w]	−	−	−	−	−	−	−
Fibrinolysin	NR	NR	−	−	−	NR	−
Heat-stable nuclease	NR	V−	V−w	−	−	V−w	−
Hemolysins (hemolysis)	−	−	−	+	V[t]	V−w	+[w]
DNase	NR	+[w]	+[w]	+[w]	−	NR	NR
Acid (aerobically) from							
L-Arabinose	−	−	−	−	A	−	A
D-Cellobiose	−	−	−	NR	V−w	−	A
β-D-Fructose	A	A	A	A	A	A	A
D-Fucose	NR	−	−	NR	−	NR	A
D-Galactose	A	V	A	NR	A	V	A
α-Lactose	A	V	A	A	V	A	V
Maltose	A	−	V	A	V	−	A
D-Mannitol	−	A	V	A[t]	A	V	A
D-Mannose	−	A	A	A	A	A	A
D-Melezitose	NR	−	−	NR	A	−	A
Raffinose	NR	−	−	NR	−	−	A
D-Ribose	NR	A	A	NR	A	V	A
Salicin	NR	−	−	NR	NR	−	A
Sucrose	V	−	A	A	A	V	A
Trehalose	V	V	A	−	A	A	A
D-Turanose	−	−	V	NR	V	NR	A
Xylitol	−	−	−	−	−	−	V
D-Xylose	−	−	−	−	A	−	A
Misc. tests[x]							
Alkaline phosphatase	−	+	+	+	+[t]	+	+[t]
Arginine dihydrolase	V	+	+	+	−	+	−
Hyaluronidase	NR	NR	−	NR	−	−	−
Ornithine decarboxylase	−	−	−	NR	−	NR	−
Pyrrolidonylarylamidase	+	+	V	NR	−	NR	−

(continued)

	S. hyicus[a,i]	S. intermedius[j]	S. kloosii[k]	S. lentus[l]	S. muscae[m]	S. piscifermentans[n]	S. sciuri[o]	S. vitulus[p]
	+	+	+	+	+	+	+	+
	−	−	−	+	−	−	+	+
	+	+	−	+	+	+	+	+
	−	−	V	V	−	−	V	+
	−							
	G	G	G	G[t]	G	G	G	G[t]
	G	G[t]	NG	V[−w]	G	G	G[t]	NG
	G	G	NR	G	NR	NR	G	NR
	G[−w]	V	NR	V[−w]	NR	NR	V	NR
	G	G	NR	V[−w]	NR	NR	G	NR
	V[−w]	G	NR	NG	NR	NT	V[−w]	NR
	V	+	−	−	−	−	−	−
	−	V	−	−	−	−	−	−
	V	−	−	NR	NR	NR	NR	NR
	+	+	−	−	−	−	NR	−
	−	V	V[t]	−	+[t]	−	−	−
	+	+	−	+[w]	NR	NR	+	NR
	−	−	V	V	−	−	V	−
	−	−	−	A	−	−	A	V
	A	A	A	A[t]	NR	NR	A	NR
	−	−	−	V	NR	NR	A	NR
	A	A	A	V	NR	NR	A[t]	NR
	A	V	V	V	−	V	V	−
	−	A[t]	V	V	−	V	V[t]	−
	−	V[t]	A	A	−	V	A	A
	A	A	−	A[t]	−	−	V	−
	−	−	A[w]	−	NR	NR	V	NR
	−	−	V[−w]	A	−	−	−	−
	A	A	A	A	NR	NR	A	NR
	−	−	NR	V	NR	NR	A	NR
	A	A	V	A	A	V	A	A
	A	A	A	A	A	A	A	V[t]
	−	V	A[w]	−	A	−	−	−
	−	−	V[−w]	−	NR	NR	−	NR
	−	−	−	V[−w]	A	−	−	V
	+	+	V	+[w]	+	+	+[w]	−
	+	V	−	−	−	+	−	−
	+	NR	−	NR	NR	NR	NR	NR
	−	−	−	−	−	NR	−	−
	−	+	V	−	NR	NR	−	−

(*continued*)

Table 43.45. Differentiation of *Staphylococcus* spp. That May Be Found in Foods or Cause Animal Infections (*continued*)

Test	*S. caseolyticus*[a,b]	*S. carnosus*[c]	*S. chromogens*[a,d]	*S. delphini*[e]	*S. equorum*[f]	*S. felis*[g]	*S. gallinarum*[b]
Esculin hydrolysis	NR	−	−	NR	V	NR	+
Urease	−	−	V	+	+	+	+
Voges-Proskauer (VP)[y]	−	+	−	−	−	−	−
β-Glucosidase	−	−	V	NR	NR	−	+
β-Glucuronidase	−	−	−	NR	+	−	V
β-Galactosidase	−	+	−	NR	V	+	V−w
Sensitivity tests							
Novobiocin resistance[z]	−	−	−	−	+	−	+
Polymyxin B resistance[aa]	−	−	+	NR	NR	NR	−

V, variable reactions; V+, variable, usually positive; V−, variable, usually negative, w, weak reaction; NR, no test result; A, positive result with acid production (+); wt/vol weight per volume; NT, not tested.
Data from 26, 33, 40.
[a]One of the primary animal species isolated from veterinary specimens.
[b]*S. caseolyticus* isolated from milk and dairy products.
[c]*S. carnosus* isolated from fermented meats; e.g., sausage and salami.
[d]*S. S. chromogens* isolated from cattle.
[e]*S. delphini* isolated from dolphins.
[f]*S. equorum* isolated from horses.
[g]*S. felis* isolated from cats and other Carnivora.
[h]*S. gallinarum* isolated primarily from poultry.
[i]*S. hyicus* isolated from pigs.
[j]*S. intermedius* isolated from dog bites, Carnivora, and certain other mammals and birds. May be misindentified as *S. aureus* if only coagulase is tested (19).
[k]*S. kloosii* isolated from a variety of mammals.
[l]*S. lentus* isolated from goats and sheep.
[m]*S. muscae* isolated from a variety of animals.
[n]*S. pisicifermentas* isolated from fish.

(*continued*)

	S. hyicus[a,j]	S. intermedius[j]	S. kloosii[k]	S. lentus[l]	S. muscae[m]	S. piscifermentans[n]	S. sciuri[o]	S. vitulus[p]
	−	−	V	+	−	V	+	V
	V	+	V	−	−	+	−	−
	−	−	V	−	−	−	−	−
	V	V	V	+	NR	+	+	+
	V	−	V	−	NR	−	−	−
	−	V+	V	−	−	V[t]	−	−
	−	−	+	+	−	−	+	+
	+	−	−	−	NR	NR	−	NR

[o] *S. sciuri* isolated from rodents and certain other mammals.
[p] *S. vitulus* isolated from ingulates and dairy and meat products.
[q] Produced by cells growing aerobically; occasional strains are catalase-negative; absent in respiratory deficient mutants.
[r] Modified oxidase test for the detection of cytochrome c. *S. caseolyticus*, *S. lentus*, *S. sciuri*, and *S. vitulus* are modified oxidase-positive.
[s] Positive means visual detection of carotenoid pigments (e.g., yellow, yellow-orange, orange) during colony development at normal or room temperature. Pigmentation is not always a reliable characteristic.
[t] If positive, may be delayed.
[u] Semisolid thioglycolate medium symbols; G, growth moderate or heavy down tube within 18–24 h; V, heavier growth in upper portion of tube and less in lower, anaerobic portion; no visible growth upper portion of tube in 48 h, but weak diffuse growth or a few scattered cells lower portion in 72–96 h.
[v] Free coagulase; tube test; rabbit plasma.
[w] Bound coagulase; slide test; rabbit or human plasma.
[x] Detected primarily by commercial, rapid, differential tests.
[y] Acetoin.
[z] Positive: MIC ≥ 1.6 μg/mL or a growth inhibition zone diameter ≤ 16 mm with 5-μg novobiocin disk.
[aa] Positive: growth inhibition zone diameter < 10 mm with 300-U polymyxin disk.

GENUS: *STOMATOCOCCUS* (26, 33, 40)

Gram-positive cocci usually arranged in clusters as pairs and tetrads
Nonsporeforming
Facultative anaerobes
Catalase variable; if positive, weak
Encapsulated
Nonmotile
Oxidase negative
O/F glucose: F (fermentative)
Optimal temperature: 37°C
Requires nutritionally enriched media; **does not** grow on nutrient agar with 5% NaCl
1 species: *S. mucilaginous* ATCC 25296, NCTC 10663
Formerly included within the genera *Staphylococcus* and *Micrococcus*

Table 43.46. Biochemical Characteristics of *Stomatococcus mucilaginous*

Nitrate reduction	−
10°C	NG
45°C	NG
6.5% NaCl	NG
Esculin hydrolysis	+
Voges-Proskauer (VP)	+
LAP (Leucine aminopeptidase or leucine arylamidase)	+
Gelatin liquefaction	+
PYR (pyrrolidonyl arylamidase)	V+
Vancomycin (30 μg)	S

V+, variable, usually positive; NG, no growth; S, sensitive (susceptible).

GENUS: *STREPTOCOCCUS* (26, 33, 40)

Gram-positive spherical or ovoid cocci arranged **in pairs and chains in liquid media**
S. pneumoniae: Gram-positive, lancet-shaped diplococci; **bile soluble**
Other *Streptococcus* spp.: Gram-positive cocci, singly, in pairs or characteristic chains (long in broth media; short on solid media); **bile insoluble**
Nonsporeforming
Facultative anaerobes
Catalase negative
Capsulae variable; virulent strains encapsulated
Nonmotile; rare exceptions; "*S. milleri*" sliding motility
Oxidase negative
Nitrate reduction negative
O/F glucose: F (fermentative)
Optimal growth temperature 37°C (range, 22–45°C)
Nutritionally fastidious; growth enhanced by addition of blood or serum to media
45 species: *S. acidominimus, S. agalactiae, S. alactolyticus, S. anginosus, S. bovis, S. canis, S. constellatus, S. cricetus, S. cristatus, S. difficile, S. downei, S. dysgalactiae* subsp. *dysgalactiae, S. dysgalactiae* subsp. *equisimilis, S. equi, S. equi* subsp. *equi, S. equi* subsp. *zooepidemicus, S. equinus, S. ferus, S. gallolyticus, S. gordonii, S. hyointestinalis, S. hyovaginalis, S. iniae, S. intermedius, S. intestinalis, S. macacae, S. mitis, S. mutans, S. oralis, S. parasanguinis, S. parauberis, S. phocae, S. pleomorphus, S. pneumoniae, S. porcinus, S. pyogenes, S. ratti, S. salivarius, S. sanguinis, S. sobrinus, S. suis, S. thermophilus, S. thoraltensis, S. uberis, S. vestibularis*
Type species: *S. pyogenes* ATCC 12344, NCTC 8198
(*Notes:* Synonym for *S. anginosus,* "*Streptococcus milleri.*" *S. constellatus* and *S. intermedius* are

subjective synonyms of *S. anginosus*. *S. difficile* is a new species: nonhemolytic, group B, type 1b streptococci; **indistinguishable** from *S. algalactiae* (19).)

Table 43.47. Biochemical Characteristics of Anaerobic *Streptococcus pleomorphus*

Lancefield serological gp(s)	NR	Lactose	−
Hemolysis, 5% SBA	γ	Mannitol	−
H_2S	+w	Salicin	−
Growth		Sorbitol	−
Aerobic	NG	Hippurate hydrolysis	−
Anaerobic[a]	G		
Growth in			
5% CO	NG		
6.5% NaCl	NR		
40% Bile	NR		
Growth at			
10°C	NG		
45°C	G		

NR, no results; G, growth; NG, no growth; : gamma (no hemolysis); SBA, sheep blood agar; +w; weakly positive.
Data from references 26, 33, 40.
[a]Thioglycolate medium.

Table 43.48. Differentiation of β-Hemolytic *Streptococcus* spp.

Test	*S. agalactiae*[a]	*S. canis*	*S. dysgalactiae* subsp. *equisimilis*	*S. equi*	*S. equi* subsp. *equi*	*S. equi* subsp. *zooepidemicus*
Classification	Pyo	Pyo	Pyo	Pyo	Pyo	Pyo
Lancefield serological gp(s)	B[d]	G	C,L	C	C	C
Hemolysis, 5% SBA	β	β	α,β,γ	β	β	β
Growth						
Aerobic	G	G	G	G	G	G
Anaerobic[f]	G	G	G	G	G	G
Growth in						
5% CO_2	G	G	G	G	G	G
6.5% NaCl	V	NG	NG	NG	NG	NG
40% Bile	V+	NG	NG	NG	NG	NG
Growth at						
10°C	V	NR	NG	NG	NG	NG
45°C	NG	NR	NG	NG	NG	NG
Carbohydrates						
Lactose	V	−	−	−	V	A
Inulin	−	−	−	−	−	−
Mannitol	−	−	−	−	−	−
Raffinose	−	−	−	−	−	−
Ribose	A	A	−	−	A	V
Salicin	V	A	A	A	NR	NR
Sorbitol	−	−	−	−	−	A
Trehalose	A	V	−	−	A	−
Misc. tests						
Alkaline phosphatase	+	+	+	+	+	+
Arginine hydrolysis	+	+	+	+	+	+
Bile solubility						
CAMP[g]	+	−	−	NR	−	−
Esculin hydrolysis	−	+	V	V−	−	V−
Hippurate hydrolysis	+	−	−	−	−	−
Voges-Proskauer (VP)	+	−	−	−	−	−
α-Galactosidase	−	V	−	−	−	−
β-Glucuronidase	V	V	+	+	+	+
β-Galactosidase	−	V	−	−	−	−
Pyrrolidonearylamidase (PYR)	−	−	−	−	−	−
Optochin	S	NR	R	R	R	R
Bacitracin	R	NR	R[h]	R[h]	R[h]	R

V, variable results; V+, variable, usually positive; V−, variable, usually negative; NR, no results; S, sensitive (susceptible); R, resistant; SBA, sheep blood agar; NG, no growth; α, alpha; β, beta; γ, gamma; Pyo, pyogenic.

Data from references 26, 33.

[a]*S. agalactiae* is encapsulated.
[b]"*S. milleri*" group composed of three former species: *S. anginosus*, *S. constellatus*, and *S. intermedius*.
[c]*S. pneumoniae* is encapsulated.

(*continued*)

	S. iniae	*S. intestunalis*	"*S. milleri*" group[b]	*S. pneumoniae*[c]	*S. porcinus*	*S. pyogenes*	*S. suis*
	Pyo	Misc.	Oral	Oral	Pyo	Pyo	Pyo
	Uncertain or F	Occ G	Occ G or F	None	E,P,U	A	D,R
	α,β	β	β	α,β[e]	β	β	α,β
	G	G	V	G	G	G	G
	G	G	G	G	G	G	G
	G	G	V	G	G	G	G
	NG	NG	NG	NG	V	NG	NR
	NG	NG	V	NG	V	NG	G
	G	NG	NG	NG	NR	NG	NR
	NG	G	V	NG	NG	NG	NR
	—	—	V+	A	V	A	A
	—	NR	V	V	—	—	A
	A	—	V−	V−	A	—	—
	—	—	V	A	—	—	—
	A	—	NR	—	A	—	NR
	A	A	V+	—	A	A	A
	—	—	V−	—	A	—	—
	A	—	V	A	A	A	A
	NR	NR	+	—	+	+	—
	NR	—	V	V+ Sol	+	NR	NR
	—	—	—	NR	NR	—	—
	+	+	V	V	V−	—	+
	—	—	—	—	—	—	—
	NR	NR	V	—	+	—	NR
	NR	NR	V	V+	—	—	+
	NR	NR	—	—	+	V−	+
	NR	NR	—	V	—	+	—
	—	—	—	V	NR	+	—
	R	NR	NR	S	R	R	NR
	NR	NR				S	

[d]*S. agalactiae* may show serologic cross-reactivity between groups B and G (40).
[e]*S. pneumoniae* occasionally exhibits β-hemolysis.
[f]Thioglycolate medium.
[g]CAMP test is a lytic phenomenon named after original authors: Christie, Atkins, and Munch-Peterson, CAMP factor is **not** specific to group B; may be positive with groups C, F, and G; a test for synergistic hemolysis.
[h]Occasional exception.

Table 43.49. Differentiation of Alpha (α)-Hemolytic and Gamma (γ)-Hemolytic *Streptococcus* spp.

Test	*S. acidominimus*	*S. agalactiae*[a]	*S. alactolyticus*	*S. bovis*[b]	*S. cricetus*	*S. downei*	*S. dysgalactiae* susp. *dysgalactiae*	*S. equinus*	*S. ferus*	*S. gordonii*	*S. hyointestinalis*	*S. iniae*	*S. macacae*
Classification	Other	Pyo	Other	Other	Oral	Oral	Pyo	Misc	Oral	Oral	Misc	Pyo	Oral
Lancefield serological gp(s).	NR	B[e]	NR	D	None	NR	C	D	None	None	None	Uncertain	NR
Hemolysis, 5% SBA	α,γ	α,β	α	α[w]	γ	NR	α	α[w]	α	α	α,β	α	β,γ
Growth													
Aerobic	G	G	G	G	V	G	G	G	V	G	G	G	G[w]
Anaerobic[f]	G	G	G	G	G	G	G	G	G	G	G	G	G
Growth in													
5% CO$_2$	G	G	G	G	V	G	G	G	V	G	G	G	G
6.5% NaCl	NR	V	G	NG	V	NG	NG	NG	NG	NG	NG	NG	NG
40% Bile	NR	V[+]	NR	G	V	V	NG	G	NR	NR	NG	NG	G
Growth at													
10°C	NG	V[-]	NR	NG	NG	NR	NG	NG	NG	NR	NR	G	NR
45°C	NG	NG	G	V	V	NG	NG	G	NG	NR	NR	NG	NG
Carbohydrates													
Lactose	A	V	–	A	A	A	A	–	NR	A	A	–	NR
Inulin	–	–	–	V	V	A	–	V[-]	A	V	–	–	–
Mannitol	V	–	V[+]	V	A	A	–	–	A	–	–	A	A
Raffinose	–	–	A	NR	A	–	–	V[-]	–	V	V	–	A
Ribose	–	A	–	–	NR	NR	NR	–	NR	NR	–	A	–
Salicin	A	V	V[+]	A	A	A	V	V[+]	A	A	A	A	NR
Sorbitol	A	–	–	V	A	–	V	–	A	–	–	–	A
Trehalose	V[+]	A	V	V	A	A	A	NR	NR	A	A	A	A
Misc tests													
Alkaline phosphatase	V[+]	+	–	–	NR	NR	+	–	NR	+	+	NR	NR
Arginine hydrolysis	V[-]	+	–	–	–	–	+	–	–	+	–	NR	–
Bile solubility													
Bile esculin				+		–							
CAMP[g]	–	+	–	–	–	–	–	–	–	–	–	–	–
Esculin hydrolysis	V[-]	–	+	+	V	–	–	+	+	+	+	+	+
Hippurate hydrolysis	V[wh]	+	–	–	–	–	–	–	–	–	–	–	NR
Voges-Proskauer (VP)	+	V	+	+	+	+	–	+	V	–	+	NR	NR
α-Galactosidase	–	–	+	V	NR	NR	–	–	NR	V	V	NR	NR
β-Glucuronidase	V	NR	–	V	NR	NR	+	–	NR	–	–	NR	NR
β-Galactosidase	V	–	–	V	NR	NR	–	–	NR	V[+]	–	NR	NR
Pyrrolidonearyl-amidase (PYR)	–	–	–	–	NR	NR	–	–	NR	NR	–	–	NR
Optochin	NR	SA	NR	S	S	R	R	NR	R	R	NR	R	R
Bacitracin					S	S	R		S				S

Pyo, pyogenic; NR, no results; NG, no growth; V, variable results; V[+], variable, usually positive; V[-], variable, usually negative; S, sensitive (susceptible); R, resistant; w, weak reaction.

Data from references 26 and 40.

[a]*S. agalactiae* is encapsulated.

[b]*S. bovis* could be renamed *S. inulinaceus* (2). Unable to grow in media with salt.

[c]"*S. milleri*" group composed of three former species: *S. anginosus*, *S. constellatus*, and *S. intermedius*.

(continued)

	"S. milleri"[c]	S. mitis	S. mutans	S. oralis	S. pneumoniae[d]	S. porcinus	S. raHi	S. salivarius	S. sanguis	S. sobrinus	S. suis	S. thermophilus	S. uberis	S. vestibularis
	Oral	Oral	Oral	Oral	Oral	Pyo	Oral	Oral	Oral	Oral	Pyo	Misc	Misc	Oral
	Occ F or G	None	None	None	None	E,P,U, or V	None	Often K	H	None	D,R, or S	Uncertain	Occ E	NR
	α	α,γ	γ	α	α,β	β,γ	γ	α,γ	α	γ	α,β	α,γ	α,γ	α
	V	G	V	G	G	G	V	G	G	V	G	G	G	G
	G	G	G	G	G	G	G	G	G	G	G	G	G	G
	V	G	V	G	G	G	V	G	G	V	G	G	G	G
	NG	NG	NG	NG	NG	V	NG	NG	NG	V	NR	NG	NG	NR
	V	V	V	NG	NG	V	V	V	V	V	G	NG	V	NG
	NG	G	NG	V−	NG	NR	NG	NG	NG	NG	NR	NG	G	NG
	V	V	V	V	NG	NG	V	V+	V	V	NR	G	NG	NG
	V+	A	A	A	A	V	A	V+	A	A	A	A	A	A
	V	V	A	−	V	−	A	A	V+	V	A	−	A	−
	V	−	A	−	V−	A	A	−	V−	A	−	−	A	−
	V	V	A	V	A	−	A	A	V	V	−	NR	V−	−
	NR	NR	NR	NR	−	A	NR	NR	NR	NR	NR	NR	A	−
	V+	V	A	−	−	A	A	A	A	−	A	−	A	A
	V−	V	A	−	−	A	A	−	V−	V	−	−	A	−
	V	V	A	A	A	A	A	V+	V+	V	A	NR	A	V
	+	V	−	V	−	+	NR	V	V	NR	−	NR	V	NR
	V	V	V−	V−	V+	+	+	−	+	−	NR	V	+	−
					Sol									
	−	−	NR	NR	NR	NR	−	−	−	−	−	−	−	−
	V	V	+	V	V	V−	+	+	V	V	+	−	+	V+
	−	−	−	−	−	−	−	−	−	−	−	−	+	V
	V	−	+	V	−	+	+	V+	−	+	NR	NR	NR	V+
	V	V+	V	V	V+	−	NR	−	V	NR	+	NR	−	NR
	−	−	−	−	−	+	NR	V	−	NR	+	NR	+	NR
	−	−	−	+	V	−	NR	−	V	NR	−	NR	−	NR
	−	−	−	NR	V	NR	NR	−	−	NR	−	NR	−	NR
	NR	NR	R	R	S	R	R	R	R	R	NR	NR	NR	R
			R				R			R				

[d]S. pneumoniae is encapsulated.
[e]S. agalactiae may show serologic cross-reactivity between groups B and G (40).
[f]Thioglycolate medium.
[g]CAMP test is a lytic phenomenon named after original authors: Christie, Atkins, and Munch-Petersen. CAMP factor is **not** specific to group B; may be positive with groups C, F, and G; a test for synergistic hemolysis.
[h]If positive, may be delayed.

GENUS: *TSUKAMURELLA* (26, 40)

Gram-positive, straight to slightly curved or short rods; can fragment into rods and cocci (19)
Nonsporeforming
Obligate (strict) aerobes
Nonmotile
Weakly to strongly acid-fast
Possess mycolic acid in cells
Partly acid-fast
5 species: *T. inchonensis, T. paurometabolum, T. pulmonis, T. tyrosinosolvens, T. wratislaviensis*
Type species: *T. paurometabolum* ATCC 8368
Not in *Bergey's Manual of Systematic Bacteriology*; created by Collins et al. (10)

GENUS: *TURICELLA* (33)

Gram-positive, long, irregular, pleomorphic rods
Nonsporeforming
Facultative anaerobic
Catalase positive
Nonencapsulated
Nonmotile
No mycolic acid in cells
Needs serum for growth
Key characteristic: CAMP positive
1 species: *T. otitidis* DSM 8821
According to Ruimy et al. (35), the validity is doubtful since *Turicella* genus clearly belongs to the genus *Corynebacterium*.

Table 43.50. Biochemical Characteristics of *Turicella otitidis*

$NO_3 \rightarrow NO_2$	−	Glucose	−
CAMP	+	Lactose	−
Esulin	−	Maltose	−
Unrease	−	Mannose	−
		Sucrose	−

GENUS: *VAGOCOCCUS* (26, 33, 40)

Gram-positive cocci, ovals, or short rods; arranged **singly, in pairs, or short chains**
Nonsporeforming
Facultative anaerobes
Catalase negative
Nonencapsulated
Motility variable, usually positive; peritrichous flagella
O/F glucose: F (fermentative)
Optimal growth temperature 25–35°C
Some species Lancefield serologic group N
Pathogenicity unclear
Genus not in *Bergey's Manual*; established by Collins et al. (8)
2 species
Type species: *V. fluvialis* ATCC 49515, NCDO 2497

Table 43.51. Differentiation of *Vagococcus* spp.

Test	V. fluvialis	V. salmoninarum
LAP	+	+
H$_2$S	−	+
Growth 40°C	G	NG
Glycerol	V	−
Sorbitol	A	−

V, variable results; A, acid production (+); G, growth; NG, no growth.

GENUS: *XANTHOBACTER* (26, 40)

Gram-positive or Gram-variable rods; pleomorphic. Cell wall Gram-negative type
Nonsporeforming
Obligate (strict) aerobes
Catalase positive
Motility variable; peritrichous flagella
Optimal growth temperature 25–30°C
Not acid-fast
4 species: *X. agilis*, *X. autotrophicus*, *X. flavus*, *X. tagetidis*
Type species: *X. autotrophicus* ATCC 35674

WARNING

When using the identification tables be aware that the results noted have been compiled from the references cited. However, living microorganisms often give conflicting results because of mutation or the type of media used for isolation, cultivation, identification, and maintenance.

Often proper identification to genus or genus and species requires considering (a) the clinical specimen/source, (b) Gram stain morphology, and (c) cultural characteristics (e.g., pigmentation, hemolysis) along with biochemical tests. In some cases, serologic and toxin testing are required for confirmation.

Be flexible when interpreting biochemical results. All microorganisms do not necessarily exhibit all the results of the battery of biochemical tests in the tables. At times "best fit" is necessary for identification. The more test results, the better the chance of correct identification.

Diagram 43.1.

Separation of the Gram-positive bacteria by shape.

Bacilli (rods)

Abiotrophia spp.[8]
Acetobacterium spp.
Actinomyces spp.
Amycolatopsis spp.
Arcanobacterium spp.[1]
Arthrobacter spp.[2,5]
Aureobacterium spp.
Bacillus spp.
Bifidobacterium spp.[3]
Brevibacillus spp.
Brevibacterium spp.[4]
Brochothrix spp.[4]
Butyrivibrio spp.
Cellulomonas (Oerskovia) spp.[4,5]
Clostridium spp.
Corynebacterium (Caseobacter) polymorphous
Corynebacterium spp.
Dermabacter hominus[5,6]
Erysipelothrix rhusiopathiae
Eubacterium spp.[5]
Falcivibrio spp.
Gardnerella vaginalis
Gordonia spp.[5]
Jonesia denitrificans[4]
Kurthia spp.[4]
Lactobacillus spp.[8]
Leuconostoc spp.[5]
Listeria spp.[9]
Microbacterium spp.
Mobiluncus spp.
Mycobacterium spp.
Nocardia spp.[7]
Paenibacillus spp.
Propionibacterium (Arachnia propionica) propionicus
Propionibacterium spp.
Rhodococcus spp.[5]
Rothia dentocariosa[8]
Tsukamurella spp.[12]
Turicella otitidis[13]
Vagococcus spp.[5]
Xanthobacter spp.[5]

See Diagram 43.2

Cocci (spheres)

Abiotrophia spp.
Aerococcus spp.
Alloiococcus spp.
Arcanobacterium spp.[1]
Arthrobacter spp.[2,5]
Bifidobacterium spp.[3]
Brevibacterium spp.[4]
Brochothrix spp.[4]
Cellulomonas spp.[4,5]
Clostridium spp.[13]
Coprococcus spp.
Corynebacterium (Caseobacter) polymorphus)
Corynebacterium spp.
Deinococcus spp.
Dermabacter hominus[5,6]
Enterococcus spp.[11]
Eubacterium spp.[5]
Exiguobacterium spp.
Gemella spp.
Globicatella sanguis
Gordonia spp.[5,8]
Helococcus kunzii
Jonesia denitrificans[4]
Kurthia spp.[4]
Lactobacillus spp.[8]
Lactococcus spp.
Leuconostoc spp.[5]
Listeria spp.[9]
Micrococcus spp.
Nocardia spp.[7]
Pediococcus spp.
Peptococcus niger
Peptostreptococcus spp.[8]
Propionibacterium spp.[10]
Rhodococcus spp.[5]
Rothia dentocariosa[8]
Sarcina spp.
Staphylococcus spp.
Stomatococcus mucilaginous
Streptococcus spp.
Tsukamurella spp.[12]
Turicella otitidis[13]
Vagococcus spp.[5]
Xanthobacter spp.[5]

See Diagram 43.32

---

[1]Older cultures of *Arcanobacterium* exhibit irregular rods and cocci and are difficult to distinguish from *Corynebacterium* spp.
[2]In the stationary stage, almost all *Arthrobacter* spp. cells are coccoid.
[3]Older cells of *Bifidobacterium* spp. are swollen coccoid shapes.
[4]Older culture cells appear coccoid.
[5]Rods and cocci forms.
[6]*Dermabacter hominus* cells are difficult to distinguish from *Corynebacterium* spp.
[7]May appear coccoid.

(continued)

[8]Cells may give a coccobacilli appearance.
[9]*Listeria* cells may appear coccoid; arranged in pairs and often confused with *Streptococcus pneumoniae* cells.
[10]Older cultures exhibit short rods with rounded ends often tapered or coccobacillary and may resemble streptococci; "anaerobic diphtheroids."
[11]Occasionally coccobacilli when cultivated and Gram stained from agar growth.
[12]*Tsukamurella* spp. can fragment into rods and cocci (19).
[13]Pleomorphic rods.

Diagram 43.2.

Differentiation of Gram-positive rods by oxygen (O_2) requirement.

Aerobic/Facultative Anaerobic	Anaerobic
Actinomyces spp.	*Arcanobacterium* spp.[2]
Amycolatopsis spp.	*Bifidobacterium* spp.[4]
Arcanobacterium spp.[2]	*Butyrivibrio* spp.[6]
Aureobacterium spp.	*Clostridium* spp.[7]
Bacillus spp.[3]	*Eubacterium* spp.[6]
Bifidobacterium spp.[4]	*Falcivibrio* spp.
Brevibacterium spp.[5]	*Lactobacillus* spp.[8,9]
Brochothrix spp.	*Microbacterium* spp.[10]
Clostridium carnis[7]	*Mobiluncus* spp.
Clostridium histolyticum[7]	*Propionibacterium* spp.[11]
Clostridium tertium[7]	
Corynebacterium spp.	See Diagram 43.16
Dermabacter hominus	
Erysipelothrix rhusiopathiae	
Gardnerella vaginalis	
Gordonia spp.	
Jonesia denitrificans	
Kurthia spp.[3]	
Lactobacillus spp.[8,9]	
Leuconostoc spp.	
Listeria spp.	
Microbacterium spp.[10]	
Mycobacterium spp.[12]	
Nocardia spp.[5]	
Propionibacterium spp.[11]	
Rhodococcus spp.	
Rothia dentocariosa	
Tsukamurella spp.[5]	

See Diagram 43.3

---

[1]Genera *Abiotrophia, Acetobacterium, Arthrobacter, Brevibacillus, Cellulomonas, Paenibacillus, Turicella, Vagococcus,* and *Xanthobacter* are **not** included any further in schemata of Gram-positive bacilli (rods).
[2]Anaerobic growth better than aerobic.
[3]Some species are obligate (strict) aerobes (e.g., *B. firmus, B. megaterium, B. sphaericus,* and *B. subtilis*) (33).
[4]Few species can grow in air with 10% CO_2.
[5]Obligate (strict) aerobes.
[6]Obligate (strict) anaerobes.
[7]Few species capable of growth in air; aerotolerant (e.g., *Cl. carnis, Cl. histolyticum,* and *Cl. tertium*).
[8]20% obligate (strict) anaerobes (33); occasionally microaerophilic. Grows poorly in air; enhanced growth with reduced oxygen tension. Isolation of some anaerobes enhanced by CO_2.
[9]Facultative anaerobic or obligate (strict) anaerobic.
[10]*Microbacterium* spp. are aerobic; weak anaerobic growth possible.
[11]Some strains aerotolerant, but growth best anaerobically.
[12]Slow growing; 2–60 days.

Diagram 43.3.

Differentiation of aerobic/facultative anaerobic Gram-positive rods (bacilli) by catalase reaction.

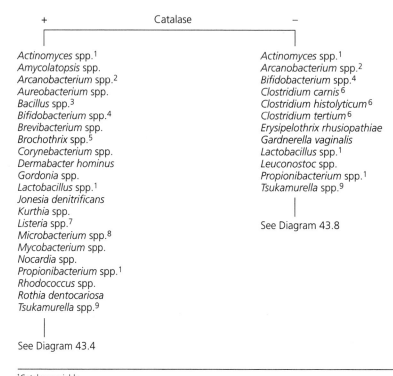

Actinomyces spp.[1]
Amycolatopsis spp.
Arcanobacterium spp.[2]
Aureobacterium spp.
Bacillus spp.[3]
Bifidobacterium spp.[4]
Brevibacterium spp.
Brochothrix spp.[5]
Corynebacterium spp.
Dermabacter hominus
Gordonia spp.
Lactobacillus spp.[1]
Jonesia denitrificans
Kurthia spp.
Listeria spp.[7]
Microbacterium spp.[8]
Mycobacterium spp.
Nocardia spp.
Propionibacterium spp.[1]
Rhodococcus spp.
Rothia dentocariosa
Tsukamurella spp.[9]

See Diagram 43.4

Actinomyces spp.[1]
Arcanobacterium spp.[2]
Bifidobacterium spp.[4]
Clostridium carnis[6]
Clostridium histolyticum[6]
Clostridium tertium[6]
Erysipelothrix rhusiopathiae
Gardnerella vaginalis
Lactobacillus spp.[1]
Leuconostoc spp.
Propionibacterium spp.[1]
Tsukamurella spp.[9]

See Diagram 43.8

---

[1]Catalase variable.
[2]Some strains of *A. haemolyticum* exhibit weak activity, but usually negative.
[3]Catalase variable, usually positive; a few species are negative, but seldom seen in a clinical laboratory.
[4]Rare positive reaction when grown in air with CO_2 (33).
[5]Catalase dependent on medium and temperature of incubation; incubation at 20°C.
[6]*Clostridium* variable, usually negative; trace amounts may be detected in some strains (27).
[7]Rare strains negative (26).
[8]Catalase not routinely performed.

+	Oxidation	+
+	Acid fast	V
−	Branching	V
−	Aerial hyphae	+

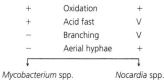

Mycobacterium spp.   *Nocardia* spp.

[9]Catalase reaction not known; treated here as variable.

Diagram 43.4.

Initial differentiation of **catalase-positive**, aerobic to facultative anaerobic, Gram-positive bacilli (rods).

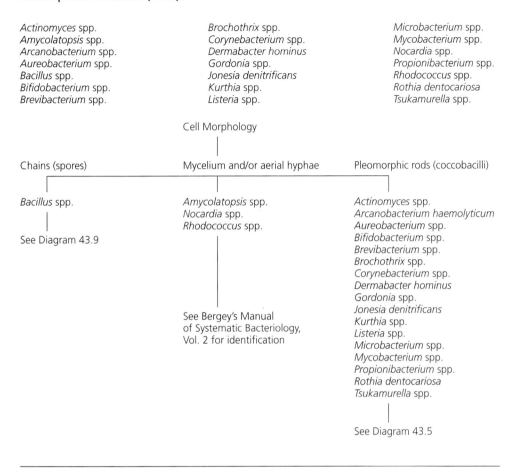

578 Biochemical Tests for Identification of Medical Bacteria

Diagram 43.5.

Differentiation of **catalase-positive**, aerobic to facultative anaerobic, Gram-positive, **nonsporeforming** pleomorphic rods (coccobacilli).

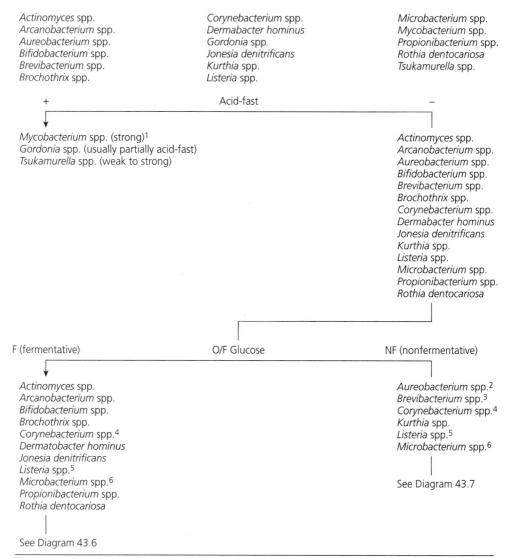

Actinomyces spp.	*Corynebacterium* spp.	*Microbacterium* spp.
Arcanobacterium spp.	*Dermabacter hominus*	*Mycobacterium* spp.
Aureobacterium spp.	*Gordonia* spp.	*Propionibacterium* spp.
Bifidobacterium spp.	*Jonesia denitrificans*	*Rothia dentocariosa*
Brevibacterium spp.	*Kurthia* spp.	*Tsukamurella* spp.
Brochothrix spp.	*Listeria* spp.	

Acid-fast

+ → *Mycobacterium* spp. (strong)[1]
Gordonia spp. (usually partially acid-fast)
Tsukamurella spp. (weak to strong)

− → *Actinomyces* spp.
Arcanobacterium spp.
Aureobacterium spp.
Bifidobacterium spp.
Brevibacterium spp.
Brochothrix spp.
Corynebacterium spp.
Dermabacter hominus
Jonesia denitrificans
Kurthia spp.
Listeria spp.
Microbacterium spp.
Propionibacterium spp.
Rothia dentocariosa

O/F Glucose

F (fermentative):
Actinomyces spp.
Arcanobacterium spp.
Bifidobacterium spp.
Brochothrix spp.
Corynebacterium spp.[4]
Dermatobacter hominus
Jonesia denitrificans
Listeria spp.[5]
Microbacterium spp.[6]
Propionibacterium spp.
Rothia dentocariosa

See Diagram 43.6

NF (nonfermentative):
Aureobacterium spp.[2]
Brevibacterium spp.[3]
Corynebacterium spp.[4]
Kurthia spp.
Listeria spp.[5]
Microbacterium spp.[6]

See Diagram 43.7

---

[1]*Mycobacterium* spp.: require special media and conditions for growth; tests not routinely performed in most laboratories. Specimens sent to Public Health and other reference laboratories for genus/species identification.
[2]Oxidative (O); slow and weak.
[3]Oxidative (O) or inert (−).
[4]Fermentative (F), oxidative (O), or inert (−).
[5]Fermentative (F) or oxidative (O).
[6]Oxidative (O) or weakly fermentative (F).

Diagram 43.6.

Differentiation of **catalase-positive**, aerobic to facultative anaerobic, Gram-positive, **nonsporeforming** pleomorphic rods (coccobacilli) that are **not acid-fast** and **ferment glucose**.

Actinomyces spp.
Arcanobacterium spp.
Bifidobacterium spp.
Brevibacterium spp.
Brochothrix spp.

Corynebacterium spp.
Dermabacter hominus
Jonesia denitrificans
Listeria spp.

Microbacterium spp.
Propionibacterium spp.
Rothia dentocariosa

```
          +              Motility                    −
  ┌───────┴──────────────────────────────────────────┴────────┐
```

Corynebacterium aquaticum
Corynebacterium matruchotii
Jonesia denitrificans
Listeria spp.[1]
Microbacterium spp.[2]

Actinomyces spp.
Arcanobacterium spp.
Bifidobacterium spp.
Brevibacterium spp.
Brochothrix spp.
Corynebacterium spp.
Dermabacter hominus
Listeria spp.[1]
Microbacterium spp.[2]
Propionibacterium spp.
Rothia dentocariosa

Actinomyces spp.: Species best differentiated by gel electrophoresis (40); however, see Table 43.1 to differentiate the most frequently isolated species.

Arcanobacterium spp.: See Table 43.3 to differentiate species. *Arcanobacterium haemolyticum* reverse CAMP-positive.

Bifidobacterium: Requires specialized techniques for strict anaerobiosis and/or metabolic studies.

Brevibacterium spp.: See Table 43.6 to differentiate the most frequently isolated species.

Brochothrix spp.: nonmotile at 22°C; see Table 43.7 to differentiate species.

Corynebacterium spp.: See Diagram 43.10 to 43.14 to differentiate species.

Dermabacter hominus: See Table 43.20 for biochemical characteristics.

Jonesia denitrificans: See Table 43.27 for biochemical characteristics.

Listeria spp.: See Diagram 43.15 to differentiate species.

Microbacterium spp.: See Table 43.33 to differentiate some species.

Propionibacterium spp.: See Table 43.20 to differentiate species.

Rothia dentocariosa: See Table 43.21 for biochemical characteristics.

---

[1]Motile when grown at 20–25°C (room temperature) in nutrient broth; characteristic end-over-end tumbling motility in wet mount.
[2]Motility variable, usually negative; only orange-pigmented species *M. imperiale* and *M. arborescens* are motile at 28°C (19).

Diagram 43.7.

Differentiation of **catalase-positive**, aerobic to facultative anaerobic, Gram-positive, **nonsporeforming** pleomorphic rods (coccobacilli) that are **not acid-fast** and are **nonfermentative**.

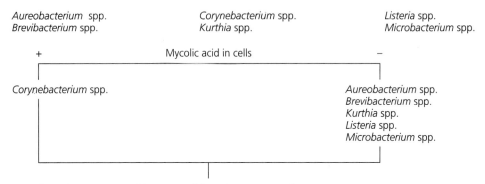

Aureobacterium spp.: See Table 43.4 to differentiate some species.

Brevibacterium spp.: See Table 43.6 to differentiate species.

Corynebacterium spp.: See Diagram 43.10–43.14 to differentiate species.

Kurthia spp.: characteristic "bird feather" growth on nutrient gelatin slants; concentration and brand critical; See Table 43.28 to differentiate species.

Listeria spp.: See Diagram 43.15 to differentiate species.

Microbacterium spp.: See Table 43.33 to differentiate species.

Diagram 43.8.

Identification of **catalase-negative**, aerobic to facultative anaerobic, Gram-positive rods (bacilli).

Actinomyces spp.[1]
Arcanobacterium spp.
Bifidobacterium spp.
Clostridium carnis[2]

Clostridium histolyticum[2]
Clostridium tertium[2]
Erysipelothrix rhusiopathiae
Gardnerella vaginalis[3]

Lactobacillus spp.
Leuconstoc spp.
Propionibacterium spp.
Tsukamurella spp.[4]

Actinomyces spp.: Species best differentiated by gel electrophoresis (25); however, see Table 43.1 to differentiate the most frequently isolated species. Catalase-negative *A. israelii*, *A. naeslundii*, and *A. odontolyticus* exhibit H_2S on TSI.

Arcanobacterium haemolyticum: Reverse CAMP-positive; see Table 43.3 to differentiate three species.

Bifidobacterium spp.: Requires specialized techniques for strict anaerobiosis and/or metabolic studies.

Clostridium carnis, *Cl. histolyticum*, *Cl. tertium*:

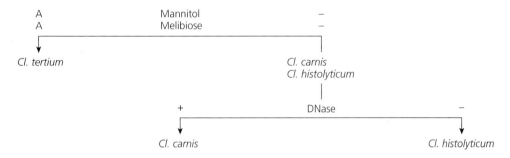

Erysipelothrix rhusiopathiae: H_2S-positive on TSI; see Table 43.22 for biochemical characteristics.

Gardnerella vaginalis: See Table 43.25 for biochemical characteristics.

Lactobacillus spp.: See Bergey's Manual of Systematic Bacteriology, Volume 2 and Table 43.29 for the differentiation of the most frequently isolated species.

Leuconstoc spp.: See Table 43.31 to differentiate the most frequently isolated species.

Propionibacterium spp.: See Table 43.20 to differentiate the most frequently isolated species.

Tsukamurella spp.: weakly to strongly acid-fast.

---

[1]Catalase variable.
[2]*Clostridium carnis*, *Cl. histolyticum*, and *Cl. tertium* are aerotolerant, but when cultivated aerobically they **do not form spores.**
[3]False-positive catalase reaction observed when growth for this test is taken from media containing human blood (e.g., Vaginalis agar).
[4]Catalase reaction not known; treated here as variable.

Diagram 43.9.

Differentiation of the most frequently isolated spore-forming *Bacillus* spp.

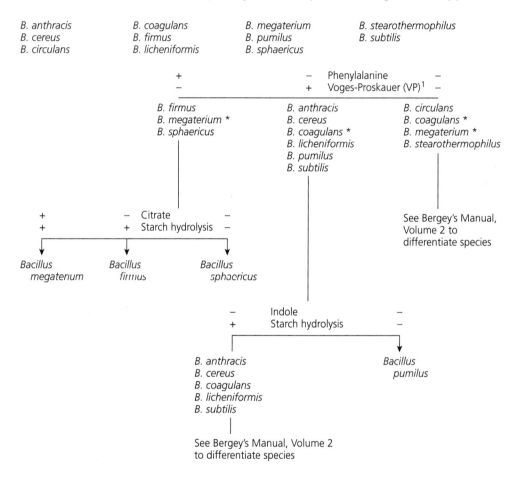

*Variable results.
[1]Incubate an additional 24 hrs at 37°C.

Diagram 43.10.

Initial differentiation of most frequent *Corynebacterium* spp. that may cause human infections.

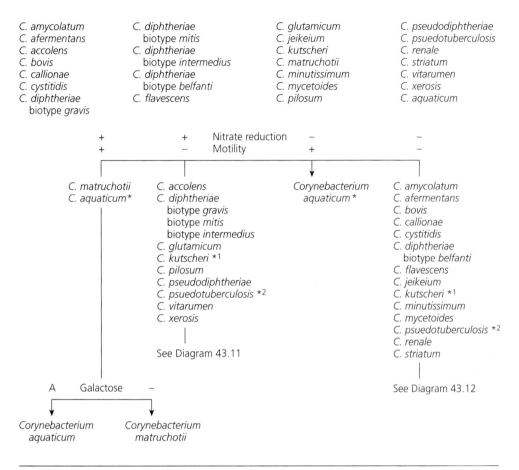

*Variable results.
[1]Nitrate reduction negative in strains from sheep and goats and positive from horses and cattle (12).
[2]Studies by Knight (28) and Biberstein and Knight (4) showed equine strains reduce nitrate while ovine strains were positive.

Diagram 43.11.

Differentiation of **nitrate reduction-positive, nonmotile** *Corynebacterium* spp.

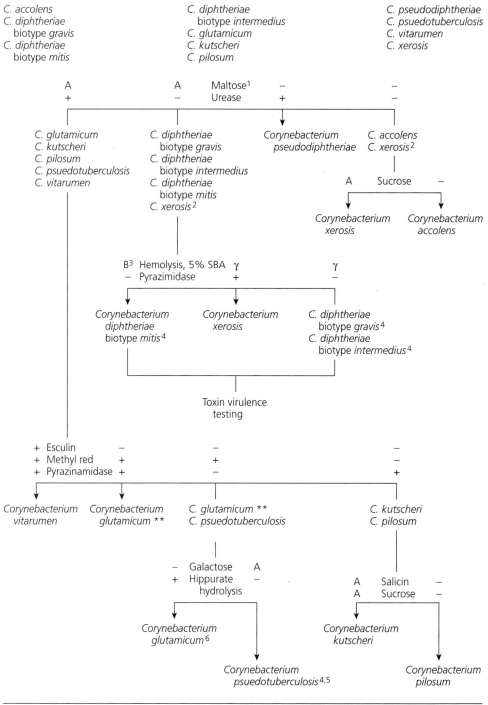

**No results; treated as variable.
[1]All corynebacteria listed here are fermenters except *C. glutamicum*; no results.
[2]Occasional strain positive.
[3]When beta (β), slight hemolysis with narrow zone.
[4]Halo on modified Tinsdale medium.
[5]Phospholipase-D-positive.
[6]CAMP-positive.

Diagram 43.12.

Differentiation of **nitrate reduction-negative, nonmotile** *Corynebacterium* spp.

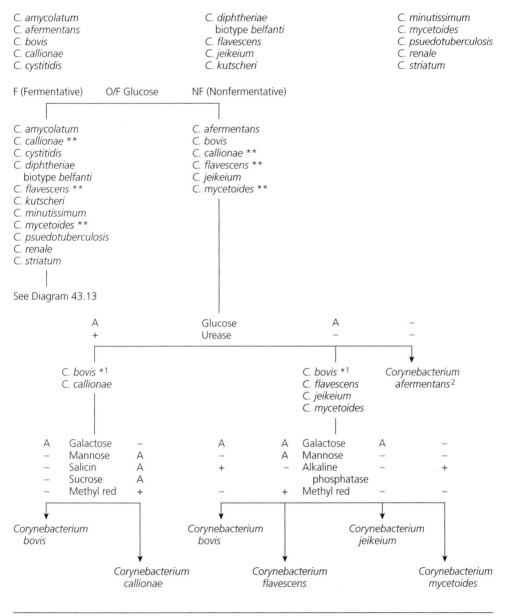

*Variable results.
**No results; treated as variable.
[1] *C. bovis* ONPG-positive and CAMP-positive.
[2] *C. afermentans* subsp. *afermentans* CAMP-variable.

Diagram 43.13.

Differentiation of **nitrate reduction-negative, nonmotile** *Corynebacterium* spp. that are **glucose fermenters**.

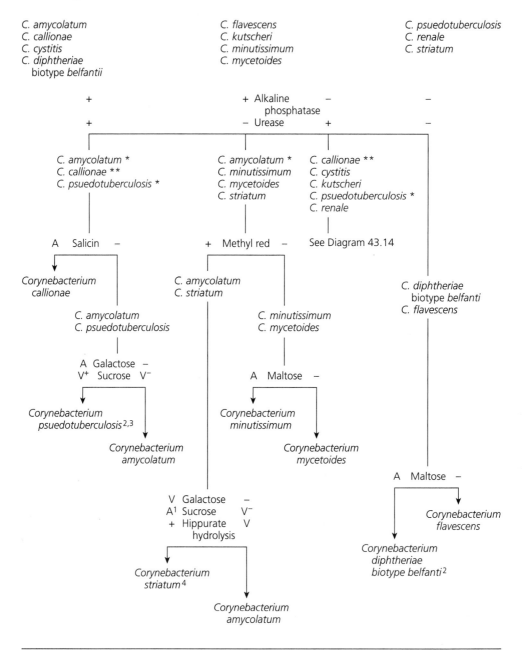

*Variable results.
**No results; treated as variable.
[1]Only aerobically.
[2]Halo on modified Tinsdale medium.
[3]Phospholipase-D-positive.
[4]CAMP-variable.

Diagram 43.14.

Differentiation of **nitrate reduction-negative, nonmotile** *Corynebacterium* spp. that are **glucose fermenters, urease-positive,** and **alkaline phosphatase-negative**.

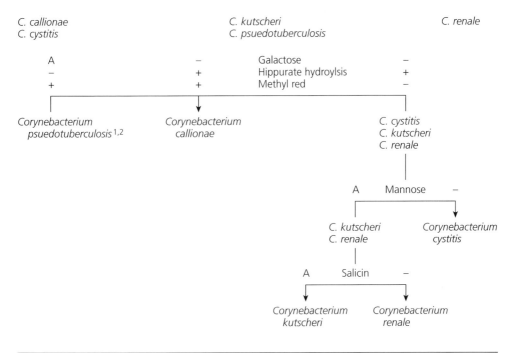

[1] Halo on modified Tinsdale medium.
[2] Phospholipase-D-positive.

Diagram 43.15.

Differentiation of *Listeria* spp.

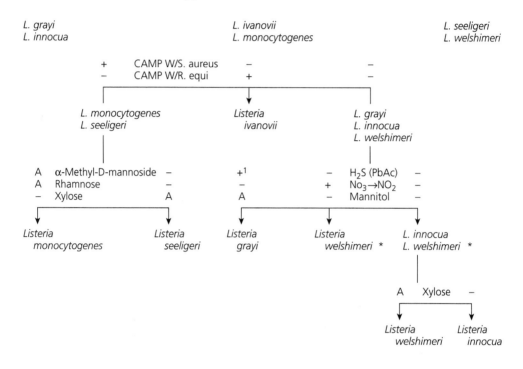

*No results on nitrate reduction; treated as variable.
[1]Small amount.

Diagram 43.16.

Initial differentiation of **anaerobic** Gram-positive rods (bacilli).

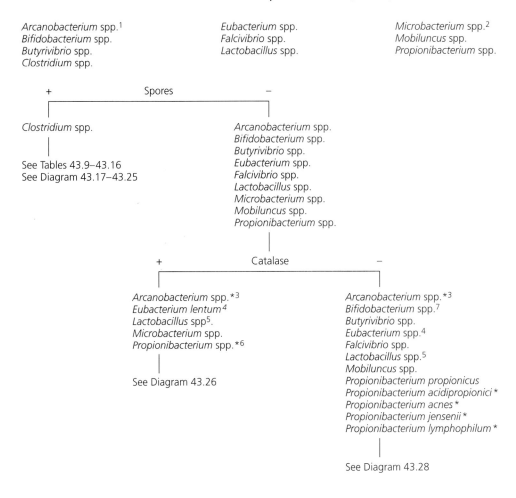

*Variable reaction.
[1]Anaerobic growth better than aerobic.
[2]*Microbacterium* spp. are aerobic; weak anaerobic growth possible.
[3]Catalase variable; usually negative; some strains exhibit weak activity.
[4]Occasional strain of *E. lentum* catalase-positive.
[5]Some positive strains (26).
[6]Catalase variable; usually positive.
[7]Catalase-negative; rare positive reaction when grown in air with CO_2.

Diagram 43.17.

Initial differentiation of anaerobic spore-forming, Gram-positive *Clostridium* spp. with **subterminal,** oval spores.

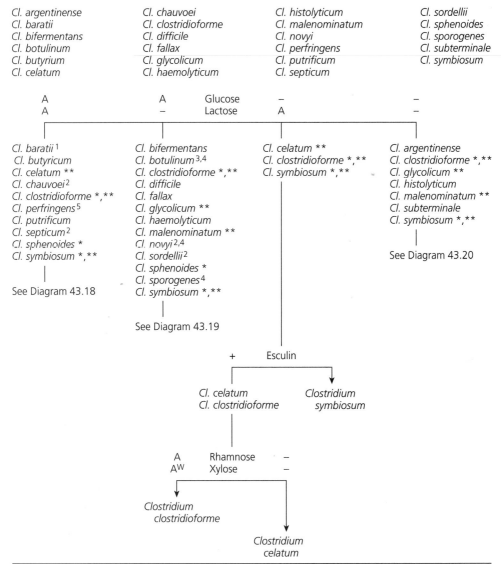

*Variable results.
**No results; treated as variable.
[1]Weak fermentation of lactose.
[2]Fluorescent antibody tests available for identification.
[3]Cultivation, isolation, and identification of *Cl. botulinum* should be attempted **only** by reference laboratories.
[4]Toxin neutralization test necessary for identification of *Cl. botulinum* and *Cl. novyi* A and B; also toxin test necessary for some *Cl. sporogenes* species which are difficult to differentiate from proteolytic *Cl. botulinum* (ABF).
[5]Most commonly isolated clostridia: *Cl. perfringens* and *Cl. ramosum*.

Diagram 43.18.

Differentiation of **glucose-positive** and **lactose-positive** *Clostridium* spp. with **subterminal**, oval spores.

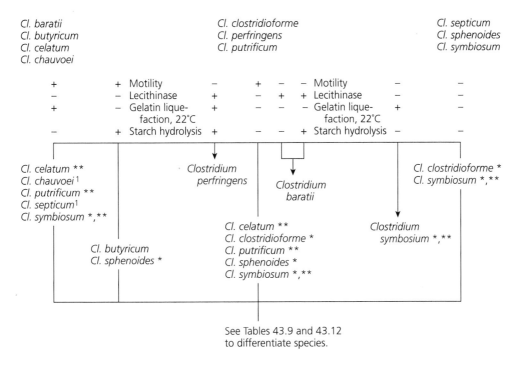

See Tables 43.9 and 43.12 to differentiate species.

---

*Variable results.
**No results; treated as variable.
[1]Fluorescent antibody tests available for identification.

Diagram 43.19.

Differentiation of **glucose-positive** and **lactose-negative** *Clostridium* spp. with **subterminal**, oval spores.

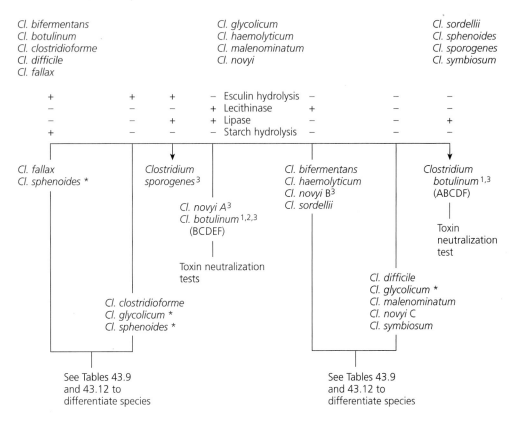

*Variable results.
[1]Cultivation, isolation, and identification of *Cl. botulinum* should only be attempted by reference laboratories.
[2]If positive lecithinase, very small amounts.
[3]Toxin neutralization test necessary for identification of *Cl. botulinum* and *Cl. novyi* A and B; also toxin test necessary for some *Cl. sporogenes* species which are difficult to differentiate from proteolytic *Cl. botulinum* (ABF).

Diagram 43.20.

Differentiation of **glucose-negative** and **lactose-negative** *Clostridium* spp. with **subterminal**, oval spores.

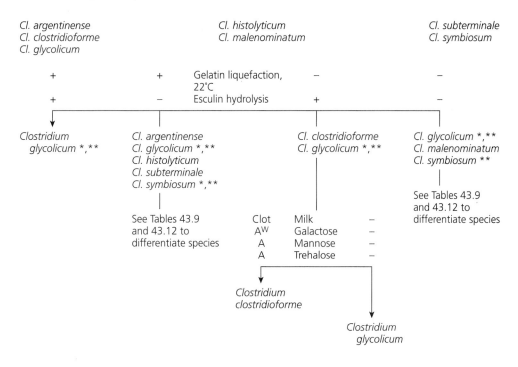

*Variable results.
**No results; treated as variable.

Diagram 43.21.

Initial differentiation of anaerobic, spore-forming, Gram-positive *Clostridium* spp. with **terminally** located spores.

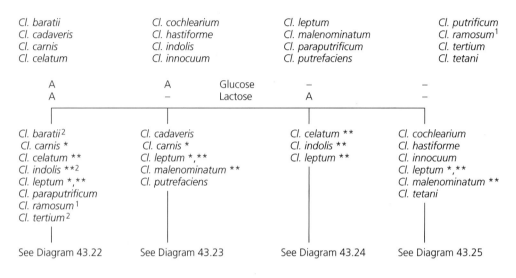

*Variable reactions.
**No results; treated as variable.
[1]Most commonly isolated clostridia: *Cl perfringens* and *Cl. ramosum*; *Cl. ramosum* resistant to standart MIC antimicrobial agents.
[2]Weak fermentation of lactose.

Chapter 43 / Gram-Positive Bacteria **595**

Diagram 43.22.

Differentiation of **glucose-positive, lactose-positive** *Clostridium* spp. with **terminal** oval or round spores.

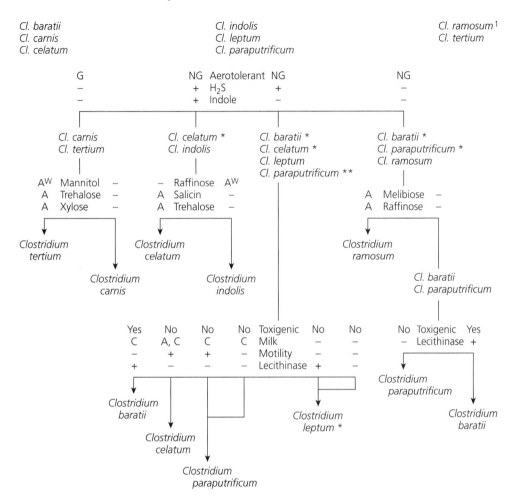

*No results; treated as variable.
[1]Most commonly isolated clostridia: *Cl. perfringens* and *Cl. ramosum*.

Diagram 43.23.

Differentiation of **glucose-positive, lactose-negative** *Clostridium* spp. with **terminal** oval or round spores.

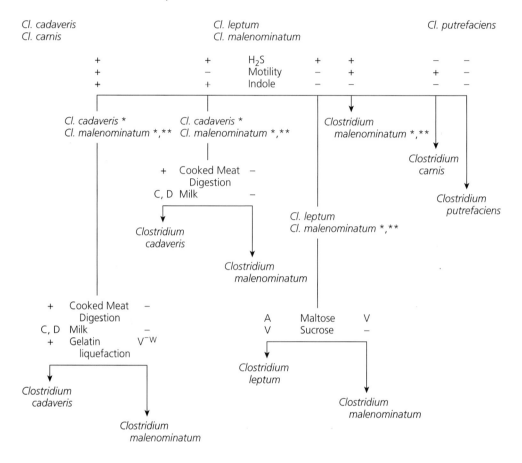

*Variable results.
**No results; treated as variable.

Diagram 43.24.

Differentiation of **glucose-negative** and **lactose-positive** *Clostridium* spp. with **terminal** oval or round spores.

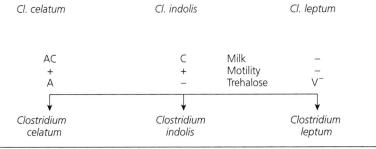

Diagram 43.25.

Differentiation of **glucose-negative** and **lactose-negative** *Clostridium* spp with **terminal** oval or round spores.

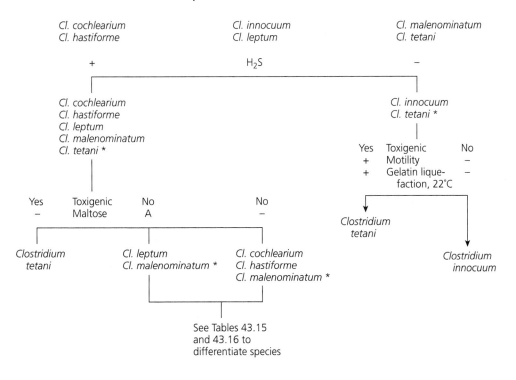

*Variable results.

Diagram 43.26.

Differentiation of **catalase-positive, anaerobic,** Gram-positive rods (bacilli).

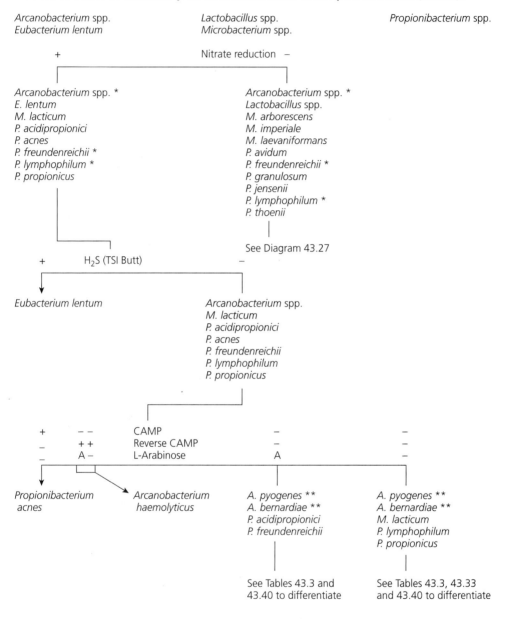

*Variable reaction.
**No results; treated as variable.

Diagram 43.27.

Differentiation of **catalase-positive, anaerobic,** Gram-positive rods (bacilli) that are **nitrate reduction-negative**.

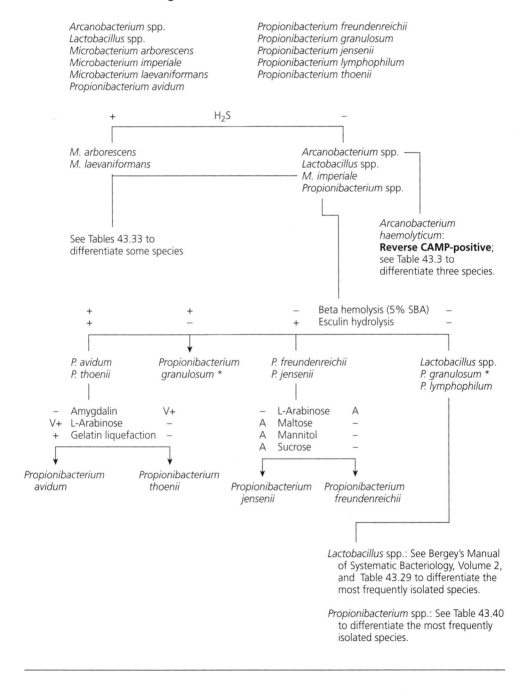

600 Biochemical Tests for Identification of Medical Bacteria

Diagram 43.28.

Differentiation of **catalase-negative, anaerobic,** Gram-positive rods (bacilli).

Arcanobacterium spp.
Bifidobacterium spp.
Butyrivibrio spp.
Eubacterium spp.
Falcivibrio spp.
Lactobacillus spp.
Mobiluncus spp.

Propionibacterium acnes
Propionibacterium acidipropionici
Propionibacterium jensenii
Propionibacterium lymphophilum
Propionibacterium propionicus

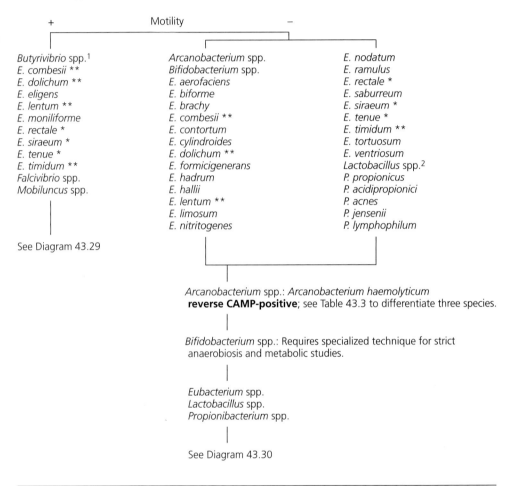

```
                    +        Motility         −
```

Butyrivibrio spp.[1]
E. combesii **
E. dolichum **
E. eligens
E. lentum **
E. moniliforme
E. rectale *
E. siraeum *
E. tenue *
E. timidum **
Falcivibrio spp.
Mobiluncus spp.

See Diagram 43.29

Arcanobacterium spp.
Bifidobacterium spp.
E. aerofaciens
E. biforme
E. brachy
E. combesii **
E. contortum
E. cylindroides
E. dolichum **
E. formicigenerans
E. hadrum
E. hallii
E. lentum **
E. limosum
E. nitritogenes

E. nodatum
E. ramulus
E. rectale *
E. saburreum
E. siraeum *
E. tenue *
E. timidum **
E. tortuosum
E. ventriosum
Lactobacillus spp.[2]
P. propionicus
P. acidipropionici
P. acnes
P. jensenii
P. lymphophilum

Arcanobacterium spp.: *Arcanobacterium haemolyticum*
reverse CAMP-positive; see Table 43.3 to differentiate three species.

Bifidobacterium spp.: Requires specialized technique for strict anaerobiosis and metabolic studies.

Eubacterium spp.
Lactobacillus spp.
Propionibacterium spp.

See Diagram 43.30

---

*Variable results.
**No results; treated as variable.
[1]Rapid and vibratory motility.
[2]Positive motility rare.

Chapter 43 / Gram-Positive Bacteria **601**

Diagram 43.29.

Differentiation of **catalase-negative, anaerobic**, Gram-positive rods (bacilli) that are **motile**.

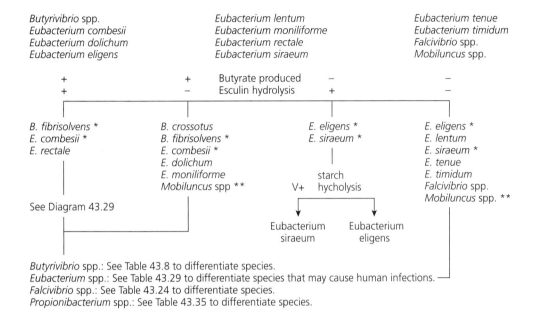

Butyrivibrio spp.: See Table 43.8 to differentiate species.
Eubacterium spp.: See Table 43.29 to differentiate species that may cause human infections.
Falcivibrio spp.: See Table 43.24 to differentiate species.
Propionibacterium spp.: See Table 43.35 to differentiate species.

---

*Variable results.
**No results; treated as variable.

Diagram 43.30.

Differentiation of **catalase-negative, anaerobic**, Gram-positive rods (bacilli) that are **nonmotile**.

Arcanobacterium spp.
Eubacterium aerofaciens
Eubacterium biforme
Eubacterium brachy
Eubacterium combesii
Eubacterium contortum
Eubacterium cylindroides
Eubacterium dolichum
Eubacterium formicigenerans
Eubacterium hadrum
Eubacterium hallii

Eubacterium lentum
Eubacterium limosum
Eubacterium nitritogenes
Eubacterium nodatum
Eubacterium ramulus
Eubacterium rectale
Eubacterium saburreum
Eubacterium siraeum
Eubacterium tenue
Eubacterium timidum

Eubacterium tortuosum
Eubacterium ventriosum
Lactobacillus spp.
Propionibacterium acidipropionici
Propionibacterium acnes
Propionibacterium jensenii
Propionibacterium lymphophilum
Propionibacterium propionicus

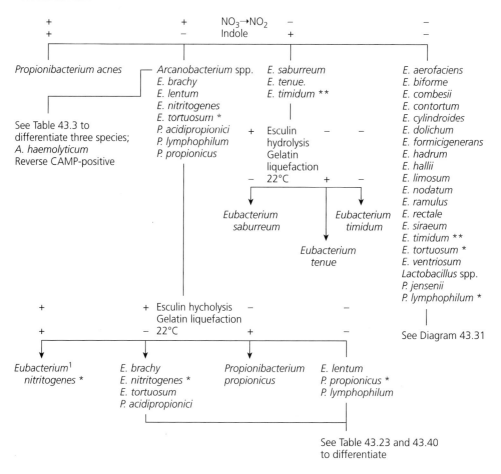

*Variable results.
**No results; treated as variable.
[1]If positive gelatin liquefaction, weak.

Diagram 43.31.

Differentiation of **catalase-negative, nonmotile, anaerobic,** Gram-positive rods (bacilli) that are **nitrate reduction-negative** and **indole-negative**

Eubacterium aerofaciens *Eubacterium formicigenerans* *Eubacterium siraeum*
Eubacterium biforme *Eubacterium hadrum* *Eubacterium timidum*
Eubacterium combesii *Eubacterium hallii* *Eubacterium tortuosum*
Eubacterium contortum *Eubacterium limosum* *Eubacterium ventriosum*
Eubacterium cylindroides *Eubacterium nodatum* *Lactobacillus* spp.
Eubacterium dolichum *Eubacterium ramulus* *Propionibacterium jensenii*
  Eubacterium rectale *Propionibacterium lymphophilum*

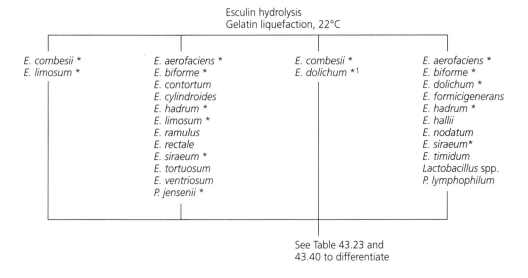

Esculin hydrolysis
Gelatin liquefaction, 22°C

E. combesii *	E. aerofaciens *	E. combesii *	E. aerofaciens *
E. limosum *	E. biforme *	E. dolichum *¹	E. biforme *
	E. contortum		E. dolichum *
	E. cylindroides		E. formicigenerans
	E. hadrum *		E. hadrum *
	E. limosum *		E. hallii
	E. ramulus		E. nodatum
	E. rectale		E. siraeum*
	E. siraeum *		E. timidum
	E. tortuosum		Lactobacillus spp.
	E. ventriosum		P. lymphophilum
	P. jensenii *		

See Table 43.23 and 43.40 to differentiate

---

*Variable results.
¹If positive gelatin liquefaction, weak.

Diagram 43.32.

Initial differentiation of Gram-positive **cocci** by oxygen (O_2) requirement.

Aerobic/Facultative Anaerobic	Anaerobic
Abiotrophia spp.	Arcanobacterium spp. *[3]
Aerococcus spp.[1]	Bifidobacterium spp.[4]
Alloiococcus otitidis[2]	Cellulomonas spp.[5]
Arcanobacterium spp. *[3]	Clostridium spp.[6,7]
Arthrobacter spp.	Coprococcus spp.[6]
Brevibacterium spp.[2]	Eubacterium spp.[6]
Brochothrix spp.	Lactobacillus spp. *[8]
Cellulomonas spp. *[5]	Peptococcus niger [6]
Clostridium spp. *[7]	Peptostreptococcus spp.
Corynebacterium spp.	Propionibacterium spp. *[9]
Deinococcus spp.	Sarcina spp.[6]
Dermatobacter hominis	Streptococcus pleomorphus
Enterococcus spp.	
Exiguobacterium spp.	
Gemella spp.	See Diagram 43.46
Globicatella sanguis	
Gordonia spp.	
Helcococcus kunzii	
Jonesia denitrificans	
Kurthia spp.[2]	
Lactobacillus spp. *[8]	
Lactococcus spp.	
Leuconostoc spp.	
Listeria spp.	
Micrococcus spp.[2]	
Nocardia spp.[2]	
Pediococcus spp.	
Propionibacterium spp. *[9]	
Rhodococcus spp.	
Rothia dentocariosa	
Staphylococcus spp.	
Stomatococcus mucilaginous	
Streptococcus spp.	
Tsukamurella spp.[2]	
Turicella otitidis	
Vagococcus spp.	
Xanthobacter spp.[2]	

See Diagram 43.33

---

*Variable results.

[1]Microaerophilic to facultative anaerobic; best growth at reduced oxygen tension; poor growth anaerobically.

[2]Strict (obligate) aerobe.

[3]Anaerobic growth better than aerobic.

[4]Few species can grow in air with 10% CO_2 (26).

[5]Some strains grow poorly anaerobically.

[6]Strict (obligate) anaerobes.

[7]A few species capable of growth in air (e.g., Cl. carnis, Cl. histolyticum, and Cl. tertium; aerotolerant.

[8]Facultative or strict (obligate) anaerobes; 20% obligate anaerobes; occasionally microaerophilic. Grows poorly in air; enhanced growth with reduced oxygen tension. Isolation of some anaerobes enhanced by carbon dioxide (CO_2).

[9]Usually strict (obligate) anaerobes; some strains aerotolerant, but grow best anaerobically.

Diagram 43.33.

Differentiation of **aerobic** to **facultative anaerobic**, Gram-positive cocci by catalase reaction.

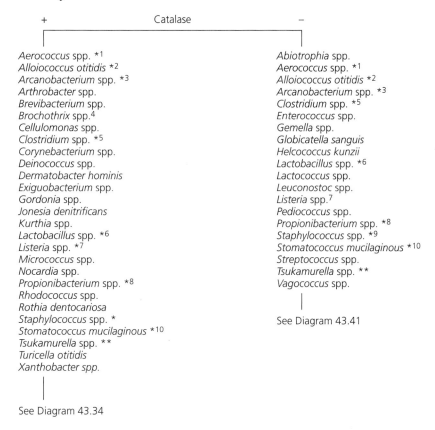

+	Catalase	−
Aerocococcus spp. *[1]		*Abiotrophia* spp.
Alloiococcus otitidis *[2]		*Aerococcus* spp. *[1]
Arcanobacterium spp. *[3]		*Alloiococcus otitidis* *[2]
Arthrobacter spp.		*Arcanobacterium* spp. *[3]
Brevibacterium spp.		*Clostridium* spp. *[5]
Brochothrix spp.[4]		*Enterococcus* spp.
Cellulomonas spp.		*Gemella* spp.
Clostridium spp. *[5]		*Globicatella sanguis*
Corynebacterium spp.		*Helcococcus kunzii*
Deinococcus spp.		*Lactobacillus* spp. *[6]
Dermatobacter hominis		*Lactococcus* spp.
Exiguobacterium spp.		*Leuconostoc* spp.
Gordonia spp.		*Listeria* spp.[7]
Jonesia denitrificans		*Pediococcus* spp.
Kurthia spp.		*Propionibacterium* spp. *[8]
Lactobacillus spp. *[6]		*Staphylococcus* spp. *[9]
Listeria spp. *[7]		*Stomatococcus mucilaginous* *[10]
Micrococcus spp.		*Streptococcus* spp.
Nocardia spp.		*Tsukamurella* spp. **
Propionibacterium spp. *[8]		*Vagococcus* spp.
Rhodococcus spp.		
Rothia dentocariosa		See Diagram 43.41
Staphylococcus spp. *		
Stomatococcus mucilaginous *[10]		
Tsukamurella spp. **		
Turicella otitidis		
Xanthobacter spp.		

See Diagram 43.34

---

*Variable results.
**No results; treated as variable.
[1] If positive, weak; pseudocatalase reaction; due to nonheme catalase (32).
[2] Catalase-positive but weak; catalase-negative **only** when cultivated on media devoid of whole blood (e.g., chocolate agar).
[3] Some strains exhibit weak activity; usually negative.
[4] Catalase dependent on medium and temperature of incubation; incubation at 20°C (12).
[5] Catalase-variable, usually negative; trace amounts may be detected in some strains (40).
[6] Some catalase-positive strains (26).
[7] Catalase-positive, cytochromes produced; rare strains negative (26).
[8] Catalase-variable; usually positive.
[9] *S. aureus* subsp. *anaerobius* and *S. saccharolyticus* are catalase-negative and usually **only** grow anaerobically.
[10] Catalase-variable; if positive, weak.

Diagram 43.34.

Differentiation of **catalase-positive**, aerobic to facultative anaerobic Gram-positive cocci.

Aerococcus spp.
Alloiococcus otitidis
Arcanobacterium spp.
Arthrobacter spp.
Brevibacterium spp.
Brochothrix spp.
Cellulomonas spp.
Clostridium spp.
Corynebacterium spp.

Deinococcus spp.
Dermabacter hominis
Exiguobacterium spp.
Gordonia spp.
Jonesia denitrificans
Kurthia spp.
Lactobacillus spp.
Listeria spp.
Micrococcus spp.

Nocardia spp.
Propionibacterium spp.
Rhodococcus spp.
Rothia dentocariosa
Staphylococcus spp.
Stomatococcus mucilaginous
Tsukamurella spp.
Turicella otitidis
Xanthobacter spp.

F	O/F Glucose	NF
Aerococcus spp. Alloiococcus otitidis ** Arcanobacterium spp. Brochothrix spp. Cellulomonas spp. *[2] Clostridium spp. Corynebacterium spp. *[3] Deinococcus spp. Dermatobacter hominis Exiguobacterium spp. Gordonia spp. ** Jonesia denitrificans Lactobacillus spp. Listeria spp. *[4] Propionibacterium spp. Rothia dentocariosa Staphylococcus spp. Stomatococcus mucilaginous Tsukamurella spp. ** Turicella otitidis ** Xanthobacter spp. **		Alloiococcus otitidis ** Arthrobacter spp. Brevibacterium spp.[1] Cellulomonas spp. *[2] Corynebacterium spp. *[3] Gordonia spp. ** Kurthia spp. Listeria spp. *[4] Micrococcus spp. Nocardia spp. Rhodococcus spp. Tsukamurella spp. ** Turicella otitidis ** Xanthobacter spp. **
See Diagram 43.35		See Diagram 43.40

---

*Variable results.
**No results; treated as variable.
[1] O (oxidative) or inert (−).
[2] F (fermentation) and O (oxidative).
[3] F (fermentation), O (oxidative) or inert (−).
[4] F (fermentation) or O (oxidative).

Diagram 43.35.

Differentiation of **catalase-positive, aerobic** to **facultative anaerobic**, Gram-positive cocci that **ferment glucose**.

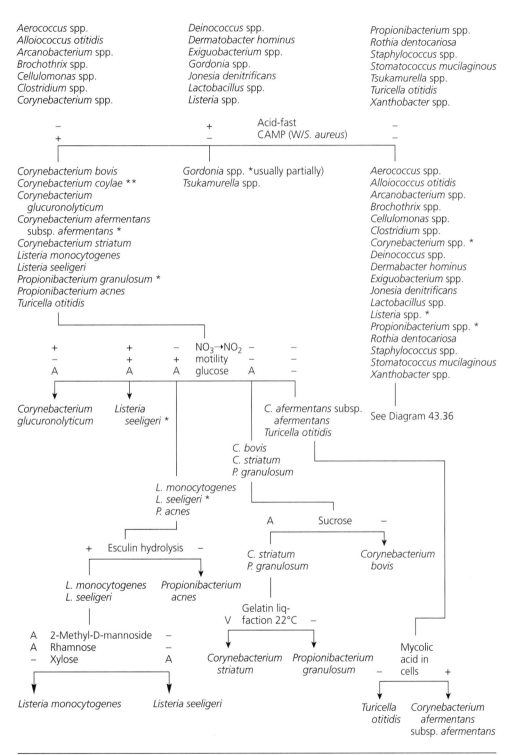

*Variable results.
**Not included in Tables.

Diagram 43.36.

Differentiation of **catalase-positive, aerobic,** to **facultative anaerobic** Gram-positive cocci that **ferment glucose**, are **not acid-fast**, and are **CAMP-negative**.

Aerococcus spp.
Alloiococcus otitidis
Arcanobacterium spp.
Brochothrix spp.
Cellulomonas spp.
Clostridium spp.
Corynebacterium spp.

Deinococcus spp.
Dermabacter hominus
Exiguobacterium spp.
Jonesia denitrificans
Lactobacillus spp.
Listeria spp.

Propionibacterium spp.
Rothia dentocariosa
Staphylococcus spp.
Stomatococcus mucilaginous
Xanthobacter spp.

+ ─────────── Motility ─────────── −

Alloiococcus otitidis **	Aerococcus spp.
Cellulomonas spp. *	Alloiococcus otitidis **
Clostridium spp. *	Arcanobacterium spp.
Corynebacterium spp. *	Brochothrix spp.[1]
Exiguobacterium spp.	Cellulomonas spp. *
Jonesia denitrificans	Clostridium spp. *
Lactobacillus spp. *	Corynebacterium spp. *
Listeria spp. *[2]	Deinococcus spp.
Xanthobacter spp. *	Dermabacter hominus
	Lactobacillus spp. *[3]
	Listeria spp. *[2]
	Propionibacterium spp.
	Rothia dentocariosa
See Diagram 43.37	Staphylococcus spp.
	Stomatococcus mucilaginous
	Xanthobacter spp.

Aerococcus spp.: See Table 43.2 to differentiate species.
Alloiococcus otitidis **: See genus description.
Arcanobacterium spp.: A. haemolyticum reverse CAMP-positive; see Table 43.3 to differentiate species.
Brochothrix spp.: See Table 43.7 to differentiate species. Usually does not grow at 35-37°C; range 20-25°C; MR-positive and VP-positive.
Cellulomonas spp.: See genus description.
Clostridium spp. *: See Diagrams 43.17 and 43.21 to differentiate aerotolerant species. cl. carnis, cl. histoluticum, and cl. tertium.
Corynebacterium spp. *: See Diagrams 43.10–43.15 to differentiate species.
Deinococcus spp.: See Table 43.19 to differentiate the most frequently encountered species.
Dermabacter hominus: See Table 43.20 for biochemical characteristics.
Exiguobacterium spp.: See genus description.
Jonesia denitrificans: See Table 43.27 for biochemical characteristics.
Lactobacillus spp. *: See Table 43.29 for differentiation of frequently isolated species from clinical specimens..
Listeria spp. *: See Diagram 43.15 to differentiate species.
Propionibacterium spp.: See Table 43.40 to differentiate species.
Rothia dentocariosa: See Table 43.41 for biochemical characteristics.
Stomatococcus mucilaginous: See Table 43.46 for biochemical characteristics.
Xanthobacter spp.: See genus description.

---

*Variable results.
**No results; treated as variable.
[1]Nonmotile at 22°C.
[2]Motile when grown in nutrient broth at room temperature (20–25°C); characteristic end-over tumbling motility in wet mounts.
[3]Rare positive motility.

Diagram 43.37.

Initial differentiation of **catalase-positive**[1] *Staphylococcus* spp. most frequently isolated from humans, other primates, food, and animals.

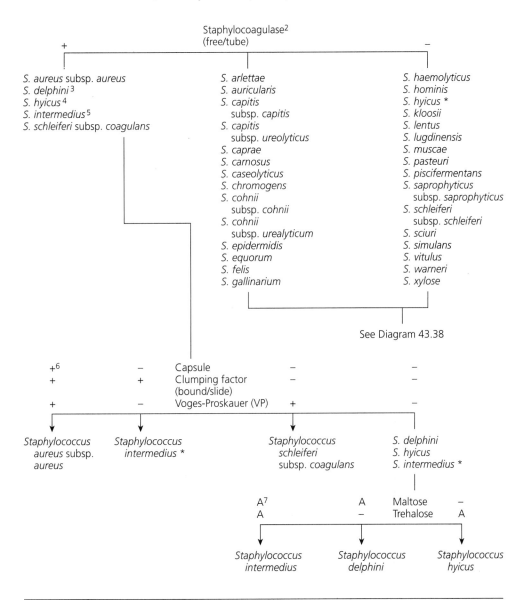

---

*Variable reactions.

[1] All *Staphylococcus* species are catalase-positive **except** *S. aureus* subsp. *anaerobius* and *S. saccharolyticus*; both exhibit growth **anaerobically only.** *S. aureus* subsp. *aureus* is variable for catalase production, usually positive.

[2] Coagulase test is the usual final criterion for *Staphylococcus* spp. differentiation; however some *S. aureus* strains lose their coagulase activity. Further criteria depend on anaerobic fermentation of glucose and mannitol.

[3] Isolated from dolphins.

[4] One of the primary animal species isolated from veterinary specimens; isolated from pigs.

[5] Isolated from dog bites, Carnivora, and certain other mammals and birds.

[6] Encapsulated strains produce colonies which are smaller and more convex than noncapsulated strains and have a glistening, wet appearance (40).

[7] Positive reaction may be delayed.

Diagram 43.38.

Differentiation of **catalase-positive, coagulase-negative** *Staphylococcus* species most frequently isolated from humans, other primates, food, and animals.

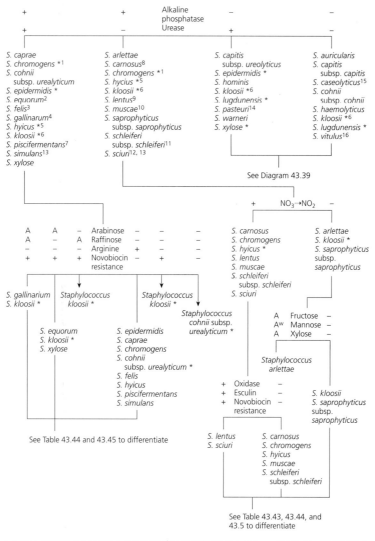

*Variable results

[1] *S. chromogens* isolated from cattle.

[2] *S. equorum* isolated from horses.

[3] *S. felis* isolated from cats.

[4] *S. gallinarum* isolated primarily from poultry.

[5] *S. hyicus* isolated from pigs.

[6] *S. kloosii* isolated from a variety of mammals.

[7] *S. piscifermentans* isolated from fish.

[8] *S. carnosus* isolated from fermented meats; e.g., sausage and salami.

[9] *S. lentus* isolated from goats and sheep.

[10] *S. muscae* isolated from a variety of animals.

[11] *S. schleiferi* subsp. *schleiferi* is a pathogen in European countries, but seldom seen in the United States (33).

[12] *S. sciuri* isolated from rodents and certain other mammals.

[13] Weak alkaline phosphatase reaction; may be delayed.

[14] *S. pasteuri* rarely encountered in clinical specimens.

[15] *S. caseolyticus* is one of the primary animal species isolated from veterinary specimens; from milk and dairy products.

[16] *S. vitulus* isolated from ingulates and dairy and meat products.

Diagram 43.39.

Differentiation of **catalase-positive, coagulase-negative, alkaline-phosphatase-negative** *Staphylococcus* species most frequently isolated from humans, other primates, food, and animals.

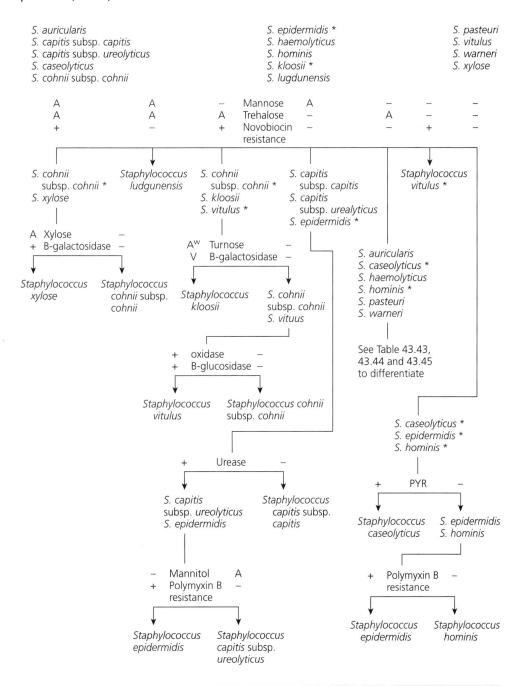

*Variable results.

Diagram 43.40.

Differentiation of **catalase-positive** Gram-positive cocci that **do not ferment glucose (NF, nonfermentative).**

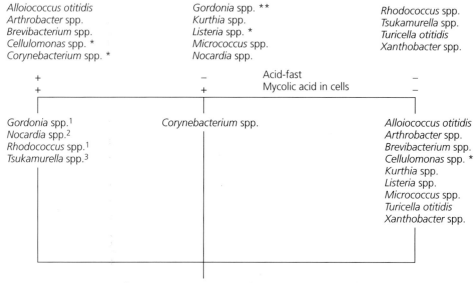

Alloiococcus spp.: See genus description.
Arthrobacter spp.: See genus description.
Brevibacterium spp.: See Table 43.6 to differentiate species.
Cellulomonas spp.: See genus description.
Corynebacterium spp.: See Diagrams 43.10–43.15 to differentiate species.
Gordonia spp.: See genus description.
Kurthia spp.: See Table 43.28 to differentiate species.
Listeria spp.: See Diagram 43.15 to differentiate species.
Micrococcus spp.: See Table 43.34 to differentiate species.
Nocardia spp.: See Table 43.36 to differentiate the most frequently isolated species.
Rhodococcus spp.: See genus description.
Tsukamurella spp.: See genus description.
Turicella otitidis: See Table 43.50 for biochemical characteristics, **CAMP-positive**.
Xanthobacter spp.: See genus description.

---

*Variable results.
**No results; treated as variable.
[1] Usually partially acid-fast.
[2] Acid-fastness variable; usually positive.
[3] Weak to strongly acid fast.

Chapter 43 / Gram-Positive Bacteria

Diagram 43.41.

Differentiation of **aerobic to facultative anaerobic** Gram-positive cocci that are **catalase-negative**.[1]

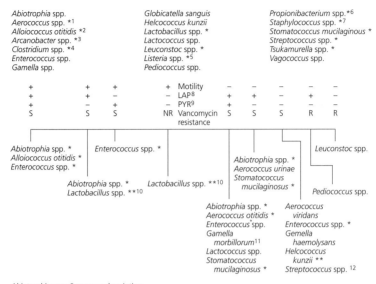

Abiotrophia spp.: See genus description.
Aerococcus spp.: See Table 43.2 to differentiate species.
Alloiococcus otitidis: See genus description.
Arcanobacterium spp.: See Table 43.3 to differentiate species.
Clostridium spp.: See Diagrams 43.17 and 43.21 to differentiate aerotolerant species.
Gemella spp.: See Table 43.26 to differentiate species.
Globicatella sanguis: See genus description.
Helcococcus spp.: See genus description.
Lactobacillus spp.: See Table 43.29 to differentiate the most frequently isolated species.
Lactococcus spp.: See Table 43.30 to differentiate species.
Leuconstoc spp.: See Table 43.31 to differentiate frequently isolated species.
Listeria spp.: See Diagram 43.15 to differentiate species.
Pediococcus spp.: See Table 43.38 to differentiate species.
Staphylococcus spp.: See Diagrams 43.37-43.39 to differentiate species.
Stomatococcus mucilaginosus: See Table 43.46 for biochemical characteristics.
Tsukamurella spp.: See genus description.
Vagococcus spp.: See Table 43.51 to differentiate species.
Enterococcus spp.: See Diagram 43.42.
Streptococcus spp.: See Diagrams 43.43–43.45.

---

*Variable reactions.
**No results; treated as variable.
[1]Catalase-negative or weak (pseudocatalase); due to nonheme catalase (32).
[2]Catalase-positive but weak; catalase-negative only when cultivated on media devoid of whole blood (e.g., chocolate agar).
[3]Some strains exhibit weak activity; usually catalase-negative.
[4]**Only** *Cl. carnis, Cl. histolyticum,* and *Cl. tertium* are aerotolerant; catalase variable, usually negative.
[5]Catalase-positive; rare strains negative (26).
[6]Some strains aerotolerant; usually strict (obligate) anaerobes; growth best anaerobically; catalase variable.
[7]*Staphylococcus aureus* subsp. *anaerobius* and *Staphylococcus saccharolyticus* catalase-negative and usually only grows anaerobically.
[8]LAP: leucine aminopeptidase.
[9]PYR: pyrrolidonylarylamidase.
[10]No results for vancomycin resistance.
[11]According to Facklam and Washington (17) in order to avoid false-negative PYR reaction a large inoculum **must be used.**
[12]Group A streptococci PYR-positive; other species are negative.

Diagram 43.42.

Differentiation of *Enterococcus* species.

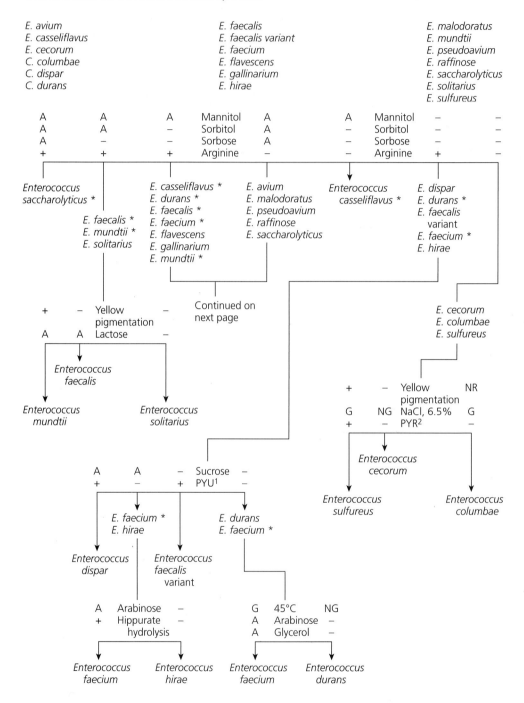

(continued)

Chapter 43 / Gram-Positive Bacteria **615**

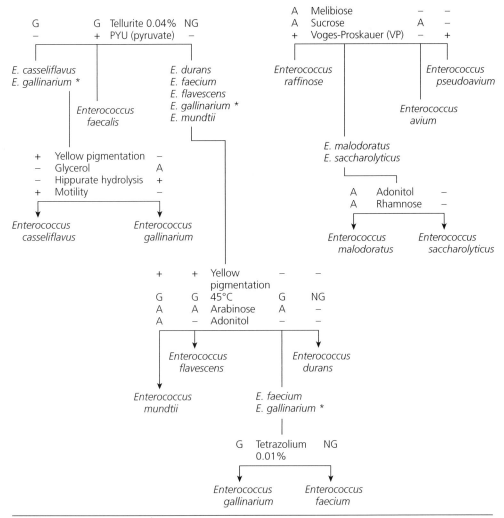

*Variable reactions.
[1]PYU: pyruvate
[2]PYR: pyrrolidonyl-B-naphthylamide (pyrrolidonylarylamidase)

Diagram 43.43.

Differentiation of beta (β) hemolytic *Streptococcus* species.

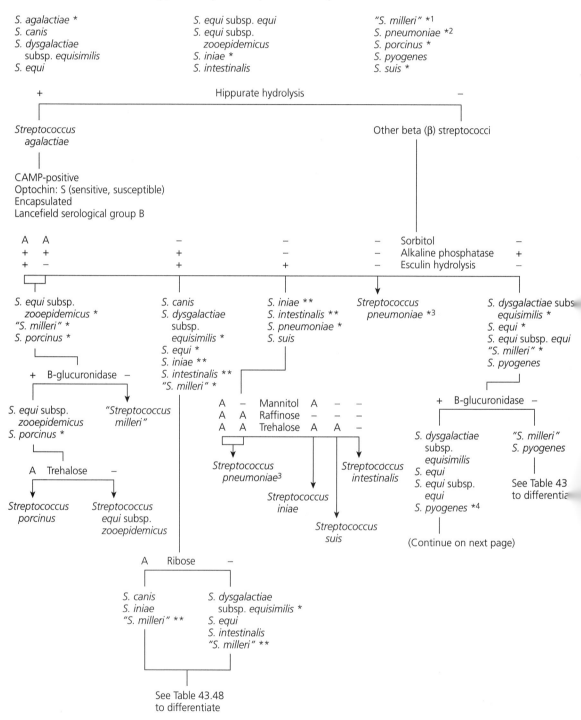

Chapter 43 / Gram-Positive Bacteria **617**

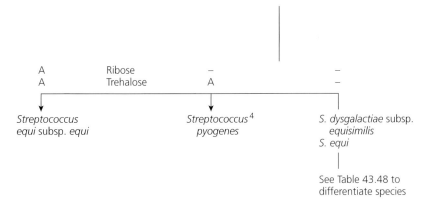

*Variable results.
**No results; treated as variable.
[1] *S. milleri* group composed of three former species: *S. anginosus, S. constellatus,* and *S. intermedius.*
[2] *S. pneumoniae* occasionally exhibits beta (β) hemolysis.
[3] *S. pneumoniae:*
    Encapsulated
    Bile soluble
    Optochin: S (sensitive, susceptible)
        |
    Colony morphology
        |
    + Large, mucoid colonies −
    + Confluent growth
    Type III   Type I or other types
[4] *S. pyogenes:*
    Optochin: R (resistant)
    Bacitracin: S (sensitive, susceptible)
    Lancefield serological group A
    Streptolysin O and S.

Diagram 43.44.

Differentiation of alpha (α) or gama (γ) hemolytic *Streptococcus* species.

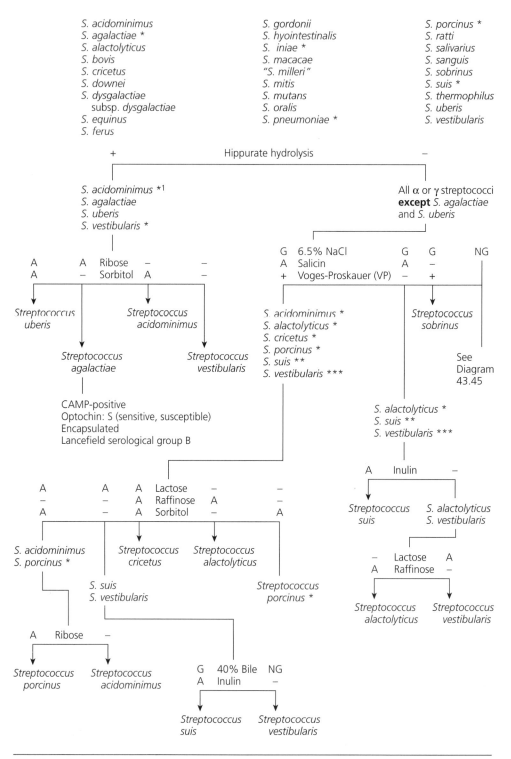

*Variable results.
**No results; treated as variable.
[1]Positive reaction may be delayed.

Diagram 43.45.

Differentiation of alpha (α) or gamma (γ) hemolytic *Streptococcus* species that are **hippurate hydrolysis-negative** and **do not grow in 6.5% NaCl**.

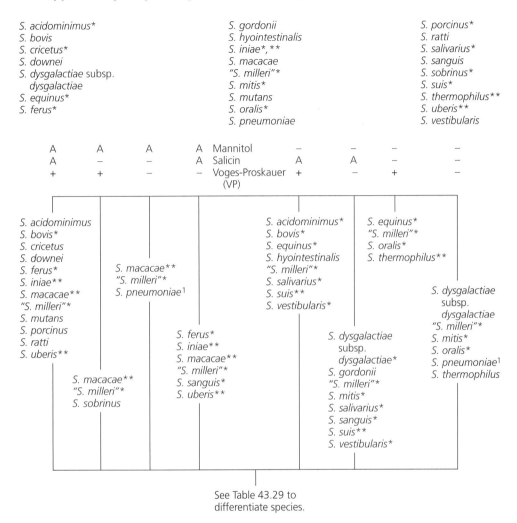

See Table 43.29 to differentiate species.

---

*Variable results.
**No results; treated as variable.
[1] *S. pneumoniae:* encapsulated; bile soluble; optochin: S (sensitive, susceptible).

620 Biochemical Tests for Identification of Medical Bacteria

Diagram 43.46.

Differentiation of **anaerobic** Gram-positive **cocci**.

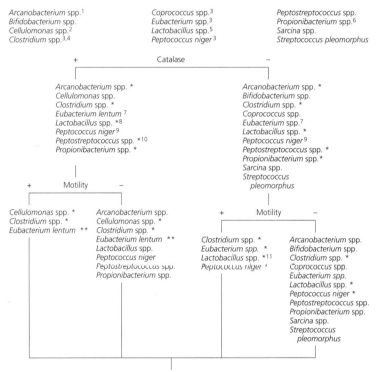

Difficult to differentiate *Bifidobacterium*, *Eubacterium*, anaerobic *Lactobacillus*, *Propionibacterium* accurately to genus without end-product analysis (19).

Arcanobacterium spp.: See Table 43.3 to differentiate three species. *A. haemolyticum* reverse CAMP-positive.
Bifidobacterium spp.: See genus description and Diagram 43.28.
Cellulomonas spp.: See genus description.
Clostridium spp.: See Tables 43.9–43.16 and Diagrams 43.16–43.25; spore-forming.
Coprococcus spp.: See Table 43.17.
Eubacterium spp.: See Table 43.23 for species that may cause human infections and Diagrams 43.28-43.31.
Lactobacillus spp.: See Table 43.29 and Diagram 43.28 for differentiation of frequently isolated species from clinical specimens.
Peptococcus niger: See genus description; H_2S-positive in SIM medium.
Peptostreptococcus spp.: See Table 43.39 for differentiation of species that may cause human infections and Diagram 43.47.
Propionibacterium spp.: See Table 43.20 and Diagrams 43.26–43.27 and 43.30–43.31 to differentiate the most frequently isolated species.
Sarcina spp.: See Table 43.42 to differentiation species.
Streptococcus pleomorphus: See Table 43.27 for biochemical characteristics; weakly $H_2S(-)$ positive.

---

*Variable results.
**No results; treated as variable.
[1]Anaerobic growth better than aerobic.
[2]Some strains grow poorly anaerobically.
[3]Strict (obligate) anaerobes.
[4]Few species capable of growth in air (e.g., *Cl. carnis*, *Cl. histolyticum*, and *Cl. tertium*); aerotolerant.
[5]Facultative or strict (obligate) anaerobes; 20% obligate anaerobes; occasionally microaerophilic; grows poorly in air; enhanced growth with reduced oxygen tension. Isolation of some anaerobes enhanced by carbon dioxide (CO_2).
[6]Usually strict (obligate) anaerobes; some strains aerotolerant, but grow best anaerobically.
[7]Occasional strain of *Eubacterium lentum* catalase-positive.
[8]Some catalase-positive strains (26).
[9]Variable, usually negative; may be weakly positive.
[10]Few strains weak or produce a pseudocatalase reaction (e.g., *P. saccharolyticus*).
[11]Motility rare.

Diagram 43.47.

Differentiation of **anaerobic** *Peptostreptococcus* species

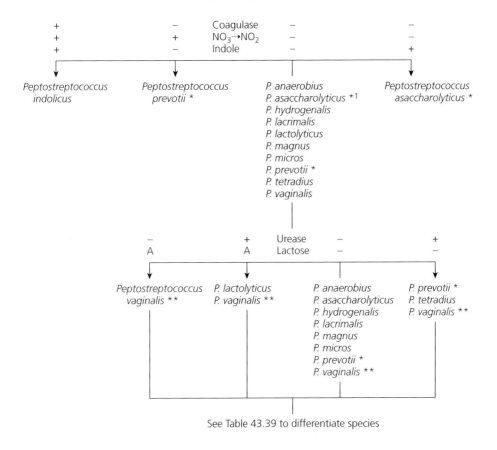

See Table 43.39 to differentiate species

---

*Variable results.
**No results; treated as variable.
[1]Occasional strains are indole (−) negative

REFERENCES

1. Barksdale L, Linder R, Sulea IT, Pollice M. Phopholipase D activity of *Corynebacterium pseudotuberculosis* (*Corynebacterium ovis*) and *Corynebacterium ulcerans*. A distinctive marker within the genus *Corynebacterium*. J Clin Microbiol 1981; 13(2):335–343.
2. Baron EJ, Peterson LR, Finegold SM. Bailey & Scott's Diagnostic Microbiology, ed 9. St. Louis: CV Mosby, 1994:505.
3. Barreau C. Bimet F, Kiredjian M, Rouillon N, Bizet C. Comparative chemotaxonomic studies of mycolic acid-free coryneform bacteria of human origin. J Clin Microbiol 1993;31(8):2085–2090.
4. Biberstein EL, Knight HD. Two biotypes of *Corynebacterium pseudotuberculosis*. Vet Rec 1971; 89:691–692.
5. Charfreitag O, Collins MD, Stackebrandt E. Reclassification of *Arachnia propionica* as *Propionibacterium propionicus*. Int J Syst Bacteriol 1988; 38(4):354–357.
6. Clewell DB. Movable genetic elements and antibiotic resistance in enterococci. Eur J Clin Microbiol Infect Dis 1990;9:90–102.
7. Collins MD, Farrow JAE, Jones D. *Enterococcus mundtii* sp. nov. Int J Syst Bacteriol 1986;36 (1):8–12.
8. Collins MD, Farrow JAE, Phillips BA, Kandler O. Validation of the publication of new names and new combinations previously effectively published outside of the IJSB. List no. 14. Int J Syst Bacteriol 1984;34(2):270–271.
9. Collins MD, Jones D, Farrow JAE, Kilpper-Bläz R, Schleifer KH. *Enterococcus avium* nom. rev., comb. nov.; *E. casseliflavus* nom. rev., comb. nov.; *E. durans* nom. rev.; comb. nov.; *E. gallinarum* comb. nov.; and *E. malodoratus* sp. nov. Int J Syst Bacteriol 1984;34(2):220–223.
10. Collins MD, Smida J, Dorsch M, Stackebrandt E. *Tsukamurella* gen. nov. harboring *Corynebacterium paurometabolum* and *Rhodococcus aurantiacus*. Int J Syst Bacteriol 1988;38(4):385–391.
11. Collins MD, Smida J, Stackebrandt E. Phylogenetic evidence for the transfer of *Caseobacter polymorphus* (Crombach) to the genus *Corynebacterium*. Int J Syst Bacteriol 1989;39(1):7–9.
12. Coyle MB, Lipsky BA. Coryneform bacteria in infectious diseases: Clinical and laboratory aspects. Clin Microbiol Rev 1990;3(3):227–246.
13. De Briel D, Couderc F, Riegel P, Minck P. High-performance liquid chromatography of corynomycolic acids as a tool in identification of *Corynebacterium* species and related organisms. J Clin Microbiol 1992;30(6):1407–1417.
14. Domenech A, Prieta J, Fernandez-Garayzabal JF, Collins MD, Jones D, Dominquez L. Phenotypic and phylogenetic evidence for a close relationship between *Lactococcus garvieae* and *Enterococcus seriolicida*. Microbiologia 1963;9:63–68.
15. Facklam R, Hollis D, Collins MD. Identification of gram-positive coccal and coccobacillary vancomycin-resistant bacteria. J Clin Microbiol 1989;27(4):724–730.
16. Facklam RR, Thacker LG, Fox B, Eriquez L. Presumptive identification of streptococci with a new test system. J Clin Microbiol 1982;15(6): 987–990.
17. Facklam RR, Washington JA II. *Streptococcus* and related catalase-negative gram-positive cocci. In: Balows A, Hausler WJ Jr, Hermaan KL, Isenberg HD, Sahadomy HJ, eds. Manual of Clinical Microbiology, ed 5. Washington, DC: American Society for Microbiology, 1991:238–257.
18. Fontana R, Canepari P, Lleo MM, Satta G. Mechanism of resistance of enterococci to beta-lactam antibiotics. Eur J Microbiol Infect Dis 1990;9: (2):103–105.
19. Forbes BA, Sahm DF, Weissfeld AS. Bailey & Scott's Diagnostic Microbiology, ed 10. St. Louis: CV Mosby, 1998:626–633, 637–671, 708–709.
20. Garvie EI, Farrow JAE. *Streptococcus lactis* subsp. cremoris (Orla-Jensen) comb. nov. and *Streptococcus lactis* subsp. *diacetilactis* (Matuszewski et al.) nom. rev., comb. nov. Int J Syst Bacteriol 1982;32(4):453–455.
21. Gruner E, Pfyffer GE, von Graevenitz A. Characterization of *Brevibacterium* spp. from clinical specimens. J Clin Microbiol 1993;31(6):1408–1412.
22. Hammann R, Kronibus A, Viebahn A, Brandis H. Validation list no. 15. Int J Syst Bacteriol 1984;34(3):355–357.
23. Hill GB, Ayers OM, Kohan AP. Characteristics and sites of infection of *Eubacterium nodatum, Eubacterium timidum, Eubacterium brachy,* and other asaccharolytic eubacteria. J Clin Microbiol 1987;25(8):1540–1545.
24. Holdeman LV, Cato EP, Moore WEC, eds. Anaerobic Laboratory Manual, ed 4. Blacksburg, VA: Virginia Polytechnic Institute Anaerobic Laboratory (VPI), 1977.
25. Holdeman LV, Moore WEC. New genus *Coprococcus*, twelve new species, and emended description of four previously described species of bacteria from human specimens. Int J Syst Bacteriol 1974;24(2)260–277.
26. Holt JG, Krieg NR, Sneath PHA, Staley JT, Williams ST. Bergey's Manual of Determinative Bacteriology, ed 9. Baltimore, Williams & Wilkins, 1994:99–100, 172, 199, 295, 525–562, 565–569, 571–596, 598–601, 611–644.
27. Johnson AP, Uttley ANC, Woodford N, George RC. Resistance to vancomycin and teicoplanin: An emerging clinical problem. Clin Microbiol Rev 1990;3(3):280–291.
28. Jones D, Collins MD. Validatum of the publication of new names and new combinations previously effectively published outside the IJSB. Int J Syst Bacteriol 1989;39(1):93–94.
29. Knight HD. Corynebacterial infections in the

horse: Problem of prevention. J Am Vet Med Assoc 1969;155:446–452.
30. Koneman EW, Allen SD, Janda WM, Schreckenberger PC, Winn WC Jr. Color Atlas and Textbook of Diagnostic Microbiology, ed 4. Philadelphia: JB Lippincott, 1992;475.
31. Moore WEC, Holdeman LV. Human fecal flora: The normal flora of 20 Japanese-Hawaiians. Appl Microbiol 1974;27:961–979.
32. Murray BE: The life and times of the *Enterococcus*. Clin Microbiol Rev 3(1):46–65, 1990.
33. Murray PR, Baron EJ, Tenover FC, Yolken RH. Manual of Clinical Microbiology, ed 6. Washington, DC: American Society for Microbiology, 1995:15, 257–366, 417–426, 574–599, 604–609.
34. Rocourt J, Wehmeyer U, Stackebrandt E. Transfer of *Listereria dentrificans* to a new genus, *Jonesia* gen. nov., as *Jonesia denitrificans* comb. nov. Int J Syst Bacteriol 1987;37(3):266–270.
35. Ruimy R, Riegel P, Boiron P, et al. Phylogeny of the genus *Corynebacterium* deduced from analyses of small-subuit ribosomal DNA sequences. Int J Syst Bacteriol 1995;45(4):740–746.
36. Schillinger U, Holzapfel W, Kandler O. Validatum of the publication of new names and new combinations previously effectively published outside the IJSB. List no. 31. Int J Syst Bacteriol 1989;39(4):495–497.
37. Schleifer KH, Kilpper-Bälz R. Transfer of *Streptococcus faecalis* and *Streptococcus faecium* to the genus *Enterococcus* nom. rev. as *Enterococcus faecalis* comb. nov. and *Enterococcus faecium* comb. nov. Int J Syst Bacteriol 1984;34(1):31–34.
38. Sherman JM. The streptococci. Bacteriol Rev 1937;1:3–97.
39. Smith LDS, William BL. The pathogenic anaerobic bacteria, ed 3. Springfield, IL: Charles C Thomas, 1984.
40. Sneath PHA, Mair NS, Sharpe ME, Holt JG, eds. Bergey's Manual of Systematic Bacteriology, vol 2. Baltimore: Williams & Wilkins, 1986:255, 1131, 1239, 1305, 1421.
41. Spiegel CA, Roberts M. *Mobiluncus* gen. nov., *Mobiluncus curtisii* subsp. *curtisii* sp. nov., *Mobiluncus curtisii* subsp. *holmesii* subsp. nov., and *Mobiluncus mulieris* sp. nov., curved rods from the human vagina. Int J Syst Bacteriol 1984;34(2):177–184.
42. Stackebrandt E, Smida J, Collins MD. Evidence of phylogenetic heterogeneity within the genus *Rhodococcus*: Revival of the genus *Gordona* (Tsukamura). J Gen Applied Microbiol 1988;34:341–348.
43. Suen JC, Hatheway CL, Steigerwalt AG, Brenner DJ. *Clostridium argentinense* sp. nov.: A genetically homogeneous group composed of all strains of *Clostridium botulinum* toxin type G and some nontoxigenic strains previously identified as *Clostridium subterminale* or *Clostridium hastiforme*. Int J Syst Bacteriol 1988;38:375.
44. Takahashi T, Fujisawa T, Tamura Y, Suszuki S, Muramatser M, Sawada T, Benno Y, Mitsuoka T. DNA relatedness *Erysipelothrix rhusiopathiae* strains representing all twenty-tree serovars and *Erysipelothrix tonsillarum*. Int J Syst Bacteriol 1987;37(2):166–168.
45. Williams AM, Rodriques UM, Collins MD. Intrageneric relationships of enterococci as determined by reverse transcriptase sequencing of small-unit rRNA. Res Microbiol 1991;142(1):67–74.
46. Williamson R, Al-Obeid S, Shlaes JH, Goldstein FW, Shlaes DM. Inducible resistance to vancomycin in *Enterococcus faecium* D 366. J Infect Dis 1989;159(6):1095–1104.

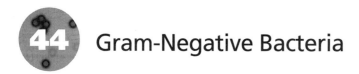

44 Gram-Negative Bacteria

Classification 624
Changes in Nomenclature of Gram-Negative Rods (Bacilli) and Gram-Negative Cocci
  (Spheres) 628
Genera Descriptions/Tables 639
Warning 705
Flow Charts
  Bacilli (Rods)
    Gram-Negative Aerobes/Facultative Anaerobes 705
    Gram-Negative Microaerophiles/Anaerobes 723
  Cocci (Spheres)
    Gram-Negative Aerobes/Facultative Anaerobes 722
    Gram-Negative Microaerophiles/Anaerobes 729
References 730

CLASSIFICATION

Proposed Outline of *Bergey's Manual of Systematic Bacteriology*, 2nd edition

Volume 2 The Proteobacteria

Kingdom: *Proteobacteria*

Section XV: The α-Proteobacteria

  Class I Rhodospirilli
    Order IV. Sphingomonadales
      Family: *Sphingomonadaceae*
        Sphingomonas: 23 species
    Order V. Caulobacterales
      Family: *Caulobacteracea*
        Brevundimonas: 7 species
    Order VI. Rhizobiales
      Family I. *Rhizobiaceae*
        Agrobacterium: 5 species
      Family III. *Bartonellaceae*
        Bartonella: 14 species
      Family IV. *Brucellaceae*
        Brucella: 1 species
        Ochrobactrum: 2 species
      Family VI. *Bradyrhizobiaceae*
        Afipia: 3 species
      Family VII. *Methylobacteriaceae*
        Methylobacterium: 10 species

Family X. *Hyphomicrobiaceae*
    Xanthobacter: 4 species

Section XVI The β-Proteobacteria

Class: Neisseriae
  Order I. Neisseriales
    Family: *Neisseriaceae*
      Neisseria: 21 species
      Kingella: 3 species
      Chromobacterium: 1 species
      Eikenella: 1 species
  Order II. Burkholderiales
    Family I. *Burkholderiaceae*
      Burkholderia: 17 species
      Ralstonia: 5 species
    Family III. *Alcaligenaceae*
      Alcaligenes: 3 species
      Bordetella: 7 species
      Taylorella: 1 species
    Family IV. *Comamonadaceae*
      Comamonas: 2 species
      Leptothrix: 1 species

Section XVII δ-Proteobacteria

Class Zymobacteria
  Order II. Xanthomonadales
    Family: *Xanthomonadaceae*
      Xanthomonas: 22 species
      Stenotrophomonas: 2 species
  Order III. Cardiobacteriales
    Family I. *Cardiobacteriaceae*
      Cardiobacterium: 1 species
      Suttonella: 1 species
  Order IV. Thiotrichales
    Family III. *Francisellaceae*
      Francisella: 5 species
  Order V. Legionellales
    Family I. *Legionellaceae*
      Legionella: 39 species
  Order VIII. Pseudomonadales
    Family I. *Pseudomonadaceae*
      Pseudomonas: 76 species
      Acidovorax: 7 species
      Chryseomonas: 1 species
      Flavimonas: 1 species
      Janthinobacterium: 1 species
      Morococcus: 1 species
      Oligella: 2 species

Family II. *Moraxellaceae*
    Moraxella: 13 species
    Acinetobacter: 7 species
    Psychrobacter: 5 species
Order IX. Alteromonadales
  Family. *Alteromonadaceae*
    Shewanella: 12 species
Order X. Vibrionales
  Family. *Vibrionaceae*
    Vibrio: 39 species
Order XI. Aeromonadales
  Family *Aeromonadaceae*
    Aeromonas: 22 species
Order XII. Enterobacteriales
  Family *Enterobacteriaceae* (see Chapter 45)
Order XIII. Pasteurellales
  Family *Pasteurellaceae*
    Pasteurella: 19 species
    Haemophilus: 17 species
    Actinobacillus: 16 species

Section XIX δ-Proteobacteria

Class Campylobacteres
  Order I. Campylobacterales
    Family I. *Campylobacteraceae*
      Campylobacter: 18 species
    Family II. *Helicobacteraceae*
      Helicobacter: 18 species
      Wolinella: 1 species

Volume 3 Bacteria: The Low G + C Gram Positives. (Low guanine-plus cytosine base content of DNA; bacteria more regular in shape)

Section XX: The Clostridia and Relatives

Class: Clostridia
  Order I: Clostridiales
    Family II. *Peptostreptococcaceae*
      Peptostreptococcus: 15 species
    Family III. *Eubacteriaceae*
      Tissierella: 3 species
    Family IV. *Lachnospiraceae*
      Butyrivibrio: 2 species
    Family V. *Peptococcaceae*
      Acidaminococcus: 1 species
      Megasphaera: 2 species
      Selenomonas: 11 species
      Mitsuokella: 1 species
      Veillonella: 7 species
      Succinivibrio: 1 species

Section XXI The Mollicutes

Class Mollicutes
    Order Mycoplasmatales
        Family I. *Mycoplasmataceae*
            Mycoplasma: 104 species
            Ureaplasma: 6 species
        Family II. *Acholeplasmataceae*
            Acholeplasma: 13 species

Section XXII The Bacilli and Lactobacilli

Class Bacilli
    Order II. Lactobacillales
        Family VIII. *Staphylococcaceae*
            Gemella: 4 species

Volume 4 Bacteria: The High G + C Gram Positives. (High guanine-plus-cytosine base content of DNA; bacteria irregular cell shape)

Section XXIII: Class *Actinobacteria*

Subclass V. Actinobacteridae
    Order I. Actinomycetales
        Suborder I. Actinomycineae
            Family. *Actinomycetaceae*
                Mobiluncus: 3 species
    Order II. Bifidobacteriales
        Family. *Bifidobacteriaceae*
            Gardnerella: 1 species

Volume 5 The Planctomycetes, Spirochaetes, Fibrobacteres, Bacteroides and Fusobacteria

Kingdom *Bacteroides*
Division I *Bacteroides*

Section XXVII The Bacteroides

Class I. Bacteroides
    Order Bacteroidales
        Family I. *Bacteroidaceae*
            Bacteroides: 25 species
            Anaerorhabdus: 1 species
            Centipeda: 1 species
            Megamonas: 1 species
            Anaerobiospirillum: 1 species
            Succinimonas: 1 species
        Family III. *Porphyromonadaceae*
            Porphyromonas: 12 species
        Family IV. *Prevotellaceae*
            Prevotella: 26 species

Section XXVIII The Flavobacteria

Class II. Flavobacteria
    Order Flavobacteriales
        Family I. *Flavobacteriaceae*
            Flavobacterium: 19 species
            Weeksella: 1 species
            Capnocytophaga: 7 species

Section XXX The Fusobacteria

Kingdom Fusobacteria
    Class Fusobacteria
        Order Fusobacteriales
            Family *Fusobacteriaceae*
                Fusobacterium: 20 species
                Propionigenium: 2 species
                Leptotrichia: 1 species
                Streptobacillus: 1 species

(*Note*: Bergey's outline of classification is listed only for those organisms covered in this chapter or new genera and species listed in New Nomenclature. Outline courtesy of Dr. George Garrity, Editor-in-Chief, Bergey's Manual Trust.)

CHANGES IN NOMENCLATURE OF GRAM-NEGATIVE RODS (BACILLI) AND GRAM-NEGATIVE COCCI (SPHERES)

(*Note:* Bergey's Manual of Determinative Bacteriology, 9th edition, was printed in 1994; therefore, references to new genera or new species are listed from 1995 to 1999.)

Definitions

Basonym: original name of a new combination
Synonym:
    Objective: more than 1 name
    Subjective: different name to different types; first published, senior; later, junior
comb. nov.: new combination; species transferred to another genus or subsp. transferred to another species
gen. nov.: new genus
sp. non.: new species
nomen dubium: doubtful name

Current name	Old name (basonym(s)/synonym(s))
Achromobacter piechaudii	*Alcaligenes piechaudii*
Achromobacter ruhlandii	*Alcaligenes ruhlandii*
Achromobacter xylosoxidans subsp. *denitrificans*	*Alcaligenes denitrificans*
Achromobacter xylosoxidans subsp. *xylosoxidans*	*Alcaligenes xylosoxidans*
Acidovorav avenae subsp. *avenae*	*Pseudomonas avenae, Pseudomonas avenae* subsp. *avenae, Pseudomonas rubrilineans*
Acidovorax avenae subsp. *citrulli*	*Pseudomonas avenae* subsp. *citrulli, Pseudomonas pseudoalcaligenes* subsp. *cirulli*
Acidovorax avenae subsp. *cattleyae*	*Pseudomonas cattleyae*

Acidovorax delafieldii	*Pseudomonas delafieldii*
Acidovorax facilis	*Pseudomonas facilis*
Acidovorax konjaci	*Pseudomonas avenae* subsp. *konjaci*, *Pseudomonas pseudoalcaligenes* subsp. *konjaci*
Actinobacillus delphinicola, sp. nov.[1]	
Actinobacillus indolicus, sp. nov.[2]	
Actinobacillus minor, sp. nov.[2]	
Actinobacillus porinus, sp. nov.[2]	
Actinobacillus scotiae, sp. nov.[3]	
Actinobacillus succinogenes, sp. nov.[4]	
Actinobacillus ureae	*Pasteurella ureae*
Aeromonas encheieia, sp. nov. emended[5]	
Aeromonas eucrenophila, sp. nov., emended[5]	
Aeromonas popoffii, sp. nov.[5]	
Aeromonas tructi	*Aeromonas trota*, incorrect name
Alcaligenes defragrans, sp. nov.[6]	
Alcaligenes denitrificans	*Alcaligenes denitrificans* subsp. *denitrificans*, *Alcaligenes xylosoxidans* subsp. *denitrificans*
Alcaligenes xylosoxidans	*Alcaligenes denitrificans* subsp. *xylosoxidans*, *Alcaligenes xylosoxidans* subsp. *xylosoxidans*, *Achromobacter xylosoxidans*
Agrobacterium tumefaciens	*Agrobacterium radiobacter*
Aminobacter aminovorans	*Pseudomonas aminovorans*
Anaerorhabdus furcosus	*Bacteroides furcosus*
Anaerobiospirillum thomasii, sp. nov.[7]	
Arcobacter butzleri	*Campylobacter butzleri*
Arcobacter cryaerophilus	*Campylobacter cryaerophilus*
Arcobacter nitrofigilis	*Campylobacter nitrofigilis*
Aureobacterium esteraromaticum	*Flavobacterium esteraromaticum*
Bartonella alsaticia, sp. nov.[8]	
Bartonella clarridgeiae, sp. nov.[9]	
Bartonella doshiae, sp. nov.[10]	
Bartonella elizabethae	*Aochalimaea elizabethae*
Bartonella grahamii, sp. nov.[10]	
Bartonella henselae	*Rochalimaea henselae*
Bartonella peromysci, comb. nov.[10]	
Bartonella quintana	*Rochalimaea quintana*
Bartonella talpae, comb. nov.[10]	
Bartonella taylorii, sp. nov.[10]	
Bartonella tribocorum, sp. nov.[11]	
Bartonella vinsonii subsp. *berkhoffii*, subsp. nov.[12]	
Bartonella vinsonii subsp. *vinsonii*	*Rochalimaeae vinsonii*
Brevundimonas alba, sp. nov., comb. nov.[13]	
Brevundimonas aurantiaca, sp. nov.[13]	
Brevundimonas bacteroides, comb. nov.[13]	*Caulobacter bacteroides*
Brevundimonas diminuta	*Pseudomonas diminuta*
Brevundimonas intermedia, comb. nov.[13]	*Caulobacter intermedius*
Brevundimonas subvibrioides, comb. nov.[13]	*Caulobacter subvibrioides*

Brevundimonas vescularis	*Pseudomonas vescularis*
Brucella melitensis	*Brucella abortus, Brucella canis, Brucella neotomae, Brucella ovis, Brucella suis*
Burkholderia, gen. non., emended[14]	
Burkholderia andropogonis, sp. nov.[14]	*Pseudomonas andropogonis*
Burkholderia caryophylli	*Pseudomonas caryophylli*
Burkholderia cepacia	*Pseudomonas cepacia*
Burkholderia cocovenenans, sp. nov.[14]	*Pseudomonas cocovenenans*
Burkholderia gladioli	*Pseudomonas gladioli, Burkholderia cocoveneans*
Burkholderia glathei, comb. nov.[15]	*Pseudomonas glathei*
Burkholderia glumae	*Pseudomonas glumae*
Burkholderia graminis, sp. nov.[15]	
Burholderia mallei	*Pseudomonas mallei*
Burkholderia multivorans, sp. nov.[16]	
Burkholderia norinbergensis, sp. nov.[17]	
Burkholderia phenazinum, comb. nov.[15]	*Pseudomonas phenazinum*
Burkholderia plantarii	*Pseudomonas plantarii, Burkholderia vandii*
Burkholderia pseudomallei	*Pseudomonas pseudomallei*
Burkholderia pyrrocinia, sp. nov.[15]	*Pseudomonas pyrrocinia*
Burkholderia thailandensis sp. nov.[18]	
Burkholderia vietnamiensis, sp. nov.[14]	
Carbophilus carboxidus	*Alcaligenes carboxydus*
Campylobacter coli	*Campylobacter hyoilei*
Campylobacter cryaerophilus	*Campylobacter cryaerophila*, incorrect name
Campylobacter curvus	*Wolinella curva*
Campylobacter gracilis, comb. nov.[19]	*Bacteroides gracilis*
Campylobacter lari	*Campylobacter laridis*, incorrect name
Campylobacter mucosalis	*Campylobacter sputorum* subsp. *mucosalis*
Campylobacter rectus	*Wolinella recta*
Capnocytophaga canimorsus	CDC group DF-2
Capnocytophaga cynodegmi	CDC group DF-2-like
Capnocytophaga gingivalis	CDC group DF-1
Capnocytophaga ochracea	*Bacteroides ochraceus*, CDC group DF-1
Capnocytophaga sputigena	CDC group DF-1
Chryseobacterium balustinum	*Flavobacterium balustinum*
Chryseobacterium gleum	*Flavobacterium gleum*
Chryseobacterium indologenes	*Flavobacterium inodologenes*
Chryseobacterium indoltheticum	*Flavobacterium indoltheticum*
Chryseobacterium luteola	*Chryseobacterium polytricha, Pseudomonas luteola*, CDC group Ve-1
Chryseobacterium meningosepticum	*Flavobacterium meningosepticum*
Chryseobacterium saccharophilum	*Cytophaga saccharophila*
Chryseobacterium scophthalmum	*Flavobacterium scophthalmum*
Comamonas acidovorans	*Pseudomonas acidovorans*
Comamonas terrigena	*Aquaspirillum aquaticum*
Comamonas testosteroni	*Pseudomonas testosteroni*
Cytophaga uliginosa	*Flavobacterium uliginosum*
Dalftia acidovorans	*Comamonas acidovorans*
Dietzia maris	*Flavobacterium maris*
Empedobacter brevis	*Flavobacterium brevis*

Flavimonas oryzihabitans
Flavobacterium branchiophilum

Flavobacterium capsulata
Flavobacterium columnare, sp. nov.[20]
Flavobacterium flevense, sp. nov.[20]
Flavobacterium halmephiluma

Flavobacterium hibernum, sp. nov.[21]
Flavobacterium hydatis, sp. nov.[20]
Flavobacterium johnsoniae, sp. nov.[20]
Flavobacterium mizutaii
Flavobacterium pectinovorum, sp. nov.[20]
Flavobacterium psychrophilum, sp. nov.[20]

Flavobacterium saccharophilum, sp. nov.[20]
Flavobacterium succinicans, sp. nov.[20]
Fluoribacter bozemanae
Fluoribacter dumoffii
Fluoribacter gormanii
Francisella philomiragia
Fusobacterium varium
Gemella bergeriae, sp. nov.[22]
Gemella sanguinis, sp. nov.[22]
Haemophilus actinomycetemcomitans
Haemophilus felis, sp. nov.[23]
Halomonas aquamarina

Halomonas cupida
Halomonas halmophila
Halomonas halodurans
Halomonas marina
Halomonas pacifica
Halomonas paradoxus
Halomonas venusta
Helicobacter acinonychis
Helicobacter bilis, sp. nov.[24]
Helicobacter bizzozeronii, sp. nov.[25]
Helicobacter cholecystus, sp. nov.[26]
Helicobacter cinaedi
Helicobacter fennelliae
Helicobacter mustelae

Helicobacter pullorum, sp. nov.[27]
Helicobacter pylori

Helicobacter rodentium, sp. nov.[28]
Helicobacter salomonis, sp. nov.[29]
Helicobacter trogontum, sp. nov.[30]
Herbaspirillum rubrisubalbicans
Hydrogenophaga flava

CDC Ve-2
Flavobacterium branchiophila, incorrect name
Flavobacterium capsulatum
Cytophaga columnaris, Flexibacter columnar
Cytophaga fevensis
Flavobacterium halmephilium, incorrect name

Cytophaga aquatilis
Cytophaga johnsoniae
Sphingobacterium mizutae
Cytophaga pectinovora
Cytophaga psychrophila, Flexibacter psychrophila

Cytophaga saccharophila
Cytophaga succinicans
Legionella bozemanii
Legionella dumoffii
Legionella gormanii
Yersinia philomoragia
Fusobacterium pseudonecrophorum

Actinobacillus actinomycetemcomitans

Alcaligenes aestus, Alcaligenes aquamarinus, Alcaligenes faecalis, subsp. *homari*
Alcaligenes cupidus
Flavobacterium halmephilum
Pseudomonas halodurans
Pseudomonas marina
Alcaligenes pacifica
Alcaligenes paradoxus
Alcaligenes venustus
Helicobacter acinix, incorrect name

Campylobacter cinaedi
Campylobacter fennelliae
Campylobacter mystelae, Campylobacter pylori subsp. *mustelae*

Campylobacter pylori, Campylobacter pyloridis

Pseudomonas rubrisubalbicans
Pseudomonas flava

Hydrogenophaga pallaronii	*Pseudomonas palleronii*
Hydrogenophaga pseudoflava	*Pseudomonas pseudoflava*
Kingella kingae	*Moraxella kingae*
Legionella lytica, comb. nov.[31]	*Sarcobium lyticum*
Legionella taurinensis, sp. nov.[32]	
Legionella waltersii, sp. nov.[33]	
Mannheimia granulomatis	*Pasteurella granulomatis*
Mannheimia haemolytica	*Pasteurella haemolytica*
Marinobacter hydrocarbonoclasticus	*Pseudomonas nautica*
Megamonas hypermegas	*Bacteroides hypermegas*
Mesoplasma lactucae	*Mycoplasma lactucae*
Methylobacterium mesophilicum	*Pseudomonas mesophilica*
Methylobacterium radiotolerans	*Pseudomonas radiora*
Methylobacterium rhodinum	*Pseudomonas rhodos*
Methylobacterium thiocynatum, sp. nov.[34]	
Microbacterium arborescens	*Flavobacterium arborescens*
Microbacterium maritypicum	*Flavobacterium maritypicum*
Mitsuokella multiacidus	*Bacteroides multiacidus*
Moraxella atlantae	CDC Group M-3
Moraxella boevrei, sp. nov.[35]	
Moraxella caprae, sp. nov.[36]	
Moraxella catarrhalis	*Branhamella catarrhalis*
Moraxella caviae	*Neisseria caviae*
Moraxella cuniculi	*Neisseria cuniculi*
Moraxella lacunta	*Moraxella liquefaciens*
Moraxella ovis	*Branhamella ovis*, *Neisseria ovis*
Moritella marina	*Vibrio marinus*
Mycoplasma adleri, sp. nov.[37]	
Mycoplasma crocodyli, sp. nov.[38]	
Mycoplasma elephantis, sp. nov.[38]	
Mycoplasma lagogenitalium, sp. nov.[39]	
Mycoplasma sturni, sp. nov.[40]	
Myroides odoratus	*Flavobacterium odoratum*
Ochrobactrum anthropi	CDC group Vd, CDC group Vd (biotype 1 and 2)
Ochrobactrum intermedium, sp. nov.[41]	
Oligella ureolytica	CDC group IVe
Oligella urethralis	*Moraxella urethralis*
Oligotrophia carboxidovorans	*Pseudomonas carboxidovorans*
Pasteurella avium	*Haemophilus avium*
Pasteurella bettyae	*Pasteurella bettii*, HB-5
Pasteurella dagmatis	CDC *Pasteurella* sp. "n. sp. 1"(*Pasteurella* "gas")
Pasteurella gallicida	Rejected name
Pasteurella langaaensis, sp. nov.	*Pasteurella langaa*, incorrect name
Pasteurella lymphangitidis	BLG group
Pasteurella trehalosi	*Pasteurella haemolytica*, biovar T
Photobacterium iliopiscarium	*Vibrio iliopiscarius*
Planococcus okeanokoites	*Flavobacterium okeanokoites*
Porphyromonas asaccharolytica	*Bacteroides asaccharolyticus*
Porphyromonas assemblage	*Bacteroides asaccharolyticus*

Porphyromonas catonia	*Oribaculum catoniae*
Porphyromonas endodontalis	*Bacteroides endodontalis*
Porphyromonas gingivalis	*Bacteroides gingivalis*
Porphyromonas levii, comb. nov.[42]	
Porphyromonas macacae	*Bacteroides melaninogenicus* subsp. *macacae*, *Bacteroides salivosus*, *Porphyromonas salivosus*
Prevotella biva	*Bacteroides bivius*
Prevotella brevis	*Bacteroides ruminicola*, *Prevotella ruminicola*
Prevotella buccae	*Bacteroides buccae*, *Bacteroides capillus*
Prevotella buccalis	*Bacteroides buccalis*
Prevotella corporis	*Bacteroides corporis*
Prevotella dentalis, comb. nov.[43]	*Mitsuokella dentalis*
Prevotella denticola	*Bacteroides denticola*
Prevotella disiens	*Bacteroides disiens*
Prevotella heparinolytica	*Bacteroides heparinolyticus*
Prevotella intermedia	*Bacteroides intermedium*, *Bacteroides melaninogenicus*
Prevotella loescheii	*Prevotella* strain DIC-20, *Bacteroides loescheii*
Prevotella melaninogenica	*Bacteroides melaninogenicus*
Prevotella oralis	*Bacteroides oralis*
Prevotella oris	*Bacteroides oris*
Prevotella oulora	*Bacteroides oulora*
Prevotella pallens, sp. nov.[44]	
Prevotella ruminicola subsp. *ruminicola*	*Prevotella brevis*, *Bacteroides ruminicola* subsp. *ruminicola*
Prevotella veroralis	*Bacteroides veroralis*
Prevotella zoogleoformans	*Bacteroides zoogleoformans*, *Capsularis zoogleoformans*
Propionigenium maris, sp. nov.[45]	
Pseudoalteromonas nigrifaciens	*Pseudomonas nigrifaciens*
Pseudoalteromonas piscicda	*Pseudomonas piscicida*
Pseudomonas abietaniphila, sp. nov.[46]	
Pseudomonas amygdali	*Pseudomonas ficuserectae*
Pseudomonas avellanae, sp. nov.[47]	*Pseudomonas syringae* pv. *avellanae*
Pseudomonas balearica, sp. nov.[48]	
Pseudomonas beteli	*Pseudomonas betle*, incorrect name; *Xanthomonas maltophila*
Pseudomonas cannabina, sp. nov.[49]	
Pseudomonas chlororaphis	*Pseudomonas aureofaciens*
Pseudomonas corrugata, sp. nov.[50]	
Pseudomonas graminis, sp. nov.[51]	
Pseudomonas hibiscicola	*Xantomonas maltophila*
Pseudomonas jessenii, sp. nov.[52]	
Pseudomonas libanensis, sp. nov.[53]	
Pseudomonas luteola	*Chryseomonas polytrichia*
Pseudomonas mandelii, sp. nov.[52]	
Pseudomonas monteilii, sp. nov.[54]	
Pseudomonas multiresimivorans, sp. nov.[46]	
Pseudomonas rhodesiae, sp. nov.[55]	

Pseudomonas savastanoi	*Pseudomonas syringae* subsp. *savastanoi*
Pseudomonas stutzeri	*Pseudomonas perfectomarina*
Pseudomonas syringae	*Pseudomonas compransoris*
Pseudomonas tremae, sp. nov.[49]	
Pseudomonas vancouverens, sp. nov.[46]	
Pseudomonas veronii, sp. nov.[56]	
Psychrobacter phenylpyruvicus	*Moraxella phenylpyruvicus*
Psychroflexus gondwanensis	*Flavobacterium gondwanense*
Ralstonia eutropha	*Alcaligenes eutrophus*
Ralstonia gilardi, sp. nov.[57]	
Ralstonia pickettii	*Pseudomonas pickettii*
Ralstonia solanacearum	*Pseudomonas solanacearum*
Riemerella anatipestifer	*Moraxella anatipestifer*
Rochalimaea	Genus eliminated
Ruegeria atlantica	*Agrobacterium atlanticum*, *Agrobacterium meteori*
Ruegeria gelatinovorum	*Agrobacterium gelatinovorum*
Selenomonas acidminovorans, sp. nov.[58]	
Selenomonas lipolytica, sp. nov.[59]	
Shewanella amazonensis, sp. nov.[61]	
Shewanella baltica, sp. nov.[62]	
Shewanella frigidimarina, sp. nov.[60]	
Shewanella gelidimarina, sp. nov.[60]	
Shewanella oneidensis, sp. nov.[63]	
Shewanella putrefaciens	*Pseudomonas putrefaciens*, *Alteromonas putrefaciens*
Shewanella violacea, sp. nov.[64]	
Shewanella woodyi, sp. nov.[65]	
Slackia heliotrinireducens	*Peptostreptococcus heliotrinireducens*
Sphingobacterium heparinum	*Flavobacterium heparinum*
Sphingobacterium multivorum	*Flavobacterium multivorum*
Sphingobacterium pophilum	*Flavobacterium pophilum*
Sphingobacterium spiritivorum	*Flavobacterium spiritivorum*
Sphingobacterium thalpophilum	*Flavobacterium thalpophilum*
Sphinomonas aromaticivorans, sp. nov.[66]	
Sphinomonas asaccharolytica, sp. nov.[67]	
Sphingomonas capsulata	*Flavobacterium capsulatum*
Sphingomonas echinoides, sp. nov.[68]	*Pseudomonas echinoides*
Sphingomonas mali, sp. nov.[67]	
Sphingomonas natatoria, comb. nov.[69]	*Blastobacter natatorius*, *Blastomonas natatoria*
Sphingomonas paucimobilis	*Flavobacterium devorans*, *Pseudomonas paucimobilis*
Sphingomonas pruni, sp. nov.[67]	
Sphingomonas rosa, sp. nov.[67]	
Sphinogomonas stygia, sp. nov.[66]	
Sphingomonas subarctica, sp. nov.[70]	
Sphingomonas suberifaciens, sp. nov.[69]	
Sphingomonas subterranea, sp. nov.[70]	
Sphingomonas trueperi, sp. nov.[71]	
Sphingomonas ursincola, comb. nov.[69]	*Erythromonas ursincola*

Stenotrophomonas maltophila	*Pseudomonas maltophilia, Xanthomonas maltophilia*
Suttonella indologenes	*Kingella indologenes*
Tatlockia maceachernii	*Legionella maceschernii*
Tatlockia micdadei	*Legionella micdadei, Legionella pittsburghensis*
Taylorella equigenitalis	Species *incertae sedis* in genus *Haemophilus*
Telluria mixta	*Pseudomonas mixta*
Tissierella creatinini, sp. nov.[72]	
Tissierella creantinophila, sp. nov.[73]	
Tissierella praeacuta	*Bacteroides praeacutus*
Variovorax paradoxus	*Alcaligenes paradoxus*
Veillonella atypica	*Veillonella parvula* subsp. *atypica*
Veillonella criceti	*Veillonella alcalescens* subsp. *criceti*
Veillonella dispar	*Veillonella alcalescens* subsp. *dispar*
Veillonella parvula	*Veillonella alcalescens* subsp. *parvula*
Veillonella ratti	*Veillonella alcalescens* subsp. *ratti*
Veillonella rodentium	*Veillonella alcalescens* subsp. *rodentium*
Vibrio alginolyticus	*Beneckea alginolytica*
Vibrio campbellii	*Beneckea campbellii*
Vibrio cholerae	*Beneckea harveyi, Lucibacterium harveyi*
Vibrio gazogenes	*Beneckea gazogenes*
Vibrio halioticoli, sp. nov.[74]	
Vibrio ichthyoenteri, sp. nov.[75]	
Vibrio iliopiscarius, sp. nov.[76]	
Vibrio logei	*Photobacterium logei*
Vibrio natriegens	*Beneckea natriegens*
Vibrio nereis	*Beneckea nereida*
Vibrio nigripulchritudo	*Beneckea nigrapulchrituda*
Vibrio parahaemolyticus	*Beneckea parahaemolytica*
Vibrio pectenicida, sp. nov.[77]	
Vibrio penaeicida, sp. nov.[78]	
Vibrio proteolyticus	*Aeromonas hydrophila* subsp. *proteolytica*
Vibrio rumoiensis, sp. nov.[79]	
Vibrio scophthalmi, sp. nov.[80]	
Vibrio splendidus	*Beneckea splendida*
Vibrio tapetis, sp. nov.[81]	
Vibrio trachuri, sp. nov.[82]	
Vibrio vulnificus	*Beneckea vulnifica*
Vogesella indigofera	*Pseudomonas indigofera*
Weeksella virosa	CDC group IIf
Weeksella zoohelcum	CDC group IIj
Wolinella succinogenes	*Vibrio succinogenes*
Xanthomonas arboricola, sp. nov.[83]	
Xanthomonas bromi, sp. nov.[83]	
Xanthomonas campestris, sp. nov.[83]	
Xanthomonas cassavae, sp. nov.[83]	
Xanthomonas codiaei, sp. nov.[83]	
Xanthomonas cucurbitae, sp. nov.[83]	
Xanthomonas hortorum, sp. nov.[83]	
Xanthomonas hyacinthi, sp. nov.[83]	

Xanthomonas melonis, sp. nov.[83]
Xanthomonas pisi, sp. nov.[83]
Xanthomonas saccari, sp. nov.[83]
Xanthomonas theicola, sp. nov.[83]
Xanthomonas translucens, sp. nov.[83]
Xanthomonas vasicol, sp. nov.[83]
Xanthomonas vesicatoria, sp. nov.[83]
Zavarzinia compransorsis   *Pseudomonas compransoris*

(Note: In 2000, the *International Journal of Systematic Bacteriology* (IJSB) will become the *International Journal of Systematic and Evolutionary Microbiology* (IJSEM).

REFERENCES

[1] Foster G, Ross HM, Malnick H, et al. *Actinobacillus delphinicola* sp. nov., a new member of the family *Pasteurellaceae* Pohl (1979) 1981 isolated from sea mammals. Int J Syst Bacteriol 1996;46(3):648–652.

[2] Moller K, Fussing V, Grimont PA, et al. *Actinobacillus minor* sp. nov., *Actinobacillus porcinus* sp. nov., and *Actinobacillus indolicus* sp. nov., three new V factor-dependent species from the respiratory tract of pigs. Int J Syst Bacteriol 1996;46(4):951–956.

[3] Foster G, Ross HM, Patterson AP, et al. *Actinobacillus scotiae* sp. nov., a new member of the family *Pasteurellaceae* Pohl (1979) 1981 isolated from porpoises (*Phocoena phocoena*). Int J Syst Bacteriol 1998;48(3):929–933.

[4] Guettler MV, Rumler D, Jain MK. *Actinobacillus succinogens* sp. nov., a novel succinic acid-producing bacterium from the bovine rumen. Int J Syst Bacteriol 1999;49(1):207–216.

[5] Huys G, Kampfer P, Altwegg M, et al. *Aeromonas popoffii* sp. nov., a mesophilis bacterium isolated from drinking water production plants and reservoirs. Int J Syst Bacteriol 1997;47(4):1165–1171.

[6] Foss S, Heyen U, Harder J. Validation list no. 67. Int J Syst Bacteriol 1998;48(3):1083–1084.

[7] Malnick H. *Anaerobiospirillum thomasii* sp. nov., an anaerobic spiral bacterium isolated from the feces of cats and dogs and from diarrheal feces of humans, and emendation of the genus *Anaerobiospirillum*. Int J Syst Bacteriol 1997;47(2):381–384.

[8] Heller R, Kubina M, Mariet P, et al. *Bartonella alsatica* sp. nov., a new *Bartonella* species isolated from the blood of wild rabbits. Int J Syst Bacteriol 1999;49(1):283–288.

[9] Lawson PA, Collins MD. Validation list no. 58. Int J Syst Bacteriol 1996;46(3):836–837.

[10] Birtles RJ, Harrison TG, Saunders NA, Molyneux DH. Proposals to unify the genera *Grahamella* and *Bartonella*, with descriptions of *Bartonella talpae* comb. nov., *Bartonella peromysci* comb. nov., and three new species, *Bartonella grahamii* sp. nov., *Bartonella taylori* sp. nov., and *Bartonella doshiae* sp. nov. Int J Syst Bacteriol 1995;45(1):1–8.

[11] Heller R, Riegel P, Hansmann Y, et al. *Bartonella tribocorum* sp. nov., a new *Bartonella* species isolated from the blood of wild rats. Int J Syst Bacteriol 1998;48(4):1333–1339.

[12] Kordick DL, Swaminathan B, Greene CE, et al. *Bartonella vinsonii* subsp. *berkhoffii* subsp. nov., isolated from dogs: *Bartonella vinsonii* subsp. *vinsonii*; and emended description of *Bartonella vinsonii*. Int J Syst Bacteriol 1996;46(3):704–709.

[13] Abraham WR, Strömpl C, Meyer H, et al. Polygeny and polyphasic taxonomy of *Caulobacter* species. Proposal of *Maricaulis* gen. nov. with *Maricaulis maris* (Poindexter) comb. nov. as the type species and emended description of the genus *Brevundimonas* and *Caulobacter*. Int J Syst Bacteriol 1999;49(3):1053–1073.

[14] Gillis M, Van TV, Bardin R, et al. Polyphasic taxonomy of *Burkholderia* leading to an emended description of the genus and proposition of *Burkholderia vietnamiensis* sp. nov. for N2-fixing isolates from mice in Vietnam. Int J Syst Bacteriol 1995;45(3):274–289.

[15] Viallard V, Poirier I, Cournoyer B, et al. *Burkholderia graminis* sp. nov., and reassessment of [*Pseudomonas*] *phenazinium*, [*Pseudomonas*] *pyrrocinia* and [*Pseudomonas*] *glathei* as *Burkholderia*. Int J Syst Bacteriol 1998;48(2):549–563.

[16] Vandamme P, Holmes B, Vancanneyt M, et al. Occurrence of multiple genomovars of *Burkholderia cepacia* in cystic fibrosis patients and proposal of *Burkholderia multivorans* sp. nov. Int J Syst Bacteriol 1997;47(4):1188–1200.

[17] Wittke R, Ludwig W, Peiffer S, Kleiner D. Validation list no. 66. Int J Syst Bacteriol 48(3):631–632.

[18] Brett PJ, Deshazer D, Woods DE. *Burkholderia thailandensis* sp. nov., a *Burkholderia pseudomallei*-like species. Int J Syst Bacteriol 1998;48(1):317–320.

[19] Vandamme P, Daneshvar MI, Dewhirst FE, et al. Chemotaxonomic analyses of *Bacteroides gracilis* and *Bacteroides ureolyticus* and reclassification of *B. gracilis* as *Campylobacter gracilis* comb. nov. Int J Syst Bacteriol 1995;45(1):145–152.

[20] Bernardet JF, Segers P, Vancanneyt M, et al. Cutting a Gordian knot: Emended classification and description of the genus *Flavobacterium*, emended description of the family *Flavobacteriaceae*, and pro-

posal of *Flavobacterium hydatis* nom. nov. (basonym, *Cytophaga aquatilis* Strohl and Tait 1978). Int J Syst Bacteriol 1996;46(1):128–148.

[21]McCammon SA, Innes BH, Bowman JP, et al. *Flavobacterium hibernum* sp. nov., a lactose-utilizing bacterium from a fresh water Antarctic lake. Int J Syst Bacteriol 1998;48(4):1405–1412.

[22]Collins MD, Hutson RA, Falsen E, et al. Validation list no. 66. Int J Syst Bacteriol 1998;48(3):631–632.

[23]Inzana TJ, Johnson JL, Shell L, et al. Validation list no. 69. Int J Syst Bacteriol 1999;49(2):341–342.

[24]Fox JG, Yan LL, Dewhirst FE, et al. Validation list no. 61. Int J Syst Bacteriol 1997;47(2):601–602.

[25]Hänninen ML, Happonen I, Saaei A, Jalava K. Culture and characteristics of *Helicobacter bizzozeronii*, a new canine gastric *Helicobacter* sp. Int J Syst Bacteriol 1996;46(1):160–166.

[26]Franklin CL, Beckwith CS, Livingston RS, et al. Validation list no. 61. Int J Syst Bacteriol 1997; 47(2):601–602.

[27]Stanley J, Linton D, Burnens AP, et al. Validation list no. 53. Int J Syst Bacteriol 1995;45(2):418–419.

[28]Shen Z, Fox JG, Dewhirst FE, et al. *Helicobacter rodentium* sp. nov., a urease-negative *Helicobacter* species isolated from laboratory mice. Int J Syst Bacteriol 1997;47(3):627–634.

[29]Jalava K, Kaartinen M, Utriainen M, et al. *Helicobacter salomonis* sp. nov., a canine gastric *Helicobacter* sp. related to *Helicobacter felis* and *Helicobacter bizzozeronii*. Int J Syst Bacteriol 1997;47(4):975–982.

[30]Mendes EN, Queiroz DM, Dewhirst FE, et al. *Helicobacter trogontum* sp. nov., isolated from the rat intestine. Int J Syst Bacteriol 1996;46(4):916–921.

[31]Hookey JV, Saunders NA, Fry NK, et al. Phylogeny of *Legionellaceae* based on small-subunit ribosomal DNA sequences and proposal of *Legionella lytica* comb. nov., for *Legionella*-like amoebal pathogens. Int J Syst Bacteriol 1996;46(2):526–531.

[32]Lo Presti F, Riffard S, Meugnier H, et al. *Legionella tuariensis* sp. nov., a new species antigentically similar to *Legionella spiritensis*. Int J Syst Bacteriol 1999;49(2):397–403.

[33]Benson RF, Thacker WL, Daneshvar MI, Brenner DJ. *Legionella waltersii* sp. nov., and an unnamed *Legionella* genomospecies isolated from water in Australia. Int J Syst Bacteriol 1996;46(3):631–634.

[34]Wood AP, Kelly DP, McDonald IR, et al. Validation list no. 69. Int J Syst Bacteriol 1999;49(2): 341–342.

[35]Kodjo A, Richard Y, TYnjum T. *Moraxella boevrei* sp. nov., a new *Moraxella* species found in goats. Int J Syst Bacteriol 1997;47(1):115–121.

[36]Kodjo A, TYnjum T, Richard Y, BYvre K. *Moraxella caprae* sp. nov., a new member of the classical moraxellae with very close affinity to *Moraxella bovis*. Int J Syst Bacteriol 1995;45(3):467–471.

[37]Del Giudice RA, Rose DL, Tully JG. *Mycoplasma adleri* sp. nov., an isolate from a goat. Int J Syst Bacteriol 1995;45(1):29–31.

[38]Kirchhoff H, Mohan K, Schmidt R, et al. *Mycoplasma crocodyli* sp. nov., a new species from crocodiles. Int J Syst Bacteriol 1997;47(3):742–746.

[39]Kobayashi H, Runge M, Schmidt R, et al. *Mycoplasma lagogenitalium* sp. nov., from the preputial smegma of Afghan pikas (*Ochotona rufescens refescens*). Int J Syst Bacteriol 1997;47(4):1208–1211.

[40]Forsyth MH, Tully JG, Gorton TS, et al. *Mycoplasma sturni* sp. nov., from the conjunctiva of a European starling (*Sturnus vulgaris*). Int J Syst Bacteriol 1996;46(3):716–719.

[41]Velasco J, Romero C, López-Goñi I, et al. Evaluation of the relatedness of *Brucella* spp. and *Ochrobactrum anthropi* and description of *Ochrobactrum intermedium* sp. nov., a new species with a closer relationship to *Brucella* spp. Int J Syst Bacteriol 1998;48(3):759–768.

[42]Shah HN, Collins MD, Olsen I, et al. Reclassification of *Bacteroides levii* (Holdeman, Cato, and Moore) in the genus *Porphyromonas*, as *Porphyromonas levii* comb. nov. Int J Syst Bacteriol 1995;45(3):586–588.

[43]Willems A, Collins MD. 16SrRNA gene similarities indicate that *Hallella seregens* (Moore and Moore) and *Mitsuokella dentalis* (Haapasalo et al.) are genealogically highly related and are members of the genus *Prevotella* emended description of the genus *Prevotella* (Shah and Collins) and description of *Prevotella dentalis* comb. nov. Int J Syst Bacteriol 1995;45(4):832–836.

[44]Könönen E, Eerola E, Frandsen EVG, et al. Phylogenetic characterization and proposal of a new pigmented species to the genus *Prevotella*: *Prevotella pallens* sp. nov. Int J Syst Bacteriol 1998;48(1):47–51.

[45]Janssen PH, Liesack W. Validation list no. 56. Int J Syst Bacteriol 1996;46(1):362–363.

[46]Mohn WW, Wilson AE, Bicho P, Moore ERB. Validation list no. 70. Int J Syst Bacteriol 1999;49 (3):935–936.

[47]Janse JD, Rossi P, Angelucci L, et al. Validation list no. 61. Int J Syst Bacteriol 1997;47(2):601–602, 1997.

[48]Bennasar A, Rosselló-Mora R, Lalucat J, Moore ERB. 16rRNA gene sequence analysis relative to genomovars of *Pseudomonas stutzeri* and proposal of *Pseudomonas balearica* sp. nov. Int J Syst Bacteriol 1996;46(1):200–205.

[49]Gardan L, Shafik H, Belovin S, et al. DNA relatedness among the pathovars of *Pseudomonas syringae* and description of *Pseudomonas tremae* sp. nov. and *Pseudomonas cannabina* sp. nov. (ex Sutic and Dowson 1959). Int J Syst Bacteriol 1999; 49(2):469–478.

[50]Sutra L, Siverio F, Lopez MM, et al. Taxonomy of *Pseudomonas* strains isolated from tomato pith necrosis: Emended description of *Pseudomonas corrugata* and proposal of three unnamed fluorescent *Pseudomonas* genomospecies. Int J Syst Bacteriol 1997;47(4):1020–1033.

[51]Behrendt U, Ulrich A, Schumann P, et al. A taxonomic study of bacteria isolated from grasses: A

proposed new species *Pseudomonas graminis* sp. nov. Int J Syst Bacteriol 1999;49(1):2297–2308.

[52]Verhille S, Baida N, Dabbousii F, et al. Validation list no, 70. Int J Syst Bacteriol 1999;49(3):935–936.

[53]Dabboussi F, Hamze M, Elomari M, et al. *Pseudomonas libanensis,* sp. nov., a new species isolated from Lebanese spring waters. Int J Syst Bacteriol 1999;49(3):1091–1101.

[54]Elomari M, Cololer L, Verhille S, et al. *Pseudomonas monteilli* sp. nov., isolated from clinical specimens. Int J Syst Bacteriol 1997;47(3):846–852.

[55]Coroler L, Elomari M, Hoste B, et al. *Pseudomonas rhodesiae* sp. nov., a new species isolated from natural mineral waters. Int J Syst Bacteriol 1997; 47(2):601–602.

[56]Elomari M, Coroler L, Hoste B, et al. DNA relatedness among *Pseudomonas* strains isolated from natural mineral waters and proposal of *Pseudomonas veronii* sp. nov. Int J Syst Bacteriol 1996;46(4): 1138–1144.

[57]Coenye T, Falsen E, Vancanneyt M, et al. Classification of *Alcaligenes faecalis*-like isolates from the environment and human clinical samples as *Ralstonia gilardii.* Int J Syst Bacteriol 1999;49(2): 405–413.

[58]Guangsheng C, Plugge CM, Roelofsen W, et al. Validation list no. 61. Int J Syst Bacteriol 1997;47 (2):601–602.

[59]Dighe AS, Shouche YS, Ranade DR. *Selenomonas lipolytica* sp. nov., an obligately anaerobic bacterium possessing lipolytic activity. Int J Syst Bacteriol 1998;48(3):783–791.

[60]Bowman JP, McCammon SA, Nichols DS, et al. *Shewanella gelidimarina* sp. nov., and *Shewanella frigidimarina* sp. nov., novel Antarctic species with the ability to produce eicosapentaenoic acid (20:5 omega 3) and grow anaerobically by dissimilatory Fe (III) reduction. Int J Syst Bacteriol 1997;47 (4):1040–1047.

[61]Venkateswaran K, Dollhopf ME, Aller R, et al. *Shewanella amazonensis* sp. nov., a novel metal-reducing facultative anaerobe from Amazonian shelf muds. Int J Syst Bacteriol 1998;48(3):965–972.

[62]Ziemke F, Höfle MG, Lalucat J, Rosselló-Mora R. Reclassification of *Shewanella putrefaciens* Owen's genomic group II as *Shewanella baltica* sp. nov. Int J Syst Bacteriol 1998;48(1):179–186.

[63]Venkateswaran K, Moser DP, Dollhopf ME, et al. Polyphasic taxonomy of the genus *Shewanella* and description of *Shewanella oneidensis* sp. nov. Int J Syst Bacteriol 1999;49(2):705–724.

[64]Nogi Y, Kato C, Horikoshi K. Validation list no. 69. Int J Syst Bacteriol 1999;49(2):341–342.

[65]Makemson JC, Fulayfil NR, Landry W, et al. *Shewanella woodyi* sp. nov., an exclusively respiratory luminous bacterium isolated from the Alboran Sea. Int J Syst Bacteriol 1997;47(4):1034–1039.

[66]Balkwill DL, Drake GR, Reeves RH, et al. Taxonomic study of aromatic-degrading bacteria from deep-terrestrial-subsurface sediments and description of *Sphingomonas aromaticivorans* sp. nov., *Sphingomonas subterranea* sp. nov., and *Sphingomonas stygia* sp. nov. Int J Syst Bacteriol 1997;47(1):191–201.

[67]Takeuchi M, Sakane T, Yanagi M, et al. Taxonomic study of bacteria isolated from plants: Proposal of *Sphingomonas rosa* sp. nov., *Sphingomonas pruni* sp. nov., *Sphingomonas asaccharolytic* sp. nov., and *Sphingomonas mali* sp. nov. Int J Syst Bacteriol 1995;45(2):334–341.

[68]Denner EBM, Kämpfer P, Bosse HJ, Moore ERB. Reclassification of *Pseudomonas echinoides* Heumann 1962, 343^AL in the genus *Sphingomonas* as *Sphingomonas echinoides* comb. nov. Int J Syst Bacteriol 1999;49(3):1103–1109.

[69]Yabuuchi E, Kosako Y, Naka T, et al. Validation list no. 70. Int J Syst Bacteriol 1999;49(3):935–936.

[70]Nohynek LJ, Nurmiaho-Lassila EL, Suhonen EL, et al. Description of chlorophenol-degrading *Pseudomonas* sp. strains KF1T, KF3, and NKF1 as a new species of the genus *Sphingomonas, Sphingomonas subartica* sp. nov. Int J Syst Bacteriol 1996: 46(4):1042–1055.

[71]Kämpfer P, Denner EBM, Meyer S, et al. Classification of "*Pseudomonas azotocolligas*" Anderson 1995, 132, in the genus *Sphingomonas* as *Sphingomonas trueperi* sp. nov. Int J Syst Bacteriol 1997; 47(2):577–583, 1997.

[72]Farrow JAE, Lawson PA, Hippe H, et al. Phylogenetic evidence that the Gram-negative nonsporulating bacterium *Tissierella* (*Bacteroides*) *praeacuta* is a member of the *Clostridium* subphylum of the Gram-positive bacteria and description of *Tissierella creatinini* sp. nov. Int J Syst Bacteriol 1995;45(3):436–440.

[73]Harms C, Schleicher A, Collins MD, Andreesen JR. *Tissierella creatinophila* sp. nov., a Gram-positive, anaerobic, non-sporeforming creatinine-fermenting organism. Int J Syst Bacteriol 1998;48(3): 983–993.

[74]Sawabe T, Sugimura I, Ohtsuka M, et al. *Vibrio halioticoli* sp. nov., a non-motile alginolytic marine bacterium isolated from the gut of the abalone *Haliotis discus hannai.* Int J Syst Bacteriol 1998;48(2):573–580.

[75]Ishimaru K, Akagawa-Matsushita M, Muroga K. *Vibrio ichthyoenteri* sp. nov., a pathogen of Japanese flounder (*Paralichthys olivaceus*). Int J Syst Bacteriol 1996;46(1):155–159.

[76]Onrheim AM, Wiik R, Burghardt J, Stackebrandt E. Validation list no. 53. Int J Syst Bacteriol 1995; 45(2):418–419.

[77]Lambert C, Nicolas JL, Cili V, Corre S. *Vibrio pectenicida* sp. nov., a pathogen of scallop (*Pecten maximus*) larvae. Int J Syst Bacteriol 1998;48 (2):481–487.

[78]Ishimaru K, Akagawa-Matsushita M, Muroga K. *Vibrio penaeicida* sp. no., a pathogen of kuruma prawns (*Penaeus japonicus*). Int J Syst Bacteriol 1995;45(1):134–138.

[79]Yumoto I, Iwaa H, Sawabe T, et al. Validation list

no. 70. Int J Syst Bacteriol 1999;49(3):935–936.

[80]Cerdà-Cúellar M, Rosselló-Mora RA, Laluca J, et al. *Vibrio scophthalmi* sp. nov., a new species from turbot (*Scophthalmus maximus*). Int J Syst Bacteriol 1997;47(1):58–61.

[81]Borrego JJ, Castro D, Luque A, et al. *Vibrio tapetis* sp. nov., the causative agent of the brown ring disease affecting cultured clams. Int J Syst Bacteriol 1996;46(2):480–483.

[82]Iwamoto Y, Suzuki Y, Kurita A, et al. Validation list no. 56. Int J Syst Bacteriol 1996;46(2):625–626.

[83]Vauterin L, Hoste B, Kersters K, Swings J. Reclassification of *Xanthomonas*. Int J Syst Bacteriol 1995;45(3):472–489.

GENERA DESCRIPTIONS/TABLES

Table 44.1. Differential Characteristics of Gram-Negative Aerobic to Facultative Anaerobic Bacteria of Medical Importance

Bacteria	Oxygen requirements	Catalase	Oxidase	MacConkey (MAC) agar	Nitrate Reduction	Motility, 37°C	O/F Glucose
Rods (coccobacilli)							
Acholeplasma	Fac	NR	NR	NR	NR	—	F
Acidovorax	Aer	V+	+	V+	+	+	O
Acinetobacter	Fac	+	—	G	—	+	O
Actinobacillus[a]	Fac	V+	V+	V[b]	+	—	F/O
Aeromonas	Fac	+	+	V	+	V+	F/O
Afipia	Fac	V−w	+	V−c	V−	+	O/−
Agrobacterium	Aer	+	V+	G	—	+	O
Alcaligenes	OAer	+	+	G	V	+	O
Bartonella	Aer	V−	V	NG	V−	V	—
Bordetella	OAer	+	V+	V+	V−	V	O/−
Brevundimonas	Aer	V+	+	V	—	+	O
Brucella[d]	Aer	+	+	NG	V+	—	O
Burkholderia	Aer	+	V+	V+	V	+	O
Capnocytophaga	Fac	V−	V	NG	V−	—	F
Cardiobacterium	Fac	—	+	NG	—	—	F
Chrombacterium	Fac	+	V[e]	G	+	+	F
Chryseomonas	Aer	+	—	G	—	+	O
Comamonas	OAer	+	+	G[c]	V+	+	O
Eikenella[f]	Fac	—	+	NG	+	—	—
Enterbacteriaceae[g]	Fac	V+	—	G	+	V	F
Flavimonas	Aer	+	—	G	—	V	O
Flavobacterium[h]	Aer	+	+	G[i]	—	—	O[j]
Francisella[k]	OAer	+w	V−	NG	NR	—	F
Gardnerella	Fac	—	—	NR	—	—	F
Haemophilus[l]	Fac	V	V	V−	+	—	F/O
Janthinobacterium	OAer	+	V+	NR	—	+	F
Kingella	Fac	—	+	NG	V	—	F
Legionella	Aer	+	V−w	NG	NR	V	—
Methylobacterium	Aer	+c	+c	V	V	+	—
Moraxella	Aer	+	+	V	V	—	−/NG
Mycoplasma	Fac	—	NR	NR	NR	V	NR
Ochrobactrum	OAer	+	+	G	NR	+	O
Oligella	Aer	+	+	V+	V	V	—

(continued)

Table 44.1. Differential Characteristics of Gram-Negative Aerobic to Facultative Anaerobic Bacteria of Medical Importance (*continued*)

Bacteria	Oxygen requirements	Catalase	Oxidase	MacConkey (MAC) agar	Nitrate Reduction	Motility, 37°C	O/F Glucose
Pasteurella[m]	Fac	V+	+[n]	V	V+	−	O
Pseudomonas	Aer	+	V	G	V	V	O
Ralstonia	Aer	NR	+	NR	V+	+	O
Roseomonas	Aer	+	V[i c]	G	V	V+	O/−
Shewanella	Aer	+	+	G	+	+	O
Sphingomonas	Aer	+	V+	NG	−	+	O
Stenotrophomonas	Aer	NR	−	G	V	+	O
Streptobacillus	Fac	−	−	NG	−	−	F
Suttonella	Fac	−	+	NG	−	−	F
Vibrio[o]	Fac	+	V+	G	V+	V+	F/O
Weeksiella	Aer	+	+	NG	−	−	−
Xanthobacter	OAer	+	+	NR	+	V	O
Xanthomonas	OAer	+	V−w	G	−	+	F
Cocci (diplococci)							
Alcaligenes	OAer	+	+	G	V	+	O
Gemella	Fac	−	−	NR	NR	−	F
Moraxella catarrhalis	Aer	+	+	NG	V+	−	−/NG
Moraxella ovis	Aer	+	+	V	+	−	−/NG
Morococcus	Aer	+	+	NR	+	−	F
Neisseria	Aer	V+	+	NR	V−	−	O[p]
Psychrobacter	Fac	+	+	G[q]	V	−	O/−

G, growth; NG, no growth; NR, no results; V, variable reactions; V+, variable, usually positive; V−, variable, usually negative; O, oxidative; F, fermentative; O/F glucose −, inert; w, weak reaction; Aer, aerobic; Fac, facultatively anaerobic; OAer, obligately (strict) aerobic.

[a]Requires serum added to basal fermentation medium to enhance growth (8).
[b]May be slight growth.
[c]Positive reaction may be delayed or weakly positive.
[d]Do not consider primary cultures negative until after 21 days incubation.
[e]Pigment may interfere with oxidase reaction; pigment only produced in presence of oxygen (O_2); use nonpigmented growth from an anaerobic culture for oxidase testing.
[f]"Pitting" of agar surface.
[g]See Chapter 45, *Enterobacteriaceae* for biochemical characteristics.
[h]Overall incubation temperature below 30°C preferable.
[i]Growth may be poor.
[j]Often inert (−) first 24–48 h incubation; best treated as an oxidizer (O).
[k]No growth in ordinary media; use a cysteine medium.
[l]No growth in ordinary media; requies X and/or V growth factors.
[m]Initial growth enhanced by use of blood or serum agar with increased carbon dioxide (CO_2).
[n]Rarely oxidase negative with Kovacs' reagent.
[o]Grows best in alkaline media.
[p]Questionable fermenters; early reaction that of an oxidizer (O).
[q]Poor growth; best growth at 20–25°C.

Table 44.2. Differential Characteristics of Gram-Negative Nonsporeforming, Microaerophilic to Obligately Anaerobic Bacteria of Medical Importance

Bacteria	Oxygen requirement	Catalase	Oxidase	MacConkey (MAC) agar	Nitrate reduction	Motility, 37°C	O/F glucose
Rods (coccobacilli)							
Anaerobiospirilum	Anaero	−	NR	NR	−	+	F
Anaerorhabdus	Anaero	−	NR	NR	−	−	F
Bacteroides	OAnaero	V−	V−	NR	V−	V+	F/−
Butyrivibrio	OAnaero	−	−	NR	−	+	F
Campylobacter	OMicro	V+	+	V+	V	+	−
Centipeda	Anaero	NR	NR	NR	NR	+	F
Fusobacterium	OAnaero	−	−	NR	−	−	Fw
Helicobacter	Micro	+	+	NR	V	+	F
Leptotrichia[a]	Anaero	−	−	NR	−	−	F
Megamonas	Anaero	NR	NR	NR	NR	−	F
Mitsuokella	Anaero	NR	NR	NR	NR	−	F
Mobiluncus	Anaero	−	−	NR	V−	+	Fw
Porphyromonas	Anaero	−	−	NR	−	−	F
Propionigenium	Anaero	−	−	NR	NR	−	F
Prevotella	Anaero	V−	−	NR	−	−	F
Selenomonas	OAnaero	−	−	NR	V	+[b]	F
Succinimonas	OAnaero	−	−	NR	−	+[b]	F
Succinivibrio	OAnaero	−	−	NR	−	+	F
Taylorella	Micro	+	+	G	−	−	O
Tissierella	Anaero	−	−	NR	NR	+	Fw/O
Ureaplasma	Micro	−	−	NR	NR	NR	
Wolinella	Micro	−	+	NG	+	+	−
Cocci (diplococci)							
Acidaminococcus	Anaero	−	−	NR	−	−	F(−)[c]
Megasphaera	Anaero	−	−	NR	−	−	F
Peptostreptococcus	Anaero	−	NR	NR	V−	−	F
Veillonella	Anaero	V	−	NG	+	−	F

NR, no results; G, growth; NG, no growth; F, fermentation; O, oxidative; −, inert; Anaero, anaerobic; OAnaero, obligately (strict) anaerobic; Micro, microaerophilic; w, weak reaction; V, variable reaction; V+, variable, usually positive; V−, variable, usually negative.
[a]May be aerotolerant; CO_2 (5%) essential for isolation; ascitic fluid, serum, or starch enhances growth; thioglycolate may inhibit some strains.
[b]Slow and progressive; may be lost on exposure to air.
[c]Weakly fermentative (F); may be inert (−).

GENUS: *ACHOLEPLASMA* (14)
Gram-negative filamentous and spherical cells bound by plasma membrane **only**; mollicutes
Nonsporeforming
Facultative anaerobic
Catalase, no results
Nonencapsulated
Nonmotile
Oxidase, no results
O/F glucose: F (fermentative)
Optimal growth temperature: 20–40°C
13 species: *A. axanthum, A. brassicae, A. cavigenitalium, A. equifetale, A. granularum, A. hippikon, A. laidlawii, A. modicum, A. morum, A. multilocale, A. oculi, A. palmae, A. parvum*

Type species: *A. laidlawii* ATCC 23206
Serum or cholesterol required for growth
Colonies on solid media have a "fried egg" appearance

Table 44.3. Differentiation of the Most Frequently Isolated *Acholeplasma* spp.

Test	*A. axanthum*	*A. equifetale*	*A. granularum*	*A. hippikon*	*A. laidlawii*	*A. morum*	*A. oculi*	*A. parvum*
Motility	−	−	−	−	−	−	−	−
Glucose	A	A	A	A	A	A	−	NR
Mannose	A	V	−	−	V	+	+	−
Esculin hydrolysis	−	V	−	+	V	−	−	NR
Arginine dehydrolase	−	−	−	−	−	−	−	−
Gelatin liquefaction, 22°C	NR	−	−	−	V	−	−	−
Casein hydrolysis	NR	−	−	−	−	−	NR	−
Urease	−	−	−	−	−	−	−	−

A, acid production (+); V, variable reactions; V, variable, usually positive; NR, no results. Data from reference 14.

GENUS: *ACIDAMINOCOCCUS* (14)
Gram-negative **cocci**, often oval or kidney-shaped diplococci
Nonsporeforming
Anaerobic
Catalase negative
Nonencapsulated
Motility, no results
Oxidase negative
O/F glucose: F (fermentative)
Optimal growth temperature: 30–37°C
Nitrate reduction: negative
Single species: *A. fermentans* ATCC 25085

GENUS: *ACIDOVORAX* (14)
Gram-negative, straight to slightly curved rods arranged singly or in short chains
Nonsporeforming
Aerobic
Catalase variable, usually positive
Nonencapsulated
Motile; single polar flagellum
Oxidase positive
O/F glucose: O (oxidative)
Optimal growth temperature: 25–37°C
7 species: *A. avenue* subsp. *avenue*, *A. avenue* subsp. *cattleyae*, *A. avenue* subsp. *citrulli*, *A. delafieldii*, *A. facilis*, *A. konjaci*, *A. temperans*
Type species: *A. facilis* ATCC 11228 (not in *Bergey's Manual*; created by Willems A, et al. (30))

Table 44.4. Differentiation of the Most Frequently Isolated *Acidovorax* spp.

Test	*A. delafieldii*	*A. facilis*	*A. temperans*
Catalase	V	+	+
Oxidase	+	+	+
$NO_3 \rightarrow NO_2$	+	+	+
MacConkey (MAC)	G[a]	NG	G[a]
Pigmentation	+[b]	−	+[b]
H_2S			
TSI	−	−	−
PbAc	+	+	+
Motility	+	+	+
Esculin hydrolysis	−	−	−
Citrate	+	−	−
Lysine decarboxylase	−	−	−
Gelatin liquefaction, 22°C	−	+	−
Urease	+	NR	NR

PbAc, lead acetate; G, growth; NG, no growth; NR, no results; V, variable reactions. Data from reference 29.
[a]Weak and late reaction.
[b]Yellow pigmentation.

GENUS: *ACINETOBACTER* (5, 14)

Gram negative but often difficult to decolorize; rods become spherical in stationary growth phase. Arranged in pairs and chains of variable length
Nonsporeforming
Aerobic
Catalase positive
Nonencapsulated
Motile: "twitching motility"; polar fimbriae
Oxidase negative
O/F glucose: O (oxidative)
Optimal growth temperature: 33–35°C; however, growth at 20–30°C
7 species: *A. baumanni*, *A. calcoaceticus*, *A. haemolyticus*, *A. johnsonii*, *A. junii*, *A. lwoffii*, *A. radioresistens*
Type species: *A. calcoaceticus*, ATCC 23055, CIP 81.08

Table 44.5. Differentiation of *Acinetobacter* species

Test	*A. baumannii*	*A. calcoaceticus*	*A. haemolyticus*	*A. johnsonii*	*A. junii*	*A. lowffii*
Catalase	+	+	+	+	+	+
Oxidase	−	−	−	−	−	−
MacConkey (MAC)	G	G	G	G	G	G
$NO_3 \rightarrow NO_2$	−	−	−	−	−	−
Growth at						
37°C	G	G	G	NG	G	G
41°C	G	NG	NG	NG	V	NG
Hemolysis, 5% SBA	−	−	+	−	−	−
Citrate (Simmons)	+[a]	+	V+	+	V	−
Esculin hydrolysis	−	−	−	−	−	−
Gelatin liquefaction, 22°C	−	−	V+	−	−	−
Malonate	V+	+	−	V	−	−
Arginine dehydrolase	V+	+	V+	V	V+	−
Lysine decarboxylase	−	−	−	−	−	−
Ornithine decarboxylase	V+	+	−	V−	−	V−
Phenylalanine deaminase	V	+	−	−	−	−
Glucose	V+	A	V	−	−	V−

V, variable reactions; V, variable, usually positive; V, variable, usually negative; SBA, sheep blood agar; G, growth; NG, no growth.
Data from reference 5.
[a]All strains except two auxotrophic strains.

GENUS: *ACTINOBACILLUS* (14, 26)

Gram-negative, irregularly staining, spherical or oval rods; mostly bacillary interspersed with coccal forms that may lie at the pole of a bacillus, giving the characteristic "**Morse code**" appearance. Arranged singly and pairs; rarely in chains
Nonsporeforming
Facultatively anaerobic
Catalase variable, usually positive
Nonencapsulated
Nonmotile
Oxidase variable, usually positive
O/F glucose: F (fermentative) and O (oxidative)
Optimal growth temperature: 37°C
16 species: *A. capsulatus, A. delphinicola, A. equuli, A. hominis, A. indolicus, A. lignieresi, A. minor, A. muris, A. pleuropneumoniae, A. porcinus, A. rossii, A. scotiae, A. seminis, A. succinogenes, A. suis, A. ureae*
Type species: *A. lignieresi* NCTC 4189
All species are capnophilic (i.e., require carbon dioxide (CO_2) for growth).
Fastidious microorganisms; require serum added to basal fermentation medium to enhance growth (26)

Table 44.6. Differentiation of Most Frequently Isolated *Actinobacillus* spp.

Test	A. capsulatus	A. equuli	A. hommis	A. ligniersi	A. muris	A. rossii	A. seminis	A. suis	A. ureae
Catalase	+	V	−	V	+	+	+	+	V
Oxidase	+	V+	+	V+	+	+	V	V+	V+
NO$_3$→NO$_2$	+	+	+	+	+	+	+	+	+
Hemolysis, 5% SBA	γ	γ	γ	γ	γ	V	−	+	+
MacConkey (MAC)	G	G	NG	G	NG	V+	NG	G	V
H$_2$S	−	V	NR	+	−	NR	NR	−	NR
Carbohydrates									
Glucose	A	A	A	A	A	A	A[wa]	A	A
Lactose	A	A	A	V[a]	−	V	−	A	−
Adonitol	−	−	−	−	−	NR	−	−	−
Arabinose	−	V−	−	V−	−	A	V[a]	V+	−
Cellobiose	A	−	−	−	A[a]	−	−	A	−
Dextrin	−	A	NR	A	−	NR	−	A	A
Dulcitol	−	−	−	−	−	−	−	−	−
Erythritol	NR	NR	NR	NR	−	NR	NR	NR	−
Fructose	A	A	NR	A	A	NR	−	A	A
Galactose	A	V	A	A	−	A	V[a]	V+	−
Glycerol	NR	V	NR	V	V	NR	−	A	−
Inositol	−	−	−	−	V	A	V	−	−
Inulin	−	−	NR	−	−	NR	−	−	−
Maltose	A	A	A	A	A	V	V[a]	A	V+
Mannitol	A	A	A	A	A	A	V[a]	−	A
Mannose	A	A	−	A	A	V	−	A	V
Melibiose	NR	NR	NR	NR	NR	−	−	A	−
Raffinose	A	A	A[a]	−	A[a]	V−	−	A	−
Rhamnose	−	−	−	−	−	NR	NR	−	−
Ribose	NR	A	NR	A	A	NR	NR	NR	A
Salicin	A	−	V	−	A	−	−	A	−
Sorbitol	A	V	−	V	−	A	−	−	V−
Sorbose	−	−	−	−	−	NR	NR	−	−
Sucrose	A	A	A	A	A	−	−	A	A
Trehalose	A	A	A	−	A	−	−	A	−
Xylose	A	A	A	A	−	A	−	A	−
Misc. tests									
Indole	−	−	−	−	−	−	−	−	−
Esculin hydrolysis	+[a]	−	V	−	+[a]	−	V	+	−
Arginine dehydrolase	−	−	−	−	−	NR	−	−	−
Lysine decarboxylase	−	−	−	−	−	NR	−	−	−
Ornithine decarboxylase	−	−	−	−	−	−	V	−	−
Gelatin liquefaction, 22°C	−	V	−	−	−	NR	NR	−	−
ONPG	+	V	+	V	−	V+	−	V+	−
Phosphatase	+	+	+	+	−	+	−	+	+
Methyl red (MR)	−	−	NR	−	−	NR	NR	−	−
Voges-Proskauer (VP)	−	−	−	V	−	NR	−	−	−
Urease	+	+	+	+	+	+	−	+	+

G, growth; NG, no growth; NR, no results; V, variable reactions; V+, variable, usually positive; V, variable, usually negative; SBA, sheep blood agar; A, acid production (+); γ, gamma (no) hemolysis.
Data from reference 14.
[a]Positive reaction delayed.

GENUS: *AEROMONAS* (14)

Gram-negative rods with rounded ends approaching spherical shape; arranged in pairs and short chains

Nonsporeforming

Facultatively anaerobic

Catalase positive

Nonencapsulated

Motility variable; usually positive; single polar flagellum; peritrichous flagella may be formed on solid media. Exception: *A. media* (−) and *A. salmonicida* (−)

Oxidase positive

O/F glucose: F (fermentative) and O (oxidative)

Optimal growth temperature: 22–28°C; however, most strains grow well at 37°C.

22 species: *A. allosaccharophila, A. bestiarum, A. caviae, A. encheleia, A. enteropelogenes, A. eucrenophila, A. hydrophila* subsp. *anaerogenes, A. hydrophila* subsp. *hydrophila, A. ichthiosmia, A. jandaei, A. media, A. popoffii, A. punctata* subsp. *caviae, A. punctata* subsp. *punctata, A. salmonicida* subsp. *achromogenes, A. salmonicida* subsp. *masoucida, A. salmonicida* subsp. *salmonicida, A. salmonicida* subsp. *smithia, A. schubertii, A. sobria, A. trota, A. veronii*

Type species: *A. hydrophila* subsp. *hydrophila* ATCC 7966, NCTC 8049.

Table 44.7. Differentiation of the Most Frequently Isolated *Aeromonas* spp.

Test	*A. caviae*	*A. eucrenophila*	*A. hydrophila*	*A. media*	*A. salmonicida* subsp. *achromogenes*	*A. salmonicida* subsp. *masoucida*	*A. salmonicida* subsp. *salmonicida*	*A. salmonicida* subsp. *smithia*	*A. schubertii*	*A. sobra*	*A. veronii*
Catalase	+	+	+	+	+	+	+	+	+	+	+
Oxidase	+	+	+	+	+	+	+	+	+	+	+
NO₃→NO₂	+	+	+	+	+	+	+	NR	+	+	+
H₂S	−	−	+	−	−	+	−	+	−	−	−
Motility	+	+	+	−	−	−	−	−	+	+	+
Brown soluble pigment	−	−	−	+	−	−	+	−	−	−	−
Carbohydrates											
Glucose	A	A	A	A	A	A	A	V⁺	−	−	A
Lactose	V	−	V	V	−	−	−	−	−	−	−
Adonitol	−	−	−	−	−	−	−	NR	−	−	−
Arabinose	A	A	A	A	−	A	A	NR	−	−	−
Cellobiose	V⁺	A	−	A	−	−	−	−	−	V	V
Dulcitol	−	−	−	−	−	−	−	NR	−	−	−
Erythritol	−	−	−	−	−	−	−	NR	−	−	−
Galactose	A	A	A	A	A	A	A	−	A	A	A
Glycerol	V	A	A	V	V	V	V	V⁻	V	V	A
Inositol	−	−	−	−	−	−	−	−	−	−	−
Maltose	A	A	A	A	A	A	A	−	A	A	A
Mannitol	A	A	A	A	−	A	A	−	−	V	A
Mannose	V	A	V⁺	A	A	A	A	NR	A	A	A
Melibiose	−	−	−	−	NR	NR	NR	NR	−	−	−
Raffinose	−	−	−	−	−	−	−	−	−	−	−
Rhamnose	−	−	−	−	−	−	−	NR	−	−	−
Salicin	A	A	A	V	V	V	V	NR	−	−	A
Sorbitol	−	−	−	−	−	−	−	V⁻	−	V	−
Sucrose	A	V	A	A	A	A	−	V	−	V	A
Trehalose	A	A	A	A	A	A	A	−	A	V	A
Xylose	−	−	−	−	−	−	−	−	−	−	−
Misc. tests											
Indole	+	+	+	V	+	+	−	−	−	+	+
DNase	+	+	+	+	+	+	+	+	+	+	+
Citrate (Christensen)	V	−	−	−	−	−	−	NR	+	−	+
Citrate (Simmons)	V	−	V	V	−	−	−	−	V	−	+
Esculin hydrolysis	+	+	+	V	−	+	+	−	−	−	+
Arginine dehydrolase	+	+	+	+	+	+	+	V⁻	+	+	−
Lysine decarboxylase	−	−	V	−	V	V	V	−	+	+	+
Ornithine decarboxylase	−	−	−	−	−	−	−	−	−	−	+
Gelatin liquefaction, 22°C	+	+	+	+	+	+	+	+	+	+	V⁺
KCN	G	G	G	G	NG	NG	NG	NR	NG	NG	V
Lipase	+	−	V	V	+	+	+	−	+	−	+
Malonate	−	−	−	−	−	−	−	NR	−	−	−
ONPG	+	V	+	V⁺	V	V	V	+	+	−	V⁺
Phenylalanine deaminase	−	V	−	V	−	−	−	−	V	+	V⁺
Methyl red (MR)	+	V	+	+	+	+	+	−	+	−	+
Voges-Proskauer (VP)	−	−	+	−	−	+	−	−	−	V⁺	+
Urease	−	−	−	−	−	−	−	−	−	−	−
Sensitivities:											
0/129	R	R	R	NR	NR	NR	NR	NR	R	R	R

V, variable reactions; V⁺, variable, usually positive; G, growth; NG, no growth; NR, no results; A, acid production (+); 0/129, vibriostatic agent, 2,4-diamino-6,7-diisopropylpteridine.

GENUS: *AFIPIA* (14, 26)

Gram-negative rods
Nonsporeforming
Faculatively anaerobic
Catalase negative or weakly positive (29)
Nonencapsulated
Motile: single polar, subpolar, or lateral flagellum
Oxidase positive
O/F glucose: O (oxidative) or inert (−)
Optimal growth temperature: 25–30°C; weak growth at 35°C, no growth 42°C
3 species: *A. broomeae, A. clevelandensis, A. felis*
Type species: *A. felis* ATCC 53690 (not in *Bergey's Manual;* created by Brenner DJ, et al. (1))
Fastidious

Table 44.8. Differentiation of *Afipia* spp.

Test	A. broomeae	A. clevelandensis	A. felis
Catalase	+[a]	−[a]	V
Oxidase	+	+	+
NO$_3$→NO$_2$	−	−	+
Hemolysis, 5% SBA	γ	γ	γ
MacConkey (MAC)	NG	NG	V[a]
H$_2$S	−	−	−
Motility	+	+	+
Carbohydrates			
Glucose	−	−	−
Lactose	−	−	−
Maltose	−	−	−
Mannitol	−	−	−
Sucrose	−	−	A[a]
Xylose	A	−	−
Misc. tests			
Indole	−	−	−
Esculin hydrolysis	−	−	−
Citrate	−	−	−
Gelatin liquefaction, 22°C	−	−	−
Phenylalanine deaminase	−	−	+
Urease	+[a]	+[a]	+[a]

NG, no growth; V, variable reactions; A, acid production (+); γ, gamma (no) hemolysis.
Data from reference 29.
[a]Delayed positive.

GENUS: *AGROBACTERIUM* (14)

Gram-negative rods arranged singly and in pairs
Nonsporeforming
Aerobic
Catalase positive
Nonencapsulated
Motile: 1–6 peritrichous flagella
Oxidase variable, usually positive
O/F glucose: O (oxidative)
Optimal growth temperature: 25–28°C

Urease positive
5 species: *A. ferrugineum, A. rhizogenes, A. rubi, A. tumefaciens, A. vitis*
Type species: *A. tumefaciens* ATCC 23308, CCM 1040, CIP B6

Table 44.9. Biochemical Characteristics of *Agrobacterium tumefaciens*

MacConkey (MAC)	G		
Catalase	+	Glucose	A
NO$_3$→NO$_2$	−	Mannitol	A
Esculin hydrolysis	+	Xylose	A
Arginine dehydrolase	−		
Urease	+		

A, acid production (+); G, growth.

GENUS: *ALCALIGENES* (14)
Gram-negative rods, coccobacilli, or cocci occurring singly
Nonsporeforming
Strict (obligate) aerobe
Catalase positive
Nonencapsulated
Motile: peritrichous flagella
Oxidase positive
O/F glucose: O (oxidative)
Optimal growth temperature: 20–37°
3 species: *A. defragrans, A. faecalis* subsp. *faecalis, A. latus*
Type species: *A. faecalis* subsp. *faecalis* ATCC 8750

Table 44.10. Differentiation of Two *Alcaligenes* spp.

Test	*A. faecalis* subsp. *faecalis*	*A. latus*
Catalase	+	+
Oxidase	+	+
MacConkey (MAC)	G	G
Motility	+	+
Yellow carotenoid pigment	−	−[a]
NO$_3$→NO$_2$	−	+
Indole	−	−
Citrate	+	+
DNase	−	−
Esculin hydrolysis	−	−
Gelatin liquefaction, 22°C	−	+
Urease	−	−
Glucose	−	A
Arabinose	−	−
Fructose	−	A
Mannitol	−	−
Mannose	−	−
Xylose	−	−

A, acid production (+); V, variable reactions.
Data from references 5 and 14.
[a] *A. latus* colonies are grayish, pink, or yellowish.

GENUS: *ANAEROBIOSPIRILLUM* (14)

Gram-negative spiral-shaped rods with rounded ends
Nonsporeforming
Anaerobic
Catalase negative
Nonencapsulated
Motile: corkscrew-like bipolar tufts of flagella
Oxidase: no results
O/F glucose: F (fermentative)
Optimal growth temperature: 37–40°C
2 species: *A. succuniciproducens, A. thomasii*
Type species: *A. succiniciproducens* ATCC 29305
Best isolation on chocolate agar
Strains from human cases of diarrhea differ in fermentation pattern from the original isolated from beagle dogs (14).

Table 44.11. Biochemical Characteristics of the Genus *Anaerobiospirillum*

$NO_3 \rightarrow NO_2$	−	Glucose	A
Indole	−	Lactose	A
Gelatin liquefaction, 22°C	−	Maltose	V
		Mannitol	−
		Sucose	A
		Xylose	−

A, acid production (+); V, variable reactions. Data from reference 16.

GENUS: *ANAERORHABDUS* (14, 26)

Gram-negative pleomorphic short or long rods; occasionally single, usually arranged in pairs and short chains. Some cells are **forked and Y- shaped.**
Nonsporeforming
Anaerobic
Catalase negative
Nonencapsulated
Nonmotile
Oxidase: no results
O/F glucose: F (fermentative)
Optimal growth temperature: 30–37°C
Single species: *A. furcosus* ATCC 25662 (not in *Bergey's Manual;* created by Shah and Collins (24)
Generally asaccharolytic
Growth stimulated by rumen fluid

Table 44.12. Biochemical Characteristics of *Anaerorhabdus furcosus*

Glucose	A	Bile, 20%	G	
Fructose	A	$NO_3 \rightarrow NO_2$	−	
Sucrose	V	Indole	−	
		Esculin hydrolysis	+	

V, variable reactions; A, acid production (+); G, growth; Bile 20%, bile concentration 20% or 2% Bacto oxgall (10× concentration bile).
Data from references 14 and 26.

GENUS: *BACTEROIDES* (14)

Gram-negative rods

Nonsporeforming

Strict (obligate) anaerobes, except *B. ureolyticus* is microaerophilic but can grow anaerobically.

Catalase variable, usually negative

Nonencapsulated

Motility variable, usually positive; *B. polypragmatus* and *B. xylanolyticus* are motile by peritrichous flagella; *B. galacturonicus* has flagella but is nonmotile; *B. ureolyticus* exhibits "twitching motility," but no true motility (14).

Oxidase variable, usually negative; *B. ureolyticus* oxidase positive

O/F glucose: F (fermentative) or inert (−)

Optimal growth temperature: 35–37°C

25 species: *B. caccae, B. capillosus, B. cellulosolvens, B. coagulans, B. distasonis, B. eggerthii, B. forsythus, B. fragilis, B. galacturonicus, B. helcogenes, B. merdae, B. ovatus, B. pectinophilus, B. polypragmatus, B. putredinis, B. pyogenes, B. splanchnicus, B. stercoris, B. suis, B. tectus, B. thetaiotaomicron, B. uniformis, B. ureolyticus, B. vulgatus, B. xylanolyticus*

Type species: *B. fragilis* ATCC 25285, NCTC 9343

Hemin and vitamin K required for growth of many species.

B. fragilis and *B. thetaiotaomicron* are of greatest clinical significance (26).

Table 44.13. Differentiation of the Most Frequently Isolated *Bacteroides* spp.

Test	*B. caccae*	*B. capillosus*	*B. cellulosolvens*	*B. coagulans*	*B. distasonis*	*B. eggerthii*	*B. forsythus*	*B. fragilis*	*B. helcogenes*
Catalase	−	−	−	−	+	+	NR	+	−
Oxidase	−	−	−	−	+	+	−	−	−
NO$_3$→NO$_2$	NR	NR	NR	−	−	−	NR	−	NR
Bile 20%	G	NG	NG	NG	G	G	NR	G	NG
Hemolysis, 5% SBA	β,γ	γ	NR	γ	α,γ	NR	NR	α,γ	β,γ
H$_2$S (SIM/TSI)	−	V$^−$	NR	+	+	NR	NR	+	−
Motility	−	−	−	−	−	−	−	−	−
Meat digestion	−	−	NR	−	−	−	NR	−	+^{w}
Carbohydrates									
Glucose	A	V$^+$	−	−	A	A	−	A	A
Lactose	A	−	−	−	A	A	−	A	A
Arabinose	A	−	−	−	−	A	−	−	−
Cellobiose	V	−	A	−	A	−	−	A	A
Glycerol	−	−	−	−	−	−	−	−	−
Maltose	A	−	−	−	A	A	−	A	A
Melibiose	A	−	−	−	A	−	−	A	A
Raffinose	A	−	−	−	A	−	−	A	A
Rhamnose	V	−	−	−	V	A	−	V	−
Ribose	A	V	−	−	A	−	−	A	−
Salicin	V	−	−	−	A	−	−	A	A
Sucrose	A	−	−	−	A	−	−	A	A
Trehalose	A	−	−	−	A	−	−	A	−
Xylose	A	V	−	−	A	A	−	A	A
Misc. tests									
Indole	−	−	−	+	−	+	NR	−	−
Esculin hydrolysis	+	+	NR	−	+	+	+	+	+
Gelatin liquefaction, 22°C	V^w	V^w	−	+	V$^{−w}$	−	NR	V$^{−w}$	−
Starch hydrolysis	−	V	NR	−	V$^+$	+	NR	V$^+$	V$^+$
Urease	−	−	−	−	−	−	NR	−	−
Isolated from									
Humans	+	+	NR	+	+	+	+	+	−
Animals	−	+	NR	−	−	−	−	−	+

G, growth; NG, no growth; NR, no results; A, acid production (+); V, variable reactions; V$^+$, variable, usually positive; V$^−$, variable, usually negative; w, weak reaction; β, beta hemolysis; α, alpha hemolysis; γ, gamma (no) hemolysis.
Data from reference 14.

(continued)

GENUS: *BARTONELLA* (5, 14, 26)

Gram-negative, small, short rods; may be slightly curved; readily stained with Gimenez stain
Nonsporeforming
Aerobic
Catalase variable, usually negative
Nonencapsulated
Motility variable; *B. bacilliformis* and *B. felis* motile by polar flagella; *B. henselae* and *B. quintana* "twitching motility" because of pili
Oxidase variable, usually negative
O/F glucose: inert (−)
Optimal growth temperature: 25–30°C, *B. bacilliformis*; others 35–37°C
14 species: *B. alsatica, B. bacilliformis, B. clarridgeiae, B. doshiae, B. elizabethae, B. grahamii,*

B. ovatus	B. polypragmatus	B. putredinis	B. pyogenes	B. splanchnicus	B. suis	B. tectus	B. thetaiotaomicron	B. uniformis	B. ureolyticus	B. vulgaris	B. xylanolyticus
V+	−	V−w	−	−	−	−	V+	−	−	−	−
−	−	−	−	NR	−	−	−	−	+	−	−
+	NR	−	NR	−	NR	NR	−	−	+	−	NR
G	Gw	NG	NG	G	NG	G	G	G	NG	NG	NR
γ	γ	γ	γ	NR	β,γ	NR	γ	NR	β,γ	γ	NR
+	+	+	V+	NR	−	NR	+	NR	+	V+	+
−	+	−	−	−	−	−	−	−	−	−	+
−	−	V+	−	−	−	−	−	−	V−	−	NR
A	A	−	A	A	A	V−w	A	A	−	A	A
A	A	−	A	A	A	−	A	A	−	A	A
A	A	−	−	A	A	−	A	A	−	A	A
A	A	−	V+	−	A	NR	A	A	−	−	A
−	A	−	A	−	−	NR	−	−	−	−	−
A	A	−	V+	−	A	V−w	A	A	−	A	A
A	A	−	V−	−	A	−	A	A	−	A	NR
A	A	−	V+	−	A	−	A	A	−	A	NR
A	A	−	−	−	−	−	A	−	−	A	A
A	A	−	Aw	−	Aw	−	A	−	−	−	NR
A	A	−	V−	−	A	V+	−	A	−	−	A
A	−	−	V+	−	A	−	A	A	−	A	−
A	A	−	−	−	−	−	A	−	−	−	A
A	A	−	−	−	A	−	A	A	−	A	A
+	+	+	−	+	−	−	+	+	−	−	−
+	+	−	V+	+	+	+	+	+	−	V+	NR
V+	−	+	−	V+	−	+	V−w	−	V+w	−	+
V+	−	−	V+	−	+	NR	+	V+	−	V+	NR
−	−	−	NR	−	−	NR	−	−	−	−	−
+	NR	+	−	+	−	−	+	+	+	+	NR
−	NR	+	+	−	+	+	−	−	−	−	NR

B. henselae, B. peromysci, B. quintana, B. talpae, B. taylorii, B. tribocorum, B. vinsonii subsp. *berkhoffii, B. vinsonii* subsp. *vinsonii*

Type species: *B. bacilliformis* ATCC 35685 (proposed neotype)

All species of *Rochalimaea* have been moved to the genus *Bartonella* and the genus *Rochalimaea* eliminated.

Highly fastidious; growth best on blood-enriched media; add 100 μg/mL hemin to media

Most common isolated species is *B. quintana*, causative agent of cat scratch disease of humans and peliosis hepatitis. *B. clarrifgeiae* also causes cat scratch disease; *B. vinsonii* subsp. *vinsonii* causes trench fever.

Identification by serologic methods that detect antibody and by indirect fluorescent antibody tests.

Table 44.14. Differentiation of the Most Frequently Isolated *Bartonella* spp.

Test[a]	B. bacilliformis	B. henselae	B. elizabethae	B. quintana	B. vinosonii
Catalase	+	V–	–	–	–
Oxidase	–	–	–	+[b]	+[wb]
Optimal temp., °C	25–30	35–37	35–37	35–37	35–37
$NO_3 \to NO_2$	–	–	–	–	NR
Hemolysis, 5% SBA	γ	γ	γ	γ	γ
Motility	+	–	–	–	–
MacConkey (MAC)	NG	NG	NG	NG	NG
Misc. tests					
Indole	–	–	–	–	–
Ornithine decarboxylase	–	–	–	–	–
Urease	–	–	–	–	–

NG, no growth; w, weak reaction; γ, (gamma) no hemolysis.
Data from references 26 and 29.
[a]Most species require 7 days or more incubation for biochemical results.
[b]Kovacs' modification weakly positive; routine method negative (29).

GENUS: *BORDETELLA* (14)

Gram-negative, minute coccobacilli arranged singly, in pairs, or more rarely in chains; often exhibits bipolar staining

Nonsporeforming

Strict (obligate) aerobic

Catalase positive

Nonencapsulated

Motility variable; peritrichous flagella

Oxidase variable; usually positive

O/F glucose: O (oxidative)

Optimal growth temperature: 35–37°C

7 species: *B. avium, B. bronchiseptica, B. hinzii, B. holmesii, B. parapertussis, B. pertussis, B. trematum*

Type species: *B. pertussis* ATCC 9797

Growth on Bordet-Gengou medium yields smooth, convex, pearly, glistening, nearly transparent colonies surrounded by a zone of hemolysis without definite periphery.

B. pertussis causative agent of whooping cough.

Table 44.15. Differentiation of Some *Bordetella* spp.[a]

Test	B. avium	B. bronchiseptica	B. pakapertussis	B. pertussis[b]
Catalase	+	+	+	+
Oxidase	+	+	−	+
MacConkey (MAC)	G	G	G	NG
Number days colonies appear on Bordet-Gengou medium	1–2	1–2	2–3	3–6
Browning on peptone agar	V	−	+[c]	−
$NO_3 \rightarrow NO_2$	−	+	−	−
Motility	+	+	−	−
Indole	NR	−	−	−
Citrate	NR	+	+	−
Gelatin liquefaction, 22°C	NR	−	−	−
Litmus milk	Alk	Alk	Alk	Alk
Urease	−	+[d]	+	+
Glucose	NR	−	−	A
Lactose	NR	−	−	A

G, growth; NG, no growth; V, variable; NR, no reaction; Alk, Alkaline; A, acid.

Data from reference 14.

[a]All species may be confirmed by serologic agglutination tests and/or immunofluorescent (FA) procedures.

[b]B. pertussis requires Bordet-Gengou medium (potato-blood-glycerol) for primary isolation; no growth on ordinary medium.

[c]B. parapertussis: brown, water-soluble pigmentation on Bordet-Gengou medium; melanin-like pigment not produced under anaerobic conditions.

[d]Positive within 4 h.

GENUS: *BREVUNDIMONAS* (5, 29)

Gram-negative, straight, slender rods
Nonsporeforming
Aerobic
Catalase variable, usually positive
Nonencapsulated
Motile; single polar flagellum
Oxidase positive
O/F glucose: O (oxidative)
Optimal growth temperature: 30–37°C
8 species: B. alba, B. auranitaca, B. bacteroides, B. diminuta, B. intermedia, B. subvibrioides, B. variabilis, B. vesicularis
Type species: B. diminuta ATCC 11568

Tabel 44.16. Differentiation of Two *Brevundimonas* spp.

Test	B. diminuta	B. vesicularis
Catalase	+	V
Oxidase	+	+
42°C	V	V
$NO_3 \rightarrow NO_2$	−	−
MacConkey (MAC)	G	NG
Arginine dehydrolase	−	−
Lysine decarboxylase	−	−
Starch hydrolysis	−	+
Urease	V	−
Glucose	V	A
Lactose	−	−
Mannitol	−	−

V, variable reactions; G, growth; NG, no growth; A, acid production (+).

Data from reference 5.

GENUS: *BRUCELLA* (14)

Gram-negative coccobacilli and short rods arranged singly; less frequently in pairs, short chains, or small groups
Nonsporeforming
Aerobic
Catalase positive
Nonencapsulated; true capsules not produced
Nonmotile
Oxidase positive
O/F glucose: O (oxidative)
Optimal growth temperature: 37°C; range 20–40°C
Single species: *B. melitensis* ATCC 23456; 6 biovars and 15 biotypes constitute the genus (26)

Table 44.17. Biochemical Characteristics of *Brucella melitensis*

Catalase	+	Carbohydrates[a]	
Oxidase	+	Glucose	A
$NO_3 \rightarrow NO_2$	V+	Arabinose	−
MacConkey (MAC)	NG	Galactose	−
Indole	−	Ribose	−
Gelatin liquefaction, 22°C	−	Xylose	−
Arginine dehydrolase	−		
Lysine decarboxylase	−		
Ornithine decarboxylase	−		
Methyl red (MR)	−		
Voges-Proskauer (VP)	−		

A, acid production (+); NG, no growth.
[a]No acid production from conventional carbohydrates.

GENUS: *BURKHOLDERIA* (26)

Gram-negative, straight or slightly curved rods
Nonsporeforming
Aerobic
Catalase positive
Nonencapsulated
Motile; one or more polar flagella; except *B. mallei*
Oxidase variable, usually positive
O/F glucose: O (oxidative)
Optimal growth temperature: 30–37°C
17 species: *B. andropogonis, B. caryophylli, B. cepacia, B. gladioli, B. glathei, B. glumae, B. graminis, B. mallei, B. multivorans, B. norinborgensis, B. phenazinium, B. plantarii, B. pseudomallei, B. pyrrocinia, B. thailandensis, B. vietnamiensis*
Type species: *B. cepacia* ATCC 25416, NCTC 10743
B. cepacia is the most common species to infect humans; *B. pseudomallei* also infects humans, causative agent of melioidosis

Table 44.18. Differentiation of the Most Frequently Isolated *Burkholderia* spp.

Test	B. cepacia	B. gladioli	B. mallei	B. pseudomallei
Catalase	+	+	+	+
Oxidase	+	−	V	+
$NO_3 \rightarrow NO_2$	V	V	+	+
42°C	V	NG	NG	G
MacConkey (MAC)	G	G	V+	G
Motility	+	+	−	+
Carbohydrates				
Glucose	A	A	A	A
Lactose	A	−	V−	A
Fructose	A	A	NR	A
Galactose	A	A	NR	A
Maltose	A	−	−	A
Mannitol	A	A	V	A
Mannose	A	A	NR	A
Rhamnose	−	−	NR	V
Sucrose	V	−	−	V
Xylose	A	A	V−	V
Misc. tests				
Esculin hydrolysis	V	−	−	V
Gelatin liquefaction, 22°C	V+	+	−	+
Arginine dehydrolase	−	−	+	+
Lysine decarboxylase	+	−	−	−
Ornithine decarboxylase	V	−	−	−
ONPG	V	+	NR	−
Phenylalanine deaminase	−	−	NR	−
Urease	V	+	V−	V

G, growth; NG, no growth; NR, no results; V, variable reactions; V+, variable, usually positive; V−, variable, usually negative; A, acid production (+).
Data from references 5 and 26.

GENUS: *BUTYRIVIBRIO* (14, 19, 26)

Gram-positive and Gram-negative curved rods arranged singly, in chains, and in filaments that may be helical. Stain Gram negative, but cell wall is Gram-positive type.
Nonsporeforming
Obligate (strict) anaerobes
Catalase negative
Nonencapsulated
Motile; few polar or subpolar flagella; rapid and vibratory
Oxidase negative
O/F glucose: F (fermentative)
Optimal growth temperature 37°C; slow <30°C
Nonpathogenic
2 species: *B. crossotus*, *B. fibrisolvens*
Type species: *B. fibrisolvens* ATCC 19171

Table 44.19. Differentiation of *Butyrivibrio* spp.

Media	B. crossotus	B. fibrisolvens
Catalase	−	−
Single polar flagellum	−	+
$NO_3 \rightarrow NO_2$	−	−
Motility	+	+
Butyrate produced	+	+
H_2 produced	−	+
Indole	−	−
Esculin hydrolysis	−	V
Glucose	A^w	A
Sucrose	−	A

A, acid production (+); w, weak reaction; V, variable reactions.

GENUS: *CAMPYLOBACTER* (5, 14, 26)

Gram-negative, faintly staining, slender rods that may have 1 or more helical turns; helical or vibrioid; **S-shaped or gull-wing shaped** when two cells form short chains. Older cultures may appear coccoid.

Nonsporeforming

Microaerophilic: one species aerotolerant; two species anaerobic (*C. curvus* and *C. rectus* (5))

Catalase variable, usually positive

Nonencapsulated

Motile in broth cultures; single unsheathed polar flagellum at one or both ends of cell; characteristic **corkscrew-like motion**

Oxidase positive

O/F glucose: inert (−)

Optimal growth temperature: 37–42°C

18 species: *C. coli, C. concisus, C. curvus, C. fetus* subsp. *fetus, C. fetus* subsp. *veneralis, C. gracilis, C. helveticus, C. hydrointestinalis* subsp. *hyointestinalis, C. hydrointestinalis* subsp. *lawsonii, C. jejuni* subsp. *doylei, C. jejuni* subsp. *jejuni, C. lari, C. mucosalis, C. rectus, C. showae, C. sputorum* subsp. *bubulus, C. sputorum* subsp. *sputorum, C. upsaliensis*

Type species: *C. fetus* subsp. *fetus* ATCC 27324, NCTC 10842

Require 3–15% oxygen (O_2) and 3–5% CO_2 for growth

Table 44.20. Differentiation of the Most Frequently Isolated *Campylobacter* spp. and *Wolinella succinogenes*

Test	*C. coli*	*C. concisus*	*C. fetus* subsp. *fetus*	*C. fetus* subsp. *veneralis*	*C. hyointestinalis* subsp. *hyointestinalis*	*C. jejuni* subsp. *jejuni*	*C. jejuni* subsp. *doylei*	*C. mucosalis*	*C. sputorum* subsp. *bubulus*	*C. sputorum* subsp. *sputorum*	*C. upsalianis*	*Wolinella succinogenes*
Catalase	+	−	+	+	+	+	+	−	−	−	V−w	−
Oxidase	+	+	+	+	+	+	+	+	+	+	+	+
25°C	NG	NG	G	G	G	NG	NG	NG	NG	NG	NG	NG
42°C	G	G	V−	NG	G	G	V+	G	G	G	G	NG
NO$_3$→NO$_2$	−	+	+	−	+	+	−	+	V	V	+	+
H$_2$S												
SIM	−	+	−	−	−	−	−	+	+	V	−	+
TSI	+	+	−	−	+	−	−	+	+	V	−	+
MacConkey (MAC)	G	G	G	G	G	G	NG	NR	NG	NR	NG	NR
Motility	+	+	+	+	+	+	+	+	+	+	+	+
Alkaline phosphatase	V	−	−	−	−	+	+	−	+	+	−	NR
Hippurate hydrolysis	−	−	−	−	−	+	+	−	−	−	+	−
Cephalothin disk, 30 μg	R	R	S	S	S	S	R	S	S	S	S	NR
Nalidixic acid, 30 μg	S	R	R	R	R	S	S	R	V−	V−	S	NR

V, variable reactions; G, growth; NG, no growth; NR, no results; w, weak reaction; SIM: sulfide-indole-motility medium; TSI, triple sugar agar; R, resistant; S, sensitive (susceptible).

Data from references 5 and 14.

GENUS: *CAPNOCYTOPHAGA* (5, 14, 29)

Gram-negative, thin, short, or elongated, flexible rods with round or tapered ends; may exhibit filaments; **may be pleomorphic**

Nonsporeforming

Facultative anaerobic

Catalase variable, usually negative

Nonencapsulated

Nonmotile; "gliding motility" (twitching)

Oxidase variable

O/F glucose: F (fermentative)

Optimal growth temperature: 35–37°C

7 species: *C. canimorsus, C. cynodegmi, C. gingivalis, C. granulosa, C. haemolytica, C. ochracea, C. sputigena*

Type species: *C. ochracea* ATCC 27872

Yellow-pigmented colonies

Fastidious; need to add serum to basal fermentation media (5)

All species capnophilic (i.e., require CO_2 for growth)

Presumptive identification to genus usually sufficient (26). The three species of CDC DF-2 group (*C. gingivalis, C. ochracea, C. sputigena*) cannot be identified by conventional tests (26). *C. canimorsus* and *C. cynodegmi* belong to CDC group DF-1.

Table 44.21. Differentiation of the Most Frequently Isolated *Capnocytophaga* spp.

	CDC DF-1		CDC DF-2		
Test	*C. canimolsus*	*C. cynodegmi*	*C. gingivalis*	*C. ochracea*	*C. sputigena*
Catalase	+	+	−	−	−
Oxidase	+[a]	+	−	−	−
MacConkey (MAC)	NG	NG	NG	NG	NG
$NO_3 \rightarrow NO_2$	−	V⁻	−	−	+
Indole	−	−	−	−	−
Citrate	−	−	−	−	−
Esculin hydrolysis	V	V	+	+	+
Gelatin liquefaction, 22°C	−	−	−	−	+
Arginine dehydrolase	+	+	−	−	−
Starch hydrolysis	NR	NR	−	+	−
Urease	−	−	V⁻	V⁻	−
ONPG	+	+	−	+	+
Lactose	A	A	−	A	V
Melibiose	−	A	−	−	−
Raffinose	−	A	A	A	A

V, variable reactions; V⁻, variable, usually negative; NR, no results; A, acid production (+); NG, no growth.
Data from references 5, 14, 26, and 29.
[a]May be weak.

GENUS: *CARDIOBACTERIUM* (14)

Gram-negative, straight rods with rounded ends. Cells may retain crystal violet in swollen cells or central portion of the cells. Occasionally long filaments; **pleomorphic;** arranged singly, or in pairs, short chains, or **rosette clusters**
Nonsporeforming
Facultatively anaerobic
Catalase negative
Nonencapsulated
Nonmotile
Oxidase positive
O/F glucose: F (fermentative)
Optimal growth temperature: 30–37°C
Single species: *C. hominis* ATCC 15826
Hemin required for aerobic growth; some strains require CO_2 on isolation.

Table 44.22. Biochemical Characteristics of *Cardiobacterium hominis*

Catalase	−	Glucose	A	Maltose	A
Oxidase	+	Lactose	−	Mannitol	A
$NO_3 \rightarrow NO_2$	−	Adonitol	−	Mannose	A
MacConkey (MAC)	NG	Arabinose	−	Melibiose	−
H_2S	−	Cellobiose	−	Rhamnose	−
Indole	+wa	Dulcitol	−	Salicin	−
Gelatin liquefaction, 22°C	−	Erythritol	−	Sorbitol	A
Ornithine decarboxylase	−	Fructose	A	Sucrose	A[b]
Esculin hydrolysis	−	Gelactose	−	Trehalose	−
Urease	−	Inositol	−	Xylose	−
Tween 20	−				
Tween 40	−				

A, acid production (+); w, weak reaction.
Data from references 5, 14, and 26.
[a]Indole production may be weak, and the small amount formed may **not** be detected by procedures that do not concentrate by xylene extraction (14).
[b]Acid production within 7 days.

GENUS: *CENTIPEDA* (14)

Gram-negative, serpentine rods
Nonsporeforming
Anaerobic
Catalase: no results
Nonencapsulated
Motile; flagella inserted in spiral line along cell body
Oxidase: no results
O/F glucose: F (fermentative)
Optimal growth temperature: 32–37°C
Single species: *C. periodontii* ATCC 35019 (not in *Bergey's Manual*; created by Lai (17))
Often confused with *Selenomonas* also isolated from the mouth of humans
Lactate utilization positive

GENUS: *CHROMOBACTERIUM* (14)

Gram-negative rods with rounded ends and occasionally slightly curved; may have barred or bipolar lipid inclusions; usually occur singly but occasionally pairs, elongated forms, or short chains
Nonsporeforming
Facultative anaerobic
Catalase positive
Nonencapsulated
Motile: both single polar flagellum and usually 1–4 subpolar lateral flagella
Oxidase variable; usually positive; with Kovac's reagent, violet pigment (violacein) may interfere with reading
O/F glucose: F (fermentative)
Optimal growth temperature: 25°C; species differ in their optimal temperature
Single species: *C. violaceum* ATCC 12472, NCTC 9757, NCIB 9131
Butyrous, **violet** colonies on solid nutrient agar; violet ring at junction of liquid surface and container wall in nutrient broth
Oxidase-negative strains can be mistaken for enteric species; oxidase-positive strains can be mistaken for *Aeromonas* and *Vibrio* spp. (26).

Table 44.23. Biochemical Characteristics of *Chromobacterium violaceum*

Catalase	+				
Oxidase	V				
Motility	+				
MacConkey (MAC)	G				
$NO_3 \rightarrow NO_2$	+	Glucose	A	Melibiose	−
H_2S	V^{-w}	Lactose	−	Raffinose	−
Arginine	V	Adonitol	−	Rhamnose	NR
Lysine	−	Arabinose	−	Ribose	NR
Ornithine	−	Cellobiose	−	Salicin	−
Gelatin liquefaction, 22°C	+	Dextrin	NR	Sorbitol	V
Indole	V	Dulcitol	−	Sorbose	NR
Phenylalanine	−	Erythritol	NR	Sucrose	V^-
Esculin hydrolysis	−	Fructose	A	Trehalose	A
DNase	−	Galactose	−	Xylose	−
KCN	G	Glycine	−		
ONPG	−	Inositol	−		
Voges-Proskauer (VP)	−	Inulin	−		
Urease	V^{-w}	Maltose	V		
O/129	R	Mannitol	−		
Benzylpenicillin	R	Mannose	V^+		

V, variable reaction; V^+, variable, usually positive; V^-, variable, usually negative; NR, no results; A, acid production (+); w, weak reaction; G, growth; R, resistant; O/129, vibriostatic agent, 2,4-diamino-6,7-diisopropylpteridine.
Data from references 14 and 26.

GENUS: *CHRYSEOMONAS* (5, 14)

Gram-negative, short to medium-sized rods with parallel sides and rounded ends
Nonsporeforming
Aerobic
Catalase positive
Nonencapsulated
Motile: multitrichous (10–12) polar flagella
Oxidase negative
O/F glucose: O (oxidative)
Optimal growth temperature 42°C
Single species: *C. luteola* JCM 3352 (not in *Bergey's Manual*; created by Holmes et al. (11)
Pale to yellow growth on solid media.

Table 44.24. Biochemical Characteristics of *Chryseomonas luteola*

Catalase	+	Carbohydrates[a]	
Oxidase	−	Glucose	A
MacConkey	G	Lactose	−
NO$_3$→NO$_2$	−	Arabinose	A
H$_2$S	−	Cellobiose	−
Indole	−	Dulcitol	−
Esculin hydrolysis	+	Fructose	A
Gelatin liquefaction, 22°C	+	Glycerol	A
Citrate	+	Insotil	A
Arginine dehydrolase	+	Maltose	A
Lysine decarboxylase	−	Mannitol	A
Ornithine decarboxylase	−	Raffinose	−
Phenylalanine deaminase	−	Trehalose	A
Phosphatase	−	Xylose	A
Malonate	+		
ONPG	+		
Starch hydrolysis	−		
Trybutyrin	+		
Tween 20	+		

A, acid production (+); G, growth.
[a]Carbohydrates in ammonium salt medium under aerobic conditions.

GENUS: *COMAMONAS* (14, 10)

Gram-negative, straight or slightly curved rods arranged singly or in pairs
Nonsporeforming
Strict (obligate) aerobic
Catalase positive
Nonencapsulated
Motile; **tuft** of 3 or more polar flagella
Oxidase positive
O/F glucose: O (oxidative)
Optimal growth temperature: 25–37°C
2 species: C. terrigena, *C. testesteroni*
Type species: *C. terrigena* ATCC 1196 (not in *Bergey's Manual*; created by De Vos et al. (3))

Table 44.25. Differentiation of *Comamonas* species

Test	C. terrigena	C. testosteroni
Catalase	+	+
Oxidase	+	+
MacConkey (MAC)	G^{wa}	G
NO$_3$→NO$_2$	+	V$^+$
H$_2$S (TSI)	−	−
Citrate	V	V
Urease	V	V
Glucose	−	−
Mannitol	−	−
Sucrose	−	−

A, acid production (+); variable reactions; V$^+$, variable, usually positive, w, weak reaction.
Data from references 14 and 29.
[a]Weak and delayed growth.

GENUS: *EIKENELLA* (14)

Gram-negative, straight rods; occasionally short filaments
Nonsporeforming
Facultative anaerobic
Catalase negative
Nonencapsulated
Nonmotile; no flagella but "twitching motility" may occur on agar surfaces
Oxidase positive
O/F glucose: inert (−)
Optimal growth temperature: 35–37°C
Single species: *E. corrodens* ATCC 23834
Colonies may appear to corrode agar surface; no hemolysis (gamma)
Plate culture has a "bleachlike" odor.
Hemin usually required for growth under aerobic conditions.

Table 44.26. Biochemical Characteristics of *Eikenella corrodens*

Catalase	−	Esculin hydrolysis	−
Oxidase	+	Gelatin liquefaction, 22°C	−
Motility	−	Citrate	−
MacConkey (MAC)	NG	Arginine dehydrolase	−
$NO_3 \rightarrow NO_2$	+	Lysine decarboxylase	+
Glucose	−	Ornithine decarboxylase	+
Indole	−	Urease	−

NG, no growth.
Data from refernces 5, 14 and 26.

GENUS: *FLAVIMONAS* (14, 26)

Gram-negative, short to medium-length rods with parallel sides and rounded ends
Nonsporeforming
Aerobic
Catalase positive
Nonencapsulated
Motility: variable; single polar flagellum
Oxidase negative
O/F glucose: O (oxidative)
Optimal growth temperature: 18–42°C
Single species: *F. orzihabitans* JCM 2952, DSM 6835 (not in *Bergey's Manual;* created by Holmes et al. (13))
Some strains exhibit dark brown diffusible melanin-like pigmentation on tyrosine agar.
Pathogenic for warm-blooded animals; occasional pathogen for humans

Table 44.27. Biochemical Characteristics of *Flavimonas oryzihabitans*

Hemolysis, 5% SBA	—	ONPG	—
H₂S	—	Lecithinase	—
MacConkey (MAC)	G	Trybutyrin hydrolysis	—
NO₃→NO₂	—	Starch hydrolysis	—
Casein digestion	—	Tween 20	—
Esculin hydrolysis	—	Tween 80	—
Indole	—	Glucose	A
Gelatin liquefaction, 22°C	—	Maltose	A
Arginine dehydrolase	—	Mannitol	V
Lysine decarboxylase	—	Sucrose	A
Ornithine decarboxylase	—	Xylose	A
Phenylalanine deaminase	—		
Urease	—		

SBA, sheep blood agar; G, growth; V, variable results; A, acid production (+).

GENUS: *FLAVOBACTERIUM* (14)

Gram-negative rods with parallel sides and rounded ends
Nonsporeforming
Aerobic
Catalase positive
Nonencapsulated
Nonmotile
Oxidase positive
O/F glucose: O (oxidative)
Optimal growth temperature: 37°C
19 species: *F. acidifgum, F. acidurans, F. aquatile, F. branchiophilum, F. columnare, F. ferrugineum, F. flevense, F. hibernum, F. hydatis, F. johnsoniae, F. mizutaii, F. oceanosedimentum, F. pectinovorum, F. psychrophilum, F. resinovorum, F. saccharophilum, F. salegens, F. succinicans, F. thermophilum*
Type species: *F. aquatile* ATCC 11947, CIP 55.141

Table 44.28. Biochemical Characteristics of Two Most Frequently Isolated *Flavobacterium* spp.

Test	E. aquatile	E. branchiophilum
Catalase	+	+
Oxidase	+	+
$NO_3 \rightarrow NO_2$	NG	−
MacConkey (MAC)	G	G
Motility	−	−
42°C	NG	NG
Casein digestion	+	+
Esculin hydrolysis	−	−
Indole (Ehrlich)	−	−
Gelatin liquefaction, 22°C	−	+
Phosphatase	+	+
Starch hydrolysis	NG	+
ONPG	−	−
Urease	−	NR
Carbohydrates[a]		
Glucose	A[b]	A
Lactose	A[b]	−
Adonitol	−	−
Arabinose	−	−
Cellobiose	−	A
Glycerol	−	NR
Maltose	A	A
Mannitol	−	−
Raffinose	−	A
Rhamnose	−	−
Salicin	−	−
Sucrose	A[b]	A
Trehalose	−	A
Xylose	−	−

A, acid production (+); NR, no results; w, weak reaction; NG, no growth.
Data from reference 14.
[a]Ammonium salts medium for carbohydrates.
[b]Delayed reaction.

GENUS: *FRANCISELLA* (5, 14, 26, 29)

Gram-negative, faintly staining, very small rods or coccoid; **often pleomorphic; Gram stain of little use; intracellular pathogens**
Nonsporeforming
Strict (obligate) aerobe
Catalase positive; weak
Capsule variable; associated with virulence
Nonmotile
Oxidase variable, usually negative; positive with Kovacs method
O/F glucose: F (fermentative)
Optimal growth temperature:
5 species: *F. novicida, F. philomiragia, F. tularensis* subsp. *holarctica, F. tularensis* subsp. *mediasiatica* (type B), *F. tularensis* subsp. *tularensis* (type A)
Type species: *F. tularensis* subsp. *tularensis* ATCC 6223
Cysteine or cytosine required for growth; **does not** grow on blood, chocolate, and MacConkey agars (6)
F. tularensis etiological agent of tularemia in humans and animals
Halophilic

F. tularensis is extremely infectious, a biosafety level 2 pathogen; level 3 for cultures. Most common laboratory-acquired infection; if suspected, send specimen to reference, state, or public health laboratory.

Identification and confirmation by slide agglutination test (26); **biochemical reactions have no particular value and do not justify risk to technicians** (26)

GENUS: *FUSOBACTERIUM* (14)

Gram-negative rods that may be spindle shaped; may be coccobacilli; **often pleomorphic; if no spindle shapes, often difficult to differentiate from other nonmotile anaerobes** (*Bacteroides*, *Clostridium*, and *Eubacterium* spp.)

Nonsporeforming

Strict (obligate) anaerobic

Catalase negative

Nonencapsulated

Nonmotile

Oxidase negative

O/F glucose: F (fermentative); weak reaction

Optimal growth temperature: 35–37°C

20 species: *F. alocis*, *F. gonidaformans*, *F. mortiferum*, *F. naviforme*, *F. necrogenes*, *F. necrophorum* subsp. *funduliforme*, *F. necrophorum* subsp. *necrophorum*, *F. nucleatum* subsp. *animalis*, *F. nucleatum* subsp. *fusiforme*, *F. nucleatum* subsp. *nucleatum*, *F. nucleatum* subsp. *polymorphum*, *F. nucleatum* subsp. *vincentii*, *F. perfoetens*, *F. periodonticum*, *F. prausnitzii*, *F. russii*, *F. simiae*, *F. suici*, *F. ulcerans*, *F. varium*

Type species: *F. nucleatum* subsp. *nucleatum* ATCC 25586

All strains susceptible (sensitive) to 300 μg phosphomycin

Table 44.29. Differentiation of the Most Frequently Isolated *Fusobacterium* spp.

Test[a]	*F. alocis*	*F. gonidaformans*	*F. mortiferum*	*F. naviforme*	*F. necrogenes*[b]	*F. necrophorum*	*F. nucleatum*	*F. perfoetens*	*F. periodonticum*	*F. prausnitzii*[c]	*F. russii*	*F. simiae*	*F. suici*	*F. ulcerans*	*F. varium*
Catalase	−	−	−	−	−	−	−	−	−	−	−	−	−	−	−
Oxidase	−	−	−	−	−	−	−	−	−	−	−	−	−	−	−
Bile 20%[d]	NG	NG	G	NG	V	V	NG	NG	NG	V+	NG	G	NG	NR	G
H$_2$S	−	+	+	+	+	+	V	+	+	+	V−	+	−	−	+
Hemolysis, 5% SBA	γ	α,γ	γ	γ	β,γ	α,β	β,γ	γ	γ	γ	β,γ	γ	γ	γ	γ
Motility	−	−	−	−	−	−	−	−	−	−	−	−	−	−	−
Carbohydrates															
Glucose	−	−	A^w	V^{-w}	A^w	V^{-w}	V^{-w}	A^w	A	V^{-w}	−	A	−	A	A^w
Lactose	−	−	A^w	−	−	−	−	−	−	V^{-w}	−	−	−	−	−
Cellobiose	−	−	V^{-w}	−	V^{-w}	−	−	−	−	V^{-w}	−	−	−	NR	−
Fructose	−	−	A	−	A	V	V	A^w	A	V^{-w}	−	A	−	−	A^w
Galactose	NR	−	−	−	NR	−	−	NR	−	V^{-w}	−	−	NR	NR	V
Maltose	−	−	V^{-w}	−	−	−	−	−	−	V^{-w}	−	−	−	−	−
Mannose	−	−	A^w	−	A^w	−	−	−	−	V^{-w}	−	−	−	V−	A^w
Melibiose	−	−	A^{-w}	−	V^{-w}	−	−	−	−	−	−	−	−	−	−
Raffinose	−	−	A^w	−	V^{-w}	−	−	−	−	−	−	−	−	−	−
Salicin	−	−	V^{-w}	−	V^{-w}	−	−	−	−	V^{-w}	−	−	−	NR	−
Sucrose	−	−	A^w	−	V^{-w}	−	−	A	−	V^{-w}	−	−	−	−	−
Trehalose	−	−	V−	−	V^{-w}	−	−	−	−	V^{-w}	−	−	−	NR	−
Misc. tests															
Indole	−	+	−	+	−	+	+	−	−	+	−	−	−	−	−
Esculin hydrolysis	−	−	+	−	+	−	−	−	−	+	−	−	−	−	+
Hippurate hydrolysis	−	V	−	V−	−	−	V−	NR	+	−	V−	+	−	NR	V
Lipase	−	−	−	−	−	+	−	−	−	−	−	−	−	−	−
Isolated from															
Humans	+	+	+	+	−	+	+	+	+	+	+	−	+	+	+
Animals	−	+	−	−	+	+	−	−	−	−	+	+	−	−	−

V, variable reactions; V−, variable, usually negative; w, weak reaction; NG, no growth; G, growth; NR, no results; α, alpha hemolysis; β, beta hemolysis; γ, gamma (no) hemolysis; SBA, sheep blood agar.

Data from references 14 and 26.

[a]A problem with identification is the general lack of reactivity in conventional tests; best for identification are fatty acid profiles using gas chromatography, electrophoretic patterns of glutamate dehydrogenase, and pyrolysis-mass spectrometry (5).

[b]Most commonly isolated *Fusobacterium* species from clinical infections.

[c]Rarely isolated from clinical specimens; however, commonly found in human feces.

[d]Bile concentration 20% or 2% Bacto oxgall (10× concentration bile).

GENUS: *GARDNERELLA* (14, 19)

Gram-positive, Gram-negative **pleomorphic** rods
Nonsporeforming
Facultative anaerobes
Catalase negative
Nonencapsulated
Nonmotile
Oxidase negative
O/F glucose: F (fermentative)
Optimal growth temperature 35–37°C
Human blood (HBT) but **not** sheep blood hemolyzed; β-hemolysis
Not acid-fast
Single species: *G. vaginalis* ATCC 14018; NCTC 10287

Fastidious in growth requirements
Major cause of bacterial "nonspecific" vaginalis

Table 44.30. Biochemical Characteristics of *Gardnerella vaginalis*

Nitrate reduction	−	H$_2$S	−
Hippurate hydrolysis	+	Indole	−
Starch hydrolysis	+	Lysine	−
ONPG	V	Phenylalanine	−
Methyl red (MR)	+	Ornithine	−
Arginine dihydrolase	−	Tween 80	−
Esculin hydrolysis	−	Urease	−
Gelatin liquefaction	−	Voges-Proskauer (VP)	−
Carbohydrates			
L-Arabinose	A	Mannitol	−
Cellobiose	−	Mannose	A
Dextrine	A	Melibiose	−
Fructose	A	Raffinose	−
Galactose	A	Ribose	A
Inositol	−	Rhamnose	−
Inulin	A	Salicin	−
Lactose	A	Sucrose	A
Maltose	A	Xylose	A

A, acid production (+); V, variable reactions.

GENUS: *GEMELLA* (6, 16, 19)

Gram-positive **or Gram-variable** (easily decolorized), spherical or elongated cells; often in pairs (**diplococci**) with flattened adjacent sides or in pairs of unequal size; Resemble *Neisseria* in morphology when Gram negative

Nonsporeforming

Facultative anaerobes

Catalase negative

Nonencapsulated

Nonmotile

Oxidase negative

O/F glucose: F (fermentative)

Optimum growth temperature 37°C; no growth at 10° and 45°C

4 species: *G. bergeri, G. haemolysans, G. morbillorum, G. sanguinis*

Type species: *G. haemolysans* ATCC 10379, NCTC 5414

Often confused with species in *Neisseria, Veillonella,* and *Streptococcus* genera

Table 44.31. Differentiation of Two *Gemella* spp.

Test	*G. haemolysans*	*G. morbillorum*
Catalase	−	−
Oxidase	−	−
10°C	NG	NG
45°C	NG	NG
6.5% NaCl	G	G
Motility	−	−
Esculin hydrolysis	−	−
PYR	+	+^{wa}
LAP	−	V
Vancomycin 30μg	S	S

NG, no growth; G, growth; V, variable results; +^{w}, weakly positive; S, sensitive (susceptible); LAP, leucine aminopeptidase; PYR, pyrrolidonylarylamidase.

[a]According to Facklam and Washington (4), to avoid false-negative PYR results, a large inoculum must be used.

GENUS: *HAEMOPHILUS* (5, 14)

Gram-negative, minute to medium-sized, spherical, oval, or rod-shaped cells; occasionally form threads or filaments; **marked pleomorphism**

Nonsporeforming

Facultatively anaerobic

Catalase variable

Capsulated; associated with virulence; e.g., *H. influenzae*

Nonmotile

Oxidase variable

O/F glucose: F (fermentative) and O (oxidative)

Optimal growth temperature: 35–37°C; except *H. ducreyi*, 33–35°C (5)

Reduce nitrate to nitrite and beyond

17 species: *H. actinomycetemcomitans, H. aegyptius, H. aphrophilus, H. ducreyi, H. felis, H. haemoglobinophilus, H. haemolyticus, H. influenzae, H. paracuniculus, H. paragallinarum, H. parahaemolyticus, H. parainfluenzae, H. paraphrohaemolyticus, H. paraphrophilus, H. parasuis, H. piscium, H. segnis*

Type species: *H. influenzae* ATCC 33391, NCTC 8143

Almost all species require preformed growth factors present in blood, especially X factor (protoporphyrin 1X, or protoheme) and/or V factor (nicotinamide adenine dinucleotide (NAD) or NAD phosphate (NADP)). X and V factors are **not definitive** requirements for *Haemophilus* spp.; *Actinobacillus* spp. and *Pasteurella* spp. require V factor.

Growth stimulated by 5–10% carbon dioxide (CO_2)

Cultures characteristic "mouse nest "odor

AO (acridine orange) staining enhances appearance of *Haemophilus* species; enhanced contrast between bacteria and background (26)

H. aphrophilus causative agent of conjunctivitis

H. ducreyi causative agent of venereal disease, soft chancre or chancroid

H. influenzae leading cause of meningitis in children

Table 44.32. Differentiation of *Haemophilus* spp.

Test	H. actinomycetemcomitans	H. aphrophilus	H. ducreyi	H. haemoglobinophilus	H. haemolyticus	H. influenzae	H. parecuniculus	H. paragallinarum	H. parahaemolyticus	H. parainfluenzae	H. paraprohaemolyticus	H. paraphrophilus	H. parasuis	H. segnis
Catalase	+	−	−	+	+	+	+	+	V	V	+	−	+	V
Oxidase	+	−	+	+	+	+	+	−	+	+	+	+	−	−
NO₃→NO₂	+	+	+	+	+	+	+	+	+	+	+	+	+	+
β-hemolysis, 5% SBA	−	−	Vᵃ	−	+	−	−	−	+	−	+	−	−	−
MacConkey (MAC)	V	V⁻	NG	NG	NG	NG	NG	NG	NG	NG	NG	NG	NG	NG
H₂S	−	−	−	V	+	−	−	NR	+	+	+	+	V	−
Carbohydrates														
Glucose	A	A	−	A	A	A	A	A	A	A	A	A	A	Aʷ
Lactose	−	A	−	−	−	−	−	−	−	−	−	A	V	−
Adonitol	−	−	−	−	−	−	−	−	−	−	−	−	−	−
Arabinose	−	−	−	−	−	−	−	NR	−	−	−	−	−	−
Cellobiose	−	−	−	−	−	−	−	−	−	−	−	−	−	−
Dextrin	V	NR	NR	NR	NR	NR	NR	NR	NR	NR	NR	NR	NR	NR
Dulcitol	−	−	−	−	−	−	−	−	−	−	−	−	−	−
Erythritol	NR	−	−	−	−	−	−	−	−	−	−	−	−	−
Fructose	A	A	−	−	Aʷ	−	A	A	A	A	A	A	A	Aʷ
Galactose	A	A	−	−	A	A	−	−	V	A	V	−	A	Aʷ
Glycerol	−	V	−	−	−	−	−	−	−	−	−	−	−	Aʷ
Inositol	−	V	−	−	−	−	−	−	−	−	−	−	V	−
Inulin	−	−	−	−	−	−	−	−	−	−	−	−	A	−
Maltose	A	A	−	A	A	A	A	A	A	A	A	A	A	Aʷ
Mannitol	V⁺	−	−	A	−	−	−	A	−	−	−	−	−	−
Mannose	A	A	−	A	−	−	NR	A	−	A	−	−	A	−
Melibiose	−	−	−	−	−	−	−	−	−	−	−	−	A	−
Raffinose	−	A	−	−	−	−	−	−	−	−	−	−	−	−
Rhamnose	−	−	−	−	−	−	NR	−	−	−	−	−	−	−
Ribose	−	A	−	V	A	A	NR	A	−	−	−	A	A	−
Salicin	−	−	−	−	−	−	−	−	−	−	−	−	−	−
Sorbitol	V⁻	−	−	−	−	−	−	A	−	−	−	−	−	−
Sorbose	−	−	−	−	−	−	−	−	−	−	−	−	A	−
Sucrose	V	A	−	A	−	−	−	A	A	A	A	A	A	Aʷ
Trehalose	−	A	−	−	−	−	−	−	−	−	−	−	A	−
Xylose	V	−	−	A	V	A	−	V	−	−	−	−	−	−
Misc. tests														
Indole	−	−	−	+	V	V	+	−	−	−	−	−	−	−
Esculin hydrolysis	−	−	−	−	−	−	−	−	−	−	−	−	−	−
Arginine dehydrolase	−	−	−	−	−	−	+	−	−	−	−	−	−	−
Lysine decarboxylase	−	−	−	−	−	V	NR	−	−	V	−	−	−	−
Ornithine decarboxylase	−	−	−	−	−	V⁺	+	−	V	V	−	−	−	−
Gelatin liquefaction, 22°C	−	NR	NR	−	NR	NR	NR	NR	NR	NR	NR	NR	NR	NR
ONPG	−	+	−	V	−	−	+	+	V	V	V	+	V	V
Phosphatase	+	+	+	−	+	+	+	+	+	+	+	+	+	+
Methyl red (MR)	−	NR	NR	NR	NR	NR	NR	NR	NR	NR	NR	NR	NR	NR
Voges-Proskauer (VP)	−	NR	NR	NR	NR	NR	NR	NR	NR	NR	NR	NR	NR	NR
Urease	−	−	−	−	+	V⁺	+	−	+	V	+	−	−	−
X factor requirement	−	−	+	+	+	+	−	−	−	−	−	−	−	−
V factor requirement	−	−	−	−	+	+	+	+	+	+	+	+	+	+

V, variable reaction; V, variable, ususally positive; V, variable, usually negative; NG, no growths, NR, no results; SBA, sheep blood agar; A, acid production (+); w, weak reaction.

Data from reference 14.

ᵃDelayed positive reaction.

GENUS: *HELICOBACTER* (5, 19)

Gram-negative, helical, curved, or straight rods with rounded ends. Older cultures appear coccoid.

Nonsporeforming

Microaerophilic; some growth anaerobically

Catalase positive

Nonencapsulated

Motile: rapid and darting; multiple sheath flagella that are unipolar or bipolar and lateral with terminal bulbs

Oxidase positive

O/F glucose: F (fermentative)

Optimal growth temperature: 37°C; growth at 30°C but not 25°C

18 species: *H. acinonychis, H. bilis, H. bizzozaronii, H. canis, H. cholecytus, H. cinaedi, H. felis, H. fennelliae, H. hepaticus, H. muridarum, H. mustelae, H. nemestrinae, H. pametensis, H. pullorum, H. pylori, H. rodentium, H. salomonis, H. trogontum*

Type species: *H. pylori* ATCC 43504, NCTC 11637 (not in *Bergey's Manual*; created by Goodwin et al. (7))

H. mustelae causative agent of peptic ulcers in humans.

H. pylori causative agent of type B gastritis in humans.

Table 44.33. Differentiation of Some *Helicobacter* spp.

Test	*H. cinaedi*	*H. fennelliae*	*H. mustelae*	*H. pylori*
Catalase	+	+	+	+
Oxidase	+	+	+	+
$NO_3 \rightarrow NO_2$	+	−	+	V
Motility	+	+	+	+
25°C	NG	NG	NR	NG
42°C	V	NG	G	G
H_2S (TSI)	−	−	−	−
Hippurate hydrolysis	−	−	NR	−
Indoxyhydrolacetate	V⁻	+	NR	−
Urease	+	−	NR	−
Cephalothin acid, 30 μg disk	V⁺	S	R	S
Nalidixic acid, 30 μg disk	S	S	S	R
DNase	−	−	−	+

S, sensitive (susceptible); R, resistant; BG, no growth; G, growth; NR, no results, V⁺, variable, usually positive, V⁻, variable, usually negative

Data from references 5 and 26.

GENUS: *JANTHINOBACTERIUM* (14)

Gram-negative rods with rounded ends; occasionally exhibit barred or bipolar staining with lipid inclusions; occur singly and occasionally pairs in short chains

Nonsporeforming

Strict (obligate) aerobic

Catalase positive

Nonencapsulated

Motile: both single polar flagellum and usually 1–4 subpolar or lateral flagella

Oxidase variable, usually positive by Kovacs' method; violet pigment may interfere with interpretation.

O/F glucose: F (fermentative)

Optimal growth temperature: 25°C; minimum 2°C and maximum 32°C

Single species: *J. lividum* ATCC 12473, NCTC 9796

Violet colonies on solid medium; violet ring at junction of liquid surface and container wall

Table 44.34. Biochemical Characteristics of *Janthinobacterium lividum*

NaCl, 6%	NG	Voges-Proskauer (VP)	−
NO$_3$→NO$_2$	−	Glucose	A
Indole	−	Benzylpenicillin, 10 µg/mL	R
Citrate	+	O/129	R
Phosphatase	+		

NG, no growth; R, resistant; O/129, vibriostatic agent 2,4-diamino-6,7-diisopropylpteridine; A, acid production (+).

GENUS: *KINGELLA* (5, 14, 26)

Gram-negative, straight rods with round or square ends that tend to resist decolorization or coccobacilli; arranged in pairs, occasionally short chains; may mimic *Neisseria gonorrhoeae* (26)

Nonsporeforming

Facultatively anaerobic; best growth aerobically but can grow weakly anaerobically on blood agar

Catalase negative

Nonencapsulated

Nonmotile; may be fimbriated (piliated) and exhibit "twitching motility"

Oxidase positive

O/F glucose: F (fermentative)

Optimal growth temperature: 33–37°C

3 species: *K. denitrificans*, *K. kingae*, and *K. oralis*

Type species: *K. kingae* ATCC 23330

Fastidious; may require special procedures for basal fermentation media (e.g., serum) to enhance growth

Capnophilic; require additional CO$_2$ for growth

Table 44.35. Differentiation of Two *Kingella* spp.

Test	*K. denitrificans*	*K. kingae*
Catalase	−	−
Oxidase	+[a]	+[a]
Motility	−	−
β-hemolysis, 5% SBA	−	+
NaCl, 4%	NG	NG
MacConkey (MAC)	NG	NG
NO$_3$→NO$_2$	+	−
Carbohydrates		
Glucose	A[b]	A[b]
Lactose	−	−
Maltose	−	A
Mannitol	−	−
Sucrose	−	−
Xylose	−	−
Misc. tests		
Indole	−	−
Casein digestion	−	+
Esculin hydrolysis	−	−
Phosphatase	−	+
Urease	−	−
Tween 40 hydrolysis	−	−
Penicillin	S	S

NG, no growth; S, sensitive (susceptible); V, variable results; A, acid production (+); NG, no growth.
[a]Positive with tetramethyl-*p*-phenylenediamine; weakly positive with dimethyl reagent.
[b]Delayed.

GENUS: *LEGIONELLA* (5, 5, 26)

Gram-negative, faintly staining, thin rods

Species not usually detected in clinical material by Gram stain (5); best is histologic examination of tissue sections using silver or Giemsa stains

Nonsporeforming

Aerobic

Catalase positive

Nonencapsulated

Motility: variable, usually positive; occasional nonmotile strain; 1 or more straight or curved polar or lateral flagella

Oxidase negative or weakly positive

O/F glucose: inert (−)

Optimal growth temperature: 35–37°C

Not acid-fast

Nitrate reduction negative

Urease negative

39 species: *L. adelaidensis*, *L. anisa*, *L. birminghamensis*, *L. brunensis*, *L. cherrii*, *L. cincinnatiensis*, *L. erythra*, *L. fairfieldensis*, *L. feeleii*, *L. geestiana*, *L. gratiana* *L. hackeliae*, *L. israelensis*, *L. jamestowniensis*, *L. jordanis*, *L. langsingensis*, *L. londiniensis*, *L. longbeachae*, *L. lytica*, *L. moravica*, *L. nautarum*, *L. oakridgensis*, *L. parisiensis*, *L. pneumophila* subsp. *fraseri*, *L. pneumophila* subsp. *pascullei*, *L. pneumophila* subsp. *pneumoniae*, *L. quateirensis*, *L. quinlivanii*, *L. rubrilucens*, *L. sainthelensi*, *L. santicrucis*, *L. shakespearei*, *L. spiritensis*, *L. steigerwaltii*, *L. taurinensis*, *L. tucsonensis*, *L. wadsworthii*, *L. waltersii*, *L. worsleiensis*

Type species: *L. pneumophila* subsp. *pneumoniae* ATCC 33152; causative agent of Legionnaires' disease or mild, febrile disease (Pontiac fever)

Do not grow on standard blood agars or other commonly used primary plate media; L-cysteine · HCl and iron salts buffered to pH 6.9 are required for optimal growth.

Identification by serologic testing for most frequently isolated species and serovars; radioimmunoassay, enzyme assay, latex agglutination or polymerase chain reaction (PCR); antisera for many species not available commercially.

L. pneumoniae is predominant human pathogen (5), followed by *L. micdadei* and *L. dumoffii* (31)

Biochemically inert; extensive biochemical testing of little use

All specimens suspected of harboring *Legionella* should be handled in a class II biological safety cabinet (BSC) (5); identification is performed by reference, state, or public health laboratories.

GENUS: *LEPTOTRICHIA* (5, 14)

Gram-negative, straight or slightly curved rods. **Very young cultures may stain Gram positive**, but organism has an atypical Gram-negative–type cell wall. Fusiform rods and long filaments may occur.

Nonsporeforming

Anaerobic; may be aerotolerant

Catalase negative

Nonencapsulated

Nonmotile

Oxidase negative

O/F glucose: F (fermentative)

Optimal growth temperature: 35–37°C; no growth below 25°C

Single species: *L. buccalis* ATCC 14201, NCTC 10249.

Table 44.36. Biochemical Characteristics of *Leptotrichia buccalis*

Hemolysis, 5% SBA	γ	Glucose	A
H$_2$S	−	Lactose	A
Indole	−	Cellobiose	A
Esculin hydrolysis	+	Fructose	A
Hippurate hydrolysis	−	Galactose	A
NO$_3$→NO$_2$	−	Maltose	A
		Mannose	A
		Melibiose	−
		Raffinose	V
		Salicin	A
		Sucrose	A
		Trehalose	A

A, acid production (+); V−, variable, usually negative; γ, gamma (no) hemolysis; SBA, sheep blood agar.

GENUS: *MEGAMONAS* (14)

Gram-negative, large rods with rounded ends or coccobacilli; usually granular appearance due to volutin
Nonsporeforming
Anaerobic
Catalase negative
Nonencapsulated
Nonmotile
Oxidase negative
O/F glucose: F (fermentative)
Esculin hydrolysis positive
Single species: *M. hypermegas* ATCC 25560, NCTC 10570 (not in *Bergey's Manual*; created by Shah and Collins (25))

GENUS: *MEGASPHAERA* (14)

Gram-negative **cocci** arranged in pairs (diplococci; kidney shaped) and occasionally short chains
Nonsporeforming
Anaerobic
Catalase negative
Nonencapsulated
Motility negative
Oxidase negative
O/F glucose: F (fermentative)
Optimal growth temperature: 15–40°C
2 species: *M. cerevisiae*, *M. elsdenii*
Type species: *M. elsdenii* ATCC 25940, NCIB 8927

Table 44.37. Differentiation of *Megasphaera* spp.

Test	*M. cerevisiae*	*M. elsdenii*
Catalase	−	−
40°C	NG	G
NO$_3$→NO$_2$	−	−
Glucose	−	A
Maltose	−	A

A, acid production (+); G, growth; NG, no growth.
Data from references 14 and 26.

GENUS: *METHYLOBACTERIUM* (5, 29)

Gram-negative or Gram-variable rods occurring singly or occasionally in rosettes; occasionally branched and **pleomorphic vacuolated rods**
Nonsporeforming
Aerobic
Catalase positive; may be weak
Nonencapsulated
Motile; single polar flagellum or lateral flagella
Oxidase positive; may be weak
O/F glucose: inert (−)
Optimal growth temperature: 25–30°C
10 species: *M. aminovorans, M. extorquens, M. fujisawaense, M. mesophilicum, M. organophilum, M. radiotolerans, M. rhodesianum, M. rhodinum, M. thiocyanatum, M. zatmanii*
Type species: *M. organophilum*, ATCC 27886 (not in *Bergey's Manual*; created by Green and Bousfield (9))
Pink-pigmented colonies

Table 44.38. Differentiation of *Methylobacterium* spp.

Test	*M. extorquens*	*M. fujisawaense*	*M. mesophilicum*	*M. organophilum*	*M. radiotolerans*	*M. rhodesianum*	*M. rhodinum*	*M. zatmanii*
Catalase	+	+	+	+	+	+	+	+
Oxidase	+	+	+	+	+	+	+	+
$NO_3 \to NO_2$	−	NR	−	NR	+	−	NR	−
MacConkey (MAC)	G	NR	G	NR	NG	NG	NR	NG
H_2S								
TSI	−	NR	−	NR	−	−	NR	−
PbAc	+	NR	+	NR	+	+	NR	+
Motility	+	+	+	+	+	+	+	+
Carbohydrates								
Glucose	−	A	A	A	−	A^w	−	−
Arabinose	−	A	A	−	A	−	−	−
Fructose	−	V	−	−	−	A	A	A
Xylose	−	A	A	−	A	−	−	−
Misc. tests								
Indole	−	NR	−	NR	−	−	NR	−
Esculin hydrolysis	−	NR	−	NR	−	−	NR	−
Citrate	−	NR	V+	NR	NR	NR	NR	NR
Gelatin liquefaction, 22°C	−	NR	−	NR	−	−	NR	−
Urease	V+	NR	V+	NR	V+	V+	NR	V+

G, growth; NG, no growth; V, variable reactions; V+, variable, usually positive; w, weak reaction; A, acid production (+).
Data from references 5 and 29.

GENUS: *MITSUOKELLA* (14)

Gram-negative, regular or ovoid rods
Nonsporeforming
Anaerobic
Catalase: no results
Capsule variable
Nonmotile

Oxidase: no results
O/F glucose: F (fermentative); often vigorously
Single species: M. multiacidus ATCC 27723, NCTC 10934 (not in Bergey's Manual; created by Shah and Collins (25))

Table 44.39. Biochemical Characteristics of *Mitsuokella multiacidus*

Bile 20%	G	Glucose	A
Pigmentation	−	Lactose	A
Indole	−	Arabinose	A
Esculin hydrolysis	+	Cellobiose	A
		Salicin	A
		Sucrose	A

A, acid production (+); G, growth; 20% bile, bile concentration 20% or 2% Bacto oxgall (10× concentration bile).

GENUS: *MOBILUNCUS* (14, 27)

Gram-variable, slender, curved rods with tapered ends; Gram variable or Gram negative, but cell wall is Gram-positive type; variable in shape and size and arranged singly, but at times in **pairs with gullwing appearance**
Nonsporeforming
Anaerobic
Nonencapsulated
Catalase negative
Motile by multilateral or subpolar flagella
Oxidase negative
O/F glucose: F (fermentative); weak
Optimal growth temperature 37°C
Mycolic acid in cells; largest and most complex (C_{60}–C_{90})
3 species: M. curtisii subsp. curtisii, M. curtisii subsp. holmesii, M. mulieris
Type species: M. curtisii subsp. curtisii ATCC 35241 (not in Bergey's Manual, established by Spiegel and Roberts (27)); Genus may be a synonym of *Falcivibrio* (27).

Table 44.40. Differentiation of *Mobiluncus* spp.

	M. curtisii		
Test	subsp. *curtisii*	subsp. *holmesii*	M. mulieris
Catalase	−	−	−
Oxidase	−	−	−
$NO_3 \rightarrow NO_2$	−	+	−
H_2S	−	−	−
Motility	+	+	+
Glucose	A^w	V^{-vw}	V
Fructose	V^{vw}	V^{vw}	V
Lactose	V^{vw}	−	V^{-vw}
Maltose	A^w	V^{-vw}	A
Mannitol	−	−	−
Ribose	−	−	V^{vw}
Starch	−	V^{vw}	V
Arginine dehydrolase	+	+	−
Esculin hydrolysis	−	−	−
Hippurate hydrolysis	+	+	−
Indole	−	−	−
Starch hydrolysis	+	+	+

A, acid production (+); w, if positive, weak reaction; vw, if positive, very weak reaction; V, variable results; V⁻, variable, usually negative. Data from reference 14.

GENUS: *MORAXELLA* (14, 26)

Gram-negative rods that resist decolorization; rods short and plump; arranged predominantly in pairs and occasionally short chains. Subgenus *Branhamella* cells approach coccus shape; shape enhanced by lack of O_2 and incubation above optimal; cocci are smaller and arranged singly, in pairs, or in tetrads with adjacent sides flattened. Resemble *Neisseria* species

Pleomorphic

Nonsporeforming

Aerobic; some strains may grow weakly anaerobically

Catalase positive except *M. bovis* (variable)

Capsule variable

Nonmotile; both rods and cocci may be fimbriated. "Surface-bound twitching motility" may be exhibited by some rods.

Oxidase positive; strong

O/F glucose: inert (−) or no growth

Optimal growth temperature: 33–35°C

Highly sensitive to penicillin

13 species: *M. atlantae, M. boevrei, M. bovis, M. canis, M. caprae, M. catarrhalis, M. equi, M. lacunata, M. lincolnii, M. nonliquefaciens, M. osloensis, M. ovis, M. saccharolytica*

Type species: *M. lacunata* ATCC 17967

Fastidious

According to Murray et al. (19), most laboratories **do not determine** the species of *Moraxella* because of the similarity in pathogenic significance of the species.

Table 44.41. Differentiation of the Most Frequently Isolated *Moraxella* spp.

Test	*M. atlantae*	*M. bovis*	*M. catarrhalis*	*M. lacunata*	*M. lincolnii*	*M. nonliquefaciens*	*M. osloensis*	*M. ovis*
Catalase	+	V	+	+	+	+	+	+
Oxidase	+	+	+	+	+	+	+	+
Cell shape								
Rods	+	+	−	+	+	+	+	−
Cocci	−	−	+	−	−	−	−	+
MacConkey (MAC)	G	NG	NG	NG	NG	NG	V	V
Hemolysis (human blood)	−	V+	−	−	−	−	−	NR
H$_2$S								
TSI	−	−	−	−	NR	−	−	NR
PbAc	V	+	V	V	NR	V	V	NR
NaCl, 6.5%	NG	NG	NG	NG	NG	NG	NG	NG
NO$_3$→NO$_2$	−	V−	V+	+	−	+	V	+
Gelatin liquefaction, 22°C	−	V+	−	V	−	−	−	−
Motility	−	−	−	−	−	−	−	−
Citrate	−	−	−	−	−	−	−	−
DNase	−	−	+	−	−	−	−	−
Indole	−	−	−	−	−	−	−	−
Esculin hydrolysis	−	−	−	−	−	−	−	−
Phenylalanine	−	−	V−	V	NR	−	V−	−
Urease	−	−	−	−	−	−	−[a]	−
Penicillin, 1.0 U/mL	S	S	V+[b]	S	NR	S	V+[c]	S
Isolation from								
Humans	+	−	+	+	+	+	−	NR
Animals	−	+	−	+	−	−	+	NR

V, variable reactions; V+, variable, usually positive; V−, variable, usually negative; NG, no growth; w, weak reaction; S, sensitive (susceptible); NR, no results; PbAc, lead acetate strips.
Data from references 5, 14, 26, and 29.
[a]Few strains weakly urease positive.
[b]Some strains are penicillin resistant on basis of β-lactamoase production; no β-lactamase-negative strains grow in the presence of 1.0 U/mL penicillin (14).
[c]Rare growth.

GENUS: *MOROCOCCUS* (14)

Gram-negative **cocci** held together firmly in tightly packed **mulberry-like** aggregates
Nonsporeforming
Aerobic
Catalase positive
Nonencapsulated
Nonmotile
Oxidase positive
O/F glucose: F (fermentative); weak reaction
Optimal growth temperature: 23–42°C
Single species: *M. cerebrosus* ATCC 33486, NCTC 11393 (not in *Bergey's Manual*; created by Long et al (18))

Table 44.42. Biochemical Characteristics of *Morococcus cerebrosus*

Catalase	+	Glucose	A
Oxidase	+	Lactose	−
NO$_3$→NO$_2$	+	Arabinose	−
H$_2$S (cysteine)	+	Dextrin	−
Litmus milk	Red	Fructose	A
Citrate	−	Gelactose	−
Indole	−	Inulin	−
DNase	+	Maltose	A
Esculin hydrolysis	−	Mannose	−
Gelatin liquefaction, 22°C	−	Melibiose	−
Malonate	−	Raffinose	−
Phosphatase	−	Rhamnose	−
Phenylalanine	−	Ribose	−
Ornithine decarboxylase	+	Salicin	−
Starch hydrolysis	−	Sorbose	−
Lecithinase	−	Sucrose	A
Methyl red (MR)	+	Trehalose	−
Urease	−	Xylose	−
Tween 80	−		

A, acid production (+); Red, reduction.
Data from reference 14.

GENUS: *MYCOPLASMA* (14)

Gram-negative, spherical, slightly ovoid or pear-shaped to **slender branched filaments; pleomorphic;** lack cell wall

Nonsporeforming

Facultatively anaerobic

Catalase negative

Motility: variable, usually positive; some species exhibit gliding motility

Oxidase: no results

104 species: *M. adleri, M. agalactiae, M. alkalescens, M. alvi, M. anatis, M. anseris, M. arginini, M. arthritidis, M. auris, M. bovigenitalium, M. bovirhinis, M. bovis, M. bovoculi, M. buccale, M. buteonis, M. californicum, M. canadense, M. canis, M. capricolum* subsp. *capricolum, M. capricolum* subsp. *capripneumoniae, M. caviae, M. cavipharyngis, M. citelli, M. cloacale, M. collis, M. columbinasale, M. columbinum, M. columborale, M. conjunctivae, M. corogypsi, M. cottewii, M. cricetuli, M. crocodyli, M. cynos, M. dispar, M. edwardii, M. elephantis, M. equigenitalium, M. equirhinis, M. falconis, M. fastidiosum, M. faucium, M. felifavcium, M. feliminutum, M. felis, M. fermentans, M. flocculare, M. gallinaceum, M. gallinarum, M. gallisepticum, M. gallopavonis, M. gateae, M. genitalium, M. glycophilum, M. gypis, M. hominis, M. hyopharyngis, M. hyopneumoniae, M. hyorhinis, M. hyosynoviae, M. imitans, M. indiense, M. iners, M. iowae, M. lagogenitalium, M. leopharyngis, M. lipofaciens, M. lipophilum, M. maculosum, M. meleagridis, M. moatsii, M. mobile, M. molare, M. muris, M. mustelae, M. mycoides* subsp. *capri, M. mycoides* subsp. *mycoides, M. neurolyticum, M. opalescens, M. orale, M. ovipneumoniae, M. oxoniensis, M. penetrans, M. phocacerebrale, M. phocarhinis, M. phocidae, M. pirum, M. pneumoniae, M. primatum, M. pullorum, M. pulmonis, M. putrefaciens, M. salivarium, M. simbae, M. spermatophilum, M. spumans, M. sturni, M. sualvi, M. subdolum, M. suipneumoniae, M. synoviae, M. testudinis, M. verecundum, M. yeatsii*

Type species: *M. mycoides* subsp. *mycoides*; NCTC 10114

Typical colony has a "fried egg" appearance

Requires cholesterol or related sterols for growth

Differentiation of many species by serologic determinations

GENUS: *NEISSERIA* (14, 26)

Gram-negative diplococci that tend to resist decolorization; arranged singly, often in pairs with adjacent sides flattened to give **characteristic kidney shape or coffee bean shape**; except *N. elongata*, short rods often arranged as diplobacilli or short chains

Nonsporeforming

Aerobic

Catalase positive except *N. elongata* and *N. mucosa*

Capsule variable

Nonmotile

Oxidase positive

ONPG positive: *N. lactamica*; used to help distinguish from *N. gonorrhea* and *N. meningitis*

O/F glucose: O (oxidative)

Optimal growth temperature: 35–37°C

21 species: *N. animalis*, *N. canis*, *N. cinerea*, *N. denitrificans*, *N. dentiae*, *N. elongata* subsp. *elongata*, *N. elongata* subsp. *glycolytica*, *N. elongata* subsp. *nitroreducens*, *N. flava*, *N. flavescens*, *N. gonorrhoeae*, *N. iguanae*, *N. lactamica*, *N. macacae*, *N. meningitidis*, *N. mucosa*, *N. perflava*, *N. polysaccharea*, *N. sicca*, *N. subflava*, *N. weaveri*

Type species: *N. gonorrhoeae* ATCC 19424

Some species produce a greenish yellow carotenoid pigment.

Some species are nutritionally fastidious and hemolytic.

Table 44.43. Differentiation of the Most Commonly Isolated *Neisseria* spp.

Test	*N. canis*	*N. cinerea*	*N. dentrificans*	*N. elongata*	*N. flavescens*	*N. gonorrhoeae*	*N. lactamica*	*N. macacae*	*N. meningitidis*	*N. mucosa*	*N. polysaccharea*	*N. sicca*	*N. subfava*
Cell shape													
Cocci	+	+	+	−	+	+	+	+	+	+	+	+	+
Short rods	−	−	−	+	−	−	−	−	−	−	−	−	−
Arrangement													
Pairs	+	+	+	+	+	+	+	+	+	+	+	+	+
Tetrads	−	−	−	−	+	−	−	−	−	−	+	+	+
Short chains	−	−	−	+	−	−	−	−	−	−	−	−	−
Yellowish pigmentation	−	V	V	+w	+	−	+	+	−	V	+	V	+
Hemolysis on blood from													
Human	−	−	−	−	−	−	−	−	−	−	NR	V	−
Horse	−	−	−	−	−	V	+	−	−	−	NR	V	−
Rabbit	V	−	−	−	−	−	+	−	−	−	NR	V	−
Sheep	−	−	−	−	−	−	−	−	−	−	−	−	−
Catalase	+	+	+	−	+	+	+	+	+	−	+	+	+
Oxidase	+	+	+	+	+	+	+	+	+	+	+	+	+
ONPG	−	−	−	−	−	−	+	−	−	−	−	−	−
Motility	−	−	−	−	−	−	−	−	−	−	−	−	−
$NO_3 \rightarrow NO_2$	−	−	+	−	−	−	−	−	−	+	+	−	−
Carbohydrates:													
Glucose	−	−	A	V	−[a]	A	A	A	A	A	A	A	A
Lactose	−	−	−	−	−	−	A	NR	−	−	−	−	−
Fructose	−	−	A	−	−	−	A	−	A	−	A	V	−
Maltose	−	−	−	−	−	−	A	A	A	A	A	A	A
Mannose	−	−	A	−	−	−	NR	−	−	NR	−	−	−
Sucrose	−	−	A	−	−	−	−	A	−	A	V−[b]	A	V

A, acid-production (+); V, variable reactions; V, variable, usually negative; w, weak reaction; NR, no results.

Data from reference 14.

[a]Few strains may form a small amount of acid from glucose; most strains are negative.

[b]Rare production of acid.

GENUS: *OCHROBACTRUM* (14, 26)

Gram-negative rods with parallel sides and rounded ends; usually arranged singly
Nonsporeforming
Strict (obligate) aerobe
Catalase positive
Nonencapsulated
Motile: peritrichous flagella
Oxidase positive
O/F glucose: O (oxidative)
Optimal growth temperature: 20–37°C
2 species: *O. anthropi* and *O. intermedium*
Type species: *O. anthropi* NCTC 12168 (not in *Bergey's Manual*; created by Holmes et al. (10))
Colonies exhibit brown melanin-like pigmentation on tyrosine agar.

Table 44.44. Biochemical Characteristics of *Ochrobactrum anthropi*

Catalase	+	Indole	−
Oxidase	+	Esculin hydrolysis	−
MacConkey (MAC)	G	Gelatin liquefaction, 22°C	−
Glucose	A	DNase	−
Arabinose	A	Gluconate	−
Fructose	A	Casein	−
Rhamnose	A	Arginine dehydrolase	+
Xylose	A	Lysine decarboxylase	−
		Ornithine decarboxylase	−
		Lecithinase	+
		Starch hydrolysis	+
		Tween 20	+
		Tween 80	+

A, acid production (+); G, growth.

GENUS: *OLIGELLA* (14)

Gram-negative, small rods to coccobacilli, often in pairs
Nonsporeforming
Aerobic
Catalase positive
Nonencapsulated
Motility: variable, usually positive; some strains of *O. ureolytica* long peritrichous flagella
Oxidase positive
O/F glucose: inert (−)
Optimal growth temperature: 25–37°C
2 species: *O. ureolytica* and *O. urethralis*
Type species: *O. urethralis* ATCC 17960 (not in *Bergey's Manual*; created by Rossau et al. (20))

Table 44.45. Differentiation of *Oligella* spp.

Test	*O. ureolytica*	*O. urethralis*
Catalase	+	+
Oxidase	+	+
MacConkey (MAC)	V	G
Pigmentation	−	−
Hemolysis, 5% SBA	γ	γ
42°C	NG	G
NO$_3$→NO$_2$	V$^+$	−
H$_2$S	−	−
Motility	V	−
Indole	−	−
Citrate	V	V
Esculin hydrolysis	−	−
Gelatin liquefaction, 22°C	−	−
Phenylalanine deaminase	+	−
Urease	+^{a}	−

G, growth; NG, no growth; V, variable reactions; V$^+$, variable, usually positive; γ, gamma (no) hemolysis; SBA, sheep blood agar.
Data from references 5, 14, and 26.
^{a}Strong positive result within minutes (26).

GENUS: *PASTEURELLA* (5, 14)

Gram-negative, spherical, oval rods; arranged singly and less frequently in pairs or short chains; **bipolar staining common**, especially in specimens from animals

Nonsporeforming

Facultatively anaerobic

Catalase positive; except *P. bettyae* (5) and *P. caballi* (26)

Nonencapsulated

Nonmotile

Oxidase positive

O/F glucose: O (oxidative)

Optimal growth temperature: 37°C

Nitrate reduction positive; except *P. lymphangitidis*

19 species: *P. aerogenes*, *P. anatis*, *P. avium*, *P. bettyae*, *P. caballi*, *P. canis*, *P. dagmatis*, *P. gallinarum*, *P. langaaensis*, *P. lymphangitidis*, *P. mairii*, *P. multocida* subsp. *gallicida*, *P. multocida* subsp. *multocida*, *P. multocida* subsp. *septica*, *P. pneumotropica*, *P. stomatis*, *P. testudinis*, *P. trehalosi*, *P. volantium*

Type species: *P. multocida* subsp. *multocida* NCTC 10322

All species are oxidase positive using tetramethyl-*p*-phenylenediamine dihydrochloric reagent; however, several subcultures **may be necessary** to obtain a positive reaction (5). According to Grehen and Müller (8), test should be performed from cultures grown on blood agar (BA) or chocolate agar; negative results may be obtained with other media.

Table 44.46. Differentiation of *Pasteurella* spp.

Test	*P. aerogenes*	*P. anatis*	*P. avium*	*P. bettyae*	*P. caballi*[a]	*P. canis*	*P. dagmatis*	*P. gallinarum*	*P. langaaensis*
Catalase	+	+	+	V	−	+	+	+	−
Oxidase	V	+w	+	−	+	+	+	+	+w
NO$_3$→NO$_2$	+	+	+	+	+	+	+	+	+
H$_2$S	+	NR	−	NR	NR	NR	NR	V+	NR
MacConkey (MAC)	G	Gw	NG	V	NG	NG	NG	NG	NG
β-hemolysis, 5% SBA	−	−	−	−	−	−	−	−	−
Carbohydrates									
Glucose	A	A	A	A	A	A	A	A	A
Lactose	V−	A[b]	−	−	A[b]	−	−	−	A[b]
Adonitol	−	NR	−	NR	−	−	−	−	−
Arabinose	−	−	−	−	−	−	−	−	−
Cellobiose	−	−	−	−	−	−	−	−	−
Dextrin	NR	NR	NR	NR	NR	NR	NR	A	NR
Dulcitol	−	−	−	−	−	−	−	−	−
Erythritol	NR	NR	NR	NR	NR	NR	NR	NR	NR
Fructose	NR	NR	A	NR	A	A	A	A	A
Galactose	A	A	A[b]	−	A	A	A	A	A
Glycerol	A	NR	NR	NR	NR	NR	NR	−	NR
Inositol	V	−	−	−	V	−	−	−	−
Inulin	NR	NR	NR	NR	−	NR	NR	−	NR
Maltose	A	−	−	V	V	−	A	A	−
Mannitol	V	A	−	−	A	−	−	−	A
Mannose	A	A	A[b]	V	A	A	A	A	A
Melibiose	V	−	−	−	NR	−	−	−	−
Raffinose	V	Aw	−	−	V	−	A	V+	−
Rhamnose	V	NR	−	NR	V	−	−	−	−
Ribose	NR	NR	NR	NR	NR	NR	NR	NR	NR
Salicin	−	−	−	−	−	−	−	−	−
Sorbitol	V−	−	−	−	V−	−	−	V−	−
Sorbose	NR	NR	−	NR	NR	−	−	−	−
Sucrose	A	A	−	−	A	A	A	A	A
Trehalose	−	A	A	−	−	V	A	A	−
Xylose	A	A	V	−	V	V−	−	V	−
Misc. tests									
Indole	V−	−	−	−	−	Vw	+	−	−
Esculin hydrolysis	−	−	−	−	−	−	−	−	−
Arginine dehydrolase	−	NR	−	NR	−	−	−	−	−
Lysine decarboxylase	−	NR	−	NR	−	−	−	−	−
Ornithine decarboxylase	V	−	−	−	V	+	−	−	−
Gelatin liquefaction, 22°C	−	NR	−	NR	−	−	−	−	NR
ONPG	V	+	−	−	+	−	−	−	+
Phosphatase	+	+	+	+	+	+	+	+	+
Methyl red (MR)	−	NR	NR	NR	−	NR	NR	−	NR
Voges-Proskauer (VP)	−	NR	NR	NR	−	NR	NR	−	NR
Urease	+	−	−	−	−	−	+	−	−
V Factor (NAD) requirement	−	−	V	−	−	−	−	−	NR
X Factor requirement	−	NR	−	NR	−	NR	NR	−	−

G, growth; NG, no growth; NR, no results; V, variable reactions; V+, variable, usually positive; V, variable, usually negative; w, weak reaction; SBA, sheep blood agar; X factor, protoporphyrin IX or protheme; V factor, nicotinamide adenine dinucleotide (NAD) or NAD phosphate (NADP).

(continued)

Chapter 44 / Gram-Negative Bacteria

P. lymphangitidis	P. mairii	P. multocida subsp. gallicida	P. multocida subsp. multocida	P. multocida subsp. septica	P. pneumotropica	P. stomatis	P. testudinis	P. trehalose	P. volantium
+	V	+	+	+	+	+	+	−	+
−	+	+	+	+	+	+	+	+	+
−	+	+	+	+	+	+	+	+	+
NR	NR	+	+	+	V+	NR	−	NR	NR
V	V	V	V	V	V	NG	V	G	NG
−	V	−	−	−	−	−	+	V+	−
A	A	A	A	A	A	A	A	A[b]	A
−	V−	−	−	−	V	−	V−	−	Vw
NR	NR	V−	V−	V−	V−	−	NR	NR	−
A	A	V	−	−	V−	−	V	−	−
−	−	−	−	−	−	−	−	V	NR
NR	NR	V	V	V	V	NR	V	NR	NR
−	−	−	−	−	−	−	−	−	−
NR	NR	V−	V−	V−	V−	NR	NR	NR	NR
NR	A	A	A	A	A	A	NR	NR	A
A	A	A	A	A	A	A	V+	−	NR
NR	NR	V	V	V	V+	NR	−	NR	NR
−	V	−	−	−	V	−	A[b]	V	NR
NR	NR	V	V−	V−	−	NR	−	NR	NR
V	V	−	−	V−	V	−	V+	A	A
A	V+	A	A	V+	−	−	V	A	A
A	A	A	A	A	A	A	−	A	NR
A	−	NR	NR	V−	V	−	A	V+	NR
−	−	−	−	−	V	−	V	−	NR
NR	NR	V−	V−	V−	V−	−	A	NR	−
NR	NR	NR	NR	NR	A	NR	NR	NR	NR
V	−	−	−	−	V−	−	V−	V	NR
A	V+	A	−	A	−	−	V	A	V
NR	NR	V−	V−	V−	−	−	NR	NR	−
A	A	A	A	A	A	A	A	A	NR
A	V−	−	A	V	V+	A	V	A	A
−	A	A	A	V	V	−	A	−	V
−	−	+	+	V+	+	+w	+	−	−
+	V	−	−	−	−	−	+	V	−
NR	NR	−	−	−	−	−	−	NR	−
NR	NR	−	−	−	−	−	−	NR	−
−	V+	+	+	V	+	−	−	−	V
NR	NR	−	−	−	V	−	−	NR	−
−	V	−	−	−	+	−	V+	−	+
+	+	+	+	+	+	+	−	+	−
NR	NR	−	−	−	−	NR	NR	NR	NR
NR	NR	−	−	−	−	NR	−	NR	NR
+	+	−	−	−	+	−	−	−	−
NR	NR	−	−	−	−	NR	NR	NR	NR
−	−	−	−	−	−	−	−	−	+

Data from reference 14.

[a]76% of strains produce a yellow pigment.

[b]Positive reaction may be delayed.

GENUS: *PEPTOSTREPTOCOCCUS* (14, 19, 26)

Gram-positive or Gram-variable **cocci** that are occasionally ovoid with variable arrangement: **pairs, tetrads, clumps, or chains**

Young cells of *P. anaerobius* are elongated in chains (26). *P. vaginalis, P. lacrimalis, P. lactolyticus,* and *P. hydrogenalis* short chains or in masses

Nonsporeforming

Anaerobic

Catalase negative; few strains weak or produce pseudocatalase reactions (e.g., *P. asaccharolyticus*)

Nonencapsulated

Nonmotile

Oxidase: no results

O/F glucose: F (fermentative)

Optimal growth temperature 37°C

15 species: *P. anaerobius, P. asaccharolyticus, P. barnesae, P. harei, P. hydrogenalis, P. indolicus, P. ivorii, P. lacrimalis, P. lactolyticus, P. magnus, P. micros, P. octavius, P. prevotii, P. tetradius, P. vaginalis*

Type species: *P. anaerobius* ATCC 27337

Require nutritionally enriched media

Table 44.47. Differentiation of *Peptostreptococcus* spp. That May Cause Human Infections

Test	*P. anaerobius*[a,b]	*P. asaccharolyticus*[b,c]	*P. hydrogenalis*	*P. indolicus*	*P. lacrimalis*	*P. lactolyticus*	*P. magnus*[b]	*P. micros*	*P. prevotii*	*P. tetradius*	*P. vaginalis*
Catalase	−	V	NR	−	NR	NR	V	−	V	V	NR
Coagulase	−	−	−	+[d]	−	−	−	−	−	−	−
Motility	−	−	−	−[d]	−	−	−	−	−	−	−
NO$_3$→NO$_2$	−	−	−	+	−	−	−	−	V	−	−
Glucose	− or A^w	−	A	−	−	A	− or A^w	−	A^w	A	A^w
Lactose	−	−	−	−	−	A	−	−	−	−	−
Cellobiose	−	−	−	−	−	−	−	−	−	−	−
Maltose	− or A^w	−	A	−	−	A	−	−	A^w or −	A	A^w
D-Mannose	−	−	NR	−	NR	NR	−	−	V	A	NR
Sucrose	− or A^w	−	A	−	−	A	−	−	− or A^w	A	NR
Indole	−	+[d]	−	+	−	−	−	−	−	−	−
Esculin	−	−	NR	−	NR	NR	−	−	− or +^{w}	− or +^{w}	NR
Urease	−	−	−	−	−	+	−	−	V	+	NR
Alkaline phosphatase	−	−	NR	+	NR	NR	V	+	+	−	NR
α-Glucosidase	+	−	NR	−	NR	NR	−	−	−	+^{w}	NR
β-Glucuronidase	−	−	NR	−	NR	NR	−	−	−	+	NR
Ammonia from											
Glutamate	−	+	NR	+	NR	NR	−	−	−	−	NR
Glycine	−	−	NR	−	NR	NR	+	+^{w}	−	−	NR

V, variable reactions; A, acid production (+); NR, no results; w, weak reaction.

Data from references 14, 19, 26.

[a] *P. anaerobius* pungently sweet odor (26).

[b] Most common (26): *P. mangus, P. anaerobius,* and *P. asaccharolyticus.*

[c] *P. asaccharolyticus* slight yellow pigmentation on blood-agar (BA) (26).

[d] Occasional strains are negative.

GENUS: *PORPHYROMONAS* (14)

Gram-negative short rods or coccobacilli
Nonsporeforming
Anaerobic
Catalase negative
Nonencapsulated
Nonmotile
Oxidase: no results
O/F glucose: F (fermentative)
Optimal growth temperature: 35–37°C
12 species: *P. asaccharolyticus, P. cangingivalis, P. canoris, P. cansulci, P. catoniae, P. circumdentaria, P. crevioricanis, P. endodontalis, P. gingivalis, P. gingivicanis, P. levii, P. macacae*
Type species: *P. asaccharolyticus* ATCC 25260 (not in *Bergey's Manual*; created by Shah and Collins (23))
Brown to black colonies on blood agar caused by protoheme production

Table 44.48. Biochemical Characteristics of the genus *Porphyromonas*

Catalase	—	Indole	+
Bile 20%	NG	Lipase	—
$NO_3 \rightarrow NO_2$	—	Urease	—

NG, no growth; bile 20%, bile concentration 20% or 2% Bacto oxgall (10× concentration bile).

GENUS: *PREVOTELLA* (14)

Gram-negative **pleomorphic** rods or coccobacilli
Nonsporeforming
Anaerobic
Catalase variable, usually negative
Nonencapsulated
Nonmotile
Oxidase-no results
O/F glucose: F (fermentative)
Optimal growth temperature: 35–37°C
26 species: *P. albensis, P. bivia, P. brevis, P. bryantii, P. buccae, P. buccalis, P. corporis, P. dentalis, P. denticola, P. disiens, P. enoeca, P. heparinolytica, P. intermedia, P. loescheii, P. melaninogenica, P. nigrescens, P. oralis, P. oris, P. oulora, P. pallens, P. ruminicola, P. ruminicola* subsp. *brevis, P. ruminicola* subsp. *ruminicola, P. tannerae, P. veroralis, P. zoogleoformans*
Type species: *P. melaninogenica* ATCC 25845 (genus not in *Bergey's Manual*; created by Shah and Collins (22))

Table 44.49. Differentiation of the Most Frequently Isolated *Prevotella* spp.

Test	*P. bivia*	*P. corporis*	*P. disiens*	*P. heparinolytica*	*P. intermedia*	*P. loescheii*	*P. melaninogenica*	*P. oralis*	*P. oris*	*P. oulora*
Catalase	−	−	−	−	−	−	−	−	−	+
Hemolysis, 5% SBA	NR	NR	NR	γ	β,γ	β,γ	α,β	β,γ	γ	β
$NO_3 \to NO_2$	−	−	−	−	−	−	−	−	−	−
Bile, 20%[a]	NG	NG	NG	NG	NG	NG	NG	NG	NG	NG
H_2S	NR	−	NR	−	V	NR	−	−	NR	NR
Meat digestion	+	V−	+	−	V+	−	−	−	−	−
Pigmentation[b]	−	−	−	−	+	+	−	−	−	−
Carbohydrates										
Glucose	A	−	A	A	A	A	A	A	A	A
Lactose	A	−	−	A	−	A	A	A	A	A
Arabinose	−	−	−	NR	−	−	−	−	V+	−
Cellobiose	−	−	−	A	−	A	−	A	V+	−
Glycerol	V+	−	−	NR	NR	NR	NR	−	NR	−
Maltose	A	−	A	A	A	A	A	A	A	A
Melibiose	−	−	−	NR	−	V+	V−	A	V	NR
Raffinose	−	−	−	−	V+	A	A	A	A	A
Rhamnose	−	−	−	NR	−	−	−	V+	V+	−
Ribose	−	−	−	NR	−	−	−	V−w	V+	NR
Salicin	−	−	−	A	−	−	−	A	A	−
Sucrose	−	−	−	A	A	A	A	A	A	A
Trehalose	−	−	−	NR	−	−	−	−	−	−
Xylose	−	−	−	A	−	−	−	−	A	−
Misc. tests										
Indole	−	−	−	+	+	−	−	−	−	−
Esculin hydrolysis	−	−	−	+	−	+	V−	+	+	+
Gelatin liquefaction, 22°C	+	+	+	−	+	+	+	+	+w	−
Starch hydrolysis	+	+	+	+	V+	+	+	+	+	−
Urease	−	−	−	−	−	−	−	−	−	−
Isolation from										
Humans	+	+	+	+	+	+	+	+	+	NR
Animals	+	−	−	+	−	−	−	−	−	NR

G, growth; NG, no growth; NR, no results; A, acid production (+); w, weak reaction; V, variable reactions; V+, variable, usually positive; V−, variable, usually negative; SBA, sheep blood agar; α, alpha hemolysis; β, beta hemolysis; γ, gamma (no) hemolysis. Data from references 5 and 14.

[a] Bile concentration 20% or 2% Bacto oxgall (10× concentration bile).

[b] *P. melaninogenica* and *P. bivia* often require prolonged incubation before pigmentation is evident (5).

GENUS: *PROPIONIGENIUM* (14)

Gram-negative, short rods with rounded ends; arranged singly, pairs, and short chains
Nonsporeforming
Anaerobic
Catalase negative
Nonencapsulated
Nonmotile
Oxidase: no results
O/F glucose: F (fermentative)
Optimal growth temperature: 33°C
2 species: *P. maris, P. modestum*

Type species: *P. modestum*: DSM 2376 (not in Bergey's Manual; created by Schink and Pfennig (21))

May be confused with genus *Propionispira*

GENUS: *PSEUDOMONAS* (14)

Gram-negative, straight or slightly curved rods; not helical
Nonsporeforming
Aerobic
Catalase positive
Nonencapsulated
Motility: variable, usually positive; rarely nonmotile; when positive, polar flagella; some species have lateral flagella
Oxidase variable
O/F glucose: O (oxidative)
Lipase positive: **only** *P. aeruginosa*
Optimal growth temperature: 30–37°C
76 species: *P. abietaniphila, P. aeruginosa, P. agarici, P. alcaligenes, P. amygdali, P. anguilliseptica, P. antimicrobica, P. asplenii, P. aurantiaca, P. avellanae, P. azotoformans, P. balearica, P. beijerinckii, P. beteli, P. boreopolis, P. cannabina, P. carboxydohydrogena, P. caricapapayae, P. chloroaphis, P. cichorii, P. cissicola, P. citronellolis, P. corrugata, P. duodoroffii, P. elongata, P. flavescens, P. flectens, P. fluorescens, P. fragi, P. fulva, P. fuscovaginae, P. gelidicola, P. geniculata, P. graminis, P. halophila, P. huttiensis, P. iners, P. jessenii, P. lanceolata, P. lemoignei, P. libanensis, P. lundensis, P. luteola, P. mandelii, P. marginalis, P. mendocina, P. mephitica, P. monteilii, P. mucidolens, P. multiresinivorans, P. nitroreducens, P. oleovorans, P. oryzihabitans, P. pertucinogena, P. pictorum, P. pseudoalcaligenes* subsp. *pseudoalcaligenes, P. putida, P. resinovorans, P. rhodesiae, P. saccharophila, P. savastanol, P. spinosa, P. stanieri, P. straminae, P. stutzeri, P. synxantha, P. syringae, P. syringae* subsp. *syringae, P. syzygii, P. taetrolens, P. tolaasii, P. tremae, P. vancouverensis, P. veronii, P. viridiflava, P. woodsii*

Type species: *P. aeruginosa* ATCC 10145

Table 44.50. Differentiation of the Most Frequently Isolated *Pseudomonas* spp.

Test	*P. aeruginosa*	*P. alcaligenes*	*P. chloroaphis*	*P. cichorii*	*P. fluorescens* biovar I	*P. fluorescens* biovar II	*P. fluorescens* biovar III
Catalase	+	+	+	+	+	+	+
Oxidose	+	+	+	+	+	+	+
NO$_3$→NO$_2$	+	−	NR	NR	+	+	+
No. of flagella	1	1	>1	>1	>1	>1	>1
4°C	NG	NR	G	NG	G	G	G
41°C	G	G	NG	NG	NG	NG	NG
MacConkey (MAC)	G	G	G	G	G	G	G
Carbohydrates							
Glucose	A	−	A	A	A	A	A
Inositol	−	−	A	V	A	A	A
Trehalose	−	−	A	−	A	A	A
Misc. tests							
Arginine dehydrolase	+	+	+	−	+	+	+
Esculin hydrolysis	−	−	−	−	−	−	−
Gelatin liquefaction, 22°C	+	V	+	−	+	+	+
Lysine decorboxylase	−	−	−	−	−	−	−
Lecithinase	−	−	V	+	+	+w	+
Lipase	+	−	−	−	−	−	−
Starch hydrolysis	−	−	−	−	−	−	−

G, growth; NG, no growth; NR, no results; A, acid production (+); V, variable reactions; w, weak reaction.
Data from reference 14.
^aLateral flagella of short wavelength may be produced under certain conditions.

(continued)

GENUS: *PSYCHROBACTER* (14)

Gram-negative, **cocci,** coccobacilli, oval-shaped rods; vary in length; short and relatively long rods may be swollen

Nonsporeforming

Facultative anaerobic

Catalase positive

Nonencapsulated

Nonmotile

Oxidase positive

O/F glucose: O (oxidative) or inert (−)

Optimal growth temperature: 35–37°C; most strains are psychrotrophic, able to grow 5–20°C and usually **no growth** at 35–37°C. Strains that can grow at 35–37°C usually cannot grow at 5°C; these strains are isolated from humans and animals.

5 species: *P. frigidicola, P. glacincola, P. immobilis, P. phenylpyruvicus, P. urativorans*

Type species: *P. immobilis* ATCC 43116 (not in *Bergey's Manual*; created by Juni and Heym (15))

	P. fuorescens biovar IV	P. fluorescens biovar V	P. gelidicola	P. mendocina	P. pseudoalcaligenes subsp. pseudoalcaligenes	P. putida biovar A	P. putida biovar B	P. saccharophila	P. stutzeri	P. syringae	P. varidiflava
	+	+	+	+	+	+	+	+	+	+	+
	+	+	+	+	+	+	+	+	+	−	−
	+	+	NR	+	+	V	V	NR	+	NR	NR
	>1	>1	>1	1[a]	>	>1	>1	1	1	>1[a]	1–2
	G	V	NG	NR	NR	V	G	NR	NR	V	NR
	NG	NG	G	G	G	NG	NG	NG	V	NG	NG
	G	G	G	G	G	G	G	G	G	G	G
	A	A	A	A	−	A	A	A	A	A	A
	A	A	A	−	−	−	−	−	−	V	A
	A	A	A	−	−	−	−	A	−	−	−
	+	+	−	+	V	+	+	−	−	−	−
	−	−	−	−	−	−	−	−	−	−	−
	+	+	+	−	V	−	−	+	−	V	+
	−	−	−	−	−	−	−	−	−	−	−
	+	V	+	−	NR	−	−	NR	−	V	V
	−	−	−	−	−	−	−	−	−	−	−
	−	−	−	−	−	−	−	+	+	−	−

Table 44.51. Biochemical Characteristics of *Psychrobacter immobilis*

Catalase	+	Glucose	A
Oxidase	+	Fructose	−
$NO_3 \rightarrow NO_2$	V	Mannitol	−
MacConkey (MAC)	G[a]	Sucrose	−
Esculin hydrolysis	−	Xylose	A
Phenylalanine	+		
Tryptophan	+		
Tween 80	+		
Urease	+		

A, acid production (+); G, growth; V, variable reactions.
Data from references 14 and 29.
[a]Poor growth; best growth at 20–25°C.

GENUS: *RALSTONIA* (14)

Gram-negative, slender, straight rods
Nonsporeforming
Aerobic
Catalase: no results
Nonencapsulated
Motile
Oxidase positive
O/F glucose: O (oxidative)
Optimal growth temperature: 30–37°C
5 species: *R. eutropha, R. gilardii, R. paucula, R. pickettii, R. solanacearum*
Type species: *R. pickettii* ATCC 27511

Table 44.52. Differentiation of the Three Biovars of *Ralstonia pickettii* (5)

Test	R. pickettii		
	Biovar 1	Biovar 2	Biovar 3
Oxidase	+	+	+
Motility	+	+	+
42°C	V	G	V
NO$_3$→NO$_2$	+	+	V
Arginine dehydrolase	−	−	−
Lysine decarboyxlase	−	−	−
Urease	+	+	+
Glucose	A	A	A
Lactose	A	−	A
Mannitol	−	−	A

A, acid production (+); V, variable reactions.
Data from reference 14.

(*continued*)

GENUS: *ROSEOMONAS* (5, 26)

Gram-negative, plump and short straight rods or coccobacilli arranged singly, in pairs, or in short chains
Nonsporeforming
Aerobic
Catalase positive
Nonencapsulated
Motility variable; single polar flagellum
Oxidase variable, usually positive; may be delayed (26)
O/F glucose: O (oxidative) or inert (−)
Optimal growth temperature: 25–37°C
3 species: *R. cervicalis, R. fauriae, R. gilardii*
Type species: *R. gilardii* ATCC 49956
Pink-pigmented colonies

Table 44.53. Differentiation of *Roseomonas* spp. and Genomospecies

Test	*R. cervicalis*	*R. gilardii*	*R. fauriae*	Genomospecies 4	Genomospecies 5	Genomospecies 6
Catalase	+	+	+	+	+	+
Oxidase	+	V	+	+	+	+
NO$_3$→NO$_2$	−	−	+	+	−	+
42°C	G	G	G	G	G	G
MacConkey (MAC)	G	G	G	G	G	G^w
H$_2$S						
TSI	−	−	−	−	−	−
PbAc	+	+	+	+	+	+
Motility	+	+	+	V	−	+
Carbohydrates						
Glucose	−	V	V	−	−	−
Lactose	−	−	−	−	−	−
Maltose	−	−	−	−	−	−
Mannitol	−	V	V	−	−	−
Sucrose	−	−	−	−	−	−
Xylose	V	V^a	V	A	V	−
Misc. tests						
Indole	−	−	−	−	−	−
Esculin hydrolysis	−	−	+	−	−	+
Citrate (Christensen's)	V^{+a}	+	+	V$^+$	+	+
Starch	+	+	+	+	+	+
Gelatin liquefaction, 22°C	−	−	−	−	−	−
Urease	V^{+a}	V^{+a}	+	V$^+$	+	+
Vancomycin 30 μg	R	R	R	R	R	R

G, growth; A, acid production (+); PbAc, lead acetate; V, variable reactions; R, resistant; w, weak reaction.
Data from reference 29.
[a]Delayed.

GENUS: *SELENOMONAS* (14)

Gram-negative, curved, usually crescent-shaped rods with ends often tapered; arranged singly, in pairs, or in short chains

Nonsporeforming

Strict (obligate) anaerobic

Catalase: negative

Nonencapsulated

Motile: tumbling because of up to 16 flagella arranged in a tuft or short line near center of concave side of cell

Oxidase negative

O/F glucose: F (fermentative)

Optimal growth temperature: 35–40°C; maximum 45°C; minimum 20–30°C

11 species: *S. acidaminovorans, S. artemidis, S. dianae, S. flueggei, S. infelix, S. lacticifex, S. lipolytica, S. noxia, S. ruminantium* subsp. *lactilytica, S. ruminantium* subsp. *ruminantium, S. sputigena*

Type species: *S. sputigena* ATCC 35185

Table 44.54. Differentiation of the Most Frequently Isolated *Selenomonas* spp.

Test	S. acidaminovorans	S. artemidis	S. dianae	S. flueggei	S. infelix	S. lacticifex	S. noxia	S. ruminatum[a]	S. sputigena[a]
Bile 20%	G	−	−	−	−	NR	NG	G	NG
H$_2$S	NR	−	−	−	−	NR	−	+	−
Esculin hydrolysis	−	−	+	−	+	NR	−	+	−
Gelatin liquefaction, 22°C	+	−	−	−	−	NR	−	−	−
Carbohydrates									
Glucose	NR	A	A	A	A	NR	V$^-$	A	A
Lactose	−	−	V$^+$	A	A	−	−	A	A
Arabinose	−	−	−	−	−	A	−	A	−
Cellobiose	−	−	−	−	−	V$^-$	−	A	−
Dulcitol	NR	−	−	−	−	−	−	A	−
Mannitol	−	V$^+$	A	A	A	−	−	A	−
Mannose	−	A	A	A	A	A	−	A	−
Melibiose	NR	V$^+$	V$^+$	A	A	A	−	A	A
Raffinose	NR	−	V$^+$	A	A	NR	−	NR	A
Salicin	−	−	−	−	−	V$^+$	−	A	−
Sorbitol	−	V$^-$	−	A	V$^+$	−	−	A	−
Sucrose	−	A	A	A	A	A	−	A	A
Trehalose	−	−	A	−	−	−	−	V$^+$	−
Xyloase	NR	−	−	−	−	A	−	NR	−

A, acid production (+); V, variable reactions; V$^+$, variable, usually positive; V$^-$, variable, usually negative; G, growth; NG, no growth; NR, no results; Bile 20%, bile concentration 20% or 2% Bacto oxgall (10× concentration bile).

Data from reference 14.

[a]

	S. ruminatum	S. sputigena
H$_2$S (Cystine)	−	+
NO$_3$→NO$_2$	+	V

GENUS: *SHEWANELLA* (14)

Gram-negative, short, long, or filamentous rods
Nonsporeforming
Aerobic
Catalase positive
Nonencapsulated
Motile; single polar flagellum
Oxidase positive
O/F glucose: O (oxidative)
Optimal growth temperature: 25–35°C
12 species: *S. algae, S. amazonensis, S. baltica, S. benthica, S. colwelliana, S. frigidimarina, S. gelidimarina, S. hanedai, S. oneidensis, S. putrefaciens, S. violacea, S. woodyi*
Type species: *S. putrefaciens* ATCC 8071, NCIB 10471

Table 44.55. Biochemical Characteristics of the Genus *Shewanella*

Catalase	+	Citrate	−
Oxidase	+	DNase	+
MacConkey (MAC)	G	Ornithine decarboxylase	+
NO$_3$→NO$_2$	+	Esculin hydrolysis	−
H$_2$S (TSI)	+	Urease	−

G, growth.

GENUS: *SPHINGOMONAS* (5, 26)

Gram-negative, medium to long rods
Nonsporeforming
Aerobic
Catalase positive
Nonencapsulated
Motile; single polar flagellum; may be slow
Oxidase variable, usually positive
O/F glucose: O (oxidative)
Optimal growth temperature: 25–35°C
23 species: *S. adhaesiva, S. aromaticivorans, S. asaccharolytica, S. capsulata, S. chlorophenolica, S. eichinoides, S. herbicidovorans, S. macrogoltabidus, S. mali, S. natatoria, S. parapaucimobilis, S. paucimobilis, S. pruni, S. rosa, S. sanguis, S. stygia, S. subarctica, S. suberifaciens, S. subterranea, S. terrae, S. trueperi, S. ursincola, S. yanoikuyae*
Type species: *S. paucimobilis* ATCC 29837, NCTC 11030

Table 44.56. Differentiation of the Two Frequently Isolated *Sphingomonas* spp.

Test	*S. parapaucimobilis*	*S. paucimobilis*
Catalase	+	+
Oxidase	+w	V
Motility	+	+
MacConkey (MAC)	NG	NG
$NO_3 \to NO_2$	−	−
H_2S		
TSI	−	+w
PbAC	−	+
Indole	−	−
Citrate	−	−
Gelatin liquefaction, 22°C	−	−
Esculin hydrolysis	+w	−
Urease	−	−

NG, no growth; V, variable reactions; w, weak reaction.
Data from reference 29.

GENUS: *STENOTROPHOMONAS* (5, 26)

Gram-negative, short to medium-sized, straight rods
Nonsporeforming
Aerobic
Catalase: no results
Nonencapsulated
Motile: polar tuft flagella
Oxidase negative
O/F glucose: O (oxidative)
Optimal growth temperature: 35–37°C
2 species: *S. africana, S. maltophilia*
Type species: *S. maltophilia* ATCC 13637, NCIB 920
Third most-frequently isolated **nonfermenting Gram-negative rods in clinical laboratories** (26)
Most strains require methionine for growth (or cystine plus glycine).

Table 44.57. Biochemical Characteristics of *Stenotrophomonas maltophilia*

Oxidase	−	Arginine dehydrolase	−
$NO_3 \rightarrow NO_2$	V	Lysine decarboxylase	+
MacConkey (MAC)	G	DNase	+
Gelatin liquefaction, 22°C	+	Tween 80	+
Esculin hydrolysis	V+	ONPG	+
		Glucose	A
		Maltose	A[a]

V, variable reactions; V+, variable, usually positive; G, growth; A, acid production (+).
[a]Rapid.

GENUS: *STREPTOBACILLUS* (5, 14, 26)

Gram-negative rods with rounded or pointed ends; arranged singly, in long wavy chains, or in filaments; **may be highly pleomorphic.** Single rods may show central swellings. Chains or filaments may have a series of swellings giving a "**string-of-pearls**" appearance.

Nonsporeforming
Facultative anaerobic
Catalase negative
Nonencapsulated
Nonmotile
Oxidase negative
O/F glucose: F (fermentative)
Optimal growth temperature: 35–37°C
Single species: *S. moniliformis* ATCC 14647
20% serum, ascitic fluid, or blood required for both isolation and biochemical tests incubation under CO_2
Causative agent of one form of ratbite fever in humans and Haverhill fever

Table 44.58. Biochemical Characteristics of *Streptobacillus moniliformis*

Catalase	−	Glucose	A[a]
Oxidase	−	Lactose	−
Motility	−	Maltose	A[a]
$NO_3 \rightarrow NO_2$	−	Mannitol	−
MacConkey (MAC)	NG	Sucrose	−
H_2S		Xylose	−
TSI	−		
PbAc	+		
Indole	−		
Citrate	−		
Gelatin liquefaction, 22°C	−		
Lysine decarboxylase	−		
Urease	−		

A, acid production (+); PbAc, lead acetate strips.
[a]Delayed.

GENUS: *SUCCINIMONAS* (14)

Gram-negative, short, straight rods with rounded ends; at times coccobacilli
Nonsporeforming
Strict (obligate) anaerobe
Catalase negative
Nonencapsulated
Motile: single polar flagellum

Oxidase negative
O/F glucose: F (fermentative)
Optimal growth temperature: 30–37°C; no growth 22°C or at 45°C
Single species: *S. amylolytica* ATCC 19206, ATCC 29987

Table 44.59. Biochemical Characteristics of *Succinimonas amylolytica*

Catalase	−	Oxidase	−
H_2S	−	Indole	−
$NO_3 \rightarrow NO_2$	−	Gelatin liquefaction, 22°C	−
Motility[a]	+	Voges-Proskauer (VP)	V
Pigmented colonies[b]	+		

V, variable reactions.
Data from reference 16.
[a]Slow and progressive; may be lost on exposure to air.
[b]Light tan.

GENUS: *SUCCINIVIBRIO* (14)
Gram-negative, curved or helical rods with pointed ends
Nonsporeforming
Strict (obligate) anaerobic
Catalase negative
Nonencapsulated
Motile: single polar flagellum; vibrating motility (16)
Oxidase negative
O/F glucose: F (fermentative)
Optimal growth temperature: 30–39°C; no growth at 22°C and 45°C (16)
Single species: *S. dextrinosolvens* ATCC 19716
Resembles *Anaerobiospirillum succiniciproducens,* but *Succinivibrio* lacks tufts of flagella at each pole

Table 44.60. Biochemical Characteristics of *Succinivibrio dextrinosolvens*

Catalase	−	Oxidase	−
$NO_3 \rightarrow NO_2$	−	Indole	−
H_2S	−	Gelatin liquefaction, 22°C	−
Pigmented colonies[a]	+	Voges-Proskauer (VP)	−
Motility[b]	+		

[a]Light tan.
[b]Slow and progressive; may be lost on exposure to air.

GENUS: *SUTTONELLA* (5, 29)
Gram-negative, small, plump rods that may stain irregularly
Nonsporeforming
Facultative anaerobic
Catalase negative
Nonencapsulated
Nonmotile
Oxidase positive
O/F glucose: F (fermentative)
Optimal growth temperature: 30–35°C
Single species: *S. indologenes* ATCC 25869

Table 44.61. Biochemical Characteristics of *Suttonella indologenes*

		Misc. tests	
Catalase	−	Indole	+
Oxidase	+	Citrate	−
MacConkey (MAC)	NG	Esculin hydrolysis	−
$NO_3 \to NO_2$	−	Casein hydrolysis	+
H_2S		Alkaline phosphatase	−
TSI	−	Tween 40	−
PbAc	+	Gelatin liquefaction, 22°	−
Carbohydrates		Arginine dehydrolase	−
Glucose	A	Lysine decarboxylase	−
Lactose	−	Ornithine decarboxylase	−
Malose	A[a]	Urease	−
Mannitol	−		
Sucrose	A		
Xylose	−		

NG, no growth; A, acid production (+); PbAc, lead acetate.
[a]Delayed.

GENUS: *TAYLORELLA* (14)

Gram-negative, small rods approaching spherical shape (cocci); occasional filaments
Nonsporeforming
Microaerophilic
Catalase positive
Nonencapsulated
Nonmotile
Oxidase positive
O/F glucose: O (oxidative)
Optimal growth temperature: 25–35°C
Single species: *T. equigenitalis* NCTC 11184 (not in *Bergey's Manual*; created by Sugimoto et al. (28))
Pathogenic for horses (mares)

Table 44.62. Biochemical Characteristics of *Taylorella equigenitalis*

Catalase	+	Gelatin liquefaction, 22°C	−
Oxidase	+	Arginine dehydrolase	−
MacConkey (MAC)	G	Lysine decarboxylase	−
$NO_3 \to NO_2$	−	Ornithine decarboxylase	−
Motility	−	Phosphatase	+
Indole	−	Urease	−
H_2S	−		
DNase	−		

G, growth.
Data from references 14 and 29.

GENUS: *TISSIERELLA* (14)

Gram-negative rods with rounded or pointed ends; at times coccobacilli and filaments
Nonsporeforming
Anaerobic
Catalase negative
Nonencapsulated
Motile: peritrichous flagella
Oxidase: no results
O/F glucose: F, weak (fermentative) or O (oxidative)

3 species: *T. creatinini, T. creatinophila, T. praeacuta*
Type species: *T. praeacuta* ATCC 25539, NCTC 11158 (not in *Bergey's Manual*; created by Collins and Shah (2))

GENUS: *UREAPLASMA* (14, 16)

Gram negative, round or coccobacillary; **variety of pleomorphic forms depending on age of culture**
Nonsporeforming
Microaerophilic
Catalase negative
Nonencapsulated
Nonmotile
Oxidase: no results
O/F glucose: no results
Optimal growth temperature: 37°C; growth at 22°C; no growth 42°C
Urease positive
Lipase positive: **only** *U. urealyticum*
6 species: *U. canigenitalium, U. cati, U. diversum* (human), *U. felinum, U. gallorale* (human), *U. urealyticum*
Type species: *U. urealyticum* ATCC 27618
Require special cultural conditions for membrane function and growth
In a group of bacteria called mycoplasma (mollicutes); smallest known free-living forms; have no cell wall (5), just cell membrane (26)
No direct method for identification in clinical specimens; PCR best method (5)

GENUS: *VEILLONELLA* (14)

Gram-negative, tiny **cocci** arranged as diplococci (kidney bean shape), masses, and short chains
Nonsporeforming
Anaerobic
Catalase variable: some strains produce an atypical (pseudocatalase, nonheme) catalase reaction lacking porphyrin
Nonencapsulated
Nonmotile
Oxidase negative
O/F glucose: F (fermentative)
Optimal growth temperature: 30–37°C
7 species: *V. atypica, V. caviae, V. criceti, V. dispar, V. parvula, V. ratti, V. rodentium*
Type species: *V. parvula* ATCC 10790

Table 44.63. Differentiation of *Veillonella* spp.

Test	*V. atypica*	*V. caviae*	*V. criceti*	*V. dispar*	*V. parvula*	*V. ratti*	*V. rodentium*
Catalase	−	−	+	+	−	+	−
Motility	−	−	−	−	−	−	−
NO$_3$→NO$_2$	+	+	+	+	+	+	+
Urease	−	−	−	−	−	−	−
Fructose	−	−	A	−	−	−	−

A, acid production (+).
Data from reference 14.

GENUS: *VIBRIO* (14, 26)

Gram-negative, straight or curved rods
Nonsporeforming
Facultative anaerobic
Catalase positive
Nonencapsulated
Motile: variable, usually positive; 1 or more polar flagella enclosed in sheath continuous with outer membrane of cell wall. Some strains produce multiple lateral flagella when grown on solid media (26).
Oxidase positive except *V. gazogenes* and *V. metschnikovii*
O/F glucose: F (fermentative) and O (oxidative)
Optimal growth temperature: all species 20°C; some growth at 30°C
Nitrate reduction positive except *V. metschnikovii*
39 species: *V. aestuarianus, V. alginolyticus, V. campbellii, V. carchariae, V. cholerae, V. cincinnatiensis, V. diabolicus, V. diazotrophicus, V. fischeri, V. fluvialis, V. furnissii, V. gazogenes, V. halioticoli, V. harveyi, V. hollisae, V. ichthyoenteri, V. logei, V. mediterranei, V. metschnikovii, V. mimicus, V. mytili, V. natriegens, V. navarrensis, V. nereis, V. nigripulchritudo, V. ordalii, V. orientalis, V. parahaemolyticus, V. pectenicida, V. penaeicida, V. proteolyticus, V. rumoiensis, V. salmonicida, V. scophthalmi, V. splendidus, V. tapetis, V. trachuri, V. tubiashii, V. vulnificus*
Type species: *Vibrio cholerae* ATCC 14035
Sodium ions (Na$^+$) stimulate growth of all species and are required by most.
Oxidase test **must** be performed on 5% sheep blood or any other media **without** fermentable sugars (e.g., MacConkey). If sugar is fermented, an acid condition exists, and a false-negative oxidase result may occur if pH is below 5.1 (26).
Suspected *V. cholerae* should be collected and transported in Cary-Blair medium; buffered glycerol saline is not acceptable because glycerol is toxic for vibrios (26).
V. cholerae causative agent of cholera.
V. vulnificus causative agent of a highly fatal septicemia.

Table 44.64. Differentiation of the Most Frequently Isolated *Vibrio* spp.

Test	*V. alginolyticus*	*V. cholerae*	*V. cincinnatiensis*	*V. fluvialis*	*V. furnissii*	*V. harveyi*	*V. hollisae*	*V. metschnikovii*	*V. mimicus*	*V. parahaemolyticus*	*V. vulnificus*
Catalase	+	+	+	+	+	+	+	+	+	+	+
Oxidase	+	+	+	+	+	+	+	−	+	+	+
MacConkey (MAC)	G	G	G	G	G	G	G	G	G	G	G
NO$_3$→NO$_2$[a]	+	+	+	+	+	−	+	−	+	+	+
Yellow pigmentation, 25°C	−	−	−	−	−	−	−	−	−	−	−
Swarming	+	−	−	−	−	V+	−	−	−	V+	−
H$_2$S	−	−	−	−	−	−	−	−	−	−	−
Motility	+	+	+	V	V+	−	−	V	+	+	+
Carbohydrates											
Glucose	A	A	A	A	A	A	A	A	A	A	A
Lactose	−	−	−	−	−	−	−	V	V−	−	V+
Adonitol	−	−	−	−	−	−	−	−	−	−	−
Arabinose	−	−	A	A	A	−	A	−	−	V+	−
Cellobiose	−	−	A	V	V	V	−	−	−	−	−
Dulcitol	−	−	−	−	−	−	−	−	−	−	−
Erythritol	−	−	−	−	−	−	−	−	−	−	−
Galactose	V−	A	A	A	A	−	A	V	V+	A	A
Glycerol	V+	V	+	−	V	−	−	A	V	V	−
Inositol	−	−	A	−	−	−	−	V	−	−	−
Maltose	A	A	A	A	A	A	−	A	A	A	A
Mannitol	A	A	A	A	A	A	−	A	A	A	V
Mannose	A	V+	A	A	A	V	A	A	A	A	A
Melibiose	−	−	−	−	V−	−	−	−	−	−	V
Raffinose	−	−	−	−	V	−	−	−	−	−	−
Rhamnose	−	−	−	−	V	−	−	−	−	−	−
Salicin	−	−	A	−	−	−	−	−	−	−	A
Sorbitol	−	−	−	−	−	−	−	V	−	−	−
Sucrose	A	A	A	A	A	V	−	A	−	−	V−
Trehalose	A	A	A	A	A	V	−	A	A	A	A
Xylose	−	−	A	−	−	−	−	−	−	−	−
Misc. tests											
Indole[a]	V+	+	−	V−	V−	+	+	V−	+	+	+
Citrate (Simmons)	−	+	V	+	+	−	−	V	+	−	V
Esculin hydrolysis[a]	−	−	−	−	−	−	−	V	−	−	V
DNase, 25°C	+	+	V+	+	+	−	−	V	V	+	V
Arginine dehydrolase[a]	−	−	−	−	−	−	−	V	−	−	−
Lysine decarboxylase[a]	+	+	+	−	−	+	−	V	+	+	+
Ornithine decarboxylase[a]	V	+	−	−	−	−	−	−	+	+	V
Phenylalanine deaminase	−	−	−	−	−	NG	−	−	−	−	V
Gelatin liquefaction, 22°C[a]	+	+	−	V+	V+	−	−	V	V	+	V
KCN	V−	NG	NG	V	V+	NG	NG	NG	NG	V−	NG
Lipase	V+	+	V	+	V+	−	−	+	V−	+	+
Malonate	−	−	−	−	V−	−	−	−	−	−	−
ONPG	−	+	V+	V	V	−	−	V	+	−	V
Tartrate	+	V+	+	V	V−	V	V	V	V−	+	V

(*continued*)

Table 44.64. Differentiation of the Most Frequently Isolated *Vibrio* spp. (*continued*)

Test	V. alginolyticus	V. cholerae	V. cincinnatiensis	V. fluvialis	V. furnissii	V. harveyi	V. hollisae	V. metschnikovii	V. mimicus	V. parahaemolyticus	V. vulnificus
Methyl red (MR)	V	+	+	+	+	+	−	+	+	V+	V+
Voges-Proskauer (VP)	+	V	−	−	−	V	−	+	−	−	−
Urease	−	−	−	−	−	−	−	−	−	V−	−
Sensitivities											
0/129	V−	Sb	V−	V	−	S	V	S	S	V−	S
Polymyxin B	V	V−	S	S	V+	S	S	S	V+	V	−

V, variable reactions; V+, variable, usually positive, V−, variable, usually negative; G, growth; NG, no growth; A, acid production (+); 0/129, vibriostatic agent, 2,4-diamino-6,7-diisopropyl-pteridine; S, sensitive (susceptible); R, resistant.
Data from reference 14.
aNaCl, 1% added to these media.
bSome *V. cholerae* 01 strains are resistant to 0/129 (5).

GENUS: *WEEKSELLA* (14)

Gram-negative rods with parallel sides and rounded ends
Nonsporeforming
Aerobic
Catalase positive
Nonencapsulated
Nonmotile
Oxidase positive
O/F glucose: inert (−)
Optimal growth temperature: 18–42°C
Single species: *W. virosa* NCTC 11634 (not in *Bergey's Manual;* created by Holmes et al. (12))
Colonies are butyrous, mucoid, and adherent, with tan to brown pigmentation.

Table 44.65. Differentiation of *Weeksella virosa*

Test	W. virosa
Catalase	+
Oxidase	+
MacConkey (MAC)	NG
42°C	V
NO₃→NO₂	−
Indole	+w
DNase	−
Esculin hydrolysis	−
Gelatin liquefaction, 22°C	+
Arginine dehydrolase	−
ONPG	−
Starch hydrolysis	−
Urease	−
Polymyxin B	S

NG, no growth; NR, no results; V, variable reactions; S, sensitive (susceptible); R, resistant; w, weak reaction.
Data from references 5, 14 and 26.

GENUS: *WOLINELLA* (14, 16)

Gram-negative, helical, curved, or straight rods with rounded or tapered ends
Nonsporeforming
Microaerophilic; growth anaerobically
Catalase negative
Nonencapsulated
Motile: rapid darting, single polar flagellum
Oxidase positive
O/F glucose: inert (−)
Optimal growth temperature: 37°C
Single species: *W. succinogenes* ATCC 29543
Although not an anaerobe, isolation methods are used for strict anaerobiosis (14).

Table 44.66. Biochemical Characteristics of *Wolinella succinogenes*

Catalase	−	MacConkey (MAC)	NG
Oxidase	+	Arginine dehydrolase	−
Motility	+	Lysine decarboxylase	−
$NO_3 \rightarrow NO_2$	+	Ornithine decarboxylase	−
H_2S (TSI/SIM)	+	Urease	−
		Hippurate hydrolysis	−

NG, no growth.
Data from reference 16.

GENUS: *XANTHOBACTER* (14)

Gram-negative or Gram-variable rods and cocci; some **pleomorphic**; cell wall Gram-negative type
Nonsporeforming
Obligate (strict) aerobe
Catalase positive
Nonencapsulated
Motility: variable; peritrichous flagella
Oxidase positive
O/F glucose: O (oxidative)
Optimal temperature: 25–30°C
Not acid-fast
4 species: *X. agilis, X. autotrophicus, X. flavus, X. tagetidis*
Type species: *X. autotrophicus* ATCC 35674

Table 44.67. Biochemical Characteristics of the Genus *Xanthobacter*

H_2S	−	Gelatin liquefaction, 22°C	−
$NO_3 \rightarrow NO_2$	+	Starch hydrolysis	−
Litmus milk	Alk	Phosphatase	+
Indole	−	Voges-Proskauer (VP)	−
Lecithinase	−	Urease	V
		Tween 20	−

V, variable reactions; Alk, alkaline.
Data from reference 16.

GENUS: *XANTHOMONAS* (14)

Gram-negative straight rods; mainly single
Nonsporeforming
Strict (obligate) aerobic
Catalase positive
Nonencapsulated
Motile: single polar flagellum
Oxidase negative or weakly positive
O/F glucose: F (fermentative)
Optimal growth temperature: 25–30°C
22 species: *X. albilineans, X. arboricola, X. axonopodis, X. bromi, X. campestris, X. cassavae, X. citri, X. codiaei, X. cucurbitae, X. fragariae, X. hortorum, X. hyacinthi, X. melonis, X. oryzae, X. phaseoli, X. pisi, X. populi, X. saccari, X. theicola, X. translucens, X. vasicola, X. vesicatoria,*
Type species: *X. campestris* ATCC 33913
Colonies are **yellow**, smooth, butyrous, and viscid.

Table 44.68. Differentiation of the Most Frequently Isolated *Xanthomonas* spp.

Test	*X. albilineans*	*X. axonopodis*	*X. campestris*	*X. citri*	*X. fragariae*	*X. phaseoli*	*X. populi*
Catalase	+	+	+	+	+	+	–
Oxidase							
NO$_3$→NO$_2$	–	–	–	–	–	NR	–
Maximum growth temperature, °C	37	35–37	35–39	38	33	38	27.5
MacConkey (MAC)	G	G	G	G	G	G	G
Maximum NaCl tolerance, %	0.5	1.0	2–5	NR	0.5–1.0	NR	0.4–0.6
H$_2$S from peptone	–	+	+	NR	–	NR	–
Motility	+	+	+	+	+	+	+
Carbohydrates							
Glucose	A	NR	A	NR	A	NR	–
Arabinose	–	–	A	NR	–	NR	–
Cellobiose	–	–	A	NR	–	NR	–
Fructose	–	–	A	NR	A	NR	A
Galactose	V	–	A	NR	–	NR	A
Mannose	A	–	A	NR	A	NR	A
Trehalose	–	A	A	NR	–	NR	A
Misc. tests							
Esculin hydrolysis	+	+	+	NR	–	NR	NR
Lysine decarboxylase	–	–	–	NR	–	NR	–
Starch hydrolysis	–	+	V	NR	–	+	+[a]

V, variable reactions; A, acid production (+); NR, no results; G, growth.
Data from reference 14.
[a]Slow.

WARNING

When using the identification tables be aware that the results noted have been compiled from the references cited. However, living microorganisms often give conflicting results because of mutation or the type of media used for isolation, cultivation, identification, and maintenance.

Often proper identification to genus or genus and species requires considering (*a*) the clinical specimen/source, (*b*) Gram stain morphology, and (*c*) cultural characteristics (e.g., pigmentation, hemolysis) along with biochemical tests. In some cases, serologic and toxin testing are required for confirmation.

Be flexible when interpreting biochemical results. All microorganisms do not necessarily exhibit all the results of the battery of biochemical tests in the tables. At times "best fit" is necessary for identification. The more test results, the better the chance of correct identification.

Diagram 44.1.

Initial differentiation of Gram-negative, **aerobic to facultative anaerobic rods (bacilli)**

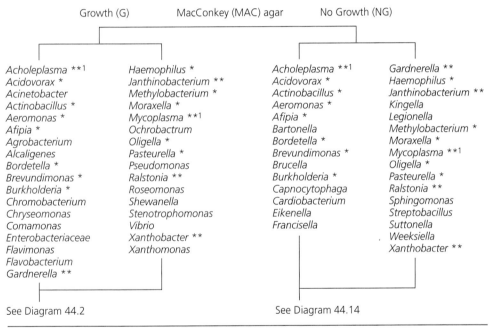

*Variable reactions.

**No results, treated as variable.

[1] *Acholeplasma* and *Mycoplasma* species have **no cell wall,** only a plasma membrane. Colonies exhibit a typical "fried-egg" appearance; however, both require cholesterol or related steroids for growth. **Not identified by conventional biochemical tests;** differentiation of many species by serological determinations. See Table 44.3.

706 Biochemical Tests for Identification of Medical Bacteria

Diagram 44.2.

Differentiation of Gram-negative, **aerobic to facultative anaerobic rods (bacilli)** that **grow on MacConkey (MAC)**

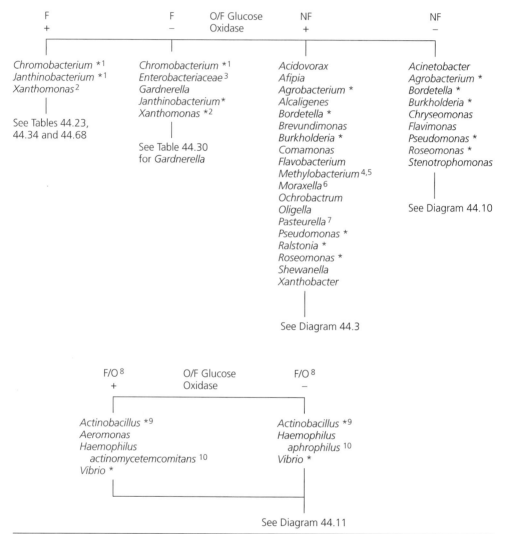

F +	F −	O/F Glucose Oxidase	NF +	NF −

F +
- *Chromobacterium* *[1]
- *Janthinobacterium* *[1]
- *Xanthomonas* [2]

See Tables 44.23, 44.34 and 44.68

F −
- *Chromobacterium* *[1]
- Enterobacteriaceae [3]
- *Gardnerella*
- *Janthinobacterium**
- *Xanthomonas* *[2]

See Table 44.30 for *Gardnerella*

O/F Glucose Oxidase NF +
- *Acidovorax*
- *Afipia*
- *Agrobacterium* *
- *Alcaligenes*
- *Bordetella* *
- *Brevundimonas*
- *Burkholderia* *
- *Comamonas*
- *Flavobacterium*
- *Methylobacterium* [4,5]
- *Moraxella* [6]
- *Ochrobactrum*
- *Oligella*
- *Pasteurella* [7]
- *Pseudomonas* *
- *Ralstonia* *
- *Roseomonas* *
- *Shewanella*
- *Xanthobacter*

See Diagram 44.3

NF −
- *Acinetobacter*
- *Agrobacterium* *
- *Bordetella* *
- *Burkholderia* *
- *Chryseomonas*
- *Flavimonas*
- *Pseudomonas* *
- *Roseomonas* *
- *Stenotrophomonas*

See Diagram 44.10

F/O [8] +
- *Actinobacillus* *[9]
- *Aeromonas*
- *Haemophilus actinomycetemcomitans* [10]
- *Vibrio* *

O/F Glucose Oxidase

F/O [8] −
- *Actinobacillus* *[9]
- *Haemophilus aphrophilus* [10]
- *Vibrio* *

See Diagram 44.11

---

*Variable results.
[1]*Chrombaterium violaceum* and *Janthinobacterium lividum* exhibit violet-pigmented colonies and a violet ring in liquid media.
[2]*Xanthomas* species exhibit yellow, smooth, butyrous, and viscid colonies.
[3]See Chapter 45.
[4]*Methylobacterium* species exhibit pink-pigmented colonies.
[5]Positive oxidase may be delayed or weak.
[6]O/F inert or **no growth.**
[7]Rarely oxidase negative with Kovacs.
[8]Both fermentative and oxidative (respiratory).
[9]*Actinobacillus* fastidious; requires serum added to basal fermentation medium to enhance growth (29).
[10]*Haemophilus actinomycetemcomitans* and *H. aphrophilus* **do not** require either X or V factors for growth; only two *Haemophilus* species to grow on MacConkey (MAC).

Diagram 44.3.

Differentiation of Gram-negative, **aerobic to facultative anaerobic rods** (bacilli) that are
> Mac-G
> Glucose-NF
> Oxidase-Pos

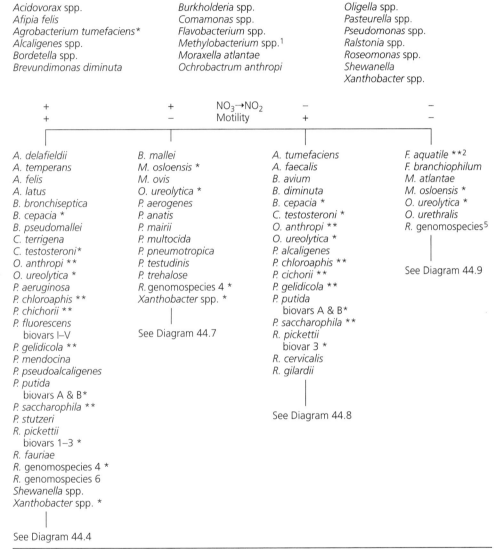

Acidovorax spp.
Afipia felis
Agrobacterium tumefaciens*
Alcaligenes spp.
Bordetella spp.
Brevundimonas diminuta

Burkholderia spp.
Comamonas spp.
Flavobacterium spp.
Methylobacterium spp.[1]
Moraxella atlantae
Ochrobactrum anthropi

Oligella spp.
Pasteurella spp.
Pseudomonas spp.
Ralstonia spp.
Roseomonas spp.
Shewanella spp.
Xanthobacter spp.

		NO$_3$→NO$_2$		
+	+	Motility	−	−
+	−		+	

A. delafieldii	*B. mallei*	*A. tumefaciens*	*F. aquatile* **[2]
A. temperans	*M. osloensis* *	*A. faecalis*	*F. branchiophilum*
A. felis	*M. ovis*	*B. avium*	*M. atlantae*
A. latus	*O. ureolytica* *	*B. diminuta*	*M. osloensis* *
B. bronchiseptica	*P. aerogenes*	*B. cepacia* *	*O. ureolytica* *
B. cepacia *	*P. anatis*	*C. testosteroni* *	*O. urethralis*
B. pseudomallei	*P. mairii*	*O. anthropi* **	*R. genomospecies*[5]
C. terrigena	*P. multocida*	*O. ureolytica* *	
C. testosteroni*	*P. pneumotropica*	*P. alcaligenes*	See Diagram 44.9
O. anthropi **	*P. testudinis*	*P. chloroaphis* **	
O. ureolytica *	*P. trehalose*	*P. cichorii* **	
P. aeruginosa	*R. genomospecies 4* *	*P. gelidicola* **	
P. chloroaphis **	*Xanthobacter* spp. *	*P. putida*	
P. chichorii **		biovars A & B*	
P. fluorescens	See Diagram 44.7	*P. saccharophila* **	
biovars I–V		*R. pickettii*	
P. gelidicola **		biovar 3 *	
P. mendocina		*R. cervicalis*	
P. pseudoalcaligenes		*R. gilardii*	
P. putida			
biovars A & B*		See Diagram 44.8	
P. saccharophila **			
P. stutzeri			
R. pickettii			
biovars 1–3 *			
R. fauriae			
R. genomospecies 4 *			
R. genomospecies 6			
Shewanella spp.			
Xanthobacter spp. *			

See Diagram 44.4

---

*Variable results.
**No results; treated as variable.
[1]*Methylobacterium* species exhibit pink-pigmented colonies, see Table 44.38 for species differentiation.
[2]*Flavobacterium aquatile* **does not** grow on nitrate medium.

708 Biochemical Tests for Identification of Medical Bacteria

Diagram 44.4.

Differentiation of Gram-negative, **aerobic to facultative anaerobic rods** (bacilli) that are

Mac-G	NO₃→NO₂-Pos
Glucose-NF	Motile
Oxidase-Pos	

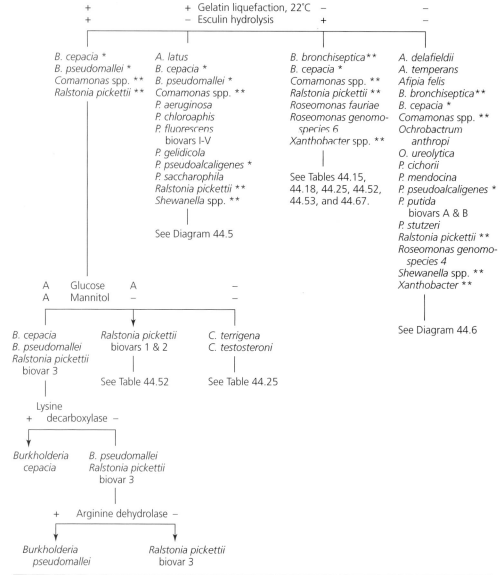

*Variable results.
**No results; treated as variable.

Diagram 44.5.

Differentiation of Gram-negative, **aerobic to facultative anaerobic rods** (bacilli) that are

Mac-G	NO₃→NO₂-Pos	Gelatin liquefaction-Pos
Glucose-NF	Motile	Esculin hydrolysis-Neg
Oxidase-Pos		

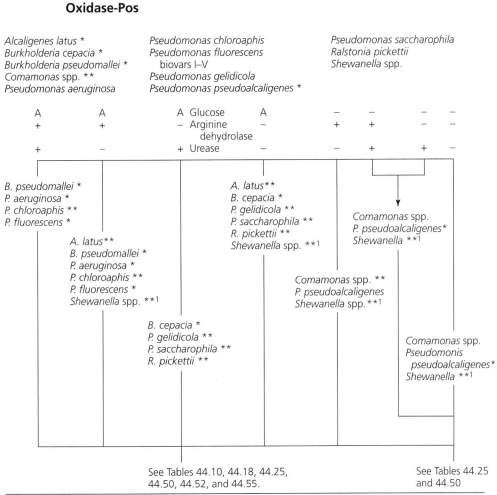

*Variable results.
**No results; treated as variable.
¹*Shewanella* species H₂S-positive.

Diagram 44.6.

Differentiation of Gram-negative, **aerobic to facultative anaerobic rods** (bacilli) that are

Mac-G	$NO_3 \rightarrow NO_2$-Pos	Gelatin liquefaction-Neg
Glucose-NF	Motile	Esculin hydrolysis-Neg
Oxidase-Pos		

Acidovorax delafieldii	Ochrobactrum anthropi	Pseudomonas stutzeri
Acidovorax temperans	Oligella ureolytica	Ralstonia pickettii
Afipia felis	Pseudomonas cichorii	Roseomans genomospecies 4
Bordetella bronchiseptica*	Pseudomonas mendocina	Shewanella spp.*
Burkholderia cepacia *	Pseudomonas pseudoalcaligenes *	Xanthobacter spp.*
Comamonas spp.*	Pseudomonas putida	
	biovars A & B	

Acidovorax delafieldii: H_2S (PbAc)-positive; see Table 44.4
Acidovorax temperans: H_2S (PbAc)-positive; see Table 44.4
Afipia felis: phenylalanine-positive; see Table 44.8
Oligella ureolytica: phenylalanine-positive; see Table 44.45
Roseomonas genomospecies 4: pink-pigmented colonies; see Table 44.53
Shewanella spp.: H_2S (TSI)-positive; see Table 44.55

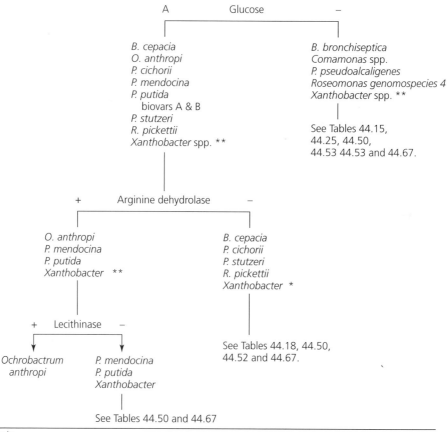

*Variable results.
**No results; treated as variable.

Diagram 44.7.

Differentiation of Gram-negative, **aerobic to facultative anaerobic rods** (bacilli) that are

Mac-G NO$_3$→NO$_2$-Pos
Glucose-NF Nonmotile
Oxidase-Pos

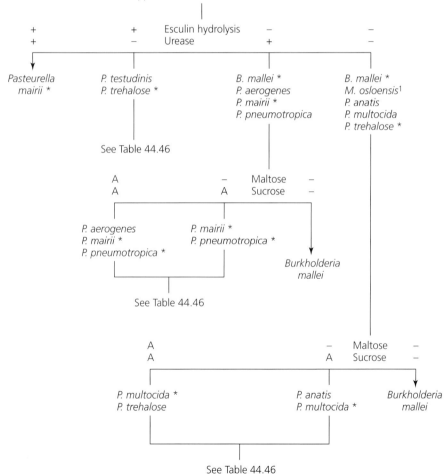

*Variable results.
[1]Few strains weakly urease positive.

Diagram 44.8.

Differentiation of Gram-negative, **aerobic to facultative anaerobic rods** (bacilli) that are

Mac-G	Oxidase-Pos	Motile
Glucose-NF	NO$_3$→NO$_2$-Neg	

Agrobacterium tumefaciens	Oligella ureolytica	Pseudomonas saccharophila *
Alcaligenes faecalis	Pseudomonas alcaligenes	Ralstonia pickettii
Bordetella avium	Pseudomonas chloroaphis *	biovar 3
Brevundimonas diminuta	Pseudomonas cichorii *	Roseomonas cervicalis
Burkholderia cepacia *	Pseudomonas gelidicola *	Roseomonas gilardii
Comamonas testosteroni *	Pseudomonas putida	
Ochrobactrum anthropi *	biovars A & B*	

Bordetella avium: animal pathogen; see Table 44.15
Oligella ureolytica: urease and phenylalanine-positive; see Table 44.45
Roseomonas spp.: H$_2$S (PbAc)-positive; see Table 44.53

	A	A	Glucose	–	–
	+	–	Arginine dehydrolase	+	–

O. anthropi	A. tumefaciens	A. faecalis **	A. faecalis **
P. chloroaphis	B. diminuta *	Comamonas	B. diminuta *
P. putida	B. cepacia	testosteroni**	Comamonas
R. pickettii	P. chichorii	P. alcaligenes	testosteroni**
biovar 3**	P. gelidicola		
	P. saccharophila		
	R. pickettii biovar 3**		

See Tables 44.10, 44.16, 44.25 and 44.50

+ Gelatin	–	+ Esculin hydrolysis	+	–	–
liquefaction		+ Gelatin liquefaction	–		+	–

Pseudomonas	O. anthropi	A. tumefaciens **	A. tumefaciens **	B. diminuta **	B. diminuta **
chloroaphis	P. putida	B. diminuta **	B. diminuta **	B. cepacia *	B. cepacia *
	R. pickettii	B. cepacia *	B. cepacia *	P. gelidicola	P. cichorii
	biovar 3**	R. pickettii	R. pickettii	P. saccharophila	R. pickettii
		biovar 3**	biovar 3**	R. pickettii	biovar 3**
				biovar 3**	

See Tables 44.44, 44.50 and 44.52

See Tables 44.16, 44.18, 44.50 and 44.52

	A	Mannitol	–

A. tumefaciens
B. cepacia
Ralstonia pickettii
biovar 3

Brevundimonas diminuta

+	Urease	–

A. tumefaciens   Burkholderia
B. cepacia *   cepacia *
Ralstonia pickettii
biovar 3

See Tables 44.9, 44.18, and 44.52

*Variable results.
**No results; treated as variable.

Diagram 44.9.

Differentiation of Gram-negative, **aerobic to facultative anaerobic rods** (bacilli) that are

        Mac-G   NO$_3$→NO$_2$-Neg
        Glucose-NF   Nonmotile
        Oxidase-Pos

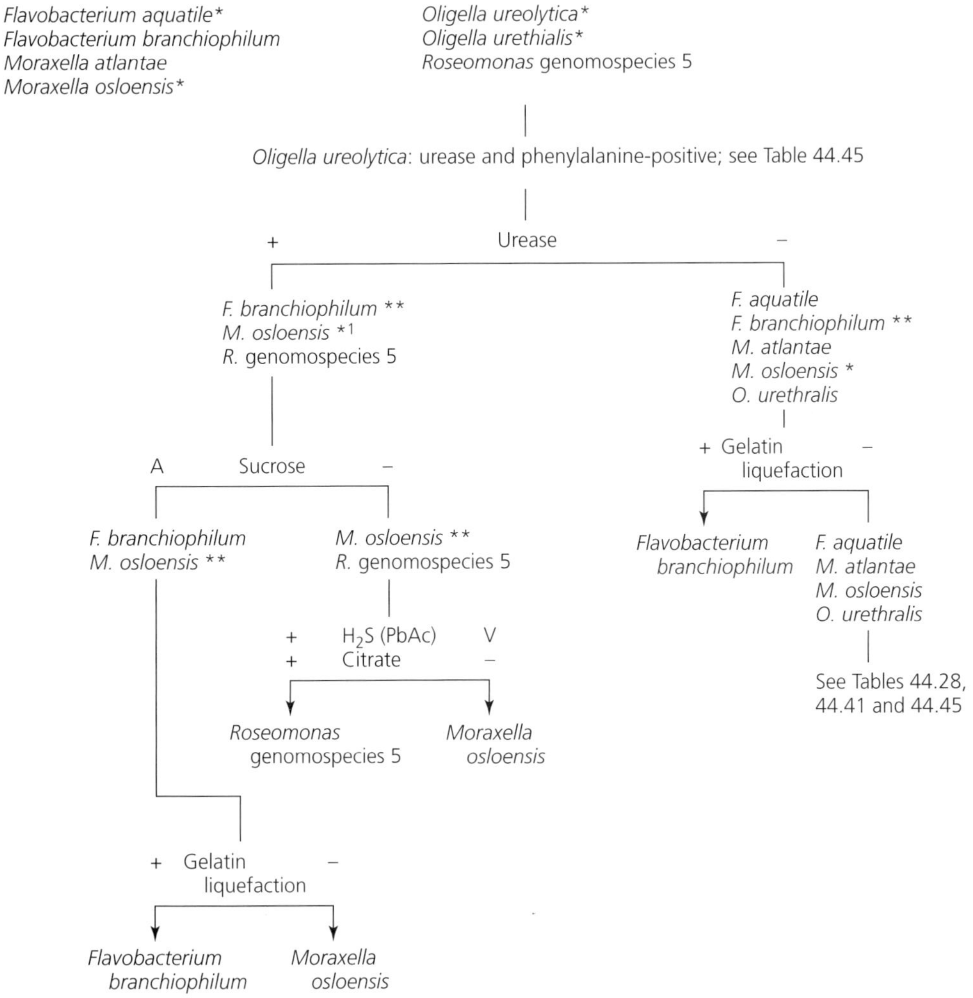

*Flavobacterium aquatile**
Flavobacterium branchiophilum
Moraxella atlantae
*Moraxella osloensis**

*Oligella ureolytica**
*Oligella urethialis**
Roseomonas genomospecies 5

Oligella ureolytica: urease and phenylalanine-positive; see Table 44.45

Urease

+
F. branchiophilum **
M. osloensis *¹
R. genomospecies 5

−
F. aquatile
F. branchiophilum **
M. atlantae
M. osloensis *
O. urethralis

Sucrose

A
F. branchiophilum
M. osloensis **

−
M. osloensis **
R. genomospecies 5

+ H$_2$S (PbAc)   V
+ Citrate   −

Roseomonas
genomospecies 5

Moraxella
osloensis

+ Gelatin liquefaction −

Flavobacterium
branchiophilum

F. aquatile
M. atlantae
M. osloensis
O. urethralis

See Tables 44.28, 44.41 and 44.45

+ Gelatin liquefaction −

Flavobacterium
branchiophilum

Moraxella
osloensis

*Variable results.
**No results; treated as variable.
¹Few strains *Moraxella osloersis* urease-positive.

714 Biochemical Tests for Identification of Medical Bacteria

Diagram 44.10.

Differentiation of Gram-negative, **aerobic to facultative anaerobic rods** (bacilli) that are
  Mac-G
  Glucose-NF
  Oxidase-Neg

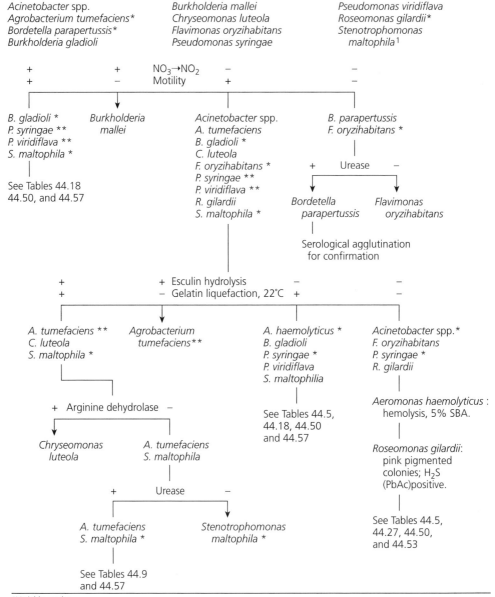

*Variable results.
**No results; treated as variable.
[1]Most strains of *Stenotrophomonas maltophila* require methiconine for growth (or cystine plys glycone).

Chapter 44 / Gram-Negative Bacteria

Diagram 44.11.
Differentiation of Gram-negative, **aerobic to facultative anaerobic rods** (bacilli) that are

      Mac-G   Glucose-F & O

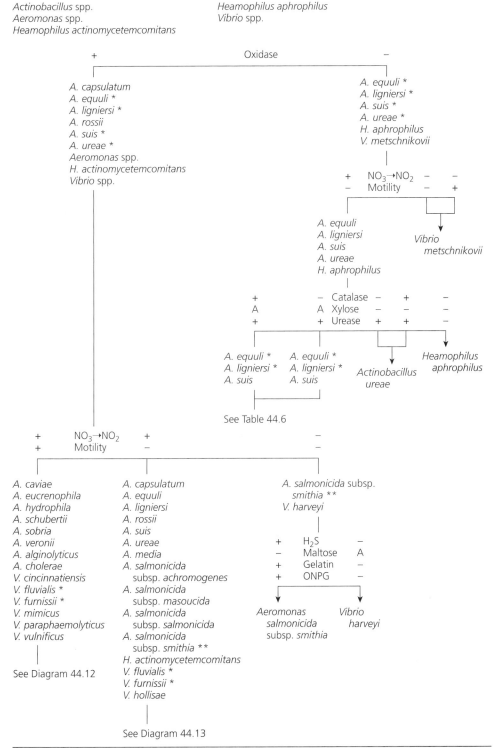

*Variable results.
**No results; treated as variable.

Diagram 44.12.

Differentiation of Gram-negative, **aerobic to facultative anaerobic rods** (bacilli) that are

        Mac-G $NO_3 \rightarrow NO_2$-Pos
        Glucose-F & O   Motile
        Oxidase-Pos

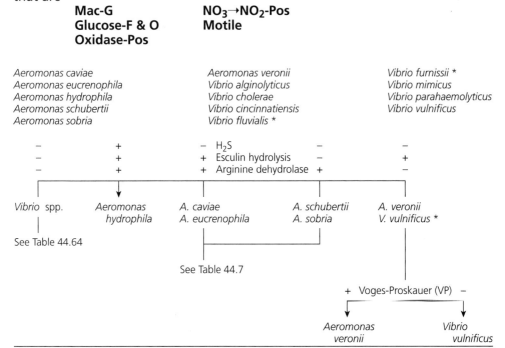

*Variable results.

Diagram 44.13.

Differentiation of Gram-negative, **aerobic to facultative anaerobic rods** (bacilli) that are **Mac-G, Glucose-F & O, Oxidase-Pos, NO₃→NO₂-Pos, Nonmotile**

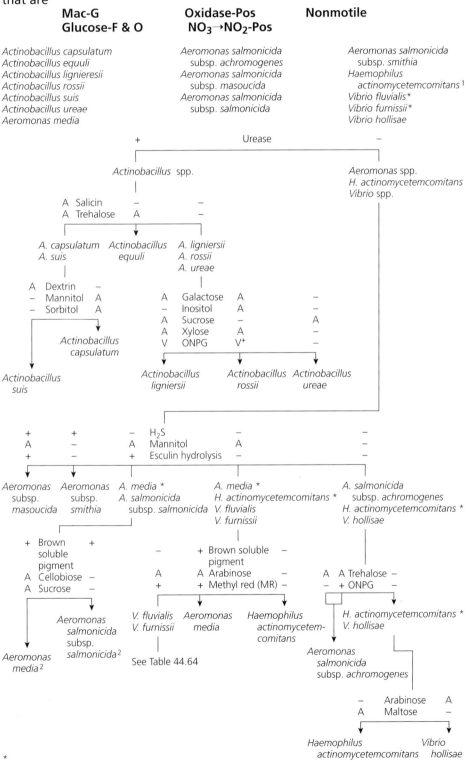

*Variable results.

[1] *Haemophilus actinomycetemcomitans* **does not** require either X or V factors for growth.

[2] *Aeromonas media* and *A. salmonicida* subsp. *salmonicida* are the only *Aeromonas* species to produce a brown, soluble pigment.

718 Biochemical Tests for Identification of Medical Bacteria

Diagram 44.14.

Differentiation of Gram-negative, **aerobic to facultative anaerobic rods** (bacilli) that **do not grow on MacConkey (MAC)**

Acholeplasma spp.[1]
Acidovorax facilis
Actinobacillus hominis
Actinobacillus muris
Actinobacillus rossii
Actinobacillus seminis
Actinobacillus ureae *
Aeromonas spp.*
Afipia spp.
Bartonella spp.
Bordetella pertussis

Brevundimonas vesicularis
Brucella melitensis
Burkholderia mallei *
Capnocytophaga spp.
Cardiobacterium hominis[2]
Eikenella corrodens
Francisella spp.[3]
Gardnerella vaginalis
Haemophilus spp.
Janthinobacterium lividum **[4]
Kingella spp.[5]

Legionella spp.
Methylobacterium spp.*
Moraxella spp.*
Oligella ureolytica*
Pasteurella spp.*
Ralstonia pickettii*
Sphingomonas spp.
Streptobacillus moniliformis
Suttonella indologenes
Weeksella virosa
Xanthobacter spp. **

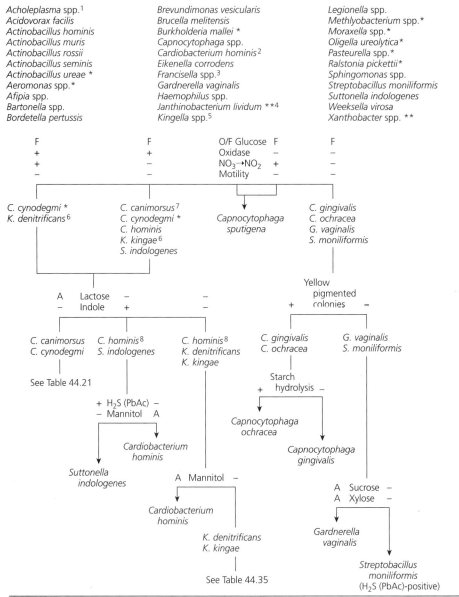

---

*Variable results.
**No results; treated as variable.
See Diagram 44.15 for above microorganisms that are **nonfermenters (NF) of glucose;** see Diagram 44.16 for above microorganisms that are **positive for both fermentation and oxidation (F & O).**

[1]*Acholplasma* species require serum or cholesterol for growth; colonies on solid media give a "fried-egg" appearance; see Table 44.3 to differentiate species.

[2]*Cardiobacterium hominis:* hemin required for aerobic growth.

[3]*Francisella* spp.: cysteine or cytosine required for growth; *F. tularensis* **extremely infectious;** identification and confirmation by slide agglutination; biochemical reactions no particular value; sent to state, reference or public health laboratory for isolation and identification.

[4]*Janthinobacterium lividum* exhibits violet-pigmented colonies on solid media and violet ring in liquid media; see Table 44.34 for biochemical characteristics.

[5]*Kingella* spp.: fastidious; may require addition of serum to basal fermentation medium to enhance growth.

[6]*Kingella* spp.: oxidase-positive with tetramethyl-*p*-phynylenediamine; weakly positive with dimethyl reagent.

[7]*Capnocytophaga canimorsus* may be weakly positive for oxidase.

[8]Indole production may be weak due to a small amount formed and may **not** be detected by procedures that **do not** concentrate by xylene extraction (14).

Diagram 44.15.

Differentiation of Gram-negative, **aerobic to facultative anaerobic rods** (bacilli) that **do not grow on MacConkey (MAC)** and are nonfermenters (O/inert)

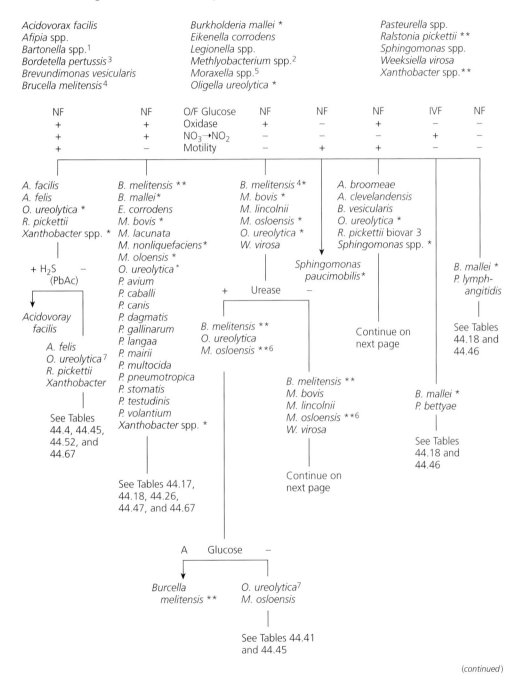

(continued)

720 Biochemical Tests for Identification of Medical Bacteria

Diagram 44.15. (*continued*)

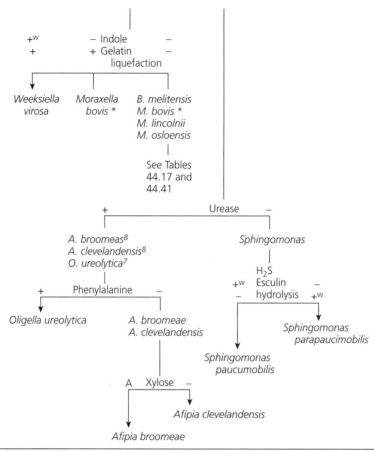

---

*Variable results.

**No results; treated as variable.

[1]*Bartonella* spp.: highly fastidious; add hemin to media; identification by serologic methods; most species require 7 days or more for biochemical results; see Table 44.14 to differentiate.

[2]*Methylobacterium* spp.: pink-pigmented colonies; see Table 44.38 to differentiate.

[3]*Bordetella pertussis* required Bordet-Gengou medium for primary isolation; no growth in ordinary media.

[4]*Brucella melitensis:* no acid production from conventional carbohydrates.

[5]*Moraxella catarrhalis* and *M. ovis* exhibit coccal and diplococcal forms; resemble *Neisseria* species, see Gram-negative cocci for biochemical differentiation.

[6]Few strains *Moraxella osloensis* weakly-urease-positive.

[7]*Oligella ureolytica* urease and phenylalanine-positive; urease strong positive, within minutes.

[8]Delayed positive.

Diagram 44.16.

Differentiation of Gram-negative, **aerobic to facultative anaerobic rods** (bacilli) that **do not grow on MacConkey (MAC)** and are **both fermenters (F) and oxidizers (O)**

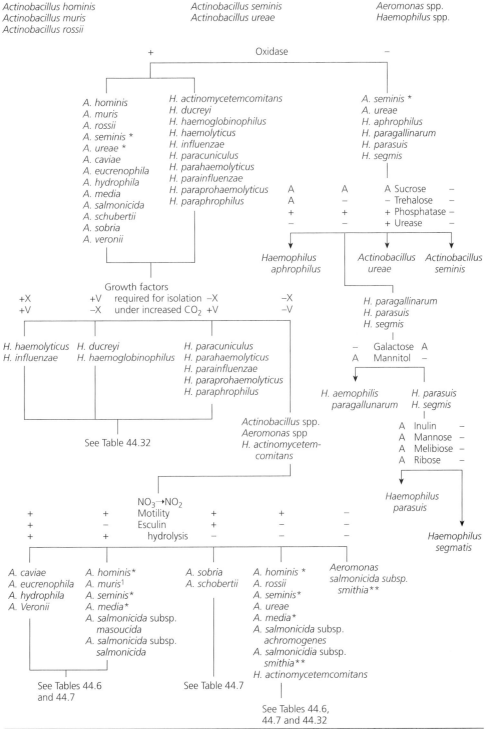

*Variable results.
**No results; treated as variable.
[1]Positive reaction delayed.

Diagram 44.17.

Differentiation of Gram-negative, aerobic to facultative anaerobic cocci/diplococci

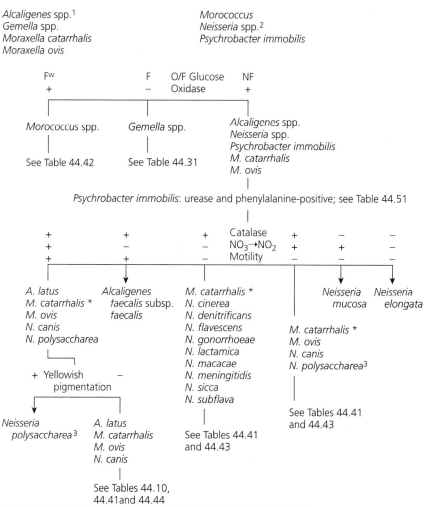

*Variable results.
[1]*Alcaligenes faecalis* and *A. latus* rods, coccobacilli, and cocci.
[2]*Neisseria elongata* exhibits short rods often arranged as diplococci or short chains.
[3]*N. polysaccharea* arranged in pairs and tetrads.

Diagram 44.18.
Differentiation of Gram-negative, **microaerophilic to anaerobic rods** (bacilli)

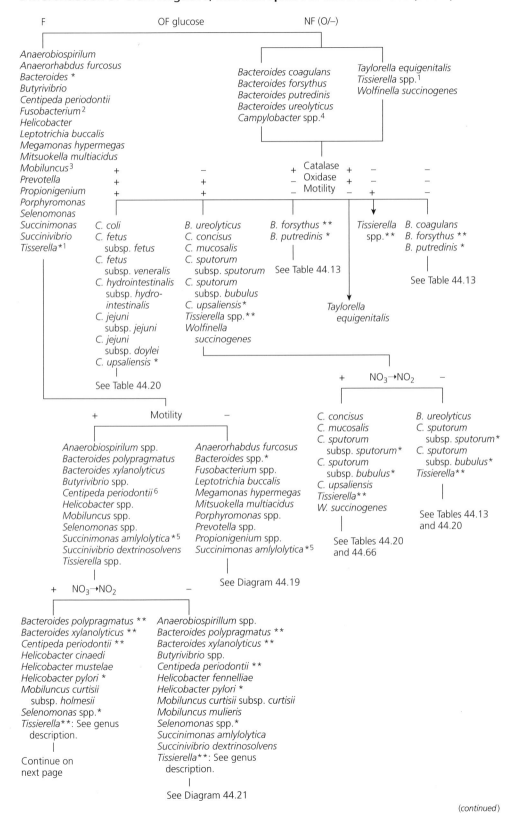

(continued)

Diagram 44.18. (continued)

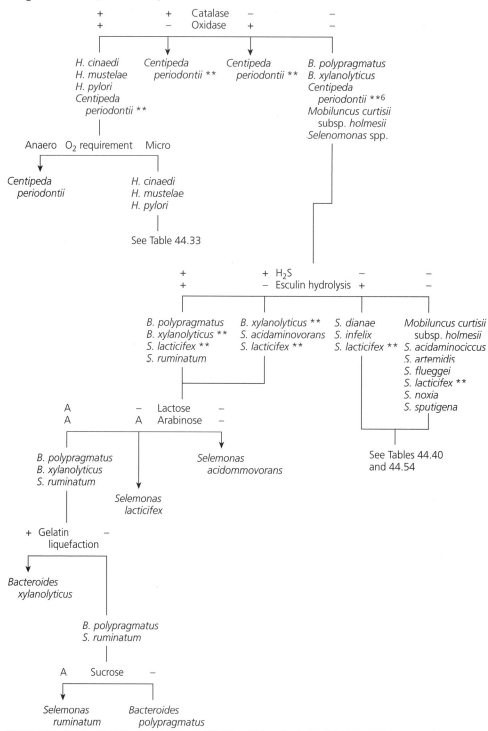

*Variable results.

**No results; treated as variable.

[1]*Tissierella* spp.: weakly fermentative (F) or oxidative (O).

[2]*Fusobacterium* weakly fermentative (F).

[3]*Mobiluncus:* Gram variable; weakly fermentative (F).

[4]*Campylobacter* spp.: require 3–15% oxygen (O) and 3–5% carbon dioxide (CO_2) for growth.

[5]*Succinimonas:* motility slow and progressive; may be lost on exposure to air.

[6]*Centipeda* colony morphology: serpentine rods; see genus description.

Diagram 44.19.
Differentiation of Gram-negative, **microaerophilic to anaerobic rods** (bacilli) that **ferment glucose** and are **nonmotile**

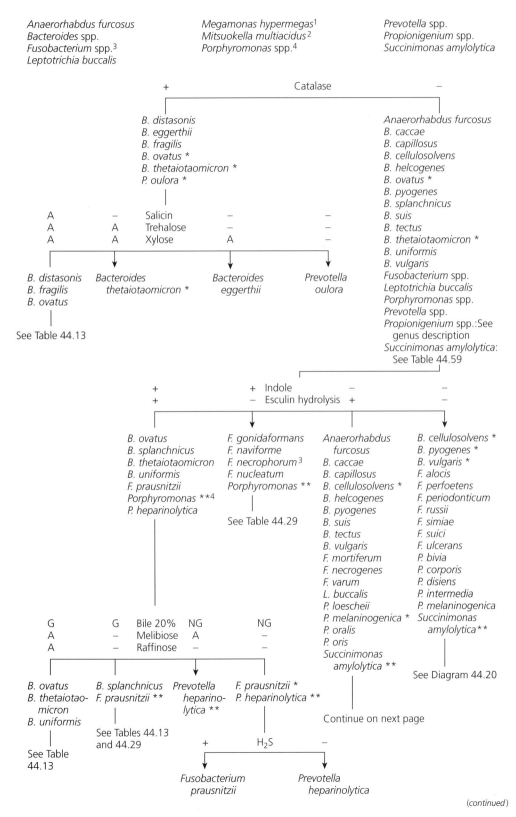

726 Biochemical Tests for Identification of Medical Bacteria

Diagram 44.19. (*continued*)

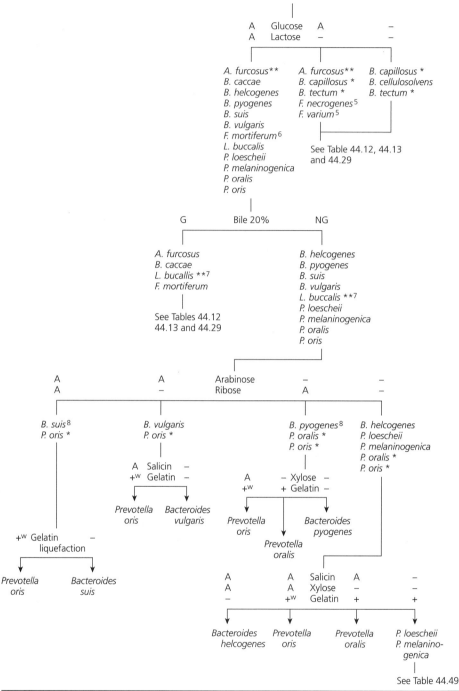

*Variable results.
**No results; treated as variable.
[1]*Megamonas:* large rods usually granular in appearance; see genus description.
[2]*Mitsuokella:* fermentation often vigorous; see Table 44.39.
[3]*Fusobacterium* spp.: identification by gas chromatography, electrophoretic patterns, and mass spectrometry; see genus footnotes.
[4]*Porphyromonas:* brown to black colonies on blood agar (BA).
[5]Glucose fermentation weak.
[6]Glucose and lactose fermentation weak.
[7]*Leptotrichia bucalis:* see Table 44.36.
[8]Ribose fermentation weak.

Diagram 44.20.

Differentiation of Gram-negative, **microaerophilic to anaerobic rods** (bacilli) that are Glucose-F Nonmotile, Catalase-Neg Indole-Neg, Esculin hydrolysis-Neg

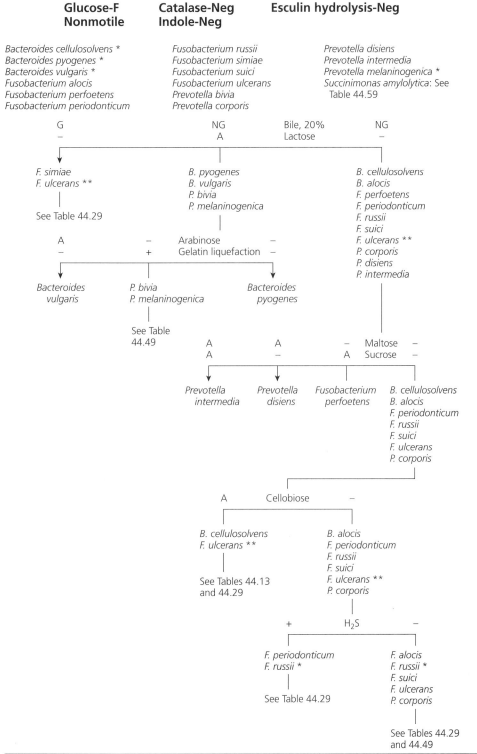

*Variable results.
**No results; treated as variable.

Diagram 44.21.

Differentiation of Gram-negative, **microaerophilic to anaerobic rods** (bacilli) that are:
   Glucose-F   NO₃→NO₂-Neg
   Motile

Anaerobiospirilum spp.   *Helicobacter pylori* *
Bacteroides polypragmatus **   *Mobiluncus curtisii* subsp. *curtisii*
Bacteroides xylanolyticus **   *Mobiluncus mulieris*
Butyrivibrio spp.   *Selenomonas* spp.*
Centipeda periodontii **¹   *Succinimonas amylolytica* *²
Helicobacter fennelliae   *Succinivibrio dextrinosolvens*

+	−	Catalase	−
+	+	Oxidase	−

H. fennelliae   *Anaerobiospirilum* **   *Anaerobiospirilum* **
H. pylori   *B. crossotus* **   *B. polypragmatus*
                          B. fibrisolvens **   *B. xylanolyticus*
See Table 44.33   *B. crossotus* **
                          See Tables 44.11   *B. fibrisolvens* **
                          and 44.19   *M. curtisii* subsp. *curtisii*
                                                        M. mulieris
                                                        Selenomonas spp.
                                                        Succinimonas amylolytica:
                                                            See Table 44.59
                                                        Succinivibrio dextrinosolvens

+	+	H₂S	−
+	−	Esculin hydrolysis	−
		+	−

Anaerobiospirilum **   *Anaerobiospirilum* **   *Anaerobiospirilum* **   *Anaerobiospirilum* **
B. fibrisolvens **   *B. crossotus* **   *B. fibrisolvens* **   *B. fibrisolvens* **
B. polypragmatus   *B. fibrisolvens* **   *S. dianae*   *B. crossotas* **
S. ruminatism   *B. xylanolyticus* **   *S. infelix*   *M. curtisii* subsp. *curtisii*
B. xylanolyticus **   *S. acidaminovorans* **   *S. lactilytica* **   *M. muliersi*
S. lactilytica **   *S. lactilytica* **   *S. dextrinosolvens* **   *S. acidaminovorans* **
                                                                              S. artemidis
                                                                              S. flueggei
                                                                              S. lactilytica **
                                                                              S. noxia
                                                                              S. sputigena *
                                                                              S. dextrinosolvens **

See Diagrams 44.11, 44.13, 44.19, 44.40, 44.54 and 44.60

*Variable results.
**No results; treated as variable.
¹*Centipeda* colony morphology serpentine rods; see genus description.
²Motility slow and progressive; may be lost on exposure to air.

Diagram 44.22.

Differentiation of Gram-negative, **anaerobic, cocci/diplococci** that are
Glucose-F   Nonmotile
Catalase-Neg

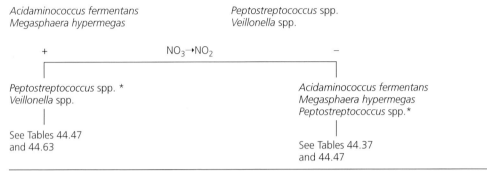

*Variable results.

REFERENCES

1. Brenner DJ, Hollis DG, Moss CW, et al. Validation list no. 41. Int J Syst Bacteriol 1992;42:327–328.
2. Collins MD, Shah HN. Reclassification of *Bacteroides praeacutus* Tissier (Holdeman and Moore) in a new genus, *Tissierella*, as *Tissierella praeacuta* comb. nov. Int J Syst Bacteriol 1986; 36:461–463.
3. De Vos P, Kersters K, Falsen E, et al. *Comamonas* Davis and Park 1962, gen. nov., nom. rev. emend, and *Comamonas terrigena* Hugh 1962, sp. nov., nom. rev. Int J Syst Bacteriol 1985;35:443–453.
4. Facklam RR, Washington JA. *Streptococcus* and related catalase-negative Gram-positive cocci. In: Balows A, Hausler WJ Jr, Hermaan KL, et al., eds. Manual of Clinical Microbiology, ed 5. Washington, DC: American Society for Microbiology, 1991:238–257.
5. Forbes BAG, Sahn DF, Weissfeld AS. Bailey & Scott's Diagnostic Microbiology, ed 10. St. Louis: Mosby, 1998.
6. Fortier AH, Green SJ, Polsinelli T, et al. Life and death of an intracellular pathogen: *Francisella tularensis* and the macrophage. Immunol Ser 1994;60:349–361.
7. Goodwin CS, Armstrong JA, Chilvers T, Transfer of *Campylobacter pylori* and *Campylobacter mustelae* to *Helicobacter* gen. nov. as *Helicobacter pylori* comb. nov. and *Helicobacter mustelae* comb. nov., respectively. Int J Syst Bacteriol 1989;39:397–405.
8. Grehn M, Müller F. The oxidase reaction of *Pasteurelaa multocida* strains cultured on Müller-Hinton medium. J Clin Microbiol 1989;9(3): 333–336.
9. Green PN, Bousfield IJ. Emendation of *Methylobacterium* Patt, Cole, and Hanson 1976: *Methylobacterium rhodinum* (Heumann 1962) comb. nov. corrig., *Methylobacterium radiotolerans* Iito and Iisuka 1971) comb. nov., corrig., and *Methylobacteium mesophilicum* (Austin and Goodfellow 1979) comb. nov. Int J Syst Bacteriol 1983;33: 875–877.
10. Holmes B, Popoff M, Kiredjian M, Kersters L. *Ochrobactrum anthropi* gen. nov., sp. nov. from human clinical specimens. And previously known as Vd. Int J Syst Bacteriol 1988;38:406–416.
11. Holmes B, Steigerwalt AG, Weaver RE, Brenner DJ. *Chryseomonas polytricha* gen. nov., sp. nov., a *Pseudomonas*-like organism from human clinical specimens and formerly known as group Ve-1. Int J Syst Bacteriol 1986;36:161–165.
12. Holmes B, Steigerwalt AG, Weaver RE, Brenner DJ. Validation list no. 23. Int J Syst Bacteriol 1987;37:179–180.
13. Holmes B, Steigerwalt AG, Weaver RE, Brenner DJ. *Chryseomonas luteola* comb. nov., and *Flavimonas oryzihabitans* gen. nov., comb. nov., *Pseudomonas*-like species from human clinical specimens and formerly known, respectively as groups Ve-1 and Ve-2. Int J Syst Bacteriol 1987; 37:245–250.
14. Holt JG, Kreig NR. Bergey's Manual of Determinative Bacteriology vol 2. Baltimore: Williams & Wilkins, 1994.
15. Juni E, Heym GA. *Psychrobacter immobilis* gen. nov., sp. nov.: Genospecies composed of Gram-negative, aerobic, oxidase-positive coccobacilli. Int J Syst Bacteriol 1986;36:388–391.
16. Kreig NR, Holt JG. Bergey's Manual of Determinative Bacteriology, vol 1. Baltimore: Williams & Wilkins, 1984.
17. Lai CH, Males BM, Dougherty PA, et al. *Centipeda periodontii* gen. nov., sp. nov., from human peridontal lesions. Int J Syst Bacteriol 1983;33:628–635.
18. Long PA, Sly I, Pham AV, Davis GHG. Characterization of *Morococcus cerebrosus* gen. nov., sp. nov., and comparison with *Neisseria mucosa*. Int J Syst Bacteriol 1981;31:294–301.
19. Murray PR, Baron EJ, Pfaller MA, et al. Manual of Clinical Microbiology, ed 6. Washington, DC: American Society for Microbiology, 1995.
20. Rossau R, Kersters K, Falsen E, et al. *Oligella*, a new genus including *Oligella urethralis* comb. nov. (formerly *Moraxella urethralis*) and *Oligella ureolytica* sp. nov. (formerly CDC group Ive): Relationship to *Taylorella equigenitalis* and related taxa. Int J Syst Bacteriol 1987;37:198–210.
21. Schink B, Pfennig N. Validation list no. 12. Int J Syst Bacteriol 1983;33:896–897.
22. Shah HN, Collins MD. *Prevotella*, a new genus to include *Bacteroides melaninogenicus* and related species formerly classified in the genus *Bacteroides*. Int J Syst Bacteriol 1990;40:205–208.
23. Shah HN, Collins MD. Proposal for reclassification of *Bacteroides asaccharolyticus*, *Bacteroides gingivalis*, and *Bacteroides endodontalis* in a new genus, *Porphyromonas*. Int J Syst Bacteriol 1988;38:128–131.
24. Shah HN, Collins MD. Validation list no. 22. Int J Syst Bacteriol 1986;36:573–576.
25. Shah HN, Collins MD. Validation list no. 10. 1983;33:438–440.
26. Sneath PHA, Mair NS, Sharpe ME, Holt JG, eds. Bergey's Manual of Systematic Bacteriology, vol 2. Baltimore: Williams & Wilkins, 1986.
27. Spiegel CA, Roberts M. *Mobiluncus* gen. nov., *Mobiluncus curtisii* subsp. *curtisii* sp. nov., and *Mobilincus mulieris* sp. nov., curved rods from the human vagina. Int J Syst Bacteriol 1984; 34(2):177–184.
28. Sugimoto C, Isayama Y, Sakazaki R, Kuramoch I. Validation list no. 16. Int J Syst Bacteriol 1984;34:503–504.
29. Weyant RS, Moss CW, Weaver RE, et al. Identification of Unusual Pathogenic Gram-Negative Aerobic and Facultatively Anaerobic Bacteria. Baltimore: Williams & Wilkins, 1996.

30. Willems A, Falsen E, Pot B, et al. *Acidovorax*, a new genus for *Pseudomonas facilis, Pseudomonas delafieldii*, E. Falsen (EF) group 13, EF group 16, and several clinical isolates, with the species *Acidovorax facilis* comb. nov., *Acidovorax delafieldii* comb. nov., and *Acidovorax temperans* sp. nov. Int J Syst Bacteriol 1990;40(4):384–398.
31. Winn WE. *Legionella* and the clinical microbiologist. Infect Dis Clin North Am 1993;7:377–392.

45 Gram-Negative *Enterobacteriaceae* and Other Intestinal Bacteria

Taxonomy 732
Changes in Nomenclature of Gram-Negative *Enterobacteriaceae* 733
Classification/Genera and Species 735
Enterobacteriaceae General Characteristics 741
Media for Isolation and Differentiation of *Enterobacteriaceae* 742
KIA/TSI Reactions of Most Enterobacteriaceae 744
Warning 747
KIA/TSI: Acid/Acid, with/without Gas
    Biochemical Reactions 748
    Diagrams/Flow Charts 758
KIA/TSI: Acid/Acid, H_2S, with/without Gas
    Biochemical Reactions 769
    Diagrams/Flow Charts 771
KIA/TSI: Alkaline/Acid, with/without Gas
    Biochemical Reactions 772
    Diagrams/Flow Charts 782
KIA/TSI: Alkaline/Acid, H_2S, with/without Gas
    Biochemical Reactions 796
    Diagrams/Flow Charts 798
KIA/TSI: Alkaline/Alkaline or Alkaline/No Change
    Biochemical Reactions 800
    Diagrams/Flow Charts 801
References 802

TAXONOMY

Many changes in taxonomy and nomenclature have occurred within the family *Enterobacteriaceae* since the last edition of this manual. Many new genera and species have been discovered, some unusual and rare, and many species have been reclassified into new genera.

   These changes in taxonomy and nomenclature have resulted from a polyphasic approach to taxonomy; the use of a wide variety of procedures such as new biochemical tests, specific species/group bacteriophages, deoxyribonucleic acid (DNA) relatedness tests, ribonucleic acid (RNA) typing (ribotyping), and polymerase chain reaction (PCR) tests. These procedures aid in definitive assignment of distinct morphologic and biochemical strains of bacteria to species and occasionally to new genera.

   Taxonomy and nomenclature of the *Enterobacteriaceae* differ among clinical microbiologists. This chapter on *Enterobacteriaceae* uses the classification as listed in the proposed 2nd edition of *Bergey's Manual of Systematic Bacteriology*.

CHANGES IN NOMENCLATURE OF GRAM-NEGATIVE *ENTEROBACTERIACEAE*

(Note: Bergey's Manual of Determinative Bacteriology, 9th edition, was printed in 1994; therefore, references to new genera or new species are listed from 1995 to 1999.)

Definitions

Basonym: original name of a new combination
Synonym:
    Objective: more than 1 name
    Subjective: different name to different types; first published, senior; later, junior
gen. nov.: new genus
sp. nov.: new species

Current name	Old name (basonym(s)/synonym(s))
Brenneria nigrifluens	*Erwinia nigrifluens*
Brenneria paradisiaca	*Erwinia paradisiaca*
Brenneria quercina	*Erwinia quercina*
Brenneria rubrifaciens	*Erwinia rubrifaciens*
Brenneria salicis	*Erwinia salicis*
Buttiauxella agrestii, sp. nov.[1]	
Buttiauxella brennerae, sp. nov.[1]	
Buttiauxella ferragutiae, sp. nov.[1]	
Buttiauxella gaviniae, sp. nov.[1]	
Buttiauxella izardii, sp. nov.[1]	
Buttiauxella noackiae, sp. nov.[1]	
Buttiauxella warmboldiae, sp. nov.[1]	
Cedecea davisae	Enteric group 15, Davis subgroup[2]
Cedecea neteri	*Cedecea* species 4
Cedecea species 3	*Cedecea* strain 001[3]
Cedecea species 5	*Cedecea* strain 002[3]
Citrobacter amalonaticus	*Levinea amalonatica*
Citrobacter koseri	*Citrobacter diversus*
Citrobacter rodentium, sp. nov.[4]	
Enterobacter aerogenes	*Klebsiella mobilis*
Enterobacter amnigenus biogroups 1 & 2	Group H3
Enterobacter asburiae	Enteric group 17
Enterobacter cancerogenus	*Enterobacter taylorae*, *Erwinia cancerogen*
Enterobacter dissolvens	*Erwinia dissolvens*
Enterobacter hormaechei	Enteric group 75
Enterobacter intermedius	Incorrect name, *Enterobacter intermedium*
Enterobacter kobei, sp. nov.[5]	
Enterobacter nimipressuralis	*Erwinia nimipressuralis*
Enterobacter sakazakii	Yellow pigmented *Enterobacter cloacae*
Erwinia alni, sp. nov.[6]	
Erwinia carnegieana	*Pectobacterium carnegieana*
Erwinia carotovora subsp. *carotovora*	*Pectobacterium carotovorum*
Erwinia chrysanthemi	*Erwinia paradisiaca*, *Pectobacterium chrysanthemi*
Erwinia cypripedii	*Pectobacterium cypripedii*

Erwinia rhapontici	Pectobacterium rhapontici
Escherichia fergusonii	Enteric group 10[7]
Escherichia hermannii	Enteric group 11[7]
Escherichia vulneris	Enteric group 1[7], API group 2[7], Alma group [17]
Erwingella	Enteric group 40
Francisella philomiragia	Yersinia philomiragia
Hafnia alvei	Enterobacter hafnia
Klebsiella ornithinolytica	Klebsiella group 47
Klebsiella oxytoca	Indole-positive strains Klebsiella pneumoniae
Klebsiella planticola	Klebsiella species 2, Enteric group 47, group K of Izard et al.[8], Klebsiella trevisanii
Klebsiella pneumoniae subsp. ozaenae	Klebsiella ozaenae
Klebsiella pneumoniae subsp. rhinoscleromatis	Klebsiella rhinoscleromatis
Klebsiella terrigena	Group L of Izard et al.[8]
Kluyvera ascorbata	Enteric group 8, API group 1
Kluyvera cochleae, sp. nov.[1]	
Kluyvera georgiana, sp. nov.[1].	
Leclercia adecarboxylata	Escherichia adecarboxylata
Leminorella	Enteric group 57
Moellerella wisconsensis	Enteric group 46
Pantoea agglomerans	Enterobacter agglomerans, Erwinia milletiae, Erwinia herbicola
Pantoea ananatis	Incorrect name, Pantoea ananas; Erwinia ananas, Erwinia ureodovora
Pantoea stewartii subsp. stewartii	Erwinia stewartii
Pectobacterium cacticida	Erwinia cacticida
Pectobacterium carotovorum subsp. atrosepticum	Erwinia carotovorum subsp. atroseptica
Pectobacterium carotovorum subsp. betavasculorum	Erwinia carotovora subsp. betavasculora
Pectobacterium carotovorum subsp. carotovorum	Erwinia carotovora subsp. carotovora
Pectobacterium carotovorum subsp. odoriferum	Erwinia carotovora subsp. odorifera
Pectobacterium carotovorum subsp. wasabiae	Erwinia carotovora subsp. wasabiae
Pectobacterium chrysanthemi	Erwinia chrysanthemi
Pectobacterium cypripedii	Erwinia cypripedii
Pectobacterium rhapontici	Erwinia rhapontici
Photorhabdus luminescens	Xenorhabdus luminescens
Proteus inconstans	Providencia alcalifaciens
Proteus morganii subsp. morganii	Proteus morganii
Providencia rettgeri	Proteus rettgeri
Providencia rustigianii	Providencia friedericiana
Salmonella choleraesuis subsp. arizonae	Salmonella arizonae; incorrect name, Salmonella cholerae-suis
Salmonella choleraesuis subsp. diarizonae	Incorrect name, Salmonella cholerae-suis
Salmonella choleraesuis subsp. houtenae	Incorrect name, Salmonella cholerae-suis
Salmonella choleraesuis subsp. salamae	Incorrect name, Salmonella cholerae-suis
Serratia proteamaculans subsp. proteamaculans	Serratia liquefaciens

Serratia rubidaea	*Serratia marinorubra*
Tatumella ptyseus	Group EF-9 (CDC)
Trabulsiella	Enteric group 90
Wigglesworthia, gen. nov.[9]	
Wigglesworthia glossinidia, sp. nov.[9]	
Xenorhabdus beddingii	*Xenorhabdus nematophilus* subsp. *beddingii*
Xenorhabdus bovienii	*Xenorhabdus nematophilus* subsp. *bovienii*
Xenorhabdus japonicus sp. nov.[10]	
Xenorhabdus poinarii	*Xenorhabdus nematophilus* subsp. *poinarii*
Yersinia aldovae	Group X2 within *Yersinia enterocolitica*
Yersinia bercovieri	*Yersinia enterocolitica* biogroup 3B
Yersinia mollaretii	*Yersinia enterocolitica* biogroup 3A
Yokenella regensburgei	*Koserella trabulsii*, Enteric group 45

(*Note:* Enteric group is a designation given to yet unnamed genera/species.)

REFERENCES

[1] Müller HE, Brenner DJ, Fanning GR, et al. Emended description of *Buttiauxella agrestis* with recognition of six new species of *Buttiauxella* and two new species of *Kluyvera*: *Buttiauxella ferragutiae* sp. nov., *Buttiauxella gaviniae* sp. nov., *Buttiauxella brennerae* sp. nov., *Buttiauxella izardii* sp. nov., *Buttiauxella noackiae* sp. nov., *Kluyvera cochleae* sp. nov., and *Kluyvera georgiana* sp. nov. Int J Syst Bacteriol 1996;46(1):50–63.

[2] Bae BH, Sureka SB, Ajamy JA. Enteric group 15 (*Enterobacteriaceae*) associated with pneumonia. J Clin Microbiol 1981;14(5):596–597.

[3] Farmer JJ 3rd, Davis BR, Hickman-Brenner FW, et al. Biochemical identification of new species and biogroups of *Enterobacteriaceae* isolated from clinical specimens. J Clin Microbiol 1985;21(1):46–76.

[4] Schauer DB, Zabel BAG, Pedraza IF, et al. Validation list no. 56. Int J Syst Bacteriol 1996;46(1):362–363.

[5] Kosako Y, Tamura K, Sakazaki R, Miki K. Validation list no. 62. Int J Syst Bacteriol 1997;47(4):915–916.

[6] Surico G, Mugnai L, Pastorelli R, et al. *Erwina almi*, a new species causing bark cankers of alder (*Alnus* Miller) species. Int J Syst Bacteriol 1996;46(3):720–726.

[7] Pien FD, Shrum S, Swenson JM, et al. Colonization of human wounds by *Escherichia vulneris* and *Escherichia hermannii*. J Clin Microbiol 1985;22(2):283–285.

[8] Izard D, Ferragut C, Gavini F, et al. *Klebsiella terrigena*, a new species from soil and water. Int J Syst Bacteriol 1981;31(1):116–127.

[9] Aksoy S. *Wigglesworthia* gen. nov. and *Wigglesworthia glossinidia* sp. nov., taxa consisting of the mycetocyte-associated, primary endosymbionts of tsetse flies. Int J Syst Bacteriol 1995;45(4):848–851.

[10] Nishimura Y, Hagiwara A, Suzuki T, Yamanaka S. Validation list no. 54. Int J Syst Bacteriol 1995;45(3):619–620.

CLASSIFICATION/GENERA AND SPECIES

Enterobacteriaceae genera and species: proposed outline of *Bergey's Manual of Systematic Bacteriology*, 2nd edition

Volume 2 The Proteobacteria

The Bacteria
Kingdom Proteobacteria

Section XVII: The δ-Proteobacteria

Class Zymobacteria
    Order XII. Enterobacteriales
        Family: *Enterobacteriaceae*

Arsenophonus

Single species, *A. nasoniae* ATCC 49151 (not in *Bergey's Manual;* created by Gherna et al. (1); occurs in wasps; fastidious microorganism, requires unusual media

Buchnera

Single species, *B. aphidicola*

Budvicia

Single species, *B. aquatica* ATCC 25567, ATCC 35567 (not in *Bergey's Manual;* created by Aldova et al. (2)

Buttiauxella: 7 species (not in *Bergey's Manual;* created by Ferragut et al. (3); phenotypically similar to genus Kluyvera; isolated from fresh waters; no human or animal isolates.

> *B. agrestis,* type species ATCC 33320
> *B. brennerae*
> *B. ferragutiae*
> *B. gaviniae*
> *B. izardii*
> *B. noackiae*
> *B. warmboldiae*

Calymmatobacterium

Single species, *C. granulomatis*

Cedecea: 3 species; similar to genus *Serratia;* infrequent opportunistic pathogen; species 3 and 5 yet unnamed

> *C. davisae,* type species ATCC 33431
> *C. lapagei*
> *C. neteri*
> *C. species 3*
> *C. species 5*

Citrobacter: 9 species; opportunistic pathogen; produce virulence factors such as endotoxins

> *C. amalonaticus;* colonizes humans or associated with human infections.
> *C. braakii*
> *C. farmeri*
> *C. freundii,* type species ATCC 8090, NCTC 9750; colonizes humans or associated with human infections; some strains resemble *Salmonella* biochemically and agglutinate in *Salmonella* polyvalent O antiserum; may be incorrectly identified as *Salmonella* spp.
> *C. koseri* (*C. diversus*); colonizes humans or associated with human infections
> *C. rodentium*
> *C. sedlakii*
> *C. werkmanii*
> *C. youngae*

Edwardsiella: 4 species; opportunistic pathogen; produces virulence factors such as endotoxins

    E. anguillimortifera
    E. hoshinae
    E. ictaluri
    E. tarda, type species ATCC 15947; colonizes humans or associated with human infections

Enterobacter: 13 species; opportunistic pathogen; produces virulence factors such as endotoxins

    E. aerogenes; colonizes humans or associated with human infections
    E. amnigenus; colonizes humans or associated with human infections
    E. asburiae
    E. cancerogenus (*E. taylorae*); colonizes humans or associated with human infections
    E. cloacae, type species ATCC 13047; colonizes humans or associated with human infections
    E. dissolvens
    E. gergoviae; colonizes humans or associated with human infections
    E. hormaechei
    E. intermedius
    E. kobei
    E. nimipressuralis
    E. pyrinus
    E. sakazakii; colonizes humans or associated with human infections.

Erwinia: 10 species; primarily colonizes plants; rarely isolated from humans.

    E. amylovora, type species ATCC 15580
    E. aphidicola
    E. billingiae
    E. carnegieana
    E. mallotivora
    E. persicinus
    E. psidii
    E. pyrifoliae
    E. rhapontici
    E. tracheiphila

Escherichia: 5 species

    E. blattae
    E. coli, type species ATCC 1175, NCTC 9001; colonizes humans or associated with human infections; *E. coli* is subdivided by virulence factors such as entotoxins, invasiness, colonization: *E. coli* (ETEC) enterotoxigenic, *E. coli* (EIEC) enteroinvasive, *E. coli* (EPEC) enteropathogenic, *E. coli* (EHEC) enterohemorrhagic, *E. coli* (EAEC) enteroaggregative
    E. fergusonii
    E. hermannii
    E. vulneris

Ewingella: (not in *Bergey's Manual;* created by Grimont PAD et al. (4); similar to genus Cedecea; infrequent opportunistic pathogen.

Single species, *E. americana;* ATCC 33852

Hafnia; opportunistic pathogen; produces virulence factors such as endotoxins

Single species, *H. alvei;* ATCC 13337, NCTC 8105

Klebsiella: 7 species; opportunistic pathogen; produces virulence factors such as endotoxins

> *K. ornithinolytica*
> *K. oxytoca;* colonizes humans or associated with human infections
> *K. planticola*
> *K. pneumoniae* subsp. *ozaenae;* colonizes humans or associated with human infections
> *K. pneumoniae* subsp. *pneumoniae,* type species ATCC 13883, NCTC 9633; colonizes humans or associated with human infections
> *K. pneumoniae* subsp. *rhinoscleromatis*
> *K. terrigena*

Kluyvera: 4 species; similar to *Buttiauxella* spp.; infrequent opportunistic pathogen

> *K. ascorbata,* type species ATCC 33433
> *K. cochleae;* colonizes humans or associated with human infections
> *K. cryocrescens*
> *K. georgiana*

Leclercia: not in *Bergey's Manual;* created by Tamura et al. (5); infrequent opportunistic pathogen

Single species, *L. adecarboxylata* (*Escherichia adecarboxylata*); ATCC 23216

Leminorella: 2 species not in *Bergey's Manual;* created by Hickman-Brenner et al. (6)

> *L. grinontii,* type species ATCC 33999
> *L. richardii*

Moellerella: not in *Bergey's Manual;* created by Hickman-Brenner et al. (6)

Single species, *M. wisconsensis;* ATCC 35017

Morganella: 2 species

> *M. morganii* subsp. *morganii;* type species ATCC 25830; colonizes humans or associated with human infections
> *M. morganii* subsp. *sibonii*

Obesumbacterium; brewery contaminant

Single species, *O. proteus*; ATCC 12841, NCTC 8771

Pantoea: 8 species not in *Bergey's Manual;* created by Gavini et al. (7); opportunistic pathogen

> *P. agglomerans*, type species ATCC 27155, NCTC 9381; colonizes humans or associated with human infections
> *P. ananatis*
> *P. citrea*
> *P. dispersa*
> *P. punctata*
> *P. stewartii* subsp. *indologenes*
> *P. stewartii* subsp. *stewartii*
> *P. terrea*

Photorhabdus

Single species, *P. luminescens*; ATCC 29999

Plesiomonas

Single species, *P. shigelloides*; ATCC 14029

Pragia: not in *Bergey's Manual;* created by Aldová et al. (8)

Single species, *P. fontium*; CDC 963–84

Proteus: 4 species; opportunistic pathogen; produces virulence factors such as endotoxins

> *P. mirabilis*; colonizes humans or associated with human infections
> *P. myxofaciens*
> *P. penneri*; colonizes humans or associated with human infections
> *P. vulgaris*, type species ATCC 13315, NCTC 4175; colonizes humans or associated with human infections

Providencia: 5 species

> *P. alcalifaciens*; type species; ATCC 9886
> *P. heimbachae*
> *P. rettgeri*
> *P. rustigianii*
> *P. stuartii*

Rahnella

Single species, *R. aquatilis*; ATCC 33071

Saccharobacter

Single species, *S. fermentatus*; WVB 8512

Salmonella: 10 species; all serotypes colonize humans or are associated with human infections

>   S. bongori
>   S. choleraesuis subsp. *arizonae*
>   S. choleraesuis subsp. *choleraesuis*, type species ATCC 13312, ATCC 13314, NCTC 5735
>   S. choleraesuis subsp. *diazonae*
>   S. choleraesuis subsp. *houtenae*
>   S. choleraesuis subsp. *indica*
>   S. choleraesuis subsp. *salamae*
>   S. enteritidis
>   S. typhi
>   S. typhimurium

Serratia: 10 species; opportunistic pathogen; produces virulence factors such as endotoxins

>   S. entomophila
>   S. ficaria
>   S. fonticola
>   S. grimesii
>   S. marcescens, type species ATCC 13880; colonizes humans or associated with human infections
>   S. odorifera
>   S. plymuthica
>   S. proteamaculans subsp. *proteamaculans* (*S. liquefaciens*); colonizes humans or associated with human infections
>   S. proteamaculans subsp. *quinovora*
>   S. rubidaea

Shigella: 4 species; overt pathogen, all species cause dysentery

>   S. boydii
>   S. dysenteriae, type species ATCC 13313
>   S. flexneri
>   S. sonnei

Tatumella

Single species, *T. ptyseos*; ATCC 33301

Trabulsiella

Single species, *T. guamensis*; ATCC 49490

Wigglesworthia; found in tsetse flies

Single species, *W. glossinidia*

Xenorhabdus: 5 species

>   X. beddingii
>   X. bovienii

X. *japonicus*
  X. *nematophilus*, type species ATCC 19061
  X. *poinarii*

Yersinia: 11 species

  Y. *aldovae*
  Y. *bercovieri*
  Y. *enterocolitica;* colonizes humans or associated with human infections
  Y. *frederiksenii;* colonizes humans or associated with human infections
  Y. *intermedia;* colonizes humans or associated with human infections
  Y. *kristensenii*
  Y. *mollaretii*
  Y. *pestis,* type species ATCC 19428, NCTC 5923; colonizes humans or associated with human infections; overt pathogen, causative agent of "black" plague.
  Y. *pseudotuberculosis;* colonizes humans or associated with human infections
  Y. *rohdei*
  Y. *ruckeri*

Yokenella: not in *Bergey's Manual;* created by Kosako et al. (9); biochemically similar to *Hafnia*

Single species, Y. *regensburgei*
(Outline courtesy of Dr. George Garrity, Editor-in-Chief, Bergey's Manual Trust)

REFERENCES

1. Werren et al. Int J Syst Bacteriol 1991;41(3): 563–564.
2. Aldova EK, et al. Zentralbl Bakteriol Parasitenkd Infektionskr Hyg Abt I. Orig, Reihe 1983; A254:95–108. Validated by Bouvet OMM, et al. Int J Syst Bacteriol 1985;35(2):60–64.
3. Ferragut CD, et al. Int J Syst Bacteriol 1982;32(2):266–268.
4. Grimont PAD, et al. Int J Syst Bacteriol 1984;34(1):91–92.
5. Tamura K et al. Int J Syst Bacteriol 1987;37(2): 179–180.
6. Hickman-Brenner FW, et al. Int J Syst Bacteriol 1984;34(3):355–357. Hickman-Brenner FW, et al. Int J Syst Bacteriol 1985;35(2):375–376.
7. Gavini F, et al. Int J Syst Bacteriol 1989;39(3): 337–345.
8. Aldová EK, et al. Int J Syst Bacteriol 1988;38(2):183–189.
9. Kosako Y, et al. Int J Syst Bacteriol 1985;35(2): 223–224.

ENTEROBACTERIACEAE GENERAL CHARACTERISTICS

  Gram-negative straight rods (bacilli)
  Nonsporeforming
  Facultative anaerobic
  Catalase variable, usually positive
  Capsule variable
  Motility variable; if positive, peritrichous flagella; **except** *Tatumella,* lateral flagella
  Oxidase negative
  O/F glucose: F (fermentative) or both F and O (oxidative)
  Optimal growth temperature: 37°C
  Nitrate reduction: variable, usually positive
  MacConkey (MAC) growth; **except** *Arsenophonus nasoniae*

MEDIA FOR ISOLATION AND DIFFERENTIATION OF *ENTEROBACTERIACEAE*

Table 45.1. Media for Isolation and Differentiation of *Enterobacteriaceae*[a]

Agar Plate Media[b]	Carbohydrate(s) Present[c]	H$_2$S Indicator	pH Indicator	Incubation (h)	Colonies LF (RLF)[e]	Colonies NLF[e]
Selective isolation						
Bismuth sulfite agar (BS, BSA)[f]	Glucose	+	None[g]	18–24	Generally inhibited; if growth: brownish green color	*S. typhi*: jet black surrounded by wide brownish black zones w/wo metallic sheen; other *Salmonella* spp. green-black colonies, no zones surrounding colonies; *Shigella* spp.: green-brown
Brilliant green (BG, BGA)[h]	Lactose, Sucrose[c]	–	Phenol red	48	Yellow–greenish yellow surrounded by an intense yellow-green zone	Red-pink-white, opaque, surrounded by an intense brilliant red zone
Salmonella-Shigella (SS)[i]	Lactose	+	Neutral red	18–24	Coliforms: colorless with pink centers; others: pink-red	Colorless w/wo black centers
Xylose-lysine-desoxycholate (XLD)[j]	Lactose,[c] Sucrose,[c] Xylose[e]	+[k]	Phenol red	18–24	Yellow, opaque	Red-pink w/wo black centers
Differential						
Eosin-methylene blue (EMB)[j]	Lactose, sucrose[c]	–	Eosin Y, methylene blue[m]	18–24	*E. coli*: dark blue-black to brownish w/wo green metallic sheen[n]; may have dark centers with amber colorless peripheries	Colorless or transparent amber (light purple) color
Desoxycholate citrate (DC) (Leifson's)	Lactose	+	Neutral red	18–24	Pink-red, opaque Often surrounded by red zone w/wo black centers	Transparent to colorless to light pink or tan, w/wo black centers
Desoxycholate citrate lactose (DCL)	Lactose	+	Neutral red	18–24		

Table 45.1. Media for Isolation and Differentiation of Enterobacteriaceae[a]

Agar Plate Media[b]	Carbohydrate(s) Present[c]	H$_2$S Indicator	pH Indicator	Incubation (h)	Colonies LF (RLF)[e]	Colonies NLF[e]
Deoxycholate citrate lactose sucrose (DCLS) (Leifson)[o]	Lactose, sucrose[c]	+	Neutral red	18–24	See DCL	See DCL
Deoxycholate citrate lactose sucrose (DCLS) (Hajna and Damon)	Lactose, sucrose[c]	+	Bromcresol purple (BCP)	18–24	Transparent, translucent, or opaque bluish colonies	Yellow to white, opaque, translucent[p]
Hektoen enteric agar (HE, HEA, HEK)	Lactose, sucrose[c] salicin[c]	+	Bromthymol blue (BTB), acid fuchsin[q]	18–24	Yellow to salmon colored	*Proteus*: blue-green to blue or salmon colored, most with black centers
MacConkey (MC, MAC)	Lactose	–	Neutral red	18–24	Brick red to pink-red	Colorless or slightly yellow

[a]Differentiation primarily by carbohydrate(s) utilization with pH changes; H$_2$S production incidental and **not** always evident on plate media: use KIA/TSI/LIA for H$_2$S results.
[b]All plate media contain various dyes that usually inhibit most Gram-positive bacteria.
[c]A non-lactose fermenter may give a false-positive indication of lactose fermentation if other carbohydrate(s) are present that can be utilized (e.g., sucrose by *Proteus vulgaris*).
[d]Possible H$_2$S indicators: iron (II) sulfate, iron (III) citrate, sodium thiosulfate, iron (III) citrate and ammonium citrate), and iron (III) ammonium sulfate.
[e]LF: lactose-fermenter; RLF: rapid lactose fermenter; NFL, non-lactose fermenter.
[f]Wilson and Blair medium; highly selective; coliforms largely inhibited and *Shigella* spp. may be inhibited; recommended for isolation of *Salmonella typhi* and other enterics.
[g]Brilliant green incorporated along with a heavy metal, bismuth sulfite, as inhibitors.
[h]Highly selective; recommended for isolation of *Salmonella* spp. **other than** *S. typhi*; also **not** for isolation of *Shigella* spp.; reddish-brown colored medium which becomes bright red during incubation and returns to normal color at room temperature (22–25°C).
[i]Generally inhibitory to coliforms.
[j]Recommended for isolation of enteric pathogens, especially *Shigella* spp. and *Providencia* spp.
[k]Incubation for 48 h increases visibility of H$_2$S black centers by *Salmonella*; however, incubation period exceeding 48 h may lead to false-positive results.
[l]Most frequently used medium of Levine contains **only** lactose; Holt-Harris and Teague medium contains lactose and sucrose.
[m]Two aniline dyes combine to form a precipitate at acid pH; dyes act both as differential indicators and inhibitors.
[n]Blue-black with transmitted light; metallic sheen by reflected light.
[o]Recommended for isolation of *Salmonella* and *Shigella* spp. and cholera vibrio; *Alcaligenes* and some *Proteus/Providencia* spp. may be inhibited.
[p]Sucrose fermenters.
[q]See Table 45.2.

Table 45.2. Andrade's Indicator

Dye	Acid	Alkaline
Acid fuchsin (Andrade's indicator)	pinkish red (pH 5.0)	Red (pH 12.0) to colorless (pH 14.0) Pale yellow (pH 8.0)
Bromcresol purple	Yellow (pH 5.2)	Purple (pH 6.8)
Bromthymol blue	Yellow (pH 6.0)	Deep Prussian blue (pH 7.6)
Neutral red	Red (pH 6.8)	Yellow (pH 8.0)
Phenol red	Yellow (pH 6.8)	Red (pH 8.4)

Table 45.3. KIA/TSI Reactions of Most *Enterobacteriaceae* (All Glucose Positive (A, Acid))[a]

Microorganism	Gas, Glu	Lac	Suc	H$_2$S	KIA	TSI
Arsenophonus nasoniae	–	–	A	–	ALK/A	A/A
Budvicia aquatica	V	V$^+$	–	V$^+$	A/A	A/A
					A/A, H$_2$S	A/A, H$_2$S
					ALK/A	ALK/A
					ALK/A, H$_2$S	ALK/A, H$_2$S
Buttiauxella agretis	+	A	–	–	A/A	A/A
Cedecea davisae	V	V$^-$	A	–	A/A	A/A
					ALK/A	
C. lapagei	+	V	–	–	A/A	A/A
					ALK/A	ALK/A
C. neteri	+	V	A	–	A/A	A/A
					ALK/A	
Cedecea species 3	+	–	V	–	ALK/A	A/A
						ALK/A
Cedecea species 5	+	–	A	–	ALKA	A/A
Citrobacter amalonaticus	+	V	V$^-$	–	A/A	A/A
					ALK/A	ALK/A
C. amalonaticus biogroup 1	+	V$^-$	A	–	A/A	A/A
					ALK/A	
C. freundii	+	V	V	V$^+$	A/A	A/A
					ALK/A	ALK/A
					A/A, H$_2$S	A/A, H$_2$S
					ALK/A, H$_2$S	ALK/A, H$_2$S
C. koseri	+	V	V	–	A/A	A/A
					ALK/A	ALK/A
Edwardsiella hoshinae	V	–	A	–	ALK/A	A/A
E. ictaluri	V	–	–	–	ALK/A	ALK/A
E. tarda	+	–	–	+	ALK/A, H$_2$S	ALK/A, H$_2$S
E. tarda biogroup 1	V	–	A	–	ALK/A	A/A
Enterobacter aerogenes	+	A	A	–	A/A	A/A
					ALK/A	ALK/A
E. amnigenus biogroup 1	+	V	A	–	A/A	A/A
					ALK/A	
E. amnigenus biogroup 2	+	V	–	–	A/A	A/A
					ALK/A	ALK/A
E. asburiae	+	V$^+$	A	–	A/A	A/A
					ALK/A	
E. cancerogenus	–	–	–	–	ALK/A	ALK/A
E. cloacae	+	A	A	–	A/A	A/A
E. dissolvens	+	V	A	–	A/A	A/A
					ALK/A	
E. gergoviae	+	V	A	–	A/A	A/A
					ALK/A	
E. hormaechae	V$^+$	–	A	–	ALK/A	A/A
E. intermedius	+	A	V	–	A/A	A/A
E. nimipressuralis	+	A	–	–	A/A	A/A
E. sakazakii	+	A	A	–	A/A	A/A
Escherichia blattae	+	–	–	–	ALK/A	ALK/A

(continued)

Table 45.3. KIA/TSI Reactions of Most *Enterobacteriaceae* (All Glucose Positive (A, Acid))[a] (*continued*)

Microorganism	Gas, Glu	Lac	Suc	H_2S	KIA	TSI
E. coli	+	A	V	−	A/A	A/A
E. coli inactive	−	V−	V−	−	A/A	A/A
					ALK/A	ALK/A
E. fergusonii	+	−	−	−	ALK/A	ALK/A
E. hermannii		V	V	−	A/A	A/A
					ALK/A	ALK/A
E. vulneris	+	V−	−	−	A/A	A/A
Ewingella americana	−	V	−	−	A/A	A/A
					ALK/A	ALK/A
Hafnia alvei	+	−	−	−	ALK/A	ALK/A
H. alvei biogroup 1	−	−	−	−	ALK/A	ALK/A
Klebsiella ornithinolytica	+	A	A	−	A/A	A/A
K. oxytoca	+	A	A	−	A/A	A/A
K. planticola	+	A	A	−	A/A	A/A
K. pneumoniae subsp. ozaenae	V	V	V−	−	A/A	A/A
					ALK/A	ALK/A
K. pneumoniae subsp. pneumoniae	+	A	A−	−	A/A	A/A
K. pneumoniae subsp. rhinoscleromatis	−	−	V+	−	Alk/A	A/A
						Alk/A
K. terrigena	V+	A	A	−	A/A	A/A
Kluyvera ascorbata	+	A	A	−	A/A	A/A
K. cryocrescens	+	A	V+	−	A/A	A/A
					ALK/A	ALK/A
Leclerica (Escherichia) adecarboxylata	+	A	V	−	A/A	A/A
Leminorella grimontii		−	−	+	ALK/A, H_2S	ALK/A, H_2S
L. richardii	−	−	−	+	ALK/A, H_2S	ALk/A, H_2S
Mollerella wisconsensis	−	A	A	−	A/A	A/A
Morganella morganii subsp. moraginii biogroup 1	+	−	−	−	ALK/A	ALK/A
M. morganii subsp. morganii biogroup 2	+	−	−	V	ALK/A	ALK/A
					ALK/A, H_2S	ALK/A, H_2S
Obesumbacterium proteus	−	−	−	−	ALK/A	ALK/A
Pantoea agglomerans	−	V−	A	−	A/A	A/A
					ALK/A	
P. dispersa	−	−	A	−	ALK/A	A/A
Plesiomonas shigelloides	−	A	−	−	A/A	A/A
Pragia fontium	−	−	−	V+	ALK/A	ALK/A
					ALK/A, H_2S	ALK/A, H_2S
Proteus inconstans	V+	−	V−	−	ALK/A	A/A
P. mirabilis	+	−	V−	+	ALK/A, H_2S	A/A, H_2S
						ALK/A, H_2S
P. myxofaciens	+	−	A	−	ALK/A	A/A
P. penneri	V	−	A	V	ALK/A	A/A
					ALK/A, H_2S	A/A, H_2S
P. vulgaris	V+	−	A	+	ALK/A, H_2S	A/A, H_2S
						ALK/A

(*continued*)

Table 45.3. KIA/TSI Reactions of Most *Enterobacteriaceae* (All Glucose Positive (A, Acid))[a] *(continued)*

Microorganism	Gas, Glu	Lac	Suc	H$_2$S	KIA	TSI
Providencia heimbachae	−	−	−	−	ALK/A	ALK/A
P. rettgeri	−	−	V$^-$	−	ALK/A	A/A
P. rustigianii	V	−	V	−	ALK/A	A/A
						ALK/A
P. stuartii	−	−	V	−	ALK/A	A/A
						ALK/A
Rahnella aquatilis	−	A	A	−	A/A	A/A
Salmonella bongori	V$^+$	−	−	+	ALK/A, H$_2$S	ALK/A, H$_2$S
S. choleraesuis subsp. *arizonae*	+	V$^-$	−	+	A/A, H$_2$S	A/A, H$_2$S
					ALK/A, H$_2$S	ALK/A, H$_2$S
S. choleraesius subsp. *choleraesuis*	+	−	−	+	ALK/A, H$_2$S	ALK/A, H$_2$S
S. choleraesuis subsp. *diarizonae*	+	V$^+$	−	+	A/A, H$_2$S	A/A, H$_2$S
					ALK/A, H$_2$S	ALK/A, H$_2$S
S. choleraesuis subsp. *houtenae*	+	−	−	+	ALK/A, H$_2$S	ALK/A, H$_2$S
S. choleraesuis subsp. *indica*	+	V$^-$	−	+	A/A, H$_2$S	A/A, H$_2$S
					ALK/A, H$_2$S	ALK/A, H$_2$S
S. choleraesuis subsp. *salamae*	+	−	−	+	ALK/A, H$_2$S	ALK/A, H$_2$S
S. choleraesuis serovar *choleraesuis*	+	−	−	V	ALK/A	ALK/A
					ALK/A, H$_2$S	ALK/A, H$_2$S
S. choleraesuis serovar *gallinarum*	−	−	−	+	ALK/A, H$_2$S	ALK/A, H$_2$S
S. choleraesuis serovar *paratyphi* A	+	−	−	V$^-$	ALK/A	ALK/A
					ALK/A, H$_2$S	ALK/A, H$_2$S
S. choleraesuis serovar *pullorum*	+	−	−	+	ALK/S, H$_2$S	ALK/A, H$_2$S
S. choleraesuis serovar *typhi*	−	−	−	+	ALK/A, H$_2$S	ALK/A, H$_2$S
Serratia entomophila	−	−	A	−	ALK/A	A/A
S. ficaria	−	V$^-$	A	−	A/A	A/A
					ALK/A	
S. fonticola	V$^+$	A	V$^-$	−	A/A	A/A
S. grimesii	+	−	A	−	ALK/A	A/A
S. marcescens	V	−	A	−	ALK/A	A/A
S. odorifera biogroup 1	−	V	A	−	A/A	A/A
S. odorifera biogroup 2	V$^-$	A	−	−	A/A	A/A
S. plymuthica	V	V$^+$	A	−	A/A	A/A
					ALK/A	
S. proteamaculans subsp. *proteamaculans*	−	−	A	−	ALK/A	A/A
S. rubidaea	V	A	A	−	A/A	A/A
Shigella spp.	−	−	−	−	ALK/A	ALK/A
Tatumella ptyseos	−	−	A	−	ALK/A	A/A
Yersinia aldovae	−	−	V$^-$	−	A/A	A/A
					ALK/A	
Y. bercovieri	−	V$^-$	A	−	A/A	A/A
					ALK/A	
Y. enterocolitica	−	−	A	−	ALK/A	A/A
Y. frederiksonii	V	V	A	−	A/A	A/A
					ALK/A	
Y. intermedia	V$^-$	−	−	−	A/A	A/A
					ALK/A	
Y. kristensinii	V$^-$	−	−	−	ALK/A	ALK/A
Y. mollaretii	−	V	A	−	A/A	A/A
					ALK/A	

(continued)

Table 45.3. KIA/TSI Reactions of Most *Enterobacteriaceae* (All Glucose Positive (A, Acid))[a] (*continued*)

Microorganism	Gas, Glu	Lac	Suc	H$_2$S	KIA	TSI
Y. pestis	−	−	−	−	ALK/A	ALK/A
Y. pseudotuberculosis	−	−	−	−	ALK/A	ALK/A
Y. rohdei	−	−	A	−	ALK/A	A/A
Y. ruckeri	−	−	−	−	ALK/A	ALK/A
Yokenella (Koserella) regensburgei	+	−	−	−	ALK/A	ALK/A
Enteric groups						
63	+	−	−	−	ALK/A	ALK/A
64	V	A	−	−	A/A	A/A
68	−	−	A	−	ALK/A	A/A

[a]Except genera *Erwinia* and *Xenorhabdus*.

KIA/TSI REACTIONS OF MOST ENTEROBACTERIACEAE

WARNING

When using the identification tables be aware that the results noted have been compiled from the references cited. However, living microorganisms often give conflicting results because of mutation or the media used for isolation, cultivation, identification, and maintenance.

Often proper identification to genus or genus and species requires considering (*a*) the clinical specimen/source, (*b*) Gram stain morphology, and (*c*) cultural characteristics (e.g., pigmentation, hemolysis) along with biochemical tests. In some cases, serologic and toxin testing are required for confirmation.

Be flexible when interpreting biochemical results. All microorganisms do not necessarily exhibit all the results of the battery of biochemical tests in the tables. At times "best fit" is necessary for identification. The more test results, the better the chance of correct identification.

ACID/ACID, WITH/WITHOUT GAS

Table 45.4. Biochemical Reactions of *Enterobacteriaceae* with a KIA/TSI Reaction of Acid/Acid, with/without Gas

Test	*Arsonophonus nasoniae*[a]	*Budvicia aquatica*[b]	*Buttiauxella agrestis*[c]	*Cedecea davisae*[d]	*Cedecea lapagei*[e]	*Cedecea neteri*	*Cedecea species 3*[f]
Catalase, 24 h	+	+	+	+	+	+	NR
Oxidase	−	−	−	−	−	−	−
NO₃→NO₂	−	+	+	+	+	+	+
O-F glucose	F	F	F	F	F	F	F
H₂S (KIA/TSI)	−	V⁺	−	−	−	−	−
KIA	ALK/A	A/A, A/A, H₂S ALK/A, H₂S	A/A	A/A ALK/A	A/A ALK/A	A/A ALK/A	ALK/A
TSI	A/A	A/A A/A, H₂S ALK/A	A/A	A/A	A/A ALK/A	A/A	A/A ALK/A
Carbohydrate fermentations							
Glucose & gas	A	Ⓐ	Ⓐ	Ⓐ	Ⓐ	Ⓐ	A
Lactose	−	V⁺	A	V⁻	V	V	−
Sucrose	A	−	−	A	−	A	V
Adonitol		−	−	−	−	−	−
L-Arabinose	−	V⁺	A	−	−	−	−
D-Arabitol	NR	V	−	−	−	−	−
Cellobiose	−	−	A	A	A	A	A
Dulcitol	−	−	−	−	−	−	−
Erythritol	NR	−	−	−	−	−	−
Glycerol	−	−	V	−	−	−	−
myo-Inositol	−	−	−	−	−	−	−
Maltose	−	−	A	A	A	A	A
D-Mannitol	−	V	A	A	A	A	A
D-Mannose	NR	−	A	A	A	A	A
Melibiose	NR	−	A	−	−	−	A
α-Methyl-D-Glucoside	NR	−	−	−	−	−	V
Mucate	NR	V⁻	A	−	−	−	−
Raffinose	−	−	A	V⁻	−	−	A
L-Rhamnose	−	A	A	−	−	−	−
Salicin	NR	−	A	A	A	A	A
D-Sorbitol	NR	−	−	−	−	A	−
Trehalose	−	−	A	A	A	A	A
D-Xylose	−	A	A	A	−	A	A
IMViC Reactions							
Indole	−	−	−	−	−	−	−
Methyl red (MR)	−	+	+	+	V	+	+
Voges-Proskauer (VP)	−	−	−	V	V⁺	V	V
Citrate (Simmons)	NR	−	+	+	+	+	+
Decarboxylase/dihydrolase reactions							
Arginine dihydrolase	−	−	−	V	V⁺	+	+
Lysine decarboxylase	−	−	−	−	−	−	−
Ornithine decarboxylase	−	−	+	+	−	−	−
Urea/phenylalanine reactions							
Urease (Christensen's)	NG	V	−	−	−	−	−
Phenylalanine deaminase 24 h	NR	−	−	−	−	−	−
Misc. reactions							
Acetate use	NR	−	−	−	V	−	V
DNase, 25°C	NG	−	−	−	−	−	−
Esculin hydrolysis	−	−	+	V	+	+	+
Gelatin liquefaction, 22°C	+	−	−	−	−	−	−
Gluconate	NR	NR	+	NR	NR	NR	NR
KCN broth-growth	NR	−	V⁺	V⁺	+	V	+
Lipase (corn oil)	NR	−	−	+	+	+	+
Malonate utilization	−	−	V	+	+	+	−
ONPG	NR	+	+	+	+	+	+
Tartrate, Jordon	NR	V	V	−	−	−	−
Motility, 36°C/flagella	−	Vp[aa]	+p	+p	Vp	+p	+p
Pigmentation	−	−	−	−	−	−	−

Chapter 45 / Gram-Negative Enterobacteriaceae

	Cedecea species 5	Citrobacter amalonaticus	Citrobacter amalonaticus biogroup 1	Citrobacter koseri	Citrobacter freundii	Edwardsiella hoshinae	Edwardsiella ictaluri	Edwardsiella taerda biogroup 1	Enterobacter aerogenes	Enterobacter amnigenus biogroup 1	Enterobacter amnigenus biogroup 2	Enterobacter asburiae	Enterobacter cloacae
	NR	+	+	+	+	+	+	+	+	+	+	+	+
	−	−	−	−	−	−	−	−	−	−	−	−	−
	+	+	+	+	+	+	+	+	+	+	+	+	+
	F	F	F	F	F	F	F	F	F	F	F	F	F
	−	−	−	−	V+	−	−	−	−	−	−	−	−
	ALK/A	A/A ALK/A	A/A ALK/A	A/A ALK/A	A/A A/A, H_2S	ALK/A	ALK/A	ALK/A	A/A	A/A ALK/A	A/A ALK/A	A/A ALK/A	A/A A/A
	A/A	A/A ALK/A	A/A	A/A ALK/A	ALK/A ALK/A, H_2S A/A A/A, H_2S ALK/A ALK/A, H_2S	A/A	ALK/A	A/A	A/A	A/A	A/A ALK/A	A/A	
	Ⓐ	Ⓐ	Ⓐ	Ⓐ	Ⓐ	Ⓐ	Ⓐ	Ⓐ	Ⓐ	Ⓐ	Ⓐ	Ⓐ	Ⓐ
	−	V	V	V	V	−	−	−	A	V	V	V+	A
	A	V−	A	V−	Vw	A	−	A	A	A	−	A	A
	−	−	−	A	−	−	−	−	A	−	−	−	V−
	−	A	A	A	A	V−	−	−	A	A	A	A	A
	−	−	−	−	−	−	−	−	A	−	−	−	−
	A	A	A	A	V	−	−	−	A	A	A	A	A
	−	−	−	V	V	−	−	−	−	−	−	−	V−
	−	−	−	A	−	−	−	−	−	−	−	−	−
	−	V	V	A	A	V	−	−	A	−	−	V−	V
	−	−	−	−	−	−	−	−	A	−	−	−	V−
	A	A	A	A	A	A	A	A	A	A	A	A	A
	A	A	A	A	A	A	−	A	A	A	A	A	A
	A	A	A	A	A	A	A	A	A	A	A	A	A
	−	−	A	−	V	−	−	−	A	A	A	−	A
	−	−	V	V	−	−	−	−	A	V	A	A	V+
	−	A	A	A	−	−	−	−	A	V	A	V−	V+
	A	−	A	−	A	−	−	−	A	−	−	V	A
	−	A	A	A	V	A	−	−	A	A	A	−	A
	Aw	Vw	−	V−x	A	V	−	−	A	A	A	A	V+
	A	A	A	A	A	−	−	−	A	−	A	A	V+
	A	A	A	A	A	A	A	−	A	A	A	A	A
	A	A	A	A	A	−	−	−	A	A	A	A	A
	−	+	+	+	−	V	−	+	−	−	V	−	−
	+	+	+	+	+	+	−	+	−	−	−	+	−
	V	−	−	−	−	−	−	−	+	+	+	−	+
	+	V+	−	+	+	−	−	−	+	V	+	+	+
	V	V+	V+	Vw	V	−	−	−	−	−	V	V−	+
	−	−	−	−	−	+	+	+	+	+	+	−	−
	V	+	+	+	V−	+	V	+	+	+	+	+	+
	−	V	V	V	Vw	−	−	−	−	−	−	V	Vw
	−	−	−	−	−	−	−	−	−	−	−	−	−
	V	V+	V+	V+	V+	−	−	−	V	−	−	V+	V+
	−	−	−	−	−	−	−	−	−	−	−	−	−
	+	−	−	−	−	−	−	−	+	+	+	−	V−
	NR	+	NR	NR	−	−	NR	NR	+	NR	NR	NR	+
	+	+	+	−	+	−	−	−	+	+	+	+	+
	V	−	−	−	−	−	−	−	−	−	−	−	−
	−	−	−	+	V−	+	−	−	+	+	+	−	V
	+	+	+	+	+	−	−	−	+	+	+	+	+
	−	V+	V+	V+	+	−	−bb	−	+	−	−	V−	V−
	+p	+p	+p	+p	+p	+p		+	+p	+p	+p	−	+p
	−	−	−	−	−	−		−	−	−	−	−	−

Table 45.4. Biochemical Reactions of *Enterobacteriaceae* with a KIA/TSI Reaction of Acid/Acid, with/without Gas (*continued*)

Test	*Enterobacter dissolvens*	*Enterobacter gergoviae*	*Enterobacter hormaechae*	*Enterobacter intermedius*	*Enterobacter nimipressuralis*	*Enterobacter sakazakii*	*Erwinia amylovora*[g]
Catalase, 24 hr	+	+	+	+	+	+	+
Oxidase	−	−	−	−	−	−	−
NO$_3$→NO$_2$	+	+	+	+	+	+	−
O-F glucose	F	F	F	F	F	F	F
H$_2$S (KIA/TSI)	−	−	−	−	−	−	−
KIA	A/A ALK/A	A/A ALK/A	ALK/A	A/A	A/A	A/A	ALK/A
TSI	A/A	A/A	A/A	A/A	A/A	A/A	A/A
Carbohydrate fermentations							
Glucose & gas	Ⓐ	Ⓐ	Ⓐ	Ⓐ	Ⓐ	Ⓐ	Ⓐ
Lactose	V	V	−	A	A	A	−
Sucrose	A	A	A	V	−	A	A
Adonitol	−	V	−	A	−	A	−
L-Arabinose	A	A	A	A	A	A	V
D-Arabitol	−	A	−	−	−	−	NR
Cellobiose	A	A	A	A	A	A	−
Dulcitol	−	−	V+	A	−	−	−
Erythritol	−	−	−	−	−	−	NR
Glycerol	−	A	−	A	A	V−	−
myo-Inositol	−	−		−	−	V+	−
Maltose	A	A	A	A	A	A	−
D-Mannitol	A	A	A	A	A	A	−
D-Mannose	A	A	A	A	A	A	−
Melibiose	A	A	−	A	A	A	−
α-Methyl-D-Glucoside	A	−	V	A	A	A	−
Mucate	A	−	A	A	A	−	NR
Raffinose	A	A	−	A	−	A	−
L-Rhamnose	A	A	A	A	A	A	−
Salicin	A	A	V	A	A	A	−
D-Sorbitol	A	−	−	A	A	−	V
Trehalose	A	A	A	A	A	A	A
D-Xylose	A	A	A	A	A	A	−
IMViC reactions							
Indole	−	−	−	−	−	V	−
Methyl red (MR)	−	−	V	+	−	−	NR
Voges-Proskauer (VP)	+	+	+	+	+	+	+
Citrate (Simmons)	+	+	+	V	+	+	+
Decarboxylase/dihydrolase reactions							
Arginine dihydrolase	+	−	V+	−	+	+	−
Lysine decarboxylase	−	+[y]	−	−	−	−	−
Ornithine decarboxylase	+	+	+	V+	+	+	−
Urea/phenylalanine reactions							
Urease (Christensen's)	+	+	V+	−	−	−	−
Phenylalanine deaminase 24 h	−	−	−	−	−	V[z]	−
Misc. reactions							
Acetate use	+	+	V	−	−	+	+
DNase, 25°C	−	−	−	−	−	−	−
Esculin hydrolysis	+	+	−	+	+	+	NR
Gelatin liquefaction, 22°C	−	−	−	−	NR	−	+
Gluconate	NR	+	NR	NR	NR	+	NR
KCN broth-growth	+	−	+	V	+	+	NR
Lipase (corn oil)	V	−	−	−	−	−	NR
Malonate utilization	+	+	+	+	+	V	−
ONPG	+	+	+	+	+	+	NR
Tartrate, Jordon	−	+	V−	+	−	−	NR
Motility, 36°C/flagella	−p	+p	Vp	+p	+p	+	+p
Pigmentation	−	−	−	−	−	+y[dd]	−

	Erwinia persicinus[g]	*Escherichia coli*[h]	*Escherichia coli* inactive[i]	*Escherichia hermannii*	*Escherichia vulneris*	*Erwingella americana*[j]	*Klebsiella ornithemolytica*	*Klebsiella oxytoca*	*Klebsiella planticola*	*Klebsiella pneumoniae* subsp. *oxaenae*	*Klebsiella pneumoniae* subsp. *pneumoniae*[k,l]	*Klebsiella pneumoniae* subsp. *rhinoscleromatis*[l]	*Klebsiella terrigena*
	+	+	+	+	+	+	+	+	+	+	+	+	+
	−	−	−	−	−	−	−	−	−	−	−	−	−
	+	+	+	+	+	+	+	+	+	V+	+	+	+
	F	F	F	F	F	F	F	F	F	F	F	F	F
	−	−	−	−	−	−	−	−	−	−	−	−	−
	A/A	A/A	A/A, ALK/A	A/A, ALK/A	A/A, ALK/A	A/A, ALK/A	A/A	A/A	A/A	A/A, ALK/A	A/A	ALK/A	A/A
	A/A	A/A	A/A, ALK/A	A/A, ALK/A	A/A, ALK/A	A/A, ALK/A	A/A	A/A	A/A	A/A	A/A, ALK/A	A/A	A/A, ALK/A
	A	Ⓐ	A	Ⓐ	Ⓐ	A	Ⓐ	Ⓐ	Ⓐ	Ⓐ	Ⓐ	A	Ⓐ
	A	A^w	V−	V	V−	V	A	A	A	V−	A	−	A
	A	V	V−	V	−	−	A	A	A	V−	A	V	A
	−	−	−	−	−	−	A	A	A	A	A	A	A
	A	A	V+	A	A	−	A	A	A	A	A	A	A
	NR	−	−	−	−	A	A	A	A	A	A	A	A
	A	−	−	A	A	−	A	A	A	A	A	A	A
	−	V	V	V−	−	−	−	V	V−	−	V	−	V−
	NR	−	−	−	−	−	−	−	−	−	−	−	−
	A	V	V	−	V−	V−	A	A	A	V	A	V	A
	A	−	−	−	−	−	A	A	A	V	A	A	V+
	A	A	V+	A	A	V−	A	A	A	A	A	A	A
	A	A	A	A	A	A	A	A	A	A	A	A	A
	A	A	A	A	A	A	A	A	A	A	A	A	A
	A	V+	V	−	A	−	A	A	A	V	A	A	A
	−	−	−	−	V−	−	A	A	A	V	A	−	A
	NR	A	V	A	V+	−	A	A	A	V−	A	−	A
	A	V	V−	V	A	−	A	A	A	A	A	A	A
	A	V+	V	A	A	V−	A	A	A	V	A	A	A
	A	V	−	V	V	V+	A	A	A	A	A	A	A
	A	A	V+	−	−	−	A	A	A	V	A	A	A
	A	A	A	A	A	A	A	A	A	A	A	A	A
	−	A	V	A	A	A	A	A	A	A	A	A	A
	−	+	V+	+	−	−	+	+	V−	−	−	−	−
	NR	+	+	+	+	V+	+	V−	+	+	V−	+	V
	+	−	−	−	−	+	V	+	+	−	+	−	+
	+	−	−	−	−	+	+	+	+	V	+	−	V
	−	V−	−	−	V	−	−	−	−	−	−	−	−
	−	+	V	−	V+	−	+	+	+	V	+	−	+
	−	V	V−	+	−	−	−	−	−	−	−	−	V−
	−	−	−	−	−	−	+	+	+	−	+	−	−
	−	−	−	−	−	−	−	−	−	−	−	−	−
	−	+	V	V+	V	−	+	+	V	−	V+	−	V−
	−	−	−	−	−	−	−	−	−	−	−	−	−
	+	V	−	V	V−	V	+	+	+	V+	+	V	+
	NR	NR	NR	NR	NR	NR	NR	NR	NR	−	NR	−	+
	−	−	−	+	V−	−	+	+	+	+	V+	V+	+
	−	−	−	−	−	−	−	−	−	−	−	−	−
	+	−	−	−	V+	−	+	+	+	−	+	+	+
	+	+	V	+	+	V+	+	+	+	V+	+	−	+
	−	+	V+	V	V	−	+	+	+	V	+	V	+
	+p	+p	−	+p	+p	Vp	−	−	−	−	−	−	−
	+r	−	−	+y	Vy	−	−	−	−	−	−	−	−

Table 45.4. Biochemical Reactions of *Enterobacteriaceae* with a KIA/TSI Reaction of Acid/Acid, with/without Gas (*continued*)

Test	*Kluyvera asorbata*[m]	*Kluyvera cryocrescens*	*Leclercia adecarboxylata*	*Moellerella wisconsemsin*	*Pantoea agglomerans*	*Pantoea anamatis*	*Pantoea dispersa*[n]
Catalase, 24h	+	+	+	+	+	+	+
Oxidase	−	−	−	−	−	−	−
$NO_3 \rightarrow NO_2$	+	+	+	+	+	+	V
O-F glucose	F	F	F	F	F	F	F
H_2S (KIA/TSI)	−	−	−	−	−	−	−
KIA	A/A	A/A ALK/A	A/A	A/A	A/A ALK/A	A/A	ALK/A
TSI	A/A	A/A ALK/A	A/A	A/A	A/A	A/A	A/A
Carbohydrate fermentations							
Glucose & gas	Ⓐ	Ⓐ	Ⓐ	A	A	A	A
Lactose	A	V	A	A	V−	A	−
Sucrose	A	V+	V	A	A	NR	A
Adonitol	−	−	A	A	−	A	−
L-Arabinose	A	A	A	−	A	A	V
D-Arabitol	−	−	A	V	V	NR	NR
Cellobiose	A	A	A	−	V	A	V
Dulcitol	V−	−	V+	−	−	−	−
Erythritol	−	−	−	−	−	NR	−
Glycerol	V	−	−	−	−	A	V−
myo-Inositol	−	−	−	−	−	A	V
Maltose	A	A	A	V	A	A	A
D-Mannitol	A	A	A	V	A	A	A
D-Mannose	A	A	A	A	A	A	A
Melibiose	A	A	A	A	−	A	−
α-Methyl-D-Glucoside	A	A	−	−	−	−	−
Mucate	A	V+	A	−	−	NR	V
Raffinose	A	A	V	A	−	A	−
L-Rhamnose	A	A	A	−	A	A	A
Salicin	A	A	A	−	A	V	−
D-Sorbitol	V	V	−	−	−	A	−
Trehalose	A	A	A	−	A	A	A
D-Xylose	A	A	A	−	A	A	A
IMViC Reactions							
Indole	+	+	+	−	−	+	−
Methyl red (MR)	+	+	+	+	V	NR	V
Voges-Proskauer (VP)	−	−	−	−	+	+	+
Citrate (Simmons)	+	V+	−	V+	+	NR	+
Decarboxylase/dihydrolase reactions							
Arginine dihydrolase	−	−	−	−	−	−	−
Lysine decarboxylase	+	V−	−	−	−	−	−
Ornithine decarboxylase	+	+	−	−	V	−	−
Urea/phenylalanine reactions							
Urease (Christensen's)	−	−	V	−	−	−	−
Phenylalanine deaminase, 24h	−	−	−	−	V+	−	−
Misc. reactions							
Acetate use	V	V+	V−	−	−	NR	NR
DNase, 25°C	−	−	−	−	−	+	−
Esculin hydrolysis	+	+	+	−	+	NR	−
Gelatin liquefaction, 22°C	−	−	−	−	−	+	−
Gluconate	NR	NR	NR	NR	+	NR	+
KCN broth-growth	+	V+	+	V	V+	−	+
Lipase (corn oil)	−	−	−	−	NR	NR	NR
Malonate utilization	+	V+	+	−	+	NR	−
ONPG	+	+	+	+	+	NR	+
Tartrate, Jordon	V	V−	V+	V	−	NR	V
Motility, 36°C/flagella	+p	+p	Vp	−	+p	+p	+p
Pigmentation	−	−	+y	−	+y	+y	Vy

Proteus inconstans[o]	Proteus myxofaciens	Proteus penneri	Providencia heumbachae	Prouldencia rettgori	Providencia rustigianii	Providencia stuartii	Rahnella aquotilis	Serratia entomophila	Serratia ficaria	Serratia fonticola
+	+	+	+	+	+	+	+	+	+	+
−	−	−	−	−	−	−	−	−	−	−
+	+	+	+	+	+	+	+	+	+	+
F	F	F	F	F	F	F	F	F	F	F
−	−	V	−	−	−	−	−	−	−	−
ALK/A	ALK/A	ALK/A ALK/A, H₂S	ALK/A	ALK/A	ALK/A	ALK/A	A/A	ALK/A	A/A ALK/A	A/A
A/A ALK/A	A/A	A/A A/A, H₂S	A/A ALK/A	A/A ALK/A	A/A ALK/A	A/A ALK/A	A/A	A/A	A/A	A/A
(A)[25]	(A)	(A)	A	A	(A)	A	(A) A	A	A	(A) A
−	−	−	−	−	−	−	−	−	V⁻	−
V⁻	A	A	V⁻	−	V	V	A	A	A	V⁻
A	−	−	A	A	−	−	−	−	−	A
−	−	−	A	−	−	−	A	−	A	A
−	−	−	A	A	−	−	−	V	A	A
−	−	−	−	−	−	−	V⁺	−	−	A
−	−	−	−	V	−	−	−	−	−	−
V⁻	A	V	−	V	−	V	V⁻	−	−	V⁺
−	−	−	V	A	−	A	−	−	V	V
−	A	A	V	−	−	−	A	A	A	A
−	−	−	−	A	−	−	A	A	A	A
A	−	−	A	A	A	A	A	A	A	A
−	−	−	−	−	−	−	A	−	V	A
−	−	V⁺	−	−	−	−	−	−	−	A
−	−	−	−	−	−	−	V	−	−	−
−	−	−	−	−	−	−	A	−	V	A
−	−	−	A	V	−	−	−	A	A	V
−	−	−	V	−	−	−	A	A	A	A
−	−	−	−	−	−	−	A	−	A	A
−	A	V	−	−	−	A	A	A	A	A
−	−	A	−	−	−	−	A	V	A	V⁺
+	−	−	−	+	+	+	−	−	−	−
+	+	+	V⁺	+	V	+	V⁺	V⁻	V	+
−	+	−	−	−	−	−	+	+	V	−
+	V	−	−	+	V	+	+	+	+	+
−	−	−	−	−	−	−	−	−	−	−
−	−	−	−	−	−	−	−	−	−	+
−	−	−	−	−	−	−	−	−	−	+
−	+	+	−	+	−	V	−	−	−	V⁻
+	+	+	+	+	+	+	+ʷ	−	−	−
V	−	−	−	V	V⁻	V	−	V⁺	V	V
−	V	V	−	−	−	−	−	+	+	−
−	−	−	−	V	−	−	+	+	+	+
−	+	V	−	−	−	−	−	+	+	−
NR	NR	NR	NR	NR	NR	NR	NR	NR	NR	NR
+	+	+	−	+	+	+	−	+	V	V
−	+	V	−	−	−	−	−	V⁻	V	−
−	−	−	−	−	−	−	+	−	−	V⁺
+	+	−	+	+	V	+	+	+	+	+
+p	+p	V⁺ p	Vp	+p	Vp	V⁺ p	−	+p	+p	+p
−	−	−	−	−	−	−	−	−	−	−

Table 45.4. Biochemical Reactions of *Enterobacteriaceae* with a KIA/TSI Reaction of Acid/Acid, with/without Gas (*continued*)

Test	*Serratia grimesii*	*Serratia marcescens*	*Serratia odorifera* biogroup 1[p]	*Serratia odorifera* biogroup 2[p]	*Serratia plymuthica*	*Serratia proteamauculans*[q]	*Serratia rubidaea*
Catalase, 24h	+	+	+	+	+	+	+
Oxidase	−	−	−	−	−	−	−
NO$_3$→NO$_2$	+	+	+	+	+	+	+
O-F glucose	F	F	F	F	F	F	F
H$_2$S (KIA/TSI)	−	−	−	−	−	−	−
KIA	ALK/A	ALK/A	A/A ALK/A	A/A	A/A ALK/A	ALK/A	A/A
TSI	A/A	A/A	A/A	A/A	A/A	A/A	A/A
Carbohydrate fermentations							
Glucose & gas	Ⓐ	Ⓐ	A	Ⓐ	Ⓐ	Ⓐ	Ⓐ
Lactose	−	−	A	A	V+	−	A
Sucrose	A	A	A	−	A	A	A
Adonitol	−	V	V	V	−	−	A
L-Arabinose	A	−	A	A	A	A	A
D-Arabitol	NR	−	−	−	−	NR	V+
Cellobiose	−	−	A	A	V+	−	A
Dulcitol	−	−	−	−	−	−	−
Erythritol	NR	−	−	−	−	NR	−
Glycerol	NR		V	V	V	NR	V−
myo-Inositol	NR	V	A	A	V	NR	V−
Maltose	A	A	A	A	A	A	A
D-Mannitol	A	A	A	A	A	A	A
D-Mannose	A	A	A	A	A	A	A
Melibiose	A	−	A	A	A	A	A
α-Methyl-D-Glucoside	−	−	−	−	V	−	−
Mucate	−	−	−	−	−	−	−
Raffinose	A	−	A	−	A	A	A
L-Rhamnose	−	−	A	A	−	V	−
Salicin	A	A	A	V	V	V	A
D-Sorbitol	A	A	A	A	V	V+	−
Trehalose	A	A	A	A	A	A	A
D-Xylose	A	−	A	A	A	A	A
IMViC Reactions							
Indole	−	−	V	V	−	−	−
Methyl red (MR)	V+	V−	+	V	+	V	V−
Voges-Proskauer (VP) 22°C 37°C	V	+	V	+	V+	V+	−
Citrate (Simmons)	+	+	+	+	V	+	+
Decarboxylase/dihydrolase reactions							
Arginine dihydrolase	+	−	−	−	−	−	−
Lysine decarboxylase	+	+	+	+	−	+	V
Ornithine decarboxylase	+	+	+	−	−	+	−
Urea/phenylalanine reactions							
Urease (Christensen's)	−	V−	−	−	−	−	−
Phenylalanine deaminase, 24h	−	−	−	−	−	−	−
Misc. reactions							
Acetate use	NR	V	V	V	V	NR	V+
DNase, 25°C	+	+	+	+	+	+	+
Esculin hydrolysis	+	+	+	V	V+	V	+
Gelatin liquefaction, 22°C	+	+	+	+	V	+	+
Gluconate	NR	NR	NR	NR	NR	NR	NR
KCN broth-growth	+	+	V	V−	V	+	V−
Lipase (corn oil)	+	+	V	V	V	+	+
Malonate utilization	−	−	−	−	−	−	+
ONPG	+	+	+	+	V	+	+
Tartrate, Jordon	NR	V	+	+	+	NR	V
Motility, 36°C/flagella	+p	+p	+p	+p	Vp	+p	V+p
Pigmentation	−	Vr[ee]	−	−	Vr	−	+r

Chapter 45 / Gram-Negative Enterobacteriaceae

Tatumella ptyseos[r]	*Xenorhabdus beddingii*[s]	*Xenorhabdus bovienii*[s]	*Yersinia aldovae*[t]	*Yersinia bercovieri*	*Yersinia enterocolitica*	*Yersinia frederiksenii*	*Yersinia intermedia*	*Yersinia mollaretti*	*Yersinia rohdei*[u]	Enteric group 64	Enteric group 68
+	−	−	+	+	+	+	+	+	+	NR	NR
−	NR	NR	−	−	−	−	−	−	−	−	−
+	−	V	+	+	+	+	+	+	V+	+	+
F	NR	F	F	F	F	F	F	F	F	F	F
−	−	NR	−	−	−	−	−	−	−	−	−
ALK/A	NR	NR	ALK/A	A/A ALK/A	AKL/A ALK/A A/A	A/A ALK/A A/A	A/A ALK/A A/A	A/A ALK/A A/A	ALK/A A/A	A/A A/A	ALK/A A/A
A/A	NR	NR	A/A ALK/A	A/A							
A	NR	A	A	A	A	Ⓐ	Ⓐ	A	A	Ⓐ	A
−	NR	NR	−	V−	−	V	V	V	−	A	−
A	NR	NR	V−	A	A	A	A	A	A	−	A
−	NR	NR	−	−	−	−	−	−	−	A	−
−	NR	NR	V	A	A	A	A	A	A	A	−
−	NR	NR	−	−	V	A	V	A	−	A	−
−	NR	NR	−	A	V	A	A	A	V−	A	−
−	NR	NR	−	−	−	−	−	−	−	−	−
−	NR	NR	−	−	V	−	−	−	−	−	−
−	V	NR	−	−	A	V+	V+	V−	V	−	V
−	NR	NR	−	−	V	V−	V−	V−	−	−	−
−	A	NR	−	A	V	A	A	−	−	A	V
−	NR	NR	V+	A	A	A	A	V	A	A	A
A	A	NR	A	A	A	A	A	A	A	A	A
V	NR	NR	−	−	−	−	V+	A	V	−	−
−	NR	NR	−	−	−	−	V	−	−	−	−
−	NR	NR	−	−	−	−	−	−	−	A	−
V	NR	NR	−	−	−	V	V	−	V	−	−
−	NR	NR	−	−	−	A	A	−	−	NR	NR
V	V+	−	−	V−	V−	A	A	−	−	A	V
−	NR	NR	V	A	A	A	A	V−	A	−	−
A	A	NR	V+	A	A	A	A	A	A	A	A
−	NR	NR	V	A	V	A	A	V+	V	A	−
−	−	V	−	−	V	+	+	−	−	−	−
−	−	NR	V+	+	+	+	+	+	V	+	+
−	−	NR	−	−	V+	−	−	22°C− 37°C−	−	−	V
−	−	NR	−	−	−	−	−	V	−	V	−
−	−	NR	−	−	−	−	−	−	−	V	−
−	−	NR	−	−	−	−	−	−	−	−	−
−	−	NR	V	V+	+	+	+	V+	V−	−	−
−	−	−	V	V	V	V	V+	V−	V	−	−
+	−	−	−	−	−	−	−	−	−	−	−
−	NR	NR	−	−	V−	V−	V−	−	−	−	−
−	NR	NR	−	−	−	−	−	−	−	−	+
−	+	NR	−	−	V−	V+	+	−	−	+	−
−	+	NR	−	−	−	−	−	−	−	−	−
NR	NR	NR	NR	NR	NR	−	−	NR	NR	NR	NR
−	+	NR	−	−	−	−	−	−	−	+	+
−	−	NR	−	−	V	V	V−	−	−	−	−
−	−	NR	−	−	−	−	−	−	−	+	−
−	NR	NR	−	V+	+	+	+	V−	V	+	−
−	NR	NR	+	+	V+	V	V+	+	+	V	−
−	+p	NR	−	−cc	22°C+p 37°C−	−	−	22°C− 37°C−	−	+p	−
−	+b	+y	−	−	−	−	−	−	−	−	−

[a]Fastidious organism; requires unusual media for growth; e.g., 1% Protease-Peptone (6). Optimal temperature 30°C; maximum, 35°C.
[b]Rarely isolated from humans; no known clinical significance (6).
[c]Phenotypically similar to genus *Kluyvera* (6) and enteric groups 63 and 64 (1).
[d]Genus ingrequently opportunistic pathogen; similar to *Ewingella* (6) and resembles species of *Serratia* in many biochemical tests but may be distinguished by DNase-negative results. Genus first thought to be intermediate between typical *Serratia* spp. and *Serratia fonticola*.
[e]Genus *Cedecea* often negative in standard (O'Meara) Voges-Proskauer test because of the small amount of 2,3-butanediol produced; except *C. lapagei* is usually strongly VP-positive with O'Meara method (3).
[f]Occurs in clinical specimens (6); unnamed species.
[g]Most tests and conditions are markedly different for genus *Ewinia* from those listed for other enterics; genus studies done mainly by phytopathologists; rarely isolated from humans.
[h]*E. coli* strains often exhibit atypical reactions in a variety of tests; e.g., H_2S, citrate, urease, KCN, adonitol, inositol, and indole; must consider overall biochemical profile rather than specific "key" reactions before eliminating *E. coli* from consideration (6).
[i]Difficult to differentiate metabolically **in**active *E. coli* strains from *Shigella* spp., especially those strains that are lactose negative, nonmotile, and anaerogenic.
[j]*Ewingella* is similar to *Cedecea* spp. and to other enterics that are arginine, lysine, and ornithine negative (6).
[k]Large polysaccharide capsule that gives rise to large mucoid colonies, especially on carbohydrate-enriched media.
[l]According to *Bergey's Manual of Determinative Bacteriology* (42), *K. ozaenae* and *K. rhinocleromatis* are the same genospecies as *K. pneumoniae*; however, most laboratories treat them as separate species.
[m]Genus closely resembles *Buttiauxella agrestis*; superficially resemble *E. coli*, *Citrobacter*, and *Enterobacter*; 4% of both species (*K. ascorbata* and *K. cryocrescens*) produce red-blue crystals in and around colonies with prolonged incubation (3).
[n]Optimal temperature, 32°C.
[o]*P. myxofaciens* produces large amount of slime in broth media when grown at 22°C; TSP, plus; swarms at 25°C but **not** at 36°C (3). Most other *Proteus* spp. swarm at 37°C.
[p]*S. odorifera* produces a pungent odor; "musty, potato-like, like crushed wild poppies", or "vegetable-like" (3); odor probably due to 2-methyl-3-isopropyl pyrpyrazine (or structurally similare compound (3); odor noted as soon as incubator is opened (3).
[q]Two subspecies: *S. quinovora* and *S. proteamaculans* (4).
[r]More active metabolically at 25°C.
[s]Genus *Xenorhabdus* optimal temperature is 25°C.; grows poorly or not at all at 36°C. Older culture cells contain crystalline inclusions (**not** poly-β-hydroxybutyrate) spheroplasts or coccoid bodies resulting from disintegration of cell wall; seen in last third of exponentail growth.
[t]Best growth at 25–28°C; delayed or variable reactions at 35–37°C. Growth at 35°C may lead to misidentification of *Y. aldovae* as a metabolically inactive species such as *Shigella* or inactive *E. coli* (2).
[u]Maximum growth at 22–25°C.
[v]Gas production variable; majority positive.
[w]May be delayed.
[x]If positive, may be delayed.
[y]Few reactions delayed.
[z]Weak phenylalanine reaction; very slight greening after addition of reagent; often overlooked and reported as doubtful or negative.
[aa]Motile at 22°C; less than half of strains are motile at 36°C (6).
[bb]*E. ictaluri* prefers a lower temperature; motile at 25°C, but not at 37°C.
[cc]Nonmotile at 36°C; 65% motile at 25°C (3).
[dd]Yellow, nondiffused; best formed at 25°C; may be lost upon subculturing.

Table 45.5. Differentiation among the Species and Subspecies of *Klebsiella*

Test	*K. ornithinolytica*	*K. oxytoca*	*K. pneumoniae* subsp. *ozaenae*	*K. pneumoniae* subsp. *pneumoniae*	*K. pneumoniae* subsp. *rhinoscleronnatis*	*K. planticola*	*K. tenigena*
Lactose	A	A	V	A	—	A	A
Indole	+	+	—	—	—	V−	—
Methyl red	+	V−	+	V−	+	+	V
Voges-Proskauer	V	+	—	+	+	+	+
Simmons citrate	+	+	V	+	—	+	V
Malonate	+	+	—	+	+	+	+
Christensen's Urease	+	+[a]	—	+[a]	—	+[a]	—
Lysine	+	+	V	+	—	+	+
ONPG	+	+	V+	+	—	+	+

[a]May be slow or delayed.

Table 45.6. Four Distinct DNA Relatedness Groups of *Y. enterocolitica*

Test Media	Group I	Group II	Group III	Group IV
Sucrose	A	A	A	—
Rhamnose	—	A[a]	A	—
Melibiose	—	A[a]	—	—
ONPG	—	+[a,b]	—	—
Simmons citrate	—	+[c]	−[d]	—

Principal Results	Report
Sucrose-positive strains	*Y. enterocolitica*
Sucrose-negative strains	Sucrose-negative biogroup of *Y. enterocolitica*
Rhamnose-positive	*Y. enterocolitica*-like rhamnose-positive melibiose-positive group

[a]May be delayed at 37°C.
[b]ONPG may be delayed at 37°C with relatedness group II.
[c]22°C.
[d]22° and 37°C.

758 Biochemical Tests for Identification of Medical Bacteria

Diagram 45.1.

Differentiation of *Enterobacteriaceae* with a KIA/TSI reaction of **ACID/ACID, WITH/WITHOUT GAS** that may cause human infections

Cedecea davisae
Cedecea lapegei
Cedecea neteri
†*Cedecea* species 3
†*Cedecea* species 5
Citrobacter amalonaticus
Citrobacter amalonaticus
  biogroup 1
Citrobacter freundii
Citrobacter koseri
†*Edwardsiella tarda*
  biogroup 1
Enterobacter aerogenes
Enterobacter amnigenus
  biogroups 1 & 2
Enterobacter asburiae
Enterobacter cloacae
Enterobacter dissolvens

Enterobacter gergoviae
Enterobacter sakazakii
Escherichia coli
Escherichia coli
  inactive
Escherichia hermannii
Escherichia vulneris
Ewingella americana
Klebsiella ornithinolytica
Klebsiella oxytoca
Klebsiella planticola
Klebsiella pneumoniae
  subsp. *ozaenae*
Klebsiella pneumoniae
  subsp. *pneumoniae*
Klebsiella pneumoniae
  subsp. *rhinoscleromatis*

Klebsiella terrigena
Kluyvera ascorbata
Kluyvera cryocrescens
Leclercia adecarboxylata
Moellerella wisconsensis
Pantoea agglomerans
Plesiomonas shigelloides
†*Proteus inconstans*
†*Proteus penneri*
†*Providencia rettgeri*
†*Providencia rustigianii*
†*Providencia stuartii*
Rahnella aquatilis
l *Serratia ficaria*
†*Serratia fonticola*
†*Serratia grimesii*
†*Serratia marcescens*
Serratia odorifera
  biogroups 1 & 2

Serratia plymuthica
†*Serratia proteamaculans*
Serratia rubidaea
†*Tatumella ptyseos*
Yersinia bercovieri
†*Yersinia enterocolitica*
Yersinia frederiksenii
Yersinia intermedia
Yersinia mollaretii
†*Yersinia rohdei*
Enteric group 64
†Enteric group 68

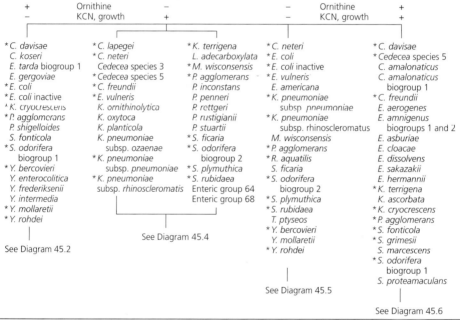

†Acid/Acid TSI **only**; KIA, Alkaline/Acid
*Variable reactions.

Diagram 45.2.

Differentiation of *Enterobacteriaceae* with a KIA/TSI reaction of **ACID/ACID, WITH/WITHOUT GAS** enterics that may cause human infections that are:

ORNITHINE-POSITIVE
KCN-GROWTH-NEGATIVE

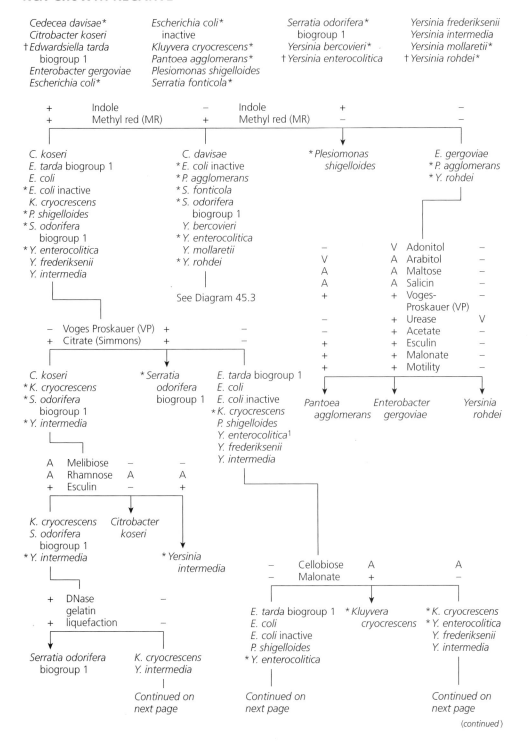

(continued)

760 Biochemical Tests for Identification of Medical Bacteria

Diagram 45.2. (continued)

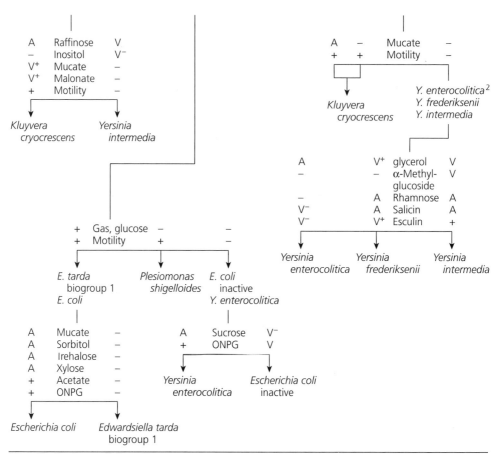

†TSI, Acid/Acid **only**; KIA: Alkaline/Acid
*Variable results.
[1]Voges-Pnoskauer negative at 37°C; variable at 22°C
[2]Motility negative at 37°C, positive at 22°C.

Diagram 45.3.

Differentiation of *Enterobacteriaceae* with a KIA/TSI reaction of **ACID/ACID, WITH/WITHOUT GAS** that may infect humans that are:

ORNITHINE-POSITIVE **INDOLE-NEGATIVE**
KCN-GROWTH-NEGATIVE **METHYL RED (MR)-POSITIVE**

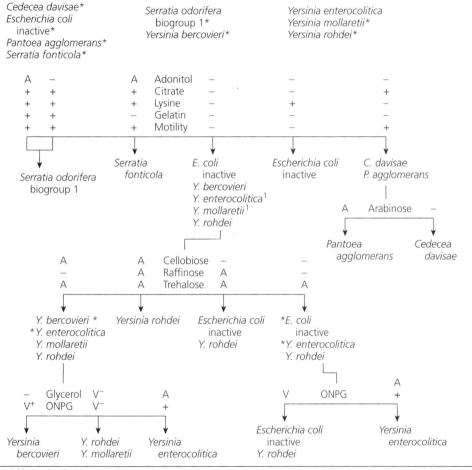

*Variable reactions/
†Motility negative at 37°C, positive at 22°C.

Diagram 45.4.

Differentiation of *Enterobacteriaceae* with a KIA/TSI reaction of **ACID/ACID, WITH/WITHOUT GAS** that may infect humans that are:

ORNITHINE-NEGATIVE
KCN-GROWTH-POSITIVE

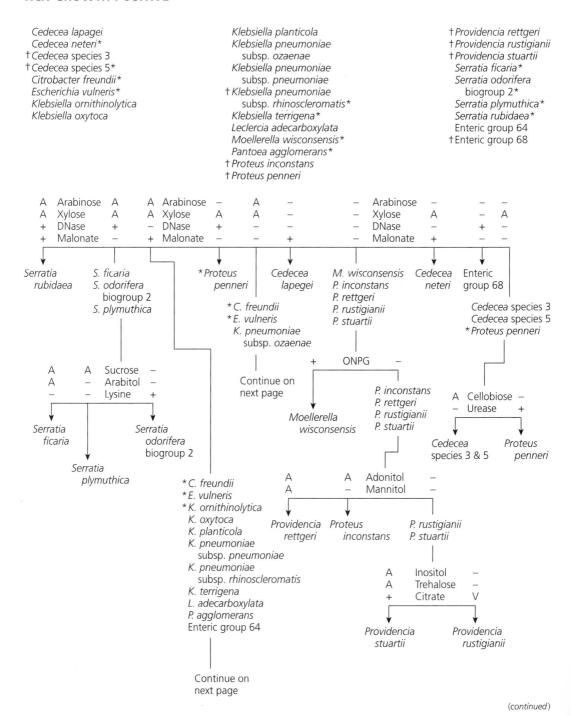

(continued)

Diagram 45.4. (*continued*)

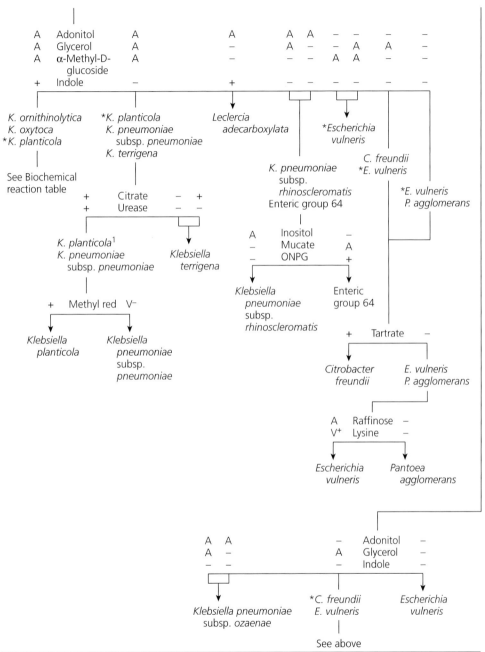

*Variable results.
†Acid/Acid, TSI **only**; KIAL: Alkaline/Acid.
¹Urease may be slowly delayed.

764 Biochemical Tests for Identification of Medical Bacteria

Diagram 45.5.

Differentiation of *Enterobacteriaceae* with a KIA/TSI reaction of **ACID/ACID, WITH/WITHOUT GAS** that may infect humans that are:

ORNITHINE-NEGATIVE
KCN-GROWTH-NEGATIVE

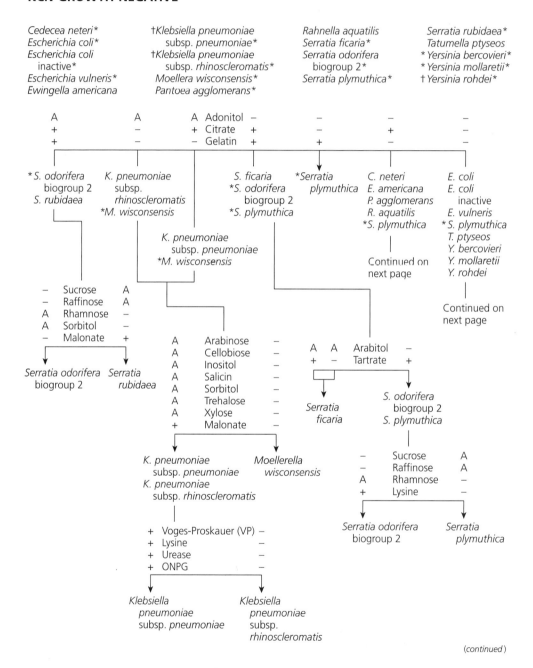

(continued)

Chapter 45 / Gram-Negative Enterobacteriaceae

Diagram 45.5. (*continued*)

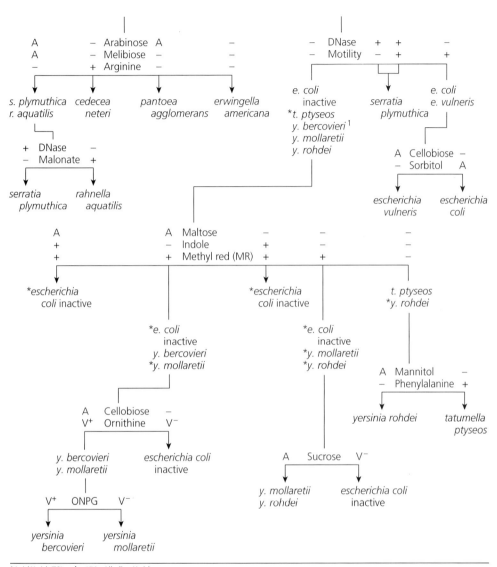

†Acid/Acid, TSI **only**; KIA: Alkaline/Acid.
*Organisms with variable reactions.
[1]Nonmotile at 36°C; 66% at 25°C (17).

Diagram 45.6.

Differentiation of *Enterobacteriaceae* with a KIA/TSI reaction of **ACID/ACID, WITH/WITHOUT GAS** that may infect humans that are:

ORNITHINE-POSITIVE
KCN-GROWTH-POSITIVE

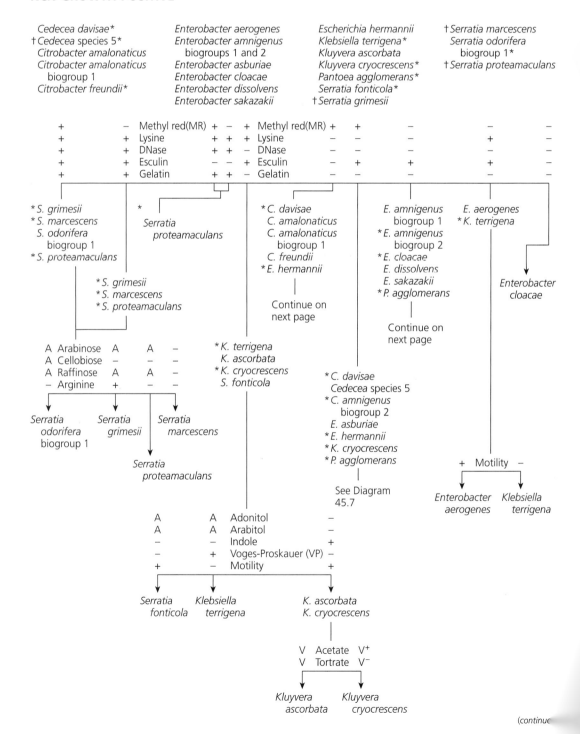

Diagram 45.6. (continued)

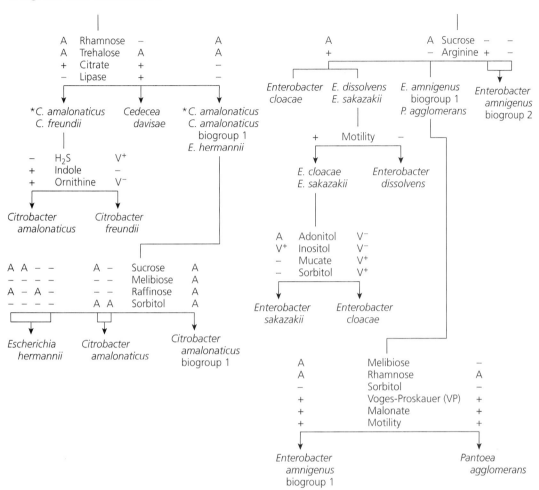

†Acid/Acid TSI **only**; KIA: Alkaline/Acid.
*Variable reactions.

Diagram 45.7.

Differentiation of *Enterobacteriaceae* with a KIA/TSI reaction of **ACID/ACID, WITH/WITHOUT GAS** that may infect humans that are:

ORNITHINE-POSITIVE   **METHYL-RED(MR)-POSITIVE**   **LYSINE-NEGATIVE**   **GELATIN-NEGATIVE**
KCN-GROWTH-POSITIVE   **ESCULIN-POSITIVE**   **DNASE-NEGATIVE**

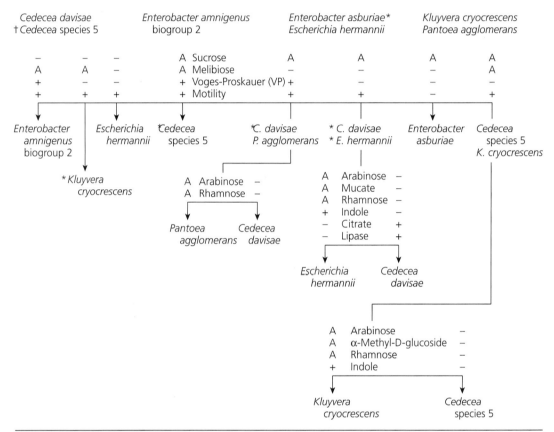

†Acid/Acid TSI **only**; KIA: Alkaline/Acid.
*Variable results.

ACID/ACID, H$_2$S, WITH/WITHOUT GAS

Table 45.7. Biochemical Reactions of *Enterobacteriaceae* with KIA/TSI Reaction of ACID/ACID, H$_2$S with/without GAS

Test	*Buduicia aquatica*	*Citrobacter freundii*	*Proteus mirabilis*	*Proteus penneri*	*Proteus vulgaris*	*Salmonella choleraesuis* subsp. *arizonae*	*Salmonella choleraesuis* subsp. *diaizonae*	*Salmonella choleraesuis* subsp. *indica*
Catalase, 24 hr	+	+	+	+	+	+	+	+
Oxidase	−	−	−	−	−	−	−	−
NO$_3$→NO$_2$	+	+	+	+	+	+	+	+
O-F glucose	F	F	F	F	F	F	F	F
H$_2$S (KIA/TSI)	V$^+$	V$^+$	+	V	+	+	+	+
KIA	A/A	A/A, A/A, H$_2$S, ALK/A, ALK/A, H$_2$S	ALK/A, H$_2$S	ALK/A, ALK/A, H$_2$S	ALK/A, H$_2$S	A/A, H$_2$S, ALK/A, H$_2$S	A/A, H$_2$S, ALK/A, H$_2$S	A/A, H$_2$S, ALK/A, H$_2$S
TSI	A/A, H$_2$S, ALK/A, H$_2$S	A/A, H$_2$S, ALK/A, H$_2$S	A/A, H$_2$S, ALK/A, H$_2$S	A/A, A/A, H$_2$S	A/A, H$_2$S	A/A, H$_2$S, ALK/A, H$_2$S	A/A, H$_2$S, ALK/A, H$_2$S	A/A, H$_2$S, ALK/A, H$_2$S
Carbohydrate fermentations								
Glucose & gas	Ⓐ	Ⓐ	Ⓐ	Ⓐ	Ⓐ ^{a}	Ⓐ ^{b}	Ⓐ	Ⓐ
Lactose	V$^+$	V^c	−	−	−	V$^−$	V$^+$	V$^−$
Sucrose	−	V	V$^−$	A	A	−	−	−
Adonitol	−	−	−	−	−	−	−	−
L-Arabinose	V$^+$	A	−	−	−	A	A	A
D-Arabitol	V	−	−	−	−	NR	NR	NR
Cellobiose	−	V	−	−	−	−	−	−
Dulcitol	−	V	−	−	−	−	−	V
Erythritol	−	−	−	−	−	NR	NR	NR
Glycerol	−	A	V	V	V	−	−	V
myo-Inositol	−	−	−	−	−	−	−	−
Maltose	−	A	−	A	A	A	A	A

(continued)

Table 45.7. Biochemical Reactions of *Enterobacteriaceae* with KIA/TSI Reaction of ACID/ACID, H_2S with/without GAS (*continued*)

Test	*Buduicia aquatica*	*Citrobacter freundii*	*Proteus mirabilis*	*Proteus penneri*	*Proteus vulgaris*	*Salmonella choleraesuis* subsp. *arizonae*	*Salmonella choleraesuis* subsp. *diaizonae*	*Salmonella choleraesuis* subsp. *indica*
D-Mannitol	V	A	–	–	–	A	A	A
D-Mannose	–	A	–	–	–	A	A	A
Melibiose	–	V	–	–	–	A	A	V+
α-Methyl-D-Glucoside	–	–	–	V+	V	–	–	–
Mucate	V–	A	–	–	–	A	V	A
Raffinose	–	V	–	–	–	–	–	–
L-Rhamnose	–	A	–	–	–	A	A	A
Salicin	–	–	–	–	V	–	–	–
D-Sorbitol	–	A	–	–	–	A	A	–
Trehalose	–	A	A	V	V	A	A	A
D-Xylose	A	A	A	A	A	A	A	A
IMViC reactions								
Indole	–	–	–	–	+	–	–	–
Methyl red (RM)	–	+	+	+	+	+	+	+
Voges-Proskauer (VP)	–	–	V	–	–	–	–	–
Citrate (Simmons)	NR	+	V	–	V–	+	+	V+
Decarboxylase/dihydrolase reactions								
Arginine dihydrolase	–	V	–	–	–	V	V	V
Lysine decarboxylase	–	–	–	–	–	+	+	+
Ornithine decarboxylase	–	V–	+	–	–	+	+	+
Urea/phenylalanine reactions								
Urease (Christensen's)	V	Vw	+	+	+	–	–	–
Phenylalanine deaminase, 24h	–	–	+	+	+	–	–	–
Misc. reactions								
Acetate utilization	–	V+	V–	–	V–	+	V+	V+
DNase, 25°C	–	–	V	V	V+	–	–	–
Esculin hydrolysis	–	–	–	–	V	–	–	–
Gelatin liquefaction, 22°C	–	–	+	V	+	–	–	–
Gluconate	NR	–	NR	NR	NR	NR	NR	NR
KCN broth-growth	–	+	+	+	+	–	–	–
Lipase (corn oil)	–	–	+	V	V+	–	–	–
Malonate utilization	–	V–	–	–	–	+	+	–
ONPG	+	+	–	–	–	+	+	V
Tartrate, Jordon	V	+	V+	V+	V+	–	V–	–
Motility, 36°C/flagella	Vp[d]	+p	+p	V+p	+p	+p	+p	+p
Pigmentation	–	–	–	–	–	–	–	–

[a]If gas produced, a slight amount.
[b]May be delayed.
[c]May be delayed.
[d]Motile at 22°C; less than half of strains are motile at 36°C. (5).

Diagram 45.8.

Differentiation of *Enterobacteriaceae* with a KIA/TSI reaction of **ACID/ACID, WITH/WITHOUT GAS H₂S** that may infect humans

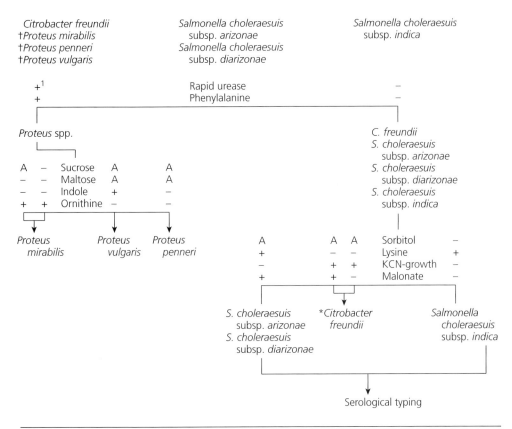

†Acid/Acid, H₂S, TSI **only**; KIA: Alkaline/Acid, H₂S.
*Organisms with variable reactions.
¹Occassional strain of *Proteus mirabilis* delayed and weak urease positive, but phenylalanine-positive.

ALKALINE/ACID WITH/WITHOUT GAS

Table 45.8. Biochemical Reactions of *Enterobacteriaceae* with a KIA/TSI Reaction of ALKALINE/ACID, with/without Gas

Test	*Arsenophonus nasoniae*[a]	*Budvicia aquatica*[b]	*Cedecea davisae*[c]	*Cedecea lapagei*[d]	*Cedecea neteri*	*Cedecea species 3*[e]	*Cedecea species 5*[e]
Catalase, 24 h	+	+	+	+	+	NR	NR
Oxidase	−	−	−	−	−	−	−
NO₃→NO₂	−	+	+	+	+	+	+
O-F glucose	F	F	F	F	F	F	F
H₂S (KIA/TSI)	−	V	−	−	−	−	−
KIA	ALK/A	A/A, A/A, H₂S ALK/A, H₂S	A/A ALK/A	A/A ALK/A	A/A ALK/A	ALK/A	ALK/A
TSI	A/A	A/A, A/A, H₂S ALK/A	A/A ALK/A	A/A	A/A ALK/A	A/A	A/A
Carbohydrate fermentations							
Glucose & gas	A	Ⓐ	Ⓐ	Ⓐ	Ⓐ	A	Ⓐ
Lactose	−	V+	V−	V	V	−	−
Sucrose	A	−	A	−	A	V	A
Adonitol	−	−	−	−	−	−	−
L-Arabinose	−	V+	−	−	−	−	−
D-Arabitol	NR	V	−	−	−	−	−
Cellobiose	−	−	A	A	A	A	A
Dulcitol	−	−	−	−	−	−	−
Erythritol	NR	−	−	−	−	−	−
Glycerol	−	−	−	−	−	−	−
myo-Inositol	−	−	−	−	−	−	−
Maltose	−	−	A	A	A	A	A
D-Mannitol	−	V	A	A	A	A	A
D-Mannose	NR	−	A	A	A	A	A
Melibiose	NR	−	−	−	−	A	A
α-Methyl-D-Glucoside	NR	−	−	−	−	V	−
Mucate	NR	V−	−	−	−	−	−
Raffinose	−	−	V−	−	−	A	A
L-Rhamnose	−	A	−	−	−	−	−
Salicin	NR	−	A	A	A	A	A[bb]
D-Sorbitol	NR	−	−	−	A	−	A
Trehalose	−	−	A	A	A	A	A
D-Xylose	−	A	A	−	A	A	A
IMViC reactions							
Indole	−	−	−	−	−	−	−
Methyl red (MR)	−	+	+	V	+	+	+
Voges-Proskauer (VP)	−	−	V	V+	V	V	V
Citrate (Simmons)	NR	−	+	+	+	+	+
Decarboxylase/dihydrolase reactions							
Arginine dihydrolase	−	−	V	V+	+	+	V
Lysine decarboxylase	−	−	−	−	−	−	−
Ornithine decarboxylase	−	−	+	−	−	−	V
Urea phenylalanine reactions							
Urease (Christensen's)	NG	V	−	−	−	−	−
Phenylalanine deaminase, 24h	NR	−	−	−	−	−	−
Misc. reactions							
Acetate use	NR	−	−	V	−	V	V
DNase, 25°C	NG	−	−	−	−	−	−
Esculin hydrolysis	−	−	V	+	+	+	+
Gelatin liquefaction, 22°C	+	−	−	−	−	−	−
Gluconate	NR	NR	NR	NR	NR	NR	NR
KCN broth-growth	NR	−	V+	+	V	+	+
Lipase (corn oil)	NR	−	+	+	+	+	V
Malconate utilization	−	−	+	+	+	−	−
ONPG	NR	+	+	+	+	+	+
Tartrate, Jordon	NR	V	−	−	−	−	−
Motility, 36°C/flagella	−	Vp[gg]	+p	Vp	+p	+p	+p
Pigmentation	−	−	−	−	−	−	−

Chapter 45 / Gram-Negative Enterobacteriaceae

	Citrobacter amalonaticus	*Citrobacter amalnaticus* biogroup 1	*Citrobacter koseri*	*Citrobacer freundii*	*Edwardsiella hoshinae*	*Edwardsiella ictaluri*	*Edwardsiella tarda* biogroup 1	*Enterobacter aerogenus*	*Enterobacter amnigenus* biogroup 1	*Enterobacter amnigenus* biogroup 2	*Enterobacter asburiae*	*Enterobacter cancerogenus*	*Enterobacter dissolvens*
	+	+	+	+	+	+	+	+	+	+	+	+	+
	−	−	−	−	−	−	−	−	−	−	−	−	−
	+	+	+	+	+	+	+	+	+	+	+	+	+
	F	F	F	F	F	F	F	F	F	F	F	F	F
								−					−
	−	−	−	V+	−	−							
	A/A ALK/A	A/A ALK/A	A/A ALK/A	A/A A/A, H₂S ALK/A ALK/A, H₂S	ALK/A	ALK/A	ALK/A	A/A	A/A ALK/A	A/A ALK/A	A/A ALK/A	ALK/A	A/A ALK/A
	A/A ALK/A	A/A	A/A ALK/A	A/A A/A, H₂S ALK/A ALK/A, H₂S	A/A	ALK/A	A/A	A/A	A/A	A/A	A/A ALK/A	ALK/A	A/A
	Ⓐ	Ⓐ	Ⓐ	Ⓐ	ⒶÄ	ⒶÄ	ⒶÄ	Ⓐ	Ⓐ	Ⓐ	Ⓐ	Ⓐ	Ⓐ
	V	V−	V	V^bb	−	−	−	A	V	V	V+	−	V
	V−	A	V	V	A	−	A	A	A	A	A	−	A
	−	−	A	−	−	−	−	A	−	−	−	−	−
	A	A	A	A	V−	−	A	A	A	A	A	A	A
	−	−	−	−	−	−	−	A	−	−	−	−	−
	A	A	A	V	−	−	−	A	A	A	A	A	A
	−	−	V	V	−	−	−	−	−	−	−	−	−
	−	−	A	A	−	−	−	−	−	−	−	−	−
	V	V	A	−	V	−	−	A	−	−	V−	−	−
	−	−	−	−	−	−	−	A	−	−	−	−	−
	A	A	A	A	A	A	A	A	A	A	A	A	A
	A	A	A	A	A	−	A	A	A	A	A	A	A
	A	A	A	A	A	A	A	A	A	A	A	A	A
	−	A	−	V	−	−	−	A	A	A	−	A	A
	−	V	V	−	−	−	−	A	V	A	A	−	A
	A	A	A	A	−	−	−	A	A	A	V−	V	A
	−	A	−	V	−	−	−	A	A	−	V	−	A
	A	A	A	A	−	−	−	A	A	A	−	A	A
	V^bb	−	V−dd	−	V	−	−	A	A	A	A	A	A
	A	A	A	A	−	−	−	A	A	A	A	−	A
	A	A	A	A	A	−	−	A	A	A	A	A	A
	A	A	A	A	−	−	−	A	A	A	A	A	A
	+	+	+	−	V	−	+	−	−	V	−	−	−
	+	+	+	+	+	−	+	−	−	V	+	−	−
	−	−	−	−	−	−	−	+	+	+	−	+	+
	V+	−	+	+	−	−	−	+	V	+	+	+	+
	V+	V+	V^bb	V	−	−	−	−	−	V	V−	+	+
	−	−	−	−	+	+	+	+	−	−	−	−	−
	+	+	+	V−	+	V	+	+	+	+	+	+	+
	V	V	V	V^w	−	−	−	−	−	−	V	−	+
	−	−	−	−	−	−	−	−	−	−	−	−	−
	V+	V+	V+	V+	−	−	−	V	−	−	V+	V	+
	−	−	−	−	−	−	−	−	−	−	−	−	−
	−	−	−	−	−	−	−	+	+	+	+	+	+
	+	NR	NR	−	NR	NR	+	NR	NR	NR	NR	NR	NR
	+	+	−	+	−	−	+	+	+	+	+	+	+
	−	−	−	−	−	−	−	−	−	−	−	−	V
	−	−	+	V−	+	−	−	+	+	+	−	+	+
	+	+	+	+	−	−	−	+	+	+	+	+	+
	V+	V+	V+	+	−	−	−	+	−	−	V−	−	−
	+p	+p	+p	+p	+p	−hh	+	+p	+p	+p	−	+p	−
	−	−	−	−	−	−	−	−	−	−	−	−	−

Table 45.8. Biochemical Reactions of *Enterobacteriaceae* with a KIA/TSI Reaction of ALKALINE/ACID, with/without Gas (*continued*)

Test	*Enterobacter gergoviae*	*Enterobacter hormaechei*	*Erwinia amylovira*[f]	*Erwinia mallotivira*[f]	*Escherichia blattae*[g]	*Escherichia coli* inactive[g]	*Escherichia fergusonii*
Catalase, 24 hr	+	+	+	+	+	+	+
Oxidase	−	−	−	−	−	−	−
NO₃→NO₂	+	+	−	−	+	+	+
O-F glucose	F	F	F	F	F	F	F
H₂S (KIA/TSI)	−	−	−	−	−	−	−
KIA	A/A ALK/A	ALK/A	ALK/A	ALK/A	ALK/AA	A/A ALK/A	ALK/A
TSI	A/A	A/A	A/A	NR	ALK/A	A/A ALK/A	ALK/A
Carbohydrate fermentations							
Glucose & gas	Ⓐ	Ⓐ	A	A	Ⓐ	A	Ⓐ
Lactose	V	−	−	−	−	V⁻	−
Sucrose	A	A	A	NR	−	V⁻	−
Adonitol	V	−	−	−	−	−	A
L-Arabinose	A	A	V	−	A	V⁺	A
D-Arabitol	A	−	−	NR	−	−	A
Cellobiose	A	A	A	−	−	−	A
Dulcitol	−	V	−	−	−	V	V
Erythritol	−	−	−	NR	−	−	−
Glycerol	A	−	−	−	A	V	V⁻
myo-Inositol	−	−	−	−	−	−	−
Maltose	A	A	−	−	A	V⁺	A
D-Mannitol	A	A	−	A	−	A	A
D-Mannose	A	A	−	A	A	A	A
Melibiose	A	−	−	−	−	V	−
α-Methyl-D-Glucoside	−	V⁺	−	−	−	−	−
Mucate	−	A	NR	NR	V	V	−
Raffinose	A	−	−	−	−	V⁻	−
L-Rhamnose	A	A	−	−	A	V	A
Salicin	A	V	−	−	−	−	V
D-Sorbitol	−	−	V	−	−	V⁺	−
Trehalose	A	A	A	A	V⁺	A	A
D-Xylose	A	A	−	A	A	V	A
IMViC reactions							
Indole	−	−	−	−	−	V⁺	+
Methyl red (MR)	−	V	NR	NR	+	+	+
Voges-Proskauer (VP)	+	+	+	+	−	−	−
Citrate (Simmons)	+	+	+	NR	V	−	V⁻
Decarboxylase/dihydrolase reactions							
Arginine dihydrolase	−	V⁺	−	NR	−	−	−
Lysine decarboxylase	+[ff]	−	−	NR	+	V	+
Ornithine decarboxylase	+	+	−	NR	+	V⁻	+
Urea/phenylalanine reactions							
Urease (Christensen's)	+	V⁺	−	−	−	−	−
Phenylalanine deaminase, 24 h	−	−	−	−	−	−	−
Misc. reactions							
Acetate utilization	+	V	+	NR	−	V	+
DNase, 25°C	−	−	−	NR	−	−	−
Esculin hydrolysis	+	−	NR	NR	−	−	V
Gelatin liquefaction	−	−	+	−	−	−	−
Gluconate	+	NR	NR	NR	NR	NR	NR
KCN broth-growth	−	+	NR	−	−	−	−
Lipase (corn oil)	−	−	NR	NR	−	−	−
Malonate utilization	+	+	−	−	+	−	V
ONPG	+	+	NR	NR	−	V	V⁺
Tartrate, Jordon	+	V⁻	NR	NR	V	V⁺	+
Motility, 36°C/flagella	+p	Vp	+p	+p	−	−	+p
Pigmentation	−	−	−	−	−	−	−

Chapter 45 / Gram-Negative *Enterobacteriaceae*

	Escherichia hermannii	*Escherichia vulneris*	*Ewingella americana*[h]	*Hafnia alvei*	*Hafnia alvei* biogroup 1	*Klebsiella pneumoniae* subsp. *ozaenae*[i]	*Klebsiella pneumoniae* subsp. *rhinoscleromatis*	*Kluyvera crejocrescens*	*Morganella morganii* biogroup 1	*Morganella morganii* biogroup 2	*Obesiumbacterium proteus*[j]	*Pantoea agglomerans*	*Pantoea dispersa*[k]
	+	+	+	+[x]	+[x]	+	+	+	+	+	+	+	+
	–	–	–	–	–	–	–	–	–	–	–	–	–
	+	+	+	+	+	V+	+	+	+	+	+	+	V
	F	F	F	F	F	F	F	F	F	F	F	F	F
	–	–	–	–	–	–	–	–	–	V	–	–	–
	A/A ALK/A	A/A ALK/A	A/A ALK/A	ALK/A	ALK/A	A/A ALK/A	ALK/A	ALK/A ALK/A	ALK/A	ALK/A ALK/A, H₂S	ALK/A	A/A ALK/A	ALK/A
	A/A ALK/A	A/A ALK/A	A/A ALK/A	ALK/A	ALK/A	A/A ALK/A	A/A ALK/A	A/A ALK/A	ALK/A	ALK/A ALK/A, H₂S	ALK/A A/A	A/A	A/A
	Ⓐ	Ⓐ	A	Ⓐ	A	Ⓐ	A	Ⓐ	Ⓐ	Ⓐ	A	A	A
	V	V–	V	–	–	V	A	V	V+	–	–	V–	–
	V	–	–	–	–	V–	V	V+	–	–	–	A	A
	–	–	–	–	–	A	A	–	–	–	–	–	–
	A	A	–	A	–	A	A	A	–	–	–	A	V
	–	–	A	–	–	A	A	–	–	–	–	V	NR
	A	A	–	V–	–	A	A	A	–	–	–	V	V
	V–	–	–	–	–	–	–	–	–	–	–	–	–
	–	V–	V–	A	–	V	V	–	–	A	–	–	V
	–	–	–	–	–	V	V	–	–	–	–	–	V
	A	A	V–	A	–	A	A	A	–	–	V	A	A
	A	A	A	A	V	A	A	A	–	–	–	A	A
	A	A	A	A	A	A	A	A	A	A	V–	A	A
	–	A	–	–	–	A	A	–	–	–	–	–	–
	–	V–	–	–	–	–	–	A	–	–	–	–	–
	A	V+	–	–	–	V–	–	V+	–	–	–	–	V
	V	A	–	–	–	A	A	A	–	–	–	–	–
	A	A	V–	A	–	V	A	A	–	–	V–	A	A
	V	V	V+	V–	V	A	A	A	–	–	–	A	–
	–	–	–	–	–	–	–	A	–	–	–	–	–
	A	A	A	A	V	A	A	A	–	–	V+	A	A
	A	A	V–	A	–	A	A	A	–	–	V–	A	A
	+	–	–	–	–	–	–	+	+	+	–	–	–
	+	+	V+	V	V+	+	+	+	+	+	V–	V	V
	–	–	+	V+	V	–	–	–	–	–	–	+	+
	–	–	+	–	–	V	–	V+	–	V	–	+	+
	–	V	–	–	–	–	–	–	–	–	–	–	–
	–	V+	–	+	+	V	–	V–	–	+	+	–	–
	+	–	–	+	V	–	–	+	+	+	+	V	–
	–	–	–	–	–	–	–	–	+[w]	+[w]	–	–	–
	–	–	–	–	–	–	–	–	+	+	–	V+	–
	V+	V	–	V–	V	–	–	V+	–	–	–	–	NR
	–	–	–	–	–	–	–	–	–	–	–	–	–
	V	V–	V	–	–	V+	V	+	–	–	–	+	–
	NR	NR	NR	NR	NR	NR	NR	NR	NR	NR	NR	+	+
	+	V–	–	+	–	+	V+	V+	+	+	–	V+	+
	–	–	–	–	–	–	–	–	–	–	–	NR	NR
	–	V+	–	V	V	–	+	V+	–	–	–	+	–
	+	+	V+	+	V	V+	V	V	V–	+	+	+	+
	V	–	V	V	–	V	V	V–	+	+	V–	–	V
	+p	+p	Vp	V+p	–	–	–	+p	+p	–	–	+p	+p
	+y	Vy	–	–	–	–	–	–	–	–	–	+y	Vy

Table 45.8. Biochemical Reactions of *Enterobacteriaceae* with a KIA/TSI Reaction of ALKALINE/ACID, with/without Gas (*continued*)

Test	*Pragia fontium*	*Proteus inconstans*	*Proteus myxofaciens*	*Proteus penneri*	*Providencia rettgeri*	*Providencia heimbachae*	*Providencia rustigianii*
Catalase, 24 hr	+	+	+	+	+	+	+
Oxidase	−	−	−	−	−	−	−
$NO_3 \rightarrow NO_2$	+	+	+	+	+	+	+
O-F glucose	F	F	F	F	F	F	F
H_2S (KIA/TSI)	V^+	−	−	V	−	−	−
KIA	ALK/A, ALK/A, H_2S	ALK/A	ALK/A	ALK/A, ALK/A, H_2S	ALK/A	ALK/A	ALK/A
TSI	ALK/A, ALK/A, H_2S	A/A, ALK/A	A/A	A/A, A/A, H_2S	A/A, ALK/A	A/A, ALK/A	A/A, ALK/A
Carbohydrate fermentations							
Glucose & gas	A	Ⓐ z	Ⓐ	Ⓐ	A	A	Ⓐ
Lactose	−	−	−	−	−	−	−
Sucrose	−	V^-	A	A	−	V	V
Adonitol	−	A	−	−	A	A	−
L-Arabinose	−	−	−	−	−	−	−
D-Arabitol	−	−	−	−	A	A	−
Cellobiose	−	−	−	−	−	−	−
Dulcitol	−	−	−	−	−	−	−
Erythritol	−	−	−	−	V	−	−
Glycerol	−	V^-	A	V	V	−	−
myo-Inositol	−	−	−	−	A	V	−
Maltose	−	−	A	A	−	V	−
D-Mannitol	−	−	−	−	A	−	−
D-Mannose	−	A	−	−	A	A	A
Melibiose	−	−	−	−	−	−	−
α-Methyl-D-Glucoside	−	−	−	V^+	V	−	−
Mucate	−	−	−	−	−	−	−
Raffinose	−	−	−	−	−	−	−
L-Rhamnose	−	−	−	−	V	A	−
Salicin	V	−	−	−	V	−	−
D-Sorbitol	−	−	−	−	−	−	−
Trehalose	−	−	A	V	−	−	−
D-Xylose	−	−	−	A	−	−	−
IMViC reactions							
Indole	−	+	−	−	+	−	+
Methl red (MR)	+	+	+	+	+	V^+	V
Voges-Proskauer (VP)	−	−	+	−	−	−	−
Citrate (Simmons)	V^+	+	V	−	+	−	V^-
Decarboxylase/dihydrolase reactions							
Arginine dihydrolase	−	−	−	−	−	−	−
Lysine decarboxylase	−	−	−	−	−	−	−
Ornithine decarboxylase	−	−	−	−	−	−	−
Urea/phenylalanine reactions							
Urease (Christensen's)	−	−	+	+	+	−	−
Phenylalanine deaminase, 24 h	V^-	+	+	+	+	+	+
Misc. reactions							
Acetate use	−	V	−	−	V	−	V^-
DNase, 25°C	−	−	V	V	−	−	−
Esculin hydrolysis	V	−	−	V	V	−	−
Gelatin liquefaction, 22°C	−	−	+	V	−	−	−
Gluconate	+	NR	NR	NR	NR	NR	NR
KCN broth-growth	−	+	+	+	+	−	+
Lipase (corn oil)	−	−	+	V	−	−	−
Malonate utilization	−	−	−	−	−	−	−
ONPG	−	−	−	−	−	−	−
Tartrate, Jordon	−	+	+	V^+	+	V	V
Motility, 36°C/flagella	+p	+p	+p	V^+p	+p	V p	V p
Pigmentation	−	−	−	−	−	−	−

Providencia stuartii	*Salmonella choleraesuis* subsp. *choleraesuis* serovar *choleraesuis*	*Salmonella choleraesuis* subsp. *choleraesuis* serovar *paratyphi* A	*Serratia entomophila*	*Serratia ficaria*	*Serratia grimesii*	*Serratia marcescens*	*Serratia odorifera* biogroup 1[m]	*Serratia plymuthica*	*Serratia proteamaculans*[n]	*Shigella dysenteriae* (A)[o]	*Shigella flexneri* (B)[p]	*Shigella boydii* (C)[q]
+	+	+	+	+	+	+	+	+	+	+	+	+
−	−	−	−	−	−	−	−	−	−	−	−	−
+	+	+	+	+	+	+	+	+	+	+	+	+
F	F	F	F	F	F	F	F	F	F	F	F	F
−	V	V[−y]	−	−	−	−	−	−	−	−	−	−
ALK/A	ALK/A	ALK/A	ALK/A	A/A	ALK/A	ALK/A	A/A	A/A	ALK/A	ALK/A	ALK/A	ALK/A
	ALK/A, H$_2$S	ALK/A, H$_2$S		ALK/A			ALK/A	ALK/A				
A/A	ALK/A	ALK/A	A/A	A/A	A/A	A/A	A/A	A/A	A/A	ALK/A	ALK/A	ALK/A
ALK/A	ALK/A, H$_2$S	ALK/A, H$_2$S										
A	(A)	(A)	A	A	(A)	(A)	A	(A)	(A)	A	(A)[aa]	A
−	−	−	−	V[−]	−	−	V	V[+]	−	−	−	−
V	−	−	A	A	A	A	A	A	A	−	−	−
−	−	−	−	−	−	V	V	−	−	−	−	−
−	−	A	−	A	A	−	A	A	A	V	V	V
−	−	−	V	A	NR	−	−	−	NR	NR	NR	NR
−	−	A	−	A	−	−	A	V[+]	−	−	−	−
−	−	−	−	−	−	−	−	−	−	−	−	−
−	−	−	−	−	NR	−	−	−	NR	NR	NR	NR
V	−	−	−	−	NR	−	V	V	NR	−	−	−
A	−	−	−	V	NR	V	A	V	NR	−	−	−
−	A	A	A	A	A	A	A	A	A	V	V	V
−	A	A	A	A	A	A	A	A	A	A	A[cc]	A
A	A	A	A	A	A	A	A	A	A	A	A	A
−	V	A	−	V	A	−	A	A	V	−	V	V
−	−	−	−	−	−	−	−	−	−	−	−	−
−	−	−	−	V	A	−	A	A	A	V	V	V
−	A	A	−	V	−	−	A	−	V	−	−	−
−	A	A	A	A	A	A	A	V	V	−	−	−
−	A	A	−	A	A	A	A	V[+]	A	V[+]	V	V
A	−	A	A	A	A	A	A	A	A	V[+]	V[+ee]	V[+]
−	A	−	V	A	A	−	A	A	A	−	−	−
+	−	−	−	−	−	−	V	−	−	V	V	V
+	+	+	V[−]	V	V[+]	V[−]	+	+	V	+	+	+
−	−	−	+	V	V	+	V	V[+]	V[+]	−	−	−
+	V[−]	−	+	+	+	+	+	+	+	−	−	−
−	V	V[−]	−	−	+	−	−	−	−	−	−	−
−	+	−	−	−	+	+	+	−	+	−	−	−
−	+	+	−	−	+	+	+	−	+	−	−	−
V	−	−	−	−	−	V[−]	−	−	−	−	−	−
+	−	−	−	−	−	−	−	−	−	−	−	−
V	−	−	V[+]	V	NR	V	V	V	NR	−	−	−
−	−	−	+	+	+	+	+	+	+	−	−	−
−	−	−	+	+	+	+	+	V[+]	V	−	−	−
−	−	−	+	+	+	+	+	V	V[+]	−	−	−
NR	NR	NR	NR	NR	NR	NR	NR	NR	NR	NR	NR	NR
+	−	−	+	V	+	+	V	V	+	−	−	−
−	−	−	V[−]	V	+	+	V	V	+	−	−	−
−	−	−	−	−	−	−	−	−	−	−	−	−
+	V[+]	−	+	V[−]	NR	V	+	+	NR	V	V	V
V[+]p	+p	+p	+p	+p	+p	+p	+p	Vp	+p	−	−	−
−	−	−	−	−	−	Vr[ii]	−	Vr	−	−	−	−

Table 45.8. Biochemical Reactions of *Enterobacteriaceae* with a KIA/TSI Reaction of ALKALINE/ACID, with/without Gas (*continued*)

Test	*Shigella sonnei* (D)[r]	*Tatumella ptyseos*[s]	*Xenorhabdus beddingii*[t]	*Xenorhabdus bovienii*	*Photorhabdus*[t,u] (*Xenorhabdus*) *luminescens*[t,u]	*Xenorhabdus nematophilus*[t,u]	*Yersinia poinari*[t]	*Yersinia aldovae*[v]
Catalase, 24 hr	+	+	−	−	+	−	−	+
Oxidase	−	−	NR	NR	−	−	−	−
NO$_3$→NO$_2$	+	+	−	V	−	V$^-$	NR	+
O-F glucose	F	F	NR	F	F	F	NR	F
H$_2$S (KIA/TSI)	−	−	−	NR	−	−	NR	−
KIA	ALK/A	ALK/A	NR	NR	ALK/A	ALK/A	NR	ALK/A
TSI	ALK/A	ALK/A	NR	NR	ALK/A	ALK/A	NR	A/A, AlK/A
Carbohydrate fermentations								
Glucose & gas	A	A	NR	A	Ⓐ	Ⓐ	NR	A
Lactose	−	−	NR	NR	−	−	NR	−
Sucrose	−	A	NR	NR	−	−	NR	V$^-$
Adonitol	−	−	NR	NR	−	−	NR	−
L-Arabinose	A	−	NR	NR	−	−	NR	V
D-Arabitol	NR	−	NR	NR	−	−	NR	−
Cellobiose	−	−	NR	NR	−	−	NR	−
Dulcitol	−	−	NR	NR	−	−	NR	−
Erythritol	NR	−	NR	NR	−	−	NR	−
Glycerol	V$^-$	−	V	NR	−	−	−	−
myo-Inositol	−	−	NR	NR	−	−	NR	−
Maltose	A	−	A	NR	V	−	NR	−
D-Mannitol	A	−	NR	NR	−	−	NR	V$^+$
D-Mannose	A	A	A	NR	A	V$^+$	NR	A
Melibiose	V	V	NR	NR	−	−	NR	−
α-Methyl-D-Glucoside	−	−	NR	NR	−	−	NR	−
Mucate	−	−	NR	NR	−	−	NR	−
Raffinose	−	V$^-$	NR	NR	−	−	NR	−
L-Rhamnose	V$^+$	−	NR	NR	−	−	NR	−
Salicin	−	V	V$^+$	−	−	−	−	−
D-Sorbitol	−	−	NR	NR	−	−	NR	V
Trehalose	A	A	A	NR	−	−	NR	V$^+$
D-Xylose	−	−	NR	NR	−	−	NR	V
IMViC Reactions								
Indole	−	−	−	V	V	V	−	−
Methyl red (MR)	+	−	−	NR	−	−	NR	V$^+$
Voges-Proskauer (VP) 22°C	−	−	−	NR	−	−	NR	−
37°C								
Citrate (Simmons)	−	−	−	NR	V	−	NR	−
Decarboxylase/dihydrolase reactions								
Arginine dihydrolase	−	−	−	NR	−	−	NR	−
Lysine decarboxylase	−	−	−	NR	−	−	NR	−
Ornithine decarboxylase	+	−	−	NR	−	−	NR	V
Urea/phenylalanine reactions								
Urease (Christensen's)	−	−	−	−	V$^-$	−	−	V
Phenylalanine deaminase, 24h	−	+	−	−	−	−	−	−
Misc. reactions								
Acetate utilization	−	−	NR	NR	−	−	NR	−
DNase, 25°C	−	−	+	NR	−	V$^-$	NR	−
Esculin hydrolysis	−	−	+	−	−	−	−	−
Gelatin liquefaction, 22°C	−	−	+	NR	V	V$^+$	NR	−
Gluconate	NR	NR	NR	NR	NR	NR	NR	NR
KCN broth-growth	−	−	+	NR	−	−	NR	−
Lipase (corn oil)	−	−	−,	NR	−	−	NR	−
Malonate utilization	−	−	−	NR	−	−	NR	−
ONPG	+	−	NR	NR	−	−	NR	−
Tartrate, Jordon	+	−	NR	NR	V	V	NR	+
Motility, 36°C/flagella 22°C	−	−[ii]	+p	NR	+p	+p	+p	−
37°C								
Pigmentation	−	−	+b	+y	+o,r,y[kk]	+y	+b	−

Yersinia bercovieri	*Yersinia enterocolitica*	*Yersinia frederiksenii*	*Yersinia intermedia*	*Yersinia kristensenii*	*Yersinia mollaretii*	*Yersinia pestis*	*Yersinia pseudotuberculosis*	*Yersinia rohdei*	*Yersinia ruckeri*[iw]	*Yokenella regensburgei*	Enteric group 63	Enteric group 68
+	+	+	+	+	+	+	+	+	+	+	NR	NR
−	−	−	−	−	−	−	−	−	−	−	−	−
+	+	+	+	+	+	V+	+	V+	V+	+	+	+
F	F	F	F	F	F	F	F	F	F	F	F	F
−	−	−	−	−	−	−	−	−	−	−	−	−
A/A	ALK/A	A/A	A/A	ALK/A	A/A	ALK/A	ALK/A	ALK/A	ALK/A	ALK/A	ALK/A	ALK/A
ALK/A		ALK/A	ALK/A		ALK/A							
A/A	A/A	A/A	A/A	ALK/A	A/A	ALK/A	ALK/A	A/A	ALK/A	ALK/A	ALK/A	A/A
A	A	(A)	(A)	(A)	A	A	A	A	A	(A)	(A)	A
V−	−	V	V	−	V	−	−	−	−	−	−	−
A	A	A	A	−	A	−	−	A	−	−	−	A
−	−	−	−	−	−	−	−	−	−	−	−	−
A	A	A	A	V	A	A	V	A	−	A	A	−
−	V	A	V	V	−	−	−	−	−	−	−	−
A	V	A	A	A	A	−	−	V−	A	A	A	−
−	−	−	−	−	−	−	−	−	−	−	−	−
−	V	−	−	−	−	−	−	−	−	−	−	−
−	A	V+	V	V	V−	V	V	V	V	−	−	V
−	V	V−	V−	V−	−	−	−	−	−	−	−	−
A	V	A	A	A	V	V+	A	−	A	A	A	V
A	A	A	A	A	A	A	A	A	A	A	A	A
A	A	A	A	A	A	A	A	A	A	A	A	A
−	−	−	V+	−	−	V	V	V	−	A	−	−
−	−	−	V	−	−	−	−	−	−	−	−	−
−	−	V	V	−	−	−	V−	V	−	V−	−	−
−	−	A	A	−	−	−	V	−	−	A	A	NR
V−	V−	A	A	V−	V−	V	V−	−	A	−	A	V
A	A	A	A	A	A	A	−	A	V	−	A	−
A	A	A	A	A	A	A	A	A	A	A	A	A
A	V	A	A	V+	V	A	A	V	−	A	A	−
−	V	+	+	V	−	−	−	−	−	−	−	−
+	+	+	+	+	+	V+	+	V	+	+	+	+
−	V+	−	−	−	−	−	−	−	−	−	−	V
	−											
−	−	−	V	−	−	−	−	−	−	+	−	−
−	−	−	−	−	−	−	−	−	−	−	−	−
−	−	−	−	−	−	−	−	−	V	+	+	−
V+	+	+	+	+	V+	−	−	V−	+	+	+	−
−	V	V	V+	V+	V−	−	+	V	−	−	−	−
−	−	−	−	−	−	−	−	−	−	−	−	−
−	V−	V−	V−	−	−	−	−	−	−	V−	−	−
−	−	−	−	−	−	−	−	−	−	−	−	+
V−	V−	V+	+	−	−	V	+	−	−	−	+	−
−	−	−	−	−	−	−	−	−	V	−	−	−
NR	NR	−	−	−	NR	NR		NR	NR	−	NR	NR
−	−	−	−	−	−	−	−	−	V−	+	−	+
−	V	V	V−	−	−	−	−	−	V	−	−	−
V+	+	+	+	V	V−	V	V	V	V	+	+	−
+	V+	V	V+	V	+	−	V	+	V	−	−	−
−	+p	−	−	−	−	−	−	−	−	+p	Vp	−
	−				−							
	−											

[a]Fastidious organism; requires unusual media for growth; e.g., 1% Proteose-Peptone (5). Optimal temperature 30°C; maximum, 35°C.
[b]Rarely isolated from humans; no known clinical significance (5).
[c]Genus infrequently opportunistic pathogen; similar to *Ewingella* (5) and genus resembles species of *Serratia* in many biochemical tests, but may be distinguished by DNase-negative results (1). Genus first thought to be intermediate between typical *Serratia* spp. and *Serratia fonticola*.
[d]Genus *Cedecea* often negative in standard (O'Meara) Voges-Proskauer test because of the small amount of 2,3-butanediol produced; except *C. lapagei* is usually strongly VP-positive with O'Meara method (3).
[e]Occurs in clinical specimens (6); unnamed species.
[f]Most tests and conditions are markedly different for genus *Erwinia* from those listed for other enterics; genus studies mainly by phytopathologists and rarely isolated from humans.
[g]Difficult to differentiate metabolically inactive *E. coli* strains from *Shigella* spp., especially those strains that are lactose negative, nonmotile, and anaerogenic.
[h]*Ewingella* similar to *Cedecea* spp. and other enterics that are arginine, lysine, and arnothine-negative (5)
[i]Large polysaccharide capsule that gives rise to large, mucoid colonies, especially on carbohydrate-enriched media.
[j]Optimal temperature, 32°C.
[k]Optimal temperature, 30°C.
[l]*P. myxofaciens* produces large amount of slime in broth media when grown at 22°C; TSP plus; swarms at 25°C but **not** at 36°C (3). Most other *Proteus* species swarm at 37°C.
[m]*S. odorifera* produces a pungent odor: "musty, potato-like, like crushed wild poppies," or "vegetable-like" (3); odor probably due to 2-methyl-3-isopyr-pyrszine (or structurally similar compound) (3); odor noted as soon as incubator is opened (3).
[n]Two subspecies: *S. guinovora* and *S. proteamaculans* (4).
[o]Subgroup A; 10 serotypes (1–10).
[p]Subgroup B; 6 serotypes (1–6) and X and Y variants.
[q]Subgroup C; 15 serotypes (1–15).
[r]Subgroup D; single serotype. *S. sonnei* may be separated biochemically; however, *S. boydii*, *S. dysenteriae*, and *S. flexneri* cannot be separated biochemically; it is necessary to confirm species identification by somatic (0) antigen typing.
[s]More active metabolically at 25°C.
[t]Genus *Xenorhabdus* optimal temperature is 25°C; grows poorly or not at all at 36°C (3). Older culture cells contain crystalline inclusions (not poly-β-hydroxybutyrate) spheroplasts or coccoid bodies resulting from disintegration of cell wall; seen in last third of exponential growth.
[u]*Photorhabdus* (*Xenorhabdus*) *luminescens* and *X. nematophilus* do not grow at all at 36°C; differentiation (7); catalase and bioluminescent: *P. luminescens* is catalase positive and bioluminescent positive; *X. nematophilus* is catalase negative and bioluminescent negative.
[v]Best grown at 25–28°C; delayed or variable reactions at 35–37°C. (Growth at 35°C may lead to misidentification of *Y. aldovae* as a metabolically inactive species such as *Shigella* spp. or inactive *E. coli* (2).
[w]Maximum growth at 22–25°C.
[x]Strong.
[y]If positive, may be weak.
[z]Gas production variable, majority positive.
[aa]*S. flexneri* serotype 6 gas production positive; slight amount.
[bb]May be delayed.
[cc]*S. flexneri* serotype 6 may be mannitol negative.
[dd]If positive, may be delayed.
[ee]*S. flexneri* serotype 6 usually trehalose positive although most are delayed positive.
[ff]Few reactions delayed.
[gg]Motile at 22°C, less than half of strains are motile at 36°C
[hh]*E. ictaluri* prefers a lower temperature; motile at 25°C, but not at 37°C.
[ii]Nonmotile at 36°C; 66% motile at 25°C (3).
[jj]Non-water-soluble; pink-red-magenta pigmentation at room temperature (22–25°C), rarely at 37°C.
[kk]Delayed.
[ll]See Table 45.9.

Table 45.9. Four Distinct DNA Relatedness Groups of *Y. enterocolitica*

Test Media	Group I	Group II	Group III	Group IV
Sucrose	A	A	A	—
Rhamnose	—	A[a]	A	—
Melibiose	—	A[a]	—	—
ONPG	—	+[a,b]	—	—
Simmons citrate	—	+[c]	—[d]	—

Principal Results	Report as
Sucrose-positive strains	*Y. enterocolitica*
Sucrose-negative strains	Sucrose-negative biogroup of *Y. enterocolitica*
Rhamnose-positive	*Y. enterocolitica*-like rhamnose-positive, melibiose-positive group

[a]May be delayed at 37°C.
[b]ONPG may be delayed at 37°C with relatedness group II.
[c]22°C.
[d]22° and 37°C.

Diagram 45.9.

Differentiation of *Enterobacteriaceae* with a KIA/TSI reaction of **ALKALINE/ACID, WITH/WITHOUT GAS** that may infect humans

†*Cedecea davisae*	*Escherichia coli*	*Morganella morganii*	†*Serratia proteamaculans*
Cedecea lapegei	inactive	biogroup 2	*Shigella* spp.
†*Cedecea neteri*	*Escherichia fergusonii*	†*Pantoea agglomerans*	†*Tatumella ptyseos*
Cedecea species 3	*Escherichia hermannii*	*Proteus inconstans*	†*Yersinia bercovieri*
†*Cedecea* species 5	*Escherichia vulneris*	*Proteus penneri*	†*Yersinia enterocolitica*
Citrobacter amalonaticus	*Ewingella americana*	*Providencia rettgeri*	†*Yersinia frederiksenii*
†*Citrobacter amalonaticus*	*Hafnia alvei*	*Providencia rustigianii*	†*Yersinia intermedia*
biogroup 1	*Hafnia alvei*	*Providencia stuartii*	*Yersinia kristensenii*
Citrobacter freundii	biogroup 1	*Salmonella choleraesuis*	†*Yersinia mollaretii*
Citrobacter koseri	*Klebsiella pneumoniae*	serovar *choleraesuis*	*Yersinia pestis*
†*Edwardsiella tarda*	subsp. *ozaenae*	*Salmonella choleraesuis*	*Yersinia pseudotuberculosis*
biogroup 1	*Klebsiella pneumoniae*	serovar *paratyphi A*	†*Yersinia rohdei*
†*Enterobacter amnigenus*	subsp. *rhinoscleromatis*	†*Serratia ficaria*	*Yokenella regensburgei*
biogroup 1	*Kluyvera cryocrescens*	†*Serratia grimesii*	Enteric group 63
Enterobacter amnigenus	*Morganella morganii*	†*Serratia marcescens*	†Enteric group 68
biogroup 2	biogroup 1	†*Serratia odorifera*	
†*Enterobacter asburiae*		biogroup 1	
Enterobacter cancerogenus		†*Serratia plymuthica*	
†*Enterobacter gergoviae*			
†*Enterobacter hormaechei*			

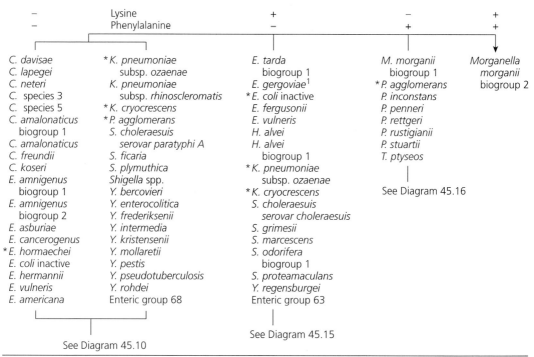

†Alkaline/Acid, KIA only; TSI: Acid/Acid.
*Organisms with variable reactions.
[1]Few reactions of *E. gergoviae* are delayed lysine-positive.

Diagram 45.10.

Differentiation of *Enterobacteriaceae* with a KIA/TSI reaction of **ALKALINE/ACID, WITH/WITHOUT GAS** that may infect humans that are:

PHENYLALANINE-NEGATIVE
LYSINE-NEGATIVE

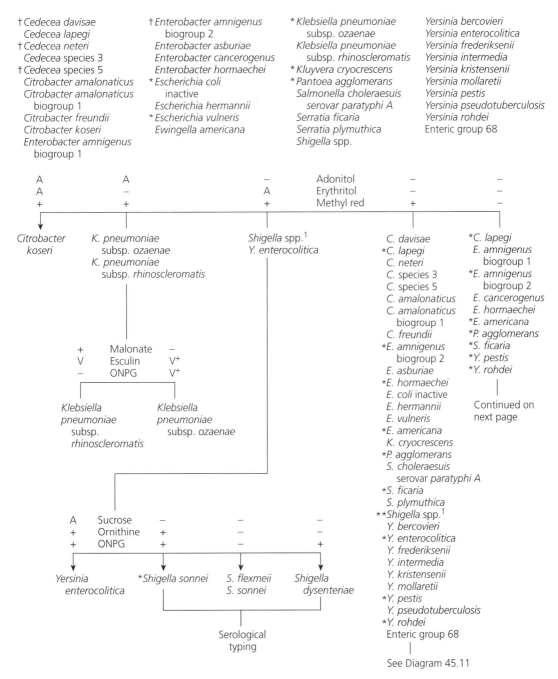

(continued)

784 Biochemical Tests for Identification of Medical Bacteria

Diagram 45.10. (*continued*)

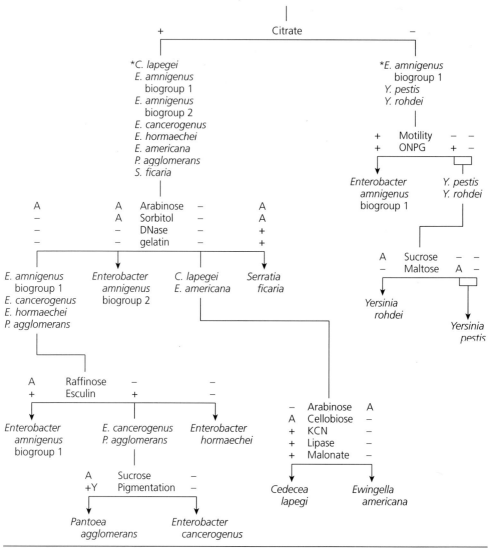

†Alkaline/Acid KIA **only;** TIS: Acid/Acid
*Variable reactions.
**No results; treated as variable.
¹No results on erythritol.

Diagram 45.11.

Differentiation of *Enterobacteriaceae* with a KIA/TSI reaction of **ALKALINE/ACID, WITH/WITHOUT GAS** that may infect humans that are:

PHENYLALANINE-NEGATIVE LYSINE-NEGATIVE	METHYL RED (MR)-POSITIVE ADONITOL-NEGATIVE		ERYTHRITOL-NEGATIVE
Cedecea davisae *Cedecea lapegi* †*Cedecea neteri* *Cedecea* species 3 †*Cedecea* species 5 *Citrobacter amalonaticus* *Citrobacter amalonaticus* biogroup 1 *Citrobacter freundii*	*Enterobacter amnigenus* biogroup 2 †*Enterobacter asburiae* †*Enterobacter hormaechei* *Escherichia coli* inactive *Escherichia hermannii* *Escherichia vulneris* *Ewingella americana*	*Kluyvera cryocrescens* *Pantoea agglomerans* *Salmonella choleraesuis* serovar *paratyphi A* †*Serratia ficaria* †*Serratia plymuthica* *Shigella* spp. *Yersinia bercovieri* *Yersinia enterocolitica*	†*Yersinia frederiksenii* †*Yersinia intermedia* *Yersinia kristensenii* †*Yersinia mollaretii* *Yersinia pestis* *Yersinia pseudotuberculosis* †*Yersinia rohdei* †Enteric group 68

+ Ornithine	+ Ornithine	+	− − − −
+ Esculin	+ Esculin	−	+ + − −
+ KCN-growth	− + KCN-growth	−	+ − + −

C. davisae
Cedecea species 5
E. amnigenus biogroup 2
E. asburiae
E. hermannii
K. cryocrescens
P. agglomerans

C. davisae
K. cryocrescens
P. agglomerans
Y. bercovieri
Y. enterocolitica
Y. frederiksenii
Y. intermedia

C. davisae
C. amalonaticus
C. amalonaticus biogroup 1
C. freundii
E. hormaechei
E. hermannii

C. davisae
E. coli inactive
S. choleraesuis serovar *paratyphi A*
S. sonnei
Y. bercovieri
Y. enterocolitica
Y. frederiksenii
Y. kristensenii
Y. mollaretii
Y. rohdei

C. lapegi
C. neteri
C. species 3
Cedecea species 5
Cedecea freundii
E. coli inactive
E. vulneris
E. americana
P. agglomerans
S. ficaria
S. plymuthica
**S. dysenteriae*
**S. flexneri*
**S. boydii*
Y. bercovieri
Y. mollaretii
Y. pestis
Y. pseudotuberculosis
Y. rohdei
Enteric group 68

Continued on next page

Continued on next page

See Diagram 45.12

See Diagram 45.13

| A | Melibiose | A | − | − |
| − | Malonate | + | + | − |

Cedecea species 5
K. cryocrescens

E. amnigenus biogroup 2
K. cryocrescens

C. davisae
P. agglomerans

E. asburiae
E. hermannii

A	Arabinose	−
A	α-Methyl-D glucoside	−
A	Rhamnose	−

Kluyvera cryocrescens   *Cedecea* species 5

| A | Arabinose | − |
| A | Rhamnose | − |

Pantoea agglomerans   *Cedecea davisae*

| − | Raffinose | A | A | Sorbitol | − |
| + | Voges-Proskauer | − | − | Motility | + |

Enterobacter amnigenus biogroup 2

Kluyvera cryocrescens

Enterobacter asburiae

Escherichia hermannii

(continued)

Diagram 45.11. (*continued*)

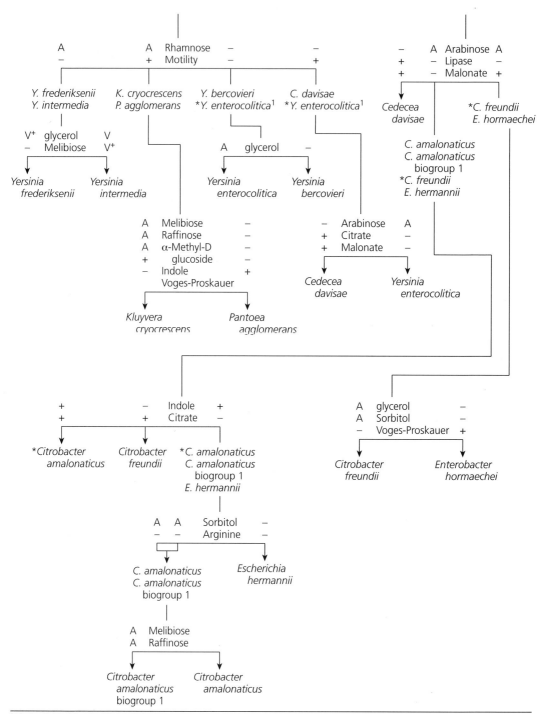

†Alkaline/Acid, KIA **only**; TSI: Acid/Acid.
*Variable reactions.
**No results; treated as variable.
[1] *Y. enterocolitica* motile at 22°C, nonmotile at 37°C.

Diagram 45.12.

Differentiation of *Enterobacteriaceae* with a KIA/TSI reaction of **ALKALINE/ACID, WITH/WITHOUT GAS** that may infect humans that are:

PHENYLALANINE-NEGATIVE   **ADONITOL-NEGATIVE**   **ESCULIN-NEGATIVE**
LYSINE-NEGATIVE   **ERYTHRITOL-NEGATIVE**   **KCN-GROWTH-NEGATIVE**
METHYL RED (MR)-POSITIVE   **ORNITHINE-POSITIVE**

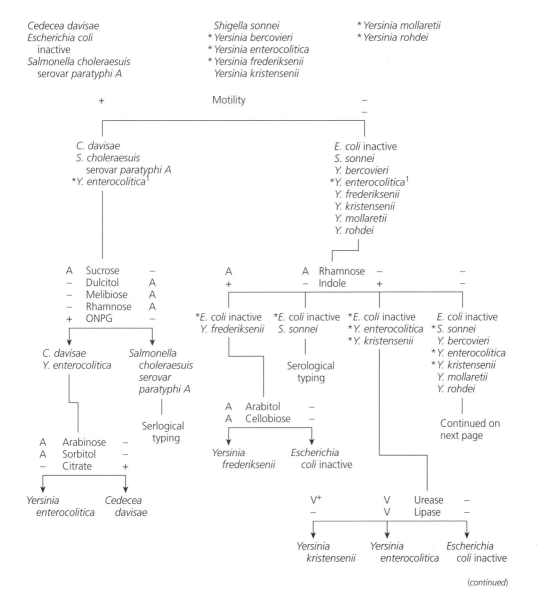

(continued)

Diagram 45.12. (*continued*)

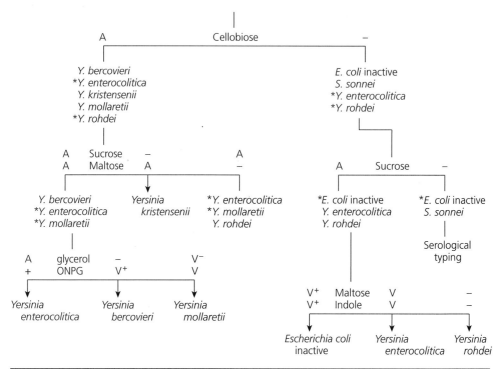

*Variable reactions.
†*Y. enterocolitica* motile at 22°C, nonmotile at 37°C.

Diagram 45.13.

Differentiation of *Enterobacteriaceae* with a KIA/TSI reaction of **ALKALINE/ACID, WITH/WITHOUT GAS** that may infect humans that are:

PHENYLALANINE-NEGATIVE   ADONITOL-NEGATIVE   ESCULIN-VARIABLE
LYSINE-NEGATIVE   ERYTHRITOL-NEGATIVE   KCN-GROWTH-VARIABLE
METHYL RED (MR)-POSITIVE   ORNITHINE-NEGATIVE

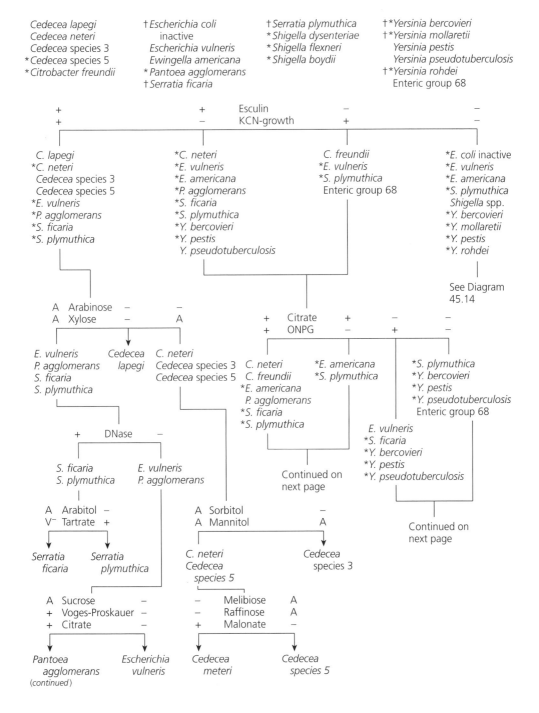

790 Biochemical Tests for Identification of Medical Bacteria

Diagram 45.13. (*continued*)

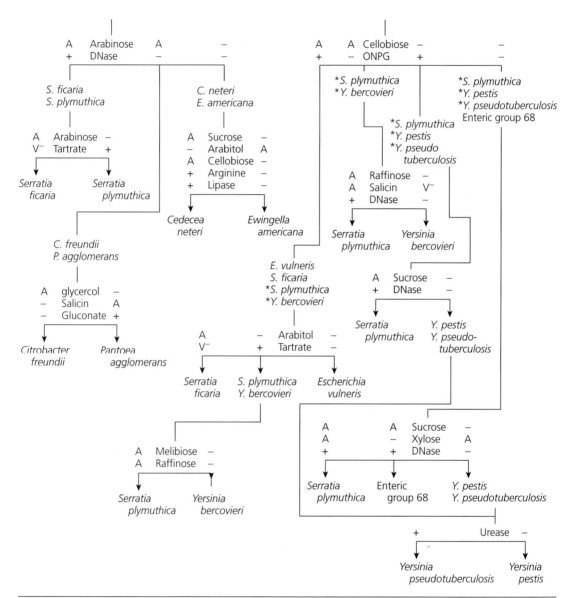

†Alkaline/Acid, KIA **only**; TSI: Acid/Acid.
*Variable reactions.

Diagram 45.14.

Differentiation of *Enterobacteriaceae* with a KIA/TSI reaction of **ALKALINE/ACID, WITH/WITHOUT GAS** that may infect humans that are:

PHENYLALANINE-NEGATIVE   ADONITOL-NEGATIVE   ESCULIN-NEGATIVE
LYSINE-NEGATIVE   ERYTHRITOL-NEGATIVE   KCN-GROWTH-NEGATIVE
METHYL RED (MR)-POSITIVE   ORNITHINE-NEGATIVE

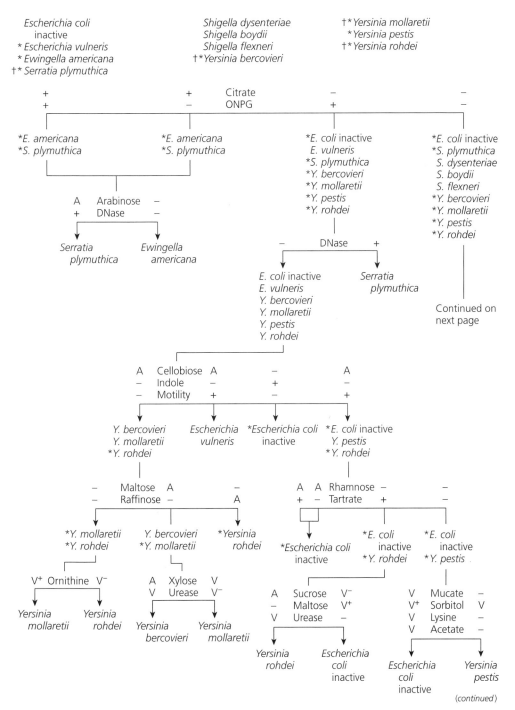

(continued)

Diagram 45.14. (continued)

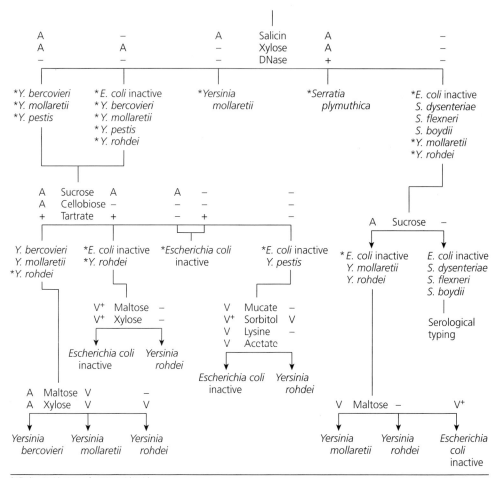

†Alkaline/Acid, KIA **only**; TSI: Acid/Acid.
*Variable results.

Diagram 45.15.

Differentiation of *Enterobacteriaceae* with a KIA/TSI reaction of **ALKALINE/ACID, WITH/WITHOUT GAS** that may infect humans and are:

PHENYLALANINE-NEGATIVE
LYSINE-POSITIVE

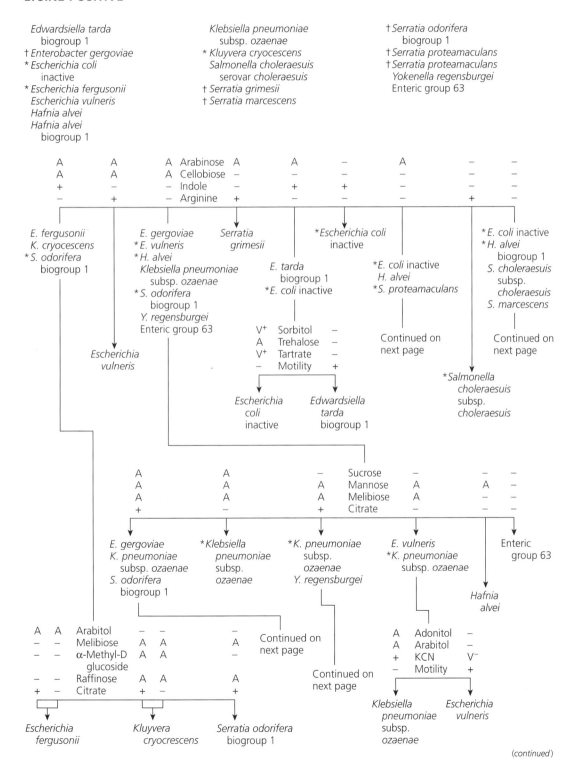

(continued)

794 Biochemical Tests for Identification of Medical Bacteria

Diagram 45.15. (*continued*)

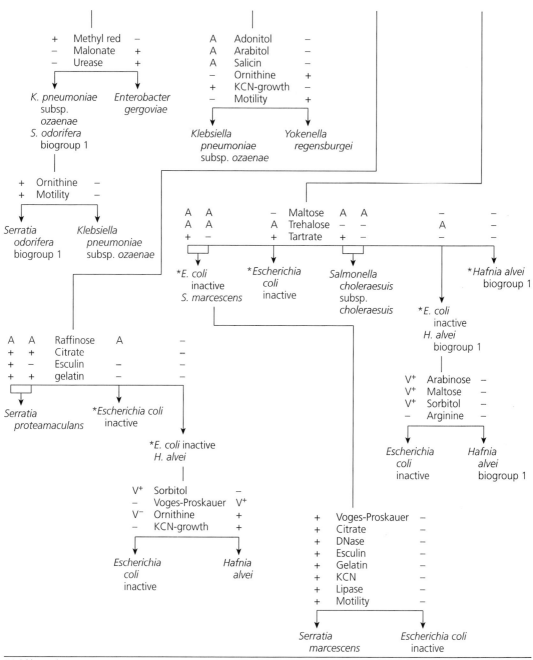

*Variable reactions.

Diagram 45.16.

Differentiation of *Enterobacteriaceae* with a KIA/TSI reaction of
ALKALINE/ACID, WITH/WITHOUT GAS that may infect humans that are:
PHENYLALANINE-POSITIVE   LYSINE-NEGATIVE

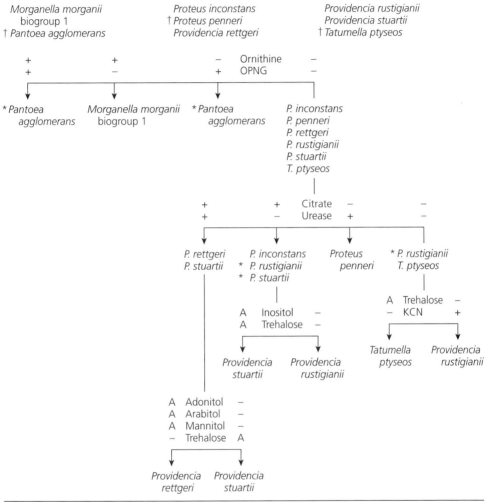

†Alkaline/Acid, KIA **only**; TSI: Acid/Acid.
*Variable reactions.

ALKALINE/ACID, H₂S, WITH/WITHOUT GAS

Table 45.10. Biochemical Reactions of *Enterobacteriaceae* with a KIA/TSI Reaction of ALKALINE/ACID, H₂S, with/without Gas

Test	*Budvicia aquatica*[a]	*Citrobacter freundii*	*Edwardsiella tarda*	*Leminorella grimontii*	*Leminorella richardii*	*Morganella morganii* biogroup 2	*Pragia fontium*	*Proteus mirabilis*	*Proteus penneri*	*Proteus vulgaris*
Catalase, 24h	+	+	+	+	+	+	+	+	+	+
Oxidase	−	−	−	−	−	−	−	−	−	−
NO₃→NO₂	+	+	+	+	+	+	+	+	+	+
O-F glucose	F	F	F	F	F	F	F	F	F	F
H₂S (KIA/TSI)	V⁺	V⁺	+	+	+	V	V⁺	+	V	+
KIA	A/A A/A, H₂S ALK/A, H₂S	A/A A/A, H₂S ALK/A ALK/A, H₂S	ALK/A, H₂S	ALK/A, H₂S	ALK/A, H₂S	ALK/A ALK/A, H₂S	ALK/A ALK/A, H₂S	ALK/A H₂S	ALK/A ALK/A, H₂S	ALK/A, H₂S
TSI	A/A A/A, H₂S ALK/A ALK/A, H₂S	A/A A/A, H₂S ALK/A ALK/A, H₂S	ALK/A, H₂S	ALK/A, H₂S	ALK/A, H₂S	ALK/A ALK/A, H₂S	ALK/A ALK/A, H₂S	A/A, H₂S ALK/A, H₂S	A/A A/A, H₂S	A/A, H₂S
Carbohydrate fermentations										
Glucose & gas	Ⓐ V⁺	Ⓐ V^f	Ⓐ −	Ⓐ −	Ⓐ −	Ⓐ −	A −	Ⓐ −	Ⓐ −	Ⓐ −
Lactose										
Sucrose	−	V	−	−	−	−	−	V⁻	A	A
Adonitol	−	−	−	−	−	−	−	−	−	−
L-Arabinose	V⁺	A	−	A	A	−	−	−	−	−
D-Arabitol	V	−	−	−	−	−	−	−	−	−
Cellobiose	−	V	−	−	−	−	−	−	−	−
Dulcitol	−	V	−	V⁺	−	−	−	−	−	−
Erythritol	−	−	−	−	−	−	−	−	−	−
Glycerol	−	A	V	V	−	A	−	V	V	V
myo-Inositol	−	−	−	−	−	−	−	−	−	−
Maltose	−	A	A	−	−	−	−	−	A	A
D-Mannitol	V	A	−	−	−	−	−	−	−	−
D-Mannose	−	A	A	−	−	A	−	−	−	−
Melibiose	−	V	−	−	−	−	−	−	−	−
α-Methyl-D-Glucoside	−	−	−	−	−	−	−	−	V⁺	V
Mucate	V⁻	A	−	A	V	−	−	−	−	−
Reffinose	−	V	−	−	−	−	−	−	−	−
L-Rhamnose	A	A	−	−	−	−	−	−	−	−
Salicin	−	−	−	−	−	−	V	−	−	V
D-Sorbitol	−	A	−	−	−	−	−	−	−	−
Trehalose	−	A	−	−	−	−	−	A	V	V
D-Xylose	A	A	−	V⁺	A	−	−	A	A	A
IMViC reactions										
Indole	−	−	+	−	−	+	−	−	−	+
Methyl red (MR)	+	+	+	+	−	+	+	+	+	+
Voges-Proskauer (VP)	−	−	−	−	−	−	−	V	−	−
Citrate (Simmons)	−	+	−	+	−	V	V⁺	V	−	V⁻
Decarboxylase/dihydrolase reactions										
Arginine dihydrolase	−	V	−	−	−	−	−	−	−	−
Lysine decarboxylase	−	−	+	−	−	+	−	−	−	−
Ornithine decarboxylase	−	V⁻	+	−	−	+	−	+	−	−
Urea/phenylalanine reactions										
Urease Christensen's)	V	V^w	−	−	−	+^w	−	+	+	+
Phenylalanine deaminase, 24h	−	−	−	−	−	+	V⁻	+	+	+
Misc. reactions										
Acetate use	−	V⁺	−	−	−	−	−	V⁻	−	V⁻
DNase, 25°C	−	−	−	−	−	−	−	V	V	V⁺
Esculin hydrolysis	−	−	−	−	−	−	V	−	−	V
Gelatin liquefaction, 22°C	−	−	−	−	−	−	−	+	V	+
Gluconate	NR	−	NR	NR	NR	NR	+	NR	NR	NR
KCN broth-growth	−	+	−	−	−	+	−	+	+	+
Lipase (corn oil)	−	−	−	−	−	−	−	+	V	V⁺
Malonate utilization	−	V⁻	−	−	−	−	−	−	−	−
ONPG	+	+	−	−	−	−	−	−	−	−
Tartrate, Jordon	V	+	V⁻	+	+	+	−	V⁺	V⁺	V⁺
Motility, 36°C/flagella	Vp^h	+p	+p	−	−	−	+p	+p	V⁺p	+p
Pigmentation	−	−	−	−	−	−	−	−	−	−

Chapter 45 / Gram-Negative *Enterobacteriaceae*

Salmonella bongori	*Salmonella choleracsuis* subsp. *arizonae*	*Salmonella cholerasuis* subsp. *choleraesuis*	*Salmonella choleraesuis* subsp. *diazonae*	*Salmonella choleraesuis* subsp. *houtenae*	*Salmonella choleraesuis* subsp. *indica*	*Salmonella choleraesuis* subsp. *salamae*	*Salmonella choleraesuis* serovar *choleraesuis*	*Salmonella choleraesuis* serovar *gallinaium*	*Salmonella choleraesuis* serovar *paratyphi* A	*Salmonella choleraesuis* serovar *pullorum*	*Salmonella typhi*	*Erwinia psidii*	*Erwinia tracheiphila*
+	+	+	+	+	+	+	+	+	+	+	+	+	+
−	−	−	−	−	−	−	−	−	−	−	−	−	−
NR	+	+	+	+	+	+	+	+	+	+	+	−	−
F	F	F	F	F	F	F	F	F	F	F	F	F	F
+	+	+	+	+	+	+	V	+	V−c	+	+wd	+	+
ALK/A, H₂S	A/A, H₂S ALK/A, H₂S	ALK/A, H₂S	A/A, H₂S ALK/A, H₂S	ALK/A, H₂S	A/A, H₂S ALK/A, H₂S	ALK/A, H₂S	ALK/A ALK/A, H₂S	ALK/A H₂S	ALK/A ALK/A, H₂S	ALK/A, H₂S	ALK/A, H₂S	ALK/A, H₂S	ALK/A, H₂S
ALK/A, H₂S	A/A, H₂S ALK/A, H₂S	ALK/A, H₂S	A/A, H₂S ALK/A, H₂S	ALK/A, H₂S	A/A, H₂S ALK/A, H₂S	ALK/A H₂S	ALK/A ALK/A, H₂S	ALK/A H₂S	ALK/A ALK/A, H₂S	ALK/A, H₂S	ALK/A, H₂S	NR	NR
Ⓐ	Ⓐ	Ⓐ	Ⓐ	Ⓐ	Ⓐ	Ⓐ	Ⓐ	A	Ⓐ	Ⓐ	A	A	A
−	V−	−	V+	−	V−	−	−	−	−	−g	−	−	−
−	−	−	−	−	−	−	−	−	−	−	−	NR	NR
A	A	A	A	A	A	A	−	V+	A	A	−	NR	−
NR	NR	NR	NR	NR	NR	NR	−	−	−	−	−	NR	NR
A	−	A	−	V	−	A	−	A	A	−	−	A	−
NR	NR	NR	NR	NR	NR	NR	−	−	−	−	−	NR	NR
−	−	−	−	−	V	V−	−	−	−	−	V−	NR	−
−	−	V	−	−	−	−	−	−	−	−	−	A	−
A	A	A	A	A	A	A	A	A	A	A	A	NR	A
A	A	A	A	A	A	A	A	A	A	A	A	A	−
V+	A	A	A	A	V+	−	V	−	A	−	A	NR	−
−	−	−	−	−	−	−	−	−	−	−	−	A	−
A	A	A	V	−	A	A	−	V	−	−	−	−	NR
−	−	−	−	−	−	−	−	−	−	−	−	A	−
A	A	A	A	A	A	A	A	−	A	A	−	A	−
A	A	−	V	−	−	−	−	−	A	A	−	−	−
A	A	A	A	A	A	A	−	V	A	A	A	−	−
A	A	A	A	A	A	A	V	−	A	V+	−	−	−
−	−	−	−	−	−	−	−	−	−	−	−	−	−
+	+	+	+	+	+	+	+	+	+	+	+	NR	NR
−	−	−	−	−	−	−	−	−	−	−	−	+	V
+	+	+	+	+	V+	+	V−	−	−	−	−	NR	NR
V+	V	V	V	V	V	+	V	−	V−	−	−	−	NR
+	+	+	+	+	+	+	+	+	−	+	+	−	NR
+	+	+	+	+	+	+	+	−	+	+	+	−	NR
−	−	−	−	−	−	−	−	−	−	−	−	−	−
−	−	−	−	−	−	−	−	−	−	−	−	NR	−
−	+	+	V+	V	V+	+	−	−	−	−	−	−	NR
−	−	−	−	−	V−	−	−	−	−	−	−	NR	NR
−	−	−	−	−	−	−	−	−	−	−	−	NR	−
NR	NR	NR	NR	NR	NR	NR	NR	NR	NR	NR	NR	NR	NR
−	−	−	+	−	−	−	−	−	−	−	−	NR	−
−	+	−	+	−	−	+	−	−	−	−	−	NR	NR
−	+	−	+	−	V	V−	−	−	−	−	−	NR	NR
−	−	+	V−	V	−	V	V+	+	−	−	+	NR	NR
+p	+p	+p	+p	+p	+p	+p	−	+p	−	+p	−	+p	+p
−	−	−	−	−	−	−	−	−	−	−	−	−	−

798 Biochemical Tests for Identification of Medical Bacteria

*a*Rarely isolated from humans; no known clinical significance (5).
*b*Most tests and conditions are markedly different from genus *Erwinia* from those listed for other enterics; genus studies mainly done by phytopathologists and Erwinia is rarely isolated from humans.
*c*If positive, may be weak.
*d*May have a ring of H_2S (mustache-like); its presence **is not** diagnostic for *S. typhi*; H_2S production may be overlooked and reported as negative or some strains fail to produce detectable H_2S on KIA, TSI, or LIA slants.
*e*If gas produced, a slight amount.
*f*May be delayed.
*g*Although rare, lactose-positive variants exist.
*h*Motile at 22°C; less than half of strains are motile at 36°C (5).

Diagram 45.17.

Differentiation of *Enterobacteriaceae* with a KIA/TSI reaction of **ALKALINE/ACID, WITH/WITHOUT GAS, H_2S** that may cause human infections:

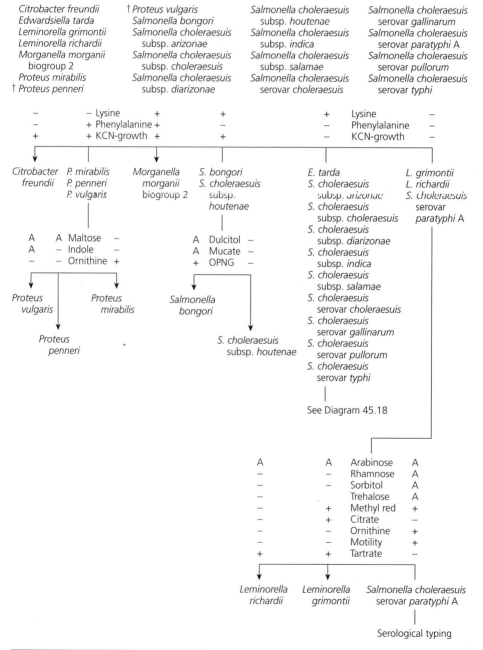

†Alkaline/Acid, H_2S KIA only; TSI: Acid/Acid.

Diagram 45.18.

Differentiation of *Enterobacteriaceae* with a KIA/TSI reaction of
ALKALINE/ACID, WITH/WITHOUT GAS, H₂S that may infect humans and are:
**LYSINE-POSITIVE   KNC-GROWTH-NEGATIVE
PHENYLALANINE-NEGATIVE**

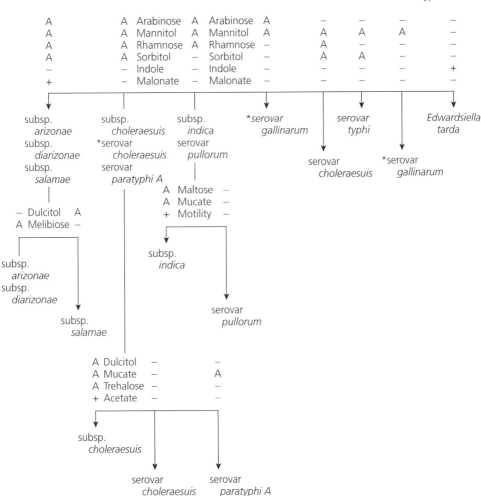

FINAL I.D. *Salmonella* spp.: Serological typing.

*Variable reactions.

ALKALINE/ALKALINE OR ALKALINE/NO CHANGE

Table 45.11. Differentiation of the Most Frequently Isolated Nonenteric Intestinal Bacteria

Test	Acinetobacter baumanni	Acinetobacter calcoaceticus	Acinetobacter lwoffii	Alcaligense faecalis	Alcaligenes latus	Alcaligenes piechaudii	Alcaligenes xylosonidans	Pseudomonas aeruginosa
Catalase	+	+	+	+	+	+	+	+
Oxidase	−	−	−	+	+	+	+	+
NO$_3$→NO$_2$	−	−	−	−	+	+	+	+
MacConkey (MAC)	G	G	G	G	G	G	G	G
41°C	G	NG	NG	NR	NR	NR	NR	G
O/F glucose	0	0	0	0	0	0	0	0
Citrate	+	+	−	+	+	+	+	NR
Gelatin liquefaction, 22°C	−	−	−	−	+	−	−	+
Glucose	V$^+$	A	V$^-$	−	A	−	A	A

Chapter 45 / Gram-Negative *Enterobacteriaceae*

Diagram 45.19.

Differentiation of the most frequently isolated **NONENTERIC** intestinal bacteria with a KIA/TSI reaction of **ALKALINE/ALKALINE** or **ALKALINE/NO CHANGE**

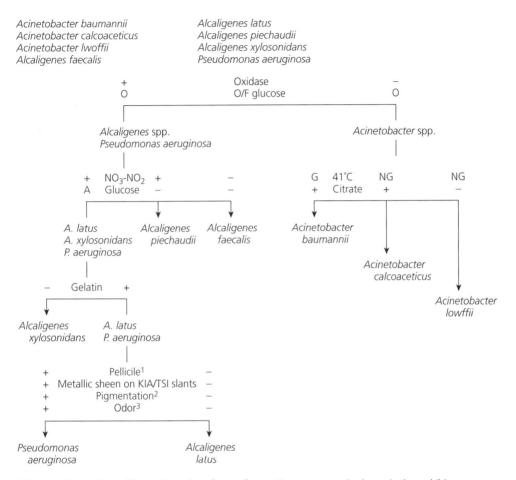

Sellers medium: tubed, differential medium for nonfermenting gram-negative bacteria that exhibit Alkaline/Alkaline or Alkaline/No Change KIA/TSI; useful for differentiating among *Acinetobacter*, *Alcaligenes*, and *Pseudomonas*.

Table 45.12

Differentiating criteria	*Acinetobacter* spp.	*Alcalgenes faecalis*	*Pseuodmonas aeruginosa*
Slant	Blue	Blue	Green
Butt	No change	Blue or change	Blue or no change
Band	Yellow/–	–	–
Fluorescent slant	–	–	Yellow-green
Nitrogen gas	–	+	+

[1]Scum on top of liquid media
[2]Bluish-green.
[3]Grape-like

REFERENCES

1. Balows A, Hausler WJ Jr, Herrmann KL, Isenberg HD, Shadomy HJ. Manual of Clinical Microbiology, ed 5. Washington, DC: American Society for Microbiology, 1991.
2. Bercovier H, Steigerwalt AG, Guiyoule A, Huntley-Carter G, Brenner DJ. *Yersinia aldovae* (formerly *Yersinia enterocolitica*-like group X2): A new species of *Enterobacteriaceae* isolated from aquatic ecosystems. Int J Syst Bacterial 1984;34(2):166–172.
3. Farmer JJ III, Davis BR, Hickman-Brenner FW, McWhorter A, Huntley-Carter GP, Asbury MA, Riddle C, Wathen-Grady HG, Elias C, Fanning GR, Steigerwalt AG, O'Hara CM, Morris GK, Smith PB, Brenner DJ. Biochemical identification of new species and biogroups of *Enterobacteriaceae* isolated from clinical specimens. J Clin Microbiol 1985;21(1):46–76.
4. Grimont PAD, Irino K, Grimont F. The *Serratia liquefaciens-S. proteamaculans-S. grimessi* complex: DNA relatedness. Curr Microbiol 1982;7:63–68.
5. Holt JG, Krieg NR, Sneath PHA, Staley JT, Williams ST. Bergey's Manual of Determinative Bacteriology, ed 9. Baltimore: Williams & Wilkins, 1994.
6. Koneman EW, Allen SD, Janda WM, Schreckenberger PC, Winn WC Jr. Color Atlas and Textbook of Diagnostic Microbiology, ed 4. Philadelphia: JB Lippincott, 1992.
7. Thomas GM, Poinar GO. *Xenorhabdus* gen. nov., a genus of entomopathogenic nematophilic bacteria of the family *Enterobacteriaceae*. Int J Syst Bacteriol 1979;29:352–360.

SECTION IV

Appendices

APPENDIX 1

Photographic Results

PHOTOGRAPHIC CREDITS

BD Biosciences
Courtesy of BD Biosciences (formerly Becton Dickinson Microbiology Systems)
7 Loveton Circle
Sparks MD 21152

REMEL, Inc.
Courtesy of REMEL
12076 Santa Fe Drive
Lenexa, KS 66215

Anaerobe Systems
Courtesy of Anaerobe Systems
15906 Concord Circle
Morgan Hill, CA 95037

JM
James O. Murray, MS, SM (AAM)
Microbiologist
Army Medical Department Center & School
Academy of Health Sciences
Department of Clinical Support Services
Fort Sam Houston, TX 78234

COLOR FIGURES

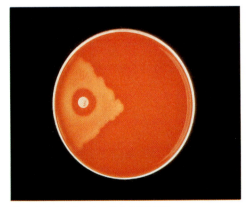

Fig. 1.1. Bacitracin disk (REMEL)

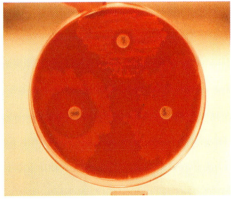

S. aureus   E. coli

Fig. 1.2. Bacitracin disk (REMEL)

806 Biochemical Tests for Identification of Medical Bacteria

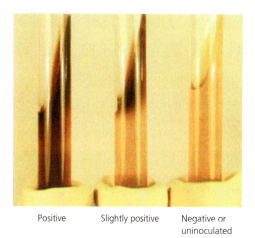

Positive   Slightly positive   Negative or uninoculated

Fig. 2.1. Bile esculin (aesculin) test

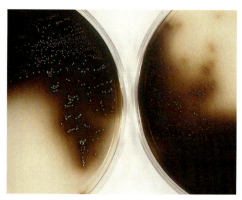

Gp. D **Non**-enterococci   Gp D. Enterococci

Fig. 2.2. Bile esculin agar (REMEL)

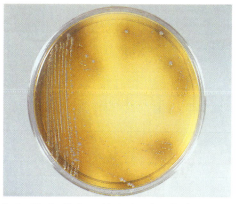

Bacteroides fragilis Group (darkening of medium)
Fusobacterium necrophorum

Fig. 2.3. Bacteroides bile esculin (BBE) agar (JM)

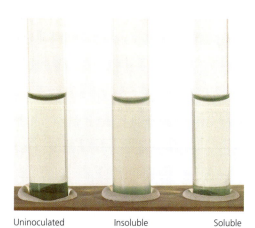

Uninoculated   Insoluble   Soluble

Fig. 3.1. Bile solubility test

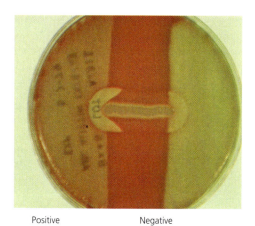

Positive   Negative
(arrowhead)

Fig. 4.1. CAMP test (reaction)

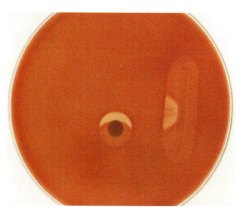

Fig. 4.2. β-Lysin disk for CAMP test for group B *Streptococcus* and *Staphylococcus* streak (REMEL)

Appendix 1 / Photographic Results **807**

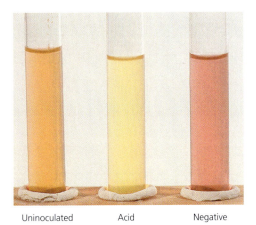

Uninoculated   Acid   Negative

Fig. 5.1. Carbohydrate fermentation test

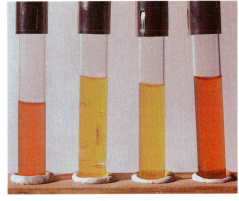

Uninoculated   Acid and gas   Acid   Negative

Fig. 5.2. Semisolid carbohydrate fermentation test

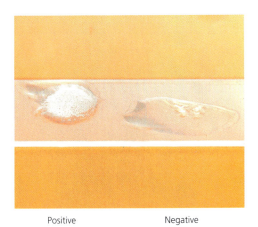

Positive   Negative

Fig. 6.1. Catalase test

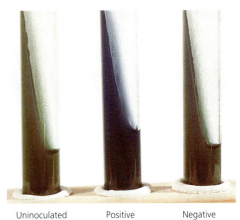

Uninoculated   Positive   Negative

Fig. 7.1. Simmons citrate test

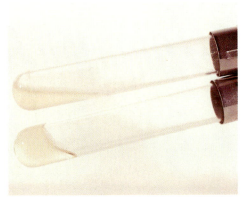

Fig. 8.1. Coagulase test

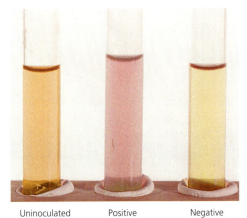

Uninoculated   Positive   Negative

Fig. 9.1. Falkow's lysine test

Biochemical Tests for Identification of Medical Bacteria

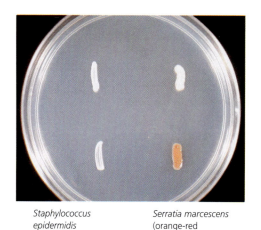

Staphylococcus epidermidis   *Serratia marcescens* (orange-red pigmentation)

Fig. 10.1. DNase test agar **before HCl added** (JM)

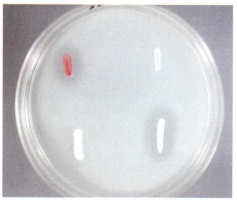

Klebsiella pneumoniae subsp. *pneumoniae* (−)   *Staphylococcus aureus* subsp. *aureus* (+)

Fig. 10.2. DNase test agar **after HCl added—intermediate** (JM)

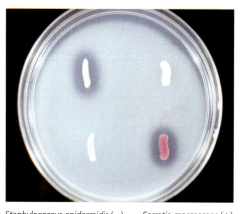

Staphylococcus epidermidis (−)   *Serratia marcescens* (+)

Fig. 10.3. DNase test agar **after HCL added—complete** (JM)

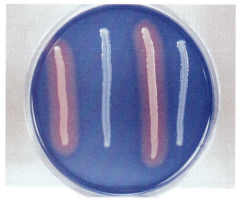

Serratia marcescens: Positive, pink
Klebsiella pneumoniae subsp. *pneumoniae:* Negative

Fig. 10.4. DNase test agar with toluidine blue O (JM)

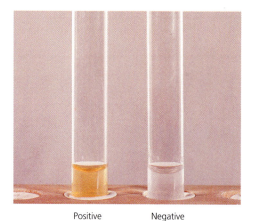

Positive   Negative

Fig. 11.1. β-Galactosidase test (ONPG)

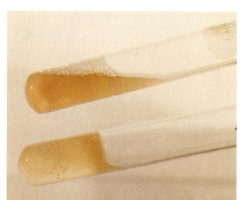

Positive (liquefied)

Negative

Fig. 12.1. Gelatin liquefaction test

Appendix 1 / Photographic Results **809**

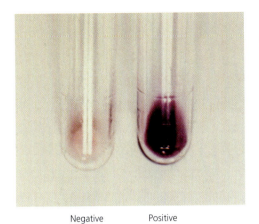

Negative   Positive

Fig. 14.1. Hippurate disk

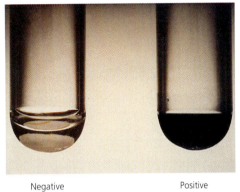

Negative   Positive

Fig. 14.2. Rapid hippurate disk test (REMEL)

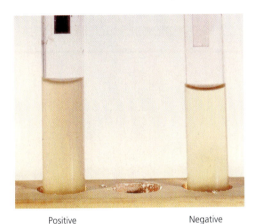

Positive   Negative

Fig. 15.1. Hydrogen sulfide lead acetate (PbAc) strip test

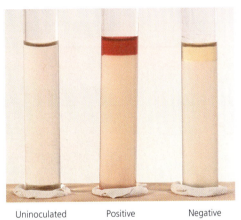

Uninoculated   Positive   Negative

Fig. 16.1. Kovacs' indole test

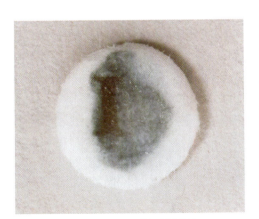

Fig. 17.1. Indoxyl acetate disk (REMEL)

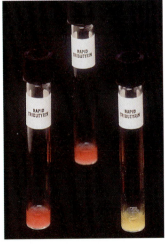

Fig. 17.2. Rapid tributyrin test (REMEL)

Biochemical Tests for Identification of Medical Bacteria

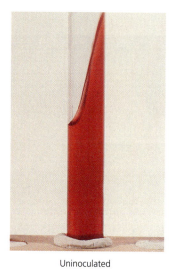

Uninoculated
Fig. 18.1. Kligler's iron agar

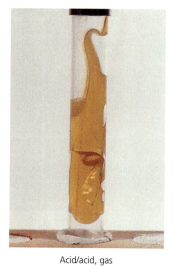

Acid/acid, gas
Fig. 18.2. Kligler's iron agar

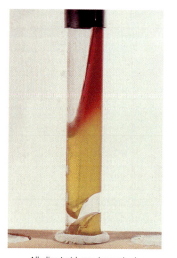

Alkaline/acid, gas (reversion)
Fig. 18.3. Kligler's iron agar

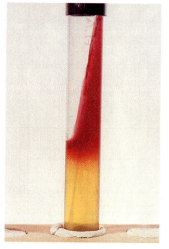

Alkaline/acid
Fig. 18.4. Kligler's iron agar

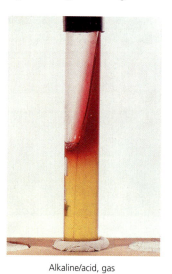

Alkaline/acid, gas
Fig. 18.5. Kligler's iron agar

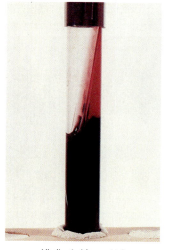

Alkaline/acid, gas, H_2S
Fig. 18.6. Kligler's iron agar

Appendix 1 / Photographic Results **811**

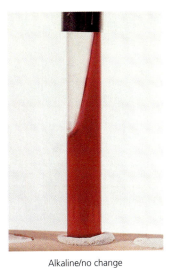

Alkaline/no change
Fig. 18.7. Kligler's iron agar

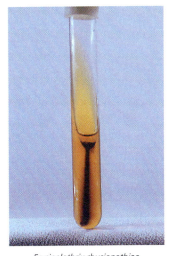

Erysipelothrix rhusiopathiae
Fig. 18.8. Triple sugar iron (TSI) agar (JM)

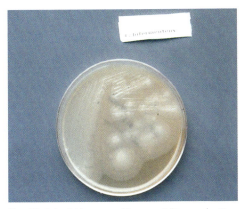

Fig. 20.1. Lecithinase positive result (Anaerobe Systems)

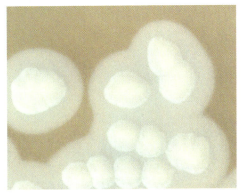

Fig. 20.2. Lecithinase positive result (Anaerobe Systems)

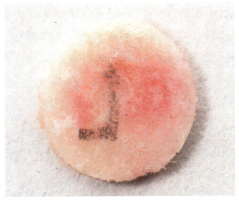

Fig. 21.1. Leucine aminopeptidase (LAP) disk (REMEL)

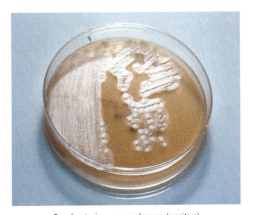

Fusobacterium necrophorum (positive)
Fig. 22.1. Lipase test (Anaerobe Systems)

812 Biochemical Tests for Identification of Medical Bacteria

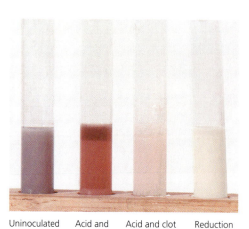

Uninoculated | Acid and digestion | Acid and clot | Reduction

Fig. 23.1. Litmus milk

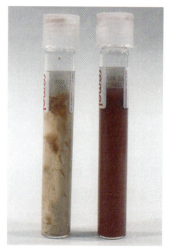

Stormy fermentation Reduction of litmus | Acid and digestion

Fig. 23.2. Litmus milk

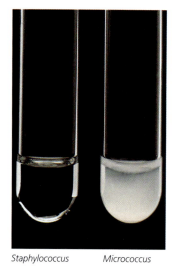

Staphylococcus *Micrococcus*

Fig. 24.1. Lysostaphin test (RE-MEL)

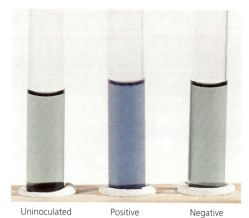

Uninoculated | Positive | Negative

Fig. 25.1. Malonate medium test

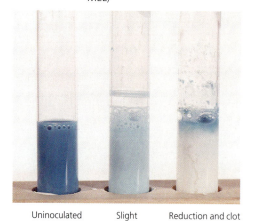

Uninoculated | Slight reduction (+) | Reduction and clot

Fig. 26.1. Methylene blue milk reduction test for enterococci

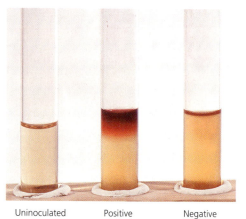

Uninoculated | Positive | Negative

Fig. 27.1. Methyl red (MR) test

Appendix 1 / Photographic Results **813**

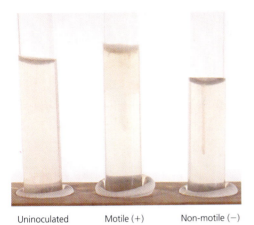

Uninoculated   Motile (+)   Non-motile (−)

Fig. 28.1. Motility test

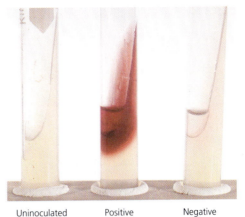

Uninoculated   Positive   Negative

Fig. 30.1. Nitrate reduction test (phase 1, no zinc)

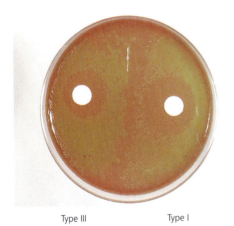

Type III   Type I

Fig. 31.1. Optochin sensitivity test (*Streptococcus pneumoniae* subsp. *pneumoniae*)

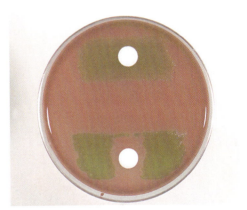

Fig. 31.2. Optochin sensitive (*Streptococcus pneumoniae* subsp. *pneumoniae*) and resistant (α-*Streptococcus* spp.) test

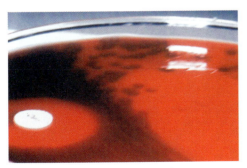

Fig. 31.3. Optochin sensitivity test (*Streptococcus pneumoniae* subsp. *pneumoniae*)

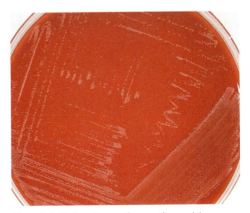

Fig. 32.1. *Neisseria* spp. (nonpathogenic)

814 Biochemical Tests for Identification of Medical Bacteria

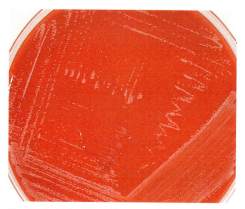

Fig. 32.2. *Neisseria* oxidase test (pink stage)

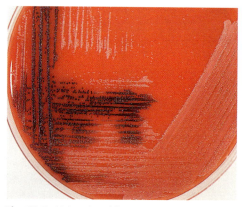

Fig. 32.3. *Neisseria* oxidase positive test (black)

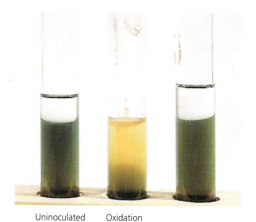

Fig. 33.1. OF Media-Oxidative Reaction

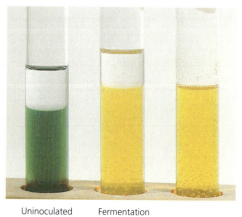

Fig. 33.2. OF Media-Fermentation Reaction

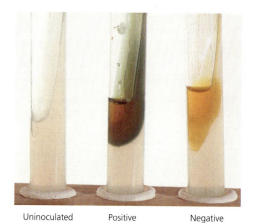

Fig. 34.1. Phenylalanine test

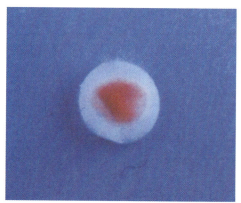

Fig. 36.1. Porphyrin-δ-aminolevoline acid (ALA) disk (REMEL)

Appendix 1 / Photographic Results **815**

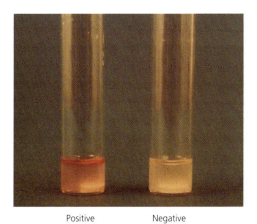

Positive   Negative

Fig. 37.1. Pyrrolidonyl-β-naphthylamide (PYR) broth (REMEL)

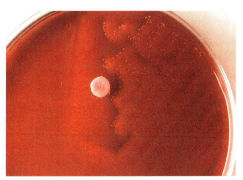

Fig. 37.2. Pyresculin disk (REMEL)

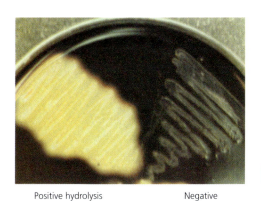

Positive hydrolysis   Negative

Fig. 38.1. Starch hydrolysis test

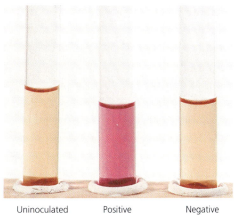

Uninoculated   Positive   Negative

Fig. 39.1. Stuart's urease test

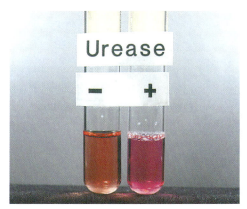

Fig. 39.2. *Mycobacterium* urease test medium (JM)

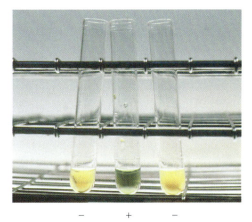

−   +   −

Fig. 39.3. Urea-phenylalanine disks (REMEL)

816 Biochemical Tests for Identification of Medical Bacteria

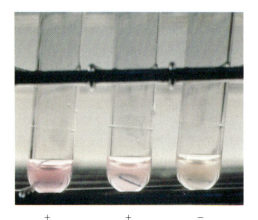

+   +   −

Fig. 39.4. Urea-phenylalanine (PDA) disks (REMEL)

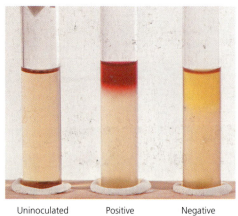

Uninoculated   Positive   Negative

Fig. 40.1. Voges-Proskauer (VP) test

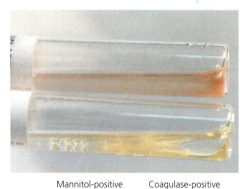

Mannitol-positive   Coagulase-positive

Fig. 42.1. Coagulase mannitol broth (Phenol Red Mannitol Broth Base) (REMEL)

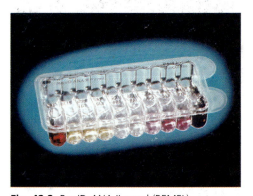

Fig. 42.2. RapID-ANA II panel (REMEL)

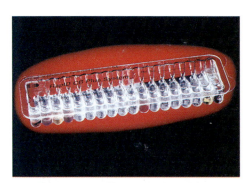

Fig. 42.3. RapID CB-Plus system (REMEL)

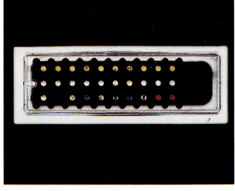

Fig. 42.4. BBL Crystal Enteric/Nonfermenter ID panel (BD Biosciences)

Appendix 1 / Photographic Results **817**

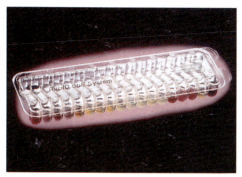

Fig. 42.5. RapID ONE system (REMEL)

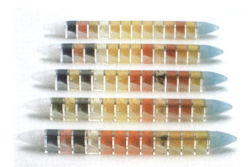

Fig. 42.6. Enterotube II (BD Biosciences)

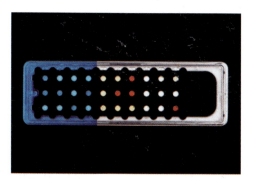

Fig. 42.7. BBL4 Crystal Gram-Positive ID panel (BD Biosciences)

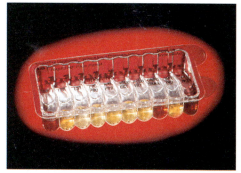

Fig. 42.8. RapID NF Plus panel (REMEL)

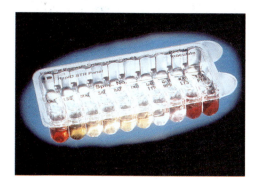

Fig. 42.9. RapID STR panel (REMEL)

APPENDIX 2

Metric System Units of Measure

Centi- (prefix): meaning 100 (1/100).
Milli- (prefix): meaning 1000 (1/1000).

UNITS OF LENGTH
Meter (m)
    1 m = 100 cm = 1000 mm
    1 m = 39.37011 inches
Centimeter (cm): one hundredth of a
    meter (10^{-2} m)
    1 cm = 0.01 m = 10 mm
    1 cm = 0.3937 inch
Millimeter (mm): one thousandth
    of a meter (10^{-3} m)
    1 mm = 0.01 cm = 0.001 m
    1 mm = 0.03937 inch
Micron (μ): one thousandth of a
    millimeter (10^{-3} mm); one millionth
    of a meter (10^{-6} m)
    1 μ = 0.001 mm = 0.000001 m
    1 μ = 1/25,400 inch
Millimicron (mμ): one thousandth of a
    micron (10^{-3} μ); one millionth of a
    millimeter (10^{-6} mm);
    one billionth of a meter (10^{-9} m)
    1 mμ = 0.001 μ = 0.000001 mm = 0.000000001 m

UNITS OF WEIGHT
Gram (g)
    1 g = 1,000 mg
    1 g = 15.43248 grains
Milligram (mg): one thousandth of a
    gram (10^{-3} g)
    1 mg = 0.001 g
    1 mg = 0.01543 grain

UNITS OF VOLUME (CAPACITY)
Liter (L)
    1 L = 1000 mL (cc)
Milliliter (mL, cc): one thousandth of a liter
    (10^{-3} L)
    1 mL = 0.0001 L
    1 mL = 0.0033815 fluid ounce

CONVERSIONS
m × 100 = cm
m × 1000 = mm

cm × 0.01 = m
cm × 10 = mm

mm × 0.1 = cm
mm × 1000 = μ

μ × 0.000001 = m
μ × 0.0001 = cm
μ × 0.001 = mm
g × 1000 = mg
mg × 0.001 = g

L × 1000 = mL (cc)
mL × 0.001 = L
inches × 2.54 = cm
inches × 25.4 = mm
inches × 25,400 = μ

APPENDIX 3

pH Indicators

Indicator	pK[a]	Acid pH	Alkaline pH	Chemical Compound
Andrade's	7.2, colorless	5.0, pink	8.0, pale yellow	Acid fuchsin
Bromcresol purple	6.3, purple	5.2, yellow	6.8, purple	Dibromo-o-cresol-sulfonphthalein ($C_{21}H_{16}O_5SBr_2$)
Bromthymol blue	7.0, green	6.0, yellow	7.6, deep Prussian blue	Dibromophenol-sulfonphthalein ($C_{27}H_{28}O_5SBr_2$)
o-Cresol red (alkaline)	8.3	7.2, yellow	8.8, red	o-Cresolsulfonphthalein ($C_{21}H_{18}O_5S$)
Litmus (pure)	6.8	4.5, red	8.3, blue	Commercial indicator: plant extract
Methyl red	5.0	4.4, red	6.0, yellow	4'-Dimethylamino-azobenzene-2-carboxylic acid ($C_{15}H_{15}N_3O_2$)
Neutral red	7.5	6.8, red	8.0, yellow	2-Methylamino-phenazine ($C_{15}H_{17}N_4Cl$)
Phenol red	7.9	6.8, yellow	8.4, red	Phenolsulfonaphthalein ($C_{19}H_{14}O_5S$)

[a] pK: symbol for the logarithm of the reciprocal of the dissociation constant of an electrolyte (pH). pK = log 1/k.

APPENDIX

4 pH Adjustment

"A worker is only as good as the tools he employs." In this case, microbiologists' tools are the media and reagents they prepare for themselves and coworkers. The ability of a microbiologist to isolate pathogenic bacteria from clinical specimens can only be as effective as the media used for cultivation. Correct pH is only one of many criteria required for proper preparation of culture media; others are discussed throughout the text.

Each individual batch of medium **must** be at its optimal pH, usually at the finished (sterilized), cooled stage. If it is too acid or alkaline, pH must be adjusted; most bacteria of medical importance prefer a neutral or slightly alkaline environment for optimal growth. The use of commercial, dehydrated media **usually** eliminates pH adjustment; however, if media are prepared from scratch, pH adjustment is almost always necessary. The major reasons for pH changes are: oversterilization, incomplete mixing, use of alkaline containers, hydrolysis of ingredients, presence of detergents in unclean glassware, repeated remelting, or improperly distilled or demineralized water use for rehydration.

The final pH required varies among commercial suppliers, even among the same type of medium; refer to the commercial label for recommended pH. Acceptable pH should be ± 0.2 unit of desired value (Table 4.1).

Table 4.1. Required pH of Isolation and Biochemical Test Media[a]

Medium	Desired pH (± 0.2)
Acid-DNase (Jeffries, Holtman, and Guse) agar	7.3
Acridine orange–deoxyribonucleate agar (ADA)	9.0
Arginine decarboxylase	6.0
Bile esculin agar (BE, BEA, BEM)	7.0
Bismuth sulfite agar (BSA)	7.6
Brain heart infusion (BHI)	7.4
Brilliant green agar (BGA)	6.9
Christensen's urea agar	6.8
Clark and Lubs (MR/VP)	6.9
Cystine Trypticase agar (CTA)	7.3
Eosine methylene blue (Levine) (EMB)	7.1
Falkow lysine decarboxylase	6.8
Gluconate peptone broth	7.0
Gonococcus identification (GCID) medium	7.5
Heart infusion (HI)	7.4
Hugh and Leifson's O-F basal medium (OFBM)	7.1
Indole-nitrate	7.2
Kenner fecal streptococcal (KF)	7.2
Kligler's iron agar (KIA)	7.4
Litmus milk	6.8[b]
Lysine iron agar (LIA)	6.7
MacConkey agar (MAC)	7.1
Malonate broth	6.7
Metachromatic agar-diffusion (DNase) (MAD)	9.0
Methylene blue milk (MBM)	6.4
Methyl red/Voges-Proskauer (Clark and Lubs)	6.9

(continued)

Table 4.1. Required pH of Isolation and Biochemical Test Media[a]

Medium	Desired pH (± 0.2)
Møller decarboxylase base	6.0
Motility (semisolid)	7.2–7.3
Mueller-Hinton	7.4
Ninhydrin broth	7.2
Nitrate broth	7.0
Nitrite broth	6.8
Nutrient gelatin (stab)	6.8
ONPG (β-galactosidase) broth	7.3
Ornithine decarboxylase broth (Fay and Barry)	5.5
Peptone iron agar (PIA)	6.7
Phenolphthalein diphosphate (PDP) nutrient broth	7.4
Phenol red broth base	7.4
Phenol red broth base with Andrade's indicator	7.1–7.2
Phenol red-carbohydrate broth	6.8
Phenol red (semisolid) base	7.5
Phenylalanine agar	7.3
Rustigian and Stuart's urea broth	6.8
Salmonella-Shigella agar (SS)	7.0
Sheep blood agar (SBA)	7.3
Simmons' citrate	6.9
Staph OF	7.0
Starch basal medium	7.2
Streptococcus faecalis broth (SF)	6.9
Sulfide-indole-motility (SIM)	7.3
Thioglycollate gelatin	7.0
Todd-Hewitt broth	7.8
Triple sugar iron agar (TSI)	7.4
Trypticase soy agar (TSA)	7.3
Tryptophan broth (indole test)	7.3

[a]Final desired pH may vary among commercial suppliers; values given here are for BBL or Difco products.
[b]Adjust with added litmus; **not** with HCl.

A. Reagents
  1. Hydrochloric acid (HCl); concentrated approximately 12 N or 36% weight in volume
      a. Hydrochloric acid (HCl), 1N
          (1) HCl, concentrated, reagent grade (R. G.) .... 8.7 mL
          (2) Distilled water . . . to bring to .... 100.0 mL
      b. HCl, 0.1 N
          (1) HCl, **1** N .... 10.0 mL
          (2) Distilled water . . . to bring to .... 100.0 mL
  2. Sodium hydroxide (NaOH)
      a. NaOH, 10 N (40%)
          (1) NaOH, carbonate-free, R. G. .... 40.0 g
          (2) Distilled water . . . to bring to .... 100.0 mL
      b. NaOH, 1 N (4%)
          (1) NaOH, **10** N .... 10.0 mL
          (2) Distilled water . . . to bring to .... 100.0 mL
      c. NaOH, 0.1 N (N/10, 1/10 N)
          (1) NaOH, **10** N .... 1.0 mL
          (2) Distilled water . . . to bring to .... 100.0 mL
  3. Method of preparation
      a. Sodium hydroxide, 10 N (40%)

(1) **Rapidly** weigh sodium hydroxide and dissolve in less than 100 mL of distilled water in a beaker. This reagent is highly in hygroscopic.
(2) Place beaker in a circulating water bath to Control temperature.
(3) Cool and transfer NaOH solution to a 100-mL volumetric flask and bring to 100 mL with distilled water.
(4) Store in a polyethylene or paraffin-lined glass reagent bottle.
(5) Label correctly.
  b. 1 N and 0.1 N NaOH and HCl solutions
    (1) Fill a 100-mL volumetric flask with approximately 50 mL of distilled water.
    (2) Use a Pro pipette (bulb) or similar apparatus attached to a volumetric pipette to withdraw acid or alkali from stock bottle (NaOH, 10 N) or concentrated acid bottle (HCl); **never pipet by mouth.**
    (3) With Pro pipette, **slowly** release desired volume of acid/alkali down side of flask and discard pipette in appropriate container. Always add acid/alkali to water, **never** water to acid/alkali, as splattering could occur. Both reagents are extremely caustic; avoid any contact with skin or eyes and if splattering occurs, flood area **immediately** with running tap water.
    (4) Bring to desired volume (100 mL) with distilled water. It is not necessary to make more than 100 mL as usually only a few drops are necessary to adjust pH.
    (5) Mix well and store in labeled, glass-stoppered reagent bottles.
B. Colorimetric comparative procedures; two choices
  1. pH test papers; paper strips impregnated with various indicators; color matched against comparator chart
    a. Two commercial types of indicator strips suitable; **do not** use litmus paper.
      (1) pHydrion test strips
      (2) Nitrazine (sodium dinitrophenolazonaphthol); **universal indicator**
    b. Procedure
      (1) Tear off approximately 1 inch of paper; have as little finger contact as possible.
      (2) Place against a white background; e.g., filter paper.
      (3) Dip **clean** glass rod into **well-mixed** flask of medium (**gently** swirl flask to mix) and place **1 drop** onto indicator strip; **avoid area touched by fingers.**
      (4) Allow color to stabilize; a few **seconds.**
      (5) Compare with comparator chart provided with indicator paper. Most Nitrazine paper has a comparator chart ranging from pH 3 to 9; however, the accurate range is only 4.5 (acid, yellow) to 7.5 (alkaline, blue).
  2. Commercial sealed-tube standards or colored disk solutions
    a. A set per each type of indicator
      (1) One set: 9 tubes.
      (2) pH range: 0.2 unit intervals between tubes; e.g., phenol red: 6.8, 7.0, 7.2, . . . 8.4.
    b. Procedure.
      (1) Mix flask of medium thoroughly by **gently** swirling the flask and by pipette (sterile if testing finished product) remove 10 mL aliquot and place in a tube the **same diameter** as the standards.
      (2) Place tubes in comparator block and compare with desired pH tube.
  3. Adjustment using paper strips or commercial standards
    a. If **Acid** (pH 0–6.9), add **measured** quantities of 0.1 N NaOH to 10-mL aliquot until color matches the desired pH (standard tube or paper strip reading) and **record** quantity used.
    b. If **alkaline** (pH 7.1–14), add **measured** quantities of 0.1 N HCl to 10-mL aliquot un-

til color matches desired pH (standard tube or paper strip reading) and **record** quantity used.
  4. Calculations
     a. The amount of HCl or NaOH used to adjust a 10-mL aliquot × 10 = the amount required to adjust 1 L of prepared medium.
     b. Example: 1.0 mL of 0.1 N NaOH is required to adjust phenol red broth base to 7.4; 1.0 × 10 = 10 mL of 0.1 N NaOH/L.
  5. With a pipette, add a calculated amount of 0.1 N acid or base to 1L of prepared medium and **mix well**; **recheck** pH and **readjust** if necessary. pH paper strips measure pH to within a few tenths of a pH unit determined.
C. pH meter; **method of choice**; most accurate
  1. Principle: two (or combined) electrodes and standard cell to measure hydrogen ion concentration
     a. As hydrogen ion concentration increases, pH decreases (becomes more acid).
     b. Acidity, pH 0–6.9; neutrality, pH 7.0; alkalinity, pH 7.1–14.
  2. Method of testing
     a. **Nonsterile** media
        (1) Place flask of prepared **liquid** medium onto a magnetic stirrer (e.g., Vortex) to mix well; if solid or semisolid preparation, keep at 45–50°C to avoid solidification. Use a flask at least twice the size of the amount of medium being prepared; e.g., a 2 L flask for 1 L of medium.
        (2) Place electrodes in flask; test total volume of prepared medium; remove from magnetic stirrer to take pH readings.
        (3) Take pH reading using a temperature converter; the dial reads pH directly in pH units.
        (4) If adjustment is necessary, return the flask to the magnetic stirrer and **drop by drop** add the appropriate reagent, **0.1** N acid or alkali, depending on the pH reading and the desired acidity or alkalinity. **Recheck** the pH and **readjust** as often as necessary to reach the desired pH. It is better to use a lower concentration of reagents (0.1 N) to avoid overcorrecting for pH; a 1 N concentration is stronger and less is needed for adjustment, but too often the end point is reached too rapidly or overshot.
     b. Cooled, **sterilized** (finished) media; **preferred** state of testing as desired pH of commercial dehydrated media (as shown on label) is for sterilized product at 25°C (room temperature)
        (1) Solid or semisolid media
           (a) 50-mL aliquot in beaker
           (b) Standard combination electrode or spear-shaped electrode: avoids necessity of melting down media and thus compensates for increased temperature
        (2) Liquid media: two surface electrodes or combination electrode
        (3) Final value: average of three separate readings; acceptable pH ± 0.2 unit of desired pH.
  3. Precautions
     a. pH meters **must** be calibrated (standardized) frequently against standard buffer of known pH and readjusted, if necessary.
        (1) Standard buffer should be as close to the pH of media being tested as possible.
        (2) Temperature of the standard buffer should be the same as media when taking readings.
     b. Temperature influences pH readings.
        (1) Where applicable, depending on type (model) of instrument used, temperature

control **must** be set at temperature of medium being tested **before** a reading is taken.
   (2) The ionization constant increases with a rise in temperature; e.g., CO_2-free distilled water at 25°C has a pH of 7.0 but at 40°C, the pH is 6.7.
 c. Keep electrodes immersed in water when not in use; **do not** allow them to dry out.
 d. Commercial meters vary in types of electrodes, circuits, and operating instructions; refer to literature accompanying instrument for standard operating procedures (SOP). The most precise pH measurements are made with pH meters; readings are usually to within 1-hundredth of a pH unit.

APPENDIX 5

McFarland's Nephelometer Standards

A. Purpose: to measure turbidity
   1. To measure bacterial densities in a liquid culture
   2. To produce a culture of a desired density
B. Preparation of standards; barium sulfate
   1. Reagents
      a. Barium chloride ($BaCl_2$), 1% aqueous solution
      b. Sulfuric acid (H_2SO_4), chemically pure (C. P.), 1% aqueous solution
      c. $BaCl_2 + H_2SO_4 \rightarrow BaSO_4 + 2\ HCl$
   2. Test tubes
      a. 10 **new** screw-capped tubes (or ampules) of equal size; thoroughly cleaned and rinsed
      b. Same diameter (size) as tubes to be compared
   3. Add reagents to appropriately labeled (1 to 10) tubes in amounts indicated below:

	Barium Sulfate Standards									
Tube Number	1	2	3	4	5	6	7	8	9	10
1% $BaCl_2$ (mL)	0.1	0.2	0.3	0.4	0.5	0.6	0.7	0.8	0.9	1.0
1% H_2SO_4 (mL)	9.9	9.8	9.7	9.6	9.5	9.4	9.3	9.2	9.1	9.0
Approx. cell density ($\times 10^8$/mL)	3	6	9	12	15	18	21	24	27	30
Approx. cell density (in millions/mL)	300	600	900	1200[a]	1500	1800	2100	2400	2700	3000[b]

[a] 1 billion, 200 million.
[b] 3 billion.

   4. Seal tubes or ampules and label.
   5. Suspended $BaSO_4$ precipitate equal approximately to homogenous *Escherichia coli* densities per milliliter throughout.
C. Method of use
   1. Shake standard tubes **gently.**
   2. **Aseptically**, add a measured aliquot of broth culture to be tested into a **sterile** tube the **same diameter** (size) as standard tubes.
   3. **Aseptically**, add a measured amount of **sterile** saline (NaCl), until turbidity matches that of desired standard tube number.
      a. To measure test culture tube density
         (1) Each tube a given multiple of 300,000,000 (million) organisms/mL
         (2) $10^8 = 100,000,000.$
         (3) Cell density standard tube no. $\times$ 300,000,000 = no. of organisms/mL

(4) Example: tube no. 3
   9×10^8 = 900,000,000 organisms/mL
   b. To produce a desired density; for example, need bacterial density of 10^5 (100,000)
      (1) Culture corresponding to tube no. 1 (3×10^8) is diluted 1:3 to equal 10^8.
      (2) Then diluted again 1:1000.
      (3) $10^8 - 10^3 = 10^5$
D. Precautions
   1. If broth culture to be tested is not clear:
      a. Subtract value of **uninoculated** medium from value of culture to get corrected bacterial density.
      b. Example: tube no. 4   −   tube no. 1   =   tube no. 3
                  (broth culture)   (incubated,   (corrected reading)
                                      uninoculated)
   2. If broth is highly colored, place **uninoculated** tube **behind** standard tube to facilitate reading.

REFERENCES

Branson D. Methods in Clinical Bacteriology, Springfield, IL.: Charles C Thomas, 1972:106.

Finegold SM, Martin WJ, Scott EG. Bailey and Scott's Diagnostic Microbiology, 5th ed. St. Louis: CV Mosby, 1978:488–489.

APPENDIX 6

Reagent Preparations

Chemical Gradin 827
Table 6.1—Data on Common Reagents Used in Media Preparation 827
Percent (%) Solutions (v/v, w/v, w/w) 828
Gram Formula Weight (GFW) 829
Mole 829
Molarity 830
Table 6.2—Positive Valences of More Commonly Used Elements in Media Preparation 831
Gram Equivalent Weight (GEW) 831
Normality (Normal Solution) 831
Stock Solution Dilutions 833
Titration 833
Concentrated Acid/Alkali Dilutions 834
Buffers 835
Dyes-Indicators 836
Enrichments 837
Table 6.3—Components of Commercial V Factor 838
Miscellaneous Reagents 839
Preparation of Sealants 841
General References 841

CHEMICAL GRADING

1. **Reagent grade (R. G.)/analytical reagent (A. R.):** high purity
2. **Chemically Pure (C. P.):** pure enough for clinical use
3. **United States Pharmacopeia (U. S. P.):** less pure than C. P.
4. **Technical, Practical, or Commercial Grade:** used primarily for industrial use; **not** usually used for clinical purposes.

Table 6.1. Data on Common Reagents Used in Media Preparation

Concentrated Reagent[a]	Formula	Positive Valence	GEW	Sp. gr.[b]	W/W%[c]	Normality[d]	No. of mL Equivalent to 1 g Pure Solute
Acetic acid, glacial	$HC_2H_3O_2$	1	60	1.06	99.5	17.6	0.96
Ammonium hydroxide as	NH_3	1	17	0.90	28.0	14.8	3.97
Hydrochloric acid	HCl	1	36.5	1.19	37.0	12.1	2.30
Nitric acid	HNO_3	1	63	1.42	70.0	15.8	1.01
Phosphoric acid	H_3PO_4	3	32.7	1.71	85.0	44.4	0.70
Sulfuric acid	H_2SO_4	2	49	1.84	98.0	36.8	0.57

[a]Commercially available as w/w solutions.
[b]At room temperature, 22–25°C.
[c]May vary over a small range; check label on commercial reagent and recalculate, if necessary. w/w% = number of grams of solute per 100 g of solution.
[d]Calculation of normality of concentrated and acid/alkali; example, HCl.

1. Gram equivalent weight (GEW) = $\dfrac{\text{Gram formula weight (GFW)}}{\text{Valence of positive ions}}$

    $= \dfrac{36.5}{1} = 36.5$

2. Normality (N) = $\dfrac{\text{Sp. gr.} \times \text{Assay (w/w\%)} \times 10}{\text{Gram equivalent weight (GEW)}}$

    $= \dfrac{1.19 \times 37.0 \times 10}{36.5} = 12.1 \text{ N}$

PERCENT (%) SOLUTIONS

1. **Weight/volume (w/v) percent (%) solution**
    a. Definition: number of grams of solute per 100 mL of solution
    b. Purpose: determination of the number of grams of a solution required to prepare a w/v% solution of a desired volume
    c. Formula:
       Grams of solute desired = $\dfrac{(\text{w/v\%})(\text{desired volume in mL})}{100}$
    d. Example: prepare 500 mL of a 10% w/v solution of NaCl

       $= \dfrac{(10)(500)}{100} = 50.0 \text{ g}$

2. **Volume/volume (v/v) percent (%) solution**
    a. Definition: number of millimeters of solute in each 100 mL of solution
    b. Purpose: determination of the number of milliliters of solute required to prepare a v/v% solution of a desired volume
    c. Formula:
       Milliliters of solute required = $\dfrac{(\text{v/v\%})(\text{desired volume in mL})}{100}$
    d. Example: prepare 250 mL of a 1.5% solution of concentrated HCl.

       $= \dfrac{(1.5)(250)}{100} = 3.75 \text{ mL}$

3. **Weight/weight (w/w) percent (%) solution**
    a. Definition: number of grams of solute per 100 g of solution; e.g., 49% H_2SO_4 in water contains 49 g of acid in each 100 g of solution.
    b. Not routinely used; used as a v/v% solution **or** must be converted to a w/v% solution
    c. To prepare a w/v% solution, there are two methods of calculation.
    d. Example: prepare a 10% w/v solution of HCl (see data in Table 2.1).
    e. **Calculation method 1.**
       (1) HCl w/w% = 37
       (2) Step 1: calculate number of grams of concentrated solution that will contain 10 g (ratio:proportion)

       $\dfrac{37.0 \text{ g pure HCl}}{100 \text{ g concentrated solution}} = \dfrac{10 \text{ g pure HCl}}{\text{X (grams of concentrated solution)}}$

       $37 \text{ X} = 1000$

       $\underline{\text{X} = 27 \text{ g}}$

       27 g concentrated HCl solution = 10 g pure HCl

Appendix 6 / Reagent Preparations **829**

(3) Step 2: Conversion of w/w% to w/v% solution
   (a) Purpose: determination of the volume of concentrated reagent that contains a desired weight of the pure compound in solution
   (b) Formula:

   $$\text{Milliliters of solution containing required weight} = \frac{\text{Grams concentrated solution required}}{\text{Sp. gr. concentrates solution}}$$

   $$= \frac{27}{1.19} = 230.0 \text{ mL}$$

   (c) 10% w/v HCl: dilute 23 mL concentrated solution to 100 mL with water.
      1 23 mL weighs 27 g.
      2 23 mL contains 10 g pure HCl.

f. **Calculation method 2**; use data from Table 2.1.
   a. Purpose: determination of the number of milliliters of a concentrated w/w% reagent required to prepare a w/v% solution of a desired volume
   b. Formula:

   Milliliters of concentrated reagent required

   $$= \frac{(\text{Milliliters equivalent to 1 g, see Table 2.1})(\text{Desired w/v\%})(\text{Volume desired in mL})}{100}$$

   $$= \frac{(2.3)(10)(100)}{100} = 23 \text{ mL}$$

   c. 23 mL of concentrated HCl diluted to 100 mL with water

GRAM FORMULA WEIGHT (GFW)

1. Also listed as gram molecular or gram molar weight (GMW) or relative formula mass
2. Definition: sum of all atomic weights of individual elements making up a molecule of the compound (chemical formula) expressed in grams
   a. Each element is calculated by number of times it occurs in a specific chemical formula.
   b. Example: Sodium carbonate, Na_2CO_3.

Element	No. atoms	×	Atomic weight of one atom	=	Total weight in formula
Na	2		23		46
C	1		12		12
O	3		16		48
					Gram formula weight = 106

MOLE (mol)

1. Definition: formula weight of a compound in grams
   1 mole = GFW (or GMW)
2. Examples:
   1 mole NaOH = 40 g NaOH
   1 mole Na_2CO_3 = 106 g Na_2CO_3
3. Millimole (mmol)
   a. Definition: 1/1000 of a mole

b. Examples:
   1 mole NaOH = 40 g; 1 mmol = 0.04 g
   1 mole Na_2Co_3 = 106 g; 1 mmol = 0.106 g

MOLARITY (M)

1. Also listed as molar solution
2. Definition: number of gram formula weights (GFW) of a compound per liter of final solution **or** number of moles per liter of final solution **or** number of moles of solute in one cubic decimeter of solution (1 dm^{-3}).
3. Two basic formulas
   a. **Formula 1**
      (1) Purpose: **determination of the weight of a compound required to prepare a solution of desired molarity and volume**

      (2) Grams of reagent = $\dfrac{\text{(Molecular weight)} \quad \text{(Desired molarity)} \quad \text{(Final volume in mL)}}{1000}$

   b. **Formula 2**
      (1) Purpose: **determination of the number of milliliters of a concentrated w/w reagent required to prepare a solution of a desired molarity and volume**
      (2) Milliliters concentrated reagent to use

      $= \dfrac{\text{(Mollecular weight)} \quad \text{(Desired molarity)} \quad \text{Final volume in ml)} \quad \text{Last column, Table 2.1)}}{1000}$

   c. Examples:
      (1) NaCl: GFW = 58.5.
         1 M = 58.5 g/L of solution.
         0.5 M = $\dfrac{58.5}{2}$ = 29.25 g/L of solution.
         3 M = 3 × 58.5 = 175.5 g/L of solution.
      (2) Prepare 1L of 2 M HCl from the concentrated acid
         $\dfrac{(36.5)\,(2\,M)\,(1000)\,(2.3)}{1000}$ = 167.9 mL

4. Alternative formulas
   a. M = $\dfrac{\text{No. moles of solute}}{\text{No. of liters of solution}}$

   b. M = $\dfrac{\text{No. of grams of solute}}{\text{GFW}} \times \dfrac{1}{\text{No. liters of solution}}$

   c. No. moles of solute = Molarity × No. liters of solution
   d. No. grams of solute = Molarity × GFW × No. liters of solution

5. Alternative ways to express a particular molarity
   a. 0.5 M = 1/2 M **or** M/2
   b. 0.2 M = 1/5 M **or** M/5

Appendix 6 / Reagent Preparations **831**

Table 6.2. Positive Valences of More Commonly Used Elements in Media Preparation

1+	2+	3+
Cu (cuprous)	Ba	Al
H	Ca	Bi
Hg (mercurous)	Cd	Fe (ferric)
K	Cu (cupric)	Mn
Li	Fe (ferrous)	
Na	Hg (mercuric)	
NH_4 (ammonium)	Mg	
Tl (thallious)	Mn	
	Zn	

GRAM EQUIVALENT WEIGHT (GEW)

1. Definition: weight in grams or mass of an element that will liberate, combine with, or replace, either directly or indirectly, 1 g atom of hydrogen.
2. Formula (also see data in Table 2.2)

$$GEW = \frac{GFW}{\text{Valence of positive ions}}$$

3. Examples:

	GFW	GEW
HCl	36.5	$\frac{36.5}{1} = 36.5$
H_2SO_4	98	$\frac{98}{2} = 49.0$
H_3PO_4	98	$\frac{98}{3} = 32.7$

4. Milligram equivalent weight = 1/1000 of a GEW

NORMALITY (NORMAL SOLUTION) (N)

1. Definition: number of gram equivalent weights (or equivalents) per liter of solution **or** the number of milliequivalents per milliliter **or** fraction of equivalent weight of a solute dissolved in one cubic decimeter ($1\ dm^{-3}$) of solution
2. Two basic formulas
   a. **Formula 1**
      (1) Purpose: **determination of the weight of a compound required to prepare a solution of a desired normality and volume**

      (2) Grams required = $\dfrac{\text{(Molecular weight) (Desired normality) (Final volume in mL)}}{\text{(Total positive valence) (1000)}}$

      or

      $= \dfrac{\text{(GEW) (Desired N) (Final volume in mL)}}{1000}$

      (3) Example: prepare 250 mL of a 2 N magnesium sulfate solution ($MgSO_4$)

(a) Molecular weight = 120; GEW = $\dfrac{120}{2}$ = 60

(b) Grams required = $\dfrac{(120)(2)(250)}{(2)(1000)}$ = 30

or

= $\dfrac{(60)(2)(250)}{1000}$ = 30

b. **Formula 2**
   (1) Purpose: **determination of the number of milliliters of a concentrated w/w reagent required to prepare a solution of a desired normality and volume**
   (2) Milliliters concentrated reagent required

$$= \dfrac{\text{(Molecular weight)} \quad \text{(Desired normality)} \quad \text{(Final volume in mL)} \quad \text{(Last column Table 2.1)}}{\text{(Total positive valence)} (1000)}$$

or

$$= \dfrac{\text{(GEW) (Desired N) (Final volume) (Last column Table 2.1)}}{1000}$$

   (3) Example: prepare 1 L of 2 N H_2SO_4 from the concentrated acid

   (a) Molecular weight = 98; GEW = $\dfrac{98}{2}$ = 49

   (b) Milliliters required = $\dfrac{(98)(2)(1000)(0.57)}{(2)(1000)}$ = 55.9

   or

   = $\dfrac{(49)(2)(1000)(0.57)}{1000}$ = 55.9

3. Alternative formulas

   a. $N = \dfrac{\text{GEW of solute}}{\text{Liters of solution}}$

   b. $N = \dfrac{\text{No. of grams of solute}}{\text{GFW/valence}} \times \dfrac{1}{\text{Liters of solution}}$

   c. $N = \dfrac{\text{No. of moles}}{\text{Valence}} \times \dfrac{1}{\text{Liters of solution}}$

   d. $N = \dfrac{\text{No. of grams of solute}}{\text{GEW}} \times \dfrac{1}{\text{Liters of solution}}$

   e. N = GEW/liters of solution
   f. N = Molarity × total positive valence

4. Alternative ways to express a particular normality
   a. 0.1 N = 1/10 N **or** N/10.

b. $0.67 \text{ N} = 2/3 \text{ N}$ or $\dfrac{2N}{3}$.

STOCK SOLUTION DILUTIONS

1. Purpose: determination of the milliliters of a concentrated stock solution required to prepare a more dilute solution
2. Formula; all units must be the same (e.g., % from %, normal from a normal solution, etc.).

   No. of milliliters concentrated stock solution to be diluted

   $= \dfrac{\text{(Milliliters diluted solution desired) (Desired concentration of solution)}}{\text{Concentration of stock solution}}$

3. Example
   a. HCl, stock solution 1 N; desire 100 mL of a 0.1 N solution

   $= \dfrac{(100 \text{ mL}) (0.1 \text{ N})}{1 \text{ N}} = 10$

   b. Add 10 mL of 1 N HCl to volumetric flask and bring to 100 mL with distilled water.

TITRATION

1. Definition: method to measure the concentration of one solution by comparison with a measured volume of a solution of known concentration (a standard solution)
   a. Quantity of hydronium ions (H^+) that will react with hydroxyl ions (OH^-) with resultant formation of a salt and water
   b. H^+ ions react with OH^- ions in molar ratio 1:1. One volume of a 1 N solution of any acid will react completely with one volume of 1 N solution of any base or vice versa.
   c. **Equivalence point:** point at which all available H^+ ions (or OH^- ions) are neutralized
      (1) **Neutralization:** equivalence point of titration (endpoint) evident by use of a specific pH indicator
      (2) **Indicator:** index of the endpoint of the reaction evident by a color change; color change depends on indicator used.
2. Purpose: to determine **exact** normality of an acid or base
3. Indicators: choice depends on solution to be titrated. See Dyes-Indicators for their preparation.

Acid/Base Combination	Examples	Indicator(s)
Strong acid/strong base	HCl, H_2SO_4/NaOH, KOH	Phenol red
Strong acid/weak base	/NH_4OH	Methyl orange[a] Methyl red
Strong acid/basic salt	/Na_2CO_3	Methyl orange[a] Methyl red
Weak acid/strong base	CH_3COOH/	Phenolphthalein[b]
Acid salt/strong base	K acid phthalate/	Phenolphthalein[b]

[a]**Do not** use with phthalate buffers.
[b]Fades in strong alkali.

4. Calculation
   a. Purpose: determination of the exact normality of an acid or base after titration
   b. Formula:
      (Volume acid used) (Normality acid used) = (Volume base used) (Normality base used)

   $$\text{or } (V_1)(N_1) = (V_2)(N_2)$$

c. Example: determine normality of a prepared 0.5 N NaOH; 18.3 mL of prepared 0.5 N NaOH neutralized 10 mL of 1.0 N HCl
   (1) Step 1: $(10)(1.0) = (18.3)(N)$
   $$N = \frac{10}{18.3} = 0.55 \text{ N}$$
   (2) Step 2: NaOH too concentrated; dilute using dilution formula.

   Milliliters stock concentrated solution to be diluted

   $$= \frac{\text{(Milliliters of dilute solution desired) (Concentration of dilute solution)}}{\text{Concentration of stock solution}}$$

   $$= \frac{(1000)(0.5)}{0.55} = 925.0 \text{ mL}$$

   = 925.0 mL of 0.55 N. NaOH diluted to 1 L with deionized water

CONCENTRATED ACID/ALKALI DILUTIONS

(*Note:* Concentrated acids and alkalies are extremely caustic, so avoid exposure to the skin as painful burns may occur. If splattering occurs, wash area **immediately** with running tap water.)
1. **Hydrochloric acid (HCl), concentrated:** Reagent grade (R. G.); equals 12.1 N or 37% weight in volume
   a. **Preparation**
      (1) Prepare in 100-mL or 1 **volumetric** flask; **add acid** to a small volume of distilled water **slowly. Do not** add water to acid, as splattering may occur.
      (2) **Slowly** bring to total desired volume with distilled water.
   b. **Concentrations**
      (1)

Desired Normality (N)	Milliliters of concentrated acid	
	per 100 mL	per 1 L
2 N	16.8 mL	167.9 mL
1 N	8.4 mL	84.0 mL

   (2) 0.1 N: Two means of preparation
      (a) 8.4 mL of concentrated HCl/1 L; 0.8 mL/100 mL distilled water
      (b) 100.0 mL of 1 N HCl brought to 1 L or 10.0 mL of 1 N HCl brought to 100 mL with distilled water

(*Note:* Store all acids and alkalies in a polyethylene or paraffin-lined glass reagent bottle. Label with name, exact normality, date prepared, and initials of preparer.)

2. **Sodium hydroxide (NaOH), concentrated:** Reagent grade (R. G.) and carbonate-free
   a. Preparation
      (1) **Rapidly** weight NaOH and dissolve in less than 100 mL of distilled water in a **beaker.** This reagent is highly hygroscopic; avoid exposure to air any longer than necessary.
      (2) Place beaker in a circulating water bath to control the temperature; a large amount of heat is generated.
      (3) Cool and transfer NaOH solution to a 100-mL **volumetric** flask and bring to 100 mL with distilled water.
   b. **Concentrations**

Desired normality (N)	% Concentration	Milliliters of Concentrated Alkali	
		per 100 mL	per 1 L
10 N	40	40	400
9 N	36	36	360
1 N (or 1 M)	4	4	40
0.1 N	0.4	0.4	4.0
N/15 (0.067)	0.67	0.67	6.7
N/20 (0.05)	0.5	0.5	5.0

BUFFERS

1. **ACES:** N-(2-acetamido)-2-aminoethane sulfonic acid, 2-(2-amino-2-oxoethyl)-aminoethane sulfonic acid
2. **Dipotassium phosphate, 1 M**

   K_2HPO_4 174.0 g
   Distilled water   1000.0 mL
3. **HCl-KCl, 0.2 M:** acid-wash; pretreatment of water samples
   a. Solution A: KCl, 0.2 M: 14:9 g/L distilled water
   b. Solution B: HCl, 0.2 M: 16.8 mL concentrated acid, bring to 1000 mL with distilled water
   c. Buffer: 50 mL of solution A and desired amount of solution B depending on desired pH; final volume **200 mL**

Soln B (mL)	Final pH
97.0	1.0
78.0	1.1
64.5	1.2
51.0	1.3
41.5	1.4
33.3	1.5
26.3	1.6
20.6	1.7
16.6	1.8
13.2	1.9
10.6	2.0
8.4	2.1
6.7	2.2

4. **Monopotassium phosphate, 1 M**

   KH_2PO_4 136.0 g
   Distilled water   1000.0 mL
5. **Phosphate buffer, M/45 (0.02 M)**

   Monopotassium phosphate, KH_2PO_4 1.17 g
   Disodium phosphate, Na_2HPO_4 4.85 g
   Distilled water   1000.0 mL
6. **Sodium bicarbonate, 1.4%**

   $NaHCO_3$ 14.0 g
   Distilled water   1000.0 mL
7. **Sodium carbonate, 2 N**

   Na_2CO_3 106.0 g
   Distilled water   1000.0 mL

8. **Sodium carbonate, 0.1 N.**
   Na_2CO_3 5.3 g
   Distilled water   1000.0 mL
9. **Sorensen phosphate pH buffer.**
   a. Solution A: disodium phosphate, M/15 (0.067 M); Na_2HPO_4, 9.47 g/L distilled water; anhydrous salt previously dried at 130°C
   b. Solution B: potassium phosphate, M/15 (0.067 M); KH_2PO_4, 9.07 g/L distilled water; anhydrous salt previously dried at 110°C
   c. Combine solutions A and B; quantities depend on pH desired

pH	Soln. A (mL) Na_2HPO_4	Soln. B (mL) KH_2PO_4
5.4	3.0	97.0
5.6	5.0	95.0
5.8	7.8	92.2
6.0	12.0	88.0
6.2	18.5	81.5
6.4	26.5	73.5
6.6	37.5	62.5
6.8	50.0	50.0
7.0	61.1	38.9
7.2	71.5	28.5
7.4	80.4	19.6
7.6	86.8	13.2
7.8	91.4	8.6
8.0	94.5	5.5

DYES-INDICATORS

1. **Alcoholic diluent, ethanol**
   a. Stock: ethanol (ethyl alcohol), C_2H_5OH, 95%
   b. Dilution calculation: $\dfrac{\% \text{ Required}}{\% \text{ Stock}} = \dfrac{x}{\text{Volume required}}$

   c. Example: prepare 100 mL of a 40% solution

   $\dfrac{40\%}{95\%} = \dfrac{x}{100 \text{mL}} = \dfrac{4000}{95} = 42.1$ mL of 95% ethanol brought to 100 mL with distilled water

(*Note:* With all alcoholic/water dye-indicator preparations, dissolve dye in ethanol, then add deionized water.)

2. **Alcoholic bromcresol purple (BCP)/bromthymol blue (BTB)**
   a. BCP: dibromo-*o*-cresol sulfonphthalein, $C_{21}H_{16}O_5SBr_2$
   b. BTB: dibromothymol sulfonphthalein, $C_{27}H_{28}O_5SBr_2$
   c. Ingredients.
      (1) Concentration: 0.04%

Dye of choice	0.04 g
Ethanol, 95% or desired percentage	500.0 mL
Deionized water	500.0 mL

      (2) Concentration: 0.04%; 0.04 g/100 mL ethanol/water diluent
3. **Methyl orange, 0.1%**
   a. Purpose: indicator for acid-base titrations
   b. Ingredients

        Methyl orange, $C_{14}H_{14}N_3O_3SNa$ 0.1 g
        Deionized water   100.0 mL
    c. Acid, orange-red; alkaline, yellow
 4. **Methyl red, 0.2%**
    a. Purpose: indicator for acid-base titrations
    b. Ingredients
        Methyl red, $C_{15}H_{15}N_3O_2$ 0.2 g
        Ethanol, 95%   100.0 mL
    c. Acid, red; alkaline, yellow.
 5. **Phenolphthalein, 1%**
    a. Purpose: indicator for acid-base tritrations
    b. Ingredients
        Phenolphthalein, $C_{20}H_{14}O_4$ 1.0 g
        Ethanol, 95%   100.0 mL
    c. Acid, colorless; alkaline red.
    d. Precaution; **always** titrate alkaline solution from a burette into acid solution; **do not** reverse.
 6. **Phenol red, 0.01 and 0.2%**
    a. Purpose: indicator for acid-base titrations
    b. Ingredients
        Phenol red, $C_{19}H_{14}O_5S$
            0.01%   0.01 g
            0.2%   0.2 g
        Ethanol, 95%   500.0 mL
        Deionized water   500.0 mL
    c. Acid, yellow; alkaline, red.
 7. **Litmus indicator**
    a. Ingredients
        Litmus, granular   250.0 g
        Ethanol, **40%**   1000.0 mL
    b. Preparation, **litmus solution**
        (1) Grind litmus to a fine powder.
        (2) Into a 2-L flask, add 500 mL of 40% ethanol and ground litmus.
        (3) Boil **1 min.**
        (4) **Carefully** decant supernatant (liquid) into another 2-L flask.
        (5) Add remaining 500 mL of 40% ethanol to residue in **initial** flask.
        (6) Boil again for **1 min.**
        (7) **Carefully** decant supernatant into flask containing the first 500-mL portion of boiled liquid.
        (8) Centrifuge supernatant (liquid) and decant into a 1-L graduated cylinder.
        (9) Centrifuge volume to 1 L with 40% ethanol.
        (10) Drop by drop, add 1 H NCl (hydrochloric acid) until solution turns **purple.**
    c. Control testing of litmus reaction
        (1) Boil 10 mL of deionized water and cool.
        (2) Add **1 drop** of litmus solution and **mix well.**
        (3) If properly prepared, the water turns **mauve.** The concentration of litmus indicator is approximately 2.5%.

ENRICHMENTS

1. **V factor:** replaces yeast autolysate and yeast dialysate
    a. Commercial preparations

b. IsoVitaleX (IVX) (BBL), Supplement VX (Difco), and Thayer-Martin Supplement II (Merck)
c. Components (see Table 6.3)

2. **GC supplement (Oxoid) with and without VCNT**

Yeast fractions	5.0 g
Glucose (dextrose)	0.75 g
Sodium bicarbonate, $NaHCO_3$	0.075 g
Optional additives	
Vancomycin (V)	1500 μg
Colistin (C)	3750 μg
Nystatin (N)	6,250 units
Trimethoprim (T)	2,500 μ

Table 6.3. Components of Commercial V Factor

Component	Bio-X/CVA/IsoVitale X/ T-M Supplement II		Supplement VX (mg)
	mg	g	
Adenine sulfate	10.0	1.0	10.0
p-Aminobenzoic acid[a]	0.13	0.013	0.26
Cocarboxylase[b]	1.0	0.1	2.0
L-Cysteine · HCl · H_2O	259.0	25.9	259.0
L-Cysteine · 2HCl	11.0	1.1	11.0
Diphosphopyridine nucleotide (DPN) (oxidized)[c]	2.5	0.25	3.5
Glucose (dextrose)	1.0	100.0	1.0 **g**
L-Glutamine	100.0	10.0	200.0
Guanine · HCl	0.3	0.03	0.3
Iron (III) nitrate[d]	0.2	0.02	
Iron (III) citrate[e]			0.3
Thiamine · HCl (B_1)[f]	0.03	0.003	0.06
Vitamin B_{12} (cyanocobalamin)	0.1	0.01	0.2
Deionized water	1000 mL	1000 mL	1000 mL

[a]PABA; $NH_2C_6H_4COOH$.
[b]Thiamine pyrophospate, $C_{12}H_{19}ClN_4O_7P_2S · H_2O$.
[c]Coenzyme I.
[d]$Fe(NO_3)_3 · 9H_2O$.
[e]$FeC_6H_5O_7 · 5H_2O$.
[f]$C_{12}H_{17}ClN_4OS$; 3-(4-amino-2-methyl-pyrimidyl-5-methyl)-4-methyl-5 or β-hydroxyethylthiazolium chloride.

3. **Kellogg supplement**

L-Glutamine	1.0 g
Cocarboxylase solution (thiamine pyrophosphate) 0.2%	1.0 **mL**
Iron (III) nitrate, $Fe(NO_3)_3 · 9H_2O$	83.47 **mg**
Deionized water	100.0 **mL**

4. **Lankford defined supplement (GCB-2DS)**

	Original	Modified
Glucose (dextrose)	20.0 g	40.0 g
L-Glutamine, 0.25%	0.5 g	1.0 g
Cocarboxylase, 0.0001%[a]	0.001 g	
0.2%		1.0 **mL**

Iron (III) nitrate, Fe(NO$_3$)$_3 \cdot$9H$_2$O	83.47 mg	
Deionized water	100.0 mL	100.0 mL

^{a}May be listed as thiamine pyrophosphate

5. **Fildes enrichment**; usually added as 25–50 ML/L base

Pepsin	6.33 g
Sodium chloride, NaCl	8.11 g
Hydrochloric acid, HCl, concentrated	38.0 **mL**
Sodium hydroxide, NaOH	19.0 g
After sterilization, add	
Sheep blood, **sterile**, defibrinated	318.0 mL

6. **Middlebrook OADC supplement**

Oleic acid	0.5 g	0.05 mg
Bovine albumin fraction V	50.0 g	5.00 mg
Glucose (dextrose)	20.0 g	2.00 mg
Beef catalase	0.04 g	0.004 mg
Sodium chloride, NaCl	8.5 g	0.85 mg
Deionized water	1000.0 mL	100.0 mL

MISCELLANEOUS REAGENTS

1. **Acetic acid 5 N (30%)**: CH$_3$COOH; 28.8 g/100 mL deionized water
2. **Egg yolk suspension**
   a. Soak fresh, raw, whole eggs 1 min in 1:100 dilution of saturated mercuric chloride (HgCl$_2$) solution.
   b. **Aseptically** crack eggs and separate yolks from the whites.
   c. Place yolks in blender and mix 5 sec with required amount of sterile physiologic saline (NaCl, 0.85%).
3. **Ferric chloride, 8 and 10%**
   Ferric chloride, FeCl$_3$
   8%   8.0 g
   10%   10.0 g
   Deionized water 100.0 mL
4. **Gram's iodine**
   a. Ingredients

Iodine, I$_2$	1.0 g
Potassium iodide, KI	2.0 g
Sodium bicarbonate solution, 5%, NaHCO$_3$ (5 g/100 mL deionized water)	60.0 **mL**
Deionized water	**240. mL**

   b. Preparation
   (1) Grind I$_2$ and KI in a mortar.
   (2) Dissolve in 5 mL deionized water; then bring to **240 mL** with deionized water.
   (3) Add NaHCO$_3$ **solution**, 60 mL.
   c. Precaution: store in a dark-colored (amber) bottle. Solution is brownish yellow; discard when color fades.
5. **Hemin stock solution, 5 µg/mL**

Hemin, C$_{34}$H$_{32}$O$_4$N$_4$FeCl	0.5 g
Sodium hydroxide, 1 N, NaOH	10.0 mL
Deionized water	bring to 100.0 mL

6. **Kovacs' reagent**

a. Purpose: indole test reagent
b. Ingredients

Pure amyl or isoamyl alcohol (butyl alcohol may be substituted)	150.0 mL
p-Dimethylaminobenzaldehyde; C. R.	10.0 g
Hydrochloric acid, HCl concentrated	50.0 mL

c. Preparation
   (1) Dissolve the aldehyde in the alcohol.
   (2) **Slowly** add the acid to the aldehyde-alcohol mixture.

7. **Nadi reagents, 1%**: indophenol oxidase reagent; N,N,N',N'-tetramethyl-*p*-phenylene-diamonium dichloride
   a. Reagent A: 1% α-naphtol ($C_{10}H_7OH$, 1-naphthol, 1-hydroxynaphthalene) in 95% ethanol
   b. Reagent B: 1% *p*-aminomethylaniline·HCl (or oxalate); $(CH_3)_2NC_6H_4NH_2 \cdot HCl$; also called dimethyl-*p*-phenylenediamine oxalate
   c. Origin of "nadi": na- from naphthol and -di from diamine

8. **Oxgall vs. bile**
   a. Oxgall, 2% = 10 × conc. of bile = 20% bile
   b. Oxgall, 1–4% = bile 10–40%

9. **Potassium hydroxide, 40% and 0.1 N**
   a. Ingredients
      (1) KOH, 40%: 40.0 g/100 mL deionized water
      (2) KOH, 0.1 N: 0.6 g/100 mL deionized water
   b. Preparation
      (1) **Rapidly** weigh KOH and dissolve in less than 100 mL of deionized water in a **beaker.** This reagent is highly hygroscopic; avoid exposure to air any longer than necessary.
      (2) Place beaker in a circulating water bath to control the temperature; a large amount of heat is generated.
      (3) Cool and transfer KOH solution to a 100-mL **volumetric** flask and bring to 100 mL with deionized water.
   c. Label and store in a polyethylene or paraffin-lined glass reagent bottle.
   d. This reagent is very caustic; avoid exposure to skin, as painful burns may occur.

10. **Potassium iodide, 0.2%**
    a. Ingredients

Potassium iodide, iodine-free, KI	2.0 g
Deionized water	100.0 mL

    b. Test for presence of iodine with a starch solution; iodine is indicated by a blue color. Discard if iodine is present or if a brown color develops upon standing.

11. **Potassium tellurite, 1%**: 1.0 g K_2TeO_3/100 mL deionized water

12. **Ringer's solution**

Sodium chloride, NaCl	8.5 g
Potassium chloride, KCl	0.2 g
Calcium chloride, $CaCl2 \cdot 2H_2O$	0.2 g
Sodium carbonate, Na_2CO_3	0.01 g
Deionized water	1000.0 mL

13. **Schiff's reagent**
    a. Also called fuchsin-sulfurous acid reagent
    b. Indicator of the presence of an aldehyde; colorless
    c. Commercial dyes may be either chloride or acetate or pure *para*-rosanlin or a mixture of the two.
    d. Ingredients

(1) Alcoholic basic fuschin dye; 1 **and** 3% concentrations, each prepared separately
(2) Sodium sulfite, anydrous, $Na_2SO_3 \cdot 7H_2O$: 0.125 g/**5 mL hot** deionized water
(3) **Separately** mix 5 mL of sodium sulfite with 1 mL of each alcoholic-dye percentage concentrations.
(4) Solution a faint pink or straw color with **no** visible precipitate

14. **Stone developer:** saturated, aqueous solution of ammonium sulfate, $(NH_4)_2SO_4$
15. **Vitamin K_1–hemin solution**

Hemin	0.5 g
NaOH	0.4 g
Vitamin K_1	0.05 g
Ethanol, 95%	10.0 mL
Deionized water	1000.0 mL

16. **Vitamin K_1 stock solution, 10 μg/mL**
    a. Ingredients.

Vitamin K_1 (phytonadione, 2-methyl-3-phytyl-1, 4-naphthoquinone), phytylmenadione, $CH_3C_{10}H_4O_{20}H_{39}$	1.09 g
Ethanol, **absolute**	99.0 mL

    b. Preparation
       (1) Weigh out vitamin K_1 on a small piece of **sterile** aluminum foil.
       (2) **Aseptically** add to 99.0 mL absolute ethanol in a **sterile** tube or bottle.
       (3) Protect from light and refrigerate, 2–8°C.

PREPARATION OF SEALANTS (1)

1. Mineral oil or paraffin
   a. To a 200-mL bottle, add 1 mL of deionized water to 100 mL mineral oil or paraffin.
   b. Sterilization; two choices
      (1) Autoclave: 121°C, 15 lb, 15 min
      (2) Hot air oven: 160–170°C, 1 h
2. Vaspar; more effective as it **does not** retract from glass as does paraffin and it is a solid, so less possibility of air diffusion.
   a. Mixture: 1:1 petroleum jelly and paraffin
   b. Too a 100-mL bottle, add 50 mL of mixture.
   c. Sterilization: for **each 50-mL aliquot,** autoclave, 121°C, 15 lb, **1 h**
   d. **After** sterilization, place in dry oven at 100°C to drive off entrapped water.

GENERAL REFERENCES

1. Branson D. Methods in Clinical Bacteriology. Springfield, IL: Charles C. Thomas, 1972:135.
2. Holum JR. Elements of General and Biological Chemistry, 4th ed. New York: John Wiley & Sons, 1975.
3. Stewart JA. Methods of Media Preparation for the Biological Sciences. Springfield, IL: Charles C. Thomas, 1974.
4. U.S. Army Technical Manual, TM 8-227-6. Laboratory Procedures in Clinical Chemistry and Urinalysis. Washington DC: Department of the Army, January, 1964.

APPENDIX 7

Common Synonymous Terminology of Media

A. Protein → proteose → peptone → amino acids
B. Peptone
  1. Protein derivative (hydrolysate) obtained by either enzymatic action or acid (or alkaline) hydrolysis
  2. Various peptones available commercially
     a. Listed in one of the following ways:
        (i) USP (United States Pharmacopeia) nomenclature; e.g. papaic digest of casein
        (ii) Trademark (brand) name; e.g., Soytone (Difco).
        (iii) Trademark name of ingredients; e.g., Soybean peptone.
     b. Trademark names

BBL	Difco
Acidicase Peptone	Bacto-Casamino Acids
Biosate Peptone	Bacto-Casitone
Gelysate Peptone	Neopeptone
Myosate Peptone	Proteose peptone
Phytone Peptone	Proteose peptone No. 3
Polypeptone Peptone	Bacto-Peptone
Thiotone Peptone	Bacto-Protone
Trypticase Peptone	Bacto-Tryptone
	Bacto-Tryptose
	Bacto-Soytone

Method of Hydrolysis/Protein	Synonyms
1. Pancreatic digest of casein, USP	Trypticase Peptone (BBL)
	Tryptone (Difco)
	Casitone (Difco)
2. Papaic digest of soy (soya) meal (bean), USP	Phytone Peptone (BBL)
	Soytone (Difco)
3. Peptic digest of animal tissues, USP	Thiotone Peptone (BBL)
	Tryptose (Difco)
	Proteose Peptone (Difco)
4. Proteose pancreatic digest of gelatin, USP	Gelysate Peptone (BBL)
	Peptone (Difco)
5. Pancreatic digest of heart muscle, USP	Myosate Peptone (BBL)
6. Pancreatic digest of casein **and** yeast, autolysate, USP	Biosate Peptone (BBL)
	Tryptose (Difco) and thiamine
7. Pancreatic digest of casein **and** peptic digest of animal tissue, USP	Polypeptone (BBL)
	Neopeptone (Difco)
	Proteose peptone No. 3 (Difco)
8. Acid hydrolysate of casein, USP	Acidicase Peptone (BBL)

APPENDIX 8

Standard Size Test Tubes for Bacteriology

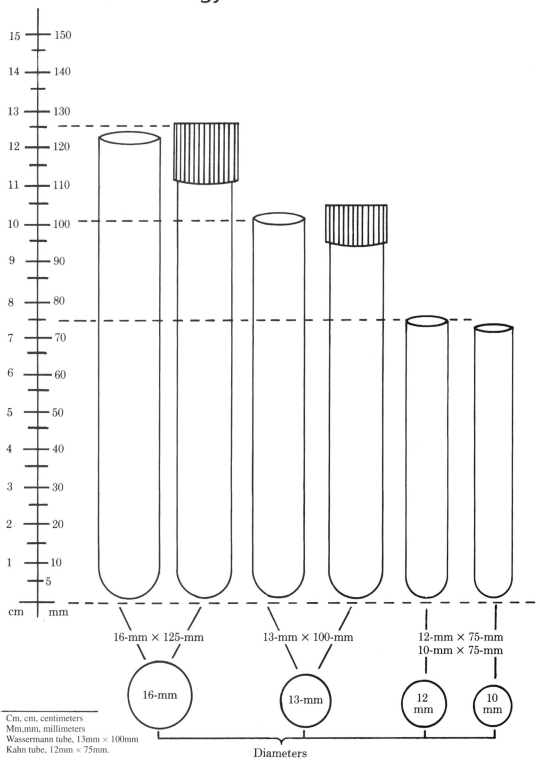

Cm, cm, centimeters
Mm, mm, millimeters
Wassermann tube, 13mm × 100mm
Kahn tube, 12mm × 75mm.

APPENDIX

Temperature Conversions

	°C	°F
Incubation temperature	37°	98.6°
Room temperature (RT)	25°	77°
Boiling point, water (b.p.)	100°	212°
Freezing point, water (f.p.)	0°	32°

°F = Fahrenheit
°F = (9/5 × °C) + 32 or (1.8 × °C) + 32

°C = Centigrade or Celsius
°C = 5/9 (°F − 32) or 0.555 (°F − 32)

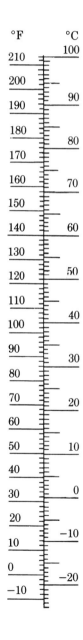

APPENDIX

Culture Collections: Reference Cultures

ACM
: **AUSTRALIAN COLLECTION OF MICROORGANISMS**
Department of Microbiology
University of Queensland
Nahan, Brisbane,
Queensland, Australia

AHU
: **LABORATORY OF CULTURE COLLECTION OF MICROORGANISMS**
Faculty of Agriculture
Hokkaido University
Sapporo, Japan

ATCC
: **AMERICAN TYPE CULTURE COLLECTION**
10801 University Boulevard
Manassas, VA 20110–2209, U.S.A.
Products & Services Order
ATCC
P.O. Box 1549
Manassas, VA 20108–1549, U.S.A.

AUCM
AUCNM
BKM
UCM
VKM
: **ALL-UNION COLLECTION OF MICROORGANISMS**
Department of Type Cultures of Microorganisms
Institute of Biochemistry & Physiology of Microorganisms
URSS Academy of Sciences
Puschino
Moscow Region 142292, Russia

AUCNM
: **ALL-UNION COLLECTION OF NON-PATHOGENIC MICROORGANISMS**
See AUCM

CBS
: **CENTRAALBUREAU VOOR SCHIMMELCULTURES**
Oosterstraat 1
3740 AG Baarn, The Netherlands

CCBAU
: **CULTURE COLLECTION OF BEIJING AGRICULTURAL UNIVERSITY**
Beijing, People's Republic of China

CCCCM
: **CHINA COMMITTEE FOR CULTURE COLLECTION OF MICROORGANISMS**
Institute of Microbiology
Academia Sinica
Beijing, People's Republic of China

CCM
: **CZECHOSLOVAK COLLECTIONS OF MICROORGANISMS**
F. E. Purkyne University of Brno
Tr. Obrancu Miru 10
66243 Brno, Czechoslovakia

CCUG	**CULTURE COLLECTION, UNIVERSITY OF GÖTEBORG** Department of Clinical Bacteriology Institute of Clinical Bacteriology, Immunology, and Virology Guldhedsgatn 10As-413 46 Göteborg, Sweden
CDC	**CENTERS FOR DISEASE CONTROL** 1600 Clifton Road Atlanta, GA 30333, U.S.A.
CECT	**COLECCIÓN ESPAGÑOLA DE CULTIVOS TIPO** Universitat de Valencia Edeficio de Investigación Campus de Burjasot 46100 Burjasot (Valencia), Spain
CFML	**COLLECTION DE LA FACULTÉ DE MÉDECINE DE LILLE** 1 Place de Verdun 59045 Lille Cedex, France
CIP	**COLLECTION DE L'INSTITUT PASTEUR** Institut Pasteur 28 Rue du Docteur Roux 75724 Paris, Cedex 15, France
CNC	**CZECHOSLOVAK NATIONAL COLLECTION OF TYPE CULTURES** Institute of Epidemiology and Microbiology Srobarova 48 Prague 10, Czechoslovakia
CNCMI **CNCM**	**COLLECTION NATIONALE DE CULTURES DE MICROORGANISMES** Institut Pasteur Rue du Docteur 75015 Paris, France
CUTEM	**COLLECTION DE L'UNITÉD ÉCOTOXICOLOGIE MICROBIENNE** Institut National de la Santé et de la Recherche Medicale 59651 Villeneuve d'Ascq, Nord, France
DSM **DSMZ**	**DEUTSCHE SAMMLUNG VON MIKROORGANISMEN UND ZELLKULTUREN** GmbH, Mascheroder Weg IB D-38124 Braunschweig, Germany
GIEM	**GAMALEYA INSTITUTE OF EPIDEMIOLOGY AND MICROBIOLOGY** Academy of Medical Sciences Moscow, Russia
HMGB	**HUNGARIAN MICROBIOLOGY GENE BANK** Microbiological Department Group of the Department of Food Technology and Microbiology of the University of Horticulture 1064 Budapest, Izabella, Hungary
HSCC	**CULTURE COLLECTION OF THE RESEARCH LABORATORY OF HIGETA SHOYU CO.** 2–8 Chuo-cho Choshi, Chiba 288, Japan
IAM	**INSTITUTE OF MOLECULAR AND CELLULAR BIOSCIENCES** The University of Tokyo Yayoi, Bunkyo-Ku Tokyo, Japan

IBPHM	**DEPARTMENT OF TYPE CULTURES OF MICROORGANISMS** Institute of Biochemistry and Physiology of Microorganisms URSS Academy of Sciences Pushchino Moscow Region 142292, Russia
ICPB	**PROFESSOR OF BACTERIOLOGY, CURATOR ICPB** International Collection of Phytopathogenic Bacteria Department of Bacteriology University of California Davis, CA 95616, U.S.A.
IFAM	**INSTITUT FÜR ALLGEMEINE MIKROBIOLOGIE** Universität Kiel Kiel, Germany
IFO	**INSTITUTE FOR FERMENTATION** 4–54 Jusonischinocho Osaka, Japan
IMET **ZIMET**	**INSTITUTE FOR MICROBIOLOGY AND EXPERIMENTAL THERAPY** (ZENTRALINSTITUT FÜR MIKROBIOLOGIE UND EXPERIMENTELLE THERAPIE) Beutenbergrasse 11 Jena 69, Germany
IMMIB	**CULTURE COLLECTION OF THE INSTITUTE OF MEDICAL MICROBIOLOGY AND IMMUNOLOGY** University of Bonn Sigmund-Freud Str. 25 D-53105 Bonn, Germany
IMRU	**INSTITUTE OF MICROBIOLOGY** Rutgers-The State University New Brunswick, NJ 08903, U.S.A.
IMSNU	**INSTITUTE OF MICROBIOLOGY** Seoul National University Seoul 151–742 Republic of Korea
IMV	**INSTITUTE OF MICROBIOLOGY AND VIROLOGY** Academy of Sciences of the Ukranian 154 Zabolotny Str. Kiev 143 252143, Ukrania
INMI	**INSTITUTE FOR MICROBIOLOGY** USSR Academy of Sciences 7 Bldg 2 Prospekt 60-letiya Oktiyabriya, Moscow GSP-7, 117811, Russia
JCM	**JAPAN COLLECTION OF MICROORGANISMS** Riken, Wako-shi Saitama 351, Japan
KCC	**CULTURE COLLECTION OF ACTINOMYCETES** Kaken Chemical Co., Ltd. 6–42 Jujodai-1-Chome Tokyo 114, Japan Collection transferred to JCM

KCTC	**KOREAN COLLECTION FOR TYPE CULTURES** Korea Research Institute of Biosciences & Biotechnology Yusong, Taejon 305–600, Korea
LIA	**MUSEUM OF CULTURES** Leningrad Research Institute of Antibiotics 23 Ogorodnikov Prospect Leningrad L-20, Russia
LMD	**LABORATORIUM VOOR MICROBIOLOGIE DER TECHNISCHE HOGESCHOOL** Delft University of Technology Julianalaan 67A 2628 BC Delft, The Netherlands
LMG	**COLLECTION OF THE LABORATORIUM VOOR MICROBIOLOGIE EN MICROBIELE GENETICA** Rijksuniversiteit Ledeganckstraat 35 B-9000, Gent, Belgium
MIM	**COLLECTION OF THE CATTEDRA DI MICROBIOLOGIA INDUSTRIALE** Universit degli Studi di Milan, Italy
MSDJ	**CULTURE COLLECTION OF THE LABORATOIRE DE MICROBIOLOGIE DES SOLS** Institut National de la Recherche Agronomique F-21304 Dijon Cedex, France
NCFB	**NATIONAL COLLECTION OF FOOD BACTERIA** AFRC Institute of Food Research Shinfield, Reading Berkshire RG2 9AT, England, United Kingdom Previously named NCDO
NCIB **NCIMB**	**NATIONAL COLLECTION OF INDUSTRIAL BACTERIA** Torry Research Station P.O. Box 31 135 Abbey Rd. Aberdeen AB9 8DG, Scotland, United Kingdom
NDDO	**SEE NCFB**
NCPPB	**NATIONAL COLLECTION OF PLANT PATHOGENIC BACTERIA** Central Science Laboratory Ministry of Agriculture, Fisheries, and Food Sand Hutton, York Y04 1LN, United Kingdom
NCTC	**NATIONAL COLLECTION OF TYPE CULTURES** Central Public Health Laboratory Collindale Avenue London NW9 5HT, United Kingdom
NIH	**NATIONAL INSTITUTES OF HEALTH** Bethesda, MD 20014, U.S.A.
NRC **NRCC**	**NATIONAL RESEARCH COUNCIL OF CANADA CULTURE COLLECTION** 100 Sussex Drive Ottawa, Ontario KIA OR6, Canada
NRL	**NEISSERIA REFERENCE LABORATORY** US Public Health Service Hospital Seattle, WA 98114, U.S.A.

NRRL	**NORTHERN REGIONAL RESEARCH CENTER** Agriculture Research Culture Collections National Center for Agriculture Utilization Research US Department of Agriculture 1815 North University Street Peoria, IL 61604, U.S.A.
NTCH	**NORTH TECHNICAL HOGSKOLLES COLLECTION** Department of Biochemistry Technical University of Norway Trondheim MTH, Norway
OGC	**OREGON GRADUATE CENTER COLLECTION** Beaverton, OR 97006–1992, U.S.A.
PDDCC ICMP	**CULTURE COLLECTION OF PLANT DISEASES DIVISION** New Zealand Department of Scientific and Industrial Research Landcare Research Private Bag 92170, Auckland, New Zealand
RML	**NATIONAL INSTITUTE OF ALLERGY AND INFECTIOUS DISEASES** Rocky Mountain Laboratories Collection Hamilton, MT 59840, U.S.A.
SABAMMRCCC	**SOUTH AMERICAN BIOTECHNOLOGY AND APPLIED MICROBIOLOGY,** Microbiological Resource Center Culture Collection (United Nations Educational, Scientific, and Cultural Organization) Tucumán, Argentina
TPH	**MICROBIOLOGICAL CULTURE COLLECTION** Public Health Laboratory Ontario Department of Health Toronto 116, Canada
UCM	**SEE AUCM**
UQM	**CULTURE COLLECTION** Department of Microbiology University of Queensland St. Lucia, Queensland 4067, Australia
UWO	**UNIVERSITY OF WESTERN ONTARIO CULTURE COLLECTION** University of Western Ontario London, Ontario N6A 587, Canada
VKM	**SEE AUCM**
VPB	**VETERINARY PATHOLOGY AND BACTERIOLOGY COLLECTION** University of Sydney New South Wales 2006, Australia
VIP	**ANAEROBE LABORATORY** Polytechnic Institute and State University Blacksburg, VA 24061, U.S.A.
WR	**QUEENSLAND WHEAT RESEARCH INSTITUTE** 13 Holberton Street, Toowocmba Queensland, Australia

WVB	**WUHAN INSTITUTE OF VIROLOGY** Academia Siniea Wuhan, Hubei People's Republic of China
WVU	**WEST VIRGINIA UNIVERSITY** Department of Microbiology Medical Center Morgantown, WV 26506, U.S.A.

APPENDIX

11 Addresses of Commercial Suppliers

MANUFACTURER

ABBOTT LABORATORIES
100 Abbott Park Road
Chicago, IL 60064-3500, USA
Tel: 847-937-6100
Fax: 837-938-6255
WEB: www.abbottdiagnostics.com/

ACCUMED INTERNATIONAL, INC.
920 North Franklin
Suite 402
Chicago, IL 60610, USA
Tel: 312-642-9200
WEB: accumed.com

Imberhorne Lane
East Grinstead
West Sussex, England
RH19 1QX
Tel: +44 (0)1342 318777
Fax: +44 (0) 1342 318666
E-mail: Accumed UK

ALDRICH CHEMICAL CO., INC.: SEE SIGMA-ALDRICH

ALLIED CHEMICAL CORP.
2217 Nicollet Avenue South
Minneapolis, MN 55404, USA
Tel: 612-874-2400
Fax: 612-874-2430
E-mail: hamspread@alliedchemical.com
WEB: www.alliedchemical.com/mail/

P.O. Box 333
Brighton BN1 2EH
United Kingdom
P.O. Box 326
Spit Junction NSW 2088
Australia

AMERICAN TYPE CULTURE COLLECTION (ATCC)
10801 University Boulevard
Manassas, VA 20110-2209, USA

Products and Service Orders
P.O. Box 1549
Manassas, VA 20108-1549, USA

PRODUCT(S)

Cx *Neisseria gonorrhoeae* assay
TestPack Plus Strep A
TestPack Plus Strep A COBC II

Sensititre Gram-Negative audio identification system

d-Dimethylaminocinnamaldehyde (DMACA)

Toluidine blue O (TBO) dye
Rhodamine B dye

Indoxyl acetate disks

AMES COMPANY
430 S. Beiger Street
Mishawaka, IN 46544, USA
Tel: 219-255-3327

Clinitest tablets

ANALYTAB PRODUCTS, INC.
P.O. Box 845
Belmont, CA 94002, USA
Tel: 415-592-1400

Rapid NFT

BALLARD MEDICAL PRODUCTS
12050 Lone Peak Parkway
Draper, Utah 84020-9414, USA
Tel: 801-572-6800
Tel: 800-528-5591 Orders
Fax: 801-572-6999
E-mail: csmock@bmed.com
WEB: www.bmed.com/contact.html

Pytest urea breath test

BAXTER MICROSCAN: SEE DADE/ MICROSCAN, INC.
One Baxter Parkway
Deerfield, IL 60015-4633, USA
Tel: 708-948-2000
WEB: www.baxter.com/

BAYER CORPORATION
Bayer Diagnostics
511 Benedict Avenue
Tarrytown, NY 10591-5097, USA
Tel: 914-631-8000
WEB: www.bayerus.com/products/medical.html

Trasylol (aprotinin)

BD BIOSCIENCES (FORMERLY BECTON DICKINSON MICROBIOLOGY SYSTEMS)
7 Loveton Circle
Sparks, MD 21152, USA
Tel: 410-316-4000
Web: www.bd.com/microbiology

BBL Crystal Anaerobe (ANR) ID Panel
BBL Crystal Enteric/Nonfermenter (E/NF) ID panel
BBL Crystal MRSA ID panel
BBL Crystal *Neisseria/Haemophilus* ID panel
BBL Crystal Rapid Gram-Positive ID panel
BBL Crystal Rapid Stool/Enteric ID panel
Bacitracin disks
Campyslide
Culturette
Directigen Meningitis test
Enterotube II tube
Furazolidone disks
Leucine
Minitek Anaerobe II
Minitek Gram-Positive test
Minitek *Neisseria* Test
Pneumoslide test
Q test strep kit
Sceptor Gram Positive MIC/ID panel
Staphyloslide test

BEHRINGWERKE AG
Dade Behring Marburg GmbH
Emil-von-Behring Str 76
35041 Marburg, Germany
Tel: 0 64 21/39-0
Fax: 0 64 21/39-3986
Web: uni-marburg.de/stadt/wifoe/behringb.html

Dipstick PADAC (b-lactamase)

BIOLOG INC.
3938 Trust Way
Hayward, CA 94545, USA
Tel: 510-785-2564
Fax: 510-782-4639
E-mail: info@biolog.com
Web: www.biolog.com

GN MicroPlate identification system—phasing out
GN2 and GP2—newer
Rainbow UTI system
Rainbow *Salmonella*
Rainbow *E.coli* 01:57

BIOMERIEUX, INC.
595 Anglum Road
Hazelwood, MI 63042-2320
Tel: 314-731-8500
Fax: 314-731-8700

69280 Marcy l'etoile
France
Tel:(33) (0) 4 78 87 20 00
Fax:(33) (0) 4 78 87 20 90
Web: www.biomerieux.com/english

bioMerieux Inc. name change reflects VITEK, VIDAS, BACTOMETER, and API

API 20 A (anaerobes)
API 20 E (enterics)
API 20 NE (Gram-negative non-enterics)
API Rapid 20 E (enterics)
ATB 32 A
API Rapid ID ANA
API An-Indent (anaerobes)
API Campy
API Coryne system
API NH system
API Staph
API 20 Strep
API Staph-IDENT
API Rapid Strep system
API QUAD-FERM (*Neisseria, M. catarrhalis*)
API-ZYM (enzyme action)
CPS ID 2
Staph ASE
Slidex Staph
Staphslide Kit
Rapid DEC Staph
Slidex Strepto Kits (A&B)
API 50 CH (carbohydrates)
Vidas *C. difficile* toxin A test
Vitek Anaerobe Identification (ANI) card
Vitek Enteric pathogen (EPS) card
Vitek HNI (Neiss-Ham-Identification) card
Vitek Gram-Positive Identification (GPI)
Vitek Gram-negative identification(GNI)

BIO-RAD LABORATORIES, INC.
Diagnostic Group
4000 Alfred Nobel Drive
Hercules, CA 94547, USA
Tel: 510-724-7000
Tel: 800-224-6723
Fax: 510-741-6373
Web: www.bio-rad.com

G.A.P. kit

BIOSTAR, INC.
6655 Lookout Road
Boulder, CO 80301, USA
Tel: 303-530-3888
Tel: 800-637-3717
Fax: 303-530-6601
Web: www.biostar.com

Strep A OIA (optical immunoassay)
Strep B OIA

BIO WHITTAKER
A Cambrex Company
8830 Biggs Ford Road
Walkersville, MD 21793, USA
Tel: 301-898-7025
Tel: 800-654-4452
Fax: 301-845-8338
Web: www.biowhittaker.com/aboutbio.html

PYLORI STAT EIA

BRISTOL-MYERS SQUIBB CO. (BMS)
225 High Ridge Road
Stamford, CT 06905, USA
Web: www.bms.com

Kanamycin

BUTYLASE LAB M CO.
England

Indoxyl butyrate strips

CALBIOCHEM-NOVIABIOCHEM CORP.
P.O. Box 12087
La Jolla, CA 92039-2087, USA
Tel: 800-854-3417
Fax: 800-776-0999
Web:www.calbiochem.com

o-Nitrophenyl-β-D-galactoside
 (o-nitrophenyl-β-D-galactopyranoside)
PADAC (pyridine-1-azo-dimethylaniline)
Cephalosporin powder (β-lactamase)

CAMBRIDGE BIO TECH

Cytoclone A&B (EIA) for *C. difficile*

CARLO ERBA REAGENTI
Strada Rivoltana Km. 6/7
20090 Rodano (Milan), Italy
Tel: 02.9523.1
Fax: 02.9523.5940
Web: www.carloerbareagenti.com/worldwide.html

Methyl green (MG) dye

CENTERS FOR DISEASE CONTROL (CDC)
1600 Clifton Road
Atlanta, GA 30333, USA
Tel: 404-639-3311
E-mail: netinfo@cdc.gov
Web: www.cdc.gov

Indoxyl acetate disks

CIBA-GEIGY AG
CIBA SPECIALTY CHEMICALS INC.
Klybeckstrasse 141
CH-4002 Basel,
Switzerland
Tel:+41 61 636 1111
E-mail: Webmaster@cibase.com
Web: www.cibase.com

Desferrioxamine (Desferal) disks

556 Morris Avenue
Summit, NJ 07901, USA
Tel: 201-277-5000

DADE/MICROSCAN INS. (DADE INTERNATIONAL)
DADE BEHRING
1584 Enterprise Boulevard
West Sacramento, CA 95691, USA
Tel: 800-677-7226 ext. 2110
Fax: 916-372-9762
E-mail: cathy_ritz@dadebehring.com
Web: www.dademicroscan.com

Haem-Neiss Identification (HNID) panel
MicroScan Pos ID panel
MicroScan Rapid Pos Combo panel
MicroScan Walkaway Auto SCAN-W/A
Rapid Anaerobic Identification system
Rapid Gram-Neg ID type 2
Rapid Gram-Neg ID type 3
Staphlatex

DELTA WEST. LTD.: SEE PHARMACIA & UPJOHN
West Australia

CLO Strip test

DIAGNOSTICS PRODUCTS CORP. (DPC)
Attn: Customer Service Department
5700 West 96th Street
Los Angeles, CA 90045-5597, USA
Tel: 310-645-8200
Fax: 310-645-9999
Fax: 800-234-4372 Orders
E-mail: info@dpconline.com
Web: www.dpcweb.com

Patho DX Tests (Strep A, Strep D, and Strep PYR)

DIFCO LABORATORIES
Division of BD Biosciences
7 Loveton Circle
Sparks, MD 21152-0999, USA
Web: www.difco.com/

Methyl green (MG) dye
MUG plus
Soluble starch

EASTMAN CHEMICAL COMPANY
100 North Eastman Road
P.O. Box 431
Kingsport, TN 37662-5075, USA
Tel: 800-327-8626
Tel: 423-229-2000
Fax: 423-229-1195
E-mail: gquillen@eastman.com
Web: www.eastman.com

Acridine orange (AO) dye
p-Dimethylaminobenzaldehyde (DMABA)
N,N-dimethyl-α-naphthylamine
Tetramethyl-p-phenylenediamine dihydrochloride (TPD)
X-ray film

ENTERIC PRODUCTS INC. (EPI)
25 East Loop Drive
Stony Brook, NY 11790-3355, USA
Tel: 800-645-6887
Tel: 516-334-1980
Fax: 516-334-0509
Web: www.enteric.com

HM-CAPELIA (HM CAP)

E-Y LABORATORIES
127 N. Amphlett Blvd.
San Mateo, CA 94401, USA
Tel: 650-342-3296

Gonochek II

FISHER SCIENTIFIC LTD.
50 Fadem Road
Springfield, NJ 07081-3193, USA
Tel: 973-467-6511
Fax: 973-376-1546

Borosilicate glass tubes
Linter starch
Methyl green (MG) dye
Toluidine blue O (TBO) dye

112 Colonnade Road
Nepean, Ontario K2E 7L6
Canada
Tel: 800-234-7437
Tel: 613-226-3273
Fax: 800-463-2996
Web: www.fishersci.ca

GEN-PROBE, INC.
10210 Genetic Center Drive
San Diego, CA 92121-1598, USA
Tel: 619-410-8000
Fax: 619-410-8625
E-mail: cindy@gen-probe.com
Web: www.gen-probe.com/tech.html

AccuProbe
Group A **Streptococcus** direct test (GASD)
PACE systems (PACE 2 and PACE 2C systems)

GLAXO WELLCOME UK LTD.
Stockley Park West
Uxbridge
Middlesex UB11 1BT
England
Tel:(0181) 990 9000
Fax:(0181)990 4321
Web: www.glaxowelcome.co.uk/about/world_locations/mn_usa.html

Nitrocefin (β-lactamase)
Chromogenic cephalosporin 87/312

GLAXO WELLCOME, INC.
Five Moore Drive
P.O. Box 13398
Research Triangle Park, NC 27709, USA
Tel: 800-437-0992
Tel: 919-248-2100
Fax: 919-248-2381
Web: www.glaxowellcome.com/index/htm

I.A.F. PRODUCTION, INC.
531 Boulevard des Prairies
Ville de Laval
Québec H7N 423
Canada
Tel: 450-687-5010

Gonobio test

INSTITUT VIRON-SERIO GMBH
Kondradstrasse 1
D-97072 Würzburg
Germany
Tel: ++49-931-309860
Fax: ++49-931-52650
Web: www.viron-seron.de/index.html

Motility kit SSM medium with cefaoperazone and trimethoprim

KARO-BIO AB
Novum
S-141 57 Huddinge
Sweden
Tel:+46 8 608 6000
Fax:+46 8 774 8261
E-mail: info@karobio.se
Web: www.Torbjorn.malmsjo@karobio.se

Phadebact GC OMNI test
Phadebact H. *influenzae* type b
Phadebact Pneumococcus

KEY SCIENTIFIC PRODUCTS
1402-D Chisolm Trail
Round Rock, TX 78681, USA
Tel: 800-843-1539
Fax: 512-218-8580
E-mail: KEYTAB@aol.com

Fluo-Card Milleri
Gelatin strips (exposed gelatinase x-ray film)
Key substrates: ONPG, nitrate disks, gluconate tablets)
LAP/LAPNA disks
NGP-Wee tabs
Oxidase disks and strips

LIOFILCHEM S.R.L.
20060 Vignate (Mi)
Via Sardegna 1
Italy
Tel: 011/39/02/95360323
E-mail: liofilchem@iol.it

Staf-Sistem 18-R

MALLINCKRODT (JT) BAKER INC.
Corporate office
16305 Swingley Ridge Dr.
Chesterfield, MO 63017, USA
Tel: 314-654-2000

Uranium acetate

Mailing address:
P.O. Box 5840
675 McDonnell Boulevard
St. Louis, MO 63134, USA
Tel: 516-93-7888
Web: www.mallinckrodt.com

Mallinckrodt Laboratory Chemicals
Division of Mallinckrodt and Baker, Inc.
222 Red School Lane
Phillipsburg, NJ 08865, USA
Tel: 800-354-2050
Fax: 908-859-6974

MERETEK
618 Grassmere Park Drive
Suite 20
Nashville, TN 37211, USA
Tel: 800-945-8252
Tel: 888-637-3835 Customer Service
Tel: 615-333-6336
Fax: 615-333-6202
E-mail: info@meretek.com
Web: www.meretek.com/info.htm

MERETEK UBT breath test for *H.pylori*

MERCK & COMPANY, INC.
P.O. Box 100
One Merck Drive
Whitehouse Station, NJ 08889-0100
Tel: 908-423-6000
Fax: 908-735-1131
Web: www.merck.com

Soluble starch

Merck GaA
Frankfurter Str.250
D-64293 Darmstadt
Germany
Tel: ++49 61 51-72-0
Fax: ++ 49 61 51-72-2000
E-mail: service@merck.de
Web: www.merck.com

MERIDIAN DIAGNOSTICS, INC.
3471 River Hills Drive
Cincinnati, OH 45244, USA
Tel: 513-271-3700
Tel: 800-343-3858 Tech Support
Fax: 513-272-5432
E-mail: sgalin@meridiandiagnostics.com
Web: www.meridiandiagnostics.com

ImmunoCard
ImmunoCard Stat
Meritec-Campy (jcl)
Meritec-GC test
Premier Cytoclone A&B
Premier EHEC
Premier Toxin A

858 Biochemical Tests for Identification of Medical Bacteria

MICROBIOLOGICS
217 Osseo Avenue North
St. Cloud, MN 56303, USA
Tel: 320-253-1640
Tel: 800-599-2847
Fax: 320-253-6250
E-mail: infor@MBL2000.com
Web: www.microbiologics.com

Lyfo-Kiwi OMI
Neisseria-Kiwi test kit

MIDI LABS, INC.
125 Sandy Drive
Newark, DE 19713, USA
Tel: 302-737-4297
Tel: 800-276-8068
Fax: 302-737-7781
Web: www.midilabs.com

Franciesella tularensus microbial identification
MIS identification system (whole cell fatty acid analysis by gas chromatography)

MILLIPORE CORP.
Attn: Order Services
80 Ashby Road
Bedford, MA 01730, USA
Tel: 781-533-6000
Tel: 800-645-5476
Fax: 781-533-3110
Web: www.millipore.com/local/US.htm

Millipore filters and membranes

MUREX DIAGNOSTICS DIVISION: SEE ABBOTT DIAGNOSTICS DIVISION
3075 Northwood Circle
Norcross, GA 30071, USA
Tel: 770-662-0666
Tel: 800-323-9100 Tech Support
Fax: 800-382-1574
WEB: www.int-murex.com

Signify Streap A
StaphAurex Plus
Streptex
Wellcogen bacterial antigen kits (Group A *Streptococcus, H. influenzae, S. pneumoniae, N. meningitidis,* and *E. coli*)

NEW HORIZONS DIAGNOSTICS CORP.
9110 Red Branch Road
Columbia, MD 21045, USA
Tel: 410-992-9357 ext. 235 or 232
Tel: 800-888-5015
Fax: 410-992-0328
E-mail: nhdiag@aol.com
Web: www.nhdiag.com

Gono Gen (chromogenic)
Gono Gen II

OMEGA DIAGNOSTICS
Omega House–Carsebridge Court
GB-FK 10 3LQ Alloa-Scotland
Great Britain
Tel: ++44 1259-217315
Fax: ++44 1259-72351

Avistaph

OXOID LTD.
Wade Road
Basingstoke
Hampshire, RG24 8PW
England Staphylase
Tel: +44 1256 841144
Fax: +44 1256 814626
E-mail: Oxoid@oxoid.com
Web: oxoid.co.uk/

β-Lactamase detection kits
MUG supplement
Staphytect Plus
StrepPlus
ONPG disk

800 Proctor Avenue
Ogdensburg, NY 13669, USA
Tel: 800-567-8378
Fax: 613-226-3728

PACIFIC BIOTECH COMPANY (PB)
Division of Bangkok RIA Card O.S.
Bangkok RIA Group
6 Ladprao 110 Ladprao Road
Bankapi, Bangkok 10310, Thailand
Tel: 662/530-2754060 530-3513-3. 530-4608-9
Fax: 530-2761, 530-4619
E-mail: brico@ksc15.th.com or info@Hlink.com

PHARMACIA & UPJOHN HUVUDKONTOR, SVERIGE
PHARMACIA & UPJOHN AB CLO strip test
Lindhagenstan 133
112 87 Stockholm
Sweden
Tel: 08 695 80 00
Web: www.pharmaciaupjohn.se (Swedish)
Web: www.pnu.com (English)

POLYSCIENCES INC.
400 Valley Road p-Phenylenediamine dihydrochloride
Warrington, PA 18976, USA
Tel: 800-523-2575
Fax: 800-343-3291
Web: www.polysciences.com/

REMEL, INC.
P.O. Box 14428 Acridine orange dye
76 Santa Fe Drive ALA disks
Lenexa, KS 66215, USA Alpha napthol 5% Anaerobic nitrate A&B reagent
Tel: 800-255-6730 An-Indent disks
Tel: 800-447-3635 Orders Bacitracin disk
Tel International: 913-888-0939 BactiCard *Neisseria*
Fax: 800-447-5750 BactiCard Strep
Fax International: 913-888-5884 Beta-lysin disk
E-mail: remel@remelinc.com Bile disk
Web: www.remelinc.com Catalase spot test
IDS RapID-ANA II
IDS RapID CB Plus
IDS RapID ONE system (*E.coli*)
IDS RapID NF Plus panel
IDS RapID NH system
IDS RapID SS/u system
IDS RapID STR
LAP disk
Microdase oxidase disks
Micro-ID
R/b Enteric Differential system
Thermonuclease agar

ROSCO A/S
Taastrpgaardsbej 30 Staph-ZYM
2630 Taastrup
Denmark
Tel: 45 43 99 33 777
Fax: 45 42 52 73 74
E-mail: info@as-rosco.dk

ROCHE DIAGNOSTICS-LABORATORY SYSTEMS
P.O. Box 50457 Oxi/Ferm (O/F) system
Indianapolis, IN 46250-0446, USA Staph RapID
Tel: 800-428-2336 Tech Service
Tel: 800-428-5030 Customer Service
Fax: 800-428-2883
E-mail: biocemts@roche.com
Web: www.roche.com

F. HOFFMAN-LA-ROCHE LTD.
CH-4070 Basel
Switzerland
Tel: ++41/61 688 11 11
Fax: ++41/61 691 93 91
Web: www.roche.com/roche/contacts/contacts.htm

SANOFI DIAGNOSTICS PASTEUR
3 Boulevard Raymond Pouncaré
92430 Marmese-La-Coquette
France
Tel:(1) 47.95.60.00
Fax:(1)47.41.84.33

Pastorex Staph-Plus

SIGMA-ALDRICH INC.
Iron Run Corporate Center
6950 Ambassador Drive
Allentown, PA 18106, USA
Tel: 610-391-9107
Fax: 610-391-9108

P.O. Box 355
1001 West St. Paul Avenue
Milwaukee, WI 53201, USA
Tel: 414-273-4979
Tel: 800-558-9160 Orders
Fax: 414-273-4979
Fax: 800-962-9591 Orders
E-mail: aldrich@sial.com
Web: www.sigma-aldrich.com

Aminolevulinic acid hydrochloride
d-Dimethylaminocinnamaldehyde (DMACA)
DNA (calf thymus)-highest grade
Indoxyl acetate
Lysostaphin
o-Nitrophenyl-β-D-galactopyranoside
   (o-nitrophenyl-β-D-galactoside) and p-(PNPG)
Phenolphthalein diphosphate (PDP)
L-Pyrrolindoxyl-β-naphthylamine
Sodium deoxynucleate
Sulfanilic acid—dry, crystalline
TRIS buffer (trizma-9/0)

SYVA INC.
405 Alberto Way
Los Gatos, CA 95032, USA
Tel: 408-356-8415
Web: www.dadebehring.com/syva.com

Fluorescent monoclonal antibody (FA) test

TECHLAB
1861 Pratt Drive
Suite 1030
Blacksburg, VA 24060-6364, USA
Tel: 540-953-1664, ext. 3012
Tel: 800-832-4522
Fax: 540-953-1665

Cambridge Bio Tech Cytoclone A&B
Tech Lab toxin A

APPENDIX 12

Glossary

PREFIXES

Definition: a syllable(s) or affix attached to beginning of a word which produces a derivative word.

A-, without.

Ana-, without.

Anti-, against.

Apo-, off, away, or from.

Aut-, auto-, self.

Aux-, auxo-, auxano-, increase in size, intensity, speed, etc.

Bi-, two, twofold; double; dual actions.

Bio-, life, living.

Bis-, twice.

Chrom-, chromo-, chromoto-, chromato-, color-producing.

De-, dehydro-, removal of atoms, radicals, water.

Deoxy- lacking an oxygen atom.

Dis-, separating, taking apart.

Ec-, out of, away from.

En-, in, on, at; appears before letters b, p, or m.

End-, endo-, within, absorbing, containing.

Ent-, ento-, inner, within.

Ex-, exo-, out of; out from; exterior, external.

Hetero-, other, different; of different species.

Homo-, similarity, same; of same species.

Inter-, between.

Intra-, within.

Iso-, alike or equal.

Lys-, lyso-, pertaining to lysis or dissolution.

Macro, large; visible with the naked eye.

Meso-, middle; mean; intermediacy.

Meta-, after, next, subsequent.

Micr-, micro-, small; visible only microscopically; one-millionth of a unit.

Mon-, mono-, one, single.

Morp-, morpho-, shape, structure.

Multi-, many.

Necr-, necro-, pertaining to death or necrosis.

Neo-, new, recent.

Non-, not.

Olig-, oligo-, few.

Ortho-, normal; straight, in proper order.

Oxa-, presence or addition of oxygen atom(s).

Oxo-, addition of oxygen.

Oxy-, oxygen in a molecule.

Path-, patho-, suffering; disease.

Philo-, affinity for.

Physi-, physio-, physical, physiologic; natural.

Pleo-, more.

Poly-, many, multiplicity.

Pro-, before, forward; precursor.

Proto-, first in a series.

Pseud-, pseudo-, false, similar to; deviation from a hypothetical parent substance.

Pyo-, suppuration, pus.

Pyr-, pyro-, heat; fever.

Radio-, pertaining to radiation.

Rib-, ribo-, root of ribose and its derivatives.

Sub-, beneath; less than normal.

Therm-, thermo-, heat.

Toxi, toxico-, poison, toxin.

Tri-, three.

Ultra-, beyond; outside certain limits.

Zym, zymo-, related to fermentation or enzymes.

SUFFIXES

Definition: a syllable(s) added to the end of a word to alter its meaning.

-ase, denotes an enzyme; name of substrate the enzyme acts upon plus the ending -ase. Example: enzyme galactosidase, substrate galactose.

-chrome, color.

-esis, condition, action, or process.

-iasis, condition or state.

-ic, denotes an acid; attached to name of element or compound; e.g., phosphoric.

-ites, itis, associated with an inflammatory disease or process.

-ose, denotes a carbohydrate.

-osis, process, condition, state; usually abnormal or diseased; any production or increase (physiologic or pathologic).

-phil, -phile, -philia, -philos, attraction or affinity for.

-ploid, multiple.

-poiesis, to make or produce.

-scope, instrument for viewing.

TERMS

Absorption, taking up a substance or substances. Compare with **Adsorption**.

Acceptor (electron), see **Electron acceptor**.

Acceptor (hydrogen), see **Hydrogen acceptor**.

Acetal, diethylacetal, 1-1-diethoxyethane, ethylidenediethyl ether, $CH_3CH(OC_2H_5)_2$.

Acetate, salt of acetic acid.

Acetoin (acetylmethylcarbinol), 3-hydroxy-2-butanone, $CH_3CHOH-CO-CH_3$. Oxidized to diacetyl. Formed from 2,3-butanediol, sugars, and pyruvic acid by acetic acid and acetone-butanol bacteria.

Acetylmethylcarbinol (AMC), see **Acetoin**.

Achroodextrin, dextrin formed from starch digested by the enzyme amylase; no color reaction with iodine reagent.

Acid, a compound that yields hydrogen ions in aqueous solution; a proton donor.

Acid curd, coagulation of casein in milk as a result of lactic acid production by microorganisms. Litmus or bromcresol purple indicators are usually incorporated in milk to show an acid reaction.

Acid dye, a dye consisting of an acidic organic grouping of atoms (anion), which is the actively staining part, combined with a metal; has affinity for cytoplasm.

Acid (sequestric), see **Ethylenediaminetetraacetate (EDTA)**.

Acidity, state of being acid; acid content of a fluid.

Acronym, a word formed from the first (or first few) letters of several words; e.g., IMViC.

Acyl, organic acid group in which the OH of the carboxyl group is replaced by another substituent (RCO-); e.g., acetyl, CH_3CO-.

Activator, cofactor, a metal ion that activates an enzyme secreted in an inactive form, e.g., the effect of magnesium and manganese on

various phases of alcoholic and lactic acid fermentation.

Adaptive enzyme (induced), an enzyme whose production requires or is markedly stimulated by a specific molecule, the inducer, which is the substrate of the enzyme or a compound structurally similar to it. The preferred term is **induced enzyme**; the inducer is the structurally similar compound responsible for evoking enzyme formation.

Adenine, part of a nucleotide, adenylic acid; a white crystalline base, 6-aminopurine, $C_5H_5N_5$ found in various animal and plant tissues.

Adenosine, a mononucleoside consisting of adenine and D-ribose; produced by hydrolysis of adenosine monophosphate; adenine riboside.

Adenosine diphosphate (ADP), consists of adenylic acid, ribose, and two phosphoric acid radicals. It is a constituent of coenzyme I, an acceptor of high-energy phosphate forming adenosine triphosphate.

Adenosine monophosphate (AMP), consists of adenylic acid, ribose, and one phosphoric acid radical. Compound is active in many energy transfer reactions by its ability to store energy and by its capacity to form adenosine di- and triphosphate.

Adenosine triphosphate (ATP), composed of adenylic acid, ribose, and three phosphoric acid radicals. It donates high-energy phosphate, forming adenosine diphosphate.

Adjuvant, that which aids or assists in immunology; a vehicle used to enhance antigenicity.

Adsorption, process by which gas molecules or small particles in solution are attracted by, and attached to, surface of another substance. Compare with **Absorption**.

Aeration, saturating a fluid with air; e.g., O_2 and CO_2.

Aerobic, requiring atmospheric oxygen or air for growth and reproduction.

Aerogenic, gas producing (CO_2 and H_2).

Aerosol, stable suspension of liquids or solids in air, oxygen, or inert gases, dispersed in a fine mist.

Aerotolerant, ability of an anaerobic organism to grow in air, usually poorly, especially after anaerobic isolation.

Affinity, attraction.

Aglycone, nonsugar moiety; hydrolytic product of a glycoside.

Agmatine, 1-amino-4-guani-dino-butane amine resulting from decarboxylation of arginine; $NH=C(NH_2)NH(CH_2)_4NH_2$.

Agar-agar, a dried polysaccharide (the sulfuric acid ester of a linear galactan) extracted from Japanese seaweed (red algae) used as a solidifying agent in biologic culture media. It dissolves in boiling water, solidifies at about 38°C, and is usually not liquefied by bacteria.

Agar slant, tube of melted agar medium permitted to solidify at an angle to give a slope or increased surface for bacterial inoculant.

Agent, anything capable of producing an effect upon an organism.

Agglutination, clumping of cells suspended in a fluid.

Agglutinin, an antibody found in immune serum which, when added to a suspension of its homologous microorganisms, causes the organisms to adhere to one another, forming clumps.

Alcohol, an organic compound containing the hydroxyl (OH) group, R-OH; a hydrocarbon derivative with one or more hydrogen atoms replaced by hydroxyl groups.

Alcohol (polyhydric), see **Polyhydric alcohol**.

Aldehyde, an organic compound containing the aldehyde (CHO) group; a hydrocarbon derivative in which two hydrogen atoms on the same carbon atom have been replaced by an oxygen atom to form the carbonyl group (C=O). Carbonyl group is attached to one carbon atom and one hydrogen atom. $R-\overset{\overset{O}{\|}}{C}-H$ This compound is an intermediate or product of bacterial fermentation formed from sugars, ethyl alcohol, pyruvic acid, and other substances by the acetic acid and acetone-butanol bacteria.

Aldose, a sugar that is a polyhydric aldehyde.

Alicyclic compound, an organic compound that exhibits aliphatic characteristics, but whose carbon atoms are in a ring rather than an open chain.

Aliphatic compound, an organic compound of open chain structure.

Aliquot, a fraction or portion.

Alkali, a water-soluble base that yields hydroxyl ions (OH) in aqueous solution.

Alkaline, having the properties of an alkali.

Alkalinity, condition of being alkaline.

Alkane, a saturated aliphatic hydrocarbon of the methane series whose carbon atoms are joined by single bonds. The carbon atoms are completely saturated with hydrogen atoms. General formula is C_nH_{2n+2}, where n represents the number of carbon atoms.

Alkene, an aliphatic hydrocarbon containing two hydrogen atoms fewer than corresponding alkane and is thus unsaturated, containing two carbon atoms joined by a double bond. The general formula is C_nH_{2n}; the compound name ends in either -ene or -ylene.

Alkyl group, a univalent radical derived from an alkane by removal of a hydrogen atom.

Amide, a derivative of an organic acid (R-COOH) in which an OH group is replaced by the amino ($-NH_2$) group. The general formula for a primary amide is: R-CO-NH_2; the compound is named according to the acid from which it is derived by changing the -ic ending to amide and dropping the word acid.

Amine, an organic derivative of ammonia in which one or more hydrogen atoms are replaced by an alkyl radical ($-NH_2$). General formula: R-NH_2; named according to alkyl groups on nitrogen with amine ending. These are basic compounds that react with inorganic acids to form salts.

Amino acid, an organic compound containing both amino ($-NH_2$) and carboxyl ($-COOH$) groups. They make up a class of organic acids characterized by substitution of an amino group in the alkyl residue R·CH(NH_2)COOH. Amino acids, the building blocks of protein molecules, provide a nitrogen source and energy to an organism. Some organisms require amino acids for growth. Amino acids important in bacterial metabolism include glycine, alanine, and serine.

Amino group, $-NH_2$ group attached to an α-carbon (i.e., the carbon atom next to the carboxyl group).

Amylase, one of a group of starch-splitting, or amylolytic, enzymes that cleave starch and glycogen.

Amylopectin, branched-chain polysaccharide (glucan) in starch.

Amylose, unbranched polysaccharide (glucan) in starch.

Anabolism, constructive metabolism in which nutrient material is assimilated by a cell to build or restore cell material and other living matter. Process by which simple chemical substances are converted into more complex substances; synthesis of material by the cell. Also called **Assimilation.**

Anaerobe, an organism that can grow and reproduce in the absence of atmospheric oxygen or air.

Anaerogenic, non–gas producing (CO_2 and H_2).

Analog, a compound that interferes with metabolism or function of another compound on the basis of a structural similarity. The two compounds are similar in function but differ structurally. Also called analogue (substrate) or **metabolic antagonist.**

Analytical (AR), grade of chemical.

Anhydride, residue of an acid after the elements of water are removed from the carboxyl groups.

Anhydrous, without water.

Anion, portion of electrolyte that carries the negative charge and travels to the anode.

Anode, positively charged electrode of an electrolytic cell. See **Pole.**

Anomer, epimer, one of two sugar molecules that are epimeric at hemiacetal carbon atom; e.g., α-D-glucose and β-D-glucose. See **Epimer.**

Antagonism, see **Competitive inhibition.**

Anticoagulant, a substance that prevents coagulation, e.g., potassium oxalate, sodium citrate, and heparin.

Antigenic, causing an animal to produce antibodies; acting as an antigen.

Antimicrobial, a biologic or chemical agent that inhibits growth of microorganisms.

Antitoxin, antibody formed in response to antigenic poisonous substance(s) of biologic origin. Substance or antibody that neutralizes or binds a toxin such as bacterial exotoxin.

Apoenzyme, the inactive protein portion of an enzyme; apoenzyme + coenzyme → holoenzyme.

Apolar, without poles or processes.

Aqueous, with water.

Aromatic acid, a compound in which one or more hydrogen atoms on a benzene ring have been replaced by carboxyl groups or in which a carboxyl group is attached to a side chain.

Aromatic amine, a compound in which an amino or substituted amino group is attached to a benzene ring.

Aromatic compound, a cyclic organic compound derived from benzene.

Artificial electron acceptor, certain synthetic dyes and other reducible substances that can serve as artificial electron acceptors when added to suspensions of living cells. Electrons derived from an oxidizable substrate are shunted from their normal pathway to reduce the dye.

Artificial medium, medium of exactly known, reproducible composition; artificial environment supports growth and reproduction of bacteria. Also known as **synthetic medium.**

Ascitic fluid, serous fluid that accumulates in the peritoneal cavity of an individual with ascites (dropsy). Used to fortify artificial culture media for the growth of fastidious organisms.

Aseptic, free of all living microorganisms capable of causing infection or contamination.

Aseptically, performing an action without permitting contamination by microorganisms.

Assay, test of purity or trial; to determine components by analysis.

Assimilation, see **Anabolism.**

Asymmetry, without symmetry; disproportion between two or more like parts.

Atom, a chemical unit made up of three kinds of particles: protons, electrons, and neutrons; the smallest part of an element, it is chemically indestructible and indivisible.

Autoclave, an apparatus that generates steam under pressure, used to sterilize equipment, materials, and products.

Autolysin, a bacterial substance capable of disintegrating the cell containing it.

Autolysis, lysis or disintegration of cells by the action of an organism's own enzymes; self-disintegration.

Autolytic, pertaining to or causing autolysis.

Autooxidation, direct combination of a substance with molecular oxygen at ordinary temperature; self-oxidation.

Auxochrome, a chemical group whose presence in a molecule containing a chromophore group enables that molecule to function as a dye. The auxochrome furnishes salt-forming properties and is responsible for transferring the color of a dye to a substance upon which it acts. See **Chromophore** and **Dye.**

Auxotroph, mutant microorganisms that can be cultivated only by supplementing a minimal medium with growth factors or amino acids not required by wild-type strains.

Azide, sodium azide (NaN_3); a substance that inhibits Gram-negative organisms; a bacteriostatic substance. Used in media because of its bacteriostatic action.

Azo-, prefix indicating presence of the group $-N:N-$.

Azo dye, a basic chromophore azo grouping $-N:N-$. A derivative of azobenzene in which a benzene or naphthalene ring is attached to each nitrogen atom.

Bacillus (pl., **bacilli**), rod-shaped bacterium; also a genus of rod-shaped bacteria of the family *Bacillaceae.*

Bacitracin, USP, BP, antibacterial polypeptide of known chemical structure; in class of antibiotics that inhibit bacterial cell wall synthesis.

Bacterium (pl., **bacteria**), minute, one-celled, microscopic organism that multiplies primarily by binary fission and lacks chlorophyll.

Bacterial filter, a filter used to separate bacteria from a fluid medium.

Bacterial strain, a pure culture of bacteria made up of descendants of a single isolate.

Bactericidal, denoting a chemical, material, agent, or substance that is lethal to bacteria; kills; is irreversible.

Bacteriology, biologic and chemical study of bacteria.

Bacteriophage, a virus with specific affinity for bacteria; e.g., corynebacteriophage.

Bacteriostatic, action of an agent inhibiting bacterial growth. Reversible reaction; when inhibitor is removed, growth and reproduction resume.

Basal medium, a medium containing all nutritional requirements needed to support bacterial growth and reproduction in an artificial environment.

Base, a compound that yields hydroxyl ions (OH) in aqueous solution; a proton acceptor.

Basic dye, a dye consisting of a basic organic grouping of atoms (cation), which is the actively staining part, combined with an acid, usually inorganic; has affinity for nucleic acids.

Beef extract, an extract of beef containing the soluble mineral components used in preparation of media such as nutrient broth.

Benzene, organic, parent aromatic compound containing a closed ring of six carbon atoms joined by alternating single and double bonds; C_6H_6.

Benzene ring,

Bile acid, organic acid that exists as a conjugate with glycine or taurine; i.e., glycocholic acid and taurocholic acid. Cholic acid, 3,7,12-trihydroxycholanic; deoxycholic acid, 3,12-dihydroxy-cholanic.

Bile salt, sodium salt of a bile acid (acid conjugate); e.g., taurocholate, glycocholate.

Bimolecular, involving two molecules; e.g., a and b reaction.

Binomial, consisting of two names; e.g., genus and species.

Biochemistry, field of chemistry that deals with the processes of living organisms, such as bacteria, and the products derived from them; the chemistry of living processes.

Biosynthesis, formation of a chemical compound by enzymes either in organism (in vivo) or by fragments or extracts of cells (in vitro).

Biotype, group of bacterial strains physiologically distinguishable from other strains of same source.

Blood agar (BA), agar enriched with blood to enhance cultivation of fastidious microorganisms and/or to differentiate hemolytic colonies. Sheep blood (5%) is preferred.

Blood plasma, fluid portion of circulating blood, as distinguished from the corpuscles, containing coagulation factors.

Blood serum, clear, watery component of blood separated by coagulation from its more solid components.

Boiling point (b.p.), temperature at which the vapor pressure of a liquid equals the ambient (surrounding) atmospheric temperature.

Bordet-Gengou medium, "cough plate"; enrichment medium for isolation and cultivation of *Bordetella pertussis,* causative agent of whooping cough.

Bound coagulase, slide test determination that measures clumping factor.

Bovine, an animal such as an ox, cow, etc.

Broad-spectrum, widely effective; denotes antibiotic effective against a variety of bacteria, both Gram-positive and Gram-negative.

Broth, a culture medium consisting of essential nutrients for heterotrophic bacteria; a liquid.

Brownian movement, irregular, rapid oscillatory movement of small particles suspended in fluid, attributable to bombardment of the particles by the kinetic movement of the molecules of the fluid. Frequently seen in liquid suspensions of bacteria. A false motility.

Bubo, an inflammation and swelling of lymphatic glands; usually in the groin or armpit.

Buffer, solution containing both a weak acid and its conjugate base. Addition to a system enables it to resist change in the hydrogen ion concentration.

Buffer action, capacity to neutralize, within limits, either acids or bases without changing the original acidity or alkalinity.

Buffer salts, salts that behave as buffers, generally salts of acids with a low dissociation constant; e.g., carbonates and phosphates.

Butt, lower portion of a slanted tubed agar medium; portion below slant.

Byproduct, substance or substances that remain after the parent compounds have been used by an organism; e.g., nitrites formed when oxygen is removed from nitrates.

Cadaverine, pentamethylenediamine, $NH_2CH_2CH_2CH_2CH_2CH_2NH_2$, a colorless liquid with a putrefactive odor formed by the decomposition of lysine or proteinaceous material by bacteria.

Capsule, thickened slime layer, primarily of carbohydrate material, that surrounds the cell wall of many bacteria. The presence of a capsule enhances bacterial pathogenicity.

Caramelize, to melt and turn sugars brown by excessive heating; degrade.

Carbamide, diamide of carbonic acid. Urea or one of its derivatives is a carbamide.

Carbinol, methyl alcohol.

Carbohydrase (cytase), enzyme that splits (hydrolyzes) carbohydrates: maltase, lactase, sucrase, amylase, etc.

Carbohydrate, large group of organic compounds containing carbon, hydrogen, and oxygen, with H and O in the proportion to form water. Carbohydrates include sugars, starches, cellulose, and glycogen. See **Monosaccharide, Disaccharide, Trisaccharide** and **Polysaccharide.**

Carbonyl group, a bivalent organic radical (−CO−) occurring in aldehydes, ketones, acids, and their derivatives.

Carboxyl group, a univalent organic radical (−COOH) that is the functional group of all carboxylic acids.

Carboxylase, enzyme belonging to the desmolases that decarboxylates α-keto acids to the corresponding aldehydes. Specifically, it acts on pyruvic acid to form acetaldehyde and carbon dioxide. Its coenzyme is cocarboxylase.

Casein, principle protein in milk; a phosphoprotein that precipitates on acidification. Milk-clotting enzymes (rennin, pepsin, and chymotrypsin), hydrolyze casein to a soluble paracasein, which in turn, in the presence of calcium ions, is converted to insoluble casein, a paracaseinate (calcium paracaseinate). Paracaseinate is called "milk curd"; the residual clear fluid is called "whey."

Catabolism, metabolic process which consists of the breakdown of complex organic molecules into simpler substances by bacteria with the liberation of energy, a part of the total process of metabolism. Also called **Dissimulation.**

Catalase, an enzyme that decomposes hydrogen peroxide (H_2O_2), liberating free oxygen.

Catalysis, the effect a catalyst exerts upon a chemical reaction.

Catalyst, a substance that accelerates or slows down a chemical or physical reaction without being destroyed or changed itself. Term generally applied to acceleration; the term *negated catalyst* is used if the reaction is retarded.

Catalytic, relating to or effecting catalysis.

Cathode, negative pole of an electrical battery or system. See **Pole.**

Cation, ion carrying a positive charge and moving toward the cathode.

Caustic, corrosive or burning.

Cell, structural unit of all plants and animals.

Cellulose, polysaccharide of the hexosan group, a polymer of glucose that is the structural material of plant walls.

Celsius, another name for centigrade.

Centigrade, temperature scale on which the freezing point of pure water is 0°C and boiling point is 100°C.

Centrifugation, separation of solids from liquids or of liquids with different specific gravities by rapid rotation.

Centrifuge, an apparatus used to separate the components or ingredients of a mixture by centrifugal force, generally by rotation in the machine.

Cephalin, member of a group of lipids called phospholipids.

Cephalosporin, one of several antibiotic substances from fungi; effective against Gram-positive and Gram-negative bacteria.

Ceramide, general term to describe any N-acetyl fatty acid derivative of sphingosine.

Cerebroside, galactolipid; class of glycosphingolipids; specifically, a monoglycosylceramide found in the myelin sheath of nerve tissue.

Characteristic, a distinguish trait or quality.

Chelate (ion), structural combination of organic compounds and metal atoms; e.g., cytochromes, hemoglobins.

Chelating agent, a substance that combines with a metal in weakly dissociated complexes in which the metal is linked to an organic ring compound by covalent links. The metallic ion is sequestered and firmly bound into a ring within the chelating molecule.

Chemical bond, linkage between different atoms or radicals of a chemical compound.

Chemical change, an alteration in the composition of a substance.

Choline, (2-hydroxyethyl)trimethylammonium ion; $HOCH_2-CH_2-N(CH_3)_3^+$; lipotropic factor, transmethylation factor. Found in most animal tissue either free or in combination with lecithin.

Chromatic, pertaining to colors.

Chromatography, absorption analysis; separation of chemical substances and particles on the basis of different movement through a two-phase system. Analytical process based on differences in the distribution ratios of the components of mixtures between a mutually immiscible mobile and a fixed phase.

Chromogen, a substance that elicits a colored product on oxidation. See **Chromophore** and **Auxochrome.**

Chromogenic, pigment producing.

Chromophore (chromatophore), a chemical group whose presence gives a specific color to a compound and which unites with certain other groups (auxochromes) to form dyes. Most common groups are quinoid, nitro, and azo. See **Auxochrome.**

Chymotrypsin, milk-clotting enzyme; an endopeptidase.

Citric acid cycle, see **Krebs' cycle.**

Cleave, split a molecule into two or more simpler molecules.

Clotting, see **Coagulation.**

Coagulant, agent that causes coagulation or clotting.

Coagulase, enzyme that causes coagulation or clotting of blood plasma.

Coagulase reacting factor (CRF), a plasma factor that combines with free coagulase in the tube coagulase test to form a substance that indirectly converts fibrinogen to fibrin, resulting in formation of a clot.

Coagulate, to clot or curdle by chemical action or fermentation.

Coagulation, separation of a colloidally dispersed material or a dissolved solid from a liquid by formation of an insoluble or gelatinous mass, such as coagulation of egg albumin, curdling of milk, or clotting of blood.

Cocarboxylase, coenzyme of carboxylase or pyruvic dehydrogenase. It is a pyrimidinethiazole pyrophosphoric acid.

Coccus (pl., **cocci**), round or sphere-shaped bacterium.

Codecarboxylase, pyridoxal phosphate; coenzyme of various amino acid decarboxylases.

Coenzyme, a low-molecular-weight, nonprotein organic substance that can attach to an enzyme and thus supplement specific active enzyme systems. The term *coenzyme* is synonymous with *prosthetic group* when used in connection with conjugated proteins that have enzyme activity.

Cofactor, prosthetic group such as heme, coenzyme, and inorganic ions such as magnesium, essential for enzyme action. Also see **Activator.**

Coliform, aerobic and facultatively anaerobic Gram-negative rods that are nonsporeforming and which ferment lactose with gas formation (*Escherichia coli* and *Klebsiella-Enterobacter* groups). They have sanitary significance in testing water, food, and milk for bacterial contamination.

Collagen, principle fibrous protein of mammalian connective tissue, tendons, and bones.

Colloid, aggregates of atoms or molecules in a finely divided state, dispersed in a gaseous, liquid, or solid medium; cannot pass through a semipermeable membrane.

Colon bacillus, See **Coliform.** Organism residing in the intestinal tract.

Colony, visible growth (macroscopic) of microorganisms, generally on a solid medium and usually derived from the multiplication of a single organism; all are the progeny of a single preexisting bacterium.

Colony morphology, macroscopic appearance of bacterial colonies on solid growth medium: size, shape, consistency, pigmentation, odor, abundance of growth are the main characteristics observed.

Colorimetric analysis, quantitative analysis of a substance by comparing the intensity of the color produced by a reagent with a standard color produced similarly in a solution of known strength.

Combination, union of two or more substances to form a new substance, or a chemical reaction in which two elements combine to form a binary compound or two binary compounds combine to form a complex compound.

Competitive inhibition, inhibition of bacterial metabolism by compounds competing with the substrate for the active group of the enzyme or with the enzyme for the substrate (**antagonism**). Competition for the same enzyme site by two different molecules with structural similarities.

Complex, relatively stable combination of two or more compounds into a larger molecule.

Complexing agent, see **Chelating agent**.

Compound, a substance composed of two or more elements united chemically in definite proportions by weight.

Concentration, the amount of a substance that exists in a unit of volume, e.g., the strength of a solution in mass of solute per unit mass of solution, or the number of moles or hydrogen ions per unit of volume or mass.

Condensation, a type of reaction in which two or more molecules of the same substance combine to form a new substance with higher molecular weight and different chemical properties.

Confirmatory, firmly establishing; proving.

Confluent (growth), bacterial growth in which colonies overlap each other and cannot be successfully picked out individually for subculture.

Conjugal transfer, conjugative transposon or "jumping gene."

Conjugate, to fuse, unit, pair, or join together. Conjugated proteins are joined to other types of molecules. Compounds containing two or more double bonds, alternating single and double bonds are called conjugated. Example: $CH_2=CH-CH=CH-CH_3$.

Conjugated proteins contain amino acid residues plus substances such as pigments (chromoproteins), carbohydrates, etc. Conjugated double bonds are two or more double bonds joined together by a single bond.

Constitutive enzyme, an enzyme produced by the cell independently of the composition of the medium in which it is grown; it does not depend upon the substrate to evoke formation.

Contamination, transfer of undesirable microorganisms to media or other materials by direct contact.

Continuity, succession without a break.

Conversion, change from one isomer to another or change from one unit or system of measurement to another.

Coordination, harmonious, integrated action of various parts and processes of an organism, test, etc.

Correlate, to bring into or be in mutual relation.

Coupling, combination of an amine or phenol with a diazonium compound to give an azo compound; reaction by which azo dyes are prepared.

Covalent bonding, type of bonding in which electrons are shared by two atomic nuclei. Range from nonpolar, involving electrons evenly shared by two atoms, to extremely polar, in which the bonding electrons are very unevenly shared.

Cross-linkage, attachment of two chains of polymer molecules by bridges composed of an element, group, or compound that joins certain carbon atoms of the chain by primary chemical bonds. Occurs in nature in substances made up of polypeptide chains joined by disulfide bonds of the cystine residue, e.g., insulin.

Cross-reaction (reactivity), a specific reaction between antiserum and an antigen complex other than the antigen complex (immunogen) that evoked the various specific antibodies in the antiserum.

Crystallization, change from the dissolved, molten, liquid, or gaseous state to a solid state of ordered and characteristic shape.

Crystalloid, resembling a crystal or being such; when in solution can pass through a semipermeable membrane.

Culture, a growth of microorganisms.

Culture medium (pl., **media**), artificial food materials upon which bacteria are cultivated.

Cupule (**cupula**, pl., **cupulae**), cup-shaped or domelike structure.

Curd, precipitated milk protein consisting mainly of casein; may result from coagulation by an acid or rennet reaction. See **Rennin curd** and **Acid curd**.

Cutaneous, relating to the skin.

Cysteine, β-mercaptoalanine, $C_3H_7O_2NS$; an amino acid derived from cystine.

Cystine, β,β'-dithiobisalanine, $C_6H_{12}O_4N_2S_2$. A sulfur-containing amino acid that can be obtained by oxidation of cysteine.

Cytase, cytohydrolytic carbohydrase enzyme.

Cytochrome, one of a group of heme protein pigments (a, b, and c) present in most living cells, with the exception of a few bacteria (e.g., *Clostridium* spp.); one of a group of reversible oxidation-reduction carriers in respiration. It can alternate oxidation and reduction.

Cytochrome oxidase, an enzyme that in the presence of molecular oxygen can oxidize cytochrome c.

Cytochrome system, a group of intracellular heme proteins produced by all aerobic bacteria, concerned with electron transfer in the major biologic oxidation-reduction pathways of metabolism.

d-, (symbol) meaning dextrorotatory. Monosaccharides and disaccharides are optically active; they rotate planes of polarized light. Those that rotate it to the right are said to be dextrorotatory.

Deaminase, enzyme that removes an amino group ($-NH_2$) from a molecule with resulting liberation of ammonia (NH_3).

Deamination, process of splitting the amino group (NH_2) from an amino acid.

Decarboxylase(s), enzyme that liberates CO_2 from the carboxyl group (−COOH) of a molecule, e.g., amino acid.

Decarboxylation, process of removing CO_2 from a carboxylic acid (−COOH), thereby removing the carboxyl group.

Decomposition, process of breaking down a substance into simpler substances.

Defibrinate, remove fibrin from blood.

Degrade, break down into simpler molecules or components.

Degree, a position or unit; a measure of temperature (e.g., °C).

Dehydrated, water removed. Usually refers to media that can be reconstituted by addition of water. See **Reconstitute.**

Dehydrogenase, conjugated protein enzymes that possess oxidation activity because of their prosthetic groups, e.g., NAD, NADP, FMN, and FAD; they effect oxidation of a substrate by accepting or transferring hydrogen by alternate reduction or oxidation. See **Prosthetic group.**

Dehydrogenation, removal of hydrogen from a molecule.

Deliquescent salt, substance capable of absorbing moisture from air and dissolving in it; e.g., $CaCl_2$.

Demineralize, eliminate minerals; e.g., demineralized water used to prepare bacterial culture media.

Denatured, changed or rendered unfit for consumption, as alcohol. Changes may be physical, chemical, or biologic such as increased digestibility, loss of enzymatic activity, changes in immunologic characteristics. Often there is no change in molecular weight. In some instances the process can be reversed. When proteins are denatured hydrogen bonds and other subsidiary linkages are broken.

Denitrification, anaerobic process by which denitrifying bacteria reduce nitrates (−NO_3) to nitrites (−NO_2) liberating free nitrogen (N_2) and ammonia (NH_3) to the atmosphere by reduction. The reverse of nitrification.

Density, mass per unit volume.

Deoxyribonucleic acid (DNA), (also spelled desoxy-). Substance in a cell that controls heredity, is specifically replicated, and bears genetic information. A polynucleotide consisting of four groups: heterocyclic nitrogenous bases of purine and pyrimidine type (adenine, guanine, cytosine, and thymine), D-2-deoxyribose, and phosphoric acid; present in the nuclei of plant and animal cells.

Deoxyribose, (also written desoxy). D-2-desoxyribose, $CH_2OH·CHOH·CHOH·CH_2·CHO$. A pentose carbohydrate constituent of desoxyribonucleic acid (DNA). See **Deoxyribonucleic acid.**

Depolymerize, depolymerization, destruction, neutralization or change in direction of polarity.

Derivative, compound, usually organic, obtained from another compound by a simple chemical process; organic compound containing a structural radical similar to that from which it is derived.

Derived protein, substance derived from simple and conjugated proteins by either hydrolysis or denaturation. Includes partially hydrolyzed proteins such as proteoses, peptones, and peptides. An example of a denatured protein is a protean.

Desiccant, drying agent; a chemical desiccant acts by **ab**sorption (i.e., reacts with water), and a physical desiccant acts by **ad**sorption (e.g., KOH, $CaCl_2$).

Desiccated, desiccation, dried, drying.

Desiccator, device for drying substances; e.g., closed glass vessel containing a deliquescent substance.

Desmolase, enzyme involved in splitting a carbon chain; e.g., β-keto carboxylase, amino acid decarboxylase, zymohexases, and aldolases.

Desorption, reverse of absorption; evolution or liberation of a volatile substance from solution.

Detergent, a purifying or cleansing agent that destroys or impairs structural organization of the cell by impairing the function of its semipermeable membrane. It is either oil- or water-soluble and helps to wet, disperse, or defloculate solid particles.

Dextran, a polysaccharide (glucose polymer) formed outside the cell by enzymatic activity of certain bacteria. A 1,6-glucosidic linkage is built up.

Dextrin, starch gum, amylin; carbohydrate intermediate between starch and sugars produced from starch by hydrolysis; reddish color with iodine and not fermentable but is converted into maltose and glucose.

Dextrose (glucose), see **Glucose.**

Diacetyl-, prefix indicating the presence of two acetyl radicals (CH_3CO). Diketobutane-CH_3CO $COCH_3$.

Diamide, amide derivative of organic acids in which the hydroxyl group (-OH) has been replaced by the amino group (NH_2). General formula for primary amide: $R-CO-NH_2$; diamide contains two NH_2 groups, NH_2-O-NH_2.

Diastase, old term. See **Amylase.**

Diastereoisomer, isomer whose molecules are partially superimposable and partially mirror images of each other. See **Isomers, Isomerization.**

Diazo compound, compound containing two azo groups: R-N:N-R-N:N-R, including many dyes.

Diazonium salt, bivalent radical −N:N- used for forming azo dyes by coupling with native phenolic compounds or coupling enzymatically with liberated compound benzene. The general type is

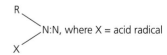

N:N, where X = acid radical

Dibasic, acids that liberate two hydrogen ions.

Differential medium, medium with certain reagents or chemicals (usually dyes) incorporated that result in a type of growth or chemical change after incubation that allows differentiation between types of bacteria. The usual results are either inhibition of certain organisms while permitting growth of others, or a pH change denoted by a specific color reaction when chemical changes occur.

Diffuse, spreading; scattered.

Diffusion, process in which unlike molecules mix; rapid in gases, slower in liquids, and very slow in solids.

Digestion, process by which a nutrient is broken down into simple soluble molecules small enough to pass through cell wall.

Diluent, a liquid used to dilute or thin another liquid.

Dilution, process of increasing the proportion of solvent to solute in any solution by addition of the same or another miscible solvent. Often used to express the amount of solute per unit volume of solution. Solute may represent bacterial cells. Antonym (opposite) of concentration. See **Concentration**.

Diphosphopyridine nucleotide (DPN); see **Nicotinamide adenine dinucleotide (NAD)**.

Diplococcus (pl., **diplococci**), cocci occurring in pairs; e.g., *Streptococcus pneumonia* (formerly classified as *Diplococcus pneumoniae*).

Diphosphopyridine nucleotide (DPN), also known as coenzyme I, cozymase, and codehydrogenase. DPN is the coenzyme of apozymase, a compound consisting of the radicals of niacinamide, ribose, two phosphoric acid units, ribose, and adenine, isolated from yeasts.

Disaccharide, sugar that yields two molecules of simple sugar on hydrolysis; composed of two monosaccharides. General formula: $C_{12}H_{22}O_{11}$.

Disk (disc), circular flat paper, usually 6 cm in diameter, impregnated with a chemical reagent(s) used to determine either biochemical or antibiotic sensitivities. See **Impregnated**.

Discernible, perceivable; evident.

Dismutation, a process in which a substance is simultaneously oxidized and reduced; changing one substance into two.

Disperse, dispersion, to scatter; dilute; to cause disappearance of.

Disseminate, scatter or distribute.

Dissimulation, also called catabolism. See **Catabolism**.

Dissociated, separated; split into simpler constituents by means such as ionization. Also used to describe substrains arising from pure bacterial strains.

Dissociation, physical breakdown of a molecule; molecule splits into simpler, less complex molecules.

Dissolution, disintegration; dissolving; autolysis.

Distilled water, water that has been vaporized and condensed.

Divalent, having a valence of two.

DL,-isomer, racemic mixture; a molecular complex of equal parts of D, and ,L forms arising during chemical synthesis. Racemization of amino acids occurs when proteins are hydrolyzed in the presence of alkali. See **d-, dextrorotatory** and **l-, levorotatory**.

Double bond, a covalent bond resulting from the sharing of two pairs of electrons; commonly represented as $CH_2=CH_2$ (ethylene).

Double-distilled water, water distilled twice; second time in a glass or platinum still.

Drop reaction, see **Spot test**.

Drops, portions of liquid; usually 0.1–0.3 mL.

Dye, material used for staining or coloring, consisting of benzene rings with chromophore and auxochrome groups. See **Auxochrome** and **Chromophore**.

Dysgonic, growing poorly (used to describe bacterial culture).

Effervescence, escape of gas from a liquid because of decreased pressure or increased temperature.

Effervescent, exhibiting bubbling because of escape of gas, not boiling.

Elaborate, to make, create, produce.

Electron, an atomic particle carrying a negative charge with a mass 1/837 that of the hydrogen atom (proton). Located in electron shells or energy levels outside the nucleus.

Electron acceptor, substance that accepts electrons (hydrogen ions) and thus becomes reduced; involved in oxidation reactions. Electron affinity is called "redox potential"; electrons are transferred from systems of lower redox potential to systems of high potential, and a coupled redox reaction occurs between two systems. Oxygen has the highest redox potential, and lowest values are for hydrogen attached to various substrates.

Electronegative, electron attracting.

Electron transport system, sequence of enzymatic reactions that mediate between oxidation of a substrate and reduction of oxygen.

Electrophoresis, migration of suspended particles in an electric field; in particular, the accelerated chromatographic separation of compounds by immersing each end of the medium in an electrolyte and applying an electrical potential.

Element, one of many fundamental forms of matter that cannot be broken down into simpler substances by ordinary chemical means.

Elution, separation, by washing, of one solid from another or removal, by means of a suitable solvent, of one material from another that is insoluble in that solvent.

Embden-Meyerhof-Parnas (EMP) pathway, main pathway of glucose fermentation. Also called *glycolysis* and *glycolytic cycle*. Concerned with phosphorylation of glucose with production of pyruvic acid and energy; pyruvic acid is possibly further degraded to lactic acid. Anaerobic form of metabolism.

Emulsion, colloidal dispersion of a liquid in another liquid.

Enantiomorph, crystal that has another crystal as a mirror image; opposite optically active substance; e.g., dextro- and levo-forms.

Endoenzyme, enzyme that is liberated only upon disintegration of the cell that produces it. See **Intracellular enzyme.**

Endogenous, endogenic, originating or produced within the organism or one of its parts.

Endonuclease, nuclease that cleaves polynucleotides (nucleic acids) at interior bonds, producing poly- and oligonucleotide fragments of various sizes.

Endothermic reaction, chemical change in which heat is absorbed.

Energy, the ability to do work in heat, light, electrical, kinetic, chemical, or nuclear terms. Unit for measuring heat energy is the calorie. Chemical energy is produced by oxidation of many different compounds.

Enolase, an enzyme belonging to the hydrases that acts on 2-phosphoglyceric acid to yield phosphopyruvic acid and water.

Enrichments, substances such as growth factors (X and V), vitamins, or materials like blood added to media to help cultivate fastidious microorganisms. See **Fastidious.**

Enteric, pertaining to the intestines.

Enterobacteriaceae, family classification of enteric, Gram-negative bacilli that are non-sporeforming and all ferment glucose. They grow well on artificial media, form acid or acid and gas from glucose, reduce nitrates, and are either motile or nonmotile and oxidase negative. They are commonly called enteric bacteria. See **Enteric.**

Enterococci, group of organisms found in the intestines; Gram-positive cocci in pairs, singly, or short chains; genus *Enterococcus.*

Enterotoxin, cytotoxin specific for cells of the mucous membranes of the intestines.

Entner-Doudoroff pathway, metabolic pathway for the breakdown of hexoses by some bacteria. The end products are pyruvate and glyceraldehyde 3-phosphate.

Enzyme, an organic, protein catalyst produced by a living cell and capable of influencing a chemical reaction without being structurally changed (altered) in the reaction. Enzymes mediate all metabolic processes.

Enzyme (exo-), see **Extracellular enzyme.**

Enzyme (induced), see **Adaptive enzyme.**

Eosin, sodium dibromodinitrofluorescein, $C_{20}H_6O_9N_2Br_2Na_2$. Used as a stain and an inhibitor of growth of some microorganisms when incorporated into media. Readily soluble in water, with green fluorescence. Also soluble in alcohol.

Epimer(ic), anomer; one of two molecules differing only in spatial arrangement about a single carbon atom. Also see **Anomer.**

Episome, class of genetic elements in bacteria that may exist either as autonomous entities that replicate independently of the bacterial chromosome or be part of the bacterial chromosome and replicate with it.

Equimolecular, denoting solutions that contain an equal number of molecules.

Equivocal (result), having two or more significations, ambiguous. Uncertain as an indication or sign; obscure. Used in recording biochemical results at times; same as a ± result.

Erythrocyte (RBC), see **Red blood cell.**

Erythrose, a four-carbon monosaccharide; a tetrose.

Esculin, a glucoside; an acetal derivative of a simple monosaccharide.

Ester, organic compound formed by a reaction between an acid and an alcohol. Acid derivative. General formula: R-CO-O-R'.

Esterase, one of a group of enzymes called hydrolases, which hydrolyze esters.

Ethanol, see **Ethyl alcohol.**

Ether, organic oxide; two alkyl radicals joined to an oxygen atom. General formula: R-O-R.

Ethyl alcohol, ethanol; CH_3CH_2OH. Produced by several microorganisms fermenting different substrates.

Ethylenediaminetetraacetate (EDTA), also called **sequestric acid.** An antiprooxidant that "sequesters" the oxidative metallic agent that increases the susceptibility of fats to oxidation. An anticoagulant that chelates ionic calcium and thus inhibits formation of a blood clot. Trade name is Versene. See **Chelating agent.**

Eugonic, describes bacterial culture growing luxuriantly.

Extracellular, outside the cell.

Extracellular enzyme, enzyme excreted into the environment. An enzyme that can be readily isolated from living cells. Also called **exoenzyme.**

Exocellular, produced outside cell in surrounding environment.

Exonuclease, nuclease that releases one nucleotide at a time, serially, beginning at one end of a polynucleotide (nucleic acid).

Exopeptidase, an enzyme that catalyzes the hydrolysis of the terminal amino acid of a peptide chain; e.g., carboxypeptidase.

Exothermic reaction, chemical change in which heat is liberated.

Exudate, to ooze or pass out gradually through the tissues; e.g., fluid or semisolid that may become encrusted or infected.

Facultative, having the power to do a thing although not ordinarily doing it; e.g., facultative anaerobes can live in the absence of atmospheric oxygen but do not ordinarily do so.

Facultative aerobe, an organism that prefers to live anaerobically but can adapt to aerobic conditions.

Facultative anaerobe, an organism that prefers to live aerobically but can adapt to anaerobic conditions.

Fahrenheit, temperature scale in which 32°F is the freezing point of water and 212°F is the boiling point.

False motility, moving involuntarily; i.e., Brownian movement. See **Brownian movement.**

Fastidious (organism), an organism that is difficult to cultivate and isolate on ordinary, synthetic, basal culture media. Requires certain enrichments for optimal growth such as blood or vitamins. See **Enrichments.**

Fermentation, oxidation of sugars and other organic compounds, mediated by enzymes secreted by microorganisms or other cells to degrade the substrates to alcohol and carbon dioxide; an anaerobic process. Incomplete oxidation in which gaseous oxygen is not involved. Fermentation produces a high energy yield.

Fibrin, insoluble protein formed during blood clotting by the union of thrombin and fibrinogen. Fibrin forms the essential portion of the blood clot.

Fibrinogen, least soluble plasma protein; a globulin. Exists in blood and other animal fluids. Fibrinogen is converted to an insoluble polymer, fibrin, forming a clot. Fibrinogen is initiated by the enzyme thrombin formed from the proenzyme prothrombin.

Fibrinolysin, substance produced by certain bacteria (mainly the group A hemolytic streptococci), which can liquefy clotted blood plasma or fibrin clots; it dissolves or destroys fibrin. Also called **streptokinase.**

Fibrinolysis, enzymatic destruction of fibrin in clotted blood resulting in dissolution of clot.

Filamentous, characterized by long threadlike structures.

Filiform, describes growth on a streak or stab culture where growth is uniform along the lines of inoculation.

Filter (Millipore), see **Membrane filter.**

Filtrate, a liquid that has passed through a filter.

Filtration, process of separating suspended particles from a liquid by means of a porous medium.

Fishtail (slant inoculum), method of inoculating tube agar slant medium. Place inoculum on slant, near slant curvature (bottom), and zig-zag up the slant. Maximum growth obtained by good use of constituents in the medium.

Flagellum (pl., **flagella**), fine, flexible, hairlike extension on certain bacteria that is the organ of locomotion (motility). May be attached to one or both ends of an organism or occur completely around it. Originates inside the cell but extends outside.

Flavin adenine dinucleotide (FAD), isoalloxazine adenine dinucleotide consisting of a riboflavin (vitamin B_2) unit and an adenosine diphosphate (ADP) unit. Compound takes part in enzymatic oxidation-reduction systems and is important in the metabolism of those organisms lacking the cytochrome system. A coenzyme.

Flavin mononucleotide (FMN), riboflavin phosphate. A three-ring system; isoalloxazine attached to the corresponding alcohol of ribose (ribitol) which in turn is phosphorylated. A coenzyme.

Flavoproteins, respiratory enzymes containing either FMN or FAD as coenzymes. See **Flavin adenine dinucleotide (FAD)** and **Flavin mononucleotide (FMN).**

Flocculation, coagulation of a finely divided precipitate.

Flocculent, clumping together of small adherent masses of bacteria in a liquid.

Fluorene, one of three classes of xanthene dyes; amino xanthenes. See **Xanthene.**

Fluorescence, emission of light (not reflected) by a substance under illumination; transmitted light.

Fluorescent, having one color by transmitted light and another by reflected light.

Fluorescein pigment, also called *fluorescein*. A fluorescent pigment that lends color (phthalein) to a living organism; a water-soluble, freely diffusible greenish yellow, fluorescent color. Produced by certain bacteria.

Formazan, product of reduction of 2,3,5-triphenyltetrazolium chloride (TTC); a water-soluble, deeply colored pigment (red).

Formula (pl., **formulae** or **formulas**), an expression of the constituents of a compound by symbols.

Fortified, strengthened; enriched.

Fragility, susceptibility, or lack of resistance, to factors able to cause disruption; e.g., against semipermeable membrane, cell fragility.

Fragment, small detached portion.

Free coagulase, tube coagulase test determination.

Functional group, a group that characterizes a molecule; its physical and chemical properties. A combination of functional groups may give the characterization.

Furanose, sugar having a furan ring as γ-glucose.

Fusiform, spindle-shaped, as in the anaerobe *Fusobacterium nucleatum.*

Galactosidase, enzyme that catalyzes the splitting of galactosides.

Galactoside, a glycoside, β-galactoside-lactose, containing the carbohydrate galactose; glucoside of galactose.

Gas chromatography, form of chromatography in which the moving phase is a mixture of gases or vapors that are separated on the basis of their different adsorption on a stationary phase (solid). See **Chromatography.**

Gas-liquid chromatography (GLC), same as gas chromatography but the stationary phase is liquid rather than solid. See **Chromatography** and **Gas chromatography.**

Gas ratio, expressing the amount of one substance or entity in relation to that of another. Gas ratio refers to carbon dioxide (CO_2) and hydrogen (H_2) gases.

Gel, a semisolid colloid.

Gelatin, an incomplete protein that lacks tryptophan and is soluble in boiling water and sets to a gel upon cooling. Used in media to determine the proteolytic activity of microorganisms and also for the preparation of peptone.

Gelatinase, extracellular (exo-) enzyme that liquefies gelatin.

Gene, functional unit of heredity. Each gene occupies a specific place, or locus, on a chromosome, can be reproduced exactly at each cell division, and may direct the synthesis of an enzyme or other protein.

Gene coding, information residing on plasmids (episomes) or the bacterial chromosome that determines such characteristics as antibiotic resistance.

Gene mutation, a change in genetic makeup that may be passed on to an offspring.

Genetic relatedness, sequences of homologous base sequences.

Genus (pl., **genera**), classification containing one or more species. Ranked below a tribe or family. A group of closely related species with many similar characteristics but some differences. The genus name is always capitalized and italicized (or underlined); e.g., *Escherichia* or Escherichia.

Geometric isomers, compounds that differ in their configuration because they lack free rotation; most commonly those involving double bonds.

Globular protein, protein composed of coiled polypeptide chains (chains of amino acid residues) held together by cross-linked groups by relatively weak bonds. They occur in cells, are soluble in aqueous solutions, and are easily attacked by enzymes because of their weak bonds.

Globulin, a simple protein but one of the most important proteins of blood plasma; antibodies produced by the body are globulins. They are insoluble in water but soluble in strong acids, alkalis, and neutral salt solutions.

γ-Globulin, fraction of blood serum protein. Contains the greatest concentration of specific antibodies.

Glucan, polyglucose; e.g., starch, cellulose, starch amylose, and glycogen amylose.

Glucose cystine blood agar, medium for *Francisella tularensis* isolation.

Glucose (dextrose), $C_6H_{12}O_6$; a monosaccharide, hexose sugar. End product of hydrolysis of many polysaccharides. Many microorganisms use glucose as an energy source.

Glycine (glycerol), glycerin, $C_3H_5(OH)_3$; a trihydric (polyhydric) alcohol.

Glycocholic acid, cholylglycine, cholic acid conjugated with glycine. $C_{26}H_{43}NO_6$. Sodium salt occurs in bile where it is formed by the combination of glycine and cholic acid.

Glycolipid, complex lipid containing sphingosine, a fatty acid, and a sugar, but no phosphoric acid.

Glycolysis, anaerobic pathway for carbohydrate metabolism in which glucose is broken down to pyruvic acid or lactic acid and ethanol. Also called Embden-Meyerhof-Parnas (EMB) pathway.

Glycolytic cycle, see **Glycolysis** or **Embden-Meyerhof-Parnas (EMP) pathway.**

Glycoside, compound containing a carbohydrate molecule and a noncarbohydrate substance that on hydrolysis yields the two separate compounds; e.g., fructosides yield fructose, galactoside yields galactose.

Glycosidic link, linkages that form polysaccharides from monosaccharide units.

Gram morphology, microscopic smear determining the color, shape, and arrangement of bacteria. Color is determined by Gram reaction; Gram positive (purple-blue) or Gram negative (red). Shapes: cocci, bacilli, coccobacilli, and spirilla. Arrangements: single cells, pairs, chains, clusters, etc.

Gram-negative bacteria, bacteria that lose the primary stain of the Gram stain procedure (crystal violet), are decolorized by alcohol, and take the color of the counterstain (safranin), resulting in a reddish pink color.

Gram-positive bacteria, bacteria that take up the primary stain of the Gram stain procedure (crystal violet), resist decolorization by alcohol, are not colored by the counterstain (safranin), and retain their initial purple-blue color.

Gram stain, differential stain incorporating two dyes of contrasting colors; devised in 1847 by Christian Gram, whence its name. Bacteria are classified as Gram positive or Gram negative, depending upon whether they retain or lose the primary stain (crystal violet) when subjected to a decolorizing agent. See **Gram-positive bacteria** and **Gram-negative bacteria.**

Gram-variable bacteria, bacteria that retain the Gram stain at times, usually when immature, but do not retain it at other times, usually in older cultures.

Granular, composed of or resembling granules; seen in many bacterial species.

Group D streptococci, those members of the genus *Streptococcus* that possess the Lancefield group D antigen, a C-specific polysaccharide contained in the cell wall.

Growth curve, graphic representation of the growth (population changes) of bacteria in phases in a culture medium: lag phase, log phase, stationary phase, and the decline or death phase. See **Lag phase** and **Log phase** for more detail.

Halophile, bacteria whose growth is accelerated by or dependent on a high salt concentration. See **Halophilic.**

Halophilic, being able to tolerate a high salt concentration; usually up to 10%.

Hanging drop technique, microscopic observation of microorganisms suspended in a drop of fluid to determine presence or absence of motility.

Haptene, specific protein-free substance that can combine with antibody in vitro but cannot stimulate antibody formation on injection. When combined with a protein carrier it acts as determinant of antigenic specificity.

Heat labile, destroyed by heat.

Heat stable, not destroyed by heat.

Helix, coiled or curved structure; e.g., DNA, Watson, and Crick helix.

Hematin; see **Heme.**

Heme, nonprotein, insoluble, iron protoporphyrin, $C_{34}H_{33}O_4N_4FeOH$, constituent of hemoglobin and various other cell respiratory pigments. Constitutes the pigment portion of the protein-free part of the hemoglobin molecule. Formerly called *hematin.*

Heme protein, a chromoprotein, pigmented because of the nonprotein prosthetic group heme-iron-proporphyrin.

Hemin, hematin, chloride of heme in which Fe^+ becomes Fe^{3+}; hematin is the hydroxide; factor X for *Haemophilus* spp.

Hemoglobin (Hg), colored compound within a red blood cell that carries oxygen. It is structurally related to chlorophyll; respiratory pigment of blood.

Hemolysin (bacterial), soluble substance elaborated by bacteria that dissolves or breaks up red blood cells with consequent liberation of hemoglobin. This phenomenon is usually exhibited by the pathogenic bacteria.

Hemolysis (α, β, and γ), presence of a zone of hemolyzed red blood cells around a colony grown on a blood agar plate. Three types of hemolysis occur. In α (alpha)-hemolysis, colonies are surrounded by a zone of incomplete (greenish) hemolysis. With β (beta) hemolysis, the colonies are surrounded by a zone of complete hemolysis (clear, transparent). Lack of hemolysis is termed γ (gamma) hemolysis.

Heparin, mucopolysaccharide acid anticoagulant. Interferes with formation of intrinsic thromboplastin and the action of thrombin; prevents the conversion of fibrinogen to fibrin, which is catalyzed by thrombin.

Heterocyclic compound, cyclic compound whose ring system contains elements other than carbon.

Heterogeneous, consisting of more than one phase and therefore not uniform; e.g., colloids; compare with **Homogeneous.**

Heterolactic fermenter, organism that ferments glucose to such compounds as acetic acid and carbon dioxide as well as lactic acid.

Heterotrophic bacteria, bacteria that depend upon organic substrates for their nutritional requirements, are unable to use carbon dioxide as the sole source of carbon, and must obtain this element from organic compounds. Most medically important bacteria fall into this classification.

Hexose, a simple sugar; a monosaccharide containing six carbon atoms.

Hippuric acid, *N*-benzoyl glycine, benzoylaminoacetic acid; benzyl derivative of glycine; an aromatic ring compound, benzoyl (C_6H_5 CO-) conjugated with amino acid glycine (NH_2CH_2COOH).

Homogeneous, composed of only parts of the same kind; having a similar structure because of descent from a common ancestor. Consisting of similar parts or elements. Compare with **Heterogeneous.**

Homolactic fermenter, organism that produces lactic acid almost quantitatively from sugar.

Homologous, the same with respect to type and species, chemically of the same type but differing by a fixed increment in certain constituents. Biologically corresponding in type of structure and in origin but not necessarily in function.

Homopolymer, polymer of a single type of residue.

Homopolysaccharide, homopolymer; saccharide polymer yielding a single substance on hydrolysis.

Hue, property of color.

Hybrid, offspring of plants and animals (bacteria) of parents who are genetically dissimilar.

Hybridization, denaturation of double-stranded (ds) DNA into single strands (ssDNA) detected with a labeled, complementary ssDNA probe. Used to demonstrate relatedness of the DNA of different organisms.

Hydrase, enzyme that adds or removes water from its substrate without causing hydrolysis.

Hydrate, a compound containing water of crystallization.

Hydrazine, a gaseous diamine; $H_2N \cdot NH_2$.

Hydrazone, a compound formed from a carbohydrate by the action of phenylhydrazine.

Hydrocarbon, any compound that contains only hydrogen and carbon.

Hydrogen, a gas; the lightest substance known. The hydrogen atom consists of just one proton and one electron.

Hydrogen acceptor, a substance that is reduced in the anaerobic oxidation-reduction process.

Hydrogenation, a chemical reaction in which hydrogen is added to a compound.

Hydrogen ion concentration, number of hydrogen ions per unit volume of a solution; is used to indicate the acidity or alkalinity of a solution and is expressed as pH. Usually designated by the symbol [H^+]. pH is the logarithm of the reciprocal of the hydrogen ion concentration, pH = log 1/[H^+].

Hydrogen peroxide; H_2O_2; strong oxidizing agent.

Hydrogen sulfide (H_2S), a gas produced by acid hydrolysis of many sulfides.

Hydrolases, enzymes that catalyze hydrolysis reactions and act on ester bonds, glycosyl compounds, and carboxylic esters. The major subdivisions of these enzymes are carbohydrases, esterases, amidases, and proteases.

Hydrolytic, referring to or causing hydrolysis.

Hydrolysis, chemical reaction in which water is added to a molecule causing subsequent splitting of the molecule and the combination of one product with the hydroxyl group and the other with the hydrogen atom.

Hydrophobic, repelling water; alkyl side chains in amino acids are hydrophobic and tend to leave the water phase and congregate in another phase.

Hydroquinone, alkaloid; organic compound characterized by content of nitrogen and the property of combining with acids to form salts. A basic substance derived from plants; a complex alkaloid containing ring systems.

Hydroxyl ion, −OH radical.

Hygroscopic, having the property of absorbing or becoming coated with moisture; changing form with changes of moisture content.

Hypothesis, theory that has not been proved by experiment. Compare with **Theory.**

Imide, suggested synonym for polypeptide; compound containing =NH group or a secondary amine, R_2NH_2, where R is an acyl radical or compound from acid anhydrides in which oxygen is replaced by NH; thus, OC:NH, carbimide.

Immiscible liquids, liquids that will not mix.

Immunofluorescence, microscopic method of determining the presence or location of an antigen (or antibody) by demonstrating fluorescence under ultra-violet light when preparation is exposed to a fluorescein-tagged antibody (or antigen).

Immunogen, antigen.

Impregnated, saturated.

IMViC test, series of tests used primarily to differentiate between *Escherichia coli* and the *Klebsiella-Enterobacter* groups. I, indole; M, methyl red; V, Voges-Proskauer; C, citrate; i for euphony.

Inactivate, destroy activity.

Incubation, holding bacterial cultures under conditions favorable to their growth (especially temperature). Incubation period is the time interval between inoculation and visible growth of bacteria on artificial media.

Indican, indoxyl-β-D-glucose; from plants. A source of indigo.

Indicator, something that renders visible the completion of a reaction; a compound that changes color with changes in the hydrogen ion concentration (pH) of a solution or medium.

Indigo (synonym, **indigo blue**), indigotin, adjectivally, a deep violet blue colored dyestuff.

Indigotin, see indigo.

Indirubin (indigo red), 2,3′-biindoline-2,3-dione; isomer of indigo; Also see **Urorosein.**

Indole, a benzopyrrole, C_6H_4NH CH:CH, produced by the decomposition of tryptophan and other related compounds by certain microorganisms.

Indophenol oxidase, an indophenolase; an oxidizing enzyme in cytochrome oxidase.

Indoxyl, product of putrefactive decomposition of tryptophan in intestines of humans through bacterial action; a heterocyclic 5-member ring fused to a benzene ring.

Induced enzyme, see **Adaptive enzyme.**

Induce, to bring on; to produce.

Inert, having no action.

Inherent, existing in someone or something as a natural and inseparable quality; see **Intrinsic.**

Inhibition, diminution or arrest of function, as prevention of growth or multiplication. Growth is inhibited by addition of chemicals such as dyes and antibiotics to culture media; see **Bacteriostatic.**

Inhibitor, substance that arrests a chemical reaction.

Inoculating loop, generally a platinum or Nichrome wire with one end fixed in a metal or glass handle and the other curved into a loop. Used to transfer drops of liquid; the amount of material transferred is termed a "loopful."

Inoculating needle, a piece of platinum or chrome alloy (Nichrome) wire approximately 3–4 inches long, fused into a glass or metal handle. Used to streak bacterial media or pick colonies for transfer.

Inoculation, introduction of an organism or inoculum into a body or animal or into/onto culture medium.

Inoculum (pl., **inocula**), material containing the microorganism to be introduced into or transferred to a medium.

Inorganic compound, a compound containing no carbon.

Insoluble, not susceptible to being dissolved.

In situ, in position.

Intersect, to divide into two parts.

Intracellular, within a cell.

Intracellular enzyme, an enzyme that catalyzes reactions within the living cell. Also called endoenzyme.

Intrinsic, innate; contained or being within; same as inherent.

Inverted, turned upside down; e.g., when referring to placement of Durham insert tube into a carbohydrate broth to trap gas produced (CO_2 and H_2) when an organism ferments a particular carbohydrate.

In vitro, outside living cells; in an artificial environment.

In vivo, within living plants, tissues, and animals, including man.

Involution forms, abnormally shaped bacterial cells occurring in an aging (old) culture.

Ion, an electrically charged atom, radical, molecule, or particle in which the charge is due to the loss or gain of one or more electrons. See **Anion** and **Cation.**

Ionize, to separate into ions; to dissociate atoms or molecules into electrically charged atoms or radicals.

Ionization, the process of being ionized.

Irreversible reaction, a reaction that cannot be reversed; a permanent one-way reaction to completion.

Isoelectric point (pK), the pH at which a substance (protein, etc.) is neutral; at a lower or higher pH it acts as an acid or a base, respectively.

Isolation, the method of obtaining bacteria in pure culture by subculturing discrete colonies, using various types of media.

Isomerization, conversion of a substrate to an isomeric form such as the conversion of an L molecule or D form to a mixture of equal amounts of both forms. See **Racemic mixture.**

Isomers, compounds that have the same molecular formula but different structural formulas; different arrangements of atoms. The structural difference may be either physical or chemical.

Isoniazide (INH), isonicotinic acid hydrazide used in the treatment of tuberculosis.

Isotonic solution, a solution in the external environment with the same osmotic pressure as the solution in a cell.

Isotopes, atoms with the same atomic number but different atomic weights; chemical properties are identical.

Keto acid, an organic acid containing a ketone carbonyl group (C=O); e.g., pyruvic acid.

Ketone, a hydrocarbon derivative; organic compound containing the carbonyl (C=O) group attached to two organic radicals. General formula:

$$R-\overset{\overset{O}{\|}}{C}-R'$$

Ketose, a simple sugar that is a polyhydric ketone.

Kinetic, pertaining to motion; dealing with forces that influence the motion of bodies.

Krebs' cycle, enzyme system that converts pyruvic acid to carbon dioxide with concomitant release of energy captured in ATP molecules; an aerobic process. Also referred to as **citric acid cycle** or the **tricarboxylic acid (TCA) cycle.**

l- (levorotatory), monosaccharides and disaccharides are optically active, i.e., they rotate the plane of polarized light. Those that rotate it to the left are said to be levorotatory.

Labeling, rendering a substance identifiable by means of radioactive isotopes; e.g., ^{14}C.

Lactalbumin, milk albumin; a water-soluble protein.

Lactoglobulin, globulin occurring in milk.

Lactose, milk sugar; $C_{12}H_{24}O_{12}$. A disaccharide used by certain organisms; on hydrolysis lactose is split into glucose and galactose.

Lag phase, second phase of the growth curve after bacterial inoculation; phase in which the rate of multiplication increases with time. No marked increase in numbers of bacteria but a considerable increase in cell size.

Latent, delayed; seemingly inactive.

Lead acetate, $Pb(C_2H_3O_2)_2 \cdot 3\ H_2O$ (PbAc), salt of the metal; indicator of H_2S production.

Lecithin, group of phospholipids; esters of oleic, stearic, palmitic, or other fatty acids with glycerophosphoric acid and choline.

Leuko base, white or colorless base; a reduced compound. Oxidized form of the dye methylene blue.

Leukocyte, a white blood cell (WBC); nucleated cell of the blood that has phagocytic activity.

Levulose (fructose), a monosaccharide; a constituent of the disaccharide sucrose or the polysaccharide inulin.

Ligand, organic molecule attached to a central metal ion by multiple coordination bonds; e.g., porphyrin portion of heme.

Ligase chain reaction (LCR), probe amplification technique.

Linear, pertaining to or resembling a line.

Lipase, enzyme belonging to the esterase group of hydrolases that split fats to fatty acids and glycerol.

Lipid, group of naturally occurring substances of the higher fatty acids; fat, oil, wax, or a derivative of these substances.

Liquefaction, transformation of a gel to a liquid by enzymatic action of certain bacteria.

Locus (pl., **loci**), a place, site.

Log phase, also called logarithmic phase. Period in the growth curve when the most rapid multiplication of bacteria occurs. The generation time (time required for doubling) may be short, about 20 min for *Escherichia coli* or long, about 60–80 min for *Lactobacillus acidophilus.*

Logarithm (space), power to which a fixed number, called the base (usually 10 or $\bar{e}$ (2.7182818)), must be raised to produce a given number.

Logarithmic (ratio, scale), marking the vertical axis of a chart in logarithms of natural numbers; the chart is known as a *semilog plot* and the vertical scale is called a *log scale.*

Lyophilized, lyophilization (biologic), prepared biologic substance in dried form by rapid freezing and dehydration in the frozen state under high vacuum. Made ready for use usually by addition of sterile distilled water. See **Reconstitute** and **Diluent.**

Lyse, dissolve.

Lysin, antibody or substance that dissolves cells and is specific in its action.

Lysis, destruction of a cell by a lysin; decomposition of a substance or a system.

Lysosome, vacuole; cytoplasmic

membrane–bound particle containing hydrolyzing enzymes.

Lysostaphin, mixture of peptidases and lysozyme.

Lysozyme, muramidase, mucopeptide, glycohydrolase enzyme that hydrolyzes 1,4-β links between N-acetylmuramic acid and N-acetylglucosamine. Destroys cell walls of certain bacteria.

m- (prefix), abbreviation; see **meta**.

Macromolecule, any molecule composed of several monomers, notably proteins, nucleic acids, polysaccharides, glycoproteins, and glycolipids.

Maltose, malt sugar; disaccharide formed by hydrolysis of starch; composed of two glucose residues.

Mammalia, class of vertebrates with milk-secreting organs (e.g., breast, udder) to nourish their young.

Mechanism, means by which an effect is obtained.

Mediate, to bring about or effect.

Medium (pl., **media**), mixture of nutrient substances in a solid, semisolid, or liquid form that meets requirements for bacterial growth and multiplication.

Melting point, temperature at which solid and liquid states of a substance are in equilibrium.

Membrane filter, a nitrocellulose disk with uniform porosity in the range of 0.03–3.0 μm used for microbiologic filtration.

Mercaptan, see **Thiol**.

Meso- (compound), diastereoisomer that contains at least two or more asymmetric carbons and which can be divided into two halves with mirror-image configuration. See **Diastereoisomer**. Mesomer is an optically inactive isomer with no effect on polarized light.

Mesophilic bacteria, bacteria who grow best at a moderate temperature of about 25–40°C. Most pathogenic bacteria have an optimal temperature range of 32–35°C.

meta- (m-), prefix indicating the 1 and 3 positions of the benzene ring.

Metabolic, pertaining to or concerning metabolism.

Metabolite antagonist, see **Analog**.

Metabolism, the sum total of all chemical changes that take place within a cell by which nutritional and functional activities are maintained. Processes by which an organism uses food to produce living protoplasm, for storage, to produce energy, and to eliminate waste products.

Metabolite, any chemical (nutrient) participating in metabolism; essential growth factor.

Metabolize, to undergo metabolism.

Metachromasia, condition in which a cell component takes on a color different from the dye solution with which it is stained.

Metachromatic, dyes that exhibit metachromasia. See **Metachromasia**.

Metal, any element marked by luster, malleability, ductility, and conductivity of electricity and heat.

Methylate, add the methyl radical (CH_3) or substitute a methyl group for another atom or radical.

Methylation, substitution of a methyl group (CH_3) for a hydrogen atom.

Microaerophilic organism, organism that grows and reproduces best under reduced oxygen tension, with a small amount of atmospheric oxygen or air.

Microbiology, science of unicellular organisms including bacteria, yeasts, molds, and viruses.

Microtechnique, handling minute objects for microscopically study; test method using smaller amounts of substrates and reagents but obtaining the same end result as routine procedures.

Migrate, to move from one area to another.

Millipore filter, see **Membrane filter**.

Mineral oil, oil derived from inorganic matter, especially petroleum and its products.

Minuscule, very small.

Mirror image, having a plane of symmetry that divides a molecule into halves; something that exhibits reverse symmetry across a plane.

Miscible, capable of being mixed or dissolved in all proportions and remaining so after mixing process ceases.

Mixed culture, growth of two or more organisms in the same medium.

Mixture, an aggregate of two or more substances that are not chemically combined and exist in no fixed proportion to each other.

Modification, change or variation.

Moiety, one of two or more parts into which something is divided.

Molecule, a chemical combination of two or more atoms that form a specific chemical substance.

Monochromatic, having one color; represented by only one wavelength.

Monomer, molecular unit that is repeated to form a large structure, or polymer. See **Polymer**.

Monosaccharide, simple sugar, $C_6H_{12}O_6$, that cannot be decomposed by hydrolysis; e.g., glucose and fructose.

Monovalent, having a valence or potency of one and capable of binding one complement only; an amboceptor.

Morphology, the study of form and structure of living organisms, principally size, shape, and arrangement of an organism. Frequently, morphology is related to biochemical reactions. See **Colony morphology** and **Gram morphology**.

Motility (false), see **False motility** and **Brownian movement**.

Mucoid, resembling the gummy, watery liquid that covers mucous membranes.

Mureins, peptidoglycans composing the sacculus, or cell casing, of bacteria. Also see **Sacculus**.

Mutant, an organism or microorganism with a changed or new gene.

NaCl, see **Saline**.

Native, natural; inborn, not inherited; not acquired.

Neonate (al), newborn in first 4 weeks after birth.

Nephelometer, instrument similar to a visual colorimeter, which uses the Tyndall phenomenon to measure the concentration density of substances in suspension.

Nephelometry, quantitative analysis by determining the amount of light scattered from a fog or suspension.

Nessler's test, delicate test for detecting ammonia (NH_3), aldehydes, and hexamethylene-amines; brown precipitates with NH_3; used for colorimetric determinations.

Neutral fat, a triester of one or more of the long-chain fatty acids and glycerol.

Neutral pH, neither acid nor basic; pH 7.0. The hydrogen ion concentration and hydroxyl ion concentration are equal.

Neutrality, state of being neutral.

Neutralization, reaction between an acid and a base to form a salt and water; the process of making a solution neutral (pH 7.0).

Niacin, official designation for nicotinic acid in its role as a vitamin.

Nichrome, trade name for a high–melting point alloy (Ni and Cr) used as a platinum substitute.

Nicotinamide adenine dinucleotide (NAD), formerly diphosphopyridine nucleotide (DPN); reduced form, NADH. A pyridine nucleotide containing nicotinic acid amide moiety derived from the vitamin niacin.

Nicotinamide adenine dinucleotide phosphate (NADP), formerly triphosphopyridine nucleotide (TPN); reduced form, NADPH.

Ninhydrin, ninidrine, trade name for triketohydrindene hydrate; reagent used for determination of amino acids and related substances.

Ninidrine, see **Ninhydrin**.

Nitrate, any salt of nitric acid or any compound containing the monovalent radical $-NO_3$.

Nitrification, oxidation of nitrogen in ammonia to nitrous and nitric acid or their salts.

Nitrifying, causing the oxidation of ammonia or atmospheric nitrogen to nitrates and nitrites; e.g., by nitrifying bacteria and nitrifying catalysts.

Nitrite, any salt of nitrous acid or any compound containing the monovalent radical $-NO_2$.

Nitrogenous, relating to or containing nitrogen.

Nomenclature, system of naming plants, animals, and organs; binomial nomenclature. See **Binomial**.

Nonchromogenic, lacking chromogens or coloring matter; producing no color.

Noncompetitive inhibitor, substance that combines with a different grouping of the enzyme molecule than does the substrate, or a substance that interferes with the breakdown of the substrate-enzyme complex.

Nonviable, dead.

Nuclease, enzyme that hydrolyzes nucleic acid or its hydrolysis products; e.g., polynucleotidase, nucleotidase, and nucleosidase. Also see **Endonuclease** and **Exonuclease**.

Nucleic acids, molecules composed of joined nucleotide complexes, involved in both synthesis of proteins and the genetic mechanisms of all cells. Organic compounds (polynucleotides) that when hydrolyzed yield nitrogenous heterocyclic bases such as purines, pyrimidines, phosphoric acid, and the carbohydrates d-ribose or D-2-deoxyribose. The principal types are deoxyribonucleic acid (DNA) and ribonucleic acid (RNA).

Nucleic acid probe, a segment of single-stranded nucleic acid that can hybridize specifically with its complementary strand via base pairing to detect DNA or RNA.

Nucleoprotein, a conjugated protein containing nucleic acids.

Nucleoside, a purine or pyrimidine base linked to ribose or deoxyribose.

Nucleotide, a phosphoriboside or phosphodeoxyribose usually obtained by hydrolysis of nucleic acids. A compound formed from one molecule of a sugar (pentose), phosphoric acid, and a purine or pyrimidine base.

Nutrient, a material or substance that can be used as a food source.

Obligate (strict), term used to describe a metabolism restricted to a single type, as in obligate anaerobe; strict or absolutely required.

Oligosaccharide, carbohydrate that yields a small number of monosaccharides on hydrolysis; e.g., disaccharides.

Opalescent, having a milky turbidity.

Opaque, impervious to light.

Optical density (O.D.), amount of light absorbed in colorimetry and photometry.

Optical isomers, stereoisomers that differ in their effect on plane polarized light, primarily those containing one or more asymmetric carbon atoms; may be either enantiomorphs or diastereoisomers. Enantiomorphs are two optical isomers in which all corresponding asymmetric atoms have mirror-image configuration. All other nonenantimorphs (or isomers) are called diastereoisomers. See **Diastereoisomer**.

Optimal temperature, temperature most favorable to growth and reproduction of a bacterial culture

Organelle (organoid), one of the specialized parts of a protozoan or tissue cell that performs some individual function. Subcellular units.

Organic acid, hydrocarbon derivative in which one or more hydrogen atoms are replaced by a carboxyl group (C=O). General formula:

$$R-COOH(\overset{O}{\overset{\|}{C}}-OH)$$

Organic compound, compound containing carbon, as distinguished from a noncarbon (inorganic) compound.

Organic salt, compound formed from acid in which the hydrogen atom of the carboxyl group has been replaced by a metal or ammonium radical, a solid.

Organism, living biologic specimen.

ortho- (o-), prefix indicating two constituents in adjacent positions on a benzene ring.

Orthochromatic, staining the same color as dye used.

Oxalate, lithium, potassium, sodium, or ammonium oxalate; an anticoagulant. Forms un-ionized calcium oxalate complex that reduces the concentration of ionized calcium below that required for coagulation.

Oxgall, BBL trade name; bile from gallbladder of oxen.

Oxidase, enzyme belonging to the group desmolases that transfers hydrogen directly from its substrate to oxygen.

Oxidation, chemical reaction in which electrons are removed from one or more atoms of a substance; combination of a substance with oxygen; an increase in valence (removal of hydrogen is dehydrogenation). In the same reaction another substance(s) gains the electrons and is reduced.

Oxidized substrate, the hydrogen donor.

Oxidizing agent, a substance that brings about oxidation of another substance and is reduced in the process; hydrogen acceptor.

Ozone, O_3 gas; oxidizing agent.

p- (prefix), abbreviation, see ***para-***.

Pancreatic digest, pancreatic secretions containing digestive enzymes: pancreatin, trypsin, amylopsin, steapsin, rennin, and invertin.

Papase, trade name for protective enzyme from *Carica papaya*: see **Papain**.

Papain, Papase, trade name; vegetable pepsin from fruit of papaya; an active proteolytic enzyme.

para- (p-), prefix indicating two constituents linked to opposite carbon atoms in the benzene ring.

Paraffin, alkane; saturated aliphatic hydrocarbon; see **Petrolatum**.

Pasteurization, process in which liquids or other materials (e.g., milk) are heated to a temperature high enough to kill pathogenic organisms if maintained for a sufficient length of time. Pasteurization of milk: 161°F (71°C) for 15 sec; not less than 143°F (61.6°C) for not less than 30 min; then immediately cooled to 50°F (10°C) or below.

Pathogenic (pathogen), term describing the ability to cause disease; (disease-producing bacteria).

Pathogenicity, disease-producing potential, depends upon the degree of virulence.

Pellicle (scum), continuous or interrupted film (scum) at the surface growth of bacteria in a liquid medium, characteristic of certain bacteria.

Penicillinase, β-lactamase I; enzyme produced by some bacterial species that inactivates certain penicillins (e.g., penicillin G).

Pentose, simple sugar; a monosaccharide with five carbon atoms in its molecule, e.g., ribose.

Pentose shunt (Warburg-Dickens pathway), alternative carbohydrate metabolism pathway used to ferment hexoses, pentoses, and several other carbohydrates in a number of organisms. It departs from the Embden-Meyerhof-Parnas pathway at the oxidation of glucose 6-phosphate to 6-phos-phogluconate, which in turn is converted to pentose phosphates.

Pepsin, digestive enzyme found in gastric juice; acts on proteins.

Peptidase, enzyme that hydrolyzes peptides to simple peptides and amino acids; liberates individual amino acids from a peptide.

Peptide (polypeptide), compound consisting of two or more amino acids. See **Polypeptide**.

Peptide bond, synonymous with **Peptide linkage,**

$$-\overset{\overset{O}{\|}}{C}-\overset{\overset{H}{|}}{N}-$$

the linkage that joins the amino acids in the protein molecule; union through carboxyl and amino group.

$$H_2N-CH_2-COOH + H-\overset{\overset{H}{|}}{N}-CH_2-COOH$$
peptide link (bond)

Peptidoglycan, glycans that have short polypeptides attached.

Peptization, change from a jelly to a liquid other than by melting.

Peptolysis, hydrolysis of peptone to amino acids.

Peptone, partially hydrolyzed protein used in culture media; soluble in water and not coagulated by heat.

Peptonization, digestion of casein in milk by proteolytic enzymes; solubilization of milk casein.

Perhydrol, see **Superoxal**.

Peritoneum, serous membrane that lines the abdominal walls and viscera.

Permeability, perviousness; ability to pass through or penetrate a substance or membrane.

Permease, specific protein in some bacterial cell membranes that facilitates passage of sugars across membrane in the direction of the concentration gradient; part of the active transport system.

Peroxidase, enzyme that catalyzes the transfer of oxygen from hydrogen peroxide or an organic peroxide to a suitable substrate, thus oxidizing the substrate.

Petri dish, circular, shallow (glass or plastic) dish used for culturing bacteria. It has a cover that fits over the top and sides. Developed by R. J. Petri, a student of Koch.

Petrolatum, Petroleum jelly, Vaseline, paraffin ointment, yellow petrolatum; purified mixture of semisolid hydrocarbons from petroleum; soluble in alcohol or chloroform; used as a lubricant, cleanser, and ointment base.

pH, symbol indicating the acidity or alkalinity of a solution; the negative log of the hydrogen ion concentration, pH = log 1/[H$^+$], the logarithm of the reciprocal of the hydrogen ion concentration. In solutions, a pH of 7.0 is the neutral point at which the concentration of hydrogen ions and hydroxyl ions are equal. When the hydrogen ion concentration exceeds the hydroxylion concentration, an acid condition exists with low pH values ranging down to 1.0 or below. Solutions in which the hydroxyl ion concentration exceeds the hydrogen ion concentration are alkaline, with pH values ranging up to 13 or 14.

Phagocyte, cell that ingests bacteria, foreign particles, or other cells.

Phagocytic action, phagocytosis; process in which particles, especially bacteria, are engulfed by certain cells, usually leukocytes (WBCs).

Phase, a stage of growth or decline of a bacterial population; solid, liquid or gaseous homogeneous substance that exists as a distinct and mechanically separate portion of a heterogeneous system.

Plasmids, episomes, extrachromosomal DNA particles; circular pieces of DNA that act independently of chromosomes.

Phenol, carbolic acid; C_6H_5OH. A general disinfectant; 5% component of antiseptics.

Phenolphthalein, compound obtained by action of phenol on phthalic acid; an anhydride; used as a hydrogen ion indicator.

Phenomenon (pl., **phenomena**), a symptom or occurrence of any sort, whether ordinary or extraordinary, in relation to a disease.

Phenotype, sum total of expressed characteristics, both external and internal (size, color, form, etc.)

Phenyl, radical C_6H_5- from benzene or phenol.

Phosphatases, a group of enzymes that catalyze the splitting of esters of phosphoric acid; split phosphate from its organic compound.

Phospholipids, fatlike substances that can be degraded to fatty acids, glycerol, phosphoric acid, and (sometimes) a nitrogenous base.

Phosphoprotein, conjugated protein in which phosphoric acid is esterified to an hydroxyl amino acid, especially serine.

Phosphorylation, esterification of a molecule with phosphoric acid; involves the addition of a phosphate group ($-H_2PO_3$) to a compound.

Photochromogenic, forming pigment consequent to light exposure.

Photometry, measurement of light intensity.

Physiologic saline, see **Saline.**

Pie plate, the bottom of a Petri dish is marked off with a grease pencil into quadrants; each quadrant is then used for a single inoculum, streaked for maximum growth. This procedure enables a single Petri dish of solid medium to be inoculated with four separate pure colonies for further studies, primarily to obtain maximum growth of an inoculum for biochemical or antibiotic sensitivity studies. It cannot be used for initial isolation. A pure culture inoculum must be used with the pie plate method.

Pigment, coloring matter of various secretions; synthesized, intracellular, nonvital product. Pigment may be retained within cell and thus color the mass of bacterial cells or it may be excreted into the medium and color the medium itself.

Plasma, fluid portion of blood, obtained by centrifuging anticoagulated blood; contains clotting factors but no erythrocytes.

Plasmin, active proteolytic enzyme derived from plasminogen; essential in blood clot dissolution (fibrinolysis).

Plasminogen, globulin present in circulating blood and within clots; inactive precursor of plasmin.

Pleomorphic, having various distinct forms or shapes exhibited by a single strain or species.

pOH, negative logarithm (base 10) of the hydroxyl (OH) ion concentration.

Polar, pertaining to a pole.

Polar bond, electrostatic union of two atoms established by the passage of one or more electrons from one to the other.

Polarity, describing a body with two poles, or different properties at terminal points.

Poles, points at opposite ends of an axis; two points with opposite physical properties. The negative pole, or cathode, is an electric terminal charged with electrons; the positive pole, or anode, becomes positively charged by loss of electrons.

Polychromatic, showing more than one color, particularly when viewed under polarized light.

Polyhydric alcohol, an alcohol (or phenol) containing more than one hydroxyl group ($-OH$); the hydroxyl groups must be on different carbons.

Polymer, compound, usually of high molecular weight, formed by combination of simpler molecules.

Polymerase chain reaction (PCR), a target amplification technique; highly sensitive technique by which minute quantities of specific DNA or RNA sequences can be enzymatically amplified to yield enough material to reach the threshold for detection.

Polymerization, linking together many like molecules to form a larger one; a polymer has the same percentage composition as the smaller unit but different properties.

Polyol, polyhydroxy alcohol, specifically, the sugar alcohols and inositols.

Polypeptide, molecule consisting of many joined amino acids. See **Peptide.**

Polysaccharide (polysaccharose), a carbohydrate formed by the combination of many molecules of monosaccharides (more than three); e.g., starch, glycogen, and cellulose.

Polysaccharose, see **Polysaccharide.**

Potentiate, potentiation, increase strength of an activity.

Precipitate, an insoluble solid deposited (settled out) in a solution after a chemical reaction caused by addition of a precipitating reagent.

Precipitation, process of clumping; forming aggregates coming out of solution.

Precursor, substance (compound) that precedes the formation of another substance (compound).

Preservative, substance that inhibits growth of microorganisms without necessarily destroying them; generally a substance that retards, hinders, or masks undesirable changes.

Presumptive diagnosis (I.D.), initial, tentative diagnosis of a disease based upon clinical evidence and often also upon first-step bacterial isolation and test results. Further studies must be conducted for confirmation.

Primary isolation, initial isolation and growth of microorganisms from a clinical specimen.

Principle, theory or assumption; a fundamental concept.

Proenzyme, inactive form of an enzyme.

Properties, characteristics by which a substance is identified; e.g., color, solubility.

Prosthetic group, the nonprotein portion of an enzyme, essential for enzyme activity. Also called **Coenzyme.**

Protease, enzyme that hydrolyzes the peptide links of proteins, releasing simpler proteins and peptides. Proteinases and peptidases are in this group of enzymes.

Proteins, complex organic compounds of high molecular weight that constitute the principal part of protoplasm and are associated with living matter. They are composed of an extremely large number of α-amino acids joined through peptide linkages.

Proteinase, enzyme that hydrolyzes proteins to polypeptides.

Proteolysis, conversion of proteins into soluble peptones by decomposition or hydrolysis.

Proteolytic, denotes something that digests or liquefies proteins or that splits proteins into simpler compounds.

Proteolytic enzyme, enzyme that hydrolyzes proteins to proteoses, peptones, etc. An exocellular enzyme secreted by many bacteria to degrade proteins.

Proteose, secondary protein derivatives that are water soluble and are not coagulated by heat; used as a component in culture media.

Prothrombin, plasma glycoprotein that is converted to thrombin by extrinsic thromboplastin during the second stage of coagulation; also called factor II.

Proton, the positive core or nucleus of the hydrogen atom with a mass of 1. A unit of positive electricity that is equivalent to the electron charge and to the hydrogen ion mass.

Prototroph, naturally occurring, or wild-type, strain that is self-sufficient nutritionally and does not require additional supplements.

Pseudocatalase, type of catalase that lacks a heme prosthetic group and is sensitive to acid pH; a false catalase.

Pteridine, a two-ring heterocyclic compound found as a component of pteroic acid and pteroylglutamic acids (folic acids, pteropterin, etc).

Pulsed-field gel electrophoresis (PFGE), specialized type of RFLP analysis (restriction fragment length polymorphism); a target amplification technique.

Pure culture, a culture containing growth of only one species of bacteria.

Purine, parent substance of some bases in nucleic acids (adenine, guanine).

Purulent, consisting of pus.

Putrefaction, bacterial decomposition of proteins that produces a disagreeable odor.

Putrescine, tetramethylenediamine $(NH_2(CH_2)_4NH_2)$ produced from the amino acid ornithine.

Pyogenic, pus producing.

Pyridine, C_5H_5N, heterocyclic compound.

Pyridoxal phosphate, codecarboxylase; an aldehyde derivative of pyridoxine; a substance with vitamin B_6 activity; coenzyme in amino acid metabolism, mediating transamination, deamination, and decarboxylation. See **Pyridoxine** and **Pyridoxal.**

Pyridoxine, 5-hydroxy-6-methyl-3,4-pyridinedimethanol; a component of the vitamin B_6 complex.

Pyrimidine, heterocyclic substance; parent substance of several bases present in nucleic acids (uracil, thymine, cytosine).

Pyrrole structure, C_4H_5N; azole heterocyclic ring compound. When warmed with acid a red precipitate is formed.

Pyruvic acid, $CH_3COCOOH$; 2-oxopropanoic acid. Occupies a central position in microbial metabolism; a key intermediate in carbohydrate metabolism. See **Embden-Meyerhof-Parnas pathway** and **Krebs' cycle.**

Qualitative test, test to identify the constituents of a compound or mixture.

Quality control, regulation and check of maintenance of a reagent, test procedure, function, action, etc. by use of known positive and negative controls.

Quantitative test, test to measure the amounts of constituents in a compound or a mixture.

Quinoidal compound, quinoid structure containing the chromatophoric group; a paraquinoid: See **Chromophore**.

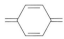

Quinone, color-producing molecular structure found in natural pigments and artificial dyes; the color produced is due to the quinoid structure. Oxidation of phenolic rings containing hydroxyl groups in the *ortho* and *para* positions forms the quinone compound. See **Quinoidal compound**.

Racemic mixture, a mixture of equal amounts of D- and L-isomers. See **Isomers** and **Isomerization**.

Radical, a group of elements or atoms that behaves as a unit in a chemical reaction; usually passing intact from one compound to another; usually incapable of prolonged existence in a free state. In chemical formulas often enclosed in parenthesis or brackets.

Radioassay, chemical analysis using radioactive indicators; e.g., ^{14}C.

Radioisotope, radioactive isotope used as a tracer in scientific research; e.g., ^{14}C.

Radiometer (radiometric), a device used to determine the penetration of x-rays.

Rate, see **Ratio**.

Ratio, rate; proportion; relation of one entity to another in respect to quantity (concentration), etc.

Reactant, original substance entering into a chemical reaction.

Reagent, substance used to produce a chemical reaction.

Reconstitute, restore a substance previously altered for preservation and storage to its original form; e.g., restore dried, stored media to a liquid state, usually involving addition of water, although other diluents may be used, such as alcohol.

Red blood cell (RBC), erythrocyte; a nonnucleated blood cell that contains hemoglobin and carries oxygen as oxyhemoglobin to other cells.

Redox indicators, certain dyes, such as methylene blue or cresol blue, that can replace cytochrome in an in vitro system, acting as hydrogen acceptors. The reduced dye is autooxidizable.

Reduce, subtract an oxygen ion from or add hydrogen to a substance; lose a positive charge or gain a negative charge.

Reducing sugar, mono- or disaccharide (e.g., glucose, fructose) that reduces copper or silver salts in hot, alkaline solution (e.g., Fehling's); indicator of free aldehyde or keto group.

Reductase, enzyme that catalyzes reduction reactions.

Reduction, removal of oxygen or its equivalent from a chemical compound or addition of hydrogen or its equivalent; the lowering of the valence of an element in combination; an interchange of electrons between atoms (the atom gaining the electron or electrons is reduced and the atom losing the electron or electrons is oxidized).

Reductive deamination, hydrolysis of amines and removal of amino group.

Rennet curd, enzymatic coagulation of milk by rennin, referred to as "sweet curd" because it is formed without altering the pH.

Rennin, rennet, an enzyme that converts the soluble casein of milk into insoluble paracasein.

Repeating unit, original structural unit of a polymer, which is repeated to form the polymer. See **Polymer**.

Replicator, device, usually automated or semiautomated, used to duplicate something.

Reproduce, duplicate; produce again; repeat.

Residual, remaining or left over at end of a process.

Residue (residuum), substance(s) remaining after completion of a physical or chemical process.

Resistant, withstanding the action or effect of.

Resonance, property of a substance that has two or more structural forms present simultaneously.

Respectively, singly, in the order designated; e.g., first, second.

Respiration, any chemical reaction in which energy is released for life processes. Energy transformation takes place either aerobically or anaerobically. An oxidation process of living cells in which oxygen is the hydrogen acceptor for hydrogen removed from the substrate.

Respiratory enzyme, enzyme that is part of oxidation-reduction system; concerned with transfer of electrons removed to oxygen.

Reversible reaction, a reaction that establishes an equilibrium; one that can proceed from right to left or from left to right: $A + B \leftrightarrow C + D$; an incomplete reaction.

Ribonucleic acid (RNA), polynucleotide consisting of phosphoric acid, *d*- ribose, heterocyclic nitrogenous bases of the purine and pyridine types (adenine, guanine, cytosine and uracil). It is found primarily in cytoplasm, with small amounts in the nucleus and in chromosomes. RNA controls the rate of protein synthesis by living cells.

Ruminant, any of various hoofed, usually horned, animals that have a stomach with four compartments and that chew a cud; e.g., cattle, goats.

Saccharide, sucrate; any of a series of compounds containing carbon, hydrogen, and oxygen in which the ratio of hydrogen to oxygen is 2:1.

Saccharolytic, capable of chemically splitting sugars.

Sacculus (pl., **sacculi**), a small sac or pouch.

Saline (NaCl), a salt; sodium chloride. Isotonic physiologic saline is 0.85% NaCl; preservative for bacterial specimens.

Salt, a compound consisting of a positive ion other than hydrogen and a negative ion other than hydroxyl; the product of the reaction of an acid with a base; positive ion derived from the base, negative ion from an acid. Salts are electrolytes.

Satellite phenomenon, growth of larger colonies of *Haemophilus* *influenzae* in the region of staphylococci or other bacteria (e.g., *Neisseria* spp.) because they synthesize the V growth factor, which diffuses into the surrounding medium; stimulation of growth of *H. influenzae* in the vicinity of colonies supplying V factor.

Saturated compound, an organic compound in which all valences are satisfied; one that has no double or triple bonds.

Saturated solution, solution in which the solute is in equilibrium with undissolved solute; solution contains all the solute it can hold at a given temperature and pressure.

Scintillation, a flash of light produced in a chemical crystal by absorption of an ionized photon; the minuscule flash of light seen on a fluorescent screen results from the spontaneous emission of charged particles across the sensitized surface.

Scintillation (liquid) counter, scintillator, device used to detect and count radioactive particles.

Scum (broth), see **Pellicle**.

Secrete, to elaborate cell products.

Seitz filter, an asbestos disk filter held into position by means of a special container; used for bacterial filtration, especially of media.

Semipermeable membrane, membrane that allows water and crystalloids to pass but holds back colloids.

Semisolid, soft and slowly flowing.

Sensitive, highly susceptible; susceptible to the action or effect of.

Sepsis, see **Septicemia**.

Septicemia (sepsis), morbid condition caused by pathogenic bacteria and their associated toxins in the blood; systemic disease.

Sequential, forming a sequence, succession, or order; number of things following one another; collectively, a series.

Sequester, remove a metal ion from a system by forming a complex ion that does not have the chemical reactions of the ion removed.

Sequestric acid, see **Ethylenediaminetetraacetate (EDTA)**.

Serotype, taxonomic subdivision of bacteria based on antigenic characteristics.

Serum, clear, amber, alkaline fluid of blood from which cellular elements have been removed by clotting; cell- and fibrinogen-free fluid.

Sheep blood agar (SBA), basal medium plus 5%, sterile, defibrinated, fresh sheep blood. Blood is both an enrichment and an indicator of hemolysis. See **Hemolysis**.

Siderophore, a macrophage containing hemosiderin found in the lung.

Simple sugar, a monosaccharide; e.g., glucose.

Simultaneous, occurring, done, or existing at same time.

Skatole, β-methylindole, $C_8H_6N \cdot CH_3$, a product of some bacterial decomposition of protein.

Slant (medium), medium hardened at an angle in a tube to increase the surface area.

Smear, preparation on a glass slide or cover slip of a thin layer of material for microscopic examination.

Soap, salt of a long-chain fatty acid.

Sodium citrate, an anticoagulant that forms an unionized complex with calcium, thus preventing coagulation.

Sodium dodecyl sulfate–polyacrylamide gel electrophoresis (SDS-PAGE), technique for analysis of soluble whole-cell proteins.

Sodium fluoride, an anticoagulant and preservative. As an anticoagulant, it forms an unionized calcium fluoride complex that prevents coagulation.

Soluble, capable of being dissolved in a fluid; no chemical change takes place; a mechanical process.

Solute; a substance dissolved in a solvent.

Solution, homogeneous mixture of two or more substances that form a single phase.

Solvent, a substance in which a solute is dissolved; a liquid.

Speciate, to identify the species of an organism of known genus.

Species (sing. and pl.), one kind of microorganism; a unit of classification in taxonomy; a subdivision of a genus. The species name is not capitalized, but it is italicized or underlined; e.g., *Escherichia* (genus) *coli* (species); Escherichia coli.

Specific gravity (sp. gr.), ratio of the weight of a given volume of a substance to the weight of an equal volume of water.

Spectrometry, measurement of wavelength of lines or bands in a spectrum and identification of the elements producing them.

Spectrophotometric analysis, determination of structure and/or quantity by light absorption at any wavelength, visible or not.

Spectrum, light separated into its component parts with the aid of a prism or grating.

Sphingomyelin, phospholipid that on hydrolysis yields fatty acid, phosphoric acid, choline, and the amino alcohol sphingosine.

Sphingosine, complex amino alcohol; constituent of cerebrosides.

Spontaneous, voluntary; occurring without external influence.

Spore, reproductive cell of bacteria, fungi, or protozoa; in bacteria, may be inactive, resistant forms within the cell.

Spot test (analysis), drop test; microchemical identification test made on a porcelain plate or impregnated filter paper.

Stab, culture in which organisms are inoculated (with an inoculating needle) into the butt of the medium to allow for possible anaerobic growth. The needle carrying the inoculum is stabbed in a straight line from the top to the bottom of the tube and removed along the same path.

Stabilizing agent, retarding agent or a substance that counteracts the effect of an accelerator; substance that preserves a chemical equilibrium.

Stable, fixed; resistant to change.

Stain, solution of a dye or dyes used to impart color to microorganisms so that they or their constituent parts may be seen and differentiated microscopically.

Standard, an established form of quality or quantity; substance used to establish the strength of volumetric solutions.

Staphylocoagulase, see **Coagulase**.

Staphylokinase (Sf), a proteinase with action similar to that of urokinase and streptokinase. See **Streptokinase** and **Urokinase**.

Staphylothrombin, see **Thrombin**.

Starch, amylum, 1,4-α-glucan; polysaccharide composed of at least two fractions: (a) amylose or α-amylose, a straight chain of 1,4-α-glucopyranose units, and (b) amylopectin or β-amylose. Starch is insoluble in cold water, alcohol, or ether and partly soluble in hot water; hydrolyzed to several forms of dextrins and to glucose.

Stationary phase, stage in growth cycle of a bacterial culture when the cell population equals the dying population.

Streptolysin O (SO), cytolysin; alters erythrocyte membranes and affects permeability of membranes; associated with subcellular organelles.

Stereoisomerism, phenomenon shown by optically active compounds having different spatial arrangement of their atoms; e.g., D-L-. See **Isomerism**.

Stereoisomers, compounds that have the same molecular formula and the same structural formula but differ in their spatial orientation. See **Geometric isomer** and **Optical isomer**.

Sterile, sterility, free from living microorganisms and their products; state of being sterile.

Sterilization, chemical or physical process used to kill all microorganisms, usually by means of heat.

Stock culture, culture of microorganisms kept as reserve for future use, known species maintained in the laboratory. They are used for quality control and various other tests and studies.

Stoichiometry, stoichiometrically, terms referring to the weight relations in chemical formulas and equations.

Stormy fermentation, reaction in litmus milk marked by rupture; characteristic of *Clostridium perfringens*. The clot previously produced by the organism is torn by the pressure of the gas produced by the organism, giving the clotted milk a rough, foamy appearance.

Strain, set of descendants that originates from a common ancestor and retains the characteristics of the ancestor. Also see **Substrain**.

Streptokinase, fibrinolysin; an extracellular enzyme found in cultures of certain strains of hemolytic streptococci which can lyse human fibrin. Cleaves plasminogen to produce plasmin, which causes liquefaction of fibrin.

Stroma, erythrocyte membrane composed of lipid-protein molecules arranged in a bimolecular leaflet.

Structural formula, formula showing the arrangement of the atoms of a molecule.

Subculture, transplant viable bacteria derived from one culture to fresh medium.

Substitution reaction, chemical reaction in which one or more elements or radicals in a compound are replaced by other elements or radicals.

Substrain, members of a strain that differ from the original isolate.

Substrate, substance upon which an enzyme acts; specific enzymes have specific substrates.

Sugars, sweet carbohydrates; generally sucrose; types include sucrose (beet or cane), glucose, fructose, arabinose, inositol, maltose, glycogen, lactose, and inositol. See **Carbohydrate**.

Sulbactam, semisynthetic 6-desaminopenicillin sulfone.

Sulfamethoxazole-trimethoprim (SXT), Gantanol; sulphamethoxazole; N^1-(5-methyl-3-isoxazoyl) sulfanilamide; cotrimoxazole, combination of two antibiotics, sulfamethoxazole and trimethoprim (TMP).

Sulfhydryl bond, univalent radical -SH. Cysteine contains a sulfhydryl bond.

Sulfonamide, compound with the typical structure RSO_2NH_2; derived from sulfanilamide; used as antiinfective agent in medicine.

Supernatant, fluid remaining after removal of suspended matter (sediment), usually after centrifugation.

Superoxal, perhydrol; 30% hydrogen peroxide (H_2O_2); known as "100 volumes," or inaccurately "100%" hydrogen peroxide because it evolves 100 times its volume of oxygen.

Superoxide, a compound characterized by the presence in its structure of the O_2^- ion. Each oxygen atom has an oxidation number of $-1/2$ instead of the -2 of a normal oxide.

Supplement, to add what is lacking; an enrichment.

Surface tension, surface particles in a liquid have strong molecular forces that tend to pull them toward the interior of the liquid; fluid acts like a stretched membrane.

Susceptibility, quality of being readily affected; easily acted upon.

Suspension, system consisting of small particles dispersed in a liquid; particles settle out slowly on standing.

Symbol, a one- or two-letter abbreviation of the name of an element.

Symmetric, symmetrical, having constituent parts arranged in a definite pattern and repeated continually in a definite direction in space.

Synergistic, synergism, combined effect of two or more agents that exceeds the sum of their individual effects.

Synovial fluid, sterile, viscid fluid secreted by the synovial membrane; found in joint cavities, bursae, etc.

Synthesis, artificial buildup of a chemical compound by the union of its elements.

Synthetic medium, medium for bacterial isolation and cultivation consisting of known chemical constituents; synonym, chemically defined medium.

System, combination of matter containing one or more phases, or organized and related group of facts, phenomena, or ideas.

Tagged, labeled; describes a compound to which a radioactive isotope has been added.

Target amplification, target sequence of DNA identified and amplified so that it can be detected; e.g., with polymerase chain reaction (PCR).

Tautomerism, form of stereoisomerism in which compounds are mutually interconvertible. Two formulas are possible, but only one stable substance is obtained. Compounds may give reactions of a carbonyl group and at other times act as if they had an alcohol group; keto and enol forms are examples.

Taxonomy (bacterial), science of the arrangement, classification, and nomenclature of bacteria; the classification is based as far as possible on natural relationships.

TCA cycle, see **Krebs' cycle.**

Teichoic acid, one of two classes of polymers constituting cell wall of Gram-positive bacteria. Also found intracellularly. Linear polymers of a polyol (ribitol or glycerol phosphate) carrying D-alanine residues esterified to OH groups and glycosidically linked sugars.

Tergitol, trade name for a group of detergents; sodium or amine salts of higher primary or secondary alkyl sulfates.

Tertiary standards, when one solution is titrated against another.

Tetrose, monosaccharide containing four carbon atoms per molecule.

Theory, reduction of data or facts to a principle and demonstration of their interrelations.

Thermolabile, destroyed by heat; broken down by temperatures below the boiling point of water.

Thermonuclease, thermostable nuclease produced by staphylococci, capable of degrading nucleic acids.

Thermostable, thermostabile, relatively resistant to heat; resistant at 100°C.

Thin-layer chromatography (TLC), chromatography through a thin-layer of cellulose or similar inert material supported on a glass or plastic plate. See **Chromatography.**

Thio- (prefix), indicates presence of sulfur in a compound, usually as a substitute for oxygen.

Thiol (mercaptan), group of organic compounds resembling alcohol but with oxygen of the hydroxyl group replaced by sulfur.

Thrombin, blood enzyme that converts fibrinogen into fibrin in blood coagulation.

Titrated (titration), determined the amount of a substance in a solution by adding a measured volume of a standard solution until the desired reaction occurs.

Toluene, hydrocarbon methylbenzene; $C_6H_5CH_3$. Also called toluol; used primarily as a chemical solvent.

Toluol, see **Toluene.**

Toxic, poisonous.

Toxin, poisonous substance released by certain bacteria; e.g., *Clostridium* spp.

Transamination, chemical reaction involving an exchange between the amino group of an amino acid and the keto group of a keto acid, resulting in the formation of a new amino acid and a new keto acid.

Transcription, (base-mediated) amplification (or nucleic acid sequence–based amplification, NASBA) or 3 SR (self-sustaining sequence amplification). Uses three enzymes in reaction mixture.

Transduction, transfer of genetic material (and first phenotypic expression) from one bacterium to another by a bacteriophage.

Transferase, transferring enzyme; enzyme that catalyzes the transfer of a chemical grouping from one substance (compound) to another.

Transformation (genetic), genetic change caused by incorporation of DNA purified from cells or viruses into another cell.

Translucent, semitransparent.

Transparent, clear; allowing the passage of light.

Transpeptidation, reaction involving the transfer of one or more amino acids from one peptide chain to another by "transpeptidase" action, or transfer of a peptide chain itself, as in bacterial cell wall synthesis.

Transposon, transposable genetic element that carries a portion of a plasmid and a piece of chromosome from one bacterium to another by **conjugal transfer.**

Transudate, similar to exudate but with low protein content; see **Exudate.**

Tricarboxylic acid cycle (TCA), see **Krebs' cycle.**

Triglyceride, any naturally occurring ester of a normal fatty acid and glycerol. General formula: $CH_2(OOCR_1)CH(OOCR_2)CH_2(OOR_3)$; chief constituent of fats and oils. R_1, R_2, R_3 usually of different chain lengths.

Trimethoprim (TMP), USP, BP, 3,4,5-trimethoxybenzyl pyrimidine); inhibits dihydrofolic acid reductase. Pyrimidine, structural analog of pteridine. 2,4-diamino-5-(3,4,5-trimethoxybenzyl pyrimidine). Antimicrobial agent; potentiates effect of sulfonamides and sulfones.

Triphenyltetrazolium chloride (TTC), monotetrazolium salt; 2,3,5-TTC; $C_{19}H_{15}N_4C_1$. On reduction it forms a deeply colored, water-soluble pigment known as formazan, used for locating oxidative enzyme systems.

Triphosphopyridine nucleotide (TPN), see **Nicotinamide dinucleotide phosphate (NADP).**

Triple sugar iron agar (TSI), medium containing glucose, lactose, and sucrose used in routine examination of stool specimens for identification of Gram-negative enterics. Hydrogen sulfide and gas production (CO_2 and H_2) can also be detected, since it is a semisolid medium.

Tris, tris(hydroxymethyl)aminomethane; buffer used in biologic preparations for in vitro enzyme studies, tests.

Trisaccharide, carbohydrate, $C_{18}H_{32}O_{16}$ that contains three sugars.

True motility, moving voluntarily. See **False motility**.

Tryptone, true peptone, as distinct from pepsin peptone; peptone produced by hydrolysis of protein by the enzyme trypsin. Used in media, especially that used to detect indole.

Tryptophan, α-amino-3-indolepropionic acid; $C_8H_6N \cdot CH_2CH(NH_2)\text{-COOH}$. Yields indole when metabolized by certain bacteria, also a nutrient required by some bacteria.

Turbid, cloudy; not clear.

Turbidimetry, determination of number of fine, suspended particles in a liquid by measuring the thickness of liquid that reduces visual transmission as much as a standard solution or standard pattern; e.g., McFarland's nephelometer. See **Nephelometry**.

Tween, ethylene oxide derivative of a sorbitan ester; an emulsifying agent that disperses fat globules and a nonionic, surface-active wetting agent. Used in microbiology to reduce surface tension, also called Tween 80.

Tyndall light phenomenon, a transverse beam of light is reflected, or dispersed, by particles suspended in a gas or liquid.

Type, term used in bacteriology to designate a subdivision of a species; e.g., *Streptococcus pneumoniae* type I, type II. Bacteria are classified by types when the differentiating characteristics are too slight to justify establishing a subspecies or variety.

Ultraviolet, portion of the spectrum just beyond violet on the short wavelength side; invisible rays that induce chemical activity and produce fluorescence.

Undissociated, existing in a nondissociated molecular form; not ionized, nonelectrolytic. See **Ionize**.

Uninoculated, having no microorganisms introduced; sterile. Often an uninoculated control is run along with known positive and negative tubes, especially when the interpretation is based on a slight color change.

Unit, a standard of measurement.

Unsaturated compound, organic compound containing double or triple bonds and capable of forming additional products.

Unstable, readily decomposing.

Urea, soluble, crystalline, nitrogenous compound; carbamide, CH_4ON_2.

Urease, enzyme that catalyzes the hydrolysis of urea with the formation of ammonium carbonate.

Urorosein, chromogen in urine that forms a red color on addition of nitric acid; increased by *Mycobacterium tuberculosis* infection (TB) and other wasting diseases.

Valence, a number indicating the combining power of an element or radical.

Variable, not constant.

Variant, an organism that varies, or differs, from the parental culture.

Variation, alteration or modification of a character in the offspring; deviation from the parent; usually a temporary change compared with a mutation.

Vaseline, see **Petrolatum**.

Vaspar, a mixture of Vaseline and paraffin, in equal weight, used to seal cover slips in the hanging drop technique and tubes of broth media inoculated with anaerobic bacteria.

Versene, trade name. See **Ethylenediaminetetraacetate (EDTA)**.

Viable, alive and able to reproduce.

Vinyl analog, a monovalent group $CH_2{:}CH\text{-}$; ethenyl, derived from the bivinyl compound ethylene; a chemical compound that is structurally similar to another but differs in a certain component and may have a similar or opposite metabolic activity.

Virulence, potential ability of an organism to cause disease; determines pathogenicity.

Viscid, viscosity, sticky, gummy, glutinous.

Viscous material, thick substance that adheres to the inoculating needle when touched; sediment that arises as a coherent swirl when liquid media is shaken.

Volatile, evaporating rapidly.

Wetting agent, substance that reduces surface tension, causing liquids to disperse more readily on a solid surface; i.e., detergents; anionic, cationic, or nonionic.

Whey, thin milk serum remaining after the curd and cream have been removed.

White blood cell (WBC), see **Leukocyte**.

Wild-type strain, strain found in nature or a standard strain; see **Auxotroph** and **Prototroph**.

Xanthene, crystalline compound that is the basic structure for many dyestuffs.

Yeast, a unicellular fungus used as a bacterial nutrient in culture media.

Zymogen, a proenzyme; inactive enzyme.

SECTION V

Indices

Index 1–General

AccuProbe
  multitest system, 460, 466
  Neisseria gonorrhoeae Culture Confirmation Test, 342
Acetalization, 414
Acetoin, 322, 325, 439–443, 447–448
Acetyl coenzyme A (acetyl-CoA), 287, 311
Acid fuchsin, 744
Acid-fast organisms, 578
Adenine, 138–140
Aesculin hydrolysis test, 8–23
Agmatine, 122
Alcoholic fermentation, 62
Alcohols
  catalase and, 81, 83
  lipids, 286–287
  sugars, 58, 73
Aldehydes, 413–414
Aldonic acids, 184
Aldose, 413
Amidases, 425
Amino acids
  cystine, 205–206
  deamination, 222–223, 283, 388–389
  decarboxylation, 120–134, 197
  glycine, 188–193, 195–198, 305–306, 308
  hydrogen sulfide test, 205–219
  leucine, 283, 284
  methionine, 205–206
  phenylalanine, 388–393
  tryptophan, 222–223
Aminocephalosporanic acid, 260
Aminolevulinic acid (ALA), 403–406
Aminopenicillanic acid, 257, 258
Ammonia, 349, 388, 398, 425
Amoxicillin, 257
Amphotericin B, 433
Ampicillin, 257
Amylase, 414–415, 422
Amylopectin, 414–417, 419–420
Amylose, 414–416, 419–420
Anaerobes
  carbohydrate fermentation media for, 69–72
  peroxidase, 79
Andrade's indicator, 64, 74–76, 744
Aniline, 373
Antibiotics
  amphotericin B, 433
  bacitracin, 3–7
  binding proteins, 256
  β-lactamase test, 254–269
  cefoperazone, 330
  cefsulodin, 433
  cephalosporins, 258–260
  cycloserine, 290
  penicillins, 256–258, 430
  plasmids and resistance, 255, 261–262
  sulfamethoxazole, 290
  sulfamethoxazole-trimethoprim, 4–7
  trimethoprim, 4–7, 290, 330, 433
  vancomycin, 433
API test systems
  multitest system, 460–467, 469
  Quad-Ferm+, 339
Aprotinin, 113–114
Arginine
  decarboxylase test
    biochemistry, 122–123
    Møller's decarboxylase, 124–125
  dihydrolase
    biochemistry, 123–124
    purpose, 120–121
    thin-layer chromatography, 132
Autolysis, 29
Auxochromes, 395
Auxotroph, 341
Azo group, 409

Bacitracin/sulfamethoxazole-trimethoprim tests, 3–7
  biochemistry of, 3–5
  interpretation, 6–7
  purpose, 3
BactiCard
  multitest system, 461, 465
  Neisseria, 341
BBL multitest system, 460, 462–464, 467
Benzoic acid, 189–193, 198
β-galactosidase (ONPG), 339–340
β-galactosidase tests, 160–168
  biochemistry, 161–164
  interpretation, 166–167
  ONPG, 160, 163–168
  PNPG, 160, 167, 168
  procedures, 165–166
  purpose, 160
  rapid tests, 167
  reagents, 164–165
β-galactoside permease, 162–164
β-hemolysin and CAMP test, 35–52
Bile esculin hydrolysis tests, 8–23
  alternate tests, 15–18

Bile esculin hydrolysis tests—*Continued*
  biochemistry of, 9–11
  interpretations, 12–13
  media, 11–12
  purpose, 8–9
  rapid tests, 13–14
Bile salts, 27–28
Bile solubility test, 27–33
  biochemistry of, 27–29
  procedure, 30–31
  purpose, 27
  rapid tests, 31–32
Bismuth sulfite agar, 742
β-lactamase test, 254–269
  biochemistry, 255–262
    β-lactamase enzymes, 255–256
      Bacteroides/Prevotella, 262
      Enterococcus faecalis, 261, 269
      Haemophilus influenzae, 262, 268
      inhibitors of, 262
      Moraxella catarrhalis, 261, 268
      Neisseria gonorrhoeae, 261, 268
      Staphylococcus, 261, 268
    cephalosporins, 258–260
    penicillins, 256–258
    plasmids and antibiotic resistance, 255
  precautions, 267–269
  purpose, 254–255
  rapid assays
    acidometric, 266, 267–268
    iodmetric slide test, 265–266, 267
    Nitrocefin (chromogenic cephalosporin), 263–265, 267
Brilliant green agar, 742
Bromcresol purple (BCP), 124, 126, 744
Bromthymol blue, 744
2,3-butanediol, 322, 440–443
Butyl alcohol (butanol) fermentation, 63
Butyrate esterase, 340–341

Cadaverine, 121–122, 130, 132
CAMP test, 35–52
  biochemistry of, 36–43
  disk test, 48
  interpretation, 45–46
  phospholipase D detection, 47–48
  purpose, 35–36
  reverse (RCT), 46–47
  spot test, 48
Carbamate kinase, 123–124
Carbohydrate fermentation tests, 57–76
  biochemistry of, 58–63
  disks, 69
  gas production, 75
  interpretation, 68–69
  media, 63–67, 69–73
  purpose, 57–58
Carbohydrates
  classification, 58–59
  disks, differential, 66
  fermentation, 59–62, 380
  gas formation, 297
  gas production, 244, 246, 248, 250–251, 322
  KIA/TSI reactions, 243–245
  lactose, 163–164, 295–297
  in media, 65–66
  methyl red test, 322
  mixed acid, 322, 439–443
    by *Neisseria,* 333–334
  tests, 57–76
  oxidation, 183–184, 380
  sterilization method, 66, 382
Casein, 295–297
Catalase test, 318, 370
  biochemistry, 79–84
  capillary tube, 90
  color reaction streak test, 91, 93
  coverslip technique, 91
  for *Enterobacteriaceae,* 89–9090
  Gram-positive cocci differentiation, 605–613
  Gram-positive rod differentiation
    aerobic/facultative anaerobic, 576–581
    anaerobic, 598–603
  interpretation, 88–89
  for *Mycobacterium* differentiation, 85–87, 88
  for *Neisseria,* 90
  precautions, 92–95
  purpose, 78–79
  slide test, 85
  tube test, 85
  whole cell test, 87, 88–89, 94–95
Cefoperazone, 330
Cefsulodin, 433
Cell wall, 28, 256, 303–305
Cellulose, 413
Cephalin, 274
Cephalosporins, 258–260
Ceramides, 37, 39–42
Cholic acid, 27–28
Chromogens, 395
Chromophores, 395
Chymotrypsin, 296
Citrate test, 98–103
  biochemistry, 99–100
  Christensen's, 101
  citrate blood test, 102
  purpose, 98–99
  Simmons, 100–101
Citrulline, 123–124
Classification
  Enterobacteriaceae, 735–741
  Gram-negative bacteria, 624–628
  Gram-positive bacteria, 483–487
Clavulanic acid, 262
Clinitest tablets, 185–186
Coagglutination test, *Neisseria,* 341–342
Coagulase mannitol agar/broth, 458
Coagulase test, 105–117
  biochemistry of, 106–108
  bound coagulase and, 106, 110–111
  coagulase-mannitol, 112, 117
  free coagulase and, 106–108, 110–111

latex agglutination, 112
pour-plate, 111–112
purpose, 105–106
slide, 110, 114
tube, 110–111, 115–117
tube coagulase-thermonuclease, 112
Coliform group fermentations, 62
Colon-dysentery-typhoid bacteria (CDT group), 62
Conjugal transfer, 255
Coordination, 192
Cresol red, 125
Curd formation, 296–297, 300–301
Cycloserine, 290
Cysteine, 70, 205–206, 353
Cysteine desulfhydrase, 205–206
Cystine, 70, 71, 205–206
Cytochromes, 79–81, 316–318, 329, 349, 369–371
Cytosine, 138–140

Deamination
  arginine, 124
  lysine, 129
Decarboxylase tests (lysine-ornithine-arginine), 120–134
  alternative tests
    lysine-iron agar (LIA), 128–129
    ninhydrin broth, 129, 134
  biochemistry, 121–124
  Falkow's, 126, 134
  media for, 124–126
  Møller's, 124–125, 134
  purpose, 120–121
  rapid tests
    lysine decarboxylase, 130–131
    ornithine decarboxylase, 131
  reagents for, 126–127
Denitrification, 349
Deoxycholic acid, 27–28
Deoxyribonuclease tests, 136–156
  acid-DNase test, 143–145, 148, 155
  alternative tests
    acidometric, 153
    Lombard-Dowell DNA agar, 153
    rapid indirect, 153
    rapid well-agar diffusion, 152
    turbidimetric assay, 152–153
  biochemistry, 137–143
  interpretation, 148
  mannitol-acid DNase test, 145, 148
  media, 143–147
  methyl green-DNase test (MG-DTA), 147, 148, 155–156
  purpose, 136–137
  thermonuclease tests, 149–152
  toluidine blue O DNase test (TBO-DTA), 145–147, 148, 155–156
Desoxycholate citrate agar, 742
Desoxycholate citrate lactose agar, 742
Desoxycholate citrate lactose sucrose agar, 743
Dextrins, 412, 416
Diacetyl, 445–446

Diisopropylfluorophosphate, 114
Direct fluorescent antibody (DFA), 460
  Neisseria gonorrhoeae identification, 341, 344
DNA (deoxyribonucleic acid), 137–140
  hybridization tests, 461
  probes, 460, 470
DNase enzymes, 141–143
  Serratia, 142–143
  staphylococcal, 141–142
  streptococcal, 143
Dyes
  acridine orange, 150–152
  auxochromes, 395
  methyl green, 147, 155–156, 399
  methylene blue, 317
  p-phenylenediamine, 373–374
  toluidine blue O, 145–147, 155–156

Egg yolk factor, 274–275
EIAs (enzyme immunoassays), 460, 465, 469
ELISA (enzyme-linked immunosorbent assay), 460
Embden-Meyerhof-Parnas pathway, 60, 62, 163, 243, 380
End product detection, 422
Endonucleases, 141
Enterobacteriaceae. (*see also specific genera* in Organism Index)
  biochemical reaction tables, 748–758, 769–770, 772–781, 796–797
  classification, 735–741
  combined test media for, 458–459
  differentiation charts, 759–768, 771, 782–795, 798–799
  general characteristics, 741
  KIA/TSI reactions, 239–243, 744–747
  media for isolation and identification, 742–744
  multitest systems, 461–463
  nomenclature changes, 733–735
  Simmons citrate reactions, 98
  taxonomy, 732
Enterotube multitest system, 462
Entner-Doudoroff pathway, 60, 62, 183, 333, 380
Enzymes
  adaptive (inducible), 121, 161
  amylase, 414–415, 422
  β-lactamase, 255–262
  caseases, 295–296
  catalase, 318
  constitutive, 190, 255, 288
  decarboxylases, 121
  DNase, 141–143
  gelatinase, 171
  hippuricase, 189–190
  inducible, 255
  lecithinases, 273–275
  leucine aminopeptidase, 283
  lipase test, 286–292
  lysostaphin, 305
  oxidase, 369–371
  permease, 162–164
  phospholipases, 288–289

Enzymes—*Continued*
  pyrrolidonase, 408
  succinic dehydrogenase, inhibition of, 310–312
  tryptophanase, 222–223, 229
  urease, 425
Eosin-methylene blue agar, 742
Episomes, 152, 255
Erythodextrins, 416, 421
Erythrocyte membranes, 38–39
Esculin, 8–23
Esculin spot test, 13
Ester linkages, 288, 340
Exonucleases, 141

FA staining and *Neisseria gonorrhoeae* identification, 341, 344
Fatty acids, 287
Fermentation
  alcoholic, 62
  butyl alcohol, 63
  carbohydrate, 57–58, 59–62
    gas formation, 297
    gas production, 322
    KIA/TSI reactions, 243–245
    lactose, 163–164
    lactose (litmus milk), 295–297
    methyl red test, 322
    mixed acid, 322, 439–443
    O/F test, 379–386
  citrate, 99
  coliform group, 62
  Embden-Meyerhof-Parnas pathway, 60, 62
  Entner-Doudoroff pathway, 60, 62
  lactic acid, 62
  malonate test, 312
  mixed acid, 62
  pentose shunt, 60, 62
  propionic acid, 62
Ferric ammonium citrate, 206–207
Fibrinogen, 106–109, 113
Fibrinolysis, 109
Flagellum, 331
Flavoproteins, 79–80, 83, 318
FLN medium (fluorescence-lactose-nitrate medium), 458
Fluorescein pigment, 359
Fluorescence, 152, 404
Fluorescent monoclonal antibody test (FA), 466
FN medium (fluorescence-denitrification medium), 458
Folic acid metabolism, 4–5
Formazan, 329
Formic acid fermentation, 62

Gas-liquid chromatography (GLC), 464
  decarboxylase tests, 132
  hippurate hydrolysis, 198
  Neisseria gonorrhoeae identification, 341
  Voges-Proskauer test, 447
Gelatin liquefaction tests, 170–181
  biochemistry, 171

interpretations, 176
Kohn gelatin, 171–173, 176, 180
mercuric chloride procedure, 176–177, 181
nutrient gelatin plate, 174, 176
nutrient gelatin stab, 173–174, 176, 180–181
purpose, 170–171
thioglycolate gelatin, 174–175, 176
x-ray film method, 177–178, 181
Gene chip technology, 470
Gluconate oxidation test, 183–187
  biochemistry, 183–184
  interpretation, 186
  media, 184–185
  purpose, 183
  reagents, 185–186
Glucosan, 412
Glucose
  KIA/TSI media, 243–248
  optical isomers, 413
  oxidation, 183–184
  starch hydrolysis, 412–417
B-glucosidic linkage, 138
T-glutamylaminopeptidase, 340
T-glutamyl-*p*-nitroanilide, 340
Glycerides, 288
Glycerol, 286, 288–289, 308
Glycerophospholipids, 38, 41–42
Glycine, 27, 188–193, 195–198, 305–306, 308
Glycogen, 415
Glycolipids, 287
Glycoside, 58
Glycosidic linkage, 161, 415–417
Glyoxylic acid cycle, 311–312
Gonobio Test, 339
Gonochek II, 340
Gonogen I test, 342
Gram-negative bacteria, 624–729
  chart
    bacilli, aerobic/facutative anaerobic
      initial differentiation, 705
      MacConkey—growth, 706–717
      MacConkey—no growth, 718–721
    bacilli, microaerophilic/anaerobic, 723–728
    cocci, aerobic/facultative anaerobic, 722
    cocci, anaerobic, 729
  genera descriptions/tables, 639–704
    differential characteristics, charts of, 639–641
  nomenclature changes, 628–639
Gram-positive bacteria, 483–623
  chart, 574–621
    bacilli, aerobic/facultative anaerobic
      Bacillus, 582
      catalase reaction, 576–581
      Corynebacterium, 583–587
      Listeria, 588
    bacilli, anaerobic
      catalase reaction, 598–603
      Clostridium, 590–597
      initial differentiation, 589
    cocci, aerobic/facultative anaerobic, 604
      catalase reaction, 605–613

Enterococcus, 614–615
Staphylococcus, 609–611
Streptococcus, 616–619
cocci, anaerobic, 620–621
Peptostreptococcus, 621
by oxygen requirement, 575, 604
by shape, 574
classification, 483–487
genera descriptions/tables, 502–573
nomenclature, 487–498
Guanidine nucleus, 445, 446
Guanine, 138–140

Hektoen enteric agar, 743
Heme, 451
Heme proteins, 79–81
Hemiacetal linkage, 414
Hemin, 403–404
Hemoglobin, 451
A-hemolysin, 46–47
Hemolysins and CAMP test, 35–52
High-pressure liquid chromatography (HPLC), 464
Hippurate hydrolysis test, 188–202
   biochemistry, 188–190
   disk test, 199
   ferric chloride reagent, 190–193, 201–202
   gas chromatography, 198
   glycine end product detection, 195–198
   interpretation, 195, 196
   MA test, 199
   media, 193–195
   ninhydrin, 196–198, 202
   precautions, 199–202
   purpose, 188
   thin layer chromatography, 198
Hirudin, 113–114
Histozyme, 190
Hydrazine, 391
Hydrogen bonds, 139
Hydrogen peroxide (H_2O_2), 79–95, 317–318, 369–370
Hydrogen sulfide test, 205–219
   biochemistry, 205–207
   interpretations, 216
   KIA/TSI media, 245, 248
   media
     lead acetate (PbAc) strip test, 213–215, 218–219
     sulfur-containing amino acid media, 208–213, 217–218
   precautions, 217–219
   purpose, 205
Hydrolysis, starch, 412–423
Hydroxylamine, 349
Hydroxyprolylaminopeptidase, 340

IDS Rapid ID multitest system, 460, 462–464, 466, 469
Immunocard multitest system, 460–461
Indole tests, 221–222
   biochemistry, 222–223
   interpretations, 227

   media, 223–224, 228–229
   multitests, 228–229
     indole-nitrite, 228–229, 231
     motility-indole-lysine (MIL), 229
     motility-indole-ornithine (MIO), 229
     MUG disk, 229
     sulfide-indole-motility (SIM), 229
   purpose, 221–222
   rapid tests, 227–228
     microtechnique, 228
     spot test, 227–228, 230–231
   reagents
     Ehrlich's, 224, 230
     Kovac's, 224–226, 230
Indoleacetic acid, 222, 230
Indole-nitrate medium, 458
Indolphenol, 370–371, 374
Indolyl, 153
Inositol, 58

Kanamycin-bile disk test, 16–17
2-ketogluconic acid, 184
Kit systems, 338–339. (*see also* Multitest systems)
   API Quad-Ferm+, 339
   API Rapid Strep, 284
   BacteriCard Neisseria, 341
   Bacti Card *Streptococcus* Test, 284
   Gonobio Test, 339
   Gonochek II, 340
   Minitek, 338–339, 344
   Neisseria-Kwik Test, 339
   Neisstrip, 341
Kligler's iron agar (KIA), 239–252
   biochemistry, 243–245
   gas production, 244, 246, 248, 250–251
   hydrogen sulfide formation, 245
   interpretations, 247–248
   media, 245–247
   precautions, 249–252
   purpose, 239–243
Krebs cycle, 243, 311–312

Lactase, 162
Lactic acid fermentation, 62
Lactose
   β-galactosidase tests, 160–168
   egg yolk media reactions, *279–280*
   fermentation, 163–164
   KIA/TSI media, 243–248
Latex agglutination, 460, 468, 469
Lead acetate, 207
Lecithin, 38–41
Lecithinase test, 273–281
   biochemistry, 273–275
   interpretations, 278–280
   media, 275–278
   precautions, 280–281
   purpose, 273
Lecithin-lactose anaerobic agar, 458
Lecithin-lipase anaerobic agar, 458
Lecithovitellin, 274

Leucine aminopeptidase (LAP) test, 282–285
   disk spot test, 284
   DMACA reagent, 283–284
   enzyme/substrate, 283
   interpretation, 285
   kit system tests, 284
   precautions, 285
   purpose, 282
Ligands, 192
Ligase chain reaction, 466, 470
Lipase test, 286–292
   biochemistry, 286–289
   egg yolk media reactions, *279–280*
   interpretation, 292
   media, 289–291
   precautions, 292
   purpose, 286
Lipids, 286–287
Liquid chain reaction (LCR), 466
Litmus milk test, 294–302
   agar, 301
   biochemistry, 295–298
   interpretations, 300–301
   litmus indicator, 298
   media, 298–300, 302
   precautions, 301–302
   purpose, 294–295
   rapid caseolysis *Enterococcus* test, 301
Lombard-Dowell (LD) media, 458
Lysine decarboxylase test
   biochemistry, 121
   Brooker-Lund-Blazevic method, 131
   Falkow's, 126
   gas chromatography, 132
   lysine-iron agar (LIA), 128–129
   Møller's decarboxylase, 124–125
   ninhydrin broth, 129–130
   purpose, 120
   spot test, 130–131
Lysine-ornithine-mannitol (LOM) agar, 458
Lysostaphin susceptibility test, 303–308
   biochemistry, 303–306
   interpretation, 307
   precautions, 307–308
   procedures, 306–307
   purpose, 303
   reagents, 306
Lysozyme, 305

MacConkey agar, 743
Malonate test, 310–315
   biochemistry, 310–312
   interpretations, 314
   media, 313
   phenylalanine-malonate broth medium, 392
   precautions, 314–315
   purpose, 310
Maltose, 343, 415–417
Media
   OF, 381–386
   anaerobic esculin broth, 15

Bacteroides Bile Esculin (BBE) agar, 8, 15–16
balanced salt solution, 434
bicarbonate (NaHCO$_3$), 337
bile esculin agar (BEA), 11, *208,* 211
bile esculin azide agar/broth, 11
bismuth sulfite agar, 742
blood, sheep, 336–337
botulinum selective medium (BSM), 290–291, 292
brain-heart infusion agar (BHIA), 451
brain-heart infusion broth (BHIB), 451
brilliant green agar, 742
calcium-cysteine solution, 275
carbohydrate fermentation, 63–67, 69–73
   for anaerobes, 69–72
   with Andrade's indicator, 63–64
   disks, differential, 65
   peptone yeast broth, 69–70
   with phenol red indicator, 63
   for staphylococci and enterics, 73
   sterilization method, 66
   for streptococci, 72–73
   thioglycolate media, 70–72, 76
casein, 224
charcoal (Kohn gelatin), 171–173
chocolate agar, 343
Christensen's citrate, 101
Clark and Lubs medium, 323
Clark and Lubs medium, modified, 443
Clostridium botulinum isolation (CBI) agar, 289–290
Clostridum difficile agar, 277
coagulase mannitol agar, 112, 117, 458
Columbia agar, 275, 399
cycloserine solution, 290
cystine trypticase agar (CTA) with carbohydrates, 334–336, 338, 343–344
desoxycholate citrate agar, 742
desoxycholate citrate lactose agar, 742
desoxycholate citrate lactose sucrose agar, 743
DNase test agar (DTA), 143–147
   with mannitol, 145, 148
   with methyl green (DTA-MG), 147, 148
   standard, 143–145, 148
   with toluidine blue O (DTA-TBO), 145–147, 148
Edwards and Ewing's medium, 331
egg yolk, 275, 290
Elrod and Braun (modified) salt solution with carbohydrates, 336, 338
enteric OF, 285, 381–383
for *Enterobacteriaceae* isolation and differentiation of, 742–744
eosin-methylene blue agar, 742
esculin, buffered, 13
esculin-based streptomycin-chloramphenicol agar, 17–18
Falkow's lysine decarboxylase, 126, 134
fluorescence-denitrification (FN), 359, 458
fluorescent lactose nitrate (FLN) medium, 359
gelatin
   aerobic low-peptone, 179
   agar plate, 179
   BCYE$_\alpha$ (buffered charcoal yeast extract), 178–179

Chapman stone agar, 178
   dilute, 179
   Kohn, 171–173
   Lombard-Dowell, 178
   metronidazole cadmium, 178
   nutrient, 173–174
   peptone yeast, 178
   Staphylococcus agar, 178
   thioglycolate, 174–175
gluconate peptone broth, 184–185
gluconate substrate test tablets, Key, 185, 186–187
gonococcus cysteine (GCC), 344
gonococcus identification medium (GCID), 336–337, 338, 344
hektoen enteric agar, 743
hemoglobin (Hb), 336
hippurate broth, 193–195
Hugh and Leifson's OF, 381–383, 385
hydrogen sulfide test, 208–215
   bile esculin agar (BEA), 208, 211
   bismuth sulfite agar, 208, 208, 217–218
   citrate sulfide agar, 208, 211
   deoxycholate agars, 208, 209, 218
   Hektoen enteric agar, 208, 210, 218
   Kligler's iron agar (KIA), 208, 208, 217
   lead acetate (PbAc) strips, 208, 213–215, 216, 218–219
   lysine iron agar (LIA), 208, 210, 218
   peptone iron agar, 208, 210
   Salmonella-Shigella agar, 208, 211
   sulfide-indole-motility (SIM) agar, 208, 210–211, 218
   table of, 208
   thiosulfate-citrate-bile salts-sucrose (TCBS) agar, 208, 211–212
   triple sugar iron (TSI) agar, 208, 208, 217
   xylose lysine desoxycholate (XLD) agar, 208, 211, 218
indole nitrate, 458
indole-nitrite, 228–229, 231
IsoVitaleX, 337, 344, 433
Kanamycin-Bile-Esculin (KEB), 8, 17
Kligler's iron agar (KIA), 245–247
lecithin solution, 275
lecithin-lactose anaerobic agar, 275–276, 458
lecithin-lipase anaerobic agar, 276–277, 458
lipase salt mannitol (LSM) agar, 291, 292
litmus milk, 298–300
litmus milk agar, 301
Lombard-Dowell (LD), 458
lysine-iron agar (LIA), 128–129
lysine-ornithine-mannitol (LUM), 458
MacConkey agar, 743
malonate broth, 313, 314
McClung-Toabe egg yolk agar, 277
methyl green phosphate, 399–400
methyl red-Voges Proskauer, 323, 443, 459
methylene blue milk medium, 318
Møller's decarboxylase base, 124–125, 134
motility, 327–329, 330
motility with tetrazolium salts, 328–329, 330
motility-indole-lysine (MIL), 229, 331, 459
motility-indole-ornithine (MIO), 229, 331, 459
motility-nitrate medium, 331, 459
motility-sulfide medium, 331, 459
MR/VP, 323, 443, 459
MUG disk, 229
ninhydrin broth, 129–130
nitrate, 350–351
nitrate disks/tablets, 358
nitrate medium for *Neisseria* spp., 357
nitrate/nitrite reduction medium, 359
nitrite test strips, 355–356
nutrient broth, 213
optochin disk, 364
peptone broth, 223, 229
pH indicators
   acid fuchsin, 744
   bromcresol purple (BCP), 124, 126, 744
   bromthymol blue, 744
   cresol red, 125
   neutral red, 744
   phenol red, 744
phenolphthalein diphosphate medium (PDP), 396–398
phenylalanine, 313, 314, 389–390
phenylalanine-malonate broth, 392
phosphate blood agar (PDPBA), 399
phosphate buffer, 356, 432
potassium nitrate, 350–351
PYR broth, 409
Salmonella-Shigella agar, 742
salt solution (Elrod and Braun), 336
semisolid selective motility (SSM), 330–331
serum glucose agar slants, 213–214
Simmons citrate, 100–101
sodium hydroxide, 64
Staph OF, 284, 382, 385
starch, 417–418
sulfide-indole-motility (SIM), 229, 331, 459
TB nitrate reduction broth, 356–357
tetrazolium salts, 328–329, 331
thioglycolate, 70–72, 76
thioglycolate gelatin, 174–175
thiopeptone broth, 213
Todd-Hewitt broth, 409
transport media, 343
trehalose-mannitol broth, 459
trehalose-mannitol-phosphate agar (TMPA), 459
triple sugar iron (TSI) agar, 246–247
trypticase nitrate broth, 228–229
trypticase soy agar (TSA), 409, 451
trypticase soy broth (TSB), 213
tryptophan broth, 223
tryptose phosphate agar (TPA), 399
urease test
   Christensen's urea agar, 427–428, 429, 436
   CLO striptest, 434
   Stuart's urea broth, 426–427, 429, 435–436
   U-9 broth, 430–431, 436–437
   urea, azide-free buffered, 432–433
   urea broth for mycobacteria, 432

Media—*Continued*
    urea disks, 432, 434
    urea R broth, 428, 429, 436
    urea-phenylalanine disks, 434
    urease test tablets, 434
  vitamin K-hemin solution, 69
  VPI salt solution, 69
  xylose-lysine-desoxycholate agar, 742
Membranes, erythrocyte, 38–39
Meritec GC test, 342
Metachromatic staining, 146–147
Methicillin, 257, 261
Methionine, 205–206
Methyl red test, 321–325
  biochemistry, 322
  interpretations, 324
  media, 323
  precautions, 324–325
  purpose, 321
  rapid microtechnique, 324
  reagent, 323–324
Methylene blue, 317
Methylene blue milk reduction test, 316–319
  biochemistry, 316–318
  interpretation, 319
  medium, 318
  precautions, 319
  purpose, 316
Methyl-red-Voges-Proskauer broth medium, 323, 443, 459
Micro-ID multitest system, 462, 464
MicroScan multitest system, 460–463, 467
Minitek
  disk system, 338–339, 344
  multitest system, 460, 462–465, 467–468
Mixed-acid fermentation, 62, 439–443
Molecular microbiology, 457–458, 470
Motility test, 327–331
  combination tests, 331
  hanging drop, 330
  interpretation, 330
  OF media, 383, 384
  motility test media (semisolid), 327–329
  precautions, 331–332
  purpose, 327
  semisolid selective motility (SSM) medium, 330–331
Motility-indole-lysine (MIL) medium, 459
Motility-indole-ornithine (MIO) medium, 459
Motility-nitrate medium, 459
Motility-sulfide medium, 459
Multitest systems, 457–470
  Accuprobe, 460, 466
  anaerobic identification, 459–460
  API, 460–467, 469
  BactiCard, 461, 465
  BBL, 460, 462–464, 467
  Bordetella pertussis identification, 460
  Brucella spp. identification, 460
  Burkholderia identification, 460
  Campylobacter spp. identification, 460
  Clostridum difficile identification, 460–461
  combined test media, 458–459
  Corynebacterium spp. identification, 460
  Enterobacteriaceae identification, 461–463
  Enterococcus spp. identification, 461
  Enterotube, 462
  fastidious Gram-negative rod identification, 464
  Francisella tularensis identification, 464
  Gram-negative bacteria identification, 463
  Gram-positive rods identification, 463–464
  Haemophilus spp. identification, 464
  Helicobacter pylori identification, 464–465
  IDS Rapid ID, 460, 462–464, 466, 469
  Immunocard, 460–461
  Lactococcus and *Leuconostoc* identification, 465
  Micro-ID, 462, 464
  MicroScan, 460–463, 467
  Minitek, 460, 462–465, 467–468
  Neisseria and *Moraxella catarrhalis* identification, 465–466
  overview, 457
  Premier, 460, 463
  RIM-H (Rapid Identification Method), 464
  Staphylococcus spp. identification, 467–469
  Streptococcus spp. identification, 469
  Ureaplasma urealyticum identification, 469
  Vibrio spp. identification, 470
  Vitek, 460, 463, 466, 467–468

NaCl tolerance, 19
Nagler test, 273
β-naphthylamines, 283–284
α-napthol, 371, 374, 375
Neisseria carbohydrate utilization tests, 333–345
  alternative tests, 341–342
  biochemistry, 333–334
  chromogenic enzyme substrate tests, 339–341
  interpretation, 338
  kit systems, 338–339
    API Quad-Ferm+, 339
    BacteriCard Neisseria, 341
    Gonobio Test, 339
    Gonochek II, 340
    Minitek, 338–339, 344
    Neisseria-Kwik Test, 339
    Neisstrip, 341
  media
    CTA/carbohydrate, 334–336, 338, 343–344
    Elrod and Braun (modified), 336, 338
    gonococcus identification medium (GCID), 336–337, 338, 344
  precautions, 342–345
  purpose, 333
Neisseria-Kwik Test kit, 339
Neisstrip, 341
Neutral red, 744
Nicotinamide adenine dinucleotide (NAD), 451
Ninhydrin, 196–198, 202
Nitrate/nitrite reduction tests, 348–361
  biochemistry, 349–350
  disk method for anaerobes, 358

interpretation, 354–355
media
fluorescence-denitrification (FN), 359
nitrate medium for *Neisseria* spp., 357
nitrite test strips, 355–356
potassium nitrate, 350–351
TB nitrate reduction broth, 356–357
for *Mycobacterium* spp., 355–357, 361
for *Neisseria* spp., 357–358
precautions, 360–361
purpose, 348
rapid tests, 358
disk/tablet, 358
spot test, 358
reagents, 351–354
Nitrocefin (chromogenic cephalosporin), 263–265, 267
Nomenclature changes
Enterobacteriaceae, 733–735
Gram-negative bacteria, 628–635
Gram-positive bacteria, 487–498
Nuclease enzymes, 141–143
Nucleic acid probes, 342, 460, 466, 470
Nucleotide, 137–140

ONPG (σ-nitrophenyl-β-D-galactopyranoside), 160, 163–168
Optical isomers, 413
Optochin disk test, 363–367
biochemistry, 363
interpretation, 365
precautions, 365–367
procedure, 363–365
purpose, 363
Ornithine decarboxylase test
biochemistry, 121–122
gas chromatography, 132
Møller's decarboxylase, 124–125
purpose, 120
rapid test, 131–132
Orthochromatic staining, 146
Oxacillin, 257, 261
Oxidase test, 368–377
biochemistry, 369–371
interpretation, 375
procedures
disks, 372–373
impregnated strips, 375
reagent solutions, 372
swab test, 373
purpose, 368–369
reagents, 371–374
Oxidation
carbohydrates by *Neisseria*, 333–334
cytochrome oxidases, 369–371
gluconate, 183–187
O/F test, 379–386
of phenylalanine, 388
of succinic acid, 310–311
Oxidation-fermentation test, 379–386
biochemistry, 379–381

fermentation, 380
oxidation, 381
interpretation of two-tube test, 384–385
media, 381–384
precautions, 385–386
procedure, standard two-tube, 383
purpose, 379
Oxidation-reduction indicator
litmus, 295
methylene blue, 317
Oxygen (O_2) requirement
Gram-positive cocci differentiation, *604*
Gram-positive rod differentiation, *575*

PACE (probe assay-chemiluminescence enhanced), 466
PACE-2NG probe, 342
PAGE (polyacrylamide gel electrophoresis), 459, 465
Paracasein, 296–297
Passive hemagglutination, 468
Penicillins, 256–258, 430
Pentose shunt, 60, 62, 333, 380
Pepsin, 296
Peptidases, 305
Peptide link, 190
Peptidoglycan, 28, 256, 303–305
Peptone
amino acid composition of, 305
hydrogen sulfide production from, 206, *208*
in KIA/TSI media, 244, 246
methyl red test, effect on, 324
Peptonization, 295–296, 301
Peroxidase test
biochemistry, 79–84
interpretation, 88–89
purpose, 78–79
whole cell test, 87, 88–89, 94–95
PH indicators. (*see* Reagents, pH indicators)
Phadebact GC OMNI Test, 342, 345
Phenol, 192, 395
Phenol red, 63, 74, 744
Phenolphthalein, 394–399, 401
Phenylalanine deaminase test, 388–393
biochemistry, 388–389
disks/tablets, 392
interpretation, 391
phenylalanine medium, 389–390
phenylalanine-malonate broth medium, 392
precautions, 393
purpose, 388
reagents, 390–391
Phenylenediamine, 373–374
Phosphatase tests, 394–401
biochemistry, 394–396
disks/tablets, 401
interpretation, 399
methyl green phosphate (MGP) procedure, 399–400
phenolphthalein diphosphate medium (PDP), 396–398
phosphate blood agar (PDPBA), 399
PNP (*p*-nitrophenylphosphate) hydrolysis, 400

Phosphatase tests—*Continued*
   precautions, 401
   purpose, 394
   reagents, 398
   spot test, 400–401
Phosphatidase D, 273–274
Phosphatidylethanolamine, 274
Phosphoglycerides, 38, 41–42, 273
Phospholipases, 288–289
   phospholipase C, 36, 39–42, 273–274, 288–289
   phospholipase D, 35, 36, 47–48
Phospholipids, 37–38, 273, 286–287
Phosphorolysis pathway, 334
Plasma clotting, 106–108
Plasmids, 255, 261–262
P-nitrophenyl-β-D-galactoside (PNPG), 160, 167, 168
Polymerase chain reaction, 459–461, 466 469–470
Polysaccharides, 58, 412–417. (*see also* Carbohydrates)
Porphyrin-δ-aminolevulinic acid (ALA) test, 403–406
   biochemistry, 403–404
   interpretations, 405–406
   precautions, 406
   procedures, 404–405
   purpose, 403
Porphyrins, 403–405
Premier multitest system, 460, 463
Propionic acid fermentation, 62
Proteases, 113
Protein catabolism by gelatinases, 171
Proteinases, 171
Prothrombin, 106–107, 113
Protoporphyrin, 80–81, 403–404, 451
Prototroph, 341
Pulsed-field gel electrophoresis, 460–461, 463, 465, 469–470
Purines, 138–140
Putrescine, 121–123, 132
Pyocyanin, 155
PYR test. (*see* Pyrrolidonyl-β-Naphthylamide hydrolysis (PYR) test)
Pyranose, 413
Pyridoxal phosphate, 125, 134
Pyrimidines, 138–140
Pyrrole structure, 225–226
Pyrrolidonyl-β-Naphthylamide hydrolysis (PYR) test, 3, 407–410
   disk spot tests, 409–410
   DMACA reagent, 408–409
   enzyme/substrate, 408
   interpretations, 410
   precautions, 410
   purpose, 407–408
   rapid tests, 409

Quinone, 226, 373, 374, 395

Reagents. (*see also* Media)
   acetic acid, 351
   acridine orange, 150–152
   p-aminodimethylaniline HCL, 371, 375
   p-aminodimethylaniline oxalate, 371, 372

δ-aminolevulinic acid (ALA) test, 404
ammonium vapor, 398
amyl alcohol, 224
Andrade's, 64, 74–76, 744
Barritt's, 444–446, 448
Benedict's, 185, 422
β-galactosidase, 339–340
β-naphthol, 339–340
β-naphthylamine, 339–340, 408
Clinitest tablets, 185–186, 422
Coblentz, 444
creatine, 444
o-dianisidine, 87
p-Dimethylaminobenzaldehyde (DMAB), 224–226, 227–228
p-Dimethylaminocinnamaldehyde (DMACA), 283, 408–409
dimethyl-*p*-aminodimethylaniline oxalate, 371, 374
dimethyl-*p*-phenylenediamine HCL, 371, 372, 374, 377
dopamine, 91
Ehrlich's indole, 224, 230
ethanol, 422, 444
ferric ammonium sulfate, 390
ferric chloride, 190–193, 201–202, 390–391
fibrinogen, 108–109
τ-glutamylaminopeptidase, 339–340
Gordon and McLeod's oxidase, 371, 372
Gram's iodine, 265, 418
Hemo-De, 230
heparin, 108–110
hydorgen peroxide, 93
hydrochloric acid, 147–148, 357
hydrogen peroxide, 79
indolphenol oxidase, 371
indoxyl butyrate, 341
iodine, Gram's, 418
iodine, Lugol's, 419, 422
isoamyl alcohol, 224–225
Kovac's indole, 224–226, 230
Kovac's oxidase, 371, 372, 375, 376
Lugol's iodine, 419, 422
lysostaphin solution, 306
M/15 phosphate buffer, 79
MAD (metachromatic agar-diffusion), 150
mercuric chloride, 177
methyl green, 147, 155–156
methylene blue, 71
α-naphthol, 444–446, 448
α-naphthylamine, 351–354, 360
Nessler's reagent, 127, 351
ninhydrin, 130, 196–198, 202
Nitrocefin (chromogenic cephalosporin), 263
N-(1-naphthyl)ethylenediamine dihydrochloride, 357
N,N-dimethyl-a-naphthylamine, 351–354, 360
O'Meara's, 444
oxidase disks, 371, 372–373
oxidation-reduction indicator, 69, 70
PADAC (pyridine-2-azo-dimethylaniline cephalosporin), 263–264, 267

penicillin G potassium, 430
pH indicators
    acid fuchsin, 744
    azolitmin, 298, 299, 302
    bromcresol purple, 744
    bromcresol purple (BCP), 74, 75, 124, 126, 382, 744
    bromthymol blue, 744
    bromthymol blue (BTB), 74, 75, 313, 336, 381, 392
    for carbohydrate media, 74
    ferric chloride, 313
    litmus, 295, 298, 299
    methyl red, 322, 323–324
    neutral red, 744
    phenol red, 63, 74, 247, 266, 334, 426, 427, 430, 744
    phenolpthalein, 395–396
phenol red, 63, 74
phosphate buffer, 164, 263, 265, 306
plasma, 108–110
p-nitrophenyl-β-D-galactoside (PNPG), 167
p-nitrophenylphosphate (PNP), 400
potassium hydroxide, 444, 446, 448
p-phenylenediamine dihydrochloride, 91
prolyl-hydroxyprolyl aminopeptidase, 340
rapid bile esculin (RBE), 14
resazurin solution, 69
rhodamine B, 199
σ-nitrophenyl-β-D-galactopyranoside (ONPG), 164–165, 167–168
sodium azide, 12
sodium deoxycholate, 29
sodium hydroxide, 29–30, 126–127, 398
sodium tauracholate, 29
starch solution, 265
sulfanilic acid, 351–354, 360
sulfanilimide, 356–357
superoxol (30% H_2O_2), 93
Taxo X, V, and XV strips/disks, 451
tetramethyl-ρ-phenylenediamine dihydrochloride, 371, 372, 373, 374
toluene, 165–166
toluidine blue O, 145–147, 155–156
Tween 80, 79, 93
uranium acetate, 199
Voges-Proskauer, 444–446
Wurster's, 374
xylene, 224, 230
zinc, 352, 360
Reduction
    of methylene blue, 317–318
    nitrate/nitrite tests, 349–350
Rennin, 295, 296–297
Reverse CAMP test, 46–47
Ribotyping, 461
RIM-H (Rapid Identification Method) multitest system, 464

Saccharopine, 129
Salmonella-Shigella agar, 742

Shandon Hemo-De, 230
Shiff base, 283–284, 408
Skatole, 222, 230
Sodium lauryl sulfate, 28
Sphingomyelin, 37–41, 43, 274, 289
Sphingomyelinase, 36, 39–42
Sphingosine, 37, 287
Staphylocoagulase, 106–108
Staphylothrombin, 114
Starch hydrolysis test, 412–423
    biochemistry, 412–417
    ethanol procedure, 422
    interpretation, 420–421, 422
    iodine test, 419–420
    media, 417–418, 422
    precautions, 422–423
    purpose, 412
    rapid micromethod, 421
    reagents, 418–420
Streptolysin, 7, 51
Sublactam, 262
Succinic acid, 310–312
Sucrose and KIA/TSI media, 243, 246–247, 252
Sulfamethoxazole, 290
Sulfamethoxazole-trimethoprim, 4–7
Sulfide indole motility medium, 459
Superoxide disumutase (SOD), 79–80, 83–84
Superoxide radical (O_2^-), 79–80, 83–84
Superoxol, 84
Synergism, 36

Taurine, 27
Tazabactam, 262
Teichoic acid, 28
Thermonuclease, 112
Thermonuclease tests
    ADA (acridine orange-deoxyribonucleate agar) overlays, 150–152, 156
    biochemistry, 137–143
    for blood cultures, 149
    MAS (metachromatic agar-diffusion) microslide technique, 150, 156
    purpose, 137
    STN (simplified thermonuclease test), 149–150
Thin-layer chromatography
    arginine dihyrolase test, 132
    hippurate hydrolysis, 198
Thiosulfate reductase, 205, 206
Thrombin, 106–107, 114
Thromboplastin, 274
Thymine, 138–140
Toluidine blue O, 145–147, 155–156
Transduction, 261
Transformation, 341
Transpeptidation, 305
Transposon, 255
Trehalose-mannitol broth, 459
Trehalose-mannitol-phosphate agar (TMPA), 459
Triglycerides, 288
Trimethoprim, 4–7, 290, 330, 433
Triple sugar iron (TSI) agar, 239–252

Triple sugar iron (TSI) agar—*Continued*
  biochemistry, 243–245
  interpretations, 247–248
  media, 245–247
  precautions, 249–252
  purpose, 239–243

Urea, 122
Urease test, 424–437
  biochemistry, 425
  Christensen's urea agar, 427–428, 429, 436
  for *Haemophilus* spp, 434
  for *Helicobacter pylori,* 432–433
  interpretation, 429
  precautions, 435–437
  purpose, 424–425
  radioisotope procedures, 434–435
  rapid tests, 434
    CLO striptest, 434
    urea disks, 434
    urea-phenylalanine disks (PDA disks), 434
    urease tablets, 434
  Stuart's urea broth, 426–427, 429, 435–436
  U-9 broth (urease color test medium), 430–431, 436–437
  urea broth for mycobacteria, 432
  urea R (rapid) broth, 428, 429, 436

urease disk test, 432
Urinary tract pathogens, multitest kits for detection, 461

V factor. (*see* X and V factors)
Vancomycin, 433
Vitek multitest system, 460, 463, 466, 467–468
Voges-Proskauer test, 439–448
  alternative tests, 447
  biochemistry, 439–443
  interpretation, 447
  media, 443
  precautions, 447–448
  procedure, 444–445
  purpose, 439
  rapid test, 447
  reagents, 444–446, 448

X and V factors, 403–406
  biochemistry, 451
  interpretation, 452
  media/reagents, 451
  precautions, 452–453
  procedure, 451–452
  purpose, 451
Xylose-lysine-desoxycholate agar, 742

Zinc reduction test, 352, 355, 360

Index 2—Microorganisms

Numbers in **bold** indicate the primary genus description. Numbers in *italics* indicate tables of test results and flow charts (ID schemas). Other entries pertaining to the organism are in normal type.

Abiotrophia, 485, **502**, 613
  adiacens, 282, 407
  dafectiva, 282, 407
Acetobacterium, 485
Acholeplasma, 627, **641–642**, 705–706, 718
  axanthum, 642
  equifetale, 642
  granularum, 642
  hippikon, 642
  laidlawii, 286, 289, 642
  morum, 642
  oculi, 642
  parvum, 642
Achromobacter, 154, 187
Acidaminococcus fermentans, 626, **642**, 729
Acidovorax, 368, 379, 625, **642–643**, 705–707
  delafieldii, 99, 171, 643, 707–708, 710
  facilis, 99, 171, 643, 718, 719–720
  temperans, 99, 171, 643, 707–708, 710
Acinetobacter, 171, 368, 379, **502**, 626, **643–644**, 705–706, 714
  baumannii, 242, 644, 800–801
  calcoaceticus, 242, 400, 644, 800–801
  equuli, 188
  haemolyticus, 171, 280, 644
  johnsonii, 644
  junii, 644
  lignieresii, 188
  lwoffii, 237, 242, 354, 644, 800–801
  ureae, 221
Actinobacillus, 327, 368, 379, 394, 424, 626, **644–645**, 705–706
  capsulatum, 645, 715, 717
  equuli, 645, 715, 717
  hominis, 645, 718, 721
  ligniersi, 645, 715, 717
  muris, 394, 645, 718, 721
  rossii, 645, 715, 717, 718, 721
  seminis, 394, 424, 645, 718, 721
  suis, 645, 715, 717
  ureae, 645, 715, 717, 718, 721
Actinomyces, 35, 160, 485, **502–503**, 576, 576–579, 581
  israelii, 503
  meyeri, 503
  naeslundii, 178, 503

  neuii
    subsp. *anitratus*, 35, 502, 503
    subsp. *neuii*, 35, 502, 503
  odontolyticismeyeri, 503
  viscosus, 178, 503
Aerococcus, 199, 485, **503–504**, 605–608, 613
  urinae, 78, 282, 321, 407, 504
  viridans, 78, 199, 282, 284, 321, 407, 504
Aeromonas, 19, 120, 136, 205, 231, 327, 368, 379, 439, 626, **646–647**, 705–706, 718
  alginolyticus, 715
  caviae, 8, 647, 715, 716, 721
  cholerae, 715
  eucrenophila, 8, 647, 715, 716, 721
  haemolyticus, 714
  hydrophilia, 8, 154, 160, 205, 321, 377, 439, 647, 715, 716, 721
  media, 327, 646, 647, 715, 717, 721
  salmonicida, 327, 646, 721
    subsp. *achromogenes*, 647, 715, 717
    subsp. *masoucida*, 205, 321, 439, 647, 715, 717
    subsp. *salmonicida*, 647, 715, 717
    subsp. *smithia*, 120, 205, 647, 715, 717
  schubertii, 647, 715, 716, 721
  sobra, 647
  sobria, 8, 439, 715, 716, 721
  veronii, 8, 120, 321, 439, 715, 716, 721
Afipia, 368, 379, 624, **648**, 705–708, 718, 719–720
  broomeae, 348, 388, 648, 719–720
  clevelandensis, 348, 388, 648, 719–720
  felis, 348, 388, 648, 710, 719–720
Agrobacterium, 368, 379, 624, **648–649**, 705–706
  tumefaciens, 649, 707, 712, 714
Agromyces, 486
Alcaligenes, 368, 379, 625, **649**, 705–707
  faecalis, 57, 171, 183, 242, 300, 348, 384, 400, 707, 712, 800–801
    subsp. *faecalis*, 649, 722
  latus, 57, 171, 242, 348, 649, 707, 708, 709, 722, 800–801
  piechaudii, 57, 171, 242, 348, 800–801
  xylosondans, 57, 171, 242, 348, 400, 800–801
Alicyclobacillus, 484
Alloiococcus otitidis, 282, 407, 485, **504**, 605–608, 612–613
Amycolatopsis, 487, **504**

Anaerobiospirillum, 627, **650**, 723, 728
Anaerorhabdus furcosus, 627, **650**, 650, 723–725
Aneurinibacillus, 484
Arachnia propionica. (see *Propionibacterium*)
Arcanobacter, 613
Arcanobacterium, 485, **505**, 576, 576–579, 581, 589, 598–600, 602, 605–608, 620
   bernardiae, 36, 505
   haemolyticum, 36, 505
   pyogenes, 36, 78, 170, 505
Arcobacter
   butzleri, 243
   cryaerophila, 233, 243
   nitrofigilis, 205, 243
Arsenophonus nasoniae, 98, 170, 240, 241, **736**, 741, 744, 748, 772
Arthrobacter, 486, **505–506**, 612
   agilis, 308, 371
Atopobium, 485
Aureobacterium, 486, **506**, 576–578, 580
   barberi, 506
   flavescens, 506
   liquefaciens, 506
   saperdae, 506
   terregens, 506
   testaceum, 506

Bacillus, 78, 141, 154, 188, 199, 221, 273, 280, 327, 412, 440, 448, 484, **506–509**, 576–577
   anthracis, 273, 327, 507, 508–509, 582
   cereus, 273, 508–509, 582
   circulans, 508–509, 582
   coagulans, 508–509, 582
   differentiation flow chart, 582
   firmus, 508–509, 582
   licheniformis, 3, 273, 508–509, 582
   megaterium, 508–509, 582
   mycoides, 273, 327, 507
   pumilis, 412, 508–509, 582
   sphaericus, 412, 508–509, 582
   stearothermiphilus, 507, 508–509, 582
   subtilis, 151, 420, 508–509, 582
Bacteroides, 14, 254, 292, 368, 458, 627, **651–653**, 723–728
   caccae, 652, 725–726
   capillosus, 652, 725–726
   cellulosolvens, 652, 725–727
   coagulans, 652, 723
   distasonis, 15, 368, 652, 725
   eggerthii, 21, 368, 652, 725
   forsythus, 652, 723
   fragilis, 8, 15–18, 21–22, 72, 94, 175–176, 254, 262, 420, 651, 652, 725
   galacturonicus, 651
   helcogenes, 652, 725–726
   melaninogenicus, 72
   ovatus, 15, 653, 725, 725–726
   polypragmatus, 651, 653, 723–724, 728
   putredinis, 653, 723
   pyogenes, 653, 725–727
   splanchnicus, 21, 653, 725–726

   suis, 653, 725–726
   tectus, 653, 725–726
   thetaiotaomicron, 15, 18, 651, 653, 725, 725–726
   uniformis, 15, 653, 725–726
   ureolyticus, 368, 651, 653, 723
   vulgatus, 15, 21, 72, 653, 725–727
   xylanolyticus, 651, 653, 723–724, 728
Bartonella, 348, 379, 424, 624, **652–654**, 705, 718, 719–720
   bacilliformis, 368, 652, 654
   clarrifgeiae, 653
   elizabethae, 368, 654
   felis, 348, 368, 424, 652
   henselae, 368, 652, 654
   quintana, 368, 652, 653, 654
   vinsonii, 368, 653, 654
Beneckea, 199
Bifidobacterium, 487, **510**, 576, 576–579, 581, 589, 600, 620
Bilophila wadsworthia, 15
Bordetella, 368, 625, **654–655**, 705–707
   avium, 327, 348, 424, 655, 707, 712
   bronchiseptica, 154, 327, 348, 424, 655, 707, 708, 710
   parapertussis, 327, 348, 368, 424, 655, 714
   pertussis, 460, 654, 655, 718, 719–720
Brevibacillus, 484, **510**
Brevibacterium, 486, **510–511**, 576–580, 605–606, 612
   casei, 188, 511
   epidermidis, 188, 511
   iodinum, 188, 511
   linens, 188, 511
Brevundimonas, 368, 379, 624, **655**, 705–706
   diminuta, 412, 655, 707, 712
   paucimobilis, 137
   vesicularis, 137, 412, 655, 718, 719–720
Brochothrix, 485, **511–512**, 576–579, 605–608
   campestris, 57, 439, 512
   thermosphacta, 57, 439, 512
Brucella, 213–214, 216, 218, 368, 427, 624, **656**, 705
   melitensis, 379, 656, 718, 719–720
   multitest system, 460
   suis, 360
Buchnera, **736**
Budvicia aquatica, 98, 160, 205, 239, 240, 241, 242, 310, 321, **736**, 744, 748, 769–770, 772, 796
Burkholderia, 460, 625, **656–657**, 705–707
   cepacia, 120, 160, 286, 368, 656, 657, 707, 708, 709, 710, 712
   gladioli, 120, 368, 657, 714
   mallei, 120, 368, 657, 707, 711, 714, 718, 719–720
   pseudomallei, 50, 120, 368, 656, 657, 707, 708, 709
Buttiauxella, 98, **736**
   agrestis, 239, 321, 744, 748
Butyrivibrio, 484, **512**, 589, 600–601, 626, **657–658**, 723–724, 728
   crossotus, 57, 512, 658
   fibrisolvens, 57, 512, 658

Caloramator, 484
Calymmatobacterium, **736**

Campylobacter, 136, 188, 198, 233, 235, 330–331, 369, 379, 626, **658–659**
 CLOs (*Campylobacter*-like organisms), 233
 coli, 78, 136, 152, 188, 195, 199, 205, 233, 659, 723
 concisus, 78, 205, 659, 723
 curvus, 658
 fennelliae, 233
 fetus, 78, 723
  subsp. *fetus, 659,* 723
  subsp. *veneralis, 659,* 723
 hyointestinalis, 78, 205, 659, 723
 jejuni, 78, 136, 152, 195, 199, 233, 237, 433
  subsp. *doylei,* 188, *659,* 723
  subsp. *jejuni,* 188, *659,* 723
 lari, 136, 152, 188, 199, 233
 mucosalis, 78, 205, 659, 723
 multitest systems for, 460
 rectus, 658
 sputorum, 78
  subsp. *bubulus,* 205, *659,* 723
  subsp. *sputorum,* 205, *659,* 723
 upsaliensis, 233, 659
Capnocytophaga, 379, 628, **659–660**, 705, 718
 canimorsus, 121, 160, 171, 348, 368, 659, *660,* 718
 cynodegmi, 121, 160, 171, 348, 368, 659, *660,* 718
 gingivalis, 121, 160, 171, 348, 368, 659, *660,* 718
 ochracea, 121, 160, 171, 348, 368, 659, *660,* 718
 sputigena, 121, 160, 171, 348, 368, 659, *660,* 718
 upsaliensis, 723
Cardiobacterium hominis, 221, 230, 231, 369, 379, 625, **660–661**, *661,* 705, 718
Carnobacterium, 485
Caseobacter. (see Corynebacterium polymorphus)
Cedecea, 8, 89, *98,* 240, 241, 310, **736**
 davisae, 239, 241, 310, 744, 748, 759–760, 761, 766–767, 768, 772, 782–788
 lapageri, 239, 241, 310, 744, 748, 762–763, 772, 782–786, 789–790
 neteri, 239, 241, 310, 744, 748, 762–763, 764–765, 772, 782–786, 789–790
 species 3, 744, 748, 762–763, 772, 782–786, 789–790
 species 5, 744, 749, 762–763, 766–767, 768, 772, 782–786, 789–790
Cellulomonas, 486, **513**, 605–608, 612, 620
 cellulans, 170
 turbata, 170
Centipeda periodontii, 627, **661**, 723–724, 728
Chromobacterium violaceum, 160, 369, 379, 625, **661–662**, *662,* 705–706
Chryseobacterium
 indologenes, 412
 meningosepticum, 412
Chryseomonas luteola, 8, 136, 160, 379, 625, **662–663**, *663,* 705–706, 714
Citrobacter, 90, *98,* 120, 160, 218, 239, 321, 386, 429, **736**
 amalonaticus, 221, 241, 310, 744, 749, 766–767, 773, 782–786
 amalonaticus biogroup 1, 744, 749, 766–767, 773, 782–786
 freundii, 20, 128, 186, 205, 215, 221, 240, 241, 242, 310, 436, 744, 749, 762–763, 766–767, 769–770, 771, 773, 782–786, 789–790, 796, 798
 koseri, 20, 221, 241, 310, 744, 749, 759–760, 773, 782–784
Classification
 Enterobacteriaceae, 735–741
 Gram-negative bacteria, 624–628
 Gram-positive bacteria, 483–487
Clavibacter, 486
Clostridium, 35, 46, 63, 78, 170, 178, 229, 255, 273, 276–277, 286, 412, 458, 484, **513–520**, 589, 605–608, 613, 620
 aminovalericum, 279
 argentinense, 279, 289–290, 294, *514, 516,* 590, 593
 baratii, 170, 273, 279, 294, 412, *514, 515, 516, 518,* 520, 590–591, 594–595
 bifermentans, 72, 273, 278, 279, 294, 420, *514, 515, 516,* 590, 592
 bijerinckii, 279, 294
 botulinum, 279, 286, 289–290, 294, *514,* 516–517, 590, 592
 butyricum, 294, 297, 300, 412, *514, 516,* 590–591
 cadaveris, 279, 294, *518, 520,* 594, 596
 carnis, 78, 279, 294, *513, 518, 520, 576, 581,* 594, 596
 celatum, 279, 294, *514, 516, 518, 520,* 590–591, 594–595, 597
 chauvoei, 279, 294, *514, 516,* 590–591
 clostridioforme, 279, 294, *514, 515, 516,* 590, 590–591, 592, 593
 cochlearium, 72, 279, 286, 294, *518, 520,* 594, 597
 difficile, 278, 279, 280–281, 294, *514, 515, 516,* 590, 592
  multitest system, 460–461
 egg yolk media reactions, 279–280
 fallax, 279, 294, 412, *515, 516,* 590, 592
 ghoni, 273, 279, 286, 294
 glycolicum, 279, 294, *515, 517,* 590, 592, 593
 haemolyticum, 273, 279, 294, *515, 517,* 590, 592
 hastiforme, 279, 294, *518, 520,* 594, 597
 histolyticum, 78, 279, 294, *513, 515, 517, 576, 581,* 590, 593
 indolis, 279, 294, *518, 520,* 594–595, 597
 innocuum, 280, 294, *519, 520,* 594, 597
 leptum, 280, 286, 294, *519, 520,* 594–596, 597
 limosum, 273, 279, 294
 litmus milk reactions, 294
 malenominatum, 279, 294, *515, 517, 519, 520,* 590, 592, 593, 594, 596, 597
 novyi, 273, 279, 286, 294, 515–517, 590, 592
 oroticum, 279, 294
 paraputrificum, 279, 294, *519, 520,* 594–595
 perfringens, 35, 46, 72, 175, 226, 273, 278, 279, 291, 294, 297, 300, 412, 420, *515, 515, 517,* 590–591
 putrefaciens, 279, 294, *515, 517, 519, 520,* 594, 596
 putrificum, 279, 294, *519, 520,* 590–591, 594
 ramosum, 279, 294, *515, 519, 520,* 594–595
 sartagoforme, 279, 294

Continued
., 154, 278, 279, 294, 515, 517, 590–591
  .tlii, 226, 273, 279, 294, 515, 515, 517, 590, 592
  phenoides, 279, 294, 412, 515, 517, 590, 590–591, 592
  spiroforme, 279, 294
  sporogenes, 278, 279, 286, 291, 294, 329, 515, 517, 590, 592
  subterminale, 280, 294, 515, 517, 590, 593
  symbiosum, 279, 280, 294, 515, 517, 590, 590–591, 592, 593
  tertium, 78, 279, 294, 513, 519, 520, 576, 581, 594–595
  tetani, 176, 280, 294, 519, 520, 594, 597
Comamonas, 369, 379, 625, **663**, 705–707, 709, 710
  acidovorans, 57, 230
  terrigena, 57, 663, 707, 708
  testosteroni, 57, 663, 707, 708, 712
Coprococcus, 484, **521**, 620
  catus, 521
  comes, 521
  eutactus, 521
Corynebacterium, 35, 47, 78, 105, 160, 199, 205, 286, 327, 394, 412, 468, 486, **521–525**, 576–580, 605–608, 612
  accolens, 521, 522, 524, 583–584
  afermentans, 583, 585
    subsp. afermentans, 35, 522, 522, 524
    subsp. lipophilum, 521
  amycolatum, 521522, 524, 583, 585, 586
  aquaticum, 327, 521, 523, 525, 583
  asperum, 521
  auris, 35, 522
  bovis, 35, 160, 522, 522, 524, 583, 585
  callionae, 522, 524
  callionaestriatum, 583, 585–587
  coylae, 35, 522
  cystitidis, 522, 524, 583, 585–587
  differentiation flow charts, 583–587
  diphtheriae, 141, 154
    subsp. belfantii, 522, 522, 524, 583, 585, 586
    subsp. gravis, 394, 412, 522, 522, 524, 583–584
    subsp. intermedius, 522, 522, 524, 583–584
    subsp. mitis, 522, 522, 524, 583–584
  flavescens, 522, 524, 583, 585, 586
  glucuronolyticum, 35, 522
  glutamicum, 522, 524, 583–584
  jeikeium, 521, 523, 525, 583, 585
  kutscheri, 523, 525, 583, 585–587
  matruchotii, 327, 521, 523, 525
  mcginleyi, 521–522
  minutissimum, 523, 525, 583, 585, 586
  multitest systems, 460
  mycetoides, 523, 525, 583, 585, 586
  pilosum, 523, 525, 583–584
  pseudodiphtheriae, 523, 525, 583–584
  pseudotuberculosis, 47–48, 170, 286, 521, 522, 523, 525, 583, 585–587
  renale, 50, 523, 525, 583, 585–587
  striatum, 35, 170, 522, 523, 525, 583, 585, 586
  ulcerans, 47–48, 286, 521, 522

  urealyticum, 522
  vitarumen, 523, 525, 583–584
  xerosis, 523, 525, 583–584
Cryptococcus, 18, 19, 22, 425
  neoformans, 8, 17–19, 22–23
Curtobacterium, 486

Deincoccus, 483, **526**, 605–608
  proteolyticus, 160, 526
  radiodurans, 160, 526
  radiophilus, 160, 526
  radiopugnans, 160, 526
Dermabacter hominus, 486, **526–527**, 576–579, 605–608
Dermacoccus nishinomiyaenis, 371, 486
Dietzia, 486

Edwardsiella, 90, 98, 120, 243, 310, **737**
  hoshinae, 240, 241, 310, 321, 327, 744, 749, 773
  ictaluri, 241, 321, 327, 744, 749, 773
  tarda, 205, 240, 241, 242, 243, 247, 327, 744, 796, 798, 799
  tarda biogroup 1, 321, 327, 744, 749, 759–760, 773, 782, 793–794
Eikenella corrodens, 221, 230, 369, 379, 420, 453, 625, **664**, 664, 705, 718, 719–720
Enteric group 63, 779, 782, 793–794
Enteric group 64, 755, 762–763
Enteric group 68, 755, 762–763, 779, 782–786, 789–790
Enterobacter, 20, 62, 89–90, 91, 98, 120, 136, 221, 251–252, 310, 313, 325, 327, 388, 424, 425, 427–428, 429, 439, 443, 448, **737**
  aerogenes, 20, 120, 128, 226, 239, 241, 314, 321, 324, 337, 440, 448, 744, 749, 766–767, 773
  amnigenus, 239, 241
    biogroup 1, 744, 749, 766–767, 773, 782–784
    biogroup 2, 744, 749, 766–767, 768, 773, 782–786
  asburiae, 239, 241, 310, 327, 424, 744, 749, 766–767, 768, 773, 782–786
  cancerogenus, 241, 744, 773, 782–784
  cloacae, 20, 127, 128, 226, 239, 310, 321, 424, 446, 744, 749, 766–767
  dissolvens, 239, 241, 327, 424, 744, 750, 766–767, 773
  gergoviae, 120, 239, 241, 424, 744, 750, 759–760, 774, 782, 793–794
  hormaechae, 240, 241, 327, 424, 744, 750, 774, 782–786
  intermedius, 239, 744, 750
  nimipressuralis, 239, 744, 750
  sakazakii, 239, 310, 744, 750, 766–767
Enterobacteriaceae, 8, 12, 20, 89–90, 91, 183, 199, 368, 705–706. (see also specific genera)
  biochemical reaction tables, 748–758, 769–770, 772–781, 796–797
  classification, 735–741
  combined test media for, 458–459
  differentiation charts, 759–768, 771, 782–795, 798–799
  general characteristics, 741

KIA/TSI reactions, 239–243, 744–747
media for isolation and identification, 742–744
multitest systems, 461–463
nomenclature changes, 733–735
Simmons citrate reactions, 98
taxonomy, 732
Enterococcus, 8–9, 19, 78, 94, 115–116, 188, 199, 200, 282, 295, 301, 316–319, 407, 485, **527–531**, *613*
  avium, 316, *528, 530, 614–615*
  casseliflavus, 316, *528, 530, 614–615*
  cecorum, 316, *529, 531, 614–615*
  columbae, *529, 531, 614–615*
  differentiation flow chart, *614–615*
  dispar, 316, *529, 531, 614–615*
  durans, 316, *529, 531, 614–615*
  faecalis, 18, 94, *201*, 215, 254, 261, 269, 284, 300, 316, 318, 365, 410, *528–531, 614–615*
  faecalis variant, *614–615*
  flaecium, 316, *528, 530*
  flavescens, 316, *528, 530, 614–615*
  gallinarum, 316, *528, 530, 614–615*
  hirae, 316, *529, 531, 614–615*
  malodoratus, 316, *528, 530, 614–615*
  multitest systems, 461
  mundtii, 316, *529, 531, 614–615*
  pseudoavium, 316, *528, 530, 614–615*
  raffinosus, 316, *528, 530, 614–615*
  saccharolyticus, 316, *529, 531, 614–615*
  solitarius, 316, *529, 531, 614–615*
  sulfureus, 316, *529, 531, 614–615*
Erwinia, 310, **737**
  amylovora, 170, *750, 774*
  cacticida, 310
  mallotivira, *774*
  persicinus, 310, *751*
  psidii, *797*
  tracheiphila, *797*
Erysipelothrix, 78, 484, **532**
  rhusiopathiae, 8, 105, 205, 243, 468, *523, 525,* 532, *576, 581*
  tonsillarum, 532
Escherichia, 57, 89–90, 91, 98, 237, 310, **737**
  blattae, 221, 242, 310, *744, 774*
  coli, 20, 62, 72, 90, 94, 98, 103, 120, 132, 154, 165, 175, 186, 215, 221, 226, 227, 233, 237, 239, 242, 247, 300, 310, 313, 314, 321, 324, 325, 327, 329, 354, 374, 384, 391, 420, 429, 439, 440, 443, 446, 448, *742, 745, 751, 759–760, 764–765*
  coli inactive, *745, 751, 759–760, 761, 764–765, 774, 782–792*
  fergusonii, 57, 221, 242, 310, *745, 774, 782, 793–794*
  hermanii, 221, 239, 242, *745, 751, 766–767, 768, 775, 782–786*
  vulneris, 221, 239, 242, 310, *745, 751, 762–763, 764–765, 775, 782, 789–794*
Eubacterium, 171, 484, **532–535**, *589, 600–601*, 620
  aerofaciens, 534, *600, 602–603*
  biforme, 534, *600, 602–603*
  brachy, 534, *600, 602*

combesii, 171, *534, 600–603*
contortum, *534, 600, 602–603*
cylindroides, *534, 600, 602–603*
dolichum, *534, 600–603*
eligens, 534
formicigenerans, *534, 600, 602–603*
hadrum, *534, 600, 602–603*
hallii, *535, 600, 602–603*
lentum, 94, *532, 535, 598, 600–602*
limosum, *535, 600, 602–603*
moniliforme, *535, 600–603*
nitritogenes, *535, 600, 602*
nodatum, *532, 535, 600, 602–603*
ramulus, *535, 600, 602–603*
rectale, *535, 600–603*
saburreum, *535, 600, 602*
siraeum, *535, 600–603*
tenue, *535, 600–602*
timidum, *535, 600–603*
tortuosum, *535, 600, 602–603*
ventriosum, *535, 600, 602–603*
Ewingella americana, 98, 239, 242, 321, **738**, *745, 751, 764–765, 775, 782–786, 789–792*
Exiguobacterium, 484, **536**, *605–608*

Falcivibrio, 487, **536–537**, *589, 600–601*
  grandis, 57, *537*
  vaginalis, 57, *537*
Filifactor, 484
Flavimonas oryzhabitans, 8, 137, 160, 379, 625, **664–665**, *665, 705–706, 714*
Flavobacterium, 369, 379, 628, **665–666**, *705–707*
  aquatile, 57, *666, 707, 713*
  branchiophilum, 57, *666, 707, 713*
Francisella, 625, **666–667**, *705, 718*
  tularensis, 464, *666–667*
Frateuria, 483
Fusobacterium, 8, 14, 21, 255, 286, 458, 628, **667–668**, *723–727*
  alocis, *668, 725–727*
  gonidaformans, *668, 725*
  mortiferum, 8, 17, 21, *668, 725–726*
  naviforme, *668, 725*
  necrogenes, 8, *668, 725–726*
  necrophorum, 286, *668, 725*
  nucleatum, 464, *668, 725*
  perfoetens, *668, 725–727*
  periodonticum, *668, 725–727*
  praunitzii, *668, 725*
  russii, *668, 725–727*
  simiae, *668, 725–727*
  suici, *668, 725–727*
  ulcerans, *668, 725–727*
  varium, *668, 725–726*

Gardnerella vaginalis, 188, 379, 464, 487, **537**, *537, 576, 581, 627,* **668–669**, *669, 705–706, 718*
Gemella, 199, 485, **538**, *613, 627,* **669**, *722*
  haemolysans, 282, 348, 407, *538, 669*
  morbillorum, 348, 407, *538, 669*
Globicatella sanguis, 282, 407, 485, **538**, *613*

..6, **538–539**, 576–578, 605–607, 612
..gative bacteria, 624–729. (*see also* Enterobacteriaceae; *specific genera*)
charts
  bacilli, aerobic/facutative anaerobic
    initial differentiation, 705
      MacConkey—growth, 706–717
      MacConkey—no growth, 718–721
    bacilli, microaerophilic/anaerobic, 723–728
    cocci, aerobic/facultative anaerobic, 722
    cocci, anaerobic, 729
  genera descriptions/tables, 639–704
    differential characteristics, charts of, 639–641
  nomenclature changes, 628–639
Gram-positive bacteria, 483–623. (*see also specific genera*)
  charts, 574–621
    bacilli, aerobic/facultative anaerobic
      Bacillus, 582
      catalase reaction, 576–581
      Corynebacterium, 583–587
      Listeria, 588
    bacilli, anaerobic
      catalase reaction, 598–603
      Clostridium, 590–597
      initial differentiation, 589
    cocci, aerobic/facultative anaerobic, 604
      catalase reaction, 605–613
      Enterococcus, 614–615
      Staphylococcus, 609–611
      Streptococcus, 616–619
    cocci, anaerobic, 620–621
      Peptopstreptococcus, 621
    by oxygen requirement, 575, 604
    by shape, 574
  classification, 483–487
  genera descriptions/tables, 502–573
  nomenclature, 487–498

Haemophilus, 27, 33, 57, 121, 221, 348, 368, 379, 394, 403, 406, 425, 434, 451–453, 452, 626, **670–671**, 705–706, 718
  actinomycetemcomitans, 452, 671, 717, 721
  aegyptius, 27
  aphrophilus, 368, 452, 670, 671, 721
  ducreyi, 57, 452, 670, 671, 721
  haemoglobinophilus, 394, 452, 452, 671, 721
  haemolyticus, 425, 434, 671, 721
  influenzae, 27, 221, 254, 262, 267, 268, 376, 405, 425, 434, 452, 452, 453, 464, 670, 671, 721
    biogroup *aegyptius*, 425, 434
    type b, 464
    multitest systems for, 464
  paracuniculus, 121, 221, 425, 452, 671, 721
  paragallinarum, 368, 452, 671, 721
  parahaemolyticus, 405, 425, 434, 452, 671, 721
  parainfluenzae, 221, 254, 425, 434, 452, 452, 453, 464, 671, 721
  paraphrophaemolyticus, 425, 434, 671, 721
  paraphrophilus, 671, 721
  parasuis, 368, 452, 671, 721
  segnis, 368, 452, 671, 721
Hafnia, 89, 98, 221, **738**
  alvei, 20, 99, 120, 154, 242, 310, 439, 443, 448, 745, 775, 782, 793–794
  alvei biogroup 1, 120, 242, 310, 745, 775, 782, 793–794
Helcococcus kunzii, 282, 407, **539**, 613
Helicobacter, 369, 379, 626, **672**, 723–724
  cinaedi, 233, 348, 425, 672, 723–724
  fennelliae, 233, 348, 672, 723, 728
  mustelae, 233, 348, 672, 723–724
  pylori, 152, 156, 233, 348, 432–433, 435, 464–465, 672, 723–724, 728

Janthinobacterium lividum, 369, 625, **672–673**, 673, 705–706, 718
Jonesia denitrificans, 486, **539**, 539, 576–579, 605–608

Kingella, 78, 221, 230, 379, 625, **673**, 705, 718
  denitrificans, 57, 78, 136, 348, 369, 673, 718
  kingae, 57, 348, 369, 673, 718
Klebsiella, 20, 62, 90, 91, 98, 120, 136, 221, 229–230, 251–252, 310, 313, 321, 325, 327, 424, 428, 429, 440, 443, 448, **738**
  ornithinolytica, 221, 239, 424, 745, 751, 757, 762–763
  oxytoca, 221, 239, 321, 424, 439, 745, 751, 757, 762–763
  planticola, 240, 424, 439, 745, 751, 757, 762–763
  pneumoniae, 20, 21, 233
    subsp. *ozaenae*, 120, 160, 240, 242, 310, 439, 745, 751, 757, 762–763, 775, 782–784, 793–794
    subsp. *pneumoniae*, 127, *128*, 148, 160, 186, 226, 237, 240, 314, 321, 424, 429, 436, 439, 745, 751, 757, 762–763, 764–765
    subsp. *rhinoscleromatis*, 120, 160, 240, 242, 439, 745, 751, 757, 762–763, 764–765, 775, 782–784
  terrigena, 240, 321, 439, 745, 751, 757, 762–763, 766–767
Kluyvera, 8, 90, 98, 240, 310, 321, **738**
  ascorbata, 745, 752, 766–767
  cryocrescens, 242, 745, 752, 759–760, 766–767, 768, 775, 782, 782–786, 793–794
Kocuria rosea, 308, 486
Kurthia, 78, 484, **539–540**, 576–578, 580, 605–606
  gibsonii, 394, 540
  sibirica, 394, 540
  zopfii, 394, 540
Kytococcus sedentarius, 308, 486

Lactobacillus, 78, 484, **540–541**, 576, 581, 589, 598–600, 602–603, 605–608, 613, 620
  acidophilus, 300, 541
  casei, 541
  plantarum, 541
Lactococcus, 120, 199, 282, 407, 465, 485, **541–542**, 613
  garviae, 120, 542
  lactis, 201

subsp. *cremoris,* 542
subsp. *holdniae,* 542
subsp. *hordniae,* 120
subsp. *lactis,* 120, 542
piscium, 542
plantarum, 542
raffinolactis, 542
Lactosphaera, 485
Leclercia adecarboxylata, 8, *98,* 240, 310, 321, **738,** 745, 752, 762–763
Legionella, 78, 87, *89,* 94, 178, 188, 255, 327, 379, 625, **674,** *705, 718, 719–720*
bozemanii, 85, *89,* 255
cincinnatiensis, 255
dumoffii, 89, 94, 674
feelei, 178, 188, 255
gormanii, 89
longbeachae, 89, 255
maceachernii, 255
micdadei, 89, 178, 255, 674
nautarum, 178
oakridgensis, 89, 327
pneumophila, 78, *89,* 94, 188
   subsp. *pneumophila,* 85, 87, 674
wadsworthii, 89
Leminorella, 205, 242, **738**
grimontii, 99, 160, 321, *745, 796, 798*
richardii, 99, 160, 321, 400, *745, 796, 798*
Leptospira
biflexa, 79, 87
interrogans, 79, 87
Leptotrichia buccalis, 628, 674, **674–675,** *723–726*
Leucobacter, 486
Leuconostoc, 8, 19, 199, 282, 407, 465, 485, **542–543,** *576, 581, 613*
carnosum, 543
citreum, 295, 543
gelidum, 543
lactis, 295, 543
mesenteroides, 295
   subsp. *cremoris,* 543
   subsp. *dextranicum,* 543
   subsp. *mesenteroides,* 543
pseudomesenteroides, 295, 543
Listeria, 8, 19, 35, 52, 57, 105, 199, 321, 439, 485, **543–544,** *576–580, 605–608, 612–613*
differentiation flow chart, *588*
grayi, 57, 188, *544, 588*
innocua, 44, 188, *544, 588*
ivanovii, 35, 44, *44,* 52, 188, *544, 544, 588*
monocytogenes, 35, 43–44, *44,* 50, 52, 78, 170, 188, 205, 327, 331, 439, 468, 523, 525, *543–544, 544, 588*
seeligeri, 35, 43, 44, 50, *544, 588*
welshimeri, 43, 44, *544, 588*

Megamonas hypermegas, 379, 627, **675,** *723–726*
Megasphaera, 626, **675**
cerevisiae, 675
elsdenii, 675
hypermegas, 729

Melissococcus, 485
Methylobacterium, 369, 379, 412, 624, **676,** *705–707, 718, 719–720*
extrorquens, 676
fujisawaense, 676
mesophilicum, 676
organophilum, 676
radiotolerans, 676
rhodesianum, 676
rhodium, 676
zatmanii, 676
Microbacterium, 486, **545,** *576–580, 589*
arborescens, 35, 205, 348, 545, *545, 598–599*
imperiale, 205, 348, 545, *545, 598–599*
lacticum, 205, 348, *545*
laevaniformans, 598–599
laevaniformis, 205, 348, *545*
Micrococcus, 78, 170, 303, 371, 379, 439, 467, 486, **545–546,** *605–606, 612*
luteus, 307, 308, 384, *546*
lylae, 546
Mitsuokell multiacidus, 626, **676–677,** *677, 723–726*
Mobiluncus, 412, 485, **546–547,** *589, 600–601,* 627, **677,** *723–724*
curtisii, 50
   subsp. *curtisii,* 121, 188, 348, *547, 677, 723, 728*
   subsp. *holmesii,* 121, 188, 348, *547, 677, 723–724*
mulieris, 50, 121, 188, 348, *547, 677, 728*
Moellerella wisconsensis, 98, 240, **738,** *745, 752, 762–763, 764–765*
Moorellaospora, 484
Moraxella, 78, 137, 368, 369, 379, 626, **678–679,** *705–707, 718, 719–720*
atlantae, 348, *679, 707, 713*
bovis, 78, 348, *678, 679, 719–720*
catarrhalis, 78, 136, 137, 146, 233, 237, 254, 261, 267, 268, 337, 340, 341, 348, 465–466, *679, 722*
caviae, 233, 349
cuniculi, 349
lacunata, 679, 719
lincolnii, 348, *679, 719–720*
nonliquefaciens, 679, 719
osloensis, 348, *679, 707, 711, 713, 719–720*
ovis, 233, 349, *679, 707, 711, 722*
Morganella, 98, 425, **738**
morganii, 20, 57, 98, 120, 242, 251, 400, 428, 435
morganii biogroup 1, *128,* 242, 286, 388, 424, 429, *745, 775, 782, 795*
morganii biogroup 2, 129, 205, 242, 286, 388, 424, 429, *745, 775, 796, 798*
Morococcus cerebrosus, 369, 625, **679–680,** *680, 722*
Mycobacterium, 85–87, 160, 167, 199, 348, 425, 432, 486, **547,** *576–578, 627*
africanum, 355
asiaticum, 88, 355
avium, 85, 88, 353, 357
bovis, 85, 88, 432
Calmette-Guerin bacillus (BCG) strains, 167
catalase reactions, *88*
celatum, 355

...*m—Continued*
...*e*, 88, 355
...*escens*, 88, 355
fortuitum, 88, 167, 348, 355, 432
gastri, 86, 88, 355
genavense, 355
gordonae, 88, 355
haemophilum, 88, 355
intracullulare-avium complex, 432
kansasii, 85, 87, 88, 348, 355, 356, 432
leprae, 547
malmoense, 88, 355
marinum, 88, 355, 432
nitrate reduction, 355, 355–357
nonchromogonicum, 88
paratuberculosis, 547
phlei, 88
scrofulaceum, 88, 167, 432
shimoidei, 355
simiae, 88, 355
smegmatis, 88
szulgai, 88, 348, 355
terrae, 88, 355
thermoresistible, 355
triviale, 88, 355
tuberculosis, 85, 86, 88, 93, 167, 348, 355, 356, 357, 361, 432
ulcerans, 88, 355
vaccae, 88
xenopi, 88, 355
Mycoplasma, **680**, 705–706
hominis, 286, 289, 437
mycoides, 286, 289
orale, 394
pneumoniae, 431
salivarium, 394
urealyticum, 424

Neisseria, 57, 78, 136, 146, 153, 160, 333–334, 348, 368, 369, 376, 625, **681**
canis, 348, 349, 681, 722
carbohydrate utilization tests, 333–345
cinerea, 465, 681, 722
denitrificans, 681, 722
elongata, 681, 681, 722
  subsp. *elongata*, 78
  subsp. *glycolytica*, 78
  subsp. *nitroreducens*, 78
flavescens, 722
gonorrhoeae, 78, 90, 254, 261, 267, 268, 333–334, 337, 338–344, 340, 348, 465–466, 681, 681, 722
iguanae, 349
lactamica, 57, 78, 160, 165, 237, 333–334, 337, 338–341, 340, 465–466, 681, 681, 722
macacae, 681, 722
meningitidis, 78, 90, 165, 333–334, 337, 338–344, 340, 465–466, 681, 681, 722
mucosa, 78, 348, 358, 374, 681, 681, 722
multitest systems, 465–466
polysaccharea, 348, 681, 722

sicca, 358, 681, 722
subflava, 681, 722
  biovar *flava*, 358
  biovar *perflava*, 358
  biovar *subflava*, 358
weaveri, 349
Nesterenkonia halobia, 371, 486
Nocardia, 486
Nocardioides, 486
Nocardiopsis, 160, 487
Nomenclature changes
  Enterobacteriaceae, 733–735
  Gram-negative bacteria, 628–635
  Gram-positive bacteria, 487–498
Norcardia, 160, 171, 179, 199, **547–548**, 576–577, 605–606, 612
  asteroides, 170, 179, 548
  brasiliensis, 170, 179, 548
  farcinia, 170, 548
  nova, 170, 548
  otididiscaviarum, 170, 548
  transvalensis, 170, 548

Obesumbacterium proteus, 98, 242, **739**, 745, 775
Ochrobactrum, 369, 624, **682**, 705–706
  anthropi, 379, 682, 707, 708, 710, 712
Oenococcus, 485
Oerskovia. (see *Cellulomonas*)
Oligella, 369, 379, 625, **682–683**, 705–707
  ureolytica, 376, 424, 682, 683, 707, 708, 710, 711, 712, 713, 718, 719–720
  urethralis, 376, 424, 683, 707, 713
Oxalophagus, 485
Oxobacter, 484

Paenibacillus, 484, **548**
  alvei, 221, 548
  macerans, 221, 548
  polymyxa, 221, 548
Pantoea, 98, 221, **739**
  agglomerans, 20, 57, 120, 170, 221, 240, 241, 310, 348, 388, 458, 745, 752, 759–760, 761, 762–763, 764–765, 766–767, 768, 775, 782, 782–786, 789–790, 795
  anamatis, 752
  dispersa, 57, 240, 241, 310, 752, 775
Pasteurella, 348, 369, 379, 394, 424, 626, **683–685**, 705–707, 718, 719–720
  aerogenes, 424, 684, 707, 711
  anatis, 684, 707, 711
  avium, 684, 719
  bettyae, 683, 684
  caballi, 683, 684, 719
  canis, 684, 719
  dagmatis, 221, 424, 684, 719
    subsp. *septica*, 221
  gallinarum, 684, 719
  haemolytica, 50, 221
  langaa, 719
  langaaensis, 684
  lymphangitidis, 348, 424, 683, 685

mairii, 424, *685, 707, 711, 719*
multocida, 50, 221, 226, *707, 711, 719*
  subsp. *gallicida*, 221, *685*
  subsp. *multocida*, 221, *685*
  subsp. *septica*, *685*
pestis, 155
pneumotropica, 221, 424, *685, 707, 711, 719*
stomatis, *685, 719*
testudinis, 394, *685, 707, 711, 719*
trehalose, *685, 707, 711*
volantium, *685, 719*
Pasteuria, 485
Pediococcus, 8, 19, 78, 121, 199, 282, 407, 485, **549**, 613
  acidilactici, 78, 121, *550*
  damnosus, *550*
  dextrinicus, *550*
  inopinatus, *550*
  parvulus, *550*
  pentosaceus, 78, 121, *550*
  urinaeequi, *550*
Peptococcus niger, 94, 484, **551**, *620*
Peptostreptococcus, 57, 105, 221, 348, 424, **551–552**, *620*, 626, **686**, 729
  anaerobius, 57, *551, 552, 621*, 686, *686*
  asaccharolyticus, 57, 221, *551, 552, 621*, 686, *686*
  differentiation flow chart, *621*
  hydrogenalis, 57, *551, 552, 621*, 686, *686*
  indolicus, 57, 105, 221, 348, *552, 621*, 686
  lacrimalis, 57, *551, 552, 621*, 686, *686*
  lactolyticus, 57, 424, *551, 552, 621*, 686, *686*
  magnus, 57, *552, 621*, 686
  micros, 57, *552, 621*, 686
  prevotii, 57, 348, 424, *552, 621*, 686
  productus, 551
  tetradius, 57, 424, *552, 621*, 686
  vaginalis, 57, *551, 552, 621*, 686, *686*
Peptostreptococcus, 484
Photorhabdus luminescens, 170, **739**, 778
Plesiomonas shigelloides, 98, 136, 160, 240, 327, 368, **739**, *745, 759–760*
Porphyromonas, 627, *723–726*
  asaccharolyticus, 221, **687**
  endodontalis, 221
  gingivalis, 221
Pragia fontium, 160, 205, 242, **739**, *745, 776, 796*
Prevotella, 78, 262, 412, 627, **687–688**, *723–726*
  bivia, 688, *725–727*
  corporis, 222, 688, *725–727*
  denticola, 222
  disiens, 688, *725–727*
  heparinolytica, 171, 688, *725*
  intermedia, 221, 412, 688, *725–727*
  levii, 222
  loescheii, 222, 688, *725–726*
  melaninogenica, 179, 222, 254, 262, 688, *725–726, 725–727*
  oralis, 254, 262, 688, *725–726*
  oris, 688, *725–726*
  oulora, 78, 171, 412, 688, *725*
Propionibacterium, 35, 50, 94, 171, 221, 301, 486, **552–553**, *576, 576–579, 581, 589, 605–608, 613, 620*
  acidipropionici, *553, 598, 600, 602*
  acnes, 35, 171, 221, 286, 295, 301, 552, *553, 598, 600, 602*
  avidium, 171, 286, 295, 301, *553, 598–599*
  freundenreichii, *553, 598–599*
  granulosum, 35, 286, 295, 301, 552, *553, 598–599*
  jensenii, *553, 598–599, 602–603*
  lymphophilum, *553, 598–600, 602–603*
  propionicus, 286, *553, 598, 600, 602*
  thoenii, *553, 598–599*
Propioniferax, 486
Propionigenium, 628, **688–689**, *723–726*
Proteus, 90, 91, *98*, 120, 129, *132*, 205, 218, 221, 388, 400, 424, 425, 427–428, 435, **739**, *743*
  inconstans, 20, 58, 221, 240, 241, 243, 286, 424, *745, 753, 762–763, 776, 782, 795*
  L forms, 436
  mirabilis, 20, 58, 120, 155, 165, 170, 205, 205, 241, 242, 243, 424, 429, 448, *745, 769–770, 771, 796, 798*
  myxofaciens, 58, 170, 240, 241, 243, 286, 424, 429, *745, 753, 776*
  penneri, 57, 58, 170, 205, 240, 241, 242, 243, 286, 424, 429, *745, 753, 762–763, 769–770, 771, 776, 782, 795, 796, 798*
  rettgeri, 20, 58, 98, 221, 240, 241, 243, 251, 424, 429, 435 (*see also Providencia rettgeri*)
  stuartii, 428, 429, 435 (*see also Providencia stuartii*)
  vulgaris, 20, 58, 90, *128*, 129, 155, 170, 175, 205, 215, 221, 231, 241, 242, 243, 246, 286, 300, 384, 391, 424, 429, 433, *745, 769–770, 771, 796, 798*
Providencia, 57, 89, 91, *98*, 120, 129, 231, 242, 286, 388, 424, **739**
  heimbachae, 424, *746, 753, 776*
  rettgeri, *746, 753, 762–763, 776, 782, 795* (*see also Proteus rettgeri*)
  rustigianii, 240, 424, *746, 753, 762–763, 776, 782, 795*
  stuartii, 20, 233, 237, 240, 400, 424, 425, *746, 753, 762–763, 777, 782, 795* (*see also Proteus stuartii*)
Pseudomonas, 120, 155, 160, 199, 286, 360, 368, 376, 379, 412, 625, **689–691**, *705–707*
  aeruginosa, 20, 91, 141, 151, 155, 183, 186, 226, 233, 242, 247, 280, 286, 292, 300, 354, 374, 384, 400, 433, 689, *690, 707, 708, 709, 800–801*
  alcaligenes, *690, 707, 712*
  aureofaciens, 183
  cepacia, 120, 187, 280
  chlororaphis, 183, *690, 707, 708, 709, 712*
  cichorii, *690, 707, 708, 710, 712*
  fluorescens, 170, 179, 183, 280, *690–691, 707, 708, 709*
  gelidicola, *691, 707, 708, 709, 712*
  maltophilia, 160, 376
  mendocina, *691, 707, 708, 710*
  pseudoalcaligenes, 120, *691, 707, 708, 709, 710*

Continued
..., 183, 691, 707, 708, 710, 712
...ophila, 412, 691, 707, 708, 709, 712
...zeri, 412, 691, 707, 708, 710
...yringae, 368, 691, 714
  viridiflava, 368, 691, 714
Pseudonocardia, 487
Pseudoramibacter, 484
Psychrobacter, 369, 626, **690**
  immobilis, 691

Rahnella aquatilis, 98, 240, 310, 388, **739**, 746, 753, 764–765
Ralstonia, 369, 379, 625, **692**, 705–707
  pickettii, 692, 707, 708, 710, 712, 718, 719–720
Rathayibacter, 486
Rhodococcus, 486, **554**, 576–577, 605–606, 612
  equi, 35, 44
Rochalimaea. (see *Bartonella*)
Roseomonas, 369, 379, 412, **692–693**, 705–707
  cervicalis, 693, 707, 712
  fauriae, 693, 707, 708
  genomospecies, 693, 707, 708, 710, 711, 713
  gilardii, 693, 707, 712, 714
Rothia dentocariosa, 486, 554, **554**, 576–579, 605–608
Rubrobacter, 485
Ruminococcus, 484

Saccharobacter, **739**
Saccharothrix, 487
Salmonella, 20, 90, 91, 98, 120, 160, 205, 217, 237, 242, 246, 310, 360, **740**, 742
  bongori, 160, 746, 797, 798
  choleraesuis, 218, 310
    serovar *choleraesuis*, 242, 746, 777, 782, 793–794, 798
    serovar *gallinarum*, 120, 133, 218, 746, 797, 798, 799
    serovar *paratyphi* A, 218, 242, 746, 777, 782–788, 797, 798
    serovar *pullorum*, 218, 746, 797, 798, 799
    serovar *typhi*, 746, 798, 799
    subsp. *arizonae*, 129, 160, 165, 215–216, 240, 310, 386, 746, 769–770, 771, 797, 798, 799
    subsp. *choleraesuis*, 746, 797, 798, 799
    subsp. *diazonae*, 160, 240, 310, 746, 769–770, 771, 798, 799
    subsp. *houtenae*, 797, 798
    subsp. *indica*, 769–770, 771, 797, 798, 799
    subsp. *salamae*, 310, 746, 797, 798, 799
  enteritidis, 740
  indica, 240
  pullorum, 217, 252
  typhi, 120, 128, 218, 251, 742, 797
  typhimurium, 128, 215
Sarcinia, 484, **555**, 620
  maxima, 57, 555
  ventriculii, 57, 555
Selenomonas, 171, 205, 626, **693–694**, 723–724, 728
  acidaminovorans, 171, 694, 723–724
  artemidis, 694, 723–724
  dianae, 694, 723–724
  flueggei, 694, 723–724
  infelix, 694, 723–724
  lacticifex, 694, 723–724
  noxia, 694, 723–724
  ocidaminococcus, 723–724
  ruminatum, 205, 694, 723–724
  sputigena, 694, 723–724
Serratia, 20, 89, 91, 98, 136, 142–143, 154, 170, 221, 286, 310, 348, 440, **740**
  DNase production, 142–143, 143, 154
  entomophila, 240, 241, 746, 753, 777
  ficaria, 240, 241, 746, 753, 762–763, 764–765, 777, 782–786, 789–790
  fonticola, 136, 142, 240, 286, 310, 746, 753, 759–760, 761, 766–767
  grimesii, 240, 241, 746, 754, 766–767, 777, 782, 793–794
  marcescens, 141, 142–143, 148, 151, 240, 241, 746, 754, 766–767, 777, 782, 793–794
  odorifera, 240
    biogroup 1, 746, 754, 759–760, 761, 766–767, 777, 782, 793–794
    biogroup 2, 746, 754, 762–763, 764–765
  plymuthica, 240, 241, 746, 754, 762–763, 764–765, 777, 782–786, 789–792
  proteamaculans, 98, 240, 241, 754, 766–767, 777, 782, 793–794
    subsp. *proteamaculans*, 136, 175, 746
  rubidaea, 240, 310, 746, 754, 762–763, 764–765
Shewanella, 369, 379, 626, **694**, 705–707, 708, 709, 710
  benthica, 243
  hanedai, 243
  putrefaciens, 21, 137, 205, 243
Shigella, 89–90, 91, 98, 120, 160, 237, 242, 246, 321, **740**, 742, 746
  boydii, 777, 782–786, 789–792
  dysenteriae, 777, 782–786, 789–792
  flexneri, 215, 247, 777, 782–786, 789–792
  sonnei, 20, 120, 160, 778, 782–788
Skermania, 486
Sphingobacterium
  multivorum, 348
  spiritivorum, 136, 348
  thalpophilum, 348
Sphingomonas, 369, 379, 624, **695**, 705, 718, 719–720
  parapaucimobilis, 205, 695, 719–720
  paucimobilis, 8, 136, 205, 695, 719–720
Sphinx multivorum, 136
Sporohalobacter, 484
Staphylococcus, 57, 78, 91, 105, 178, 199, 280, 303, 371, 379, 394, 401, 408, 439, 448, 485, **555–556**, 605–608, 613
  arlettae, 57, 558, 560
  aureus, 94, 112–113, 233, 467, 468
    subsp. *anaerobius*, 78, 105, 105, 555, 556–557
    subsp. *aureus*, 35–37, 57, 85, 105, 105, 116, 136, 137, 141–142, 145, 148, 149–151, 154, 156, 170, 176, 178, 254, 267, 268, 273, 280, 286, 289, 291, 292, 303, 305, 307, 330, 384, 394, 398, 400–401, 431, 440, 555, 556–557

auricularis, 558, 560
β-lactamase, 261, 268
capitis, 308
   subsp. *capitis,* 558, 560
   subsp. *ureolyticus,* 558, 560
caprae, 558, 560
carnosus, 156, 562, 564
caseolyticus, 371, 555, 562, 564
chromogens, 562, 564
cohnii, 305
   subsp. *cohnii,* 558, 560
   subsp. *urealyticum,* 558, 560
delphini, 105, 562, 564
DNase production, 141–142, 154
epidermidis, 136, 137, 141–142, 145, 148, 149, 154, 156, 170, 178, 291, 292, 307, 308, 398, 400–401, 459, 467, 468, 555, 556–557
equorum, 562, 564
felis, 562, 564
gallmarium, 562, 564
haemolyticus, 305, 308, 408, 555, 556–557
hominis, 305, 308, 398, 468, 559, 561
hyicus, 105, 117, 400, 563, 565
intermedius, 105, 116, 400, 408, 563, 565
kloosii, 563, 565
lentus, 371, 555, 563, 565
lugdunensis, 105, 105, 408, 468, 555, 556–557
lutrae, 555
multitest system, 467–469
muscae, 563, 565
pasteuri, 559, 561
piscifermentans, 563, 565
saccharolyticus, 78, 555, 559, 561
saprophyticus, 267, 305, 307, 379, 398, 400–401, 459, 467, 468
   subsp. *saprophyticus,* 555, 556–557
schleiferi, 400, 408
   subsp. *coagulans,* 105, 105, 556–557, 559, 561
   subsp. *schleiferi,* 105, 105, 468, 556–557, 559, 561
sciuri, 371, 555, 563, 565
simulans, 156, 305, 559, 561
vitulus, 371, 555, 563, 565
warneri, 308, 559, 561
xylosus, 57, 305, 401, 559, 561
Stenotrophomonas, 379, 625, **695–696**, 705–706
   maltophila, 130, 137, 160, *696,* 714
Stomatococcus mucilaginosus, 170, 467, 486, 566, **566**, 605–608, 613
Streptobacillus moniliformis, 628, **696**, *696,* 705, 718
Streptococcaceae, 4–7
Streptococcus, 8–9, 27–33, 49, 72, 78, 79, 91, 94, 155, 188, 199–201, 282, 412, 485, **566–571**, 613
   acidominimus, 200, *201,* 570, 618, 619
   agalactiae, 6, 35, 43, 188, 195, 199, 200, *201,* 410, 568, 570, 616, 618
   alactolyticus, 570, 618
   avium, 319
   bovis, 23, *201,* 295, 319, 410, 412, 439, *570,* 619
   canis, 568, 616
   constellatus, 19
   cricetus, 7, 570, 619
   differentiation flow charts, *616–619*

   DNase production, 143
   downei, 7, 570, 619
   dysgalactiae
      subsp. *dysgalactiae,* 200, *201,* 570, 619
      subsp. *equisimilis,* 568, *616,* 616–617
   equi, 568, *616–617*
      subsp. *equi,* 568, *616–617*
      subsp. *zooepidemicus,* 568, *616*
   equinus, 295, 319, *570,* 619
   ferus, 7, 570, 619
   gordonii, 570, 619
   group A, 4, 6, 7, 46, 49–51, *50,* 137, 141, 143, 155–156, 188, 200, 407
   group B, 7, 35, 39, 46, 49, *50,* 78, 188, 195, 199–201
   group C, 46
   group D, 8–9, 19, 188, 316, 319, 412
   group G, 46
   hyointestinalis, 570, 619
   iniae, 569, 570, 616, 618–619
   intermedius, 19
   intestinalis, 569, 616
   macacae, 7, 570, 619
   milleri, 23, 439, 566, 568, *571, 616,* 618–619
   mitis, 30, *571,* 619
   multitest systems, 469
   mutans, 19, 72, 439, *571,* 619
   oralis, 571, 619
   pleomorphus, 567, 620
   pneumoniae, 14, 23, 27–33, 282, 363–367, 407, 469, 569, *571, 616,* 618–619
   porcinus, 569, *571, 616,* 618–619
   pyogenes, 6, 19, 43, 85, 90, 137, 148, 155–156, 215, 282, 318, 407, 410, 569, *616–617*
   ratti, 571, 619
   salivarius, 195, 425, 439, *571,* 619
   sanguis, 19, 72, *571,* 619
   sobrinus, 571, 619
   suis, 569, *571, 616,* 618–619
   thermophilus, 571, 619
   uberis, 19, 200, *201, 571,* 619
   vestibularis, 425, *571,* 619
   viridans, 363, 366, 425, 439
Streptomyces, 160, 171, 179, 199, 487
Succinivibrio dextrinosolvens, 379, 626, **696**, *696,* 723, 723–724, 728
Succinomonas amylolytica, 627, 723–728
Suttonella indologenes, 221, 230, 231, 369, 379, 625, **697–698**, *698,* 705, 718
Syntrophospora, 484

Tatumella ptyseos, 98, 240, 241, 388, **740**, 741, 746, 755, 764–765, 778, 782, 795
Taylorella equigenitalis, 369, 379, 625, **698**, *698,* 723
Terrabacter, 486
Tetragenococcus, 282, 407, 485
Thermoanaerobacter, 484
Tissierella, 626, **698–699**, 723, 723–724
Trabulsiella, **740**
Tsukamurella, 486, **572**, 576, 576–578, 581, 605–607, 612–613
Turicella otitidis, 35, 487, 572, **572**, 605–607, 612

..6, 289, 436, 437, 627, **699**
..m, 280, 286, 430, 431, 437, 469, 699

..occus, 282, 407, 485, **572–573**, 613
..fluvialis, 205, 573
..salmoninarum, 205, 573
Veillonella, 94, 626, **699–700**, 729
  atypica, 700
  caviae, 700
  criceti, 700
  dispar, 700
  parula, 700
  ratti, 700
  rodentium, 700
Vibrio, 141, 155, 327, 348, 368, 379, 626, **700–702**, 705–706
  alginolyticus, 701–702, 716
  cholerae, 160, 700, 701–702, 716
  cincinnatiensis, 701–702, 715, 716
  fluvialis, 701–702, 715, 716, 717
  furnissii, 701–702, 715, 716, 717
  gazogenes, 368, 700
  harveyi, 348, 701–702, 715
  hollisae, 701–702, 717
  metschnikovii, 321, 348, 368, 700, 701–702, 715
  mimicus, 701–702, 715, 716
  parahaemolyticus, 215, 425, 701–702, 715, 716
  vulnificus, 8, 21, 700, 701–702, 715, 716

Weeksella, 628, 705
  virosa, 369, 379, 424, **702**, 702, 718, 719–720
  zoohelcum, 424
Weissella, 485
Wigglesworthia, **740**
Wolinella, 626, **703**
  curva, 233
  recta, 233

succinogenes, 205, 233, 369, 379, 659, 703, 723

Xanthobacter, 369, 379, 483, **573**, 605–608, 612, 624, 703, 705–707, 708, 710, 711, 718, 719–720
Xanthomonas, 379, 625, **704**, 705–706
  albilineans, 704
  axonpodis, 704
  campestris, 704
  citri, 704
  fragariae, 704
  phaseoli, 704
  populi, 704
Xenorhabdus, 78, 98, 170, 242, **740**
  beddingii, 755, 778
  bovienii, 755, 778
  nematophilus, 778
  poinari, 778

Yersinia, 89, 90, 98, 321, 327, 348, **741**
  aldovae, 240, 242, 755, 778
  bercovieri, 240, 241, 755, 759–760, 761, 764–765, 779, 782–792
  enterocolitica, 98, 240, 241, 243, 327, 331, 439, 755, 757, 759–760, 761, 779, 781, 782–788
  frederiksenii, 240, 241, 755, 759–760, 779, 782–788
  intermedia, 240, 241, 755, 759–760, 779, 782–786
  kristensenii, 242, 779, 782–788
  mollaretii, 240, 241, 755, 759–760, 761, 764–765, 779, 782–792
  pestis, 242, 243, 779, 782–786, 789–792
  pseudotuberculosis, 98, 242, 243, 779, 782–786, 789–790
  rohdei, 240, 241, 755, 759–760, 761, 764–765, 779, 782–792
  ruckeri, 170, 242, 779
Yokenella regensburgei, 98, 99, 242, **741**, 779, 782, 793–794